Contents

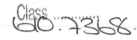

Foreword

This century has seen monumental changes both in the work of mental health nurses and the way in which they are trained. As we approach the next millennium it is important to reflect upon these changes. The editors of this book and many of the contributors have either worked at, or trained within, the Bethlem Royal and Maudsley Hospitals. It is significant that this book is first published in a year when the Bethlem Royal Hospital celebrates 750 years of caring for the mentally ill. It is the oldest psychiatric hospital in the world and, with its sister the Maudsley Hospital, has always sought to be at the leading edge of advances in mental health care provision.

Although the Bethlem's intention was to cure the insane, 750 years ago treatment often consisted of little more than patients being physically restrained or confined. Even at the beginning of this century there was little effective treatment for mental illnesses such as schizophrenia. Psychiatric patients were incarcerated in large Victorian asylums where they would often remain for the rest of their lives. Since the mid-1950's mental health services have undergone radical changes. New and effective treatments have been developed, many of the old asylums have been closed, and the majority of patients are now cared for while living in their homes. It is in this context of a rapidly changing health care system that this practical and authoritative text is published.

The role of the mental health nurse has changed dramatically over the centuries. The first nurses had little in common with today's highly skilled professionals. In the 13th Century, they were referred to as basket men because one of their responsibilities was to leave the hospital to collect food donated from the tables of rich Londoners for the patients. Today, mental health nurses are expected to fulfil a variety of roles, working in different settings with people suffering from a range of disorders. This book examines many of the key roles in contemporary mental health nursing, including the treatment of symptoms and the management of disability; for example, the use of case management involves the nurse in using modern evidence-based approaches including psycho-social and pharmacological interventions. Important advances in our understanding of mental illness are considered including biological and psychological models as well as a range of social and environmental factors.

This book will be an essential companion for practising mental health nurses. Student nurses undertaking Project 2000 courses in particular will find it an invaluable source of information and inspiration. Dramatic changes in the way nurses are trained have taken place since the late 1980s when nurse training began to be moved into higher education. Giving nurses a solid academic base is vitally important both for the profession and for service users. However, it should not be forgotten that nursing is essentially a practical discipline, and the editors and contributors must be congratulated on providing a textbook which is clearly based on good practice, and links research and nursing care throughout.

The book is written in such a way that chapters can be read in isolation. However, key themes can be seen to run through the book. Among the most important themes which emerge from the book are: the involvement of service users in developing and evaluating services and also in the provision of education to mental health nurses. The importance of multi-disciplinary working and interagency collaboration are also highlighted. It is clear that if we are to provide effective care for people with mental health problems then service users as well as health and social services must work together.

I was delighted to be asked to write this foreword as Principal of Somerville College in Oxford and as the immediate past President of the Royal College of Psychiatrists. I have always taken a keen interest in the nursing profession and am eager to see it progress and develop. As we look back over 750 years of psychiatric care and look to a new millennium I am confident that this book reflects on a long tradition of caring for the mentally ill and looks to the future with enthusiasm.

Fiona Caldicott DBE
Principal
Somerville College
Oxford

(Immediate Past President of the Royal College of Psychiatrists)

Preface

Based on the successful US text *Principles and Practice of Psychiatric Nursing* this book has been adapted by a team of 37 specialist contributors from the UK in order to meet the needs of students on the mental health branch component of diploma and degree level courses, post-graduates, nurses working in specialist or generic practice, research or academia. Anyone seeking to understand the current underpinning of effective mental health nursing in all its diversity, will find this book interesting and informative. The diversity of approaches detailed in each chapter reflects the changing role of the mental health nurse. The text endeavours to help the reader understand complex human needs from a variety of contemporary view-points.

Contributions from education, clinical practice, research, the user and carer worlds make this a widely informed and comprehensive tome for modern day mental health nurses. It offers a detailed account of biological, psycho-social and behavioural models which seek to ascribe understanding to the development and experience of mental illness and psychological distress. It provides the reader with an opportunity to take an educational tour of mental health nursing from a range of specialist services.

THE CONTENT OF THE BOOK

The text, while based on the US authors' work, reflects the legislation, culture, nursing practice terminology and health care systems currently in operation in the UK. With the addition of chapters on user perspective, quality standards, supervision and complementary medicine, it provides the reader with a comprehensive guide to mental health nursing. Each chapter integrates theory and clinical management, while demonstrating evidence based care.

STRUCTURE OF THE BOOK

Unit 1: Principles of Mental Health Nursing Care. This unit covers the fundamental and wide ranging issues facing mental health nurses today and also provides the reader with a comprehensive view of biological, psycho-social, cultural and legal issues which influence mental health. It also reflects the increasing trend towards user involvement and the importance placed on the relationships which nurses build with users.

Unit 2: Principles of Organising Care. This unit discusses the organisation of nursing practice in various settings. It details the diversity of mental health care delivery and reflects the recent emphasis on community care. Contributors highlight a range of services provided to meet the needs of people with mental health problems, including crisis intervention, acute in-patient care and continuing care. Although much of the unit concentrates on the very real problems and pressures of caring for the mentally ill it recognises the crucial role nurses have in striving to promote mental health.

Unit 3: Applying Principles in Nursing Practice. This unit concentrates on the clinical management of the main mental health problems. The chapters have been written by nurses working in clinical practice who are committed to constantly improve patient care through implementing research findings and building up a knowledge base of best practice. It is the ability to base clinical practice on sound and, whenever possible, evidence-based principles which gives this unit its strength.

The final chapter addresses the future of mental health nursing, recognising the importance of the change process, which is the most consistent, enduring and predictable factor shaping the future of mental health nursing.

THE FORMAT OF THE CHAPTERS

The chapters are designed to aid effective student learning and to assist readers in quickly finding particular subjects.
Each chapter contains:
- Learning outcomes – the main concepts which can be learned from the chapter are outlined in order to reinforce student learning.
- Boxed highlights – to extract and emphasize important issues and points for the reader, pertinent to the chapter including boxed information in the form of case studies.
- Illustrations – there are clear tables, diagrams and photographs to illustrate the text, and enhance the understanding of the text.
- Key concepts – located at the end of each chapter, these help the reader to summarize and assimilate key information.
- References – to give full citations of the literature and research on which the chapter is based in order to provide the reader with the opportunity to gather further information if required.
- Further reading – recommendations for further resources both general and related to specific conditions.

We hope you enjoy using your *Stuart and Sundeen's Mental Health Nursing: Principles and Practice*. Should you have any comments about the book, please write to us care of the Publishers – we'll be pleased to hear from you.

B Thomas
S Hardy
P Cutting

Contributors

The following people edited and contributed new chapters to this book:

Jonathan Ash
RMN, ENB 650
Clinical Nurse Leader
Behavioural Psychotherapy Unit
The Bethlem and Maudsley NHS Trust
London
Chapters 5 and 29

Jaysheree Bakrania
BSc(Hons), RMN, ENB 603, Dip (Family Nursing)
Clinical Nurse Specialist
Child and Adolescent Department
The Bethlem and Maudsley NHS Trust
London
Chapter 23

Lisa Barcan
BA
Member of Communicate User Group
The Bethlem and Maudsley NHS Trust
London
Chapter 4

Anne Benson
MA, BEd(Hons), RGN, RMN, RNT
Senior Lecturer
The Nightingale Institute
King's College
London
Chapter 6

Geoff Brennan
BA(Hons), RMNH, RMN
National Schizophrenia Fellowship
(LASER)/Harringay Healthcare NHS Trust
Tynemouth Road Health Centre
London
Chapter 32

Fran Bristow
MSc, RGN, RMN, DPSN
Quality and Audit Co-ordinator
Quality and Audit Team
The Bethlem and Maudsley NHS Trust
London
Chapter 9

Jane Bunclark
RMN, RGN
Clinical Nurse Leader
CRASSH Unit
The Bethlem and Maudsley NHS Trust
London
Chapter 13

Chris Burford
RGN, RMN, DipNS
Assistant Community Directorate Manager
Community Directorate
The Bethlem and Maudsley NHS Trust
London
Chapter 11

Sarah Burleigh
BEd(Hons), RGN, RMN, DipNurs(Lond)
Clinical Practice Development Nurse
Old Age Directorate
The Bethlem and Maudsley NHS Trust
London
Chapters 24 and 28

Patrick Callaghan
BSc, MSc, RN
Assistant Professor
Department of Nursing
The Chinese University of Hong Kong
Shatin
New Territories
Hong Kong
Chapter 9

Chris Chaloner
MSc, RMN, RGN, Dip Healthcare Ethics, FETC
Lecturer/Practitioner
Pathfinder Mental Health Services NHS Trust
Shaftesbury Clinic
Springfield University Hospital
London
Chapter 8

Adrian Childs
MSc, RMN, RGN, DipN(Lond)
Assistant Director of Quality and Nursing Practice
Kingston District Commmunity NHS Trust
Roseland Clinic
New Malden
Surrey
Chapter 12

Janet Cockerell
MA, BSc, RMN, RNT
Senior Lecturer
The Nightingale Institute,
King's College
London
Chapter 6

Penny Cutting
BSc(Hons), RGN, RMN
Women's Service Manager
Croydon Mental Health Services
The Bethlem and Maudsley NHS Trust
London
Chapters 2, 3 and 19

Stephen Firn
MSc, BSc, RMN
Director of Nursing
Oxleas NHS Trust
Bexley Hospital
Kent
Chapter 22

Catherine Gamble
BA(Hons), RMN, RNT, RGN
Lecturer - Mental Health
Royal College of Nursing Institute
Chapter 31

Sue Glazier
BSc, RMN, RGN, BTA
User Liaison and Support Worker
The Bethlem and Maudsley NHS Trust
London
Chapter 4

Kevin Gournay
MPhil, PhDC Psycho, AFBPsS, RN
Professor of Psychiatric Nursing
Section of Psychiatric Nursing
Institute of Psychiatry
University of London
London
Chapter 7

Richard Gray
BSc(Hons), RN, DipHE
Research Nurse, Fitzmary 2 Ward
The Bethlem and Maudsley NHS Trust
London
Chapters 16 and 18

Helen Hally
MSc(Econs), SRN, RMN, DipCPN
Executive Nurse Director
Guy's and Lewisham Trust
London
Chapter 1

Sally Hardy
MSc, BA(Hons), DPNS, RMN, RGN
Lecturer
School of Health
University of East Anglia
Norwich
Chapters 1, 3, 10, 17, 28, and 30

Amanda Hobson
BSc, RMN
Police Liaison Community Psychiatric Nurse
West End Community Mental Health Team
London
Chapter 11

Stephen Kirby
RMN
Research and Practice Development Nurse
The Huton Centre
St Luke's Hospital
Middlesborough
Cleveland
Chapter 26

Karina Lovell
MSc, BA(Hons), RMN, ENB 650,
Psychological Treatment Unit
The Bethlem and Maudsley NHS Trust
London
Chapter 25

Nigel McGuire
RMN, DMS
Executive Director of Nursing Services
The State Hospital
Carstairs, Lanark
Scotland
Chapter 26

Edana Minghella
BSc(Hons)
Senior Researcher - Development Initiative
Service Evaluation
The Sainsbury Centre for Mental Health
London
Chapter 17

Alistair Park
MSc, RMN
Lecturer Practitioner
King's College
London
and The Bethlem and Maudsley NHS Trust
London
Chapter 10

David Richards
BSc(Hons), RN, ENB 650
Research and Development Manager
Leeds Community and Mental Health Services
Teaching NHS Trust
Leeds
Chapter 25

Dawn Robinson
RMN
Case Manager
Lambeth Health Care NHS Trust
Lewin Road Community Mental Health Centre
London
Chapter 16

Ken Sampson
RGN, RMN, ENB 603
Child Mental Health Nurse
Child and Family Centre
Treliske Hospital
Truro
Cornwall
Chapter 23

Jane Sayer
MSc, BA(Hons), RMN
Lecturer
Professional Development Centre
The Bethlem and Maudsley NHS Trust
London
Chapter 11

Malcolm Sinclair
RMN, DipHRD, MIPD, ENB 616
Operations Manager
Community Mental Health/Drug and Alcohol Services
St Mary's Hospital
Newport
Isle of Wight
Chapter 20

Nicola Smedley
BSc(Hons)
Clinical Audit Researcher
Quality and Audit Team
The Bethlem and Maudsley NHS Trust
London
Chapters 16 and 18

David Taylor
MSc, BSc, MRPharmS
Chief Pharmacist
The Bethlem and Maudsley NHS Trust
London
Chapter 27

Ben Thomas
MSc, BSc(Hons), RMN, RGN, DipN, RNT
Director of Clinical Services/Chief Nurse
The Bethlem and Maudsley NHS Trust
London
Chapters 14 and 27

Gill Todd
BA(Hons), RMN
Clinical Nurse Leader
The Eating Disorders Unit
The Bethlem and Maudsley NHS Trust
London
Chapter 21

Janet Treasure
PhD, MRCP, FRCPsych
Consultant Psychiatrist
The Eating Disorders Unit
The Bethlem and Maudsley NHS Trust
London
Chapter 21

Robert Tunmore
MA, BSc(Hons), REN, RMN, PEDip Ed
Senior Tutor
Section of Psychiatric Nursing
Institute of Psychiatry
University of London
London
Chapters 15 and 32

Gary Winship
MA(Lond), RMN, DipGpPsych, ENB 616
Psychoanalytic Nurse Psychotherapist
Psychotherapy Department
Reading
Berkshire
Chapter 30

Acknowledgements
The Editors and Publisher gratefully acknowledge the following people for their assistance with this book.

Damian Black, Barbara Bromley, Peter Campbell, Bashir Dauharry, Kay Harwood, Steve Howarth, Sophia McKinnon, Michael Lamb, Annette Pateman, Alan Pringle, John Robertson, Bernie Stoddart, Cheryl Tringham, Dennis Turner.

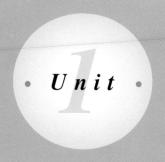

Unit *1*

Principles of
Mental Health Nursing Care

• Chapter •

1

Competent Caring:
Roles of the Mental Health Nurse

Learning Outcomes

After studying this chapter you should be able to:

- Describe the historical development of psychiatric and mental health nurses.

- Analyse the major influences on development of these roles.

- Discuss the significance of developments in training, examinations and education.

- Identify areas of importance for future developments.

CHAPTER OUTLINE

- *Historical influences*

- *Training and examinations*

- *Influences of the changing role*

- *Organizational influences*

- *Role identification*

- *Social context*

- *Contemporary practice*

*T*he terms *'psychiatric nurse' and 'mental health nurse'* are not used indiscriminately in this chapter but arise from differences in the roles and how they have evolved. The psychiatric nurse is defined as the nurse whose main focus is within the institutional setting of a hospital. The term also implies the close connection that nursing had with the medicalization of madness and mental illness. Mental health nurse is a more contemporary term that has derived from the shift of emphasis from illness to health and the changes made to service delivery. The term suggests more positive attitudes towards mental health problems through strategies of prevention and intervention.

This chapter focuses upon the influences surrounding the evolutionary role of the mental health nurse. The authors have not aimed to provide a step-by-step guide to mental health nursing, but hope that this first chapter will offer the reader an overview of where this type of nursing has come from as a basis for considering where it is heading.

Some might be led to believe that mental health nursing only came into being in the late 1970s. To lose sight of mental health nursing's history, roots and heritage may be ideologically liberating but it is a high-risk strategy. At a time when role definition in the field of mental health nursing is becoming more crucial, if it turns away from its roots nursing must be very sure of itself in the present.

The fundamental concepts of medicine, health, disease and sickness cannot be understood without a historical perspective; concepts of madness and unreason have been described as effects of political, economic and sociological systems of discourse and the distribution of power (Turner, 1987).

HISTORICAL INFLUENCES

The mind has been of considerable interest to scholars such as scientists, artists, philosophers and lawyers for many years. Madness raises important questions about society and how it is organized. The distribution of land and property, as well as an individual's level of responsibility and criminal tendencies, were all considered to be disrupted once a person was deemed insane.

Before the 1830s the mentally ill were dealt with in a relatively contained manner. They would be nursed in their own homes and attended by physicians at a level they could afford. Rich families' eccentric relatives would be cared for by domestic servants, while paupers' care would be shared among the villagers or parishioners.

Only a small minority of people, mainly women with illegitimate children, were confined to mental institutions.

The situation changed greatly after the introduction of the Poor Law in 1834. The Poor Law was the consolidation of a number of Acts passed by Elizabeth I which demanded that parish officers obtain taxes to pay for treatment for those in need within their parish. Treatment involved providing 'outdoor relief', which was money given to people in their own homes, or 'indoor relief', which involved the provision of a workhouse. The needy included orphans, the elderly, the mentally disordered, the unemployed and the physically ill.

Nursing then was not a separately identifiable occupation. Anybody could describe themselves as a nurse and call their work nursing. Only in 1923, when the General Nursing Council (GNC) register came into operation, was any discrimination made between who could and could not nurse.

ASYLUMS

The Oxford Dictionary (1990) defines asylum as:
1. Sanctuary, protection, especially for those pursued by the law
2. Any of various kinds of institution offering shelter and support to distressed or destitute individuals, especially the mentally ill.

Although asylums were distinct from workhouses they were run in the same Victorian manner. In 1859 asylums catered for 16 000 patients throughout England, while in 1939 public authorities were providing 132 000 places for lunacy patients as well as 32 500 for mental defectives.

Given the isolation of the asylums, the level of care was dependent on the character, values and beliefs of their medical superintendents and ranged from physical brutality, public humiliation and physical restraint through to high moral and religious standards.

The care of the mentally ill was under considerable review from theorists, sociologists and philosophers in the late 1800s. Public attitudes to mental illness ranged from seeing it as spiritual possession, through to eccentricity and genius. The Lunacy Act in 1890 took the view that society needed protection from those who might disturb or damage it. The Act defined the responsibility of local authorities to provide care for certified patients, free of charge. Certified patients were deprived of liberty and rights of citizenship. Asylums were geographically distant from towns and cities where the able-bodied toiled in order to provide and maintain a civilized society. Many patients once certified were disassociated from their families and remained all their lives inside the asylums' self-contained communities.

In asylums the role of the attendant or nurse involved working in the kitchen or laundry, on the farm or in the vegetable gardens. The least able inmates were cared for by some of the more able inmates, while the nurses were involved in maintaining order and carrying out the medical superintendent's instructions.

The York Retreat

William Tuke (*c*.1800) is considered to have been responsible for the official ethos of the Victorian asylums. His work derived from *The Retreat*, a Quaker community house in York.

He introduced the concept of madness being a passion that needed nurturing, which would respond to kindness and moral restraint. He stressed self-discipline and provided a regime that removed any possible stimulus of the passions, thus giving patients the opportunity to regain control of their minds. He also subscribed to the general opinion that society needed to be protected from any disturbance caused by inmates of mental institutions.

Asylum staff were called attendants, keepers or superintendents indiscriminately and subjected to the same sorts of discipline and restrictions as the domestic staff of any large household. In pauper asylums, attendants would share accommodation with the patients. Staff levels were in the region of one attendant for between 15 and 25 patients. Creative developments of the role were limited, despite the desire to employ intelligent, kind and industrious attendants. Emphasis was given to the attendants' physical ability to carry out the disciplined approach demanded by the moral treatments offered.

Towards the end of the 19th Century, moral treatments gave way to the rise of physical treatments, such as baths, medical electrotherapy and drugs. This dramatic alteration in treatment brought a change in the demands on attendants. Medical superintendents began to introduce the general hospital approach to asylums. 'The Retreat' introduced uniformed nurses in 1890, along with the nursing hierarchy of a general hospital.

NURSES AS CARE PROVIDERS

Nursing's historical roots can be traced through domestic service, the church and the armed forces. Many asylum attendants were working class men. They were employed largely for their physical strength (required to forcibly restrain inmates) but also for the agricultural and practical skills needed to maintain the asylum community and supervise asylum labour. The decline in the need for agricultural workers meant most of the able-bodied were seeking work in the towns and cities during the boom of industrialization. Nurses' wages remained modelled on those of agricultural and domestic staff.

After the First World War, modernization of asylums became fashionable under a policy of social reconstruction. Replacing or renewing asylums was impossible due to economic constraints. The term 'mental hospital' replaced asylum and demobbed men joined both as in-patients and attendants, depending on their level of fitness.

Nurses' work became more closely modelled on the general hospital, with nurses working as doctors' aides and undertaking physical treatments. Training and qualification became tools by which promotion could be earned.

TRAINING AND EXAMINATIONS

Attendants at Springfield Hospital in south London were possibly the first to receive a course of lectures from their medical superintendent, in 1843. Lectures covered what were deemed important principles and the conduct to be followed while caring for the afflicted. Most medical superintendents had begun to introduce training for attendants by 1845, which eventually culminated in a national certificate qualification in 1890. The certificate was controlled by the Medico–Psychological Association (MPA) made up of medical superintendents. Most of the material taught related to anatomy and physiology.

In 1885 a group of Scottish superintendents produced a 64-page handbook (adopted and expanded by the MPA in 1896), which became the standard text for the national certificate. Regularly updated under the title *The Handbook for Mental Nurses* (reflecting the new designation of staff of both sexes) it was used for many years. Known as the *Red Handbook* from its standard red cover, it remained central to mental nurse training until 1954.

By 1934 only 30% of all staff in mental institutions had gained the national certificate, which was seen as a path to career advancement and preferred to the General Nurse certificate. Asylum attendants were the first section of the nursing profession with a relatively uniform system of training and examination. In addition the first central record, a list of certificate practitioners, was held by the MPA.

Despite these changes, pay remained low, working conditions poor and the working day long and arduous. The status of care for the mentally ill remained below that of the physically sick in the more prestigious general hospitals. Conditions of service failed to attract educated women and men, who were drawn towards general hospitals. Senior female nurses were brought into mental hospitals with the aim of improving standards but instead caused resentment from male attendants, who saw their promotional prospects blocked.

Following the First World War, the view that mental disorder was a specialist branch of general nursing became common. Nursing patients with malaria or providing insulin therapy to diabetics required skills of cleanliness, hygiene and asepsis, all associated with general nursing practices. Dual qualifications became a requirement for senior nursing positions in mental institutions.

The interwar period was marked by a prolonged debate between the MPA and the GNC over whether mental and general nursing should become separate branches of a common occupation. The Nurses' Registration Act in 1919 created a supplementary register for mental nurses. Finally the GNC and the MPA became the Royal Medico–Psychological Association (RMPA) in 1925. The RMPA claimed its examinations had a proven value and were designed specifically to meet the special needs of mental nurses. In reality the examination was easier and cheaper than the GNC's (Nolan, 1986). It feared an influx of general nurses into mental hospitals, which would decrease the wages of staff.

By 1951, the RMPA (soon to become the Royal College of Psychiatrists) was persuaded to relinquish training in favour of the GNC. The National Health Service was introduced, but with little effect on mental institutions. Changes were made to the syllabus for mental nurse training, which reduced its general nursing content and increased the amount of psychology and psychiatry. Student nurses made up 80% of direct patient care in 1971, despite a White Paper, *Better Services for the Mentally Ill*, which set a target of 60% qualified staff.

INFLUENCES OF THE CHANGING ROLE

Mental nursing in the first half of the 1800s was a combination of domestic and agricultural labour. As medical treatments were introduced, greater technical content was added to nurses' work. Nurses increasingly took on doctors' duties. Doctors came to appreciate their helpers and used their help in administering medically prescribed treatments.

Apothecaries were responsible in the hospitals for compounding and supplying medicines and for offering advice and guidance with diagnosis. Although considered socially inferior, they joined forces with surgeons and physicians in what became the medical profession.

Apothecaries were also responsible for daily bleeding and blistering, preparations for baths and for surgery and electrical treatments. Eventually this work was taken over by medical students. Although the nurse's role was to prepare the dressings, they principally helped by fetching and carrying. If simple poultices were needed, the nurse would apply them but if any lotion or liniment was prescribed, the medical student or pupil would take over. The nurse's role in attending to the physical and spiritual comfort of patients was therefore similar to that of any other domestic servant. In the asylums, the nurse's role was also one of providing basic physical care and some rudimentary comfort.

As doctors became more interested in symptomatology and disease, they began to rely on nurses to observe and report changes in physical and mental conditions of patients. This necessitated improving nurses' education. The nurse gradually became distinguishable from other servants. This medicalization, however, did not infiltrate the workhouses and asylums until the late 1860s, where nursing was carried out by other inmates, with the nurse's role concentrated on maintaining a sense of order.

THE CRIMEAN WAR

Florence Nightingale's influence on the sanitation and organization of hospital care brought about a major change in nursing and health care. The war exposed the disorganization of medical supplies and their delivery, which was compounded by epidemics of cholera and dysentery. Nursing was carried out by able bodied male orderlies who were often recalled for armed combat, leaving the less able bodied to care for the sick. Orderlies spent a great deal of time away from patients, queuing for food, queuing for it to be cooked, queuing for medical supplies.

These problems led to parties of female, general nurses being sent out from England. One such party was under the supervision of Miss Nightingale. The behaviour and demeanour of the nurses were of considerable concern to the Victorian ladies who dictated the values and behaviour expected of them. Although contact with soldiers was severely restricted, several nurses lost their posts for misconduct and were sent back to England. Female nurses were allowed to fan patients, place ice in their mouths and help them turn in bed but they could not wash anything but the men's faces. Improvements in sanitation and the generally civilizing influence of these Victorian ladies helped to reinforce the view back in England that nursing was indeed a vocation.

PSYCHOSOCIAL NURSING

The two World Wars produced further changes to society's view of sickness in general and mental illness in particular. Army officers suffering from shell shock were sent to military hospitals to recover and regain their mental stability. Often these hospitals were large country houses in extensive grounds. Officer patients took to their beds on admission and were treated in a traditional bedside doctor relationship. However, evening mealtimes became social events. The officers would dress for dinner and once the housemaids and other orderlies had gone, the patients were left to prepare their own meals and clean up afterwards. When Dr T F Main became medical director at the Menninger Clinic in October 1946 he introduced lectures for patients. These soon turned into question and answer sessions discussing personal issues and concerns. Group therapy had emerged and with it the concept of psychosocial care.

Changes in treatment from rest to activity, regression to self-reliance, once again demanded new ways of thinking for staff. The Cassel Hospital in Richmond introduced formal training for nurses who were interested in working with patients suffering neurotic disturbances. One major task was to convince nurses of the existence of the unconscious. Standard texts were the *Psychopathology of Everyday Life* Freud (1914) and, later, Klein and Riviere's *Love, Hate and Reparation* (1936). The aim was to encourage nurses to recognize their own life experiences to help them understand how patients might feel. Nurses were given a great deal of psychopathological information which was of little practical use. While both doctors and nurses were pleased with the level of academic success, nurses became increasingly dissatisfied with their nursing role and confusion emerged between roles.

By 1955, the Cassel training had been renamed and nurses were encouraged to interview patients and relatives in their own homes. This training eventually became the family-centred nursing course.

Weddell (1968) identified the nurse as a group member and showed how nurses might lead a group and seek to understand the tensions and anxieties the group might be expressing. The nurse was encouraged to examine and criticize the group's techniques and to adapt to change as the occasion demanded.

The nurse had to be tolerant and understand the intricacies of a relationship. The patient might not need the nurse and patients' behaviour towards nurses would be coloured by emotional needs. The nurse was responsible to the doctor, to whom they reported and kept informed of their work. As a member of the nursing team, the nurse was expected to make observations and to contribute to the patient's overall management. Nurses were expected to write reports on patients and group activities, observe any change in patients' situations together with others as required by the doctor.

A ROAD LESS TRAVELLED

Providing containment and care, often in that order, for people with mental health problems is not new. As previously outlined, the provision of hospital based care for mentally ill people became a Victorian concern. This resulted in the establishment of large, self-contained communities, close to all of our major towns and cities. These county asylums have now fallen into disrepute and disrepair but were the nurseries of contemporary mental health nursing in this country. A published history of one of these hospitals describes a visit by the then Minister of Health, and quotes him as reporting, 'I have ... seen wards in which 186 patients were in the care of four nurses' and yet he praised the quality of care available. This visit took place as recently as 1956. The challenges facing nurses working in such environments, including the organization and supervision of patients, were very different from the concerns of nurses today.

Other chapters will discuss in more detail nursing environments, skills, philosophies and interventions. Discussions of the benefits of having hospital based care provision, or the ethics of transferring in-patients from different county asylums to meet the shortfall of patient labour on the hospital farms are not irrelevant; they give a sense of the living experience of the asylum system and the culture from which contemporary mental health nursing has sprung. Developments in the profession over a relatively brief 10-yard period were major. In 1965, the listing for nursing in a careers encyclopedia (Edmonds, 1965) began thus:

> A girl who enters the nursing profession undertakes work of the highest importance and adopts a career of absorbing interest ... The nursing profession is now one of the most attractive open to women; it is satisfying, full of interest and has a natural appeal to those who enjoy being of service to others.

Mental health nursing only receives two specific comments, firstly as the preserve of male nurses and secondly that 'the training allowances and salaries are considerably higher and residential accommodation is sometimes available'.

When considered against this backdrop, mental health nursing is a young profession. Professor Tony Butterworth (1990) refers to community psychiatric nursing's development as 'from an uncertain beginning, through a period of gauche, confident adolescence to a current state of more mature adulthood' (Butterworth, 1990). Arguably this is true for all areas of mental health nursing, although even as it reaches adulthood the search for identity continues. Issues of role definition, skills, competencies, scope and responsibilities are all concerns for nursing. The purpose of this next section is to explore some of the factors that have influenced the development of nursing to its current position, to consider the factors that might influence future development from this point and to capture some of the essential aspects of the role of the nurse in mental health.

POLITICAL INFLUENCES

The impact on the nursing profession of the challenge to asylum care as the dominant ideology cannot be over emphasized. Excellent examples of innovative approaches to mental health care existed well before Enoch Powell's 'water tower' speech. That speech, delivered at the 1961 MIND conference, marked a dramatic change in the way that mental health care was conceptualized. Powell called for:

> nothing less than the elimination of by far the greater part of this country's mental hospitals as they stand today. This is a colossal undertaking, not so much in the physical provision which it involves as in the sheer inertia of mind and matter which it requires to be overcome. There they stand, isolated, majestic, imperious, brooded over by the gigantic water tower and chimney combined, rising unmistakably and daunting out of the countryside – the asylums which our forefathers built with such solidity.

> *(Powell, 1961)*

In 1962 *A Hospital Plan for England and Wales* was laid before Parliament. This drew attention to the deficits of the then obsolescent and overcrowded provision and described the official closure programme. The death-knell for the asylums had been sounded.

CONTINUING CARE

Prior to this point the focus of nursing endeavours, in relation to people with continuing care needs, had been to develop a high quality range of activities based upon daily life in a hospital setting. The need for work, recreation, structured and unstructured social time was recognized. Hospitals had grand halls regularly used for patients' activities, such as dances and concerts. Local shops would be invited in, to hold sales. Sunday services were held in the hospital chapel throughout the year, with special services at Christmas and Easter. Work schemes were many and varied; most hospitals had industrial therapy units that would secure external contracts for largely unskilled and repetitive work, such as packing sterile supplies, assembling safety goggles and packing Christmas cards. Almost invariably there would be some form of market gardening where patients' labour was translated into produce for the hospital and for staff. Within this context, firmly located in the hospital setting, many excellent nurses struggled to create a high quality living environment for the people in their care. Only rarely was consideration given to alternatives to hospital care provision.

The publication of *A Hospital Plan* challenged this view (Wolsey, 1990). It recognized that acute admission and treatment areas would still be required, although these were to be resited in district general hospitals. Continuing care (the *raison d'être* of the asylums) was no longer to be a hospital, or even a health function. The plan was for a network of supported accommodation, day care, sheltered workshops and social work support to be provided by the local authority.

FROM MENTAL ILLNESS TO MENTAL HEALTH

Some parts of the system responded more rapidly than others to the proposed changes. The 1970s saw an explosion of treatment options for people with acute mental health problems. These included admission units attached to district general hospitals, day hospitals, therapeutic communities, day centres, community psychiatric nursing services, specialist services for drug and alcohol related problems and specialist out-patient groups. Aspects of all of these had been in existence for some time, but the 1970s saw the migration of these services from the periphery to the centre of mental health strategy.

These developments produced a near mortal wounding of the nursing profession. A chasm opened up between nurses who were part of the asylum culture and those of a community background. The former were unashamedly hospital focused. They believed that, for their patients, quality care and quality living could only be achieved in a traditional hospital setting. Community care was seen as tantamount to abandoning such patients and as being run by nurses who rejected all that the asylums stood for. Community based nurses believed in early intervention and health promotion as key principles in mental health. There was an implicit belief that if high quality interventions were delivered in a community setting, then serious mental illness could be eradicated. The focus of care, particularly for community psychiatric nurses, moved from people with continuing care needs, towards what some considered were the trendy therapies including self-referral systems for anyone in distress.

Nurses in the community undertook a range of specialist training, from behavioural therapy to psychotherapy. As the skills of community nurses became more specialized, their practice base narrowed and the gap between them and traditional hospital based nurses grew. There was a marked difference in the status of hospital and community nursing staff. With the advent of clinical grading, the implicit status differential was made explicit, with community nurses achieving significantly higher grades. Anecdotal evidence suggests that there were also issues of ethnicity, gender and age with community nursing becoming disproportionately the province of the young white male.

ORGANIZATIONAL INFLUENCES

Alongside the changes in social understanding of mental health came a radical change in thinking about how care should be organized and provided. At a critical time for the development of forward looking, comprehensive and integrated mental health strategy, mental health nursing was caught up in an internal struggle from which it has yet to fully recover. From the opposite sides of the chasm, the analysis of the flaws in mental health provision, and therefore the ideas about possible solutions, looked very different.

HOSPITAL VERSUS COMMUNITY CARE PROVISION

From the traditional hospital vantage point, community nurses had turned their backs on the prime client group, people with continuing care needs. Instead they were getting involved in more immediately rewarding work with people who had mental health difficulties in the context of an otherwise healthy lifestyle. The few people with severe mental health problems that community nurses accept, receive little more than regular injections and, if they become difficult, are either admitted to hospital or discharged from the community nurse's case load (Wooff, Goldberg and Fryers, 1988; Brooker, 1990).

From the community vantage point, hospital nursing staff were perceived as doing little more than acting as custodians. Communication was very poor; community nurses were often not informed when one of their patients was admitted or discharged. Hospital nurses were seen as lacking skills or vision because if they had either they would be working in the community. They were also seen as wedded to the 'medical model', regarding the patient as a condition not a person.

Clearly, both of these are exaggerated and distorted views. They do, however, contain a grain, or several grains, of truth. The drift of community nurses away from people with continuing care needs was clearly demonstrated in the first three quinquennial surveys carried out on behalf of the Community Psychiatric Nurses Association (CPNA). The last of these was carried out prior to the substantial political, professional and policy initiatives that refocused attention onto those with severe mental health problems (CPNA 1981, 1985, 1990). A 1996 survey might well demonstrate a reversal of the trends of previous years but perceptions change slowly.

The skills base of nurses who worked for many years in large traditional hospitals may not be appropriate for today's acute admission or community work. Skills can, however, be acquired. To change attitudes is more difficult and, indeed, many nursing staff from traditional hospital settings have attitudes that would enrich any acute or community setting. Such nurses often have an immense capacity to contain anxiety and to communicate a sense of safety, and have a commitment to continuity and change without disruption. Numerous examples, throughout the country, of hospital based nurses who have effected major resettlement and hospital closure programmes are clear testimony to the flexibility and competencies of staff all too frequently dismissed as anachronisms.

Nurses in acute admission areas may be criticized justifiably for not communicating fully or early enough with community colleagues. Community nurses who plan out their week in advance, who work to allocated, timed appointments, can be greatly inconvenienced when they are given short notice of care planning meetings, or when the meeting time clashes with a regular appointment. For ward staff working under the pressure of a 100%-plus bed occupancy rate, planning is a rare luxury.

INTEGRATING PRACTICE

The problems are easy to state; the real challenge comes in finding a way to bridge the divide, real or perceived, between hospital and community nursing staff. The status issue is an important one, for while the community is seen as fertile ground for the most highly skilled staff, it will become increasingly difficult to retain high calibre staff in hospital settings. If, however, the hospital is where people in the most acute distress, with the greatest need for a containing environment, are treated, arguably that is where the most highly skilled staff are required. Community mental health nursing, far from being a specialist area, should be seen as mainstream nursing. The specialist area of nursing is in-patient care and additional training should be available to enable nurses to meet the particular demands of that type of work.

What is a Nurse?

The questions 'What is a nurse?', 'What is the role of the nurse?' and 'What does a nurse do that cannot be done by a generic mental health worker?' are increasingly heard. Throughout this book there will be various responses to those questions. The Report of the Mental Health Nursing Review Team (1994) has also made a significant contribution to the debate, even going so far as to list and categorize nursing skills. However, for mental health nursing to grow and develop, it is not enough to have a text to turn to for validation. Nor is it enough to define ourselves by what we are not.

Nurses themselves must be able to answer these questions clearly and with confidence. The issue has taken on increased prominence as a result of two separate but related influences: first, the move from professional management to general management, and second the move from unidisciplinary to multidisciplinary working. The role and function of a nurse is affected by the considerable health care changes imposed by political and societal influences.

Task versus Team Nursing

During the 1970s and 1980s there was a considerable move away from task allocation, which had become the standardized system of nursing care delivery. This system, by which practical tasks were given to nurses of various hierarchical levels, was derived from delegation deemed appropriate for a particular nurse's rank during World War II. Activities or tasks were issued as orders and expected to be carried out without question. The nurse's rank or level dictated the type of activity to be carried out. Any new nursing student could expect to clean out the sluice and hope to work up the ranks to Sister, whose prestige was confirmed when allowed to accompany the doctors on the ward round and then join them for afternoon tea.

Primary Nursing

Primary nursing was first discussed in the UK by Kratz (1979) and Lee (1979). Manthey (1980) states that primary nursing was being used in the USA in the 1960s. Writers have subsequently described it both as a method of organizing care delivery and also a philosophy of nursing in itself. References to concepts of holism and individuality were becoming more frequent in the writings of nurses and to exert a significant effect on how nursing was to be organized.

Primary nursing presented a means of re-evaluating nursing care. Black (1992) suggests that how nurses interpret their individual role within the nurse–patient relationship is most crucial in primary nursing. Primary nursing can take on many guises but Black summarizes the concept as a partnership between the primary nurse and their patient. This partnership should be based on trust,which cannot exist unless the relationship is a shared one. She also identifies the skills required for nurses who wish to work as primary nurses. Primary nurses are described as confident practitioners who are able to use reflection and assertiveness in the exploration of the nurse-patient relationship.

Specific roles of the primary nurse are identified as:

1. Responsibility for the assessment, planning, delivery and evaluation of nursing care for the patient. Although the primary nurse is accountable and responsible on a daily basis, an associated nurse accepts the responsibility when the primary nurse is not on duty.
2. Carrying out patient care most of the time, acting as primary care provider.
3. Responsibility for communicating relevant information necessary for the patient to receive their full nursing care provision.

The primary nurse also:

4. Accepts and acts with authority to make decisions about the patient's care.
5. Manages a defined patient case load.
6. Acts as a mentor to associate nurses caring for the patient case load.
7. Is the primary point of communication for the patient.
8. Acts as the patient's advocate if the patient or the relatives are unable or unwilling to speak for themselves.

These roles are further defined by Zander (1980) as 12 key elements of the primary nurse's role, which are accountability, advocacy, assertiveness, authority, autonomy, continuity, commitment, collaboration, contracting, co-ordination, communication and decentralization.

Whether this system of nursing is what both nurse and patient actually want remains open to question. Numerous studies have looked at the effects of primary nursing, but little work has been carried out in the mental health care setting, where interpersonal relationships have often been considered more of an inherent skill than an advance in nursing practice.

The Named Nurse

The system of primary nursing is being superseded by the named nurse concept. Once again underpinned with the philosophy of primary nursing and holism, this requires that patients have a qualified nurse allocated to them for the duration of their hospitalization or treatment. The named nurse concept became a political diktat and was set out in the *Patient's Charter* (Department of Health, 1991, 1995). Its aim is to improve consistency of care while also extending the rights of the patient as a health consumer (Royal College of Nursing, 1992).

An increase in the level of responsibility (and therefore authority) of the nurse has developed alongside these changes. With increased responsibility and accountability has come the need for adequate training and competence. Nursing is currently in a state of transition, reinforced by political changes such as the reduction in junior doctors' hours, by nurse prescribing and by the increased technical and academic achievements of nurses. Yet nurses are still keen to remain at the patient's side and be involved in the more mundane tasks. It is nurses who make sure a patient is dressed and eats a meal, while also managing their welfare rights and dealing with their psychological distresses. These roles have to be carried out in conjunction with running a ward or department and other organizational demands.

Extending or Expanding the Nurse´s Role

There appears to be an increasing risk of nurses taking on additional tasks and technicalities but without either the accompanying authority to make decisions, or the respect for these additional practices. Wainwright (1994) describes the real test for nurses as the extent to which additional responsibilities and additional tasks are accepted with adequate amounts of authority.

GENERAL MANAGEMENT

The Griffiths' Report (DHSS, 1983) into management organization within the NHS signalled a move away from traditional managerial arrangements (where for example, occupational therapists would be managed by occupational therapists and nurses managed by nurses) towards a general management framework. The professional background of the manager became less important than managerial competence. For nursing, the upper tiers of the traditional hierarchy were swept away. By the end of the 1980s, senior nurse management positions were rare. There were many nurses in management positions, but they were there as managers, not nurses. Nursing's career progression entered a cul-de-sac providing little beyond ward manager level. Initially, this presented few problems to clinical nurses, for although their managers now had different titles, they were for the most part nurses and so had a shared understanding of the role, function and responsibilities of the mental health nurse. Gradually, however, managers from other professional backgrounds started taking on these roles and nurses found themselves being managed by non-nurses. No assumptions could be made about a shared understanding of the role. Questions about skills mix, competencies, functions and responsibilities are increasingly being asked and responses will be demanded.

The Department of Health (DoH) suggested that although nurses share common skills with other mental health professionals, they also have some that are particular to their profession:

> Nursing staff are the largest group of trained staff dealing with people with mental health problems. They work in residential settings, including psychiatric units and nursing homes and as community psychiatric nurses. Their training equips them with counselling as well as caring, rehabilitation and medication supervision skills

(DoH, 1993)

If that is the essence of nursing, it would be hard to make a case for a discrete three year training. Counsellors, social workers, occupational therapists, psychologists, care assistants, general practitioners, could all lay claim to some or all of these competencies. However, within a general management framework, it is essential that the nursing role is clear. A responsible manager, from any discipline, will ask with justification about any post 'what are the skills required to deliver the service that the client needs and from what profession are they most likely to come?'

Working in Partnership

In *Working in Partnership* (Mental Health Nursing Review Team, 1994), a more detailed attempt is made:

> It is difficult to lay any exclusive claim to the possession of these skills [English National Board taxonomy of skills], as other professional groups also operate from related knowledge and skills bases. However it is the combination of these particular skills, together with the values and practice common to the nursing profession as a whole, which provides the unique expertise of mental health nurses enabling them to:

- Establish a therapeutic relationship which rests in a respect for others and skilled therapeutic use of self.
- Sustain such relationships over time and respond flexibly to the changing needs of those with mental health problems.
- Construct, implement and evaluate a care programme.
- Provide skilled assessment, ongoing monitoring.
- Make risk assessments and judgements.
- Monitor the dosage, effects and contra-indications of medication.
- Detect early signs of deteriorating mental health including potential self harm and suicide risk, worsening physical conditions and potential threats to others.
- Prioritise work in order to respond to those most in need.
- Collaborate with members of the multi-disciplinary team.
- Network effectively, setting appropriate boundaries to professional input.
- Manage the therapeutic environment, determined by a clear awareness of such issues as safety, dignity partnership.

On such a foundation a strong case for the centrality of nursing to high quality mental health care can be built. This is important in response to the following two points:

1. Cultural changes resulting from the development of general management.
2. Adoption of multi-disciplinary and multi-agency working as the most effective route towards comprehensive mental health care.

All this has put pressure on nurses to be able to articulate clearly and confidently the unique contribution that is made by their profession.

ROLE IDENTIFICATION

Fitzpatrick, While and Roberts (1992) carried out an extensive literature search into the role of the nurse in providing high quality care. It seemed that nothing new had been written about the role and function of a psychiatric nurse to challenge the writings of theorists such as Peplau (1952) or Henderson (1966). In fact Peplau's model of nursing has been reprinted (1988), which indicates that it remains as pertinent for many nurses today as when it was written. So much has changed however with both subtle and major influences affecting the role of the mental health nurse but little seems to have affected the basic elements of what a mental health nurse is trying to achieve.

IDENTIFYING THE MULTIFACETED ROLE OF THE NURSE

When attempting to define the roles and functions of a nurse the literature confuses more than clarifies. The table listing nurse's roles (Table 1.1) is presented with the aim more to stimulate discussion and debate than as a definitive model. All items included have been taken from the nursing literature. Any nurse will recognize the scale of the task in attempting to fulfil the majority, let alone all, of these activities. What is fascinating is the variety and extreme range of activities with which nurses are dealing, which makes answering the question 'What is a nurse?' far from easy.

Research into the helping relationship between nurses and their patients reveals a large diversity of activities identified by both parties as helpful aspects of the nurse's role. Some studies identify the nurse's ability to solve problems as most helpful, while others perceive that the nurse is able to make changes in the whole treatment procedure. The overriding majority, however, said that it was being able to talk to the nurse that proved most helpful (McIntyre, Farrell and David, 1989; Carson and Sharma, 1993; Hardy, 1995).

Broad categories have deliberately been used in Figure 1.1 and therefore headings should be taken as starting points for debate rather than definitive statements.

A Personal Journey

The primary concerns of the nurse under the heading *Nursing* in Figure 1.1 are the most commonly associated words found in the literature. Each word may have several definitions which can be broad and/or specific. The reader is left to decide whether or not they agree with some or all the categories listed. What does appear to be evident is that the answer to the question 'What is a nurse?' depends on that nurse's personal

attributes. More importantly, perhaps, is what the nurse is willing to explore, reveal and work with in their interpersonal relationships. Rogers (1961) describes this as a journey in search of 'the good life'. He describes the constant struggle of trying to understand the crucial dynamics of human relationships. Perhaps this is why nursing is often described as both an art and a science; an art because of the very personal style, perceptions and interpretation nurses bring to the role that cannot be captured in words and a science because there are aspects of the role that can be systematically tested and are common to all nurses.

Scientific means of observation and investigation are increasingly elements of a nurse's work. This should not obscure recognition of the environment and its effect on what is observed. Nursing research is gradually embracing an approach that allows for the integration of many different methods. Nursing research should concentrate on the nurse, the patient and what goes on between them.

THE NURSE AS A MULTIDISCIPLINARY TEAM MEMBER

Nurses often work in collaboration with other health professionals. This not only provides a wide range of services for patients but also maximizes opportunities for educational interchange. A multidisciplinary team may comprise members from many different disciplines, such as occupational therapists, psychologists, doctors and educationalists.

Evers (1977) looked at the role of the nurse in the hospital setting and concluded that, to provide total patient care, the

'Nursing is both an art and a science' *The multifaceted role of the nurse*	
Nursing	Enabling Assisting Caring Serving
Subroles	Facilitator Teacher Counsellor Supervisor Evaluator Planner Carer Advocate Surrogate Health promoter Health educator Negotiator
Quality care provision	Ability Behaviour Knowledge Performance Judgement Skills Competence Decision maker Attitudes
Philosophical foundation	Theoretical underpinning Identifying/expressing needs Promotion of self-care Humanitarianism Health concepts Critical thinking
Skills	Communication Technical Negotiation Observation Interpersonal Research Measurement Teaching Creative

Figure 1.1 The multifaceted role of the nurse

Case study: Interdisciplinary collaboration

A student nurse had been working closely with a man who attended the ward as a day patient. She had arranged to meet the patient twice each week specifically to discuss his daily activities but also to help monitor his mood and, in particular, to ask about his persecutory voices. Once a month the consultant would ask for a review of all the day patients and the student nurse had been asked to write a summary report. She spent many hours considering what to write and finally prepared a report covering all aspects of the patient's nursing care and treatment, with the help of the supervisor.

The ward round was held in a separate room off the main ward area and the nurse was called in by the clinical charge nurse to discuss the patient. The charge nurse introduced the student to the consultant, who was holding court to a room full of people. She began to deliver the summary report but was soon interrupted by the consultant firing questions at the registrar about the patient's medication. The student sat patiently for a few minutes and then asked whether to continue. The consultant looked up for the first time that morning and said, 'A lot of people who get involved with this man get seduced into believing they are the ones who can make him better'. The student retorted that they were offering the patient time and interest, and if that helped, they were doing a good job.

nurse needed to be an integrated member of the multi-disciplinary team. This involves not only having to communicate effectively with a wide range of professionals, but also establishing the line of responsibility. According to Ritter (1989) the consultant psychiatrist is often falsely credited with sole responsibility for the patient under their care though any member of the team can be called upon to account legally for their part in the treatment process.

In the multidisciplinary setting, nurses can benefit from the approaches brought to patient care by different disciplines, including collaborative research. Each discipline will have different views and opinions on the most suitable treatment plan, assessment techniques or psychological intervention and how these are best measured or monitored. The nurse can provide important information about the patient. This will help the team develop an informed overview of the patient's mental health and physical condition on which to base the treatment plan. However, interdisciplinary collaboration does not always come easily.

The problems of working in a team have often been discussed. Benfer (1980) identified three specific problems related to team functioning:
1. Problems identifying roles and functions
2. Difficulties in resolving overlapping roles
3. The communication process.

If these issues remain unresolved, resentment, confusion and difficulties easily arise.

The Risks of Role Ambiguity

Not only are nurses no longer necessarily managed by nurses but, increasingly, they are no longer working in exclusively nursing teams. This is particularly noticeable in community nursing where Community Psychiatric Nursing (CPN) teams are rapidly giving way to multidisciplinary and multi-agency teams, known variously as community mental health teams, crisis intervention services, early intervention teams, community support teams or even assertive outreach teams. Many more varieties could be listed but all share common features. Referrals tend to be assessed by two people from different professional backgrounds. This assessment is brought back to an allocation meeting where someone from the team is identified as the key worker.

The choice of key worker is influenced by many things (e.g. capacity, skills, orientation, gender and ethnicity) although the professional background (i.e. nurse, doctor, social worker, occupational therapist, psychologist) is less relevant. This increasingly begs the questions 'if the profession does not determine the client allocation, what is the added value in having discrete professional groups and training?' and 'if we are all doing the same work, why not have a single, unified generic mental health worker?' To be able to participate in this debate, nurses must develop a clear sense of their own professional identity; they must be able to recognize their commonality with other disciplines but, crucially, they must also be able to recognize their differences. *Working in Partnership* attempts to do this:

The uniqueness of nursing is not essentially concerned with definitions which centre on professional prerogative: it should be based on a client-centred philosophy, the synthesis of knowledge upon which it draws, and, most importantly, its flexibility and responsiveness to individual needs.

PRIMARY CARE

In addition to the introduction of general management and the adoption of multidisciplinary working as the model of choice for mental health, there is a third organizational factor that will have increasing significance for the role of the mental health nurse. This is the move towards a primary care led National Health Service (NHS) and particularly, general practitioner (GP) fundholding. In June 1995, the NHS Executive published *Priorities and Planning Guidance for the NHS, 1996/97*. One of six medium-term priority areas is stated as:

Work towards the development of a primary care led NHS, in which decisions about the purchasing and provision of health care are taken as close to the patient as possible.

Key result areas are described and these include 'a significant increase in the numbers of GPs directly involved in purchasing, particularly through the expanded fundholding options'.

The growth of fundholding has already had considerable impact on the role of mental health nurses, particularly in community settings. The long running debate about the appropriate client group at whom community nursing services should be targeted (people with long-term mental health problems or people with acute distress in the context of an otherwise healthy life) has been both re-energized and sidestepped by the emergence of GP fundholders. GPs now influence what service is provided to which clients through their purchasing decisions. While as a principle this may be broadly supported, in mental health there are particular factors that make this approach problematic at times. Generally GPs will be aware of their patients' needs for specialist intervention as a result of the patients' actions in seeking help. Someone who is physically ill will generally contact the family doctor initially. In mental health, and particularly in the area of severe mental health problems, this is far less likely to occur. Analysis of referral patterns from general practice to almost any community mental health team will show a high proportion of presenting difficulties that do not fall into the severe and enduring mental health problem category. This does not mean that the people referred do not have real problems. Debate continues about the most effective way of addressing these problems while ensuring that specialist mental health services retain sufficient capacity to offer a service to people whose problems clearly fall within the high priority area. Where the GPs are fundholders this debate is stifled but does not have to create an impasse. A variety of creative schemes already exists in which mental health nurses perform a triage assessment in the primary care setting. The triage nurse will discuss potential referrals with the referrer and, if indicated, will follow this with a full client assessment. On the basis of this assessment the client may be:

- speedily referred to the specialist mental health team, or
- taken on by the triage nurse for brief, focused intervention, or
- referred to an external agency, for example Relate, or
- referred back with continuing guidance about primary care led intervention.

This follows closely the model given in the Health Advisory Service (HAS) report on child and adolescent mental health services *Together We Stand* (HAS, 1995). This tiered approach both recognizes the specialist function and puts emphasis on the need for skilled outreach, assessment and facilitation of intervention by non-specialist teams. It also offers a way forward that meets the needs of the primary care team, protects the capacity for specialist work by the core team and, most importantly, provides a flexible and responsive framework for providing high quality mental health care. In such a model the opportunity for nursing to be at the centre of assessment, intervention and coordination is at its greatest. Yet again, however, this depends on the ability of nurses to articulate the role of the mental health nurse with clarity and confidence.

SOCIAL CONTEXT

So far, attention has been given to organizational factors that have shaped the development of nursing. These factors do not occur in isolation but are themselves shaped and influenced by the social context within which they originate and operate. To explore this the hospital closure programme must be returned to oncen again.

A Hospital Plan for England and Wales addressed the development of a range of community alternatives to long stay hospital care but these were extremely slow to materialize. In 1987 Baroness Trumpington, the Health Minister, stated, 'Our policy is not to close hospitals, our policy is to build up alternative services and only then to close hospitals that are no longer needed'.

This bold claim was made a quarter of a century after the plans had been first announced. Yet only a decade after the publication of *A Hospital Plan* concerns were being expressed that community care was not working:

> What began as a brave new clarion call to liberate the chronically institutionalised and neglected patients in grim Victorian buildings miles from nowhere, has ended in a situation where staff morale in these same hospitals is even lower, large numbers of patients are adrift in a community that manifestly does not care and many more patients are finding that they have swapped their long stay hospital for a long stay prison... Patients' relatives are carrying an increasingly difficult and often unrewarding burden with inadequate support from overwhelmed, under-financed, and insufficiently staffed social services.

(Kenny and Whitehead, 1973)

Although many years have passed since these concerns were expressed, the themes are still current today. In England dedicated hospital places for people with long-term mental illness have declined from 149 000 in 1955 to 50 278 in 1992 (HMSO, 1994). In 1960 there were 130 large psychiatric hospitals in England. By March 1993 this number had dropped to 89 and further planned closures will leave only 22 open by the year 2000 (HMSO, 1994). However, provision of the community residential and day care facilities that were expected to offer appropriate alternatives to long stay hospitals has consistently fallen well below the targets set out in the White Paper *Better Services for the Mentally Ill* (1975).

CARE PROVISION AND CARE NEEDS

Several factors have contributed to this discrepancy between provision and need, including lack of status ascribed to people with mental illness and hence lack of priority that is given to the providing appropriate services. The Seebohm Report (HMSO, 1988) led to the loss of specialist mental health social workers in the move to generic working. In addition the rising awareness of child abuse and consequent priority given by social services to child protection work took large resources. However, perhaps the most significant factor that inhibited the development of community based services was finance. Community services were intended to be developed with money that would be saved as a result of closing the large, crumbling Victorian buildings, but that money was required to keep hospitals running until alternative services were available. Some attempts have been made by Central Government to address this but little progress was made until the NHS and Community Care Act 1990. The results of this legislation, which came into effect in April 1993, began to be seen 3 years later. The consequences of the years of neglect have been with us for some time.

Had community services been developed in advance of hospital closure, the transition from asylum care to community care would have required changes in attitudes and expectations on the part of patients, staff and the wider community. Patients used to controlled life in institutions had to learn new skills; staff required a period of rehabilitation and adjustment; the community would have benefited from a measure of education about mental health and some support in adjusting to new neighbours. In some areas this was dealt with extremely well. In most, hospital closure took place with little or no concern for preparation and provision. Consequently local communities felt threatened by the appearance of mentally ill people, previously hidden away in rural asylums, who were now to be seen on the streets. These changes occurred against a background of ever increasing demands on services, overstretched mental health professionals and, all too often, a lack of clarity about priorities and orientation of services. These factors converged towards the end of 1992 when, within a fourteen day period, two high profile events occurred which involved people with severe mental health problems.

The Community Reels

On 17 December 1992 Jon Zeto was fatally stabbed by Christopher Clunis, a psychiatric patient, on a London Underground platform. Two weeks later Ben Silcock, another psychiatric patient, climbed into a lion's cage at London Zoo and was badly mauled. There have been many tragedies, before and since, involving people with severe mental health problems but the impact of the two cases mentioned above on social policy and public perception has been unsurpassed. Within 13 days of the second incident, the then Health Secretary, Virginia Bottomley, announced the establishment of an internal review into the legal powers in relation to the care of mentally ill people in the community. Through the media and pressure groups (SANE (Schizophrenia: A National Emergency) in particular) there was popular clamour for new powers for the compulsory treatment of people with mental health problems.

IMPACT OF LEGAL AND POLICY CHANGES

The 1983 Mental Health Act was a piece of liberal legislation that made great strides in the defence of the rights of the individual but did it not provide for compulsory treatment in the community. This opened up a long-running debate about individual choice as opposed to the duty to comply with treatment. Several attempts at introducing new, more restrictive legislation were blocked by alliances between user groups, some voluntary organizations and some professional organizations, notably some nursing ones. Ben Silcock's climb into the lion's den triggered off renewed calls for community powers. Each successive event involving mentally ill people that has reached the national media since then has reinforced this demand. Mental Health Act amendments under Supervised Discharge Orders will allow for discharge from hospital under certain restrictions. Department of Health guidance requires the establishment of 'At Risk' registers for people who are deemed to be vulnerable or dangerous as a result of a mental illness. There is a plethora of working groups currently reviewing various aspects of mental health care provision. Regular public inquiries into tragedies involving people with severe mental health problems take place.

Effects on Staff

Together, these factors have a significant effect on the work of mental health nurses. Public opinion about the effectiveness or otherwise of mental health services has an undeniable influence on the way that people working in the field perceive themselves to be valued, and in turn, on how they value themselves. The changing policy framework produces pressures concerning ethical considerations for staff and also purely practical ones about implementation and monitoring. The increased media and political attention paid to mental health services has the potential to induce a defensive reaction; this and its concomitant inhibition of creativity would be a major loss to the practice of mental health nursing.

These increased pressures adversely affect recruitment and retention of high quality staff. Fewer nurses are being trained to become mental health nurses and the length of time staff remain in-post is decreasing. A near crisis has been identified by the Royal College of Nursing. Nurses are no longer willing or able to deal with the pressures of their role within the health care field. It has been estimated that over 170000 working days each year are lost through certified sickness, costing the health service billions of pounds (Allen, 1993). Litigation involving stress at work is commonplace in the USA.

Mental health nursing has been affected by the NHS changes, which have contributed to the increases in stress, absenteeism and staff turnover. Dawkins *et al.* (1985) listed six categories considered stressful to nurses:

1. Administrative and organizational issues.
2. Staff conflict.
3. Resources.
4. Scheduling issues.
5. Negative patient characteristics.
6. Staff performance.

Other research has produced similar results, with additional stressors identified as lack of supervision, lack of feedback, lack of education and training, violent incidents and potential suicides (Callaghan, 1991; Carson *et al.*, 1991, 1993; Schafer, 1992; Sullivan, 1993). Other studies have described work stress as affecting the quality and quantity of care delivery and thus constituting a potential threat to the entire working life of the NHS (McCarthy, 1985; Dawkins *et al.*, 1985; Dolan, 1987; Handy, 1991).

Staff Support

Jan Long pioneered a staff support service in Swindon and has shown that caring for staff has positive economic benefits (Long, 1993). She states that the philosophy of the service begins with the belief that the health of the whole organization is reflected in that of the staff, that proactive health promotion goes hand in hand with physical and mental well-being, job satisfaction and commitment. In the health professions a level of stress is essential to survive and deal with emergencies and cope with the heavy demands of the job, yet retain the energy to enjoy work and a social life. Stress becomes unhealthy when these pressures are unrelenting, which leads to frustration, anxiety, disordered thinking and reduced level of functioning. Distracted and distressed staff are twice as likely to become unwell, misuse alcohol and make mistakes (Long, 1994).

The service in Swindon, recognized as an NHS exemplar, works at both corporate and service provision levels offering training, debriefing and support to all staff.

CONTEMPORARY PRACTICE

As shown in this chapter, the nurse's role is affected by numerous extraneous circumstances. Throughout history nurses themselves appear to have initiated little to change, challenge or develop the role of the mental health nurse. The main tasks of the past (to keep wards and patients clean, quiet and tidy) were achieved by strict regimes in small, closed communities.

Professionally, many nurses knew little else than hospital life, with its long working days and staff family network (Clarke, 1993). In 1947, the Ministry of Health working party believed 'the average intellectual calibre of the nursing staff in mental hospitals to be significantly lower than in other types of hospitals'. Yet Clark, Hooper and Oram (1962) considered this more a consequence of nurses' failure to change in the face of innovations than limited intellectual ability.

Mental health nurses have done little to better themselves or their situations, with many nurses passionately opposed to any changes, such as opening the locked asylums (Clarke, 1993). They were effectively more disturbed by the introduction of therapeutic innovations in care provision than were the patients (Ramon, 1985).

As the 21st Century approaches, the future for nursing is probably as difficult to explore as it is to define nursing itself at present. It is the authors' opinion that nurses will remain central to the provision of care, if they are able to keep pace with the societal changes and political influences permeating the health service. What will not change is the very centre of nursing, human interaction.

Despite the widespread introduction of computer based techniques in psychiatry, in assessment, interviews and treatment schedules, nothing can replace face to face contact (Woolley, 1991), although these systems should not be overlooked and are now considered an essential part of everyone's education (Bouchard Ryan *et al.*, 1992). The computer's incursion into psychiatry is another example where nurses have been slow to become interested and involved in computer applications.

However, nurses are developing key roles in education, clinical specialties, management and purchasing. Such variety of career paths open to nurses should continue to be expanded and explored. Although clinical practice remains rooted in the provider units it is important for nurses to recognize their potential influence on the purchasing of health care. This would stimulate high quality services that are patient focused and relevant to patients' needs. Who better than the nurse to recognize those needs, from the very basic to the highly specialized? Such knowledge and skill are valuable instruments to help shape the future of the health service.

SUMMARY

Within the first chapter, the historical developments of understanding and handling mental health problems in society have been presented alongside the emergence of a body of professionals to look after those suffering from them. It is all too easy to suppose that prior to modern intervention and conceptions people suffering from these problems were treated cruelly. Yet there remains much about mental health and well being that still needs to be learnt, especially how best to care.

The mental health nurse has emerged through history striving to find the means to reason with the unreasonable and manage the unmanageable. The effects of economic, cultural and political changes can be traced and are presented as a means of helping to envisage where mental health nursing is heading in the next millennium.

KEY CONCEPTS

- The role of the mental health nurse has emerged alongside vast medical and social reforms.
- Education and training continues to influence the status of the mental health nurse within the health care field.
- When describing the multifaceted role of the nurse, regard must be paid to personal and professional skills and attributes.
- Service care provision and the change in emphasis from illness to health, and from hospital to community has further changed the role of the mental health nurse.
- Contemporary practice remains dynamic and interpersonally orientated while also providing increased stress and rewards.
- The patient, and how the nurse is willing to utilize their personal attributes in working with the patient, is central to nursing.
- Mental health nursing continues to respond to external and internal changes, which should be used to help shape the future of health care delivery and the role the mental health nurse has within it.

REFERENCES

Allen D: News. *Nurs Standard* 7(18):11, 1993.

Benfer BA: Defining the role and function of the psychiatric nurse as a member of a team. *Perspect Psychiatri Care* 18(4):166–177, 1980.

Black F: *Primary nursing: an introductory guide.* London, 1992, Kings Fund Centre.

Bouchard Ryan E, Szechtman B, Bodkin J: Attitudes toward younger and older adults learning to use computers. *J Gerontol* 47(2):96–101,1992.

Brooker C, editor: *Community psychiatric nursing.* London, 1990, Chapman & Hall.

Butterworth T: In: Brooker C, editor: *Community psychiatric nursing*, London, 1990, Chapman & Hall.

Callaghan P: Organisation and stress amongst mental nurses. *Nurs Times* 87(34):50, 1991.

Carson J, Barteltt H, Croucher P: Stress in community psychiatric nursing: a preliminary investigation. *Community Psychiatr Nurs J* April 8–12, 1991.

Carson J, Sharma T: In-patient psychiatric care: What helps? Staff and patients' perspectives. *J Ment Health* 3(2):99–104, 1994.

Clark DH, Hooper DF, Oram EG: Creating a therapeutic community in a psychiatric ward. *Hum Relat* 15(20):123–147, 1962.

Clarke L: The opening of doors in British mental hospitals in the 1950s. *History of Psychiatry* 4:527–551, 1993.

Community Psychiatric Nurses Association: *Community Psychiatric Nursing Services Survey.* PLACE OF PUBLICATION? 1981, CPNA.

Community Psychiatric Nurses Association: *The 1985 CPNA National Survey Update.* PLACE OF PUBLICATION?,1985, CPNA.

Community Psychiatric Nurses Association: *Community psychiatric nursing. The 1990 National Survey.* PLACE OF PUBLICATION? 1990, CPNA.

Dawkins JE, Depp FC, Selzer NE: Stress and the psychiatric nurse. *J Psychosoc Nurs* 23(11):9–15, 1985.

Department of Health: *The Patient's Charter.* London, 1991 and 1995, HMSO.

Department of Health: *Mental illness, What does it mean?* London, 1993, HMSO.

Department of Health and Social Security: *Better services for the mentally ill.* London, 1975, HMSO.

Department of Health and Social Security: *NHS Management enquiry (Griffiths report).* London, 1983, HMSO.

Dingwell R, Rafferty AM, Webster C: *An introduction to the social history of nursing.* Worcester, 1988, Routledge Billington & Sons.

Dolan ND: The relationship between burnout and job satisfaction in nurses. *J Adv Nur* 12(1):3–12, 1987.

Edmonds PJ: *1965–1966 Careers encyclopedia.* London, 1965, Macmillan & Cleaver Ltd.

Evers HK: The patient care team in the hospital ward: the place of the nursing student. *J Adv Nurs* 2(2):589–596,1977.

Fitzpatrick JM, While AE, Roberts JD: The role of the nurse in high quality patient care: a review of the literature, *J Adv Nurs,* 17:1210–1219, 1992.

Freud S: *Psychopathology of everyday life,* 2 ed. Vol 6, London, 1914, (reprinted 1960, Hogarth).

Handy J: The social context of occupational stress in a caring profession. *Int J Nurs Stud* 819–830, 1991.

Hardy SE: *The application of an empirical method to investigate the helping relationship between mental health nurses and their allocated patients.* MSc dissertation, 1995, The Institute of Psychiatry, London.

Health Advisory Service: *Child and adolescent mental health services: Together we stand.* London, 1995, HMSO.

Henderson V: *The nature of nursing. A definition and its implications for practice, research and education.* New York, 1966, Macmillan.

HMSO: *A Hospital Plan for England and Wales.* London, 1962, HMSO.

HMSO: *Report of the committee on local authority and allied social services* (chairman Lord Seebohm). London, 1988, HMSO.

Kenny T, Whitehead O: *Insight: a guide to psychiatry and psychiatric services: Together we stand.* London, 1973, HMSO.

Klein M, Riviere J: *Love, hate and reparation.* Psychoanalytical Epitomes No. 2. London. 1936, Hogarth.

Kratz C: Letter from Australia (2). Primary Nursing. *Nurs Times* 75(42):1790–1791, 1979.

Lee M: Towards better care: Primary nursing, *Nurs Times* 75(33):133–135, 1979.

Long J: *Staff support service: History and service report.* 1993, East Wiltshire Health Care (unpublished).

Long J: Changing the culture for carers. *Nurs Stand* 30(9):20–22, 1994.

Mental Health Nursing Review Team: *Working in partnership: a collaborative approach to care: report of the Mental Health Nursing Review Team* (chairman Professor T Butterworth). London, 1994, HMSO.

Manthey M: *The practice of primary nursing.* Boston, 1980, Blackwell.

McCarthy P: Burnout in psychiatric nursing. *J Adv Nurs* 10:305–310, 1985.

McIntyre K, Farrell M, David A : In-patient psychiatric care: The patient's view. *B J Med Psychol* 62:249–255, 1989.

NHS Executive: *Priorities and Planning Guidance for the NHS, 1996/97.* London, 1995, NHS Executive.

Nolan P: Mental nurse training in the 1920s. *Bulletin of the history of the nursing group* 15–23, Spring 1986.

Oxford Dictionary (Concise), 8 ed. Oxford, 1990, Oxford University Press.

Peplau H: *Interpersonal relations in nursing.* New York, 1952, JP Putman.

Powell E: In: *Emerging patterns for the mental health services and the public.* Proceedings from a conference. London, 1961, MIND.

Ramon S: *Psychiatry in Britain: Meaning and policy.* London, 1985, Croom Helm.

Ritter S: *Bethlem and Maudsley Hospital manual of clinical psychiatric nursing principles and procedures.* London, 1989, Harper & Row.

Rogers CR: *On becoming a person. A therapist's view of psychotherapy.* London, 1961, Constable.

Royal College of Nursing: The named nurse: effects on practice. *Nurs Stand* 6(45):31, 1992.

Schafer T: CPN stress and organisational change: a study. *Community Psychiatr Nurs J* Feb 16–23,1992.

Sullivan PJ: Occupational stress in psychiatric nursing. *J Adv Nurs* 18:591–601, 1993.

Turner BS: *Medical power and social knowledge.* London,1987, Sage Publications.

Wainwright P: *Professionalism and the concept of role extension.* In: Hunt G, Wainwright P, editors: *Expanding the role of the nurse. The scope of professional practice.* Oxford, 1994, Blackwell Scientific Publications.

Weddell D: *Outline of nurse training.* In: Barnes E, editor: *Psychosocial nursing: Studies from the Cassel Hospital.* Norfolk, 1968, Cox & Wyman Ltd.

Wolsey P: In: Brookes C, editor: *Community psychiatric nursing: a research perspective.* London, 1990, Chapman & Hall.

Wooff D, Goldberg D, Fryers T: The practice of community psychiatric nursing and mental health social work in Salford: some implications for community care. *Bri J Psychiatry* 152:783–792, 1988.

Woolley N: An expert to help you give the right care. Expert systems in clinical decision making. *Prof Nurse* 431–436, May 1991.

Zander K: *Primary nursing: development and management.* Maryland, 1980, Aspen Systems Co.

FURTHER READING

Babin RM: *Management teams, why they succeed or fail.* Oxford, 1981, Butterworth-Heinemann Ltd.
> *A classic text for people interested in organizations. It outlines some interesting aspects about teams and what affects their success or failure.*

Barlow DH, Hayes SC, Nelson RO: *The scientist practitioner. Research and accountability in clinical and educational settings.* Boston, 1984, Allyn & Bacon.
> *A book written for psychology students but useful for nurses who are interested in and keen to develop clinical research. It gives some history on the model described and some useful chapters on different practical methods for research. A challenge to the developing role of the nurse in the health services today.*

Department of Health and Social Security: *Organisational and management problems of mental illness hospitals (The Nodder Report).* London, 1980, DHSS.
> *A well-written document, full of insight. Although it appears a dry document, it is in fact a valuable historical text.*

Doyal L, Pennel I: *The political economy of health.* Wiltshire, 1979, Pluto Press Ltd.
> *An interesting book for anyone interested in the politics behind health care developments.*

Farrington A: Intuition and expert clinical practice in nursing. *Bri J Nurs* 2(4):228–233, 1993.
> *This article outlines the concept of intuition and expert nursing, but fails to capture the essence of what makes a skilled expert.*

Goffman I: *Asylums. Essays on the social situations of mental patients and other inmates.* Reading, 1961, Cox & Wyman Ltd.
> *A classic text that should be read by any nurse concerned about the treatment of patients with long-term mental illness and the effect upon the patient of their surroundings.*

Ham C: *Health policy in Britain.* London, 1985, Macmillan Education Ltd.
> *This small book covers health policy in Britain up to the beginning of the health reforms.*

Handy CB: *Understanding organisations.* Harmondsworth, 1976, Penguin Books.
> *A must for all those interested in the working of organizations, it gives a useful insight to all nurses working in teams and in institutions.*

Hirschhorn L: *The workplace within, psychodynamics of organisational life.* London, 1988, MIT Press.
> *A complicated concept explained and explored. This book shows how an individual can influence the environment in their workplace by considering their personal influence and concept of self.*

Jones M: Social change and the therapeutic community. *Bethlem and Maudsley Gazette* 12(3):16–19, 1971.
> *The pioneer of therapeutic communities, Maxwell Jones, here writes about the developments which brought them about. It highlights how external influence is often greater than intent.*

McGowen M, Whitcher S: *Altschul's psychiatric and mental health nursing.* 7 ed. London, 1994, Balliere Tindall.
> *A handy textbook covering some areas and influences on the role of the mental health nurse. Too small to offer much of a challenge, but a useful quick reference.*

Menzies–Lyth I: *Containing anxiety in institutions.* London, 1988, Free Association Books.
> *This book is becoming more talked-about than read. It explores and tries to explain how nurses and people in other institutional settings (ie, schools) are affected by and respond to daily stressors.*

Menzies–Lyth I: *The dynamics of the social,* London, 1989, Free Association Books.
> *More of the same but with more confidence!*

MIND (The National Association for Mental Health), Granta House, 15–19 Broadway, Stratford, London E15. Tel: 0181 519 2122
> *MIND is a charity campaigning to improve services for people with mental distress and their families with the aim of promoting an increased understanding of mental health issues.*

Ministry of Health: *Sub-committee on mental nursing and the nursing of the mentally defective.* London, 1945, HMSO.
> *A historic but sound document, it made recommendations which are only now being realized.*

Ministry of Health: *Communication between doctors, nurses and patients: an aspect of human relations in the hospital services.* London, 1963, HMSO.
> *Another historic document, it has received little attention.*

Ministry of Health: *Joint sub-committee of the standing mental health and the standing nursing advisory committees (Psychiatric nursing: Today and tomorrow).* London, 1968, HMSO.
> *Slightly heavy going but it portrays nursing clearly. It puts forward some interesting and sensible suggestions, although these are quickly forgotten.*

Onyett S: *Case management in mental health.* London, 1992, Chapman & Hall.
> *One of the first books to be written specifically for case management.*

Porter R: *Mind forg'd mannacles: a history of madness in England from the Restoration to the Regency.* London, 1987, Penguin Books.
> *An excellent historical overview of madness and the rise of psychiatry.*

Rushton A: Community-based versus hospital-based care for acutely mentally ill. *Bri J Soc Work* 20:373–383, 1990.
> *Alan Rushton, a social worker, puts forward a good argument for community care, while not ignoring its pitfalls.*

SANE (Schizophrenia: A National Emergency), 2nd floor, 199–205 Old Marylebone Road, London NW1. Tel: 0171 724 6520.
> *SANE is a fundraising and campaigning organization, aiming to fund social and medical research. SANELINE (0171 724 8000 and 0345 678000) is an out-of-hours phone service offering support and information to anyone involved in mental health issues.*

Schon DA: *The reflective practitioner. How professionals think in action.* USA, 1983, Basic Books.
> *A useful book outlining the concepts of reflection that have been used to structure and theoretically underpin clinical supervision.*

Townsend P, Davidson N: *Inequalities in health. The Black report.* Harmondsworth, 1986, Penguin Books.
> *This report was initially distributed over a Bank Holiday weekend and this is thought to be the reason that it did not receive much media attention. It is still relevant today and gives research evidence of health inequalities between classes.*

Concepts, Models and Theories in Psychiatric and Mental Health Nursing

Learning Outcomes

....

After studying this chapter you should be able to:

- Identify the importance of concept clarification within mental health nursing.

- Discuss the development of theory within mental health nursing.

- Describe the associated theories used by mental health nurses to guide their practice including:

  - The psychoanalytical model.

  - The interpersonal model.

  - The social model.

  - The existential model.

  - The supportive therapy model.

  - The medical model.

- Critically discuss the method of theory development outlined in this chapter

CHAPTER OUTLINE

- *The historical context of mental health nursing theory development*

- *Theories used in mental health nursing*

- *Borrowed or shared?*

- *Contradictions in mental health nursing*

Many patients, if allowed free rein, will talk only about themselves and their symptoms. In such cases attentive listening for long periods is prohibited...Probably you will have to tell such patients that you do not talk on such subjects because you do not understand enough to be of any real help, but each time refer the patient to his physician.

Render, 1947

This quote, taken from an early mental health nursing text that outlines the parameters of nurse–patient relationships, clearly demonstrates the tradition of mental health nursing as a service which was used to assist the 'physician', rather than the dynamic, responsive and independently thinking profession that it now strives to do (Royal College of Nursing, 1993).

Thankfully, mental health nursing has come a long way since the instructions above were written. Today the mental health nurse is seen to have a psycho-therapeutic function in her or his own right and is encouraged to develop nursing interventions and methods of care that are research based and to test the application of theories 'borrowed' from other disciplines for their applicability to mental health nursing practice (Reynolds and Cormack, 1990).

The need to develop theories that are unique to mental health nursing has been in part stimulated by authors such as Dickoff *et al.* (1968) whose writings appear to be considered useful years later:

In a practice discipline like psychiatric nursing it is not enough to describe what is happening. Psychiatric nurses must also prescribe actions (Dickoff et al., 1968). In order to do this mental health nurses must be able to identify the service users' needs/problems and prescribe nursing interventions that will result in expected outcomes of such interventions.

Thomas, 1992

The above quote highlights one of the many changes taking place in the field of mental health nursing in relation to the emphasis on the use of nursing theory in the day-to-day work of the mental health nurse.

THE HISTORICAL CONTEXT OF MENTAL HEALTH NURSING THEORY DEVELOPMENT

Historically mental health nursing has been governed by medicine and mental health nursing has had to fight off the idea that it is inferior to general nursing (Nolan, 1993). In turn, this has had a detrimental effect on the independent development of theories by mental health nurses for mental health nursing.

Despite what she says in the opening quote of this chapter, Render (1947) was a pioneer in her field. It was a great achievement for a nurse to be published so early in the history of mental health nursing, for in the 1940s and 1950s it was considered radical for a nurse to publish without the backing of a doctor. Even Peplau had to postpone the publication of her book *Interpersonal Relations in Nursing* (Peplau, 1952) for a year because she did not have such backing (O'Toole and Welt, 1989).

Over the years the role of the mental health nurse and, more specifically, what it is that mental health nurses do, has been a topic for discussion and debate. (See for instance Gullberg, 1989; Peplau, 1989; White, 1990; and most recently the Department of Health (DoH), 1994).

This is once again a topical issue. With the changes in mental health policy and the rise of the 'user movement' mental health nursing and consequently the theories that guide its practice have come into question. These changes have exposed mental health nursing to much public scrutiny and consequently have raised its profile, which in turn has catalysed recognition of the need for re-examination of the theory base that mental health nurses use.

There have been many factors that influenced theory development in mental health nursing, including e.g. the industrial revolution, world wars, the advent of the asylum, the humanitarian movement, de-institutionalization, societal changes such as increases in poverty and homelessness, changing governments, the anti-psychiatry movement, the availability of training and education for nurses and changes in the National Health Service.

More recently, legislation, reports and inquiries have raised the profile of theory based interventions being used by mental health nurses. These include the *Health of the Nation* document (DoH, 1992), which targets mental health as one of its concerns, the Community Care Act (DoH, 1990), which outlines case management as a mode of care intended to provide services based on individual need and enforces a move to community care for people with mental health problems, the Reed Report (DoH/Home Office, 1992), which calls for the reassessment of treatment for the mentally ill offender and the Ashworth Inquiry by the DoH in 1992 together with the review into mental health nursing (DoH, 1994).

It has been shown that Finnish mental health nurses have great difficulty in identifying the theoretical basis from which they work (Lindstrom, 1995). This may also be true among some mental health nurses in the UK. One cause may be that what is relevant for nurses to know is diverse and ever changing. This is shown in part by the opposite stances taken by two of the UK's professors of psychiatric nursing. One believes that health professionals should be informed about 'the advances in molecular genetics, epidemiology, neurochemistry, brain imaging and behavioural approaches' (Gournay, 1994) while the other does not believe that health professionals can 'fix' people with a variety of psychotechnology and that their focus ought to be a more humanized partnership with service users, paying more attention to the 'lived' experience of people with mental health problems (Barker, 1995).

KNOWLEDGE

One approach to expressing the nurse's knowledge base is provided by Carper (1978) and latterly adapted by White (1995), who suggest that this consists of five interrelated patterns, namely:

1. Empirics – the 'scientific' development of models and theories.
2. Ethics – knowledge of ethical theory, principles and guidelines.
3. Personal knowledge of self and how your 'self' impacts upon others.
4. Aesthetics – the 'art' of nursing.
5. Sociopolitics – the sociopolitical context of nurse and client, society's understanding of nursing and nursing's understanding of society and its politics.

Chinn and Kramer (1991) suggest that no one area of knowing is more important than another and that all patterns are interrelated and cannot be separated. For instance scientific knowledge alone is not able to provide answers or solutions to ethical dilemmas. Being able to identify one's knowledge base and to express this in understandable terms is vital to the development of theory that is relevant to the practice of the mental health nurse. It is also important to recognize that theory development is strongly related to and influenced by the sociopolitical values of the day.

CONCEPTS

Many mental health professionals practise within the framework of a conceptual model of care, i.e., a set of 'global ideas about the individuals, groups, situations and events of interest to a discipline' (Fawcett, 1992). A model is a way of organizing

a complex body of knowledge, such as concepts related to human behaviour.

Concepts are 'abstract cognitive representations of perceptible reality formed by direct or indirect experience' (Morse, 1995). In other words, they are the way the mind grasps and then labels the essence of some 'thing', experience or belief. Concept analysis is important in clarifying and developing the concepts relevant to mental health nursing so that theories for practice can be developed.

Models can help clinicians by suggesting:
1. Reasons for observed behaviour.
2. Therapeutic treatment strategies.
3. Appropriate role enactment for both service user and therapist.

Models also provide for the organization of data. This allows the clinician to measure the effectiveness of the treatment process and facilitates research into human behaviour. It would be arrogant to imagine that any one model will provide all that is needed to address the complex human difficulties experienced by users of mental health services and encountered by mental health nurses. Despite this, some nursing theorists have tried to do just this with the production of the 'nursing model'. Many of these nursing models have developed their own language, which only serves to alienate the service user, the less informed nurse and the other people within the multidisciplinary team.

THEORY

A theory in this context is 'a systematic abstraction of reality (usually conveyed by words) that represents perceptual experiences of objects, properties or events which serves some purpose'; a theory represents an ideal of reality but not the reality itself (adapted from Chinn and Kramer, 1991). There are many levels of theory and the wide ranging and generally very abstract 'nursing theories' currently available to mental health nurses provide a confusing array of information that many find unrelated to the reality of their day-to-day practice (one exception to this rule is the work of Peplau (1952) which will be discussed later). Hence many nursing theories are rejected as unworkable and inappropriate. This leaves mental health nurses often adapting the theories developed in other disciplines to guide their practice.

This chapter presents an overview of some of the many models used by mental health nurses, including the psycho-analytical, interpersonal, social, existential, supportive, and medical models. It is beyond the scope of this chapter to address the many 'nursing models' available and the reader will be directed to suitable texts. The issue of the appropriateness of using one nursing model will be addressed throughout the chapter.

THEORIES USED IN MENTAL HEALTH NURSING

Reynolds and Cormack (1987) suggest that if mental health nurses do not have a theory base they will be forced to rely upon 'trial and error, precedent, or the authority of others'. In mental health nursing, relying on the authority of others to some extent comes in the form of using theories developed in other disciplines and applying them to mental health nursing practice. For example, aspects of Peplau's work on therapeutic interaction (Peplau, 1952) are based in the work of Carl Rogers (1951). What follows are some of the major influencing theories for the mental health nurse as described by Gail Stuart and Sandra Sundeen (1995).

PSYCHOANALYTICAL MODEL

Psychoanalytical theory was developed by Sigmund Freud (Figure 2.1) in the late 19th and early 20th Centuries. It focused on the nature of deviant behaviour and proposed a new perspective on human development. Many of Freud's ideas were controversial, particularly in the Victorian society of that time. Objective observation of human behaviour was a great contribution of the psychoanalysts, as was the identification of a mental structure. Such concepts as id, ego, super-ego and ego defence mechanisms are still widely used. Most people also accept the existence of an unconscious level of mental functioning, first proposed by Freud (Freud, 1953).

Psychoanalysts trace disrupted behaviour in the adult to earlier developmental stages. Each stage of development has a task that must be accomplished. If too much emphasis is placed on any stage or if unusual difficulty arises in dealing with the associated conflicts, psychological energy (libido) becomes fixated in an attempt to deal with anxiety.

Psychoanalysts believe that neurotic symptoms arise when so much energy goes into controlling anxiety that it interferes with the individual's ability to function. They believe that everyone is neurotic to some extent. Everyone carries the

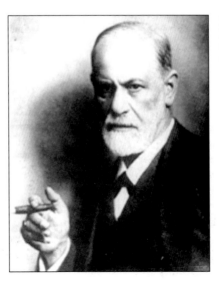

Figure 2.1 Sigmund Freud 1856–1939 (courtesy of Corbis/Bettmann)

burden of childhood conflicts and is influenced in adulthood by childhood experiences. Psychoanalysts in training must undergo personal analysis so that their own neurotic behaviour does not hinder their objectivity as therapists.

According to psychoanalytic theory, symptoms are symbols of the original conflict. For instance, compulsive hand washing may represent the person's attempt to cleanse the self of impulses that a parent labelled as unclean during the anal stage of development. However, the meaning of the behaviour is hidden from the conscious awareness of the person, who is usually upset about these uncontrollable thoughts, actions and feelings.

Freud (1953) developed most of his theories around neurotic symptoms. His theory is less well developed in the area of psychosis. However, other psychoanalytical theorists such as Frieda Fromm–Reichmann have successfully worked with psychotic service users (Fromm–Reichmann, 1950). They believe that the psychotic symptom occurs when the ego must invest most or all of the libido to defend against primitive id impulses. This leaves little, if any, energy to deal with external reality and leads to the lack of reality testing seen in psychosis.

Psychoanalytical Therapeutic Process

Psychoanalysis uses free association and analysis of dreams to reconstruct the personality. Free association is the verbalization of thoughts as they occur without any conscious screening or censorship. Of course, there is always unconscious censorship of thoughts and impulses that threaten the ego. The psychoanalyst searches for patterns in areas that are unconsciously avoided. Conflictual areas that the client does not discuss or recognize are identified as resistances. Analysis of the client's dreams can provide additional insight into the nature of the resistances, since dreams symbolically communicate areas of intrapsychic conflict.

The therapist helps the client recognize intrapsychic conflicts by interpretation, which involves explaining to the client the meaning of dream symbolism and the significance of the

issues that are discussed or avoided. However, the process is complicated by transference, which occurs when the client develops strong positive or negative feelings toward the analyst. These feelings are unrelated to the analyst's current behaviour or characteristics; they represent the client's past response to a significant other, usually a parent. Strong positive transference causes the client to want to please the therapist and to accept the therapist's interpretations of the client's behaviour. Strong negative transference may impede the progress of therapy as the client actively resists the therapist's interventions. Countertransference, or the therapist's response to the client, can also interfere with therapy if the analyst is unaware of it or unable to deal with it.

Since the therapist can temporarily replace the significant other of the client's early life experience, previously unresolved conflicts can be brought into the therapeutic situation. These conflicts can be worked through to a healthier resolution. This releases previously invested libido for mature adult functioning. Psychoanalytical therapy is usually long term. The client is often seen five times a week for several years. This approach is, therefore, time consuming and expensive.

Roles of Client and Psychoanalyst

The roles of the client and the psychoanalyst were defined by Freud. The client was to be an active participant, freely revealing all thoughts exactly as they occurred and describing all dreams. The client often lies down during therapy to induce relaxation, which facilitates free association.

The psychoanalyst is a shadow person. The client is expected to reveal all private thoughts and feelings and the analyst reveals nothing personal. The analyst is usually out of the client's sight to ensure that non-verbal responses do not influence the client. Verbal responses are brief and noncommittal for the most part to prevent interference with the associative flow. For instance, the analyst might respond with, 'Uh huh', 'Go on', or 'Tell me more'.

The therapist changes this communication style when interpreting behaviour. Interpretations are presented for the client to accept or reject, but rejections suggest resistance. Likewise, frustration that the client expresses toward the analyst is interpreted as transference. By the end of therapy, the client should be able to view the analyst realistically, having worked through conflicts and dependency needs.

Other Psychoanalytical Theorists

Much of Freud's theory is still used by psychotherapists. Theorists who followed him have modified and built on the original psychoanalytical theories. Box 2.1 presents a list of several contemporary psychoanalytical theorists and a brief statement identifying their major contributions.

INTERPERSONAL MODEL

The theorist most representative of the interpersonal model is Harry Stack Sullivan (1953), a 20th Century American therapist. In addition, attention is drawn to the interpersonal nursing theory of Hildegard Peplau (1952) (Figure 2.2). Her work

---

> **Box 2.1**
>
> ## *Contemporary psychoanalytic theorists*
>
> • Erik Erikson (1963) Expanded Freud's theory of psychosocial development to encompass the entire life cycle.
> • Anna Freud (1966) Expanded psychoanalytical theory in the area of child psychology.
> • Melanie Klein (1949) Extended the use of psychoanalytical techniques to work with young children through development of play therapy.
> • Karen Horney (1937–40) Focused on psychoanalytical theory relative to cultural and interpersonal factors; rejected Freud's view of feminine sexuality.
> • Frieda Fromm-Reichmann (1950) Used psychoanalytical techniques with psychotic individuals.
> • Karl Menninger (1963) Applied the concepts of dynamic equilibrium and coping to mental functioning.

represents a milestone in the conceptualization of the psycho-therapeutic role of the nurse in the context of the interpersonal relationship.

Interpersonal theorists believe that behaviour evolves around interpersonal relationships. While Freudian theory emphasizes a person's intrapsychic experience, interpersonal theory emphasizes social or interpersonal experience. Sullivan, like Freud, traces a progression of psychological development. Sullivan's theory states that the person bases behaviour on two drives: the drive for satisfaction and the drive for security. Satisfaction refers to the basic human drives, including hunger, sleep, lust and loneliness. Security relates to culturally defined needs such as conformity to the social norms and value system of the individual's ethnic group. Sullivan states that when the nature of a person's self-system interferes with the ability to attend to the need for either satisfaction or security, the person will become mentally ill.

When Peplau defined nursing as an interpersonal process, she also discussed the importance of basic human needs. Needs must be met if a healthy state is to be achieved and maintained. For Peplau, the two interacting components of health are physiological demands and interpersonal conditions. These may be viewed as parallel to the drives of satisfaction and security identified by Sullivan, as evident in the following case study.

Interpersonal Therapeutic Process
The interpersonal therapist, like the psychoanalyst, explores the client's life history. The crux of the therapeutic process is the corrective interpersonal experience. The idea is that by experiencing a healthy relationship with the therapist, the client can learn to have more satisfying interpersonal relationships. The therapist actively encourages the development of trust by relating authentically to the client. The therapist must share feelings and reactions with the client. The process of therapy is a process of re-education.

The therapist helps the client identify interpersonal problems and then encourages attempts at more successful styles of relating.

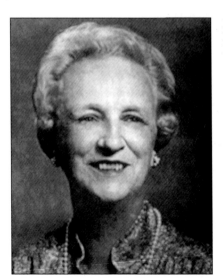

Figure 2.2 Hildegard E. Peplau (courtesy Hildegard E. Peplau)

For example, clients often have a fear of intimacy. The therapist allows the client to become close while clearly showing that there is no threat of sexual involvement. It is believed that closeness within the therapeutic relationship builds trust, facilitates empathy, enhances self-esteem and fosters growth toward healthy behaviour. Peplau (1952) describes this process as 'psychological mothering', which includes the following steps:

1. The client is accepted unconditionally as a participant in a relationship that satisfies needs.
2. There is recognition of and response to the client's readiness for growth, as initiated by the client.
3. Power in the relationship shifts to the client, as the client is able to delay gratification and to invest energy in goal achievement.

Therapy is completed when the client can establish satisfying human relationships, thereby meeting basic needs. Termination is a significant part of the relationship that must be experienced and shared by both the therapist and the client. The client learns that leaving a significant other involves pain but can also be an opportunity for growth.

Roles of Client and Interpersonal Therapist
The client–therapist dyad is viewed as a partnership in interpersonal therapy. Sullivan describes the therapist as a 'participant observer' whose role is to engage the client, establish

---

> *Case study:* **The Interpersonal Theory approach**
>
> Ms Y, a 26-year-old woman, appeared at a psychiatric clinic requesting therapy. She described her problem as, 'I can't get close to people'. She said that her childhood was happy and that she had loving parents and liked her sister. Her family were very religious, so most of her activities were church related. She had many friends during childhood and then one close girl friend in early adolescence. She thought that her fear of closeness began when she spent the night at her friend's house. During the night her friend began to fondle her in a way that she interpreted as sexual. She became very frightened and felt guilty about this. She did not tell her parents because of her guilt and, in fact, had told no one before entering therapy. Although she attended college, she never dated and would participate only in superficial social contacts. She realized that this was not healthy young adult behaviour and, as the behaviour continued into her twenties, Ms Y decided that she needed to seek help.
>
> From an interpersonal perspective, Ms Y was unable to fulfil her needs for friendship and sexual love. Interpersonal theorists would view the unfulfilled sexual love dynamism as a lack of satisfaction and her fear that she had deviated from the norm as a lack of security. Her anxiety stemmed from her conviction that her parents would disown her if they heard what had happened. This belief was based on their earlier responses to childhood sexual play. The therapist decided that Ms Y first needed to experience intimacy on a nonsexual level. This was approached in therapy. When she began to feel comfortable sharing closeness with the therapist, Ms Y was able to develop healthy relationships.

trust and empathize. There is an active effort to help the client realize that other people have similar perceptions and concerns. An atmosphere of uncritical acceptance encourages the client to speak openly. The therapist interacts as a real person who also has beliefs, values, thoughts and feelings. The client's role is to share concerns with the therapist and to participate as fully as possible in the relationship. The relationship itself is meant to serve as a model of adaptive interpersonal relationships. As the client matures in the ability to relate, life experiences with people outside the therapeutic situation can be enhanced.

Interpersonal nursing roles have been identified by Peplau (1952) and are listed in Box 2.2. These roles may be assumed by the nurse or assigned to others. The therapist helps the client meet the goals of therapy–need satisfaction and personal growth. In addition, through role performance the nurse also experiences growth and self-discovery. Self-awareness is essential to success as an interpersonal therapist.

SOCIAL MODEL

The two preceding models focused on the individual and intrapsychic processes and interpersonal experiences. The social model moves beyond the individual to consider the social environment as it affects the person and the person's life experience. Psychoanalytical theory has been criticized for not extending to other cultures and times. For example, Freud's view of women has been repeatedly challenged, particularly by feminists. Some theorists such as Thomas Szasz (1961, 1987, 1993) and Gerald Caplan (1964) believe that the culture itself is useful in defining mental illness, prescribing the nature of therapy and determining the client's future. The Community Care Act (1990) could be seen to be a governmental effort to respond to the philosophy of the social theorists (though there are many who would argue money was the driving force!)

According to the social theorists, social conditions are largely responsible for deviant behaviour. Deviancy is culturally defined. Behaviour considered normal in one cultural setting may be eccentric in another and psychotic in a third. With this point of view, Szasz (1961) writes of the 'myth of mental illness'. He believes that society has to find a way of managing 'undesirables' so it labels them as mentally ill. People who are so labelled are usually unable, or refuse, to conform to social norms and this behaviour usually leads to institutionalization. If these individuals then conform to social expectations, they are considered to be recovered and are allowed to return to the community. Institutionalization, then, performs the dual function of removing deviant members from the community and exerting social control over their behaviour.

Szasz (1961) believes that people are responsible for their behaviour. The person has control over whether to conform to social expectations. Those labelled as mentally ill may be scapegoats but they participate in the scapegoating process by inviting it or by allowing it to occur. Szasz objects to describing deviant behaviour as 'illness'. He believes that illness can occur in the body and that diseases of the body can influence behaviour (e.g., brain tumours), but that no physiological disruption can be demonstrated to cause most deviancy. He distinguishes between the biological condition that is central to illness and the social role that is the focus of deviancy.

Caplan (1964) has also studied deviant behaviour from a social perspective. He has extended the public health model of primary, secondary and tertiary prevention to the mental health field. He has focused particularly on primary prevention, since much attention has been given in the past to the secondary and tertiary levels. Lack of understanding of the cause of deviant behaviour has hindered the development of primary prevention techniques.

Caplan believes that social situations can predispose a person to mental illness. Such situations include poverty, family instability and inadequate education. Deprivation throughout the life cycle results in limited ability to cope with stress. The person has few available environmental supports. The result is a predisposition to maladaptive coping responses.

Social Therapeutic Process

Szasz advocates freedom of choice for psychiatric clients. People should be allowed to select their own therapeutic modality and therapists. This also implies a well-informed consumer who can base this decision on knowledge of available modes of therapy. Szasz does not believe in involuntary hospitalization

---

Box 2.2 *Interpersonal nursing roles identified by Peplau*

1. Stranger — the role assumed by both nurse and service user when they first meet.
2. Resource person — provide health information to a service user.
3. Teacher — assist the service user as learner to grow and learn from experience with the health-care system.
4. Leader — assist the service user as follower to participate in a democratically implemented nursing process.
5. Surrogate — assume roles that have been assigned by the service user, based on significant past relationships, similar to the psychoanalytical concept of transference.
6. Counsellor — help the service user integrate the facts and feelings associated with an episode of illness into the service user's life experience.

Case study: **An example of the Social Model approach**

A female refugee from Guyana was found outside a church, screaming in her native tongue and is deemed by a British police officer to be 'psychotic'. She is taken to the nearest psychiatric hospital under Section 136. She is only able to speak a small amount of English and, when seen by a doctor, says that she has been possessed. She is diagnosed as having experienced a psychotic breakdown. When a Guyanan interpreter is found they interview the women and convey to the medical team that her beliefs are quite consistent with her cultural background, in that she believes that her husband has put a curse on her and she was at the Church to get spiritual help but the church was locked.

of the mentally ill. He questions whether any psychiatric hospitalization is truly voluntary. Szasz disapproves of the community mental health trend to place mental health care within the reach of every citizen. He questions government involvement in what he views as a private concern.

Caplan, on the other hand, supports community psychiatry. He sees the mental health professional as using consultation to combat societal problems. He believes that future psychiatric clients would benefit indirectly from positive social change.

Roles of Client and Social Therapist

Szasz believes that a therapist can help the client only if the client requests help. The client, then, initiates therapy and defines the problem to be solved. The client also has the right to approve or reject the recommended therapeutic intervention. Therapy is successfully completed when the client is satisfied with the changes made in lifestyle. The therapist collaborates with the client to promote change. This includes making recommendations to the client about possible means of effecting behavioural change but it does not include any element of coercion, particularly the threat of hospitalization if the client does not agree with the therapist's recommendations. The therapist's role also may involve protecting the client from social demands for being treated unwillingly.

Caplan believes that society itself has a moral obligation to provide a wide range of therapeutic services covering all three levels of prevention. The client has a consumer role and selects the appropriate level of help from a wide array of available services. Ideally, effective primary preventive services would decrease the need for secondary or tertiary care.

According to this model, therapists may be professionals or non-professionals with professional consultation. People such as clergy, police, bartenders and beauticians can be trained to listen and to refer people who need professional help to appropriate resources. The therapist in the social context is not tied to the office but is involved in the community. Activities may include home visits, lectures to community groups, or consultation with other agencies. The rationale for this approach is that the more involved therapists are in the community, the greater the impact on the community's mental health. Community involvement also enhances the therapist's understanding of clients who live in that environment.

EXISTENTIAL MODEL

The existential model focuses on the person's experience in the here and now, with much less attention to the person's past than in other theoretical models.

Existentialist theorists believe that problems arise for the person when the individual is out of touch with the self or the environment. This alienation is caused by self-imposed restrictions. The individual is not free to choose from among all alternative behaviours.

The person who is self-alienated feels helpless, sad and lonely. Self-criticism and lack of self-awareness prevent participation in authentic, rewarding relationships with others.

Theoretically, the person has many choices in terms of behaviour. However, existentialists believe that people tend to avoid being real and instead give in to the demands of others.

Existential Therapeutic Process

There are several existential therapies, all of which assume that the client must be able to choose freely from what life has to offer. Although the approaches are somewhat different, the goal is to return the client to an authentic awareness of being.

The existential therapeutic process focuses on the encounter. The encounter is not merely the meeting of two or more people; it also involves their appreciation of the total existence of each other. Through the encounter the client is helped to accept and understand personal history, to live fully in the present and to look forward to the future. Table 2.1 presents an overview of several existential therapies.

Roles of Client and Existential Therapist

Existential theorists emphasize that the therapist and the client are equal in their common humanity. The therapist acts as a guide to the client, who has gone astray in the search for authenticity. The therapist is direct in pointing out areas where the client should consider changing. However, caring and warmth are also emphasized. The therapist and the client are to be open and honest. The therapeutic experience is a model for the client; new behaviours can be tested before risks are taken in daily life.

The client is expected to assume and accept responsibility for behaviour. Dependence on the therapist generally is not encouraged. The client is treated as an adult. Frequently, illness is de-emphasized. The client is viewed as a person alienated from the self and others but for whom there is hope if the therapist is trusted and directions are followed. The client is always active in therapy, working to meet the challenge presented by the therapist.

SUPPORTIVE MODEL

The supportive model differs from other models in that it is not dependent on any overriding concept or theory. Instead, it uses many psychodynamic theories to understand how people change. The aims of supportive psychotherapy include the following:
- Promote a supportive client–therapist relationship.
- Enhance client's strengths, coping skills and ability to use coping resources.
- Reduce the client's subjective distress and maladaptive coping responses.
- Help the client achieve the greatest independence possible based on the specific psychiatric or physical illness.
- Foster the greatest amount of autonomy in treatment decisions with the client.

Controlled studies have shown it to be effective in treating schizophrenia, borderline conditions, affective and anxiety disorders, post-traumatic stress disorder, eating and substance abuse disorders and the psychological component of a variety of physical illnesses (Rockland, 1993).

Supportive therapists are psychodynamically based and they describe problems as neurotic, borderline or psychotic. They subscribe to the concepts of id, ego and superego and emphasize the important role of psychological defences in adaptive functioning (Rockland, 1989). Compared with other models of psychiatric treatment, however, their focus is more behaviour oriented. They emphasize current biopsychosocial coping responses and the person's ability to use available coping resources.

Supportive Therapeutic Process

Supportive therapy is an eclectic form of psychotherapy; that is, it is not based on a particular theory of psychopathology. Rather, it can draw as needed from other models and may address different symptoms with different therapeutic methods. The methods and goals of supportive therapy are equally applicable to high-functioning clients in crisis and low-functioning clients suffering from psychosis or persistent mental illness. Its emphasis is on improving behaviour and subjective feelings of distress, rather than on achieving insight or self-understanding. Principles of supportive therapy include the following:

- Giving immediate help to the client that may include a variety of treatment modalities.
- Family and social support system involvement.
- Focus on the present and not the past.
- Anxiety reduction through supportive measures and medication if necessary.

- Clarification of the client's current problem using a variety of approaches including advice, supportive confrontation, limit setting, education and environmental change.
- Assisting the client to avoid future crises and seek help early when under stress.

Roles of Client and Supportive Therapist

In supportive therapy the therapist plays an active and directive role in helping the client improve social functioning and coping skills. The setting for supportive therapy should allow for a moderate to high level of activity in both the client and therapist. Communication is viewed as an active two-way process and the use of medications or other treatments and therapies is encouraged.

The therapist is involved and is willing to contribute to a true therapeutic alliance with the client. Expressing empathy, concern and nonjudgmental acceptance of the client are important therapist qualities. The therapist supports the client's healthy adaptive efforts, conveys a willingness to understand, respects the client as a unique human being and takes a genuine interest in the client's life activities and well-being. Finally the therapist regards the client as a partner in treatment and encourages the client's autonomy to make treatment and life decisions. In turn, the client is expected to demonstrate a willingness to talk about life events, to accept the therapist's supportive role, to participate in the therapeutic programme and to adhere to the therapeutic structure.

TABLE 2.1 Overview of existential therapies

Therapy	Therapist	Process
Rational–emotive therapy (RET)	Albert Ellis (1989)	An active–directive, cognitively oriented therapy. Confrontation is used to force patient to assume responsibility for behaviour. Patients are encouraged to accept themselves as they are and are taught to take risks and to try out new behaviour.
Logotherapy	Viktor E. Frankl (1959)	A future-oriented therapy. The search for meaning (logos) is viewed as a primary life force. Without a sense of meaning, life becomes an 'existential vacuum'. The aim of therapy is to help patients to assume personal responsibility.
Reality therapy	William Glasser (1965)	Central theme is the need for identity, which is reached by loving, feeling worthwhile and behaving responsibly. Patients are helped to recognize life goals and ways by which they keep themselves from accomplishing goals.
Gestalt therapy	Frederick S. Perls (1969)	Emphasizes the here and now. The patient is encouraged to identify feelings. The increased awareness makes the patient more sensitive to other aspects of existence. Self-awareness is expected to lead to self-acceptance.
Encounter group therapy	Carl Rogers (1970)	Focuses on the establishment of intimate interactions in a group setting. Therapy is oriented to the here and now. The patient is expected to assume responsibility for behaviour. Feeling is stressed; intellectualization is discouraged.

MEDICAL MODEL

The medical model refers to psychiatric care that is based on the traditional physician–client relationship. It focuses on the diagnosis of a mental illness and subsequent treatment is based on this diagnosis. Somatic treatments, including pharmacotherapy and electroconvulsive therapy, are important components of the treatment process. The interpersonal aspect of the medical model varies widely, from intensive insight-oriented intervention to brief sessions involving medical management of medications.

Much of modern psychiatric care is dominated by the medical model. Other health professionals may be involved in interagency referrals, family assessment and health teaching but psychiatrists are viewed as the leaders of the team when this model is in effect. Elements of other models of care may be used in conjunction with the medical model. For instance, a client may be diagnosed with schizophrenia and treated with medication. This client may also be participating in a behavioural programme to encourage socially acceptable behaviour.

A positive contribution of the medical model has been the continual exploration for causes of mental illness using the scientific process. Recently, great strides have been taken in learning about the functioning of the brain and nervous system (see Chapter 7). This progress has led to a beginning of understanding of the probable physiological components of many behavioural disorders and increasingly specific and sophisticated approaches to psychiatric care.

The medical model proposes that problems are a symptom of a central nervous system disorder (Guze, 1989). As Andreasen (1984) writes 'Mental illness is truly a nervous breakdown–a breakdown that occurs when the nerves of the brain have an injury so severe that their own internal healing capacities cannot repair it'. She lists several types of brain disorders that could lead to mental illness: loss of nerve cells, excesses or deficits in chemical transmission, abnormal patterns of brain circuitry, problems in the command centres and disruptions in the movement of messages along nerves.

Currently, the exact nature of the physiological disruption is not well understood. It is thought that the psychotic disorders such as bipolar disorder, major depression and schizophrenia involve an abnormality in the transmission of neural impulses. It is also thought that this difficulty occurs at the synaptic level and involves neurochemicals such as dopamine, serotonin and norepinephrine (see Chapter 7).

Currently, much research is taking place so that the brain's involvement in emotional response can be better understood. Another branch of research focuses on stressors and the human response to stress. Researchers are asking, 'Why do some people seem to tolerate great stress and continue to function well and others fall apart when a small problem arises?' These researchers suspect that humans may have a physiological stress threshold that may be genetically determined. These areas of research are intriguing but currently are not able to provide definitive guidelines for therapy.

Medical Therapeutic Process

The medical process of therapy is well-defined and familiar to most clients. The physician's examination of the client includes the history of the present illness, past history, social history, medical history, review of body systems, physical examination and examination of mental status. Additional data may be collected from significant others and past medical records are reviewed if available. A preliminary diagnosis is then formulated, pending further diagnostic studies and observation of the client's behaviour.

The diagnosis is stated and classified according to the *Diagnostic and Statistical Manual of Mental Disorders* of the American Psychiatric Association, fourth edition (American Psychiatric Association, 1994). The names of the various illnesses are accompanied by a description of diagnostic criteria, associated general medical and psychiatric features, diagrams showing the longitudinal course of the disorder and specific gender, age and cross-cultural aspects of each illness. Changes in the manual reflect changes in the medical model of psychiatric care. (The first edition was published in 1952; the fourth, published in 1994, is the most up-to-date).

After the diagnosis is formulated, treatment is instituted. The physician—client relationship is developed to foster trust in the physician and compliance with the treatment plan. Other health team members may contribute their expertise. Response to treatment is evaluated on the basis of the client's subjective assessment and on the physician's objective observations of symptomatic behaviour. Therapy is terminated when the client's symptoms have remitted. For instance, some people who experience depression may be able to return to usual lifestyle after a course of medication and supportive therapy. Other clients may require long-term therapy, including the long-term use of medication.

Roles of Client and Psychiatrist

The roles of physician and client have been well defined by tradition and apply in the psychiatric setting. The psychiatrist, as the healer, identifies the client's illness and institutes a treatment plan. The client may have some say in the plan, but the psychiatrist prescribes the therapy.

The role of the client involves admitting being ill, which can be a problem in psychiatry. Clients sometimes are not aware of their disturbed behaviour and may actively resist treatment. This is not congruent with the medical model. The client is expected to comply with the treatment programme and to try to get well. If observable improvement does not occur, care-givers and significant others often suspect that the client is not trying hard enough. This can be frustrating to a client who is trying to get well and is disappointed with the lack of progress. The client also may have difficulty letting people extend care while at the same time being self-sufficient.

BORROWED OR SHARED?

The models outlined above provide mental health nurses with a range of theories to use in their day-to-day practice. However, to use theories from other disciplines uncritically can cause problems if such theories are not tested for their validity and applicability to mental health nursing. Many theorists mentioned have been criticized because it is considered that the development and testing of their theories have not been sufficiently rigorous. In many cases the theories have been developed by men for women and as such their moral implications have been questioned.

These arguments must be borne in mind when considering the applicability of theories. It is important that mental health nurses 'come clean' to service users and their carers about the theory bases they are using. This ensures that service users and their carers are given information which may increase their ability to choose what is most appropriate for them. It may be that the nurse might want to work in a particular way that would harm the service user because the proposed theory stems from a philosophy which is fundamentally different from the service user's own.

Dickoff *et al.* (1968) proposed that 'mental health nurses need to do more than just describe what they see', that 'they must also prescribe actions'. Taken in historical context, this statement is probably relevant. In the 1960s and 1970s mental health nurses were still in the position of being assistants to the psychiatrist (Nolan, 1993). Therefore their role was that of reporting their observations to the psychiatrist, not of prescribing actions. Currently, however, mental health nurses are doing far more than just describing what they see. (See for example Tissier, 1986; Dawson *et al.*, 1988; Matthew, 1990; among others).

Because nursing is a skills based profession Dickoff and James (1968) thought that the theory that underpinned those skills should be 'practice theory', i.e. theory that is generated in practice for practice. They saw practice theory occurring on four levels that increase in complexity, namely:

1. Factor isolating theory – identifying concepts.
2. Factor relating theory – linking concepts.
3. Situation relating theory – testing the linked concepts.
4. Situation producing theory – prescribing, predicting and controlling outcomes.

Factor isolating theory refers to isolating concepts that are relevant to nursing and describing them in detail in terms that can be understood by others. For example, in mental health nursing it is useful to have a common understanding of the concept of 'hallucinations' in order to understand what is needed from the nurse.

However, this poses a theoretical difficulty in that mental health nursing views each person as unique (Ward, 1992). To reduce a concept to its component parts may detract from the subjective or personal meaning it has for the individual. Overall though it may be seen to be useful to have a shared understanding of a concept; the translation of the use of the concept is dependent on the individual nurse not being too narrow in their focus and on ensuring that the concept makes sense to the service user.

Factor relating theory involves the identification of possible relationships between concepts. For example, there appears to be a relationship between the experience of childhood sexual abuse and the development of suicidal behaviour in later life (Mullen, 1993).

When a link such as this is borne out and tested by research it provides a valuable piece of knowledge for nurses to use. However, there is a danger in suggesting links that are not confirmed by research. For instance, when the author asked the ward nurses why they were not providing clients with regular access to, or a copy of, their care plans, the nurses responded that they thought that the clients would leave the care plans 'lying around' and that this would lead to a breach of the person's confidentiality.

The issue to do with confidentiality was an admirable one. However, there was no evidence to suggest that this would happen and it underlined the paternalistic approach to care that was occurring on the ward. This served to alienate the service users from the nurses and displayed a lack of trust in, respect for and understanding towards the service users.

Situation relating theory aims to predict the outcome when concepts are related. For example it may be predicted that when devising a plan of care for a person, the more they are involved in that plan of care, the more they will be likely feel in control of what is happening to them.

Situation producing theory is considered to be the most sophisticated level of theory development by Dickoff and James. This level of theory is to do with controlling the outcome of interventions. For example, in the treatment of phobias, graded exposure of a person to the feared object will eventually result in a decrease in fear (Marks *et al.*, 1978). This level of theory development is most appropriately applied in the fields of behavioural and cognitive therapy, where the focus is on determining outcomes of care. However, it would be inappropriate to consider this approach applicable to all areas of enquiry as it would be grandiose to suggest that nurses

---

Case study: **An example of factor isolating theory**

During a group discussion about care planning, the group supervisor suggested that the nurses would be more in tune with service users and their perceptions of their needs or problems by using the service user's language in the written formulation of care plans. (Care plan in this context is a written document by nurse and service user to guide the care needed that is delivered during contact with the nurse.)

This was met with an indignant response by one nurse who said, 'Everybody knows what hallucinations mean so why can't I write that the patient is suffering from hallucinations?'. The nurse went on to say that she thought it 'unprofessional' to use the service user's words on a care plan. Underlying her argument was that she thought that nurses needed to use medical language to be on a par with the medical staff.

have the power to determine the outcome of interventions. (It is the service user who should be determining this). Any attempt at 'manipulation' in this way increases the imbalance of power that exists between professionals and users of the mental health service.

Another difficulty with this approach to theory building is that it can be seen to be reductionist. If one uses terms which are understood by all, then there is a risk of being 'blinkered' by the term, the reality being that one person's experience and understanding is rarely exactly the same as another's. The use of medical terms in mental health nursing, particularly diagnoses, seems to be gaining interest. What is of concern is that nursing diagnosis can be seen to be a forerunner to 'core care plans'. These are a type of menu of interventions to use for service users who present with a particular set of 'symptoms'. Apart from obvious shortcomings, i.e. the lack of individualized care and the medical model type approach being used, there appears to be little substantiated evidence that these improve care. Indeed, Wright (1990) using a mental health problem as an example for a core care plan, cited that a valid reason for using core care plans was so that 'a legible and comprehensible form to which clients could also have access' was produced. This is concerning; if nurses are unable to devise and write a plan of care that is legible and comprehensible then surely they are not fulfilling an important aspect of their role!

SITUATION-PRODUCING THEORY IN MENTAL HEALTH NURSING

Situation-producing theory 'makes it possible to prescribe actions that will bring about desired goals' (Leddy and Pepper, 1989).

Dickoff *et al.* (1968) suggest that theory must come from practice, for practice. This implies inductive reasoning, i.e. observing multiple examples of a situation and then combining those situations into a larger whole (Chinn and Kramer, 1991). Other authors such as Beckstrand (1980) and Fry (1989) suggest that this oversimplifies nursing theory.

Inductive logic is limited because it is not possible to observe all instances of a specific event. This is not to say that inductive reasoning is wrong; it is not adequate to develop theories for all that is of importance to mental health nursing. This approach stems from the scientific paradigm of the 'received view', i.e. one that espouses 'reductionism, quantifiability, objectivity and operationalisation' (Watson, 1981).

Mental health nursing is concerned with complex human emotions, which because of their nature are not necessarily amenable to scientific enquiry of the received view. Meleis (1991) believes that nursing has moved beyond this view and that it would be more appropriate to focus on nursing theory from the 'perceived view' i.e. a view which encompasses such ideas as subjectivity, multiple truths, discovery, description and understanding, patterns, holism, individuation and historicism. This involves using approaches such as phenomenology or grounded theory.

Theory in Practice

The complexity of this argument, the confusion it causes and the lack of clarity about which philosophical viewpoint is more appropriate for mental health nursing can be seen in the following example. The Practice Development Nurse (PDN) was first asked to become involved in the ward because the nurses said they were having trouble formulating care plans which met the criteria for the nursing audit tool (Russell, 1992) being used.

On investigation, it was found that, in response to criticism from the auditors, the nurses had implemented a framework for assessing service users' needs (Roy, 1984) practically overnight. They were extremely proud of their achievements and at this stage the PDN felt it prudent not to add to their difficulties by saying that this was a questionable approach.

It was clear from what the nurses were saying that they felt disempowered to change their position, a common feature of the health service (Jolley and Brykczynska, 1993) due to the hierarchy and medical domination of the organization. This in turn was being transmitted to the service users, in the form of medical jargon on care plans and a lack of collaboration in care. This in itself may expand the imbalance of power that exists between service users and nurses, a process that should be avoided (Brearly, 1990).

To facilitate empowerment of the nurses (so that they in turn could help facilitate empowerment of the service users) the PDN provided access to information that would enable them to make informed choices about the care they provided. This approach is generally thought appropriate for service users (Morgan, 1993). However, it is equally applicable to nurses.

Regular sessions were established where the PDN offered group tutorials (a method of promoting the integration of theory and practice suggested by McCaugherty (1992)) in service user care and issues to do with care planning. It became apparent that the nurses were focusing on what the nursing hierarchy wanted, rather than on what was best for the service user. This served to limit their view of what they should do and meant that they were keen to get their care plans 'right' without considering any other issue.

Ward (1992) states that 'service users must be involved' in the process of care planning as it is 'this process of defining and agreeing on the problems with the nurse that may well constitute the first stage of a service user actually learning to tackle problems for himself'.

CONTRADICTIONS IN MENTAL HEALTH NURSING

The problems encountered by the nurses in the example above reflect those outlined by Thomas (1992): on the one hand mental health nursing is being guided to adopt scientific enquiry of the received type, while at the same time being told that it must become more 'user friendly' and listen to the user movement. which espouses freedom of information, holism and the right to be informed (Butler, 1993). These tenets are in sharp contrast to the current paternalistic approach to psychiatric care (Barham, 1992).

This lack of agreement between different views of the world will serve only to confuse mental health nurses further. To reduce this effect, it is essential that mental health nurses focus their attention to develop theories which are thought important by service users and which will enhance the care that service users receive.

Barker (1993) has underlined this point by coining the term 'trephotaxis', i.e. the conditions necessary for the promotion of growth and development. Although the author does not welcome the creation of a new language that may alienate service users and colleagues in other disciplines, the idea underlying this term, i.e. 'helping people to identify and meet their own unique needs on their own unique terms' (Barker, 1993) is essential to develop theory that is important to mental health nurses and the people they work with. In a later paper (Barker, 1995) he suggests that nurses need 'to develop more sophisticated ways of helping people to tell us about their experiences', rather than just focus on diagnosis.

To do this nurses need to re-examine their philosophy. It is within the philosophy that values and beliefs about the four main constructs in nursing reside, i.e. nursing, health and ill health, the environment and the individual (Johnston and Baumann, 1990). However, they would be wise not to revisit their philosophy alone. Involvement of service users in this stage of guiding practice is essential if mental health nursing is to redress the imbalance of power that currently exists.

When a joint approach to developing a working philosophy is made then evaluating the outcomes of the service becomes a more meaningful exercise for those involved.

SUMMARY

Mental health nursing has undoubtedly come a long way since Render (1947) talked about deferring to the physician. However, it has been suggested that there is a need to move on from using theories borrowed from other disciplines, such as psychology, sociology, psychoanalysis and psychiatry, to produce theory which is unique to mental health nursing (Thomas, 1992).

In order to do this Thomas (1992) suggests that nurses base their theory development on the work of Dickoff *et al.* (1968) and develop theory that prescribes, controls and predicts outcomes of interventions.

The many influences on mental health nursing (from mental health policy and legislation to the DoH (1994) review into mental health nursing and the upsurge in the service user movement) have all rendered mental health nursing open to public scrutiny. This has given added emphasis to the need for mental health nurses to be able to articulate and develop the theories that underpin their practice.

The method of developing theory as proposed by Dickoff *et al.* (1968) has been examined for its suitability for mental health nursing. It has been found to take a reductionist view of theory development, which in turn forces the service user to relinquish power and control over their own care. This was shown in the clinical example where medical domination and the use of labels were identified as problems.

Thomas's suggestions (about nurses being able to identify service users' problems and needs and to prescribe nursing interventions that will result in expected outcomes) have been questioned. This type of approach, if not carried out in complete collaboration with the service user, will perpetuate the imbalance of power that exists in nurse–service user relationships.

The contradictions of working from a philosophy that espouses scientific empiricism, as Dickoff *et al.* (1968) propose, were considered in relation to the need for a collaborative approach to care (Brearly, 1990). This was thought to be confusing for mental health nurses and may inhibit their attempts to develop theory.

The way forward suggested here is to develop theories using approaches such as phenomenology and grounded theory and by empowering nurses, who would then be in a position to empower service users (as outlined by Morgan, 1993). It is suggested that mental health nurses need to re-examine their nursing philosophies in collaboration with service users, so that future theories developed will be directed by what the service user thinks important and not by the nurses in isolation.

KEY CONCEPTS

- The theoretical base from which mental health nurses work needs to be fully understood and made clear to people receiving care.
- Nurses need to be clear about their knowledge base. This may be achieved by using the framework of Carper (1978) and White (1995) who provide a means of expressing the range of nursing knowledge.
- The building blocks of nursing knowledge are concepts, models and theories.
- In terms of theory development, concept clarification is often considered the first step.
- Models provide the nurse with a range of ideas about the service user, situations and events and can be used as a guide to practice. However, no one model can be 'applied' to every situation and the reality is that we draw from many models during the course of our work.
- Theories present an ideal picture of reality but not the reality itself. This means that many theories appear useless because they are far too abstract to be of practical use.
- Theories can be devised at many differing levels, from simple to very abstract. This is useful since with the right support and encouragement all nurses can be involved in theory development.
- Many theories currently used by mental health nurses have been developed by other disciplines and are not necessarily congruent with the philosophical bases of the nurse's practice. It is important therefore that nurses do not use these theories without first examining them for their applicability.
- Developing theories simply because we are interested in a particular area is no longer acceptable. In future, theories need to be developed in collaboration with the service user and used to explore issues that are of real importance to the service user, rather than thought grant-worthy by academics!

REFERENCES

American Psychiatric Association: *Diagnostic and statistical manual of mental disorders.* Washington DC, 1994, American Psychiatric Association.

Andreasen NC: *The broken brain.* New York, 1984, Harper & Row.

Barham P: *Closing the asylum: the mental 'service user' in modern society.* Middlesex, 1992, Penguin Books.

Barker P: Preparing mental health nurses for practice: International perspectives – UK, (paper given to the 5th International Congress on Mental Health Nursing – Nursing Around the World) 1993, Manchester.

Barker P: Psychiatry's human face. *Nurs Times* 91(18), 1995.

Beckstrand J: A critique of several conceptions of practice theory in nursing. *Res Nurs Health* 3:69, 1980.

Brearly S: *Service user participation: the literature.* Middlesex, 1990, Royal College of Nursing.

Butler T: *Changing mental health services: the politics and policy.* London, 1993, Chapman & Hall.

Caplan G: *Principles of preventive psychiatry.* New York, 1964, Basic Books.

Carper BA: Fundamental patterns of knowing in nursing. *Adv Nurs Sci* 1(1)13–23, 1978.

Chinn PL, Kramer MK: *Theory and nursing: a systematic approach,* 4 ed. St. Louis, 1991, Mosby Year Book.

Dawson J, Johnson M, Kehiayan N: Responses to patient assault. *J Psychosoc Nurs Ment Health Ser* 26:8–15, 1988.

Department of Health: *The community care act.* London, 1990, HMSO.

Department of Health: *The health of the nation.* London, 1992, HMSO.

Department of Health/Home Office: *Review of health and social services for mentally disordered offenders and others requiring similar services–final summary report.* London, 1992, HMSO.

Dickoff J, James P: A theory of theories: a position paper. *Nurs Res* 17(3),:197–203, 1968.

Dickoff J, James P, Wiedenbach E: Theory in a practice discipline. *Nurs Res* 17(5):415–435, 1968.

Erikson E: *Childhood and society.* New York, 1963, WW Norton.

Fawcett J: Contemporary conceptualisations of nursing: philosophy or science? In: Kikuchi J, Simmons H, editors: *Philosophic inquiry in nursing.* Newbury Park CA, 1992, Sage Publications.

Freud A: *The ego and the mechanisms of defense.* New York, 1966, International Universities Press.

Freud S: In: Strachey J, editor: *The standard edition of the complete psychological works of Sigmund Freud.* London, 1953/74, Hogarth Press.

Fromm–Reichmann F: *Principles of intensive psychotherapy.* Chicago, 1950, The University of Chicago Press.

Fry ST: Toward a theory of nursing ethics. *Adv Nurs Sci* 11(4):9–22, 1989.

Gournay K: Redirecting the emphasis to serious mental illness. *Nurs Times* 90(25):40–41, 22, June 1994.

Gullberg PL: A mental health nurse's role, *J Psychosoc Nursi Ment Health Serv* 27:9–13, 1989.

Guze S: Biological psychiatry: is there any other kind? *Psychol Med* 19:315, 1989.

Horney K: *The collected works of Karen Horney* (Vols 1 and 2). New York, 1937/50, WW Norton.

Johnston NE, Baumann A: Selecting or developing a nursing model for use on clinical practice: a process-oriented approach. In: Baumann A, Johnston NE, Antai–Otong D, editors: *Decision making in psychiatric and psychosocial nursing.* Toronto, 1990, BC Decker Inc.

Jolley M, Brykczynska G: *Nursing: its hidden agendas.* London, 1993, Edward Arnold.

Klein M: *The psychoanalysis of children.* London, 1949, Hogarth Press.

Leddy S, Pepper J M: *Conceptual bases of professional nursing.* Philadelphia, 1989, JB Lippincott Company.

Lindstrom UA: The professional paradigm of qualified psychiatric nurses. *J Adv Nurs* 22:655–662, 1995.

Matthew L: A role for the CPN in supporting the carer of patients with dementia. In: Brooker C, editor: *Community mental health nursing: a research perspective.* London, 1990, Chapman & Hall.

Marks IM, Bird J, Lindley P: Behavioural nurse therapists. Developments and implications. *Behav Psychother* 6, 1978.

McCaugherty D: Integrating theory and practice. *Senior Nurse.* 12(1):36–39, 1992.

Meleis AI: *Theoretical nursing: development and progress.* Philadelphia, 1991, JB Lippincott Company.

Menninger KA: *The vital balance.* New York, 1963, Viking Press.

Morgan S: *Community mental health: practical approaches to long term problems.* London, 1993, Chapman & Hall.

Morse JM: Exploring the theoretical basis of nursing using advanced techniques of concept analysis. *Adv Nurs Sci* 17(3):31–46, 1995.

Mullen PE: Childhood sexual abuse and mental health in adult life. *BJP* 163:721–732, 1993.

Nolan P: *A history of mental health nursing.* London, 1993, Chapman & Hall.

O'Toole AW, Welt SR: *Interpersonal theory in nursing practice: selected works of Hildegard E. Peplau.* New York, 1989, Springer Publishing Co.

Peplau HE: *Interpersonal relations in nursing.* New York, 1952, GP Putnam's & Sons.

Peplau HE: Future directions in mental health nursing from the perspective of history. *J Psychosoc Nurs* 27:18–29, 1989.

Perls FS: *In and out of the garbage pail.* Lafayette, CA, 1969, Real People Press.

Render HW: *Nurse patient relationships in psychiatry.* New York, 1947, McGraw-Hill Company Inc.

Reynolds W, Cormack D: Teaching mental health nursing: interpersonal skills. In: Davis B: *Nursing education: research and developments.* London, 1987, Croom Helm.

Reynolds W, Cormack D: *Psychiatric and mental health nursing: theory and practice.* London, 1990, Chapman & Hall.

Rockland L: *Supportive therapy: a psychodynamic approach.* New York, 1989, Basic Books.

Rockland L: A review of supportive psychotherapy. 1986-1992, *Hosp Community Psychiatry* 44:1053, 1993.

Roy C: *Introduction to nursing: an adaptation model.* New Jersey, 1984, Prentice-Hall.

Royal College of Nursing: *Evidence to the national review of mental health nursing.* London. 1993, Royal College of Nursing.

Russell D: *Mental health nursing practice standards and audit.* London, 1992, Bethlem Royal and Maudsley Hospital Special Health Authority.

Stuart GW, Sundeen SJ: Conceptual models of psychiatric treatment. In: Stuart G,

Sundeen J: *Principles and practice of psychiatric nursing.* St Louis, 1995, Mosby.

Sullivan HS: *The interpersonal theory of psychiatry.* New York, 1953, WW Norton & Co.

Szasz T: *The myth of mental illness.* New York, 1961, Hoeber-Harper.

Szasz T: *Insanity: the idea and its consequences.* New York, 1987, Wiley.

Thomas BL: Theory development. In: Brooking JI, Ritter SAH, Thomas BLT, editors: *A textbook of psychiatric and mental health nursing.* London, 1992, Churchill Livingstone.

Tissier J: The development of a mental health nursing assessment form. In: Brooking J, editor: *Mental health nursing research.* Chichester, 1986, Wiley.

Ward M: *The nursing process in psychiatry.* London, 1992, Churchill Livingstone.

Watson J: Nursing's scientific quest. *Nurs Outlook* 29(7):413–416, 1981.

White E: *The future of mental health nursing by the year 2000*: a Delphi study. Manchester, Department of Nursing Studies, 1990, University of Manchester.

White JW: Patterns of knowing: review, critique and update. *Adv Nurs Sci* 17(4):73–86, 1995.

Wright S: *Building and using a model of nursing.* London, 1990, Edward Arnold.

FURTHER READING

Chinn PL, Kramer MK: *Theory and nursing: a systematic approach,* 4 ed. St Louis, 1995, Mosby Year Book.
A detailed overview with useful principles and concepts for theory development.

Marriner–Tomey A: *Nursing theorists and their work,* 3 ed. London, 1994, Mosby.
This book provides in-depth knowledge of a wide range of nursing theories. It details theory development from Florence Nightingale through to the present day. There are extensive reference lists which will prove invaluable to the reader.

Masson J: *Against therapy.* London, 1988, Fontana Paperbacks.
Masson challenges the efficacy and ethics of all 'therapeutic' relationships. This work provides a challenging insight into the dangers of 'therapy'.

White JW: Patterns of knowing: review, critique and update. *Adv Nurs Sci* 17(4):73–86, 1995.
An excellent paper which helps the reader conceptualize knowledge in nursing.

Therapeutic Nurse–Patient Relationship

<table>
<tr><td>

Learning Outcomes

After studying this chapter you should be able to:

- State the philosophy of care behind the nurse–patient relationship.

- Identify aspects of the therapeutic relationship.

- Critically discuss and apply a psychodynamic understanding to the therapeutic relationship.

- Explore the different phases of the relationship.

- Discuss tools for monitoring and measuring the therapeutic relationship.

- Discuss personal safeguards in working therapeutically.

</td><td>

CHAPTER OUTLINE

- *The philosophy of care*

- *The therapeutic environment*

- *Psychodynamic understanding*

- *Change and participation in the therapeutic relationship*

- *The nurse–patient dyad*

- *Phases of the relationship*

- *Measuring and monitoring the relationship*

- *Personal risks and safeguards*

</td></tr>
</table>

*T*hroughout their lifetime many people experience periods of despair, anxiety, frustration and great confusion. These are, after all, aspects of life that seem inevitable and 'normal'. How we cope with these experiences varies from individual to individual but the common thread that binds us all is the need to talk about them. Talking to someone who shows genuine interest can make problems seem more manageable. In mental health nursing, effective communication is the tool of the trade. Whether we work from a behavioural, pyschodynamic, existential or cognitive theoretical stance, no approach is effective if we cannot communicate our thoughts and feelings clearly.

An important part of nursing practice is to understand the most beneficial elements of the helping relationship and, in particular, what goes on between a nurse and a patient. Within mental health nursing the concept of the therapeutic relationship has been recognized as central to the care process (Altschul, 1972; Cormack, 1983). Peplau (1994) states that the most therapeutic potential is when a nurse and patient meet together for regular individual interaction sessions. These sessions allow the patient to talk through difficulties within a sustained environment, with a competent listener, whose aim is to help the patient better understand themselves. The capacity of the nurse to demonstrate the ability to listen attentively and to understand is considered pivotal to the therapeutic process (Gould, 1990).

However, research studies within the health care setting have consistently identified that nurses tend not to communicate effectively with patients (Hays and Larson, 1963; Peitchinis, 1972; McLeod Clark, 1982; Morrison and Burnard, 1989) but are more concerned with the day-to-day business of running a ward or department and maintaining order (Porter, 1993). Keeping busy with these routine activities might be considered easy work compared to providing consistent and thoughtful verbal therapeutic interactions (Peplau, 1994).

The terms 'patient' and 'nurse' are used throughout this chapter. 'Patient' has been chosen above other terms not because of the passive stereotype it has assumed but more as an expression of the vulnerability and dependency patients need to be allowed to express in order to seek and obtain the help they require. These qualities are not considered passive and weak but are recognized for the personal strength and courage needed in order to come forward and seek help.

THE PHILOSOPHY OF CARE

If we take the view that people have discrete mental illnesses which can somehow be 'fixed' by one psycho-technology or another, this philosophy of care may put a comforting distance between the patient and the professional. Alternatively if we take the view that people are presenting human responses to complex human situations we may acknowledge the common ground between ourselves and those in our care.

(Barker, 1994)

It may be a frightening experience to see 'patients' as being like yourself (Barker, 1994). One way in which mental health nurses can protect themselves from this notion is to use the medical language of illness. This chapter takes the view that people are people. Some have different problems from others but fundamentally we are all people coping with day-to-day living. Mental health nurses help people they come into contact with by working with them to meet their needs. It is important, however, to remember that, when it comes to identifying their problems or needs, the patient is the expert, not the nurse or any other 'professional'. This means that the most important thing that the mental health nurse can do is to *listen* and hear what the patient is saying. The language used by the patient will always have a meaning but can all too often be dismissed or misinterpreted as psychotic nonsense. This will result in poor communication from the start of the relationship, which inhibits understanding.

BOUNDARIES

To work therapeutically with a patient does not mean that the nurse and patient engage in a deep psychoanalytic relationship. In the current health care system where in-patient stays are very brief, it would be unwise (and possibly damaging) to foster such a relationship. It is also necessary to state that most mental health nurses do not work, and are not trained to work, as psycho-therapists. Psychotherapy cannot take place without considerable training, regular supervision and (usually) personal therapy. However, mental health nurses do utilize counselling *skills* in the course of their work of helping and caring for people. The issue of distinguishing the psychotherapeutic work of the mental health nurse and that of psychodynamic counselling or therapy may in some part be clarified by Cawley's (1977) classification of the levels of psychotherapeutic technique (see Box 3.1).

Ritter (1989) applies this classification to the work of mental health nurse and states 'It is essential that psychiatric nurses are clear about the distinction between being a psycho-therapist and behaving in a psychotherapeutic way'.

Rogers (1951) was the first to identify and research the characteristics of a therapeutic relationship. In this chapter Rogers' work is presented as an adaptable theory applicable to the helping and caring role of the mental health nurse. It is, however, at the discretion of each practitioner to test and decide whether the points listed in Box 3.2 provide a useful

Box 3.1 *Levels of psychotherapeutic technique*

Levels of psychotherapeutic technique
(proposed by Cawley, 1977)

Outer (support and counselling)
This includes the person being able to talk about problems to a sympathetic listener, to be able to ventilate feelings within a supportive relationship and to discuss problems with a non-judgemental helper.

Intermediate
This involves gaining clarification of the nature and origins of one's problems within a deepening relationship and confrontation of defences.

Deeper (exploration and analysis)
This involves the interpretation of unconscious motives and transference; regression to less adult state and less rational functioning; repetition, remembering and reconstructing the past; and resolution of conflicts by re-experiencing and working through within the therapeutic relationship.

(Brown and Pedder ,1991)

Box 3.2 *Characteristics of a helping relationship*

- 'The helper aims to participate completely in the patient's communication.
- The helper's comments are always in line with what the patient is trying to convey.
- The helper recognizes the patient as a co-worker on a common problem.
- The helper and the patient are considered equal.
- The helper struggles to understand the patient's feelings.
- The helper follows the patient's line of thought.
- The helper's tone of voice conveys the ability to share the patient's feelings.'

(Rogers, 1951)

and meaningful framework for their clinical practice.

Rogers (1951) identified the importance of interpersonal skills and their therapeutic effect in humanistic psychology. Emphasis is placed upon the therapist's need for self-understanding in regard to personality functioning, emotional patterns and character strengths as prerequisites for a successful therapeutic encounter, with conditions of genuineness, caring and empathy as integral elements.

THE THERAPEUTIC ENVIRONMENT

ETHICS

Ethically the work of the mental health nurse is guided by the United Kingdom Central Council (UKCC) Code of Conduct (1992). The fundamental principles are to do good (benefi-cence) and to do no harm (non-maleficence). In terms of the relationship that develops between the patient and the nurse, these principles need to be borne constantly in mind. The nature and context of mental health problems makes the over-stepping of boundaries a constant and potential problem for the mental health nurse. Mental health nurses work with some of the most vulnerable people in society. Many who use the mental health services have experienced abuse (either sexual or physical) at some stage of their lives and as such are particularly vulnerable within a relationship (Sayce 1995).

Despite the fact that the nurse and patient need to work as equal partners to resolve problems, it is the nurse's responsibility to ensure that no abuse takes place. Under no circumstances should a friendship be entered into that extends beyond the boundaries of the working relationship. The respect and consideration of the patient's well-being are always foremost.

PHYSICAL CONTACT

The purpose of any physical contact must be made clear to the patient and occur only with the patient's permission. An exception is in an emergency, for example where the patient is harming themselves or another person. Even so, the fact that physical holding or restraint may be used must be made clear to the patient when they first come into contact with the service. A sexual relationship is not to be entered into, even after the patient has been discharged from care. The nurse always ensures that this boundary is not crossed and must be the one who makes the boundaries of the relationship very clear. Using clinical supervision will clarify for the nurse any confusion over the boundaries of the developing relationship with the patient and offer insights that can help prevent difficult or embarrassing situations from arising.

This may seem rather harsh and not in keeping with a collaborative and equal partnership approach to care. It does not mean, however, that patients do not have a responsibility to keep themselves safe or not expose themselves to unsafe situations. At the point of receiving care the patient's ability to protect themselves may be compromised and it is the nurse who bears a legal responsibility to ensure patients are not exploited or harmed.

KNOWLEDGE AND POWER

The nurse holds a position of trust and responsibility, bringing with it a certain amount of power. This power must be used wisely, which includes ensuring the patient is able to make informed choices about the type of care they receive.

MIND (1992) clearly state the importance of patients being fully informed of the type of psychological approach taken in their care process. It is equally important that mental health nurses are clear about their own values and beliefs (a personal philosophy) because this has a direct bearing on communi-cation style and the overall way in which they work. While it may be useful to be 'eclectic' in approach, the mental health nurse might be using theories which are inconsistent with one another. For example, it would be incongruent to use the principles of behavioural therapy when your philosophical beliefs are guided by existential thought. It is important that whatever type of approach is used, the basis of such an approach is congruent and applicable to the current situation. Research has been carried out specifically for this purpose, to provide both clinical and empirical evidence to guide prac-titioners in the most appropriate approach to use.

It is worth noting, however, that there has been much criticism of the theories that underpin a psychodynamic approach to care. Some of these are outlined here:

- Masson (1988) views 'therapy' in any form as coercive in nature and based upon the helper's own beliefs about how the patient should change.
- Eichenbaum and Orbach (1983) remind us that psycho-dynamic theories concentrate on psychosexual development and have all been drawn from a male point of view. Female sexuality is identified as merely tied to reproduction and for the gratification of male sex impulses in order to maintain 'control and the subjugation of women'.
- In a similar vein, Erikson's (1965) theory of psychosocial development may be seen to equate healthy adaptation with heterosexuality, which is not consistent with current opinion (Kitzinger, 1987).

Despite these criticisms, it is undeniable that these theories offer the mental health nurse a variety of theoretical explanations about human behaviour and motivation. How the nurse utilizes them in practice is often dependent on the type of education and training they have received. It is also guided by the philosophy of care advocated in their particular area of work.

PSYCHODYNAMIC UNDERSTANDING

The very basic principles of psychodynamic understanding is that there needs to be an environment where change can occur – essentially this environment is the relationship between the key helper and the person seeking help.

A PSYCHOTHERAPEUTIC PERSPECTIVE OF THE THERAPEUTIC RELATIONSHIP

The key helper, whether a psychiatrist, nurse or occupational therapist, who works in a psychodynamic way, is primarily interested in gaining an understanding of the patient from the inside out, in other words, in looking at what lies behind observable behaviour and recognizing the effect of the patient's background, life experiences and personal development.

Brown and Pedder (1991) identify the basic concepts as:

1. Conflict—where people seek help with symptoms or problems that are a result of conflict over unacceptable aspects of themselves and how this manifests itself in their relationships with others.
2. Anxiety or psychic pain—a result of conflict, which produces a sense of disturbance for the patient and can be consciously ignored, so becoming largely unconscious.
3. Defence mechanisms—we all use different defence mechanisms to help block out unpleasant feelings and experiences; some are indeed helpful, while others can become harmful and prevent personal change, growth and development.
4. Motivational drives—despite there being theoretical debate over which drives are the most important, concern is mainly over how these drives are satisfied and the conflicts they can cause. Drives include those associated with eating, sex, aggression and attachment.
5. Phases of development— how a person manages their drives begins to be determined in childhood and develops through a process of learning from the responses from others, at first from parents or other people of emotional significance.

Other terms widely used in psychodynamic thinking will be considered in more detail than for the above principles. They are thought to be of importance when working within the therapeutic relationship. They may help to bring about a greater understanding of the patient and the relationship the nurse forms with the patient and, in particular, serve as a means of recognizing the struggles and conflicts that arise from working in this way.

Transference

In general people respond to relationships with behaviour patterns they have picked up in the past. Feelings and attitudes are transferred and developed through experiences throughout life and can be unconsciously re-enacted in similar situations. For some reason this is intensified when a person is feeling unwell or particularly anxious. Within the nurse–patient relationship, there can be a re-enactment of a past experience where feelings resurface towards the nurse, often unknown to either nurse or patient. When the nurse can help the patient to recognize the relationship these past experiences have to their present situation, change can begin.

However helpful the interpretation of transference in the context of the relationship can be, it should be handled with extreme care. Pasquali *et al.* (1989) note that the nurse should not interpret transference to the patient because the patient may not be emotionally ready to receive this interpretation and increased anxiety or exacerbation of symptoms may result; the interpretation may be wrong and any interpretation offered to the person who is experiencing a thought disorder may hint at mind reading and may enforce delusional thinking and frighten the patient.

Countertransference

This describes the feelings that can be evoked in the nurse by the patient. For example, a patient tells the (female) nurse about being sexually abused as a child and she does this in a soft tone of voice that displays little or no emotion. The nurse may notice a feeling of anger while listening to the patient's story. This anger may in fact belong to the patient who is unable to recognize or express it, as it has been repressed. This aspect of countertransference is similar to empathy where the nurse 'picks up' the feelings behind what the patient is saying. However, this needs to be used with care as it may be the nurse's own unresolved feelings that are interfering with what she believes are the client's feelings. In the above example, for instance, the nurse may have been sexually abused herself and as such she may have unresolved feelings which resurface when confronted with an abused patient. Countertransference can be a useful tool for helping to understand the relationship as it currently stands and can be used as starting point to improving the nurse's ability to tolerate and react therapeutically to the patient. Strong feelings of guilt, pain and even hatred can be produced and it is therefore essential that the nurse receives regular clinical supervision of her or his work.

Supervision

The authors believe that to have a psychodynamic understanding of the therapeutic relationship helps clarify a complicated situation. During the course of the relationship, by drawing on psychodynamic literature and knowledge and through clinical supervision, there is the opportunity to develop a greater understanding of yourself in parallel to that of the patient.

Clinical supervision should provide the nurse with the opportunity to discuss and reflect on the therapeutic relationship with another, normally more experienced, clinician. Supervision provides time and space for the nurse to talk freely about their interactions with patients, without the fear of recrimination or embarrassment. It allows for a clearer understanding of some of the unconscious elements and the difficult emotions that can be aroused through working personally and closely with a distressed individual or group. Davis (1995) states that what nurses want above anything else is to understand how to overcome the difficulties they face daily in their encounters with patients. Supervision can help achieve this, if it is focused on helping the nurse to examine her or his practice carefully and on helping the nurse to develop solutions and plans of action to help the patient's recovery.

SELF CONCEPT

Being affected by, and affecting, others is a fundamental aspect of nursing care. To care, according to Tschudin (1987), one must be able to relate to others. Several factors contribute to the way in which we relate. One factor in particular is that of the self concept. The self concept develops through a person's interaction with their environment, the person's own experiences and the introjection of the values and beliefs of others (Rogers, 1951).

A person's self concept, therefore, relates to how they see themselves and how they believe other people see them. This results in the person having a self concept that is able to distinguish their 'I' (the thinking, feeling and knowing self) from the 'me' (the self as seen by others). Rogers (1951) believed that freedom from inner tension exists when the self concept is roughly congruent with the experiential world of the person. He also believed that for a positive self concept to develop, the person must be unconditionally accepted by others.

ACCEPTANCE

It is important to clarify the concept of acceptance since, as Peplau (1952) states 'Where there is a relationship of acceptance, plans may be formulated together that will be in the interest of the patient's growth and the solution of his problem'. In this context, then, acceptance is the key factor in the success or otherwise of a collaborative approach to care.

What follows are definitions of acceptance selected from the vast range available. These were picked by the authors as representative of most other definitions.

- Acceptance according to Rogers (1951) involves putting aside one's own preoccupations, evaluative nature and tendency to guide the individual and to accept the person as they are now. This includes valuing and prizing all aspects of the person, even those that may seem wrong in the eyes of society (Rogers, 1951). Acceptance has been suggested to be the key factor in the development of trust between the nurse and the patient (Robinson, 1983).
- Pasquali *et al.* (1989) describe acceptance as seeing a person as 'a worthwhile human being'. However, acceptance is seen as not including automatic acceptance of all the patient's behaviour, which may be aggressive or self-destructive.
- Nurse (1980) defines acceptance as 'perceiving the client as she really is, her strengths and weaknesses, congenial and uncongenial qualities, constructive and destructive attitudes, all the while maintaining a sense of someone of worth and dignity as a human being'.
- Morrison (1991) outlines what she believes are accepting behaviours in nursing, these being 'showing respect for rights, expressing dignity and individuality, a non-judgemental manner and accepting the attitudes and beliefs of others'.

There are many other definitions in the nursing, psychotherapy and counselling literature. To clarify the concept, what can be deduced from the above definitions is that acceptance can be seen as:

A skill An ability to really understand the other person's communication and to convey this understanding to the person both verbally and nonverbally.

A quality Involving warmth, i.e. a caring, favourable and approachable quality.

An attitude A positive attitude that conveys respect for the person, the ability to be objective, i.e. provide a 'neutral' stance which is free from emotional response or judgement.

A behaviour A receptive behaviour, i.e. being able to 'take' and 'hold' what a patient brings.

A belief A belief in the innate value of the patient, seeing them as a worthy human being.

See Box 3.3 for an example of acceptance in practice.

CHANGE AND PARTICIPATION IN THE THERAPEUTIC RELATIONSHIP

In the next section, two primary elements of the therapeutic relationship are presented; consideration will be given as to how they are best able to come together in order to discover common ground with the ultimate aim of therapeutic effectiveness and change.

THE NURSE AS CHANGE AGENT

'True nursing is about helping people consolidate their experience of themselves, their own lives, the pleasure and the pain. True nursing involves helping people to need nurses much less' (Barker, 1990).

Within the nurse–patient relationship, the primary nurse—the term used most frequently in an in-patient area (Manthey, 1988)—or Key Worker—more commonly used in the community setting—is of considerable importance. They will be responsible for the delivery of care throughout the patient's period of care, whether that be in hospital or the community.

Peplau (1952) saw the nurse as the fundamental tool for change. The nurse comes to the relationship with knowledge and experience obtained personally throughout their lives but also through their training and work. Usually, it is considered that the more training and work experience a nurse has, the

Box 3.3 *Acceptance in practice*

Lucy (a Registered Nurse in an acute admission ward) was talking with Sidney, one of her allocated patients, when he said, 'I hate you'. Lucy, in a calm tone of voice, responded, 'That's a strong feeling to have about me. I wonder if you can tell me what you mean by the word "hate"'. Sidney said, 'Why don't you just bugger off and leave me alone'. Lucy, sensing that Sidney was troubled by something, remained calm and sitting by him said, 'You are asking me to leave you alone, which I will do. However, if you would like to talk later, then you can find me in the office'.

Critical reflection activity
How would you have handled this situation? Spend some time considering what you would do if Sidney had made a sexist or racist remark to Lucy. Would this affect your ability to be accepting?

more therapeutically effective they are likely to be but this does not always follow. There are many unconscious influences on the relationship that can both hinder and help it. These issues will be touched upon and will be considered further from a psychodynamic, theoretical perspective.

The qualities needed to be therapeutically effective, and who has them, have been of considerable interest to researchers for many years. Nursing, however, remains far behind other helping disciplines in the search for specific characteristics within the nurse–patient relationship. As a result, the literature applies largely to research on psychologists and psychiatrists and is not always easily adapted to the nurse–patient relationship, mainly because it is the nurse who spends most time with patients, carrying out activities that are intimate and sometimes distasteful. It is a nurse who will ensure that a patient's dirty clothes have been washed while also contacting welfare services and offering psychological support and counselling. A multitalented person is required to fulfil all these roles, which arise with little time between to reflect on the process and longer term therapeutic effect.

Barnes (1968) recognized that being available for patients and responding to their needs offered benefits for the nurse as well as the patient. Essentially, the patient's needs complement those of the nurse. The nurse and patient develop a bond of attachment that often results in the nurse being identified as the only person who can help. However, regressive behaviour often occurs with attachment. This can show in behavioural disturbance (such as temper tantrums), with the nurse falling into the trap of responding to every demand. Some demands may seem reasonable, while others amount to an endless request for things such as special dietary needs, or extra medication at unusual times of the day or night. The circle of trying to satisfy the patient's unquenchable demands and the nurse's own need to fulfil their unique helping role is soon all too often complete. Balint (1964) and Bowlby (1973) discuss the concept of attachment in the therapeutic relationship in detail and are reviewed by Pedder (1976) who concludes that attachment is valuable as a basic need for unity with another human being and therefore a necessary part of any therapeutic intervention.

THE PATIENT AS PARTICIPANT

Any person coming into contact with the psychiatric services and seeking help is considered a patient. The term has become linked with the passive and meek role played by someone troubled by a disturbed mind or body function. Who the patient is and how they receive help have a bearing on the outcome of the encounter. The relationship the patient forms with their principal carer, the social field split between them and the influence of other patients and carers have all been documented as affecting the relationship's development (Caudill *et al.*, 1952; Luborsky *et al.*, 1983; Gerstley *et al.*, 1989).

One researcher was deliberately admitted to a psychiatric ward and treated as any other patient. The researcher reported that pressure was exerted by other patients to behave in what were later identified as four different ways:

1 To act in certain ways towards other patients.
2 To adhere to certain attitudes towards self.
3 To adhere to attitudes towards their therapy and therapist.
4 To adhere to certain attitudes towards the nursing staff (Caudill *et al.*, 1952).

The importance of others within the therapeutic arena as an influence on therapeutic outcome has often been neglected as it is difficult to quantify. Ward atmosphere studies invariably produce only localized findings that are difficult to replicate, as situations between two or more people rarely remain unchanged. Whether a patient has voluntarily approached services for help or is forcibly maintained under the Mental Health Act 1983 will influence how the patient approaches the relationship.

Patients and their previous life experiences also influence the relationship they form with the principal carer (i.e. nurse). Marziali et al. (1981) report that the patient is the primary influence on how the relationship will develop and the patient's contribution to the relationship should be the starting point of all therapeutic endeavours. The ability of the nurse to understand, and to demonstrate this understanding to the patient, is central to a caring profession, especially at a time when nursing is striving to establish its worth within the health services.

In a study of general and surgical patients Webb and Hope (1995) found that patients wanted their nurses to be friendly, warm and sympathetic in manner, able to listen to patients' concerns and worries, to teach them about their illnesses and to relieve pain. Previous studies carried out in mental health care consistently have found that patients identified talking to the nurses as the most highly rated activity (McIntyre *et al.*, 1989; Carson and Sharma, 1994; Hardy, 1995).

THE NURSE–PATIENT DYAD

Freud (see Strachey, 1958) was first to discuss the value of having a 'serious interest' in the patient and showing them 'sympathetic understanding'. He described these elements as providing the appropriate environment for a healthy and positive attachment to occur between the patient and their helper or therapist. As a result of a supportive attitude, the patient likens the experience to that involving other people for whom they have had similar feelings in the past. Freud later described this as a positive or beneficial transference.

The interpersonal relationship between the patient and their helper is considered the primary instrument for change. The relationship becomes a necessary, but not the only, condition for successful therapeutic outcome. If the patient distrusts their nurse they are less likely to accept help, neither will they listen nor experience any hope of success.

Discussion on how to improve therapeutic effectiveness first appeared in the nursing literature in the 1950s (Peitchinis, 1972) yet only in the last decade has there begun to be experimental evidence on which to base practice. Interpersonal training is used in nurse training courses today but despite the increasing wealth of literature, possessing the knowledge and carrying out the skills remain two separate entities (Reid and Long, 1993).

Menzies (1960) proposed that nurses tend to develop intricate defence mechanisms to protect themselves from the extreme anxiety aroused in caring for someone in a highly stressful environment. According to Jourard (1961) anxiety prevents both the expression of feelings and the ability to recognize distress in others, resulting in a reduced ability to communicate effectively.

Most relationships involve both positive and negative aspects. According to Gross (1987), relationships are based upon rewards and profits. The greater the personal reward, the lower the cost and thus the larger is the attraction. Gross goes on to state that people admire and respect someone who they consider competent but that admiration is most often shown for someone who is willing to admit to being fallible. Therefore, if nurses are able to consider both the positive and negative aspects of the therapeutic relationship through supervision (or even through their own personal therapy) they are more likely to provide the important element of understanding.

The nurse–patient relationship as a therapeutic tool has been in use since the 1940s (Lego, 1980). Lego emphasizes the inter-personal relationship as opposed to physical nursing care. More recently, this lack of attention to the physical well-being of the patient has been questioned (Gournay, 1994). The nurse needs to remember that, when caring for a patient, it is inappropriate to divorce physical and psychological care as the person is a 'whole', and not separate entities of mind and body.

PHASES OF THE RELATIONSHIP

The phases of the therapeutic relationship have previously been identified by Peplau (1952) and latterly refined by Forchuk and Brown (1989). However, the framework which follows is based upon the authors' clinical experiences and, while the phases are similar to those of the authors cited above, new headings are used for each phase in an attempt to reflect its phenomenology.

OPENING PHASE

The first element of any relationship involves getting to know one another, setting out the boundaries and limits of the relationship and, to a certain extent, testing the validity of those boundaries. As the nurse relates with the patient, the main concern at this time is to establish a climate of trust and acceptance and to gain an understanding of what has brought the patient to seek help. An explanation of what is to be expected on both sides of the relationship helps reduce the anxiety of not knowing. Elements of nurse–patient contact during the opening phase might include:

- Names of both individuals and what is agreed by both as acceptable.
- Roles of the nurse.
- Role of the patient.
- Purpose of the relationship.

Case study: **Grace – phases of the relationship (part 1)**

Grace is a 32-year-old woman who is 7 months pregnant. She was brought into hospital under Section 2 of the Mental Health Act after being found wandering the street in her nightdress, shouting and screaming at passers-by. Her speech is garbled and chaotic, making it difficult for others to follow and make sense of it. On admission, she appeared very scared and was uncooperative. She would shout abuse and walk away, or flatly refuse to speak to anyone and sit staring out of the window, occasionally laughing and muttering to herself. The nurse allocated as primary nurse was not on duty for the day of Grace's admission. When she came on duty the following day, all the other staff breathed a sigh of relief and happily handed Grace over as the nurse's main problem for the day.

The nurse first went to Grace and introduced herself by name. Grace looked out of the window. The nurse said she would like to meet Grace to hear her side of the story. Grace flashed her a glance and asked whose story had she been listening to. The nurse said that other nurses had described that Grace appeared frightened and was not able to talk to anyone about it. She hoped that this could be their first opportunity to meet and discuss the issues surrounding Grace being brought into hospital. Grace began to shout about her admission and how she felt tricked by the doctor into coming to hospital, that she was pregnant and the ward was not a place for such a woman. The nurse listened and said she could understand Grace's concern and would like to talk more, and arranged to meet Grace later that morning.

When the time came for the meeting, Grace was sitting by the window. The nurse went over to her, to remind her of the meeting. Grace shouted that she was not going to meet anyone. The nurse replied that she would wait in the room. After 5 minutes Grace had not come to the door, which the nurse had left open in anticipation. The nurse went to find Grace, who this time was lying on her bed and pretending to be asleep. The nurse spoke quietly to her that she had a further 20 minutes in which to wait for Grace in the interview room and that this was Grace's opportunity to talk about her situation. Grace grunted. The nurse returned to the empty room. A few minutes later, she could see Grace walk past and look into the room through the corner of her eye. She was making for the front door, as if to leave the ward. The nurse followed her and asked her again to join her in the interview room for the remaining ten minutes. Eventually Grace came in and sat down. The nurse thanked her for coming and asked her to continue explaining how she had come into hospital. At the end of the meeting, the nurse thanked Grace again and they arranged to meet the following day to continue getting to know each other and discussing how Grace could best use her time in hospital . When the nurse said she had to now go to her next meeting, Grace admitted she was worried for the safety of her baby and that she had had thoughts of sacrificing a previous child to the devil.

Exploration and negotiating

By now Grace had met her nurse several times, called her by name and often waited at the ward door for her to come on duty. Their meetings had now turned to exploring Grace's fears of harming her baby and negotiating how best to spend her time on the ward. A relationship had soon developed between the two that allowed the nurse confidence to approach the multidisciplinary team about allowing Grace out for walks in the hospital grounds and to be accompanied down to the local shops, though not without waiting anxiously for her return!

• Expectations of the relationship.
• Meeting locations.
• Time of meetings, both duration and frequency.
• Conditions of termination.
• Confidentiality within the team.

It may prove more difficult to establish this level of contractual agreement with patients who are withdrawn or psychotic. The following case study offers some clarification on how a nurse needs to be consistent in approach and remain respectful of the patient's needs at all times during the relationship.

EXPLORATION AND NEGOTIATING

During this phase of the relationship both the nurse and the patient may still be feeling anxious and uncomfortable. The nurse has to remain focused on the purpose of the developing relationship and this may still revolve around developing an environment of trust and mutual respect. Anxiety has many manifestations for both the nurse and patient, with the nurse unsure of where the relationship is heading or what can be offered to the patient, while the patient is coming to terms with new insights and can test the nurse's intent and the consistency of the team.

MAPPING AND TARGETING

This phase has previously been referred to by Peplau (1952) as the exploitation phase. The term 'exploitation' has become more widely associated in English with a negative connotation of the word 'exploit', meaning to utilize for one's own ends. We have, therefore, changed the words to mapping and targeting, which have been drawn from both cognitive and neuro-linguistic terms (Beck, 1976 and Kostere and Malatesta, 1989).

Our internal map of the world is derived from our experiences, culture, language, beliefs, values, interests and assumptions; each individual lives in their unique reality built upon these elements. Map making, or cartography, is a good analogy to use for how the mind helps us to make sense of the complex world around us. Maps are selective and leave things out, as well as offering invaluable information on how to recognize landmarks and, most importantly, find our way around. The type of information stored on one's map is created from that which an individual notices or disregards and which thus forms their own particular map. This filtering system is necessary to help us make sense of the world but can also act as a way of distorting reality, depending on what we wish to take notice of or wish to ignore. Language is one way in which we can learn more about someone's filtering system and get some clues as to how their internal map may look (O'Connor and Seymour, 1990). This process can be used to help the nurse further create a picture of how the patient sees the world and themselves within it. Understanding some of the filters or distortions can be the starting point of therapy. Once these filters or distortions have been identified, mutually agreed targets can be set to help alter these filters and to add new dimensions to the patient's view of the world and add new and more detailed information to their map.

By setting targets, the nurse and patient will be able to monitor and measure change as it occurs. Therapy with any one patient can be seen as a single case experiment with much of the therapy subject to measurements taken during the treatment process. Such measurements can not only supply the nurse with evidence of change, but allow the patient to observe and notice the level of progress achieved. A target should only be set that is believed to be achievable. One patient suffering from agoraphobia set a target of getting to Egypt for a holiday, which was not something obtainable during her hospital stay. The target needed to be broken down further into achievable targets, such as obtaining a passport and getting brochures from the travel agents. Targets will also often turn out to be very different from the original, and precipitating problems uppermost during the earlier phases of the relationship.

WORKING

Probably the most challenging part of the relationship, the working phase is where new insights are translated into action with new knowledge and experiences adopted into new behaviours, thoughts and actions. However, resistance and testing are also most apparent at this time, as both nurse and patient have to realize the need to change aspects of themselves that have taken years to develop. The patient also begins to recognize their sense of dependence on the nurse and fear

---

Case study: **Grace – phases of the relationship (part 2)**

Towards the end of each day and first thing in the morning, the nurses had noticed that Grace did not sleep and subsequently slept most of the afternoon. She was also likely to be disturbed at night, shouting and pacing about the ward causing a disturbance, which invariably resulted in Grace having to be offered medication and a confrontation ensuing.

The nurse asked Grace about this observation and Grace was able to explain that she felt the devil was around her in the dark and asking for the baby. She only fell asleep in the afternoon because she was so tired and frightened but felt safer when other people were awake around her. Grace and her nurse decided to plan out each hour during the night and, in particular, to spend the early evening trying to do things that would be comforting to Grace and help her to relax in preparation for sleeping. Grace was not keen to keep taking sedatives for the effect they might have on the baby, so the nurse arranged for the doctor and pharmacist to send information to Grace about side effects of the medication she was taking and to discuss her fears with the doctor. Grace said she took herbal medicines at home and the doctor agreed to prescribe them for her in hospital. The nurse and Grace discussed some activities she would like to do, such as having a bath, drawing and reading a magazine before the lights were put out. Each night, one of the nurses would explain to Grace where they would be sitting should she want them in the night and that a nurse would always come round every half hour to check that she was alright. Grace appeared visibly reassured by this plan and began to negotiate activities to keep herself awake during the afternoons. She joined art and pottery classes in the Occupational Therapy Department and once she was happy and knew where to go, would take herself off to the art room most afternoons.

of this coming to an end should they progress too well. For the nurse this time can prove frustrating as they have developed a keen understanding of the patient's problems and formulated ideas of how things should be progressing, but it is important to remember to go at the patient's pace and not work at any other predetermined rate.

FUTURE STRATEGIES

As stated, going at the patient's pace for change does not always apply when considering the end of the relationship and developing future strategies for the patient to continue maximizing their health potential, once the nurse–patient relationship is over. Therefore, future strategies need to be considered throughout the relationship and discussed as a pre-requisite of the relationship from the opening phase.

Ending the relationship is both difficult and rewarding. It is when nurse and patient can review the work they have done together and recognize the changes and developments each has made. It can also be when all the time and effort spent developing honesty and trust in the relationship manifests itself as feedback and evaluation is highlighted.

Case study: **Grace – phases of the relationship (part 3)**

Grace and her nurse had established a programme of activities for almost 16 hours of the day. Some activities brought pleasure to Grace, while others she found more difficult and challenging. Every week Grace and her nurse would meet at least three times to discuss and review how things were going. Grace enjoyed these sessions and would be ready and waiting for the nurse to meet her. Two weeks into the programme, Grace left the ward without telling anyone and did not return to the ward all day. The staff had reported her missing and had tried to make contact at her home address. At 10 o'clock that evening the night staff opened the ward door to a dishevelled Grace, who sheepishly went to her room and got into bed. The next morning Grace was not ready for the nurse's meeting. The nurse went to Grace's room and tried to rouse her from her sleep. The room smelt of alcohol and Grace was snoring blissfully.

The ward round was scheduled for the next day and the nurse asked to attend and speak about Grace and how to manage this behaviour. She had still not been able to re-establish contact with Grace and to ask her what had happened. The ward staff discussed the case and decided that nothing should be altered, that the planned programme should carry on and to start talking to Grace about life after the baby, rather than concentrating on what was happening to her day by day.

Grace finally made contact with one of the night staff who had let her on to the ward on the night of her absence. She confessed to feeling dependent on the ward and everyone on it and that she was scared of leaving and having to resume life on her own. She admitted drinking a lot and said she had hoped to put herself back so that she would not have to leave the hospital.

The nurse continued to meet Grace and stated the need to discuss life outside of hospital and what that would mean to Grace. They discussed their own relationship and how they felt things were going. Grace said she could not imagine not being able to talk to her nurse and all the other people in the ward. Plans began to be drawn up for Grace's support networks outside of hospital.

The ending of the therapeutic relationship can affect how a patient will establish contact with the next person they enter into a relationship with. This is a significant responsibility and often overlooked by nurses, who may meet and say goodbye to many people in one day. Letting the patient know how many more sessions are expected and reiterating the loss that it might signify for them are all worth noting and discussing in supervision.

MEASURING AND MONITORING THE RELATIONSHIP

To understand what occurs between a nurse and a patient that is considered most beneficial or helpful is an important part of nursing practice and research. The basis of this is a successful helping relationship, enhanced, developed and sustained through effective communication. The interpersonal relationship between the nurse and patient is the primary instrument to change. It is through this relationship that the patient is able to use the nurse's communication to gain insight into patterns of behaviour, thoughts and feelings as they recur. Bordin (1979) identified that it is the patient's contribution to the relationship that enables them to collaborate with the nurse in the fight against their conflicts, anxiety and unconscious use of defence mechanisms whereas Rogerian theory argues that the patient will automatically respond to the nurse's positive attitudes (Horvarth and Luborsky, 1993).

Psychotherapy research has largely focused upon distinguishing one therapy technique from another but interest more recently has been on identifying specific features common to all therapy techniques. During the 1970s and 1980s social influence was considered an important element of the patient's judgement of the therapeutic process. Attributes such as attractiveness, expertise and trustworthiness were considered influential to therapy outcome. Differences in cultural

---

Case study: **Grace – phases of the relationship (part 4)**

Grace was by now spending alternate weekends at home and had been attending antenatal classes at the local hospital. Her nurse had discussed with the team the possibility of Grace returning to the ward to meet people weekly for her first four weeks at home, until she had met her community nurse a few more times. This also allowed Grace and her nurse to say their goodbyes and evaluate their work together. The nurse brought some of the old care plans to the meetings and Grace was able to laugh at some of the things they had agreed to do to help her sleep at night rather than through the daytime. 'I'd forgotten a lot of all that', was a frequent exclamation. At their last meeting, Grace gave the nurse a painting she had completed and asked for it to be put up on the ward some-where.

By now Grace had a list of contact numbers of people she could ring for different situations and had met her Community Psychiatric Nurse and been to the centre a couple of times, which was only a

---

upbringing, social class and age were all considered to have a negative effect. Client centred therapy (Rogers, 1951) stimulated much research into personal traits of the therapist with scales being developed, probably the most notable being those from Truax and Carkhoff (1967) and Carkhoff (1967). These scales aimed to measure the degree to which the therapist provided facilitative conditions of warmth, empathy and genuineness. Carkhoff (1967) suggests that there is an ever increasing array of therapist communication skills, which enhances the therapeutic communication and relationship process, some of which he identified as disclosure, concreteness, confrontation and immediacy. Heron (1977) produced similar facilitative conditions and has taken the therapist's side in how the relationship can be administered. However, little empirical evidence exists to reveal a causal effect of the therapist's style or skill on the outcome of a therapeutic relationship (Lambert *et al*, 1978).

Instead of identifying individual traits, research has begun to focus more on the relationship in (what is called in the literature) the helping, working or therapeutic alliance (Horvath, 1981; Hartely and Strupp, 1983; Marziali, 1984; Alexander and Luborsky, 1986; Gaston and Ring, 1992). Research findings from the literature of psychotherapy, where most of this work is being carried out, show that a positive alliance between patient and therapist is associated with a process of specific change and a positive care outcome. The literature is largely concerned with differing measurements of the alliance and to operationalize aspects of the relationship. What also emerges is that there are different levels of alliance at different stages of the relationship. Although a patient's contribution at the start of care can be used as a prediction of how they will respond, it does not remain consistent throughout the care process.

Monitoring the alliance or relationship has been found to be helpful in the following ways:
1 In helping to maintain patient's interest and collaboration in their care programme.
2 As a predictor of positive care outcomes;
3 As an effective training method.

Yet how this information will translate into clinical practice remains to be seen. Despite the increased importance placed on interpersonal skills training and what actions, behaviour, attributes and responses are best received by patients, this does not easily translate into the clinical skill of relating to another person on such a level that will produce change.

PERSONAL RISKS AND SAFEGUARDS

Jourard (1961) reviews the therapeutic effectiveness of nurses and discusses the depersonalizing effect training has on those who enter the health professions. The pressures for efficiency and effectiveness placed on people today changes the emphasis on them from being fallible human beings to competent doctors and nurses who must carry out activities to the best of their ability under the most difficult circumstances. This change in people's roles jeopardizes not only their personality but also their physical and mental well-being.

Much psychological disturbance can arise from the unconscious processes of working closely with patients in the nurse–patient relationship. Winship (1995) offers an explanation of this, suggesting that the nurse internalizes the patient's distress believing it to be the nurse's own.

A staff nurse on a ward dealing with patients who had suffered abusive relationships and were now exhibiting self-mutilating behaviour, came to supervision with a disturbing and recurrent dream. In her dream she described rampaging through the ward with a knife, chopping the patients' heads off, one by one. When she found the courage to reveal the dream to her supervisor, they were able to discuss it. They recognized the severe frustration and anger her patients were experiencing and the murderous rage the patients felt at being confronted with their thoughts and feelings, which had been repressed for years. These powerful feelings were being transferred onto the nurses and she was only able to consider and contemplate them in a dream.

Such negative feelings originate from the patient and, through the therapeutic relationship, begin to affect the nurse, invariably leaving the latter feeling denigrated and helpless (Fabricius, 1991; Dartington, 1993; Shur, 1994).

SUMMARY

Do not let unwholesome talk come out of your mouths, but only what is helpful for building others up according to their needs, that it may benefit those who listen.

(Ephesians 4:29)

The relevance to nursing of therapeutic communication and a therapeutic relationship is important to enable the helping process. The relationship itself is the vehicle through which the nurse uses communication skills to develop and utilize an understanding of the patient. Working therapeutically is both difficult and draining work, which requires constant consideration for what is being said and done. The text above from the Bible puts a heavy load on the mental health nurse. It is easy to fall into criticism, cynicism and anger when trying to deal with someone who has spent a lifetime developing defence mechanisms to keep people out of their life, rather than readily allow someone like a nurse to enter their personal world with the intention of removing these defences. For the nurse too, the experience can provide insight and information about their own ways of interacting with others and cause the nurse to change and develop alongside the patient. Aspects of self-awareness are imperative for therapeutic work as is the need for supervision, which allows for difficulties to be explored in a caring, safe and objective environment.

KEY CONCEPTS

- The therapeutic nurse–patient relationship is considered central to the treatment process.
- Several phases of the relationship have been identified and can be used to help or hinder the treatment process.
- The nurse needs to understand the use of effective communication skills in order to maximize the relationship's potential.
- At all stages of the relationship, the nurse needs to consider the well-being of the patient.
- There are certain ethical and legal requirements of the relationship that need to be made clear to both parties at the outset.
- Monitoring and measuring the relationship can help clarify change and progress.
- Supervision is essential for the nurse to remain objective and for additional insight into the unconscious process that is taking place.
- A psychodynamic, theoretical perspective of the therapeutic relationship enables the nurse to further understand some of the complexities of human interactions and relations.

REFERENCES

Alexander LB and Luborsky L: The Penn Helping Alliance Scales. In: Greenberg LS and Pinsof WM, editors: *The psychotherapeutic process; a research handbook*. New York, 1986, Guildford Press.

Altschul A: *Patient–nurse interaction*. Edinburgh, 1972, Churchill Livingstone.

Balint, M: *The doctor, the patient and the illness*. Avon, 1964, Churchill Livingstone.

Barker P: The philosophy of psychiatric nursing, *Nurs Stand* 5(12), 12 December, 28–33, 1990.

Barker P: Psychiatry's human face, *Nurs Times* 91(18), May 3, 58-59, 1994.

Barnes E: *Psychosocial nursing. Studies from the Cassell Hospital*. London, 1968, Tavistock Publications Ltd.

Beck AT: *Cognitive therapy and emotional disorders*. New York, 1976, International Universities Press.

Bordin ES: The generalisability of the psychoanalytical concept of working alliance. *Psychotherapy, theory and practice research*.16:252–260, 1979.

Bowlby J: *The making and breaking of emotional bonds*. London, 1973, Tavistock.

Brown D, Pedder J: *Introduction to psychotherapy: an outline of psychodynamic principles and practice*. London, 1991, Tavistock/Routledge Publication.

Carkoff R: Towards a comprehensive model of facilitative interpersonal processes. *J Counsel Psychology* 14:76–71, 1967.

Carson J, Sharma T: In-patient psychiatric care: What helps? Staff and patients' perspectives. *J Ment Health, 3*:99–104, 1994.

Caudill WA, Redlick F, Gilmore HR *et al.*: Social structure and interaction process in a psychiatric ward. *Am J Orthopsychiatry* 22:314–334, 1952.

Cawley RH: The teaching of psychotherapy. *Association of University Teachers of Psychiatry Newsletter* 19–36, January 1977.

Cormack D: *Psychiatric nursing described*. Edinburgh, 1983, Churchill Livingstone.

Dartington A: Where angels fear to tread. Idealism, despondency, and inhibition in thought in hospital nursing. *Winnicott Studies* 7:21–41, 1993.

Davis JD: Psychotherapy Research. Functions and functionality. *Psychother Res* 5(2):121–124, 1995.

Eichenbaum L, Orbach S: *Understanding women*. London, 1983, Penguin Books Ltd.

Erikson E: *Childhood and society*. Harmondsworth, 1965, Penguin Books Ltd.

Fabricius J: Running on the spot or can nursing really change? *Psychoanal Psychother* 5(2):97–108, 1991.

Forchuk C, Brown B: Establishing a nurse–client relationship. *J Psychosoc Nurs* 27(2):30–34, 1989.

Freud S (1921): In: Strachy J, editor: *The standard edition of the complete psychological works of Sigmund Freud 1905/1953*. London, 1958, Hogarth Press.

Gaston L, Ring JM: Preliminary results on the inventory of therapeutic strategies. *J Res Practi* 1:1–13, 1992.

Gerstley L, McLellan T, Alterman AI, Woody GE, Luborsky L, Prout M: Ability to form an alliance with the therapist; a possible marker of prognosis for patients with antisocial personality disorder. *Am J Psychiatry* 146(4):508–512, 1989.

Gould D: Empathy: a review of the literature with suggestions for an alternative research strategy. *J Adv Nurs* 15:1167–1174, 1990.

Gournay K: Redirecting the emphasis to serious mental illness. *Nurs Times* 90(25), 22 June, 40–41, 1994.

Hardy SE: *The application of an empirical method to investigate the helping relationship between mental health nurses and their allocated patients [Dissertation]*. London, 1995, The Institute of Psychiatry.

Hartely D, Strupp HH: The therapeutic alliance. Its relationship to outcome in brief psychotherapy. In: Masling J, editor: *Empirical studies in analytic theories*. New Jersey, 1983, Hullside.

Hays JS, Larson KH: *Interacting with patients*, New York, 1963, Macmillan Co.

Heron J: *Dimensions of facilitator style*. 1977, Human Potential Resource Group, University of Surrey.

Horvath AO: *An explanatory study of the working alliance. Its measurement and relation to outcome [Dissertation]*. University of British Columbia, 1981.

Horvath AO, Luborsky L: The role of therapeutic alliance in psychotherapy. *J Consult Clin Psychol* 61(4):561–573, 1993.

Jourard SM: Roles that sicken, transactions that heal. *Can Nurse* 57:623–634, 1961.

Kitzinger C: *The social constructionism of lesbianism*. London, 1987, Sage.

Kostere KM, Malatesta LK: Get the results you want. A systematic approach to neurolinguistic programming. Portland, 1989, Metamorphosis Press.

Lambert MJ, DeJulia SS, Stein MM: Therapist interpersonal skills: process outcome, methodological considerations and recommendations for future research. *Psychological Bulletin* 85(3):464–489, 1978.

Lego S: The one to one nurse–patient relationship. *Perspect Psychiatr Care*, 18(2):67–89, 1980.

Luborsky L, Crist–Christoph P, Alexander L, Margolis M, Cohen M: Two helping alliance methods for predicting outcome in psychotherapy. A counting signs versus global rating method. *J Nerv Ment Dis* 171:480–492, 1983.

Manthey M: Myths that threaten what primary nursing really is. *Nursing Management* 19:54–56, 1988.

Marziali E, Marmar C, Krupnick J: Therapeutic alliance scales: development and relationship to psychotherapy outcome. *Am J Psychiatry* 138:361–364, 1981.

Masson J: *Against therapy*. London, 1988, Fontana Paperbacks.

McIntyre K, Farrell M, David A: In-patient psychiatric care. The patient's view. *Brit J Medi Psychol* 62:249–255, 1989.

McLeod Clark J: *Nurse patient interaction. An analysis of conversations on surgical wards [Thesis]*. London, 1982, University of London.

Menzies IEP: A case study in the functioning of social systems as a defense against anxiety. *Hum Relations* 13:95–121, 1960.

MIND (National Association for Mental Health): *Being informed and giving consent – a check list for users of mental health services*. London, 1992, MIND

Publications.

Morrison RS: Teaching acceptance in nursing. *Nurse Educ* 16(5), Sept/Oct, 37, 1991.

Morrison P, Burnard P: Students and trained nurses' perceptions of their own interpersonal skills. A report and comparisons, *J Adv Nurs* 14:321–329, 1989.

Nurse G: *Counselling and the nurse.* Aylesbury, 1980, HM & M Publishers.

O'Connor J, Seymour J: Introducing neuro-linguistic programming: the new psychology of personal excellence. Chatham, Kent, 1990, Mandala.

Pasquali EA, Arnold HM, DeBasio N: *Mental health nursing: a holistic approach.* St Louis, 1989, Mosby.

Pedder J: Attachment and new beginnings. *Int J Psychoanal* 3:491–497, 1976.

Peitchinis JA: Therapeutic effectiveness in counselling by nursing personnel. *Nurs Res* 21(2):138–148, 1972.

Peplau H: *Interpersonal relations in nursing.* New York, 1952 (reprinted1988), GP Putnam's Sons.

Peplau H: Psychiatric mental health nursing: challenge and change. *J Psychiatr Ment Health Nurs* 1:3–7, 1994.

Porter S: The determinants of psychiatric nursing practice. A comparison of sociological perspectives. *J Adv Nurs* 18:1559–1566, 1993.

Reid W, Long A: The role of the nurse providing therapeutic care for the suicidal patient. *J Adv Nurs* 18:1369–1376, 1993.

Ritter S: *Bethlem Royal and Maudsley Hospital Manual of Clinical Psychiatric Nursing Principles and Procedures.* London, 1989, Harper & Row.

Robinson L: *Psychiatric nursing as a human experience.* Philadelphia, 1983, WB Saunders.

Rogers CR: *Client-centred therapy.* London, 1951, Constable.

Sayce L: Response to Violence. In: Crichton J, editor: *Psychiatric patient violence: risk and response.* London, 1995, Duckworth.

Shur R: *Countertransference enactment. How institutions and therapists actualise primitive internal worlds.* Northvale NJ, 1994, Jason Aronsons Inc.

Truax CB, Carkhoff R: *Towards effective counselling and psychotherapy.* Chicago, 1967, Aldine.

Tschudin V: *Counselling skills for nurses.* Eastbourne, 1987, Bailliere Tindall.

United Kingdom Central Council (UKCC): *Code of professional conduct.* London, 1992, UKCC.

Webb C, Hope K: What kind of nurse do patients want? *J Clin Nurs* 4:101–108, 1995.

Winship G: The unconscious impact of caring for acutely disturbed patients; a perspective for supervision. *J Ment Health Nurs* 2:227-231, 1995.

FURTHER READING

Masson J: *Against therapy.* London, 1988, Fontana Paperbacks.
A powerful argument against 'therapeutic' behaviour; a must for every mental health nurse.

Meteyard B: *Community Care Key Worker manual.* Brighton, 1994, Pavillion.
Excellent, clear outline of Key Worker role in worker–patient relationships and the extended role in context of community care and Care Programme Approach.

Wilson G, editor: *Community Care: asking the users.* London, 1996, Chapman & Hall.
Explores methods for measuring service user input and satisfaction with community services; useful insight into service user perspectives on type of service and differences in power between users and 'professionals'.

User Issues and Critical Theories

Learning Outcomes

After studying this chapter you should be able to:

- Describe the dangers inherent in the psychiatric system for the service user.

- Give a brief overview of the mental health user movement and its aims.

- Recognize nursing practice that is potentially empowering or disempowering to the service user.

- Understand the different forms of advocacy available to service users.

- Reflect critically on the notion of partnership and discuss its ideals.

- Understand what it means to be a user ally.

*T*his chapter puts mental health users and their rights at the forefront of the debate, rather than as objects of mental health practice.

ASSUMPTIONS, HISTORY AND CRITICISM

This section is written from a user perspective, and is informed both by the user's unique position in the psychiatric system and by on-going sociological debate about the domain and role of psychiatry.

MEDICAL DISEASE VERSUS HUMAN DISTRESS

There are many well documented critical approaches to the science of 'mental illness' called psychiatry, the most famous of which are by Laing (1965), Szasz (1961), and Foucault (1967) that question the capacity of psychiatry to deal with problems of the mind and spirit when its basis lies in positivistic Western medicine. These critics are from within psychiatry itself or from philosophical academia. Also, many fears have been expressed about the compulsive and coercive basis of psychiatry and consequent abuses of human rights (Szasz, 1963; Gostin, 1983). Again, these critiques come from within psychiatry itself or from human rights activists.

Much less attention has been given to work published by those who have been directly on the receiving end of psychiatric treatment. Today, with the implementation of the Community Care Act 1990 and the encouragement of consumerism in the NHS, it has become a government requirement for service providers to listen to those who have experienced psychiatry at first hand. Nevertheless, much consultation is often seen by service users as tokenistic and having minimal impact on the system. For instance, service users may be consulted on such matters as the colour of the paint on in-patient wards, i.e. on the fabric not the framework of psychiatry.

However, much discussion has taken place among users (sometimes called survivors) about the deeper philosophical critique that has become their own. Although every user is an individual, there are many common threads which run through people's experiences, their narratives and their poetry. Many of these start at the foundation of psychiatry — the medical model.

Once a distressed person becomes involved at any level with psychiatric services they are immediately deemed to be already on the road to 'mental illness' and the search is on for 'diagnosis'. As Szasz (1961) very eloquently argues, making human distress into a psychiatric diagnosis, i.e. a medical entity, is more to do with an implicit moral code and social control than with treatment or therapy.

Nobody is told when admitted to a psychiatric unit that the premise on which the hospital or unit rests is open to question. Users are not given histories of Victorian asylums (i.e. histories of social engineering on a massive scale) to read, which in many ways could clarify and place their present treatment in context (see Showalter, 1987; Scull, 1982). That is, they would see that benevolence is not a psychiatric, caring response to an 'illness' but a historically and socially constructed approach to people suffering from psychological distress. This construct assumes that mental distress is both to do with biology and moral failing (Foucault, 1967). Thus the approach is a medical form of social control. For most, this control is very effective and obscures the environmental failures such as neglect, abuse, oppression and deprivation, which have caused their distress in the first place (Jacobs, 1994). Most sinisterly, psychiatric concepts can be used as a weapon against those who challenge society's injustices in what Read (1987) calls 'medicalising dissent'.

Interestingly, the groups within society likeliest to be diagnosed with a mental illness and treated by psychiatry are the most deprived and disadvantaged: women, black people and the working class (Mercer, 1986; Showalter, 1987; Ussher, 1991). This suggests that psychiatry is more to do with social control of human misery than with real biological disease.

DIAGNOSIS AND IDENTITY DAMAGE

Many users who have reflected on their experiences believe that being diagnosed was the start of damage to their identity, both internally and in the wider world. A diagnosis brings stigma (Goffman, 1968), fear and mistrust from the undiagnosed. A diagnosis often devalues the individual and an already fragile self-esteem is lowered even further. Once labelled, the client you see from then on, becomes part of the symptoms of the diagnosis (Rosenhan, 1973). Less emphasis is placed on who the client is and where he or she has come from (which is, of course, part of the distress); the diagnosis becomes paramount. The client is no longer a normal person with the same needs, fears, joys or hopes as anyone else. Anything said or done by the client can be interpreted as 'pathological'. So begins the slippery slope into mental patienthood (Goffman, 1961; Barnham, 1992, 1993). Service users believe that acknowledging their distress, with its real historical and social causes, provides a basis for growth and development that is far more beneficial to them than 'diagnosis'.

PROGNOSIS AND IATROGENIC DISABILITY

Prognosis is also extremely problematic. In Western psychiatry the presence of psychotic symptoms is usually thought to signify a serious illness with no cure. The symptoms are not seen metaphorically, as a language that points to critical disturbance, injustice or oppression in the immediate social relationships of the user (Laing and Esterson, 1964). Instead, they are assumed to signify the presence of some biochemical illness, the organic basis of which has yet to be established (Littlewood, 1991). With its medical bias psychiatry then diagnoses 'schizophrenia' or 'manic-depressive psychosis' or 'schizo-affective state' and often tells the user that their prognosis is poor and that they will need to remain on antipsychotic medication for the rest of their life. Psychiatry's own role in this poor prognosis is not examined. The World Health Organization study of schizophrenia (WHO, 1979) found that prognosis was worse in Western, highly urbanized societies that have a great deal more psychiatric intervention and much better in rural Developing World societies that have less (Fernando, 1991).

Breggin (1991) argues that treatment also leads to a poor prognosis for people diagnosed with a serious psychiatric illness. He and others (Goffman, 1961; Szasz, 1961; Barnham, 1992, 1993) argue that treatment, far from helping people, does increasing damage. Expressly, Breggin argues that neuroleptic medication, which is said to remove psychotic symptoms, in fact has no specific action on them. Neuroleptics have a major tranquillizing effect, however, which Breggin likens to a chemical 'straight jacket'. The danger, he says, lies in the fact that long-term (or sometimes even short-term) neuroleptics cause brain damage. Tardive dyskinesia, a disorder characterized by involuntary movements including tics, spasms and tremors, facial grimaces, tongue protrusions and chewing movements, is the most frequent manifestation of this brain damage. Breggin argues that a drop in IQ and cognitive abilities is also common, leading at times to dementia. Interestingly, it took professionals a long time before they would acknowledge the existence of tardive dyskinesia (Brown and Funk, 1986). Breggin also criticizes other psycho-active drugs for their chemical interference, with the potential for this to be disastrous in the long term, in such a delicate organ as the brain. Electroconvulsive therapy (ECT), another highly controversial treatment, is acknowledged by psychiatry itself to cause memory loss and to cause other forms of serious long-term brain damage (Frank, 1990; Cameron, 1994).

UNDERLYING ASSUMPTIONS OF PROFESSIONALS

Assumptions are made about the service user by mental health workers when he or she arrives at a crisis unit or centre. These, often based on appearance, age, gender, class, culture, marital status and sexuality, further serve to alienate the client from the services. For instance, there is a strong association among mental health professionals between black skin and dangerousness. The incidence of black men being labelled schizophrenic (in isolation from their cultural background) and treated in the most restrictive ways by psychiatry is well documented (Department of Health, Home Office, 1992). There is also a common assumption that women in distress are 'attention-seeking', especially women who harm themselves (Pembroke, 1994). Services tend to be Eurocentric and homophobic. It is assumed that English will be the first language, that a partner is a husband or wife and that they will be of the opposite sex. Junior doctors seem to have little life experience or training enabling them to deal sensitively with these issues. There is evidence to show that some groups, e.g. lesbians, will avoid the system at all costs because of the fear of mistreatment and their sexuality being pathologized (Williams *et al.*, 1993).

TREATMENT AND LACK OF CHOICE

The chances are that, once within the psychiatric system and despite the rhetoric to the contrary, the user will be offered little or no choice in treatment. It is also most likely that what is offered or given is a physical treatment (usually a drug or drugs). The Mental Health Nursing Review Team heard evidence from people who had been 'unable to convince staff of the validity of their concerns about particular drugs or therapies' (Department of Health, 1994b). Usually, little information will be given to the user and their families about specific treatments, and therefore they could refuse treatment if they are legally able to. For example, if ECT is the treatment proposed, it is unlikely that a client will be given details of its dangers (Cameron, 1994; Lindow, 1994a). The treatment plan is also likely to be governed by the particular interests and specialism of the consultant psychiatrist. For example, if a consultant has a research interest in lithium many of his patients are likely to be taking it (Barcan, 1996). The same applies to 'talking treatments' (psychological interventions or psychotherapy). It is well known among users that, if the consultant is biased against these, it is unlikely the client will get one of them. It is assumed that people with 'psychotic disorders' will not benefit from psychotherapy (Breggin, 1991). For users it really does appear that 'your life is in their hands'.

As with choice of treatments, so with choice of mental health workers. It is unlikely that the client will choose who will become the Key Worker, Community Psychiatric Nurse, doctor, etc. This issue is especially pertinent to women service users (Williams *et al.*, 1993). According to the psychiatric literature, approximately 70% of women admitted to psychiatric hospital will have a history of childhood sexual abuse (Batcup, 1995). It is usual for this not to be addressed at all within the psychiatric system; neither are women given the choice of a woman worker as standard practice. Some women, admitted after being raped, do not want to be nursed by men. Others, because of their cultural backgrounds, may find close contact with males very inhibiting (MIND, 1992a). Despite a campaign by MIND and a raised profile for this issue, the goal, of choice of a woman worker by women, still appears unattainable.

A serious and related issue is that rapes and sexual assaults on women within psychiatric services have been coming to light in recent years. This has received some attention in the nursing journals (Copperman and Burrows, 1992; Batcup and Thomas, 1994) and there have been efforts to make 'women only' spaces and lounges on wards. Nevertheless, despite a long-running campaign from MIND (1992a) women-only wards are not widely available. In fact, with the recent reduction in psychiatric beds nationwide, it appears that a higher proportion of very disturbed men are being admitted to acute psychiatric wards, leaving the distressed women there in a very vulnerable position (Batcup D, 1996, personal communication). In addition to lack of choice and possible threat of assault, many users lose basic rights when entering the system even if they are not subject to the Mental Health Act. The rights lost may appear minor (such as having prescribed times for meals) but will also include pressure to participate in, for example, groups and occupational therapy. These subtle forms of social control result in the professional production of dependency (as described by Illich (1976) in his book *The Limits to Medicine*), institutionalization and setting the user on the road to becoming a chronic mental patient (see also Silverman, 1987). Because psychiatry constructs itself as a science, it is contrived and prescriptive, making self-determination for users increasingly difficult. Psychiatry's claim to scientific objectivity is effective in silencing alternative arguments and obscuring the real power relations in the situation (Szasz, 1961; Johnstone, 1994). On discharge, users often feel scared of the outside world and worried about functioning again on their own. With a little wider help in the community it may be easier for the user to be readmitted and undergo the process again.

> Nobody ever tried to explain what the nurses were for and I never worked it out. They seemed to me to spend most of their time trying to retain their rank in the hierarchy, trying to prove that they were coping and that we patients were somehow broken up and in need of their guidance.
>
> *(Galloway, 1991)*

Nowadays, with the growth of mental health teams in the community, some users are not admitted as in-patients. Nevertheless, the possibility of becoming depersonalized and 'institutionalized' in the community system is similar, with the same loss of autonomy and self-determination. For every service user in the community the spectre of the hospital still looms large as the ultimate sanction, if their behaviour does not match up to what society expects (Bean and Mounser, 1993).

CRITIQUES AND REACTIONS

Those who react to present or past social injustice or abuse with acute mental distress often have this distress compounded by the mental health system. Because of this, many users are angry.

This anger and the diverse criticisms of psychiatry (concerns over human rights, the medicalization of mental distress, identity damage and institutionalization) have over the years stimulated resistance and brought about attempts either to abolish or to change the system. These forms of group resistance and action are known collectively as the 'mental health user movement'.

THE MENTAL HEALTH USER MOVEMENT

> To me the truth of a movement is when people who have never heard of each other, from as far away as New Zealand, England and Canada, are thinking the same thing. Then you know it's true.
>
> *(O'Hagan, 1993)*

The start of a critical approach to the incarceration and institutionalization of the mentally distressed dates back to the mid 19th Century. Then the Alleged Lunatics' Friends Society was set up in Britain by John Percival (a former inmate of an asylum) to protect the interests of those improperly confined (Porter R, 1987). From 1868 Elizabeth Packard in the USA wrote several books and pamphlets challenging her committal by her husband, to an Illinois asylum and by the 1970s around 200 auto-biographical accounts of madness had been published (O'Hagan, 1993). 'Common ground can be found between the Alleged Lunatic's Friend Society, the Mental Patients' Union and the current self-advocacy movement' (Survivors Speak Out, nd).

The mental health user or survivor movement became active in Western society in the early 1970s; at that time there was a drive towards democracy, libertarian policies and the pursuit of individual freedom and fulfilment in society generally (illustrated by the rise of the US civil rights movement and the women's movement, for example). There are now users working together in many parts of the world, mainly in liberal Western countries. Although dominated by white users there is now recognition that some are more oppressed by the system than others. Consequently there are now self-organized black user groups and lesbian and gay user groups. The user movement has drawn heavily on the anti-psychiatry movement, the social sciences and the 'nurture versus nature' debate (O'Hagan, 1993). Some users are concerned with reclaiming madness and question why psychosis has less meaning and credibility than dreams (O'Hagan, 1993). (See section below on Hearing Voices Network.)

THE USA

In the USA, a criticism of psychiatry began to develop with people fighting specific areas of injustice, who then moved on to the idea of abolishing psychiatry. This led to self-help groups and the beginnings of user-led alternative mental health facilities. Since the 1980s there has been a split between those who want to reform the existing system and those who want to build self-help alternatives. Self-help alternatives are most developed in the USA, largely because of funding opportu-

nities which are less prevalent in Europe (O'Hagan, 1993). Nevertheless, there has been a backlash in the form of a growing family movement led by the National Alliance for the Mentally Ill (NAMI) which organizes relatives and carers rather then users themselves and which strongly endorses the medical model and supports psychiatry. NAMI, which has a powerful voice, resists the movement of psychiatric survivors and consistently opposes any form of psychosocial research (Breggin, 1991).

EUROPE

Italy

Italy is noteworthy for the work of Franco Basaglia, a radical psychiatrist who practised in the 1960s and 1970s and who inspired other psychiatrists and mental health workers to press for reforms in the psychiatric system. A professional-led movement was formed called the Psichiatria Democratica. Basaglia took his own hospital in Gorizia from a backward, custodial institution to firstly, an open hospital with freedom of movement and then into the era of community care and self-determination for the former patients. Because of pressure from Psichiatria Democratica, Italy was the first country to put community care into practice (Sheper–Hughes and Lovell, 1986). Nevertheless, this activity of professionals somehow stifled the user movement itself and it never became well established. Currently, there are a number of cultural activities and working cooperatives involving users, although initiatives are still isolated (van Hoorn, 1991).

Holland

Patients' councils (user groups in hospitals with some influence on how things are run) began being set up in Holland in 1970. In 1971 a user group was formed calling itself the Clients' Association. The Clients' Association became very active and eventually demanded that powers of the patients' councils be legally specified. A National Foundation of Patients' Councils was set up in 1981, subsidized by the government. These councils are now independent from service providers and have a strong voice (Haafkens *et al.*, 1986).

UK

The thinker and psychiatrist, R.D. Laing, stimulated criticism of psychiatry in Britain. He qualified as a psychiatrist in the early 1950s and quickly began developing a critique of theory and practice. Like Szasz in the USA, Laing refuted the notion that schizophrenia was any kind of medical entity and saw 'psychotic' communication as intelligible when viewed in the context of the patient's situation (1965). He and Esterson (Laing and Esterson, 1964) did a great deal of work exploring disordered communication in families that put the 'psychotic' person in an impossible existential position. The 'psychosis' was both a protest and an attempt to communicate with their intimate relations in an ambiguous code.

The work of Szasz, Laing and Goffman (a US sociologist who spent two years covertly researching an asylum while working as a fitness instructor there; Goffman, 1961) emerged at around the same time and contributed to a movement in Britain known as anti-psychiatry (Cooper, 1967). Goffman's work was particularly damning of institutional life and the dehumanization and 'warehousing' of people in long-term custodial care. In more recent years, a feminist critique of anti-psychiatry has developed noting Laing's lack of analysis of women's oppression within the family (Showalter, 1987).

In the mid-1970s the Mental Patients' Union and the British Network of Alternatives to Psychiatry were established, which took an abolitionist stance (Rogers and Pilgrim, 1991). In 1988 there was a campaign against proposed changes to the 1983 Mental Health Act to bring about Community Treatment Orders where service users could be compulsorily treated in the community, against their will. These changes had been recommended by the Royal College of Psychiatrists. User organizations and the Community Psychiatric Nurses' Association successfully opposed these changes at the time. Nevertheless, the victory was short-lived; in 1995 the Mental Health (Patients in the Community) Bill was passed. From April 1996 this Act gives a nominated 'supervisor' (i.e. a mental health professional) the power to 'take and convey' a service user subject to the Act, to a place for medical treatment, occupation, education or training. Thus, under this Act, certain mental health professionals are given the powers of arrest.

USER ORGANIZATIONS IN BRITAIN TODAY

Relatives' Organizations

In the 1980s, user groups opposed the work of SANE (a relatives' organization supporting the medical model) and, in particular, a poster they produced stereotyping people with mental health problems as dangerous. SANE campaigns for increased hospital and psychiatric provision and is acutely concerned with the issue of 'dangerousness'; it is in favour of enforced detention and medication.

Another relatives' organization in Britain is the National Schizophrenia Fellowship, which also supports the medical model. Nevertheless, it has a branch of its organization for users (called Voices) which may have the potential to be more emancipatory.

Survivors Speak Out

Survivors Speak Out was established in 1986, largely influenced by the Dutch Patients' Councils and Psichiatria Democratica in Italy (Survivors Speak Out, nd) and following the World Federation of Mental Health/MIND conference in 1985 (Rogers and Pilgrim, 1991). They saw their main task as improving communication between individuals and groups in the self-advocacy movement. In September 1987 their conference in Edale was attended by over 100 people, system survivors and their allies. Survivors Speak Out never saw itself as a national voice but a coming together of like minds. Nevertheless, like minds make for productive dialogue and in the mid 1990s it is active in making its voice heard by national

health policy makers, such as the Department of Health.

MIND

MIND has been in existence for 50 years as a mental health charity. Its membership consists of equal proportions of professional mental health workers, voluntary workers or bodies and service users (Clements, 1995). When it started, it supported the medical model but by the 1980s, with the influence of the service users in its ranks, it had begun to direct itself more towards advocacy. Its 1985 conference is seen by many as a watershed in the user movement. It was given over to the consumer viewpoint with users speaking from the platform.

MINDLINK

MINDLINK is 'a national network of users who give MIND a greater understanding of users' views' (MIND, 1992b). It has a newsletter called *Mindwaves*. MIND has seven regions and each one has a MINDLINK group. Representatives from MINDLINK serve on MIND's Regional Councils and MIND's Consumer Advisory Panel.

Hearing Voices Network

This developed out of the work of Dutch psychiatrist Marius Romme and medical writer Sandra Escher. Romme was persuaded by one of his patients that, though she heard voices, this was not necessarily a symptom of 'psychiatric illness'. Through a television programme they canvassed people in the general population for their experiences of voice hearing and subsequently organized a congress. The main conclusion was that 'the reduction of hearing voices to the status of mere pathology is not very fruitful in helping patients to deal with these experiences. It may also be an inaccurate analysis. Outside the world of psychiatry, there are many people who hear voices and manage to live with the experience; some, indeed, find it an enrichment to their lives' (Romme and Escher, 1993). A movement was started that questioned the validity of voice hearing as a psychiatric symptom. There is a Hearing Voices network in the UK and Holland where people are encouraged to share experiences.

UKAN

UKAN was set up after a national user conference in Nottingham in 1990. It is a federation of advocacy groups run by people who use or have used mental health services. It helps to develop self-advocacy through patients and users councils, and peer advocacy. Its key aim is to empower people who use services and to protect their rights as citizens (Department of Health, 1994a).

Other developed movements exist in Canada, Germany, France and Japan (Rogers and Pilgrim, 1991). In 1985 the first World Federation of Mental Health/MIND conference was held, which included a World Federation of Mental Health Users.

SELF-HELP ALTERNATIVES

There is also a growing interest in self-help alternatives to mental health services, which are user controlled and independent of mental health workers and funders. Lindow (1994b, 1994c) has extensively researched this subject and has also looked at how purchasers can buy-in these services.

THE DEVELOPING WORLD

There have also been developments in non-Western countries. O'Hagan (1993) reports an informal network of 'usuarios' in Mexico fostered by wealthy, influential women with a social conscience. O'Hagan says that in the West this would be viewed with suspicion but even fewer resources are available to users in the developing world, such as access to people in power and tools of literacy, and this may be the first step for users in these countries to access some power and control.

EMPOWERMENT

Although most nurses will have encountered the word empowerment, it is important to look at what it really means for the service user or psychiatric survivor in the mental health system (Box 4.1).

As has already been seen here, power in psychiatry is often held by the professionals and not the recipients; it can be said

Box 4.1 *Principles underlying user empowerment*

1. A basic question to ask of any service (including advocacy projects) is 'Who is being empowered by this service?'
2. Services should recognize and seek to enhance people's abilities and not simply concentrate on their difficulties.
3. Services need to recognize the existence of power relations and conflicts of interest between service providers and service users.
4. Services should be person centred and not category centred.
5. Service users have a right to their own emotional response to their life situation and the provision of services within this.
6. Service users have a right to their own advocate or access to an independent advocate who will support them in clarifying their own needs and wants and pressing for these to be responded to.
7. Service users (and their advocate) have a right of access to all information and records relating to their case.
8. Service providers should be prepared to learn from service users and their experiences.
9. Services should question and re-evaluate any areas of compulsion that exist within their practice.
10. Service users have a right to discuss issues of concern to them in a user-only context should they so wish.
11. Service users should be involved in planning, delivering and monitoring advocacy projects.
12. Services should be accessible and responsive to all users and potential users, whatever their disability, gender, sexuality or ethnic background.

(Reproduced with the permission of Dave Lowson from personal communication)

that power is taken away from individuals when they come into the system. Campbell (1992) points out that 'amongst all the groups with a vested interest in the system, the pharmaceutical industry, respected professionals, voluntary agencies, nurses and auxiliary workers, it is the interests of the recipients that should be declared paramount. Our distress fuels the system.' Users often say that there would be no psychiatry without them but they are frequently ignored as the main stake-holders. Campbell (1992) also points out that 'the principal criterion against which services must be examined is their effectiveness in enabling individuals to gain or regain control of their lives'.

PERSONAL EXPERIENCE OF EMPOWERMENT

How can users regain power in society or become empowered? For an illustration of how this has taken place in Western society see the section on the History of the User Movement. This can also be illustrated by giving an example from the personal experience of Kate, a service user.

> My early experiences as a psychiatric patient were dominated by issues such as the lack of information and choice and not being listened to, which led to me feeling very confused about my place in the world. Later, I suffered a major breakdown or crisis and I was sectioned and placed on a secure unit. The treatment within the unit was often abusive and very painful to live through. Eventually, when my life began to come together again, I was moved to a new ward which I found far more sympathetic. I was then able to consider my negative experiences within the psychiatric system and later decided to try and use them as a way of taking control over my life by speaking out against injustice. From my largely positive experiences on the new ward I also now had some idea of what sort of things constituted 'good practice' and felt that these needed to be promoted.

> So my passage through the psychiatric system had first taken my power as an individual away ([that is] my dignity, self-respect, control over my world and being valued as a person), but later I was able to use these very negative experiences in a meaningful way, to regain my power and to try to be of use to others. For me, this was an empowering experience. Additionally when I discovered that there was a whole international movement that felt similarly to me, that I could join forces with and communicate with, that was committed to building our voice into the system or forming alternatives, I felt even more powerful.

SHARING EXPERIENCES AND CONSCIOUSNESS RAISING

Kate's experience is not uncommon. People become empowered in different ways (and within a continuing process or struggle), but a major force that aids empowerment is that of sharing experiences and consciousness raising. Personal empowerment can begin in a small way. Users can set themselves achievable tasks like asking questions of their doctor, if this is something they have never done before. Chamberlain (1988) says people need confidence in their own abilities to build their self-esteem (Figure 4.1). She goes on to say that stereotypes about users in the system become internalized by the users themselves. Stereotypes include being labelled as 'weak', 'incapable', 'untrustworthy', 'sick', 'crazy' and this psychological assault teaches users to believe these things about themselves and to hate themselves. Chamberlain also cites the consciousness raising that has gone on in other groups such as the women's movement, the lesbian and gay movement and the disability lobby, where groups of people facing oppression from society will share their experiences for mutual satisfaction and growth.

EMPOWERMENT THROUGH SELF-ADVOCACY

There are many examples of user groups up and down the country meeting for mutual support. 'A bi-product of empowerment is that of self-advocacy' and 'Self-advocacy is about taking positive action for change' (Survivors Speak Out, nd) and speaking up for yourself.

Crisis Cards

Users are developing ways of advocating for themselves even when they are in a very distressed state or crisis. One involves having their wishes for care and treatment written down on a 'crisis card' that can be given to the mental health professional involved at this time.

An 'advance directive' or 'living will' written into the user's case notes 'allows someone to make decisions before they become ill about their future treatment. These decisions cannot be ignored by a doctor unless the advance directive does not apply to the particular situation that arises, the advance directive is not clear or if the Mental Health Act is used to override a person's intentions regarding treatment' (Halpern, 1995).

A development of the idea of crisis cards and advance directives, called *Direct Power* (Leader, 1995), is a resource pack for people wanting to develop their own care plans and support networks.

CONSTRAINTS ON EMPOWERMENT

The Wider Society

It is not only mental health services that disempower users. Users have to contend with unemployment, bad housing, poverty and significant stigmatization and marginalization by society. In re‍ coverage of co‍ stigmatizing a‍ of countering this include more government resourcing of housing, social, education and employment projects and campaigns aimed at changing public and media attitudes.

Opposition from Professionals

Although affirming for users themselves, unfortunately user empowerment has been seen as a threat to the system by professionals. Beeforth *et al.* (1990) say that users making attempts to gain power can be viewed in a negative light by professionals, who feel their own power will be lost. In such situations professionals can be obstructive and uncooperative. Beeforth *et al.* go on to point out that as one group becomes more powerful it does not follow that the other loses out. They argue that power can be increased for users and professionals by cooperation in service planning and provision, where roles are not adversarial.

ADVOCACY

Advocacy involves speaking up on one's own or someone else's behalf, to exert rights or secure interests. It can involve arguing a case. If advocating for someone else, a clear instructional relationship exists; the advocate will only act in accordance with the service user's wishes (Bateman, 1995).

TYPES OF ADVOCACY

The MIND Guide to Advocacy in Mental Health (1992b) highlights three major forms of advocacy. These are self-advocacy, citizen advocacy and legal advocacy. More recently, paid, non-legal advocates and peer advocates have been recognized.

Self-Advocacy

This is defined as 'a process in which an individual, or a group of people, speak or act on their own behalf in pursuit of their needs and interests' (MIND, 1992b). There is a long tradition

Figure 4.1 Degrees of user participation. (Reproduced with permission from Dean C, Freeman H, editors: *Community Mental Health Care*. London, 1993, Gaskell & Royal College of Psychiatrists.

increasing participation		
Neglect		
Paternalism		
Tokenism	'unacceptable' to service users
Partnership	acceptable to service users
Self-help	

in Britain of collective action to secure the rights of oppressed minorities and such action can often have surprisingly successful results. Self-advocacy in hospitals can include Patients' Councils (Robinson and Collins, 1995) which work to provide better facilities and treatment for in-patients.

Citizen Advocacy

Citizen advocacy originated in the USA from experience of learning difficulties and is a mixture of advocacy and befriending. The unpaid citizen advocate is paired with a disempowered service user (often someone who has been in long-term care). The advocate forms a supportive relationship with the client and helps them to self-advocate when necessary or, if the service user requests, will speak for them. Although this sounds good in theory, there are concerns that it may make conflicting demands on the advocate, placing the advocate in too many roles at once (Bateman, 1995).

Legal Advocacy

Legal advocacy uses the services of trained solicitors who specialize in the mental health field to advocate for service users on the many legal issues that beset them. Apart from representing users at Mental Health Review Tribunals and Managers' Hearings, legal advocates can deal with employment and housing issues, custody battles or other serious problems with a legal dimension. If not dealt with adequately these sorts of problems will affect the user's quality of life and, ultimately, mental health. Today in Britain there is only one Law and Advice Centre situated on a hospital site (at Springfield Hospital, London). However, the Law Society has a Mental Health Subcommittee with a national list of members who can be called upon for tribunal work.

Paid Non-Legal Advocates

Advocacy projects with paid non-legal advocates are now springing up in many mental health units. These projects are usually independently funded, often by the Health Authority and independent of the mental health provider's power structures. Such advocates will act in a range of issues, such as welfare benefits and accompanying service users to ward rounds to help them to get their voices heard by clinicians. There are numerous situations that may call for the services of an advocate; some of these are listed in *Advocacy – A Code of Practice* (Department of Health, 1994a). These projects will often have access to legal back-up should the service user need it. Many projects employ, as peer advocates, former users who know what it feels like to be on the receiving end of the system and who may have valuable experience in negotiating some of the obstacles. Other projects have volunteers working as peer advocates.

ADVOCACY IN PRACTICE

Because of the trust the service user places in the advocate, the one-to-one helping relationship and the delicacy of many of the issues, it is essential that the advocate operates within a strict ethical code. Bateman (1995) offers a number of ethical

principles, including 'Act in the client's best interests', 'Act in accordance with the client's wishes and instructions' and 'Carry out instructions with diligence and competence'. From *Advocacy – A Code of Practice* comes the following principle: 'People using advocacy services have the right to expect advocates to uphold and defend their human rights as citizens at all times. This includes their rights to be self-determining and their right to define their own needs, even their needs for advocacy' (Department of Health, 1994a). Bateman's book gives much practical guidance in the skills necessary for advocacy: interviewing, the constructive use of aggression, negotiation, self-management and legal research. He describes advocacy problems as 'bounded' and 'unbounded' and discusses advocacy styles appropriate to each. 'Bounded' problems are easy to define with laws, policies or guidelines on the user's rights and a clear procedure for ensuring a successful outcome. 'Unbounded' problems are more nebulous; rights are not enshrined in rules and guidelines and therefore it is less clear how to obtain a satisfactory outcome. In the first instance, Bateman advises an assertive approach, while in the second he recommends negotiation (Bateman, 1995).

For formal advocacy to work effectively it should be autonomous and independent of service provision. Given this, what options are open to service professionals who wish to see users empowered? *Working in Partnership* (Department of Health, 1994b) is a way forward that seems to be ethically and philosophically 'right' to many present-day service users and professionals. It is also an approach being encouraged by Government. Nevertheless, it is not without its obstacles, highlighted in the next section.

WORKING IN PARTNERSHIP

The nursing ethic is moving more and more towards valuing people, openness, and honesty as expressed in truth-telling, informing patients, and obtaining consent. More and more nurses are viewing the client/nurse relationship as a partnership.

(Bergman, 1981)

Nurses need to treat all people who use services as equal partners and stake-holders in the service, recognising that they are people first – and 'clients' second.

(Department of Health, 1994b)

SOCIAL POLICY BACKGROUND

Recent welfare legislation in the United Kingdom, such as The Children Act 1989 and the NHS and Community Care Act 1990, require service users and carers to have better information and higher levels of participation. The NHS and Community Care Act introduced a quasi-market in health care and divided up functions into the 'purchasing' and 'providing' of care. With the 'commoditization' of health care in this way a consumerist ethos developed. If health care is a commodity then the consumer has 'rights' to expect a good quality product. The State, by seeing mental health service users as 'consumers', gave some support to the user movement and encouraged the development of user participation in health care decision making. So the ground was laid for a more equitable relationship between mental health service users and health professionals, such as nurses, and 'working in partnership' has become an admirable ideal. The team that reviewed mental health nursing in Britain in 1994 called their report *Working in Partnership* (Department of Health, 1994b). However, this ethic calls for a real change in attitudes and working practice among mental health nurses, which is much easier said than done.

THE CONTRADICTORY POSITION OF NURSES

People enter nursing usually through a desire to help people and to be of service to the community. Once within the system, though, the constraints of hierarchical working conditions (Coxon, 1990), lack of resources, high case loads and lack of autonomy and discretionary power make it very difficult for nurses to maintain their vision and ideals (Smith, 1992). Mental health nurses in particular find themselves placed in a very contradictory role (Handy, 1991). The source of the contradiction can found in the parent discipline to mental health nursing, psychiatry. Mental health nursing arose out of psychiatry (Nolan, 1993) and to a large extent is subordinated to its thinking and practice. Mental health nurses are also involved in legally detaining and treating users under the Mental Health Act. So are mental health nurses really helping people or are they agents of social control?

THE CONSTRAINTS ON PARTNER-SHIP

As nurses do not have the power of diagnosis, prognosis and treatment within their remit, they have to work within the framework given to them by psychiatry. Admittedly, nurses do have some level of autonomy. They make another level of diagnosis and treatment, i.e. of the patient's nursing needs and of goals and interventions and are taught in their training to strive to 'make a relationship' with their patient, which many do. However, working under pressure in a bureaucracy (Lipsky, 1980) within a fixed world-view of biochemical dysfunction, often feeling disturbed by disturbing behaviour, sometimes physically threatened and often anxious about being accountable for decisions usually leaves nurses very little room for reflection (Menzies, 1960; Coxon, 1990; Smith, 1992).

All these things militate against the mental health user being seen as an equal and as a partner. To progress the idea of working in partnership with users takes a willingness to reflect on the constraints of present practice. Once the constraints are recognized they become open to change to some degree. When working with individual users it is important that the nurse tries to develop some understanding of expres-

sions of mental distress, not as symptoms of pathology but as manifestations of metaphorical or symbolic significance for the user that reflect internal and external realities. Such expressions cannot then be dismissed as pathological. The nurse must acknowledge their meaningfulness and strive to understand it. This is crucial to partnership at an individual level. In addition, a mental health nurse may wish to become acquainted with the user discourse in general. Eventually, the nurse may become allied to the user cause and work to support self-advocacy among users.

BEING A USER ALLY

In the situation where a psychiatric nurse can identify with the user position or at least recognize some of these critiques as valid, what can be done do to try to rectify some of the injustices and damage done to service users in the name of 'help' (Lindow, 1994a)?

There are things the nurse can do, both at an individual and a group level. Some of this takes courage, as the system is very resistant to change and can punish those who challenge it (Weick *et al.*, 1989). Therefore, challenges have to be made in a way that takes risks into account and minimizes them.

SEEING USERS' STRENGTHS

Mental health practitioners can consciously avoid the negative stereotyping of service users. They can refuse to take part in this and can challenge their colleagues when the latter do. In a reverse psychological operation, they can focus on the service user's strengths and, in partnership with the user, aim to facilitate the further development of the client (Weick *et al.*, 1989). Thy can acknowledge to service users that they are human too, that they have their own areas of weakness and fear and that they are in no way superior to their clients. Mental health practitioners can let clients know that they are willing to learn from them and to assist them, where possible, in the user cause and in empowering themselves.

QUESTIONING

At the most basic level, practitioners can question whether accepted practice embodies the principles of empowerment (see Box 4.1). Then they can ask these questions of their colleagues. Franco Basaglia working in Italy in the 1960s and 1970s had the concept of the 'negative worker'. The negative worker looks critically at the practice situation and continually raises the questions: 'What is *wrong* here?', 'What is the *real* problem?', 'Whose needs are being served – whose are being *neglected*?' (Sheper-Hughes and Lovell, 1986; original emphasis). These questions give practitioners an ethical baseline to their work and help them to analyze any situation. Once they start to ask these questions, the true power relations in the situation become exposed and the circumstances become more amenable to change.

Such questions, asked with tact and diplomacy or, sometimes, with outrage, will stimulate thinking among practitioners' colleagues. Ideally, the psychiatric team will then be concerned to engage service users in a dialogue about these questions.

FACILITATING USER INVOLVEMENT

To avoid service user involvement from being tokenistic (see Figure 4.1) it is important to ensure that real resources, training and funding are provided for users so that they can take their place in the decision-making processes as equals to professionals.

Wallcraft (1994) calls for nurses to facilitate user participation with funding, training and emotional support. She shows that many successful projects have involved professionals giving enough support to allow users to develop themselves. Once the users are established on their chosen path, sensitive professionals stand back.

THE NURSE AS ADVOCATE

Although, ideally, independent advocates should be available to mental health service users, there is a sense in which advocacy is integral to the everyday practice of the nurse. The UKCC Code of Professional Conduct states: 'Act always in such a manner as to promote and safeguard the interests and well-being of patients and clients' (UKCC, 1992).

There may be times when service users ask practitioners directly for help to promote their interests or when practitioners perceive that what is being done is not in the users' best interests. Under these circumstances there is a range of options available, which include giving users basic information, giving them information on their rights, encouraging and supporting them to speak up for themselves (self-advocacy) and referring them to an independent advocate. If no independent advocate is available, practitioners may feel morally obliged to advocate for users in accordance with the latter's wishes.

There is debate (Porter S, 1987) as to whether nurses can be sufficiently independent of their power structures to ever act as advocates. Nevertheless, in a less formal way and in many everyday situations, nurses are obliged by their code of ethics to promote the interests of their patients. *Working in Partnership* (Department of Health, 1994b), the report of the Mental Health Nursing Review Team, recommends that 'Nurses should speak out on behalf of the people in their care, but service-users should also have access to advocates on wards or in the community, who can express their wishes and views unreservedly.' Unfortunately, independent advocates are currently not always available.

Nurse advocacy can be an everyday intervention or it can be a very difficult task, depending on the circumstances. Where it involves real moral dilemmas and taking an oppositional role to the rest of the multidisciplinary team, it will take courage. *Exercising Accountability* (UKCC, 1989) emphasizes that advocacy does not necessarily have to be adversarial and there may be many opportunities to negotiate rather than take a more vigorous stand. Sometimes other clinicians may welcome or be ready to take on the user's perspective. At times conflict is inevitable and taking a stand may require 'a strong personal belief in the moral rightness of what one is doing' (Carpenter, 1992). As said earlier, it is important to act in accordance with the user's wishes and instructions at all times.

EXPOSURE TO THE USER DISCOURSE

As a professional worker there are many opportunities to be involved in the user discourse and to be allied to user groups. Such workers can join a number of user-run organizations as a professional ally, Survivors Speak Out being the most notable. Or they can join a user-focused organization such as MIND, which produces a magazine called OPEN MIND. Most user groups produce newsletters, which will keep the practitioner informed. Professional workers can read some of the numerous critiques of the psychiatric system. Belonging to a user group as an ally – if possible – is a way of demonstrating commitment to change, as is working on projects alongside users. (Note that not all user groups will tolerate the presence of allies.) Nevertheless, it is a public commitment and requires a willingness to stand by one's principles and to challenge or educate other staff.

SUMMARY

There has been a long tradition of criticism of psychiatric care coming from some psychiatrists themselves, academics, human rights activists and service users. Much of this criticism has been about the application of the medical model to states of human distress, which, in the process, obscures the basis of distress in environmental failure or oppression. Since the 1960s there has developed a worldwide mental health service user movement, the members of which share many common experiences. The aim of the user movement is to abolish or reform the present system. Most energy has gone into attempting reform, although many users have organized self-help groups or projects. There are numerous ways by which users lose their personal power within the mental health system. Empowerment comes about through users sharing their experiences with other users and by taking a critical stance on what the system provides. Gaining confidence and pressing for one's own rights and interests is an important part of taking power back. Advocacy is needed to help users gain control over their lives and over what happens to them in the system. Advocates are in an instructional relationship to users and act in accordance with users' wishes. Self-advocacy in groups is a very powerful way of users pressing for common aims and goals. Users and professionals 'Working in Partnership' is seen by Government and professional bodies as a way of making health care more responsive to needs and more accountable. For nurses there are many constraints that militate against them forming true partnerships with service users. Progress may come about through identifying these constraints to overcome them. Becoming an ally to the user cause may be an option that some nurses wish to take. This will involve the nurse in acquainting him- or herself with the user discourse and encouraging user participation at the practice level. It may involve some level of personal risk for the nurse and the ability to challenge accepted practice.

KEY CONCEPTS

- Nurses should acquaint themselves with the critique that psychiatry is part of the social control mechanism of the state and can be damaging to mental health users.
- The user movement is attempting to reform psychiatry to provide more sensitive care or to replace it with self-help alternatives.
- Empowerment comes about through users taking more control over their own lives and management of their personal distress.
- Advocacy or 'speaking out' is needed to press for users' rights and preferences.
- Nurses can aid the empowerment process by working in partnership with users as equals or by becoming allies to the user cause.

REFERENCES

Barcan L: personal communication, 1996.

Barnham P: *Closing the asylum: the mental patient in modern society.* Harmondsworth, 1992, Penguin.

Barnham P: *Schizophrenia and human value.* London, 1993, Free Association Books.

Batcup D: *Mixed sex wards: evaluating their safety and effectiveness for women* [Final Report for the Bethlem and Maudsley NHS Trust]. London, 1995, [unpublished].

Batcup D: personal communication, 1996.

Batcup D, Thomas B: Mixing the genders, an ethical dilemma: how nursing theory has dealt-with sexuality and gender. *Nurs Ethics* 1(1):43, 1994.

Bateman N: *Advocacy skills: a handbook for human service professionals.* Aldershot, 1995, Arena.

Bean P, Mounser P: *Discharged from mental hospital.* London, 1993, Macmillan Press.

Beeforth M *et al.,* editors: *Whose service is it anyway?* London, 1990, Research and Development for Psychiatry.

Bergman R: Accountability — definition and dimensions. *Int Nurs Rev* 28(2):53–59, 1981.

Breggin P: *Toxic psychiatry.* New York, 1991, St Martin's Press.

Brown P, Funk SC: Tardive dyskinesia: barriers to professional recognition of iatrogenic disease *J Health Soc Behav* 27(June):116–132, 1986.

Cameron DG: Sham statistics, the myth of convulsive therapy, and the case for consumer misinformation. In: Cohen D, editor: *Challenging the therapeutic state: further disquisitions on the mental health system J Mind Behav (special issue)* 15(1&2):177–198, 1994.

Campbell P: A survivor's view of community psychiatry. *J Mental Health* 1(1):117, 1992.

Carpenter D: Advocacy part (ii): the 'how of advocacy', professional development module. *Nurs Times* 88(27):i–viii(supplement), 1992.

Chamberlan J: *On our own.* London, 1988, MIND.

Children Act. London, 1989, HMSO.

Clements J: From her speech at 1995 MIND conference, Blackpool (unpublished).

Cooper D: *Psychiatry and anti-psychiatry.* Harmondsworth, 1967, Penguin.

Copperman J, Burrows F: Reducing the risk of assault. *Nurs Times* 88(6):64–65, 1992.

Coxon T: Ritualised repression. *Nurs Times* 86(31):35–37, 1990.

Department of Health: *Advocacy — A code of practice.* London, 1994a, HMSO.

Department of Health: *Working in Partnership. Report of the mental health nursing review team,* London, 1994b, HMSO.

Department of Health, Home Office: *Services for people from black and ethnic minority groups: issues of race and culture — review of health and social services for mentally disordered offenders and others requiring similar services.* London, 1992, HMSO.

Fernando S: *Mental health, race and culture.* London, 1991, Macmillan Education.

Foucault M: *Madness and civilization: a history of insanity in the age of reason.* London, 1967, Tavistock.

Frank LR: Death, brain damage, memory loss and brainwashing. In: Cohen D, editor: *Challenging the therapeutic state: critical perspectives on psychiatry and the mental health system. J Mind Behav* 11(3&4):489–512, 1990.

Galloway J: Brought to book. *Nurs Times* 26(87):16–17, 1991.

Goffman E: *Asylums.* Harmondsworth, 1961, Penguin.

Goffman E: *Stigma — notes on the management of spoiled identity.* Harmondsworth, 1968, Penguin.

Gostin L: The ideology of entitlement: the application of contemporary legal approaches to psychiatry. In: Bean P, editor: *Mental illness: changes and trends.* London, 1983, John Wiley.

Haafkens J, Nuhof G, Van der Poel E: Mental health care and the opposition movement in the Netherlands. *Soc Sci Med* 22(2):185, 1986.

Halpern A: *Advance directive [handout].* London, 1995, Survivors Speak Out.

Handy J: Stress and contradiction in psychiatric nursing. *Hum Relati* 44(1):39–53, 1991.

Illich I: *Limits to medicine.* London, 1976, Marion Boyars.

Jacobs DH: Environmental failure — oppression is the only cause of psychopathology. In: Cohen D, editor: *Challenging the therapeutic state, part 2: further disquisitions on the mental health system, J Mind Behav* 15(1&2), 1–18, 1994.

Johnstone L: Psychiatry: are we allowed to disagree? *Asylum* (newsletter) Summer, 35–37, 1994.

Laing RD: *The divided self.* Harmondsworth, 1965, Penguin.

Laing RD, Esterson A: *Sanity, madness and the family.* Harmondsworth, 1964, Penguin.

Leader A: *Direct power.* London, 1995, CSN/BCS/MIND/Pavillion.

Lindow V: Now is your chance to help undo some wrongs. *Ment Health Nurs* 14(1):6–8, 1994a.

Lindow V: *Purchasing mental health services.* London, 1994b, MIND.

Lindow V: *Self help alternatives to mental health services.* London, 1994c, MIND.

Lipsky M: *Street level bureaucracy — dilemmas of the individual in public services.* New York, 1980, Russell Sage Foundation.

Littlewood R: Against pathology — the new psychiatry and its critics. *Br J Psychiatry* 159(November):696–702, 1991.

Menzies I: A case study in the functioning of social systems as a defence against anxiety. *Hum Relati* 13(2):98–121, 1960.

Mercer K: Racism and transcultural psychiatry. In: Millar P, Rose N, editors: *The power of psychiatry.* Cambridge, 1986, Polity Press.

NHS and Community Care Act. London, 1990, HMSO.

MIND: *Stress on women [campaign pack].* London, 1992a, MIND.

MIND: *The MIND guide to advocacy in mental health.* London, 1992b, MIND.

Nolan P: *A history of mental health nursing.* London, 1993, Chapman & Hall.

O'Hagan M: The international user-movement. In: Dean C, Freeman H, editors: *Community mental health care.* London, 1993, Gaskell and the Royal College of Psychiatrists.

Pembroke LR: *Self-harm: perspectives from personal experience.* London, 1994, Survivors Speak Out.

Porter R: *A social history of madness — stories of the insane.* London, 1987, Weidenfeld & Nicolson.

Porter S: Siding with the system. *Nurs Times* 84(41):30–31, 1987.

Read J: To be ourselves — challenging the abuses of psychiatry. *Peace News* 3 July:13, 1987.

Robinson DK, Collins M: Working in partnership — consumer views of the patient council. *Psychiatr Care* 2(3):101–104, 1995.

Rogers A, Pilgrim D: Pulling down the churches: accounting for the British Mental

Health Users' Movement. *Sociol Health Illn* 13(2):129–148, 1991.

Romme M, Escher S, editors: *Accepting voices*. London, 1993, MIND.

Rosenhan D: On being sane in insane places. *Science* 179(19 January): 250–258, 1973.

Scull A: *Museums of madness: the social organisation of insanity in nineteenth-century England*. Harmondsworth, 1982, Penguin Education.

Sheper–Hughes N, Lovell AM: Breaking the circuit of social control: lessons in public psychiatry from Italy and Franco Basaglia. *Soc Sci Med* 23(2):159, 1986.

Showalter E: *The female malady; women, madness and English culture, 1830–1980*. London, 1987, Virago Press.

Silverman D: *Communication and medical practice — social relations in the clinic*. London, 1987, Sage.

Smith P: *The emotional labour of nursing*. London, 1992, Macmillan.

Survivors Speak Out: *Self advocacy pack*. London, nd, Survivors Speak Out.

Szasz T: *The myth of mental illness*. New York, 1961, Hoeber/Harper.

Szasz T: *Law, liberty and psychiatry*. New York, 1963, Macmillan.

UKCC: *Exercising accountability*. London, 1989, UKCC.

UKCC: *Code of professional conduct*. London, 1992, UKCC.

Ussher J: *Women's madness: misogyny or mental illness?* London, 1991, Harvester Wheatsheaf.

van Hoorn E: Users in Europe unite. *OPENMIND*, 54: December 1991/January 1992.

Wallcraft J: Empowering empowerment: professionals and self-advocacy projects. *Ment Health Nurs* 14(2):6–9, 1994.

Weick A *et al.*: A strengths perspective for social work practice. *Soc Work* 34(4)350–354, 1989.

Williams J *et al.*: *Purchasing effective mental health services for women: a framework for action*. London, 1993, MIND.

World Health Organization: *Schizophrenia: an international follow-up study*. London, 1979, Wiley.

FURTHER READING

Chesler P: *Women and madness*. New York, 1989, Harcourt Brace Jovanovich.
A classic study of the psychiatric oppression of women.

Farber S: *Madness, heresy and the rumours of angels. The revolt against the mental health system*. Illinois, 1993, Open Court.

Frame J: *Faces in the water*. London, 1980, The Women's Press.

Frame J: *An autobiography*. London, 1990, The Women's Press.
These two volumes by Janet Frame are beautifully written. They deal with her life in general, her experiences of mental distress and her experiences in the psychiatric system in New Zealand. Faces in the water is a semi-fictional, poetic but revealing account of being on the receiving end of institutional life and psychiatric treatment.

Galloway J: *The trick is to keep breathing*. London, 1991, Minerva.
A fictional but semi-autobiographical account of a young teacher who loses her grip on the world and is admitted to a psychiatric hospital.

Gotkin J, Gotkin P: *Too much anger, too many tears: a personal triumph over psychiatry*. New York, 1992, Harper Perennial.
Jenny and Paul Gotkin's personal accounts of the medicalization of Jenny's distress and her 13 years of treatment in the mental health system. It deals with Jenny's miraculous 'recovery' and her successful attempts to rebuild her life once she had rejected psychiatry's definition of her.

Mason, JM: *Against therapy: emotional tyranny and the myth of psychological healing*. New York, 1988, Atheneum.
A critique of psychotherapy and an examination of the power relations involved.

Millett K: *The loony bin trip*. London, 1991, Virago Press.
An autobiographical account of Kate Millett's attempts to withdraw from lithium (a drug she was told she would need for the rest of her life) after seven years of medication for 'manic depression', her friends fearful reaction to this and her recommittal to mental hospital. Eventually after 13 years Kate managed to secretly decrease and successfully stop her lithium intake.

O'Hagan M: *Stopovers on my way home from Mars*. London, 1993, Survivors Speak Out.
A survivor's exploration of her experiences in the mental health system and an overview of user projects in a number of countries.

OPENMIND: Published bi-monthly by MIND, Granta House, 15–19 Broadway, London.
Essential reading for up-to-date thinking, news and articles around user issues.

Plath S: *The Bell Jar*. New York, 1971, Harper and Row.
A novel which depicts some of Sylvia Plath's own experiences in the mental health system.

Rogers A, Pilgrim D, Lacey R: *Experiencing psychiatry*. London, 1993, Macmillan.
This book is the outcome of a qualitative research study done with 516 users who had received at least one period of in-patient treatment in a psychiatric hospital and whose needs would be perceived as being on the severe end of the continuum. The users voices come through very strongly in this book questioning accepted practice.

Rose SM, Black BL: *Advocacy and empowerment. Mental health care in the community*. London, 1985, Routledge and Keegan Paul.
A radical critique of community psychiatry.

Psychological Assessment and Measurement

Learning Outcomes

After studying this chapter, you should be able to:

• Describe the nature and purpose of the interview process.

• Describe the observations and clinical implications of each category of the mental state examination.

• Identify other methods of information collection.

• Discuss the use of psychological measures in psychiatric nursing practice.

---

*I**n the past, psychological assessment has been the** domain of the psychiatrist and the psychologist. However, in recent years there has been a move by the nursing profession towards the nurse taking increasing responsibility for psychological assessment and measurement of 'client needs'. With the development of nursing models of care and the nursing process, as well as the drive towards professionalism and education, nurses have been able to prove their worth as assessors of 'client needs'. Coupled with this is the development of clinical specialist courses and posts that offer nurses more autonomy in their practice. These have proved successful and nurses are accepted as therapists in their own right in many specialties (Marks, 1985; Newell and Gournay, 1994).

The psychological assessment of 'client needs' is an essential part of the nursing process and, with only a little training, most nurses can learn the techniques required. Nurses should possess the necessary knowledge of human behaviour, psychodynamics, psychotherapy and pathology, as well as the ability to use their communication skills in interviewing and assessing clients. The skills can be learned through practice under supervision, through role-play situations of different presenting problems and histories and through clinical practice. Some of the structure and techniques may be new and awkward to use at first but this should not impede learning.

Though nurses will have differing roles within a clinical area and in differing specialties, depending on their grades and job descriptions, it is probably safe to say that, at least in in-patient settings, the initial contact with the client will be by a nurse. With this being the case it would seem to make sense to have nurses trained in assessing clients' problems and mental state.

THE ASSESSMENT INTERVIEW

The nursing assessment is the systematic collection of data about the client's present problem and history, including measurement of these problems. Decisions about care can be made on these data by the multidisciplinary team. The usual way to collect these data is by the assessment interview. This will involve detailed analysis of the client's presenting problem, taking the client's history and the mental state examination.

To minimize the client's anxieties and increase their likelihood of cooperation with the interview, the nurse should prepare. For the client to be at ease, the interview environment should be selected carefully. A comfortable, quiet, naturally lighted room will help to give a sympathetic atmosphere. The nurse should ensure that there are no interruptions, if possible, so that the interview flows well and the client's train of thought is not broken. Some clinical areas are open-plan without offices. Here the nurse can try to gain privacy by selecting a quieter area or by using a group of chairs to close off some space. The presence of an advocate, who may be a carer, relative, friend or a nominated professional who is aware of the client's problem, can help the client in expressing their rights and needs. Clients should also have access to interpreting services. If clients have to give information in their second language they may lack the necessary vocabulary to express themselves and the assessment may not be accurate.

The purpose of the interview will vary. In some cases the interview will be used to determine whether a particular type of therapy is suitable. In others, it will be used to gather information before drawing up a plan of care with the client. If clients are aware of the purpose, then they are less likely to feel threatened by being questioned.

INTERVIEWING SKILLS

It is often assumed that the nurse will establish a rapport with the client and that all nurses have this 'innate' gift. However, though this may generally be true, there are things to be considered when trying to establish rapport, such as respect and awareness of the client's sense of security. Clients who feel threatened are less likely to offer information and more likely to react to questioning with hostility. The nurse should try to convey a warm, open and caring attitude, take time to listen to the client and let the client know that they are listening. This can be done through use of verbal and nonverbal communication skills, an open, relaxed posture and calm, clear verbal communication. Further skills in listening and attending, such as nods, smiles, reflecting, open-ended questions and verbal prompts, will also encourage as they act as positive reinforcements. Empathic statements and responses to cues given by the client will further promote trust and rapport. Observation skills will register information that the client does not or cannot verbalize, such as a nervous manner or depressive states. Prejudices, stereotypes and sociocultural factors can interfere with communication and nurses should be aware of their existence.

To establish rapport quickly, assume that the client is being honest, wishes to collaborate and is presently trying to cope with their problem. This assumption may be reviewed at a later date in the light of new information but must be a starting point for the therapeutic relationship.

The interviewer should clearly establish the client's name, their own name and role, the time scale of the interview and the objectives of the session. Consent for the presence of cameras or supervisors should be sought and any distractions identified. The agenda should be agreed and feedback sought from the client through comments or questions. This will ensure that the aims and objectives of the interview are clear and will, hopefully, avoid misunderstandings (Richards and McDonald, 1990).

PRESENTING PROBLEM

The initial focus of the assessment will be on the client's present problem and the impact it has on their life, as well as a history of the presenting problem. A clear account of the problem is needed and most clients are able to give this. However, where the client is not forthcoming or lacks insight and understanding of their problem, the nurse will have to use a more directed interviewing approach to elicit information.

By questioning in a progressively more focused manner the nurse can gain increasingly specific information. To start, open questions should be used. An example might be, 'Please tell me about your present problem in your own words.' From here the questions can become more specific, e.g. 'Where does the problem occur? Who makes the problem better or worse? Are there any variations in the problem during the day? Why do you feel the problem occurs?' Finally, the questions can be much more specific, e.g. 'How often do you get this problem? How long does it last? How does it make you feel?' When the present problem has been described, questions can be asked about its development, e.g. 'When did you first notice it? Has it changed over time? Are there times when it has disappeared? What factors may have influenced this?' These sorts of questions appear in many textbooks, which can be used as guidelines when interviewing (Ritter, 1989; Hawton *et al.*, 1991).

Anything that may modify the problem needs to be noted, such as medication, cigarettes, alcohol, caffeine intake and good luck talismans. These may be used as coping methods but may not be appropriate long-term solutions and may increase the risks to the client and others.

Finally, the impact the problem is having on the client's life should be noted (e.g. effects on work and social life, private leisure time and family relationships) as well the client's views of the problem. Do they feel it exists? Does it need to be changed? Who should be responsible for the change? Who caused the problem to exist in the first place? These and other questions will give insight into motivation for treatment. For instance, have these clients sought referral and admission to the service, have their family pushed them into it or have they been detained under the Mental Health Act or been ordered to undergo treatment by the courts?

HISTORY TAKING

The second stage of the interview focuses on the client's life to date. Previous events in their life may have affected how their present problems developed and, consequently, the problem may have had an effect on how their life is now. Evidence of psychological and emotional disruption and the effects of maladaptive coping strategies can often have surfaced in the past. To the client, some questions may seem irrelevant and a rationale for exploring these may be given to help with compliance. For instance, how does a fear of spiders interfere with someone's sexual life? It may not but in some cases anxiety can lead to sexual problems and this must be investigated.

Medical History

This stage can vary in length, depending on the client's age and physical state. What is essential is to note chronic problems or persistent episodes of medical care that may influence the treatment offered (e.g. use of antidepressants in epilepsy may increase the likelihood of fits occurring, as the threshold is lowered by the medication). The nurse should find out whether there are any medical problems or illnesses needing attention now or whether there have been in the past, when these illnesses occurred and the treatment given, the outcome of the treatment, any current treatment and how the problems have affected the client's mental state.

Psychiatric History

Enquire what treatment the client has had for this problem. Where did they get treatment, when did they receive it and how much did they have, what was its nature and what were the results? Have they had psychiatric treatment for other problems? It may be that two problems interact and both will need to be dealt with. Check the duration of psychiatric episodes as this will give a clue to the length of treatment needed as well as identify specific interventions that have been useful in the past.

Forensic History

Check whether the client has a criminal record or history of aggression or violence. This might influence the care provided if the client is felt to be at risk or a risk to others. What were the crimes? What were the reasons for the criminal activity? These may give clues to emotional or psychological disturbances in the past.

Personality

It is useful to get the client's account of how they think their personality has changed. To get an idea of their pre-morbid personality, ask the client to describe their personality before the problem arose and ask how the problem has changed them. This will give a picture of their present assessment of their personality. Personality changes such as reduction in self-esteem, increased nervousness and social withdrawal will give some idea of the impact of the problem and also of how the client's present personality may be affecting it.

Social and Family History

The social history consists in the client's present social conditions and contacts. Ask where the client lives and with whom, the type of residence and whether it is rented or owned. Their present financial status should be established and any social contacts, hobbies or private leisure activities. Their problem may be responsible, in part, for these social conditions and a brief outline of their past social habits may make this clearer.

Family history should include details of the ages, health and occupations of all immediate family and any dates and causes of death. Ask the client about family relationships and any known family psychiatric history. This is important as it may reflect learned behaviours or genetically inherited conditions.

Personal History

The personal history will give the nurse an impression of the emotional environment in which the client's personality developed. The content of this stage of the interview may be determined by the purpose and by the length of time that the client can participate. A good starting point is to ask where they were born and raised. The nature of their birth may relate to future emotional development. Milestones such as reading, walking and writing will give clues to developmental problems and the client should be asked generally about their childhood and whether it was happy or distressing. Questions about school (primary and secondary) will allow impressions to be formed of social and emotional interactions, lifestyle, educational ability and personality. How did they get on? Did they have friends? Did they get on with the teachers? Were they studious or did they get into trouble? Did they gain qualifications? If so how many and what type? If they went on to further education the same areas should be questioned.

Work history may give indications of mental state in the past. For instance, there may be periods of employment history where the client was sacked or had to leave a number of jobs. This may coincide with reduced mental functioning. The nurse should ask about the client's last job, the number of jobs they have had and how long they lasted, what the longest job was, if they were dismissed from any jobs and the reasons for dismissal.

For many clients, sexual history remains a taboo area and the nurse should try to reassure the client by presenting a rationale for enquiring about this. Clients should be asked to volunteer the information but should be able to refuse if they wish. Rules of confidentiality frequently need to be explained as clients often ask 'Will only you see the notes?' It should be explained that the team will have access to the notes but they still remain confidential. The sexual development of the client may give insight into their problems. This time of life is filled with physical and emotional changes. The nurse should ask at what age puberty occurred or when periods started. Were they prepared for this or did they find the change difficult to accept? The ability to form and maintain relationships can be determined by asking how many relationships have been entered into and how long they lasted. During the longest relationships, did they experience any problems? Did their problems affect the relationships?

Their first sexual encounters may have occurred during these relationships. The nurse should ask during which relationship sex first occurred and at what age. The client's present sexual habits and relationships may reveal the extent of their psychological problems. How often do they have intercourse? Do they have one partner or more? Is sex enjoyable? Are they able to achieve orgasm? Do they masturbate and how often? Does their problem have an effect on their sex life or libido?

MENTAL STATE EXAMINATION

The mental state examination is a cornerstone in the evaluation of any client with a medical, neurological or psychiatric disorder that affects thought, emotion or behaviour. It is used to detect changes or abnormalities in a person's intellectual functioning, thought content, judgement and mood that affect and can indicate possible neurological problems. It represents a cross-section of the client's psychological life and the nurse's observations and impressions at the moment. It also gives a basis for future comparison to track the progress of the client. The elements of the examination depend on the client's clinical presentation, as well as their educational and cultural background. It includes observing the client's behaviour and describing it in an objective, non-judgemental manner.

The examination itself is usually divided into several parts. These can be arranged in different ways, so long as the nurse covers all the areas. Much of the information needed for the mental state examination can be gathered during the course of the routine nursing assessment. It should be integrated into the assessment in a smooth and flowing manner. Some parts of the mental state examination are completed through simple observation of the client, such as by noting the client's clothing and facial expressions. Other aspects require specific questions, such as those related to memory and attention span. Most of all, the nurse should remember that the mental state examination does not reflect how the client fared in the past or will fare in the future; it is an evaluation of the client's current state and will, therefore, need to be repeated throughout their care.

Information obtained during the examination of mental state is used along with other objective and subjective data. These include findings from the physical examination, laboratory test results, client history, description of the presenting problem, psychological questionnaires and information obtained from family, care givers and other health professionals. With this the nurse is able to design the plan of care with the client.

Eliciting Clinical Information

The mental state examination requires a clinical rather than social approach to the client. The nurse listens closely to what is said and reflects on what is not said, structuring the process in a way that allows for broad exploration of many areas for potential problems, as well as for more detailed exploration of obvious symptoms or maladaptive coping responses. Behaviours that the nurse might not normally attend to in more general situations must be carefully observed and described. Global and judgemental statements are not acceptable. The skilled nurse attends to both the content (the overtly communicated information) and the process (how the communication occurs including feelings, intuition and behaviours that accompany speech and thought) of the client's communication. The content and process may not always be congruent. For example, a client may deny feeling depressed and yet appear sad and cry. In this case, the stated message does not match the process and the nurse should record this incongruity. It is also important for nurses to monitor their own feelings and reactions during the mental state examination. A nurse's

instinctive reactions may signal subtle emotions being expressed by the client. For example, a depressed client may make the nurse feel sad and a hostile client may make the nurse feel threatened and angry. The nurse's feelings are useful information for the mental state assessment. The nurse needs to be aware of these feelings and to respond in a therapeutic manner towards the client regardless of them. The nurse should remain calm throughout the interview and simply reflect observations back to the client. These observations should be related in an objective and non-threatening manner, for example, 'You are obviously quite upset about this' and 'Do you feel safe here?' By conveying a sense of calm, the nurse will also demonstrate being in control, even if the client is not. The nurse should try to blend specific questions into the general flow of the interview. Questions about orientation, arithmetic problems or proverbs may be introduced by soliciting client comments about potential problems with concentration, memory or understanding of written material. The nurse might then suggest that the client try answering a few questions to determine if such problems are evident. Finally, as with any other skill, nurses need to practise performing the mental state examination to gain proficiency and confidence. The nurse might start by observing a colleague conduct the examination. Videotapes of client interviews and role-playing are particularly effective teaching–learning tools. The nurse should then be observed undertaking the mental state examination by a colleague or supervisor who can provide helpful feedback and identify ways to further enhance the nurse's competency.

Content of the Examination

In completing this examination it is essential that the nurse be aware that sociocultural factors can greatly influence its outcome. Biological expressions of psychiatric illness may also be evident in the interview process.

Appearance

In the mental state examination the nurse takes note of the client's general appearance. This part of the examination provides an accurate mental image of the client. The following physical characteristics should be included: apparent age, manner of dress, cleanliness, posture, unusual gait, facial expressions, eye contact, pupil dilation or constriction and general state of health and nutrition. Dilated pupils are sometimes associated with drug intoxication, whereas constriction may indicate narcotic addiction. Stooped posture is often seen in depression.

Speech

This is usually described in terms of rate, volume and characteristics. Rate refers to the speed of speech and volume to how loudly the client talks. Speech can be described as follows: rate (rapid or slow), volume (loud or soft), amount (paucity, mute, pressured) and characteristics (stuttering, slurring of words). Speech disturbances are often caused by specific brain disturbances or anxiety. For example, mumbling may occur in clients with Huntington's chorea, stuttering in anxious clients and slurring of speech in intoxicated clients. Manic clients often show pressured speech and people suffering from depression often say little.

Motor Activity

This concerns the client's physical movements. The nurse should record the following: level of activity (lethargic, tense, restless or agitated), type of activity (tics, grimaces or tremors) and unusual gestures or mannerisms (compulsions). Excessive body movement may be associated with anxiety, mania or stimulant abuse. Little body activity may suggest depression organicity, catatonic schizophrenia or drug-induced stupor. Tics and grimaces may suggest adverse effects of medication or stress-related phenomena. Repeated motor movements or compulsions may indicate obsessive–compulsive disorder.

Interaction during the interview

How does the client relate to the nurse during the interview? This part of the examination relies heavily on nurses' emotional subjectivity and nurses must carefully examine their responses against their personal and sociocultural biases. They must guard against over-interpreting or misinterpreting clients' behaviour through social or cultural differences. Observations should include: has the client been hostile, unco-operative, irritable, guarded, apathetic, defensive, suspicious or seductive? The nurse may explore this area by asking, 'You seem irritated about something. Is that an accurate observation?' Suspicion may be evident in paranoid psychosis and irritability may suggest an anxiety disorder.

Mood

The client's self-report of their present emotional state is a reflection of their life situation. Mood can be evaluated by asking a simple, non-leading question such as, 'How are you feeling today?' Does the client report feeling sad, fearful, hopeless, euphoric or anxious? Asking the client to rate mood on a scale of 0 to 10 can help provide the nurse with an immediate reading of the client's mood and can be valuable for comparing changes that occur during treatment. The nurse should enquire into the client's thoughts about self-harm if the client is thought to be potentially suicidal. Suicidal or violent thoughts must be addressed directly. Has the client had the desire to inflict personal harm or injure someone else? Have any previous attempts been made and, if so, what events surrounded them? To judge a client's suicidal or violence risk, the nurse should assess the client's plans and ability to carry them out (such as the availability of medication for overdose) the attitudes to death and the availability of support systems.

Most people with depression describe feeling hopeless and 25% of those with depression have suicidal ideation. Elation is most common in mania.

Affect

The client's statements of emotions and the nurse's empathic responses provide clues to the appropriateness of affect. Affect can be described in terms of the following: range, duration, intensity, appropriateness. Does the client report significant life events without any emotional response, indicating flat affect? Does the client's response appear restricted or blunted in some way? Does the client demonstrate great lability in expression by shifting from one affect to another quickly or is the client's response incongruent with speech content? (For example, a client who reports being persecuted by the police and then laughs.) Labile affect is often seen in mania and a flat, incongruent affect is often evident in schizophrenia.

Perceptions

There are two major types of perceptual problems: hallucinations and delusions. Hallucinations are defined as false sensory impressions or experiences. Delusions are false perceptions or false responses to a sensory stimulus. Hallucinations may occur in any of the five major sensory modalities including: auditory (sound), visual (sight), tactile (touch), gustatory (taste) and olfactory (smell).

Command hallucinations are those that tell the client to do something, such as to kill oneself, harm another and join someone in the afterlife. The nurse might enquire about the client's perceptions by asking, 'Do you ever see or hear things or do you have strange experiences as you fall asleep or upon awakening?' Auditory hallucinations are the most prevalent and often suggest schizophrenia. Visual hallucinations suggest organic problems. Tactile hallucinations suggest organic mental disorder, cocaine abuse or delirium tremors. It is important to note the word 'suggest', as the same symptoms can be experienced in a variety of 'mental illnesses'.

Thought content

This refers to the specific meaning expressed in the client's communication, the 'what' of the client's thinking. Although the client may talk about a variety of subjects during the interview, several content areas should be noted in the mental state examination. They may be complicated and often concealed by the client. Tactful questioning by the nurse is needed to explore these areas. Does the client have recurring, persistent thoughts? Is the client afraid of certain objects or situations or excessively worried about body and health issues? Do they ever feel that things are strange or unreal? Have they ever experienced being outside of their body? Does the client ever feel singled out or watched or talked about by others or that thoughts or actions are being controlled by an outside person or force? Do they claim to have psychic or other special powers or believe that others can read their mind? Throughout this part of the interview it is important that the nurse obtain information and not dispute the client's beliefs. Obsessions and phobias are symptoms associated with anxiety disorders. Delusions that are incongruent with mood suggest schizophrenia.

Thought process

Thought process relates to how clients express themselves. A client's thought process is observed through speech. The patterns or forms of verbalization rather than the content are assessed. A number of problems can be assessed about a client's thinking. The nurse might ask a number of questions to evaluate the client's thought process. Does the client's thinking proceed in a systematic, organized and logical manner? Is the client's self-expression clear? Is it relatively easy for the client to move from one topic to another? Circumstantial thinking may be a sign of defensiveness or of paranoid thinking. Loose associations and neologisms suggest schizophrenia or other psychotic disorders. Flight of ideas indicates mania. Perseveration is often associated with brain damage and psychotic disorders.

Level of consciousness

Examinations of mental state routinely assess a client's orientation to the current situation. Deciding whether or not a client is properly oriented involves evaluating some basic cognitive functions. A variety of terms can be used to describe a client's level of consciousness, such as confused, sedated and stuporous. In addition, the client should be questioned regarding orientation to time, place and person. Typically, the nurse can determine this by the client's answers to three simple questions:
1. What is your name?
2. Where are you today? (such as in what city or in what particular building)
3. What is today's date?

If the client answers correctly the nurse can note 'oriented in time, place and person'. Level of orientation can be pursued in greater depth but this area may be confounded by socio-cultural factors. Fully functioning clients may be offended by questions about orientation, so the skilled nurse should integrate questions pertaining to this area in the course of the interview and develop other ways of assessing this category. Clients with organic mental disorder may give grossly inaccurate answers, with orientation to person remaining intact longer than orientation to time or place. Clients with schizophrenic disorders may say that they are someone else or somewhere else or reveal a personalized orientation to the world.

Memory

A mental state examination can provide a quick screen of potential memory problems but not a definitive answer to whether a specific impairment exists. Neuropsychological assessment is required to specify the nature and extent of memory impairment. Memory is broadly defined as the ability to recall past experiences, and an indication of difficulties with memory is often identified by the client or the client's carers. Normal memory recall will differ from person to person and changes in the ability to remember events will be individual to each client. The following areas must be tested: remote memory (recall of events, information and people from the distant past), recent memory (recall of events, information and people from the past week or so) and immediate memory (recall of information or data to which a person was just exposed). Recall of remote events involves reviewing information from the client's history. This part of the evaluation can be woven into the history-taking portion of the assessment. This involves asking the client questions about time and place of birth, names of schools attended, date of marriage, ages of family members and so forth. The problem with evaluation of the client's remote memory is that the nurse is often unable to tell if the client is reporting events accurately. This brings about the possibility of confabulation, which is when the client makes up stories in response to situations or events that cannot be remembered. Therefore the nurse may need to call on past records or the report of family or friends to confirm this historical information. Recent memory can be tested by asking the client to recall the events of the past 24 hours. A reliable informant may be needed to verify this information. Another test of recent memory is to ask the client to remember three words (an object, a colour and an address) and then to repeat them 15 minutes later in the interview. Immediate recall can be tested by asking the client to repeat a series of numbers either forwards or backwards within a 10-second period. The nurse should begin with a short series of numbers and proceed to longer lists. Loss of memory occurs with organicity, dissociative disorder, anxiety and conversion disorders. Clients with dementia retain remote memory longer than recent memory. Anxiety and depression can impair immediate retention and recent memory.

Level of concentration and calculation

This relates to the client's ability to pay attention during the course of the interview; calculation is the person's ability to do simple mathematics. These and other areas of cognitive functioning may vary in expected and unexpected ways. The nurse should note the client's level of distractibility. Calculation can be assessed by asking the client to do the following:
1. Count from 1 to 20 rapidly.
2. Do simple calculations, such as serially subtract 7 from 100.

If clients have difficulty subtracting 7 from 100, they can be asked to subtract 3 from 20 in the same way. Finally, more functional calculation skills can be assessed by asking practical questions. The clinical implications of this part of the mental state examination must be carefully evaluated. Many psychiatric illnesses impair the ability to concentrate and to complete simple calculations. It is particularly important to differentiate among organic mental disorder, anxiety and depression.

Information and intelligence

Information and intelligence are controversial areas of assessment and the nurse should be cautious about judging intelligence after the brief, limited contact typical of the mental state examination. The nurse should also remember that information in this category is highly influenced by socio-cultural factors of the nurse, the client and the treatment setting. The nurse should assess the last year of school completed, and the client's general fund of knowledge and use of vocabulary. It is also important to assess the client's level of literacy.

The ability to conceptualize and abstract can be tested by having the client explain a series of proverbs. The client can be given an example of a proverb with its interpretation and then asked to explain what several proverbs mean. Most adults are able to interpret proverbs as symbolic of human behaviour or events. However, sociocultural background should be considered when assessing client information and intelligence. If the client's educational level is below average, asking the client to list similarities between a series of paired objects may better help the nurse assess the ability to abstract. A higher-level reply would address function, while a description of structure would indicate more concrete thinking.

To determine a client's fund of general knowledge, the nurse can, for example, ask the client to name the last five prime ministers, five large cities or the occupation of a well-known person. The client's educational level and any learning disabilities should be carefully evaluated. Learning difficulties should be ruled out whenever possible. Although the client's level of literacy may be a general assessment, it will be an important factor in any health guidance or other didactic information that is offered to the client.

Judgement

Making decisions that are constructive and adaptive involves the ability to understand facts and draw conclusions from relationships. Judgement can be evaluated by exploring a client's involvement in activities, relationships and vocational choices. For example, is the client regularly involved in illegal or dangerous activities or frequently engaged in destructive relationships with others? It is also useful to determine if the judgements are deliberate or impulsive. Finally, several hypothetical situations can be presented for the client to evaluate; for example:
- What would you do if you found a stamped, addressed envelope lying on the ground?
- How would you find your way out of a forest in the daytime?
- What would you do if you entered your house and smelled gas?
- If you won £10, 000 what would you do with it?

Judgement is impaired in organic mental disorders, schizophrenia and intoxication.

Insight and motivation

Insight refers to the client's understanding of the nature of the problem or illness. It is important for the nurse to determine if the client accepts or denies the presence of a problem or illness. In addition, the nurse should enquire whether the client blames the problem on someone else or on external factors. Several questions may help to determine the client's degree of insight. What does the client think about the current situation? What does the client want others, including the nurse, to do about it? Insight is impaired in organic mental disorder, or psychosis. Whether or not a client sees the need for treatment also critically affects the therapeutic alliance, setting of mutual goals and implementation of the treatment plan and future adherence to it.

Documenting and reporting clinical information

Information from the mental state examination may be recorded in various ways. Some clinicians write a descriptive report. Written reports should be brief, clear and concise and address all categories of information. Others use an outline format that is completed with short answers, others a format compatible with computerized information systems. Regardless of format, important findings should be documented and verbatim responses by the client recorded whenever they add important information and support the nurse's assessment. It is useful to write a summary of the client's presenting problem and its impact, and of the mental state of the client, for other nurses to be able to read at a glance.

This, however, is not the nurse's only responsibility. Simply recording the information is not always sufficient. The data from the assessment and the mental state examination are essential to all members of the team and to other agencies involved. If there are any doubts about a person's mental state or if the assessment interview reveals new information that presents their case in a new light, then the need to disseminate this information to appropriate agencies should be considered. The United Kingdom Central Council for Nursing, Midwifery and Health Visiting (UKCC) *Code of Professional Conduct* gives guidance for nurses on the disclosure of information and the occasions when confidentiality may be broken (UKCC, 1992). Generally, this is when it is felt that the person presents a danger to themselves or others or where the law has been broken. Nurses are responsible and accountable for their practice and must use guidelines such as those given by the UKCC and local Trust policies when making decisions. Recently, reports of investigations following serious incidents have revealed how lack of communication among staff and agencies results in poor quality care with potential danger to the client and the public (Ritchie, 1994).

ADDITIONAL RESOURCES

The psychiatric interview provides the structure for obtaining pertinent information about the client. Additional resources are often used to complete a comprehensive assessment. It is important that all aspects of the client's presenting problems are assessed, including the behavioural, cognitive, affective and physiological dimensions. Measurement should cover all these dimensions to gain a full picture of the client's situation. For example, a depressed client may have physiological symptoms of depression but may be able to mask or deny negative cognitions and low mood. A full assessment of all aspects of the client's condition would address the detection of depression from different perspectives and thus reveal symptoms in a variety of areas.

Often it may be more effective to measure psychological problems using methods other than a straightforward interview technique. Various methods of measurement, effective during the assessment, treatment and evaluation stages of a client's care, are available to provide a rounded view of problems, efficacy of treatment and progress. Measurement may be made by the nurse, client or carer; measures used may be standardized or assembled by the nurse; a range of techniques may be employed or just one form of measurement used.

PSYCHOLOGICAL MEASUREMENTS

There are clear advantages to using psychological measures, both at the assessment stage and beyond; for example:

- During the interview process, the client will usually give a description of the current problem but this may be unreliable and inaccurate. The use of direct measurement provides a more accurate description of the situation (Barlow *et al.*, 1984). Direct measurement is also a more reliable indicator of change than the subjective reporting of a nurse who is delivering the treatment interventions.
- Measurements during assessment and treatment allow the nurse to judge the effectiveness of interventions and modify treatment if necessary.
- The use of direct measurement during the treatment phase can act as reinforcement and a confidence booster for clients, particularly if the results are presented graphically.

SELF-MONITORING

Client self-monitoring is often used in the assessment phase and during treatment. The technique has benefits of enhancing the working relationship between the nurse and the client, by empowering the client to be active in their own treatment process. Carried to its furthest extreme, clients become 'personal scientists', who are skilled in the analysis of their own illness (Mahoney, 1974).

Often, client self-reporting is the only way in which the nurse is able to gain access to information about covert and non-observable problem behaviours. The nurse works with the client, explaining the process of self-monitoring techniques. The process of self-monitoring involves the client realizing that the behaviour or occurrence has occurred and recording this (Barlow *et al.*, 1984). Accuracy of self-monitored data is enhanced if the amount of data to be recorded is small, specific and fully explained to the client (Hawton *et al.*, 1991). Specific strategies enhance the self-monitoring process generally (Mahoney, 1977; Barlow *et al.*, 1984). These include:

- Asking the client to make a verbal or written commitment to the self-monitoring process.
- Training the client in the use of self-monitoring techniques before starting to keep records.
- Letting the client know that the accuracy of the records will be checked by the nurse and when accuracy is positively reinforced.
- Counting the frequency of a behaviour or problem can be tedious if it is a regular occurrence and clients may prefer to record for short, specified time periods.
- Recordings should be made as soon as possible after the

phenomenon has occurred, to maintain accuracy. A notebook may be used to record information when occurrence is frequent.

- Ensuring that the phenomenon to be measured is specific and clearly defined and that the recording measures are as simple and relevant as possible.
- Ensuring that the client has the means to record occurrences. For example. the nurse should provide record sheets, diary sheets or counting devices.
- Using a range of measures that are both sensitive to small changes and also able to detect overall patterns of change.

Information gathered during the self-monitoring process is recorded in a number of ways, as follows.

FREQUENCY COUNTS

Frequency counts are used to measure problems or behaviours that occur in discrete units. Records can be kept simply by keeping a tally on a piece of paper or by using a counting device. Frequency counts can be used to measure a number of phenomena such as: intrusive or negative thoughts, auditory hallucinations, ritual behaviours, sexual fantasies and headaches. They are useful for keeping a record of cognitions or private behaviours which could not be monitored by a third person. Figure 5.1 illustrates an example of a record sheet that could be used to record the frequency of checks made on her baby's breathing by a new mother, obsessed with thoughts that her baby will stop breathing.

The nurse requires data collected over several days to determine if there are patterns of frequency of checking at particular times of the day or on particular days.

In Figure 5.2 the client with post-traumatic stress syndrome records the frequency of three intrusive thoughts related to the traumatic incident. The client identifies three of the most common intrusive thoughts or images, and each time the thought occurs the client marks the record sheet and keeps a daily tally. In this way the nurse and the client can discover which thoughts are occurring most frequently and treat this situation accordingly.

DIARIES

Diaries are often used during assessment to clarify specific circumstances of occurrence of the problem or behaviour. The information collected using the diary format usually consists of that about the actual occurrence, what was happening before the event (antecedent) and what happened afterwards (consequence). Figure 5.3 shows an example of how a diary might be used to collect information about auditory hallucinations in the form of voices.

The diary format, therefore, not only collects information regarding frequency and duration of the voices but also indicates the situations in which auditory hallucinations are likely to occur and which coping strategies might be effective in reducing the frequency and duration of the voices. Additional self-monitoring would also be effective and would provide a clearer picture of the problem. For example, the

	Mon	Tue	Wed	Thu	Fri	Sat	Sun
Midnight – 2.00am							
2.00am – 4.00am							
4.00am – 6.00am							
6.00am – 8.00am							
8.00am – 10.00am							
10.00am – Noon							
Noon – 2.00pm							
2.00pm – 4.00pm							
4.00pm – 6.00pm							
6.00pm – 8.00pm							
8.00pm – 10.00pm							
10.00pm – Midnight							
Daily total							

Figure 5.1 Frequency of checking record sheet

Intrusive thought	Mon	Tue	Wed	Thu	Fri	Sat	Sun
1.							
2.							
3.							

Figure 5.2 Frequency of intrusive thoughts record sheet

Date						
What time did you start to hear the voices?	Where were you?	Who were you with?	What were you doing?	What did you do while you were hearing the voices?	Did you do anything to stop the voices? If so, what?	Was there a time when you stopped hearing the voices?

Figure 5.3 Diary for auditory hallucination data collection

client might also record information by using self-rating scales regarding the content of the voiced material, the intensity of the voices and the degree of distress experienced.

SELF-RATING SCALES (VISUAL ANALOGUE SCALES)

Self-rating scales are used by the client to measure specific needs, problems or behaviours. Used in conjunction with validated broad-based measures, they provide a record of overall and specific progress. In conjunction with the nurse, the client identifies a specific dimension to be measured, constructs a rating scale – often a visual analogue scale – and records ratings at specific intervals. In the example (Figure 5.4), the client receiving bereavement therapy uses a visual analogue scale to rate the level of distress experienced during a therapy session.

Over a number of sessions the client and the nurse should see a change in the ratings for distress experienced, which should indicate efficacy of treatment.

In Figure 5.5, a client with depression rates overall level of mood twice daily using a visual analogue scale. Visual analogue scales should be constructed so that the client understands the rating process and the terminology is familiar.

The use of self-rating measures is common in the area of behavioural psychotherapy, where specific problems and targets (goals) are measured on assessment, during treatment and at follow-up intervals (see Chapter 29 for further details). However, the use of such measures need not be restricted to clients with behavioural problems. For example, the client with auditory hallucinations may be encouraged to use the principles of problem and target setting in the following manner (Figure 5.6) (Marks, 1986).

SELF-REPORTING

Self-reporting is another type of measurement made by the client, usually in the form of retrospective assessment rather than recording a problem or behaviour at the time that it occurs, as with self-monitoring procedures. By using self-reporting, it is possible for the client to measure objective, observable phenomena and also subjective states, such as mood and anxiety. The results of self-reporting do not always agree with direct observations of behaviour (Lang and Lazovik, 1963). Inaccuracy may be caused by the content of the measure (for example, ambiguous wording of questionnaires) or may result from a lack of understanding on the part of the client. Self-report measures are useful for gaining understanding of trends in the efficacy of treatment, although they would not be used when accurate quantitative data are required (McCleod *et al.*, 1986).

Self-report questionnaires

The most frequently used self-reporting measure is the questionnaire. Two types of questionnaire are commonly used:

1. A form of questionnaire that covers a broad aspect of mental health. Examples of this are the GHQ 28 (General Health Questionnaire; Goldberg, 1981) the SCL 90-R (Symptom Checklist; Derogatis, 1992) and the MMPI (Minnesota Multiphasic Personality Inventory; Hathaway and McKinley, 1951). These questionnaires assess various areas of the client's state and provide data that measure broad changes over the course of treatment.

2. Often the nurse requires a more specific measure of a particular aspect of the client's state. More specialized questionnaires are available, covering a range of problems and behaviours, from anxiety and depression to measures of quality of life. Table. 5.1 lists a number of these questionnaires.

0	1	2	3	4	5	6	7	8	9	10
not at all distressed		slightly distressed			moderately distressed		severely distressed		extremely distressed	

Figure 5.4 Distress rating scale

0	1	2	3	4	5	6	7	8	9	10
not at all low		slightly low			moderately low		severely low		extremely low	

Date	Morning	Evening

Figure 5.5 Mood rating scale

Figure 5.6 Problem and target ratings for auditory hallucinations

Problem

Hearing voices when with other people, leading me to become angry and avoid contact with friends and family and thus resulting in loneliness.

This problem upsets me and/or interferes with my normal activities:

	0	1	2	3	4	5	6	7	8
does not	slightly/ sometimes		definitely/ often		markedly/ very often		very severely/ continuously		

Target

To visit my parents for 1 hour three times a week.

Progress towards achieving each target regularly without difficulty. Discomfort/behaviour:

	0	1	2	3	4	5	6	7	8
None/ complete success	slight/ 75% success		definite/ 50% success		marked/ 25% success		very severe/ no success		

TABLE 5.1 Self-Report and observational scales

Content Area	Self-Report and Observational Scales
Affective Disorders	Beck Depression Inventory (BDI) Hamilton Depression Scale Zung Self-Rating Depression Scale
Anxiety Disorders	Beck Anxiety Inventory (BAI) Maudsley Obsessional Compulsive Inventory Impact of Events Scale (IES) Spielberger Anxiety State Trait Yale–Brown Obsessive Compulsive Scale (YBOC)
Psychotic Disorders	Brief Psychiatric Rating Scale (BPRS) Beliefs About Voices Questionnaire (BAVQ) Self-Report Insight Scale for Psychosis
Eating Disorders	Eating Disorders Inventory (EDI) Body Attitudes Test
Organic Disorders	Clifton Assessment Procedure (CAPE) Behaviour Assessment Scale of Later Life (BASOLL)
Substance Use Disorders	Alcohol Problem Questionnaire (APQ) Severity of Alcohol Dependence Questionnaire (SADQ) Severity of Drug Dependence Questionnaire (SDDQ)
Child /Adolescent Disorders	Yale–Brown Obsessive Compulsive Scale for Children (YBOCSC) Weschler Intelligence Scale for Children (WISC)
Social Functioning	Ways of Coping Checklist (WCCL) Quality of Life Scale (QLS) Global Assessment Scale (GAS)

A useful reference for selecting questionnaires is the *Mental Measurements Yearbook* (Kramer and Conoley, 1992). Reports on validated questionnaires usually contain details of the 'normal' range of scores. This information can be useful in determining the severity of the client's condition in relation to a given population.

OBSERVATION

Direct and indirect observation methods are used to collect data about the client's behaviour by the nurse, other professionals or significant others, such as relatives or carers. Various techniques are used and occasionally by-products of behaviour are measured, rather than the actual behaviour itself. For example, weight is measured in the treatment of clients with anorexia.

Many global rating scales are available, and are included in Table 5.1. Scales are completed during or following either a structured interview with the client or a period of observation. An example of a commonly used rating scale is the Brief Psychiatric Rating Scale (BPRS) (Lukuff *et al.*, 1986) which includes ratings for 18 symptom categories. The use of such scales is often straightforward if staff have been trained in their application. Standardized scales provide information that can be compared to established 'norms'. However, they are subject to bias, as the person rating the client's behaviour has to make inferences that may be affected by the observer's preconceptions, attitudes and skills.

Specific behaviours may be measured by a number of techniques. Simple frequency counts may be made when behaviours such as smoking are not occurring constantly, whereas the observer may need to measure at specified intervals for a period of time (time sampling) when the behaviour is of a high frequency or continual, for example, when the client is experiencing intrusive thoughts. Behaviours may occur in response to a particular stimulus, and the length of time or latency period between the stimulus and its behavioural response can be monitored. Duration of a behaviour may need to be recorded in addition to its frequency; for example, with a client who compulsively hand-washes.

Some behaviours occur naturally within the clinical environment, such as compulsive hand-washing, whereas other behaviours may need to be artificially stimulated. An example of this is the use of role-play to measure a client's social skills. Occasionally, situations need to be contrived to measure behaviour, such as the use of behavioural avoidance tests. In this case, the client with a phobia is presented with an example of the feared stimulus, such as a spider, to measure the level of avoidance behaviour. Often, these methods are the only way in which behaviour can be measured, although the creation of contrived or artificial stimuli may bias results obtained in such a test. The client's family or carers may also be asked to record behaviour occurring at home to measure it in its natural setting.

PHYSIOLOGICAL MEASUREMENTS

The range of physiological measures available to the majority of psychiatric nurses is limited, mainly because specialist equipment is prohibitively expensive. However, basic physiological measures may be used to provide information on clinical phenomena. This is particularly the case with anxiety disorders, where blood pressure, respiratory rate and temperature changes are measured to gauge the extent of an anxiety response. Clients who report disturbed sleep can be asked to keep a diary of their sleep patterns. Those who report somatized pain can keep records of pain levels.

Specialized tests, such as electroencephalograms (EEGs), computed tomography (CT) scans and magnetic resonance imaging (MRI) scans are used mainly to assist medical diagnosis. An awareness of these procedures is useful for the psychiatric nurse but simpler, less expensive measures are often appropriate for nursing assessment and evaluation.

FORMULATION

After the initial stages of assessment, which should include both interview and other forms of measurement, the nurse is able to prepare a summary. This summary, or formulation, should include a description of the current problem, with a history of its development and exploration of factors that maintain it. Formulations should not be seen as static but rather as changing commentaries, which are subject to re-evaluation in the presence of new information. A formulation will suggest areas where further information is necessary and will indicate treatment possibilities. As the nurse constructs a formulation, the client is invited to give feedback and to comment on accuracy.

DSM IV (American Psychiatric Association, 1994) provides a useful framework for summarizing an assessment. The multi-axial assessment approach offers five axes along which a wider definition of the problem may be formulated. The five axes are:

1. Axis I – Clinical Disorders. Other disorders that may be a focus of clinical attention.
2. Axis II – Personality Disorders.
   Mental Retardation.
3. Axis III – General Medical Conditions.
4. Axis IV – Psychosocial and Environmental Problems.
5. Axis V – Global Assessment of Functioning.

See the case study and its associated multiaxial assessment record (Table 5.2).

Case study: **Use of multiaxial assessment record**

Robert was a 23-year-old, single man, admitted to his local psychiatric in-patient unit on Section 2 after his neighbours reported to police that he had started to make a lot of noise at night and was not looking after himself. On admission, he appeared unkempt, was wearing dirty clothes and seemed hostile when staff approached him. His relatives told staff that he had started to withdraw from them over the past year and had accused several family members of planning to harm him.

On interview assessment, Robert said that he thought there was a conspiracy to kill him. He knew that there was a conspiracy because he had heard the voice of his dead father telling him that his brothers wanted him dead. As a result, he had avoided leaving his flat and had built a safe room at home to protect himself. He had avoided contact with his brothers specifically. This had resulted in them becoming angry with him, which he interpreted as further evidence for his theory about a conspiracy. He expressed anger about being in hospital but did not seem low in mood. His primary nurse decided to assess his symptoms further and asked him to keep a record of hearing his father's voice. The nurse measured his level of social functioning, using the Global Assessment of Functioning Scale and measured insight using the Self-Report Insight Scale for Psychosis.

TABLE 5.2 Multiaxial assessment

Axis	Multiaxial assessment
Axis I	295.30 – Schizophrenia, paranoid type
Axis II	None
Axis III	None
Axis IV	Social isolation Damp, unheated housing Problems with DSS benefits
Axis V	GAF = 39 (current)

Information from single case studies based on empirical knowledge, rather than traditional research methods involving large numbers of subjects, can be applied on a client by client basis, with single case findings having more direct clinical application. When nurses use measurement regularly they are adding to their knowledge base, improving direct client care and potentially expanding professional boundaries.

PSYCHOLOGICAL CONTEXT – BEYOND ASSESSMENT

The assessment of a client should continue throughout treatment, with efficacy of care evaluated on a regular basis and interventions modified according to the client's needs. Traditionally nurses have used a wide range of interventions, yet have often failed to evaluate their usefulness (Peplau, 1989). As nurses, as providers of a service, come further under the scrutiny of purchasers, it is necessary to evaluate critically the usefulness of each intervention, to justify actions and provide the best possible care for the client.

Many nurses make interventions based on prior experience and instinct, rather than relying on research findings. Often, the findings of research studies seem to bear little relationship to the realities of the clinical area and research results are difficult to reproduce in practice (Schon, 1983). Yet each time nurses use an intervention and assess its success, they are adding to their knowledge base and conducting personal research. This is particularly the case when interventions are evaluated in a quantitative manner, using rating scales and questionnaires on a regular basis throughout treatment to record progress. Mahoney (1974) advocates that clinicians should apply their own personal research on an individual client basis to evaluate interventions and account for their actions. The Scientist Practitioner model (Barlow *et al.*, 1984), applied originally in the field of psychology and later adapted by social workers, advocates these principles and also suggests that clinicians should disseminate their findings to other practitioners to add to the range of clinical knowledge.

FUTURE TRENDS

Many behavioural rating scales and measurement tools have been designed to help clinicians carry out the following:
1. Measure the extent of the client's problems.
2. Track the client's progress over time.
3. Document the efficacy of treatment.

Each one of these points is very important to the psychiatric nurse. The knowledge base for psychiatric care is expanding rapidly and increased emphasis is being placed on describing clearly the nature of the client's problems and the extent of the client's progress towards obtaining the expected outcomes of treatment. Thus, nurses must be able to demonstrate in a reliable and valid way what problems they are treating and what effect their nursing care is having on attaining the treatment goals.

Most psychiatric nurses have not routinely used rating scales in their clinical practice. Nevertheless, this is a critical area for contemporary psychiatric nursing practice. Nurses should become familiar with the many different forms of psychological measurement available. Many of the self-report rating scales may be used by nurses to involve clients in the monitoring of their progress and to measure efficacy of treatment.

These tools should not replace required nursing documentation. Rather, they can be used to complement nursing care and provide measurable indicators of treatment outcomes. The increasing focus on high quality, efficiency and documented effectiveness requires that psychiatric nurses be able to demonstrate the value of the services they provide. The psychological context of nursing care suggests both the tools and the process nurses can use to meet this challenge.

KEY CONCEPTS

• The nurse is in a position to make use of psychological assessment and measurement.
• The assessment interview involves systematic collection of data.
• The nurse should remain open and receptive to the client during the assessment process.
• All assessment data must be clearly documented.
• Additional psychological measurement may be used to enhance assessment.
• Evaluation should be a continuing process.
• The use of psychological measurement benefits the client and the field of psychiatric nursing.

REFERENCES

American Psychiatric Association: *Diagnostic and statistical manual of mental disorders*, ed 4. Washington DC, 1994, American Psychiatric Association.

Barlow DH, Hayes SC, Nelson RO: *The scientist practitioner: research and accountability in clinical and educational settings*. Boston, 1984, Allyn & Bacon.

Derogatis LR: SCL-90-R: *Administration, scoring and procedures manual* II. Towson, 1992, Clinical Psychometrics Research.

Goldberg D: *The General Health Questionnaire*: GHQ 28. Windsor, 1981, NFER-Nelson.

Hathaway SR, McKinley JC: *MMPI manual*. New York, 1951, Psychological Corporation.

Hawton K, Salkovskis PM, Kirk J, Clark DM: *Cognitive behaviour therapy for psychiatric problems: a practical guide*. Oxford, 1991, Oxford University Press.

Kramer JJ, Conoley JC, editors: *The 11th mental measurements yearbook*. Lincoln, 1992, University of Nebraska.

Lang PJ, Lazovik AD: Experimental desensitization of a phobia. *J Abnor. – Soc Psychol* 66(6):519, 1963.

Lukuff D, Neuchterlain KH, Ventura J: Appendix A: manual for the expanded Brief Psychiatric Rating Scale (BPRS). *Schizophr Bull* 12(3):578, 1986.

McCleod DR, Hoehn–Saric R, Stefan RL: Somatic symptoms of anxiety: comparison of self-report and physiological measures. *Biol Psychiatry* 21(4):301, 1986.

Mahoney MJ: *Cognition and behavior modification*. Cambridge MA, 1974, Ballinger.

Mahoney MJ: Some applied issues in self monitoring. In: Cone JD, Hawkins RP, editors: *Behavioral assessment: new directions in clinical psychology*. New York, 1977, Brunner/Mazel.

Marks IM: *Nurse therapists in primary care*. London, 1985, RCN Publications.

Marks IM: *Behavioural psychotherapy: The Maudsley pocket book of clinical management*. Bristol, 1986, Wright.

Newell R, Gournay KM: British nurses in behavioural psychotherapy: a 20 year follow-up. *J Adv Nurs* 20(1):53, 1994.

Peplau HE: Future directions in psychiatric nursing from the perspective of history, *J Psychosoc Nurs* 27(2):18, 1989.

Richards D, McDonald B: *Behavioural psychotherapy: a handbook for nurses*. Oxford, 1990, Heinemann Nursing.

Ritchie JH: *The report of the inquiry into the care and treatment of Christopher Clunis*. London, 1994, HMSO.

Ritter S: *Manual of clinical psychiatric nursing*. London, 1989, Harper & Row.

Schon DA: *The reflective practitioner: how professionals think in action*. New York, 1983, Basic Books.

UKCC: *Code of Professional Conduct*. London, 1992, UKCC.

FURTHER READING

Barlow DH, Hayes SC, Nelson RO: *The scientist practitioner: research and accountability in clinical and educational settings*. Boston, 1984, Allyn & Bacon.

Although becoming rather elderly, the scientist-practitioner model continues to appeal to many health care professions. This book contains a very clear rationale for the use of assessment tools, and places them in the context of both clinical and research considerations.

Hawton K, Salkovskis PM, Kirk J, Clark DM: *Cognitive behaviour therapy for psychiatric problems: a practical guide*. Oxford, 1991, Oxford University Press.

This contains a clear and concise description of the assessment process with a useful checklist to enhance thorough assessment. Although written from a cognitive behavioural perspective, the assessment procedure can be adapted to suit the needs of the individual. It also contains details of self-assessment rating scales.

Newell R: *Interviewing skills for nurses and other health care professionals*. London, 1994, Routledge.

A thorough, readable and invaluable guide to assessment procedures, using interview and other techniques. This book addresses interpersonal issues alongside the minutiae of assessment procedures and encourages the reader to reflect on the practice of interviewing.

Streiner DL, Norman GR: *Health measurement scales: a practical guide to their development and use*. Oxford, 1989, Oxford Medical Publications.

For clinicians who wish to develop and validate their own measurement scales, this is an essential guide to the issues and processes involved.

Sociocultural Context of Mental Health Nursing Care

Learning Outcomes

After studying this chapter you should be able to:

- Critically examine the need for mental health nurses to be culturally aware.

- Explore the sociocultural determinants of mental health and illness.

- Discuss how sociocultural awareness can be translated into socioculturally sensitive individualized nursing care.

- Explain how sociocultural factors can be addressed to provide culturally sensitive services.

CHAPTER OUTLINE

- *Ethnicity*

- *Gender*

- *Socio-economic factors*

- *Age*

- *Implications for mental health nursing*

---

*W*hen the Mental Health Nursing Review Team* reported its work, they suggested that 'mental health nursing should re-examine every aspect of its policy and practice in the light of the needs of people who use services' (Butterworth, 1994). For mental health nurses to know, understand, plan for and respond to the needs of service users, it is essential that they have a working knowledge of the sociocultural context in which those needs arise. 'Sociocultural context' refers to sociostructural (e.g. the family), cultural and socio-economic factors. Although this chapter will focus on sociocultural factors, they need to be seen in relation to each other and in a further relationship with physiological, psychological and sociopolitical.

The sociocultural context of any society is dynamic and ever-changing, and inevitably impacts on the mental health of the population. In this chapter we will not be addressing the impact of social policies upon the mentally ill specifically. However, it is important to identify briefly recent policy changes that influence the context in which mental health nurses work. These include closure of large psychiatric institutions in the move towards care in the community. This has led to reports of increasing numbers of homeless people with mental health problems and increasing numbers of people with serious and enduring mental health problems living in the community (Gournay, 1995). In turn, these changes have radically transformed the working practices of nurses in the community. These practices include adopting the care programme approach and supervised discharge, together with an increased emphasis on interagency and multidisciplinary working.

Using the philosophy of empowerment, this chapter will explore how an understanding of sociocultural issues can be used to maintain and promote the mental health of people using services. Tones *et al.* (1990) discuss health promotion in relation to four factors: the health and medical services, genetic endowment, individual behaviours and the socio-economic and physical environment. Tones' framework suggests that empowering and mental health promoting interventions need to be made at several levels, i.e. those of the individual groups and society. For the purposes of this chapter the 'group' is seen as larger than an individual but smaller than society as a whole, e.g. the family, peer group or ethnic community group. In service provision terms it is seen at a local level, e.g. a ward, a day centre, a community project.

In each instance sociocultural awareness provides a starting point. However, this in itself is insufficient. To translate awareness into action a knowledge of the effects of sociocultural factors and the implication of these for practice is also needed. The above discussion provides a matrix within which sociocultural issues will be discussed (Figure 6.1).

In this chapter, sociocultural awareness is explored in its broadest sense, incorporating the major cultural divisions in our society, i.e. age, gender, ethnicity and socio-economic factors. Taking this stance, sociocultural awareness can be seen as an understanding of those sociocultural factors which contribute to each person's individuality. This implies that each person is different. The recent review into mental health nursing (Butterworth, 1994) emphasizes the need for mental health nurses to understand and work with difference. It also recommends that mental health nurses develop skills to meet the culturally specific needs of their clients and to deal sensitively with issues of race and gender.

Nurses themselves also have a unique sociocultural identity with values, beliefs and attitudes that may at times come into conflict or harmonize with those of their clients. To develop skilled therapeutic relationships with clients it is essential that nurses have an awareness of their own sociocultural identity and how this may influence their work with others. As the matrix shown in Figure 6.1 demonstrates, its formation goes beyond the individual to incorporate values, beliefs and attitudes influenced by groups such as family or peer groups and wider society. When all these issues are considered and combined, understanding and working with difference becomes a complex and frequently political task.

ETHNICITY

Ethnicity is increasingly used as a means of defining social, cultural and historical differences between groups of people in a multiracial and multicultural society such as found in Britain (Box 6.1). The term refers to that sense of self and collective identity formed in relation to nationality (or regional) racial identity, tribe, religion, language and inherited culture (traditions, values and beliefs). There are potential pitfalls to be avoided when categorizing people into 'ethnic groupings', including the overgeneralization of cultural attributes to specific ethnic groups, leading to stereotyping; and the denial of marked differences within such groupings.

Throughout this chapter the term 'black and minority ethnic group' will be used. We offer these definitions suggested by MIND (1992), which include:

the 'black' experience of people of Asian, African and Caribbean descent, that is, being a visible minority in our society, by virtue of their skin colour, and thus particularly susceptible to racism, discrimination, inequality and disadvantage.

those less frequently seen as ethnic minorities due to their 'white skin' e.g. Polish and Irish people.

	Awareness	Effects	Implications
Individual			
Group			
Society			

Figure 6.1 Sociocultural matrix
(Crown copyright is reproduced with permission of the Controller of Her Majesty's Stationery Office)

Box 6.1 *Ethnicity in Britain*

An estimated 3 062 634 people from minority ethnic groups live in England, Wales and Scotland.
- The minority ethnic proportion of the population is calculated to be:
  6% in England and Wales
  1.3% in Scotland
- The largest minority ethnic populations currently living in England and Wales are:
  1. Irish 840 000
  2. Indians 830 000
  3. Caribbeans 499 000
  4. Pakistanis 455 000
  5. Africans 210 000

- The largest minority ethnic groups living in Scotland are Pakistani peoples followed by Chinese and Indians. The minority ethnic population is concentrated in the four major cities of Aberdeen, Dundee, Edinburgh and Glasgow.
- The highest concentrations of minority ethnic groups are found in England, primarily in London, followed by the West Midlands, West Yorkshire and Greater Manchester. In some London boroughs (Newham, Brent) the minority ethnic population exceeds 40%; in the West Midlands it is 20% and lower in all other areas.
- There is no area of Britain where the local minority ethnic population exceeds the numbers of the local ethnic majority.

Source: 1991 Census; Balarajan and Soni Raleigh (1993)

As Doolin (1994) states, 'Because of British society's tendency to focus on the colour of a person's skin in defining ethnicity, rather than cultural practices and traditions, the experiences of Irish people tend to get lost or overlooked when attempts to investigate or ameliorate discrimination and disadvantage are made'.

Our knowledge of the interrelationship of ethnicity and mental health is, in itself, cause for concern. The researched data concentrate upon records of in-patient admissions (notoriously poor indicators of mental health in the wider community). Further material focuses upon the experiences of a particular minority ethnic group, black African–Caribbeans. Information pertaining to the largest minority ethnic group, Asian peoples (Indians, Pakistanis and Bangladeshis) is patchy and often conflicting, while there is an almost total absence of published material examining other communities such as the Chinese, Vietnamese, Cypriots, Turks, Greeks, and Middle Eastern peoples. However, all the literature available suggests that significant differences exist between the mental health of black and minority ethnic groups and that of the majority ethnic population of the UK.

THE MINORITY ETHNIC EXPERIENCE OF MENTAL HEALTH SERVICES

The minority ethnic populations experience of mental health service provision differs from the majority ethnic group in the following areas:

Pathways into the Mental Health Services

Evidence suggests that from their earliest point of contact with the mental health system, black people, especially young African–Caribbean men, tend to share a particular experience. The nature of their contact is predominantly crisis led, via the police (through the use of Section 136 of the Mental Health Act 1983) or non-health service agencies (Sashidharan, 1994a). It is also suggested that African–Caribbean people are more likely than 'whites' to make contact with mental health services via the courts or prison (Pilgrim and Rogers, 1993) and that police (or legal system) involvement is likely to lead to a negative first impression of mental health services (Moodley and Perkins, 1990). Within special hospitals, black mentally disordered offenders are reported to be detained under higher security for longer periods (DoH, 1992).

Once contact has been made, African–Caribbean people are much more likely to be detained compulsorily under the Mental Health Act 1983 (Dunn and Fahy, 1990). Conversely, in terms of voluntary-help-seeking behaviour for mental health problems, black people are under-represented in self-referral services (Littlewood and Cross, 1980). They have a lower than average uptake of out-patient services; low referral rates of black people to mental health services by GPs are found (Hitch and Clegg, 1985).

The Minority Ethnic Experience of the Mental Health System

Despite the moves to community-based mental health care provision, a disproportionately high number of black people are admitted to psychiatric hospitals as in-patients (Cope, 1989). The institutional nature of these initial contacts is confirmed by reports (Sashidharan, 1994b) of inadequate community-based options available to black people. Even when accounting for diagnostic differences, further evidence suggests that black people in psychiatric hospitals receive more physical treatments in the form of psychotropic drugs and ECT (Littlewood and Lipsedge, 1982) and higher doses of these drugs (Chen *et al.*, 1991) They are also more likely to be formally detained or nursed in locked ward environments (Noble and Rodger, 1989). Concern has also been expressed that the treatment of black clients rarely includes counselling, or psychotherapeutic or psychological 'talking therapies' (Kareem and Littlewood, 1992).

Discrepancies in Diagnosis

A high incidence of diagnosis of schizophrenia has been reported among certain minority ethnic populations living in the UK, most noticeably the African–Caribbeans (Harrison *et al.*, 1988; Cochrane and SinghBal, 1989). Hospital admission rates for schizophrenia are five to six times higher for African–Caribbeans living in the UK than for those living in Jamaica (Hickling, 1991). For second generation African–Caribbeans, rates are even higher (McGovern and Cope, 1987).

There are conflicting and inconsistent findings about the mental health problems of Asian minority groups. Beliappa (1991) challenges the view that Asians have a low prevalence of mental health problems. She finds evidence of significant mental distress in a sample from Haringey, London. Further, Soni Raleigh *et al.* (1990) reports particularly high suicide levels (especially by burning) among young Indian women and increased suicide rates in young East Africans of Indian origin.

Marked differences in diagnosis have been recorded for Irish people living the UK, which includes having the highest overall rate of hospital admission for all mental health problems. In addition, Cochrane and SinghBal (1989) report high suicide rates and higher than average rates of diagnoses for schizophrenia and alcohol-related problems. They also show that Scottish migrants have higher than average rates of admission for alcohol and drug-related problems and that there is increased likelihood of of schizophrenia in Polish people.

EXPLANATIONS FOR INEQUALITIES IN MENTAL HEALTH

For mental health nurses to understand how and why inequalities in the mental health treatment of minority ethnic groups persist, we need to examine differing explanations that have been proposed.

Essentially, the main explanations focus on two separate but related areas:

1. The impact of individual and, particularly, institutional racism upon ethnic minorities, including racism in the mental health system.

2. The lack of 'ethnocultural awareness', which would enable mental health nurses to understand cultural differences in communication, values, beliefs and expression.

Racism and Discrimination

This perspective argues that the existence and manifestations of racism are extensive in British society. Racism in this context extends beyond the racial prejudices, stereotypes and negative attitudes of individuals to actions taken on the basis of false beliefs that some races are 'superior' to others or that physical characteristics like skin colour make some people 'better' than others. Crucially, racism also refers to the generation and perpetuation of racial inequality, disadvantage and discrimination by those social institutions (the education system, mental health system, employment structures etc.) that constitute our society.

The effects of racism upon mental health operate at individual, social and institutional levels. Fanon (1986) observes that victims of racism and oppression suffer significant mental distress including detrimental effects upon the individuals' self-esteem and self-image. He also points to distress associated with feelings of inferiority, fear, anxiety states, powerlessness, despair, disaffection, despondency, trauma and depersonalization. Feelings of being persecuted, threatened and victimized are frequently reported by ethnic minority clients.

The impact of institutionalized racism is highlighted when the relationship between socio-economic or social institutional factors and mental health is examined alongside ethnicity. D'Ardenne and Mahtani (1989) quote Burke:

> Racism (Burke, 1986 argues), maintains social and economic deprivation, limited access to care, subordination and social control by the majority culture. In this way, other cultures, particularly black ones, are made more vulnerable to physical ailments, and enter a further cycle of disadvantage. What is being criticized here, of course, is not just mental health professionals or their approach to problems with ethnic clients, nor even the lack of appropriate and adequate services for them. The criticism is of an entire political and social system whose laws and practices enable personal and institutional racism to flourish.

Littlewood and Lipsedge (1989) warn against discussing social disadvantage as disease–in this instance, mental illness–and point to the disproportionately high levels of social stress and deprivation faced by minority ethnic communities. Social factors such as low income and poverty, poor housing conditions (dampness, overcrowding) and 'ghettoization' in areas of urban decay (with high crime rates, high population density and environmental degeneration) have been associated with mental distress. For further discussion of these issues see Socio-Economic Factors.

Sashidharan (1994b) argues that we still operate under the 'ideological legacy of racist 18th Century and 19th Century science' which constructed 'black' people as mentally primitive, inferior and more liable to 'emotional' disturbance of the mind (Fernando, 1991). African–Caribbean patients are especially prone to being labelled deviant, mentally ill and schizophrenic. Hence African–Caribbean beliefs in the spirits of the dead, vivid conceptions of God and religious or magical visions and perceptions (Donovan, 1984) are judged by the norms of white British society, rather than those of the Caribbean and can be misconstrued for the hallucinations, delusions and 'voices' associated with the diagnosis of schizophrenia.

In contrast with the diagnosis of schizophrenia, African–Caribbean people are under-represented in other diagnostic categories. Littlewood and Lipsedge (1989) suggest that we fail to notice depression in African–Caribbeans because our society constructs them as 'psychotic' and thus our experiences of working with them are as 'psychotics'. They link this partly to the history of racism inherent in Western scientific thinking where stereotypes of 'black' people as happy-go-lucky, as unburdened by responsibility, with irrepressible high spirits and little self-control have prevailed.

Littlewood and Lipsedge (1989) find 'no simple explanations for the different rates of mental illness applicable to all minority groups'. Rather it depends upon who emigrates, why and with what internal resources and external supports. They do find, however, that those who as refugees are forced to leave their homes and cannot return have higher diagnosed rates of mental illness. Migrants who suffer a reduction in financial and social status appear also to have higher rates of mental illness (Littlewood and Lipsedge, 1989). Those with traumatic pre-migration experiences of war, loss, torture and persecution bring obvious psychological distress and vulnerability with them to Britain. The process and stresses of adapting to a new culture may in themselves lead to mental distress. These are compounded when found in conjunction with other factors, e.g. high unemployment, social, economic and material deprivation, and racial harassment and discrimination.

Ethnocultural Awareness

This perspective is concerned to raise awareness of the influence of ethnicity and culture upon human beliefs, behaviour and interaction, including the form and presentation of mental distress. Helman (1990) defines culture as 'an inherited "lens", through which individuals perceive and understand the world they inhabit and learn to live within it'. Culture, Helman proposes, determines how we view the world, how we experience it and how we behave in it.

It is impossible for mental health nurses to know every individual client's cultural background. Rack (1982) stated that 'in observing and defining the culture of another, you are making a statement about your own cultural beliefs and practices'. Therefore any serious attempt at ethnocultural awareness requires an examination of, and reflection upon, the relative values of both the mental health nurse and client.

POTENTIAL BARRIERS IN CROSS-CULTURAL COMMUNICATION

Effective communication is a vital part of the mental health nurses role. In order to maximise cross cultural communication, nurses need to be aware of the potential barriers that can occur.

Verbal Communication and Language

The acquisition of the socially dominant language has been found to be the single most important aspect of integration for those arriving in another culture (Littlewood and Lipsedge, 1989). Great problems are faced by those who cannot speak English. The solution usually proposed is the use of translation or interpretation services. However, Stokes (1991) notes that, in the NHS, these are usually overstretched and inadequately resourced. MIND (1992) stress the importance of heavy investment in these services. Crowley (1991) demonstrates how different languages offer a wide or narrow range of words to describe aspects of the corresponding cultural life. For example, in English a variety of words can be used to describe mood, e.g. despondent, despairing, depressed, gloomy and miserable. He argues that Asian and African languages may have no direct equivalents and this poses potential barriers in cross-cultural communication.

Attention has also been drawn to not just the ability to speak English, but to do so in a certain way. D'Ardenne and Mahtani (1989) demonstrate how regional accents and 'alternative forms' of English, e.g. 'street talk' and the speech forms of African–Caribbean cultures, can elicit prejudice and disadvantage and raise barriers to communication.

Non-Verbal Communication

Signals of non-verbal communication vary across cultures in terms of posture, gesture, distance, spacing, eye contact and volume and tone of speech. D'Ardenne and Mahtani (1989) cite the example of high levels of eye contact found in some Arabic and Latin American cultures that Europeans may find uncomfortable. Cross-culturally, notions of 'comfortable distance' between individuals vary widely and point to the need for our awareness of how we frequently interpret the non-verbal conventions of other cultures by our own norms.

Western Bias Inherent in Counselling-Style Approaches

Katz (1985) argues that the fundamental components of a 'counselling-style' approach, with its emphasis upon individualism, self-disclosure and 'talk therapy' is inherently linked to the values and beliefs of 'white' Euro-American culture. The concept of 'talking through problems' as a method of solving individual or group difficulties can be seen as culture-bound; consequently it may seem strange to those from non Euro-American cultures. Likewise, the focus upon 'self' or 'individual' through self-exploration, self-awareness and self-disclosure can also be seen as a cultural preoccupation of 'individualistic' Western societies. D'Ardenne and Mahtani (1989) suggest that Western cultural attention given to the 'self', 'I' and 'me' may raise barriers to those from 'collectivist' cultures who view the individual as an integral part of a wider social group or community.

Non-Directedness

In many health settings a non-directive, client centred approach is seen as desirable and facilitative. Again, such action is an expression of Western cultural norms, values and beliefs and can be experienced as disabling and a barrier to communication in non-Western cultures. D'Ardenne and Mahtani (1989) suggest that Asian peoples may not respond well to reflective approaches which focus on feelings, that Chinese and Indian peoples may prefer a logical, rational, structured approach and that in some cultures individual members may experience high levels of anxiety from an unstructured, reflective approach. Direct or personal questions can violate cultural etiquette and thus be greeted by silence or at best a deflecting answer.

Cultural Expressions of Distress

Much attention has been given to the cultural expression of mental distress, featuring most notably in the language of 'depression'. Crowley (1991) states that depressed Asian men who visit psychiatric clinics often seem to present their problems as physical complaints such as changes in sexual potency. Asian women frequently complain of sweating, headaches and a 'spinning head'. It is proposed that these clients deny feeling depressed or having personal or family problems and 'somatize' their mental distress into physical symptoms, such as 'tired all the time', headaches, palpitations, weight loss, dizziness and vague aches and pains. Despite the client's verbal expressions of generalized bodily aches and pains, indications of mood may be given by non-verbal communication.

POTENTIAL BARRIERS IN CROSS-CULTURAL UNDERSTANDING

An appreciation of the importance of cultural diversity is essential to the delivery of effective and individual nursing care. It is crucial that mental health nurses are aware of how barriers in cross-cultural understanding can be created through the universal application of Western cultural norms.

Religious and Spiritual Beliefs and Practices

Britain is a multireligious society, in which the well-known world religions (Christianity, Islam, Judaism, Buddhism and Hinduism) are practised alongside the lesser known (Jainism, Taoism, Sikhism). Smart (1989) stresses, however, that these labels themselves encompass a great variety of subtraditions and beliefs. Further, regional variations exist in religious practices and expression, individual differences exist in belief and levels of adherence and religions themselves are impacted upon by history, politics and sociocultural forces. Animal, ancestor or other supernatural spirits can influence an individual's beliefs and actions, either as an independent spiritual value system or in co-existence with other religious beliefs.

Littlewood and Lipsedge (1989) describe how aspects of religious expression have the potential to be confused with psychiatric symptoms of mental illness, e.g. glossolalia, or 'speaking in tongues' in Pentecostal religions. Another area of potential cross-cultural misunderstanding concerns beliefs in spiritual forces. Boddy (1989) and Lewis (1971) describe beliefs in spirit possession afflicting mainly women and known as the Zar throughout Islamic Africa. Zar spirit is seen to cause certain mental states, e.g. depression, while 'cure' involves the victim ascending into a dissociative trance to 'enable the malign spirit to speak through them'. Lewis shows that in this context such beliefs are accepted as part of a wider religious system. He suggests it is a culturally normative way of presenting and explaining physical and mental distress and should not be confused with Western notions of mental illness, i.e. psychoses, delusions, hallucinations or hearing voices.

Diet and Nutrition

The food people eat is tied closely into systems of cultural beliefs, which in turn influences what is viewed as edible, what foods are defined as 'good for us' and how they are prepared, served and eaten. Mental health nurses need to be aware of clients' nutritional requirements while also observing dietary needs that are culturally or religiously determined.

Family Structure

Despite being the primary social grouping across cultures, family structure, kinship networks, moral codes of behaviour, gender roles and the influence of generational members vary widely and are themselves impacted by socio-economic factors. D'Ardenne and Mahtani (1989) highlight problems that can arise when clients and families from 'collectivist cultures' (where the family or community may have a high level of influence on and participation in the individual member's life) are confronted by the 'individualistic' expectations of white health care professionals. Strict or restricted visiting times and limits on family involvement and participation in care may conflict with cultural values of family life. The notion that an individual is responsible for dealing with his or her problems or illness without the active intervention of the family is also a culturally specific Western one. Traditional mental health care environments may violate cultural traditions of gender roles if they are mixed-sex with no secluded 'women only areas'. The issue of intergenerational conflict between original migrant parents and their second generation children draws attention to the difficulties faced by those 'born between two cultures'. Particular stresses may be faced by children who, while growing up under the forces of a dominant Western culture with experiences of institutional racism, are also socialized into a potentially conflicting set of cultural norms, beliefs and values.

Concepts of Mental Health and Mental Distress

Fernando (1991) proposes that all cultures have a way of conceiving of a departure from health. However, Western culture is unusual in that it distinguishes the mind from the body in its conceptualization of mental illness. The implications of non-Western ethnocultural concepts of health, illness and mental distress are far reaching for mental health nurses. First, they present a challenge to the way in which mental illness is defined, explained, managed and treated in the traditional western psychiatric system. Second, they confirm that the mental distress of minority ethnic groups is unlikely to be presented and articulated in the explanatory framework of Western psychiatry. Finally, they point to the inadequacy of traditional mental health services to offer flexibility of alternatives that recognize minority ethnic accounts of mental distress and acceptable treatment methods. The latter may include the use of traditional healers, herbs and protective objects, and consultation with religious or spiritual leaders.

GENDER

As Ussher (1991) comments, it is naïve to view any experience of mental illness purely in relation to gender. Factors such as socio-economic status, ethnicity and sexuality are also influential. However, statistical, epidemiological and empirical evidence indicates that mental illness can be seen as a gendered experience. In other words, there are differences in the ways in which men and women experience mental illness and mental health service provision. These differences present themselves in a variety of ways.

THE GENDERED EXPERIENCE OF MENTAL ILLNESS

Pathways into Services

There are gender differences that are influential in determining who comes into contact with mental health services in the first place. One issue that is assuming increasing importance is that of abuse. Researching any form of abuse is problematic and it is generally assumed that more remains hidden than is reported (Gillham, 1991). Gillham also comments that this is more likely to be true in the case of men and boys reporting instances when they have been the victims of such abuse. Pilgrim and Rogers (1993) and Gillham urge caution in assuming inevitable causal links between abuse and subsequent mental illness or that all abusers are male. Mental disorder is not the outcome in all instances of sexual or physical abuse and there is evidence of female abusers (Gillham, 1991). However, research does indicate that women had been more frequently the victims of abuse, that victims of abuse have increased likelihood of developing mental illness and that abused children are more prone to mental disorder in later life than their non-abused counterparts.

Surveys conducted in Britain and the United States estimated that between 25% and 40% of women had been subject to sexual abuse before the age of 16 (Finkelhor, 1991). In a British study, Palmer *et al.* (1992) found that up to 50%

of women consulting a psychiatrist have been sexually abused as children. In the Ashworth Report (1992), 80% of the women interviewed reported having been sexually abused as children. Doyal (1995) quotes studies by Levinson (1989) and Campbell (1992) that indicate that physical violence inflicted on one partner by the other within an intimate relationship is commonplace and that in 90% of cases it is inflicted by a man on a woman.

The interface between the criminal justice and psychiatric systems provides another point where gender seems to influence future pathways. This is frequently posed as the mad or bad question. Statistics indicate that men greatly outnumber women in every type of crime, including violent crimes (Burns, 1992). As will be discussed below, females outnumber males, although not to such a great extent, in psychiatric statistics. The point to be made here concerns societal views of violence. Pilgrim and Rogers (1993) argue that violent men are perceived as 'bad' whereas violent women are perceived as 'mad'. This is clearly an oversimplification. However, they suggest that this differentiation is based on social judgement concerning rule breaking and is influential in determining that females and males enter psychiatric and criminal justice systems respectively.

The relationship that women have to others can also affect their pathways into services in ways that do not occur for men. For example, women are more likely than men to be placed under a Section of the 1983 Mental Health Act if they are deemed possibly harmful to children (Miles, 1988).

Gendered Difference in Diagnosis

The majority of statistical analyses and epidemiological suggest that more females than males are diagnosed as being mentally ill (see Table 6.1).

Table 6.1 illustrates an overall greater representation of females. It also shows that the statistical representation of males and females is different for different diagnoses.

Females are twice as likely as males to be diagnosed as suffering from clinical depression (Paykell, 1991; Gorman, 1992). Clinically diagnosed eating disorders are ten times more common in females than males (Krahn, 1991), and females are over-represented in those with a diagnosis of senile dementia (Allen, 1986). Self-harm is also far more common in females than males (MIND, 1992). Neuroses such as obsessional disorders and phobias, for example goraphobia, are far more prevalent among females. Certain psychiatric diagnoses by their very definition can only be applied to females, such as post-natal depression or puerperal psychosis. Brockington (1987) cited by Thurtle (1995) suggests that up to 20% of females suffer from postnatal depression.

Some diagnoses have an over-representation of males e.g. those relating to problem drug and alcohol use. Gomez (1991) reports that 95% of children taken to a psychologist for sexually inappropriate behaviour are boys and that effective suicide in all age groups is highest in males. Psychiatric referrals under Section 136 of the Mental Health Act 1983 are higher for males than females (Pilgrim and Rogers, 1993). There is little overall gender difference in the diagnosis of

TABLE 6.1 Gender differences in admission rates

	Rates / 100 000		Excess %
	Male	Female	Female / Male
All diagnoses	567	611	8
Schizophrenia/ Paranoia	89	55	(-38)
Affective psychoses	65	117	80
Senile / Presenile dementia	79	140	77
Alcoholic dependence syndrome and alcoholic psychosis	120	45	(-63)
Other psychoses	37	46	24
Neurotic disorders	11	17	55
Personality and behavioural disorders	18	18	
Mental retardation	20	10	(-50)
Depressive disorders, non-psychotic	55	103	87
Mental Illness, diagnosis unknown	38	42	11

All admissions to mental illness hospitals and units in Scotland by diagnostic category and sex of patient / 100 000 population in 1990. Scottish Health Statistics, 1991, Edinburgh HMSO

schizophrenia. However, if this is broken down by age, the occurrence is twice as great for males between 15 and 24 than for females in the same age group (Pilgrim and Rogers, 1993).

Experience of Service Provision

There is evidence that, once in the mental health care system, the experience itself is also a gendered one. Women are prescribed over twice as many psychotropic drugs as men (Ashton, 1991). Doyal (1995) cites studies by Glantz and Backenheimer (1988) and Taylor (1987) which indicate that, in the UK, 60% of benzodiazepines are prescribed to women over 40. Many women themselves comment on the abusive nature of some of the treatment approaches, e.g. seclusion and force-feeding of women with anorexia (MIND, 1992). Indications that a woman is 'getting better' are frequently associated with the adoption of socially defined feminine roles and attractiveness, e.g. visiting the hairdresser and using make-up.

There is increasing awareness and reporting of abuse and sexual harassment of women using mental health services (Lambeth, Southwark and Lewisham Health Commission, 1994; Darton *et al.*, 1994). This is usually, although not exclusively, by men (MIND, 1992). Masson (1988) and Edwards and Fasal (1992) report on the abusive relationships that counsellors or therapists may develop with their female clients. These experiences frequently reflect, or remind women of, earlier abusive episodes in their lives.

EXPLANATIONS FOR GENDER DIFFERENCES

It is important to explore possible explanations of the gendered experience of mental illness. Although this chapter is concerned primarily with sociological explanations, these should be considered and criticized alongside psychological and physiological explanations. The main focus for discussion has been the over-representation of females among those labelled mentally ill. For clarity of understanding, the various explanations are given under discrete subheadings. In some instances the explanations contradict, in others they are influenced by, and dependent on, each other.

Social Causes

The central point of this argument is that more women than men are mentally ill because society makes them so. Women are oppressed, stressed and depressed. Brown and Harris (1978) in their study of the social origins of depression, identified a wide range of factors that, when found together in various combinations, were likely to produce the preconditions for the development of psychiatric disorder. They named three groups of aetiological factors:

1. Vulnerability factors such as the loss of a mother before the age of 11, the lack of a confiding relationship, lack of employment outside the home and three or more children aged under 15.
2. Provoking factors such as bereavement, marriage breakdown or serious illness.
3. Symptom formation factors such as previous psychiatric illness.

These aetiological factors are also linked to psychological variables such as low self-esteem. Pilgrim and Rogers (1993) offer a critique of this study, suggesting that it does not provide an explanation as to why more women than men are depressed because it studies only women, thus excluding male experiences of depression. However, it could be argued that Brown and Harris do not claim to explain why more women than men are depressed but highlight the necessary preconditions for depression. At the time of this study, these preconditions were more likely to be present for women. Given the changing political and economic climate, further research is required to establish if this is still the case, or, indeed, in the presence of the same preconditions, whether men would be equally prone to depression.

Other arguments used to support the social causation theory include poverty and differing societal expectations of the roles of men and women. There are established links between poverty and the incidence of mental ill health, addressed later in the section on socio-economic factors. Social indicators demonstrate that women experience more poverty than men (Pilgrim and Rogers, 1993). More women than men are dependent on social security benefits and those who are employed earn significantly less than men. In 1990, women's average earnings were 68% of men's (MIND, 1992).

The role of motherhood provides an example of how societal expectations can cause mental distress. Thurtle (1995) argues that contemporary society holds contradictory views in relation to motherhood, which place the woman in a double bind situation and can lead to mental distress. Motherhood is an admired and sought-after experience. Indeed, one is an incomplete woman unless one is a mother. However, society can be harsh on mothers, for example the poor provision of child care and recent debates on single mothers and lesbian parents. For many the experience of motherhood is not wholly positive and yet it is difficult for women to express negative feelings. Many women feel the pressure of trying to be perfect mothers, perfect partners and perfect performers in the workplace. Women who choose not to or who are unable to become mothers may find themselves stigmatized or pitied.

Much of the debate concerning gender has been led by feminists who have obviously focused on the concerns of women. In recent years increasing attention has been paid to men and masculinity (see, for example Segal, 1990; Gomez, 1991 and Frosh, 1992). Societal causation is cited as a reason for mental distress in both men and women. This is usually connected to societal expectations related to gender role and an individual's gender identity. Most societies have norms concerning appropriate gender behaviour (gender role). Gender identity is the extent to which an individual takes on the gender role of his or her culture or community (Savage, 1987). When an individual experiences incongruence between gender identity and the gender role of society, conflict will occur either within the individual or between the individual and his or her community or both. This conflict can lead to mental distress.

Patriarchal Labelling

This argument is voiced by many feminists. It is based on the idea that society is organized in a way that gives men power and dominance over women. This is called patriarchy. On an individual level both men and women can sustain or undermine this position. However, in broad terms society remains patriarchal and it is within this context that the individual behaviours of women and men are judged (Chesler, 1972; Showalter, 1987). This situation is sometimes referred to as institutionalized sexism.

In relation to mental health, the argument suggests that throughout history women have been seen as weak and vulnerable and have been labelled as mentally ill. It is suggested that this is one of the ways through which patriarchal dominance is maintained. Chesler's book *Women and Madness* is frequently cited as being one of the first to formulate and articulate this hypothesis. Showalter (1987) presents a comprehensive historical study of how women who stepped outside the boundaries of prescribed feminine behaviour were defined as mentally ill:

> Mental breakdown, then, would come when women defied their 'nature', attempted to compete with men instead of serving them, or sought alternatives or even additions to their maternal functions.

> *(Showalter, 1987)*

There are many examples of women being confined to mental institutions for having illegitimate babies or in other ways transgressing 'normal' female behaviour. Many writers highlight the fact that characteristics of a mentally healthy person such as assertiveness and independence are also perceived as male characteristics (Broverman *et al.*, 1970). Their opposites such as passivity and dependence on others are perceived as female. This leaves women in a no-win situation. A 'typical' woman, simply by being a woman, does not meet the criteria for being mentally healthy. If she behaves in an atypical way she is deemed mentally ill.

The ideas outlined above have their critics both inside and outside feminist circles. Ussher (1991) suggests that to argue that women are labelled as mad when they step out of line is ultimately unhelpful. She argues that many of the critics of the psychiatric system stop at criticism and offer nothing, or nothing accessible to vast numbers of women, in its place. This is of little help to women suffering very real experiences of despair and distress. Allen also takes the view that this argument is fundamentally unhelpful. She suggests that sexism is an integral part of psychiatry but not constitutive of it. In other words, sexism does exist within psychiatry. However, to argue that psychiatry exists to create and sustain gender differentiation is hard to justify (Allen, 1986). Both Ussher and Allen are concerned about the number of women in the psychiatric system but argue that the challenge lies not in overthrowing psychiatry as the bastion of female oppression but working on and challenging the sexism within it at both an individual and societal level.

Help-Seeking Behaviour

This explanation is based on the idea that women are more likely than men to seek help for their emotional problems or describe their problems in emotional terms. Therefore they are more likely to receive a psychiatric diagnosis and be over-represented in mental health statistics. This argument is influenced by the debates concerning social expectations, sexism and gender differentiation in diagnosis and is linked to pathways into the system (see above). It is suggested that women are more able, or it is more acceptable for them, to talk about emotional or psychological difficulties. Men, on the other hand, are socialized into non-expressive, non-asking-for-help and 'cope alone' type behaviours (Williamson, 1995)

There is also evidence to suggest that when women and men approach GPs they are likely to receive different diagnoses and treatment, sometimes for the same presenting symptoms. Sheppard (1991) reported that GPs were more likely to refer women for compulsory admission than men. Many of the female referrals following assessment by approved social workers were deemed not to require such admission. Busfield (1982) suggests that on many occasions abnormality and aspects of defined 'feminine' behaviour converge in such a way that it is allowable and expected that women be diagnosed as mentally ill. For example it is allowable and expected that women express fear and anxiety; they are therefore more likely than men to receive a psychiatric diagnosis such as a phobic disorder.

Social Constructionist Theory

This theoretical explanation has been increasingly influential over the last 20 years and is based on the work of the French philosopher Michel Foucault. It differs from theories of social causation and patriarchal labelling in the way in which it perceives society and individuals within society. It does not view concepts such as sexism or mental illness as fixed external truths that act upon individuals in inevitable and unchanging ways. Rather it views them as changing social constructs dependent on individuals creating and sustaining them. Prior (1993) in taking this approach, argues that rather than analysing the causes of neurotic depression in women and alcoholism in men we should be analysing:

> the assumptions and frameworks surrounding the concepts of neurosis and dementia themselves and the changing significance and interpretation of 'sex' in twentieth Century psychiatric epidemiology.

> *(Prior, 1993)*

In other words, rather than focusing on why society makes women, or men and women, mentally ill in different ways, we should be looking at how concepts such as 'neurosis', 'gender' and 'mental illness' are created and sustained and how they operate within our society. An example of such an analysis is provided by Smith (1990) in her account of how a group of people come to define a friend as mentally ill.

SOCIO-ECONOMIC FACTORS

The relationship between mental illness, low socio-economic status and environmental stresses is well documented (Bruce, 1990; Harrison *et al.*, 1995). Socio-economic status refers to a number of complex interrelated factors, which most - frequently encompass employment, occupational grouping, education, income, wealth and type of housing tenure. Implicit in the classification of socio-economic status are statements regarding social prestige as well as material circumstances. Therefore Bond and Bond (1994) emphasize aspects such as lifestyle, standard of living, prestige in the community, power and influence over others and the perceived value to society of different social groups.

SOCIO-ECONOMIC STATUS AND MENTAL HEALTH

Lundberg (1991) proposes that four main socio-economic factors are important in explaining inequalities or differences in rates of mental illness in the population. These factors are physical working conditions, economic hardship during upbringing, risk-related health behaviours and weak social networks, all of which are concentrated in the living and working conditions of lower social-economic groups. The factors of social isolation, poverty and 'social disorganization' are found to have a negative impact upon mental health in a review by Thornicroft (1991).

Multiple studies (Thornicroft, 1991; Jarman *et al.* 1992; Harrison *et al.*, 1995) point to the relationship between indices of low socio-economic status, social deprivation and mental health problems. The positive risk relationship between deprivation, low socio-economic status and the diagnoses of schizophrenia is a constant finding. Some also report an increased risk of 'neurotic diagnoses', especially for women of low socio-economic status (Rodgers, 1991).

Bruce (1990) in the USA found that those who met the federal criteria of poverty had an increased risk of recurrence for schizophrenia, bipolar depression, alcohol and drug related problems, depression, phobias and obsessive–compulsive problems. In an analysis of what seems to be a correlation between the diagnoses of schizophrenia and urban living, Freeman (1994) demonstrated the flaws in proposing simple cause and effect relationships. He demonstrated how 'deprived inner city living' itself cross-related with measures of low social economic status, low social class and social and material deprivation. Therefore it may be impossible or certainly over-simplistic to try to identify any one factor, e.g. 'urban living', as a risk to mental health. Those socio-economic factors constantly shown to pose a risk to mental health are listed in Box 6.2.

JOB LOSS, UNEMPLOYMENT AND MENTAL HEALTH

An aspect of socio-economic status that has been extensively researched is the link between unemployment and poor mental health (Owen and Watson, 1995). Findings correlate unemployment with minor psychological disorders and a reduction in psychological well-being, including worry, dissatisfaction and low levels of confidence and self-esteem. Further evidence points to the increased likelihood of depression, anxiety, physical ill health and increased tobacco and alcohol consumption and substance misuse after the onset of unemployment (Wilson and Walker, 1993). The risk of family related breakdown problems and psychological stress has also been linked to unemployment by Friedmann and Webb (1995). Platt *et al.* (1992) show the positive correlation between unemployment and suicide and Hawton and Rose (1986) demonstrate a 12–15 times greater risk of unemployed men committing acts of parasuicide. Contrary to previous conclusions, that a plateau of mental ill health is reached after a 3–9 month period, Winefield and Tiggeman (1990) suggest that prolonged unemployment can lead to a continuing decline in mental health.

Social groups particularly vulnerable to the negative impact of unemployment include men, especially those of middle age and beyond (Broomhall and Winefield, 1990). Lehelda (1992) proposes that the relationship between unemployment and psychological distress is less significant in women. However, other researchers show women without paid employment to have high measures of mental distress (Brown and Harris, 1978) or suggest that for single women the relationship between unemployment and mental distress is similar to that for men (Warr and Parry, 1982). Despite a lack of specific

> **Box 6.2**
>
> ### *Socio-economic factors that are risks to mental health*
>
> - Social isolation/weak social networks or extreme overcrowding and over stimulation.
>
> - Poverty/low income.
>
> - Low socio-economic status/low social class.
>
> - Job loss/unemployment.
>
> - High score on indices of 'social deprivation', e.g. The Jarman '8' indices includes:
>   - (i) Being alone and elderly: over 65 for men and 60 for women.
>   - (ii) Having a high percentage of children under the age of 5 in the household.
>   - (iii) Being a single parent.
>   - (iv) Where the head of the household is in an unskilled occupation.
>   - (v) Unemployment.
>   - (vi) Overcrowded living conditions.
>   - (vii) Recent change of address, i.e. moved house.
>   - (viii) Ethnic minority status.

evidence of the impact of unemployment upon the mental health of minority ethnic groups, we can hypothesize that this would be significant. 'Black' African–Caribbeans face particularly high levels of long-term employment, 15.8% compared to 4% in the 'white' population (Social Trends, 1995).

The impact of re-employment upon mental health has been found to be overwhelmingly positive (Lehelda, 1992). Scheid (1993) describes the beneficial impact of opportunities for skill development, social contact, increased self-esteem and income, together with higher levels of functioning in the community, for clients with mental health problems who have been able to gain employment.

HOMELESSNESS AND MENTAL HEALTH

The noticeable number of homeless mentally ill people living on our streets is a cause for serious concern. The term 'homeless' covers a range of situations and can be extended to those also living in 'temporary accommodation'. Marshall (1989) shows that up to 40% of hostel dwellers in Oxford were experiencing psychosis-related problems. Lister (1991) quotes Shelter in estimating that 15 000 people with mental health problems are sleeping rough, 3000 in London. Single homeless people are much more likely to suffer from severe mental illness, especially schizophrenia, than the average population (Connelly and Crown, 1994). Self-reports from street dwellers suggest that many (37–41%) also experience depression and anxiety (Bines, 1994). Other mental health problems include a high incidence of drug and alcohol use and an increase in suicide and self-harm (Hardy and Rees, 1994).

Studies show that there is no relationship of cause and effect between the closure of large psychiatric hospitals and an increase in the homeless mentally ill. Leff (1993) suggests that while many homeless people have had brief admissions to psychiatric hospitals, few have been long stay patients. Neither can the extremely high rates of severe mental illness be adequately explained by the 'trauma' of homelessness, although some have suggested that this can be the cause of problems of depression and anxiety (Westlake and George, 1994). Rather, Connelly and Crown suggest that 'factors associated with schizophrenia, combined with social and economic difficulties increase the chance of a housing crisis which precipitates homelessness' (Connelly and Crown, 1994). They also point to the need for housing policies to be integrated with social, health and community care policies and programmes.

WHY POOR MENTAL HEALTH AND LOW SOCIO-ECONOMIC STATUS ARE RELATED

There are two main explanations for the link between mental illness and low socio-economic status.

Social Drift Hypothesis

This suggests that mental illness itself precipitates a cycle of decline in the individual's level of social competence and functioning and consequently their ability to work, earn a living wage, afford quality housing etc. It is proposed that those with mental health problems are therefore more likely to 'drift down the social scale' in terms of their socio-economic status and become ghettoized in socially deprived inner city areas.

Social Stress Hypothesis

This proposes that material differences between groups of people in our society mean that some are more regularly exposed to socio-economic stressors than others. Thus, those of low socio-economic status are more likely to struggle with less money, less reliable employment, poorer working conditions, poor housing conditions, overcrowding, noise, pollution, high crime rates etc. Further, their physical health and diet may be negatively affected. The combination of these social factors can result in stressors that impact upon self-worth, self-esteem and ability to cope and ultimately upon the individual's mental health.

AGE

Age is another factor that mental health nurses need to consider to provide socioculturally sensitive care to their clients. As with any single issue, age must be seen in relation to other factors within the sociocultural matrix. (More about working with children and adolescents and with older people can be found in Chapters 23 and 24.)

From a sociocultural point of view, age is of particular relevance in relation to the accepted norms and expectations that groups or communities within society have of people at specific ages. Pilgrim and Rogers (1993) discuss the notion of social competence. They suggest that social competence is achieved if an individual is able to control his or her body and emotions to perform competently in the presence of others. Individuals themselves may judge that they have failed in this competence (e.g. a depressed person feels too sad to participate) or they lack the confidence in their ability to perform competently, which could present itself in anxiety or phobic states. This competency can also be seen to have failed if others judge it so, usually because a person does not conform to socially accepted norms and expectations. In this situation society may judge a person to be 'mad' (usually receiving the diagnosis of a psychotic condition such as schizophrenia), 'sick' (as is sometimes the case with homosexuality), 'bad' (and enter the criminal justice system) or 'eccentric'. The age of the individual will usually be considered when making the judgements outlined above. For example, a 2-year-old boy shouting and stamping in a supermarket will be viewed very differently from a 45-year-old man exhibiting the same behaviour.

Haralambos (1991) identified childhood as being the time when individuals learn the social rules and mores of the society to which they belong, in other words what it means to be socially competent, a process called primary socialization. In white Western culture the 'nuclear family' is upheld as the context within which this primary socialization does and should take place. The notion of the family as the foundation unit of society has been the topic of much recent political debate, e.g. the Conservative Government's 'Back to Basics' campaign and the call for a return to 'traditional family values'. When considering the sociocultural perspective of mental health and illness, whatever one's political affiliation, it is important to recognize that 'traditional families' vary from culture to culture and that many people do not live in a 'nuclear family'.

The focus on the nuclear family has attendant problems in relation to mental health. Pilgrim and Rogers (1993) suggest that mainstream psychoanalytic thought is guilty of viewing the nuclear family group as being of greatest importance in the emotional development of children and, in so doing, ignore the influence of other factors such as socio-economic status, race and gender. It also neglects the child's experiences outside the family, such as those of school or child care.

If a particular type of family is seen as the foundation unit of society, then policies that support the creation and maintenance of that type of family will be developed and implemented, therefore, for example, the current debate concerning divorce laws, the recently established Child Support Agency and the controversy concerning the right of homosexual couples to adopt children. Developments such as these have far-reaching implications, which may include the material deprivation and social marginalization of people who do not live, or were not brought up, in the 'right' type of family. Both of these factors are connected with increased levels of mental distress.

Closely linked to the idea of social competence is the idea of age-specific tasks. Rutter and Rutter (1992) and Torkington (1995) discuss tasks which face individuals at particular points through their lives. As with norms and expectations, these tasks are imbued with a sociocultural bias. For example, Krauss and Slavinsky (1982), cited by Torkington, identify four tasks of adulthood:
1. Separating from the family of origin.
2. Establishing a family of orientation.
3. Establishing an occupational role.
4. Facing the realities of ageing.

The first two tasks can be seen to reflect notions of the nuclear family, which, as previously discussed, is not a reality for many living in Britain today. However, these tasks provide a useful benchmark since they reflect the expectations of the dominant culture. Therefore, consequently adults not achieving them may be deemed, or feel, failures and thus are more likely to come into contact with the mental health system.

Another important aspect of age is the social construction of 'old age'. Regardless of personal abilities, life circumstances, past experiences or physical and mental health, older people are frequently seen in white Western cultures as frail, weak, asexual, childlike and often stupid (Victor, 1992). This overriding negative view, based on assumptions rather than individual knowledge of a person, is sometimes called 'ageism'. As with sexism and racism discussed earlier in this chapter this prejudice can lead to marginalization and be detrimental to a person's mental health. (Working with older people is discussed in more detail in Chapter 24.)

A final aspect of age to be considered here is adolescence. It is important to note that adolescence can be seen as a socially constructed phenomenon. In many cultures it is not recognized as a stage of the human life span. Adolescence, where it exists, is frequently seen and experienced as a time of emotional turmoil and disturbance. Torkington (1995), citing Rutter *et al.* (1976), suggests that the relationship between this and psychiatric morbidity has been overestimated, with adolescent trauma being misinterpreted as mental illness. Rutter and Rutter (1992) see one of the primary tasks of adolescents as 'the ability to conceptualise, to think about the meaning of their experiences and to establish concepts about themselves as distinctive individuals'. This includes establishing themselves as sexual persons. As with other tasks, failure or perceived failure to do this could result in mental health difficulties.

Peer groups are seen as being particularly influential in the shaping of values, attitudes and behaviours during adolescence. Rutter and Rutter (1992) suggest that to think of one peer group is an oversimplification. They argue that adolescents are influenced by friends rather than the rather nebulous concept of a single peer group and that many young people are part of several groups. They further suggest that:

the influences tend to be interactional rather than normative. That is teenagers are influenced by friends whom they choose and with whom they discuss ideas and exchange confidences, rather than by overall social pressures from their age group as a whole to conform to a particular pattern of behaviour

(Rutter and Rutter, 1992)

This is significant for mental health nurses, both for understanding and working with adolescents.

As is suggested, adolescence may be a time when individuals explore different life experiences such as using drugs or alcohol and the development of sexual relationships. It is easy for adolescents to be seen to be transgressing moral codes and norms at this point in their lives. As previously discussed any transgression of societal norms increases the chances of involvement with mental health services. It is particularly important therefore that adolescent behaviour be seen within its sociocultural context both to avoid unnecessary contact with mental health services and to provide the most appropriate help for those in mental distress.

IMPLICATIONS FOR MENTAL HEALTH NURSING

Implications for mental health nursing will be addressed within the framework of empowerment and health promotion, mentioned at the beginning of this chapter. In keeping with current theoretical approaches, we consider empowerment to be fundamental to the process of health promotion. To promote and maintain people's mental health, nurses need to engage with their clients in a process of empowerment. Mason *et al.* (1991) identify three dimensions of empowerment:

1. Developing a positive and potent self-esteem.
2. Developing self-efficacy with skills needed to attain personal and collective goals.
3. Consciousness raising regarding the web of political and social realities that provide a context for one's life circumstances or situation.

'When people are "depowered" they feel powerless, helpless, apathetic, alienated' (Hopson and Scally, 1981). The evidence in this chapter suggests that many who come into contact with mental health services find themselves in this position because of their marginalized and stigmatized social status. A central feature of empowerment is that, to empower others, nurses need to be empowered themselves. Therefore by implication both nurses and clients will be engaged in the same process, possibly at different points at different times but each learning from the other. We argue that both nurses and clients need to be empowered through the development of critical socio-cultural–cultural awareness and the development of self-efficacy skills.

Empowering and health promoting interventions are possible at several levels, i.e. the individual, group and society. Therefore, in the sociocultural context of mental health nursing, what has been said so far implies that nurses work within the three dimensions of empowerment at different levels. Returning to the sociocultural–cultural matrix

discussed at the beginning of the chapter, we have examined mental health and illness in relation to sociocultural differences, thus exploring the 'effects' and 'awareness' components of the matrix. To help translate awareness into action, we will address the 'implications' component.

INDIVIDUAL

To be effective therapeutically, nurses cannot afford merely to learn about the sociocultural matrix of their clients. They also need to examine the values, beliefs and attitudes inherent in their own sociocultural matrix and understand the impact that these will have in enhancing or constraining the therapeutic nurse–client relationship.

Nurses' sociocultural matrices will include the impact of the professional culture of nursing. Lea (1994) argues that, through their professional socialization, nurses absorb the values of the dominant culture of white, middle class society, together with the biomedical system which shapes nursing culture and practice. Likewise, the sociocultural matrix of many clients will be influenced by their marginalized social position, including the social stigma of mental illness, the adoption of the patient role and notions of powerlessness, low self, esteem and passivity. A framework that nurses could use for developing critical sociocultural awareness is suggested in Box 6.3.

Nurses need to develop an awareness of the institutionalized nature of the divisions in society. Such awareness may help to alleviate the feelings of guilt that many individuals have for being part of a dominant, oppressive group. This guilt can prevent people from exploring their own prejudices, which therefore remain unchallenged. Many nurses are themselves members of groups that have traditionally been oppressed. An awareness of the mechanisms through which this is achieved may help in understanding self and others and in challenging such mechanisms. It is important to recognize that, whatever one's own sociocultural identity, all people live in a context of institutionalized racism, sexism, ageism and so on. This may cause someone to expect to be treated in a particular way, based on previous experience or assumptions, taking little regard of the actual individuals in the situation; for example, a distressed black client shouting at a white nurse she has just met, 'Who do you think you are? You f****** whites are all the same!' This is obviously distressing for the white nurse and could leave her feeling misunderstood and misjudged, particularly if she does not view herself as racially prejudiced. Acting on these feelings, the nurse may avoid the client or pass on information concerning the client's 'racist' attitudes. A knowledge of the concept of institutionalized racism may lead to greater understanding and increase the likelihood of a therapeutic relationship developing. The very nature of institutionalized modes of discrimination means that they are not readily recognizable; awareness is needed, both to identify and challenge such inequalities.

In addition to awareness of sociocultural–cultural differences and the effects these have, nurses need to develop specific skills to translate this into action. These could be

---

Box 6.3 *A framework for sociocultural awareness*

- How would I describe my sociocultural matrix ?
- Are there particular sociocultural–cultural beliefs and attitudes that conflict with my own?
- What are my beliefs and expectations of women and men in society?
- How would I describe my ethnicity?
- What are my perceptions of people from different ethnic groups?
- How would I describe my socio-economic position?
- What are my perceptions and expectations of those from different socio-economic positions?
- How do I expect people to behave who are older, younger or the same age as myself?
- How do I relate to people of different ages?
- How would I deal with sociocultural differences between myself and clients with whom I am working?
- How might my sociocultural matrix shape the way I view mental distress and mental illness?
- What are my beliefs about the cause, presentation and treatment of mental distress and mental illness?
- How might my beliefs about mental distress create barriers for my relationships with clients of different sociocultural backgrounds?

described as self-efficacy skills and include assertiveness, therapeutic confrontation, problem solving and negotiation skills. Increasingly nurses are working with people from other disciplines and with multiple agencies. Therefore, development of skills for multidisciplinary teamwork is also essential. Anger is many people's response to the inequalities they face in their lives. Nurses should be aware of this and develop skills that enable the expression of anger, its subsequent management and constructive use. As both nurses and clients should be involved in the empowerment process, nurses need to develop these skills themselves and help clients to develop the same skills. Part of this process may involve assisting clients to locate aspects of their distress in social inequality and not merely in terms of their individual psychology.

As demonstrated earlier, it can be argued that many people's mental health problems are caused, or at least exacerbated, by their socio-economic position. Nurses need to be aware of how to access the various systems that may help alleviate some of the problems or improve the situation, e.g. the social security system, immigration services, and neighbourhood housing. This does not mean that nurses have to become experts in DSS benefits or the complexities of immigration law but they do need to work with clients to develop the skills and knowledge to access these services.

GROUP

Implications for mental health nursing at a group level include the recognition that individual clients' lives are shaped by their own families, communities and subcultures as well as by wider social forces. The relationship between group and individual is dynamic and of mutual influence. Through assessment nurses need to establish to what extent and how the sociocultural–cultural attitudes and expectations of the group or community influence the mental health of individuals. For example, consider the potential sociocultural issues and conflicts for a young, second generation Irish Catholic woman who has taken a paracetamol overdose following an abortion. This is not to suggest a simplistic cause and effect relationship—rather that, to be most effective, each situation must be viewed in its specific sociocultural–cultural context. Such an assessment will enable nurses to plan appropriate, culturally sensitive care for individual clients.

In addition to taking into account how the sociocultural beliefs and values of a group affect an individual, nurses can also intervene at a group or community level by, for example, consulting and educating local residents concerned about the opening of a group home for 'ex-psychiatric patients' in their street or running stalls at local community events to raise awareness of service provision and educate local people about the relationship between sociocultural factors and mental health. Part of the nurse's role also involves interaction and liaison with other care providers or services on the individual's and family's behalf.

Mental health nurses need to be involved in the provision of culturally sensitive services at a local level. By this we mean actively addressing sociocultural–cultural issues such as race

and gender, rather than ignoring them or seeing them as irrelevant. As Ussher and Nicholson (1993) and Allen (1986) point out, when these issues are neglected, services tend towards a white, male, middle class bias in their values and attitudes, rather than the neutrality that is frequently assumed or claimed.

Most services in Britain today have a statement of intent concerning equal opportunities. The challenge for nurses and others is to translate this statement into meaningful policies and practices that ensure equality of access and appropriateness of service provision. Sociocultural–cultural issues should be considered in relation to equal opportunity statements. Consideration could be given to such issues as the provision of child care, the opening hours of services, the food provided, the image of the service portrayed including the gender, age, ethnicity and position of employees.

To provide accessible and appropriate services, potential and actual service users need to be consulted. In planning consultation, care should to be taken to ensure that the voices of those frequently marginalized are heard, for example, accessing the views of user-led groups and groups established to represent the views of minority communities such as black and Asian groups or religious groups. For nurses to be able to do this they need to be aware of which groups exist in their locality. Seeking the views of isolated people who have no affiliation with a specific group, e.g. homeless people or people whose past or current mental health state means that they find participation in any structured activity difficult, presents particular challenges. One of the aims of outreach work is to establish contact with people in such extreme positions of social isolation.

Care must be taken to avoid tokenism, e.g. having one woman, a black person or one user on a committee to represent all minority interests. More creative ways of engaging in consultative processes can be developed, such as establishing discussion forums or giving draft plans and policies to local groups for critical reading and comment. Such tokenism can also be avoided if those engaged in consultation are prepared to review and change existing policies and practices in response.

The provision of separate services for specific groups in society is always controversial. However, this issue should be considered both in terms of 'specialist' service provision, e.g. by the Afro-Caribbean Mental Health Association in Brixton, and specific provision within general services, e.g. women only 'drop ins' and an Irish group in a Day Centre. Recent reports on good practice in mental health care (MIND, 1992; Butterworth, 1994) recommend that clients should be offered choice in the gender of their primary nurse and that single sex accommodation with women-only spaces should be available. Butterworth further recommends that codes of practice be developed covering the issues of sexual or racial harassment and abuse. These recommendations have obvious implications in relation to recruitment of staff and the organization of the physical environment.

When planning services for specific groups it is important

not to view issues concerning the inequalities in society as the 'problem' of the group most affected. For example, gender is not an issue solely for women. If this view is taken, women are likely to remain marginalized and the difficulties and issues concerning men and gender will go unaddresssed, e.g. the issue of men and violence and the difficulties faced by men who do not fit the accepted norms of masculinity. Much can be gained by a group of white people thinking about what it means to be white. Similarly it should not be left to women, black people or older people to challenge discriminatory practices or behaviour.

SOCIETY

The authors of this chapter challenge the view sometimes expressed by nurses that they have little to offer in this area or that their work is essentially apolitical. Nurses, individually or working in larger groups or organizations, can and should be encouraged to add their professional voice. Hopton (1995) challenges the nursing profession to become more actively involved in sociopolitical activity that aims to tackle inequality and disadvantage in our society. The Butterworth Report (1994) recommends that mental health nursing input be included 'when formulating, implementing and monitoring health care strategies'. This implies an increasing obligation for nurses to become involved in groups that will influence policy either through the process of lobbying or at a strategic planning level.

Opportunities to get involved at a societal level include seeking out the chance to engage in debate and ensuring that sociocultural issues are part of that debate by, for example, attending conferences, responding to articles in the media and joining professional organizations or local interest groups. Once again, nurses need to be aware of organizations in their area that have an interest in or impact upon mental health. With increasing emphasis on outcomes and the monitoring of services, nurses have an essential part to play in developing and implementing measurement tools that take account of sociocultural factors. In the current consumer culture, many Health Service Trusts and Provider Units put out plans and policy papers for consultation. Mental health nurses should respond to and engage in such consultation processes.

SUMMARY

The authors have explored the sociocultural context of mental health nursing and identified the major sociocultural determinants that influence mental health, i.e. gender, ethnicity, age and socio-economic factors. These factors are influential at an individual, group and societal level and exist in a dynamic relationship, with each level and factor influencing the others. The complex interrelationship of these multiple factors means that every individual has their own unique sociocultural identity.

The ways in which these sociocultural factors may affect people's mental health and the experiences that they may have of services have been discussed. Specifically, attention has been given to the inequalities that exist within our society based on sociocultural differences. These inequalities can lead to the marginalization of particular groups. Using a framework of empowerment we have examined the implications for mental health nursing. The authors have argued that nurses need to develop a critical awareness of sociocultural issues, including an awareness of their own sociocultural identity and how this may enhance or inhibit the development of therapeutic relationships with clients. To provide socioculturally sensitive, individualized care, nurses need to develop an understanding of the sociocultural identity of their clients. Awareness needs to be translated into action. This requires the development of particular skills and can involve intervention at an individual, group and societal level.

KEY CONCEPTS

- Sociocultural awareness
- Working with difference
- Ethnicity
- Gendered experience of mental illness
- Culturally sensitive nursing practice
- Marginalisation
- Inequalities in the provision of mental health services

REFERENCES

Allen H: Psychiatry and the construction of the feminine. In: Miller P, Rose N, editors: *The power of psychiatry.* Cambridge, 1986, Polity Press.

Ashton H: Psychotropic drug prescribing for women. *Br J Psychiatry.* 158 (supplement 10)30–35, 1991.

Ashworth Report: *Report of the committee of inquiry into complaints about Ashworth Hospital.* London, 1992, HMSO.

Balarajan R, Soni Raleigh V: *Ethnicity and health. A guide for the NHS [The Health of the Nation].* London, 1993, DoH.

Beliappa J: *Illness or distress? Alternative models of mental health.* Newcastle upon Tyne, 1991, Confederation of Indian Organizations.

Bines W: *The health of single homeless people.* York, 1994, Centre for Housing Policy.

Boddy J: *Wombs and alien spirits: Women, men and the Zar cult in Northern Sudan.* 1989, University of Wisconsin Press.

Bond J, Bond S: *Sociology and health care.* Edinburgh, 1994, Churchill Livingstone.

Brockington IF: Puerperal emergencies. In: Politt D, editor: *Psychiatric emergencies and family practice.* Lancaster, 1987, MIT Press.

Broomhall H, Winefield A: A comparison of the affective well-being of young and middle-aged men, matches for length of unemployment. *Br J Med Psychol* 63(1):43–52, 1990.

Brown G, Harris T: *Social origins of depression.* London, 1978, Tavistock Publications.

Broverman D, Clarkson F, Rosenkratz P: Sex roles stereotypes and clinical judgements of mental health. *J Counsel Clin Psychol* 34:1–7, 1970.

Bruce M: Socio-economic status and psychiatric disorders. *Curr Opin Psychiatry* 3:696–699, 1990.

Burke AW: Attempted suicide among Asian immigrants in Birmingham. *Br J Psychiatry* 128:528–533, 1986.

Burns J: Mad or just plain bad? Gender and the work of forensic clinical psychologists. In: Ussher J, Nicolson P, editors: *Gender issues in clinical psychology.* London, 1992, Routledge.

Busfield J: Gender and mental illness. *Int J Ment Health* 11(1&2):46–66,1982.

Butterworth T: *Working in partnership: the collaborative approach to care [Report of the Mental Health Nursing Review Team].* London, 1994, HMSO.

Campbell J: Wife battering: cultural contexts versus western social sciences. In: Counts D, Brown J and Campbell J, editors: *Sanctions and sanctuary: cultural perspectives on the beatings of wives.* Boulder, 1992, West View Press.

Census (1991): Outline statistics for England and Wales derived from County Monitors. National Monitor CEN 91 CM58. O.P.C.S. London, 1992, HMSO.

Chen E, Harrison G, Standen P: Management of first episode psychotic illness in Afro-Caribbean patients. *Br J Psychiatry* 158:517–22, 1991.

Chesler P: *Women and madness.* New York, 1972, Doubleday.

Cochrane R, Singh Bal S: Mental hospital admission rates of immigrants to England: a comparison of 1971 and 1981. *Soc Psychiatry Psychiatr Epidemiol* 24:2–11, 1989.

Connelly J, Crown J, editors: *Homelessness and ill-health [Report of a working party of the Royal College of Psychiatry].* London, 1994, Royal College of Psychiatry.

Cope R: The compulsory detention of Afro-Caribbeans under the Mental Health Act. *New Community* 15(3):343–356, 1989.

Crowley J: Races apart. *Nurs Times* 87(10)44–45, 1991.

D'Ardenne P, Mahtani A: *Transcultural counselling in action.* London, 1989, Sage Publications.

Darton K, Gorman J, Sayce L: *Eve fights back: The successes of MIND's Stress on Women Campaign.* London, 1994, MIND Publications.

DoH/Home Office: *Review of health and social services for mentally disordered offenders and others requiring similar services.* London, 1992, HMSO.

Donovan JC: Ethnicity and health: a research review. *Soc Sci Med* 19(7):663–670, 1984.

Doolin N: The luck of the Irish? *Nurs Times* 8(46) 1994.

Doyal L: *What makes women sick. Gender and the political economy of health.* London, 1995, Macmillan Press Ltd.

Dunn J, Fahy TA: Police admissions to a psychiatric hospital: demographic and clinical differences between ethnic groups. *B J Psychiatry* 156:783–78, 1990.

Edwards M, Fasal J: Keeping an intimate relationship professional. *OPENMIND* 57, 1992.

Fanon F: *Black skins, white masks.* London, 1986, Pluto Press.

Fernando S: *Mental health, race and culture.* London, 1991, MIND.

Finkelhor D: Child sexual abuse. In: Rosenberg M, Feinley M, editors: *Violence in America: a public health approach.* Oxford, 1991, Oxford University Press.

Freeman H: Schizophrenia and city residence. *Br J Psychiatry* 164:39–50, 1994.

Friedemann M, Webb A: Family health and mental health six years after economic stress and unemployment. *Issues Ment Health Nurs* 16(1)51–66, 1995.

Frosh S: Masculine ideology and psychological therapy. In: Ussher J, Nicolson P, editors: *Gender issues in clinical psychology.* London, 1992, Routledge.

Gillham B: *The facts about child sexual abuse.* London, 1991, Cassell Educational Ltd.

Glantz H, Backenheimer M: Substance abuse among elderly women. *Clin Geron* 8(1)3–26, 1988.

Gomez J: *Psychological and psychiatric problems in men.* London, 1991, Routledge.

Gorman J: *Out of the shadows.* London, 1992, MIND Publications.

Gournay K: Mental health nurses working purposefully with people with serious and enduring mental illness: an international perspective. *Int J Nurs Stud* 34(4)341–351, 1995.

Haralambos M: *Sociology: Themes and perspectives,* 2 ed.. London, 1991, Collins.

Hardy B, Rees C: Meeting the mental health needs of homeless people. *Ment Health Nurs* 14(6):8–10, 1994.

Harrison G, Owens D, Holton A, Neilson D, Boot D: A prospective study of severe mental disorder in Afro-Caribbean patients. *Psychol Med* 18:643–657, 1988.

Harrison J, Barrow S, Creed F: Social deprivation and psychiatric admission rates among different diagnostic groups. *Br J Psychiatry* 67:456–462, 1995.

Hawton N, Rose K: Unemployment and suicide in Oxford. *Health Trends* 18:29–32, 1986.

Helman C: *Culture, health and illness.* London, 1990, Butterworth–Heinemann.

Hickling FW: Psychiatric hospital admission rates in Jamaica 1971 and 1988. *Br J Psychiatry* 159:817–821, 1991.

Hitch P, Clegg P: Modes of referral of overseas immigrant and native born first admissions to psychiatric hospital. *Soc Sci Med* 14a:369–374, 1985.

Hopson B, Scally M: *Life skills teaching.* London, 1981, McGraw Hill.

Hopton J: The application of the ideas of Franz Fanon to mental health nursing. *J Adv Nurs* 21:723–728, 1995.

Jarman B, Hirsh A, White P: Predicting psychiatric admission rates. *Br Med J* 304:1146–1151, 1992.

Kareem J, Littlewood R: *Intercultural therapy: Theory and practice.* Oxford, 1992, Blackwell.

Katz JH: The socio-political nature of counselling. *The Counselling Psychologist* 13(4):615–624, 1985.

Krahn D: The relationship of eating disorders to substance abuse. *J Subst Abuse* 3:239–253, 1991.

Krauss J, Slavinsky A: *The chronically ill psychiatric patient and the community.* Boston, 1982, Blackwell.

Lambeth, Southwark and Lewisham Health Commission: *With need in mind: A five year commissioning strategy for health services in South East London.* London, 1994, Lambeth and Southwark Health Commission.

Lea A: Nursing in today's multicultural society: a transcultural perspective. *J Adv Nurs* 18:602–612, 1994.

Leff J: All the homeless people–where do they come from? *BMJ* 306:669–70, 1993.

Lehelda E: Unemployment and mental well being. *Int J Health Ser* 22:261–274, 1992.

Levinson D: *Family violence in cross cultural perspective.* California, 1989, Sage.

Lewis IM: *Ecstatic religion.* London, 1971, Penguin Books.

Lister J: At the sharp end of care. In: Page M, Powel R, editors: *Homelessness and mental illness: The dark side of community care.* London, 1991, Concern Publications.

Littlewood R, Cross S: Ethnic minorities and psychiatric services. *Sociol Health Illn* 2:194–201, 1980.

Littlewood R, Lipsedge M: *Aliens and alienists: Ethnic minorities and psychiatry.* Harmondsworth, 1989, Pelican.

Lundberg O: Caused explanations for class inequality in health–an empirical analysis. *Soc Sci Med* 32(4):385–393, 1991.

Marshall M: Collected and neglected: are Oxford's hostels for the homeless filling up with disabled psychiatric patients? *Br Med J* 299:706–709, 1989.

Mason D, Costello–Nickitas D, Scanlan J, Magnuson B: Empowering nurses for politically astute change in the workplace. *J Contin Educ* 22(1):5–10, 1991.

Masson J: *Against Therapy.* London, 1988, Fontana/Collins.

McGovern D, Cope RV: First psychiatric admission rates of first and second generation Afro-Caribbeans. *Soc Psychiatry* 22:139–49, 1987.

Miles A: *Women and mental illness.* London, 1988, Wheatsheaf Books.

MIND: *Stress on women. Policy paper on women and mental health.* London, 1992, MIND Publications.

Moodley P, Perkins R: Blacks and psychiatry. A framework for understanding access to psychiatric services, *Bull R Coll Psychiatrists* 14:1990.

Noble P, Roger S: Violence by psychiatric in-patients. *Br J Psychiatry* 155:384–390, 1989.

Owen K, Watson N: Unemployment and mental health. *J Psychiatr Ment Health Nurs* 2:63–71, 1995.

Palmer R, Chaloner D, Oppenheimer R: Childhood sexual experience with adults reported by female patients. *Br J Psychiatry* 160:261–265, 1992.

Paykell E: Depression in women. *Br J Psychiatry* 158 (supplement 10):22–29, 1991.

Pilgrim D, Rogers A: *A sociology of mental health and illness*. Buckingham, 1993, Open University Press.

Platt S, Micciolo R, Tansella M: Suicide and unemployment in Italy. *Soc Sci Med* 34:1191–1201, 1992.

Prior L: *The social organisation of mental illness*. London, 1993, Sage.

Rack P: *Race, culture and mental disorder*. London, 1982, Tavistock Publications.

Rodgers B: Socio-economic status, employment and neurosis. *Soc Psychiatry Psychiatr Epidemiol* 26(3):104–114, 1991.

Rutter M, Graham P, Chadwick O, Yule W: Adolescent turmoil: fact or fiction. *J Child Psy and Psych* 17:35–56, 1976.

Rutter M, Rutter M: *Developing minds. Challenge and continuity across the life span*. London, 1992, Penguin Books.

Sashidharan S: Opposing and resisting. *Asylum* 8(1):31–34, 1994a.

Sashidharan S: The need for community based alternatives to institutional psychiatry. *Share Newsletter* Issue 7. Jan 1994, Kings Fund Centre, 1994b.

Savage J: *Nurses, gender and sexuality*. London, 1987, Heinemann Nursing.

Scheid TL: An investigation of work and unemployment among psychiatric clients. *Int J Health Ser* 23(4):763–782, 1993.

Segal L: *Slow motion. Changing masculinities, changing men*. London, 1990. Virago.

Sheppard M: General practice, social work and mental health sections: The social control of women. *Br J Soc Work* 21:663–683, 1991.

Showalter E: *The female malady*. London, 1987, Virago.

Smart N: *The world's religions*. Cambridge, 1989, Cambridge University Press.

Smith D: *Texts, facts and femininity. Exploring the relationships of ruling*. London, 1990, Routledge.

Social trends, ed 25. Central Statistics Office London, 1995, HMSO.

Soni Raleigh V, Bulusu L, Balarajan R: Suicides among immigrants from the Indian subcontinent. *Br J Psychiatry* 156:46–50, 1990.

Soni Raleigh V, Balarajan R: Suicide and self burning among Indians and West Indians in England and Wales. *Br J Psychiatry* 161:365–368, 1992.

Stokes GA: Transcultural nurse is about. *Senior Nurse* 11(1):40–42, 1991.

Taylor D: Current usage of benzodiazepines in Britain. In: Freeman H, Rue Y, editors: *Benxodiazepines in current clinical practice*. London, 1987, Royal Society of Medicine.

Thornicroft G: Social deprivation and rates of treated mental disorder: developing statistical models to predict psychiatric service utilization. *Br J Psychiatry* 158:474–484, 1991.

Thurtle V: Post-natal depression: the relevance of sociological approaches. *J Adv Nurs* 22(3):416–424, 1995.

Tones K, Tilford S, Robinson Y: *Health education. Effectiveness and efficiency*. London, 1990, Chapman & Hall.

Torkington S: Perspectives in mental health. In: Martin P, editor: *Psychiatric nursing*. Harrow. 1995, Scutari.

Ussher J: *Women's madness: misogyny or mental illness*. London, 1991, Harvester Wheatsheaf.

Ussher J, Nicolson P, editors: *Gender issues in clinical psychology*. London, 1993, Routledge.

Victor C: *Old age in modern society*. London, 1992, Chapman & Hall.

Warr P, Parry G: Paid employment and women's psychological well-being. *Psychol Bull* 91:298–316, 1982.

Westlake L, George SL: Subjective health status of single homeless people in Sheffield. *Public Health* 108(2):111–119, 1994.

Williamson P: Their own worst enemy. *Nurs Times* 29(91):24–22, 1995.

Wilson S, Walker G: Unemployment and health: A review. *Public Health* 107(3):153–162, 1993.

Winefield A, Tiggeman M: Length of unemployment and psychological distress. *Soc Sci Med* 31:461–465, 1990.

FURTHER READING

D'Ardenne P, Mahtani A: *Transcultural counselling in action*. London, 1989, Sage Publications.

> *Focuses on issues in the provision of culturally sensitive counselling, and is illustrated with case examples.*

Darton K, Gorman J, Sayce L: *Eve fights back: The successes of MIND's Stress on Women Campaign*. London, 1994, MIND Publications.

> *Reports on MIND's Stress on Women campaign. Makes recommendations in relation to sexual harassment, gender of key worker, child care and monitoring services and treatment.*

Fernando S: *Mental health, race and culture*. London, 1991, MIND.

> *Explores the influence of racism upon psychiatry and the contruction of mental illness. Draws upon global and non-western perspectives and views of mental health.*

Helman C: *Culture, health and illness*. London, 1990, Butterworth–Heinemann.

> *Examines the impact of cultural factors upon health and illness, including perceptions of causation, explanation and treatment.*

Kareem J, Littlewood R: *Intercultural therapy: Theory and practice*. Oxford, 1992, Blackwell.

> *Identifies issues in psychotherapeutic practice across cultures and explores the theory and technique of intercultural therapy.*

Littlewood R, Lipsedge M: *Aliens and alienists: Ethnic minorities and psychiatry*. Harmondsworth, 1982, Pelican.

> *An analysis of mental illness in Black and minority ethnic groups.*

Pilgrim D, Rogers A: *A sociology of mental health and illness*. Buckingham, 1993, Open University Press.

> *Useful text examining sociological perspectives on mental health and illness. A critical analysis of key issues in race, age and gender is offered.*

Showalter E: *The female malady*. London, 1987, Virago.

> *A critical history of women and mental illness in England 1830–1980. Focuses on patriarchal practices in psychiatry and the ways in which society has shaped feminine norms of behaviour.*

Tones K, Tilford S, Robinson Y: *Health education. Effectiveness and efficiency*, London, 1990, Chapman & Hall.

> *Discusses various approaches to and strategies of health education with an analysis of their effectiveness.*

Ussher J: *Women's madness: Misogyny or mental illness*. London, 1991, Harvester Wheatsheaf.

> *A radical critique of why so many more women than men suffer from depression. Opposing viewpoints are analyzed and a new understanding of womens' mental distress is proposed.*

Ussher J, Nicolson P, editors: *Gender issues in clinical psychology*. London, 1993, Routledge.

> *An edited book containing 10 chapters. The book begins from the premise that clinical psychology has traditionally ignored gender issues. The individual chapters demonstrate the effects of this omission on service users and practitioners. Examples of theory, research and practice which incorporate gender issues are offered.*

• *Chapter* •

The Biological Context of Mental Health Nursing

<table>
<tr><td>

Learning Outcomes

After studying this chapter you should be able to:

- Relate the importance of understanding the structure and function of the brain to mental health nursing practice.

- Describe the neuro-imaging techniques used in psychiatry.

- Discuss the current status of genetic information related to psychiatric illness.

- Appreciate the biological perspectives of mental health problems in general.

- Understand the clinical implications of recent neuroscientific research related to schizophrenia, mood disorders, anxiety disorders and the dementias.

</td><td>

CHAPTER OUTLINE

- *Anatomy of the brain*

- *Neuro-imaging*

- *Neurotransmitters*

- *Genetics and mental illness*

- *Other methods of studying human inheritance*

- *Schizophrenia*

- *Mood disorders*

- *Anxiety states*

- *Dementias*

</td></tr>
</table>

*T*he majority of today's mental health nurses were trained when the study of the brain was advancing slowly, in the way that it had done for many decades. However, in the last 15 years or so, because of new techniques, we have been able to study the brain more effectively and to appreciate many of its complexities. These rapid advances in knowledge have come about through the development of new technologies, for example:
- Advances in the technology of brain imaging, which have led to our ability to see the brain more clearly and to image it continuously while the person is carrying out various functions.
- Advances in molecular biology, which have allowed us to study genetic structure and function.
- Advances in computer technology, which help both biochemical and neuro-imaging research.

The anatomy and physiology of the brain can now be studied from several perspectives and, importantly, the findings can now be integrated with those from psychology and sociology, the human being thereby being revealed in a much broader and holistic light. This is not to say that knowledge of the brain is complete. There are still many mysteries concerning the structure and function of the central nervous system and it will probably be many years before comprehensive and all-embracing knowledge can be claimed.

Mental health nursing in the UK has not kept abreast of developments. Even recent graduates have little knowledge of these advances. This situation is changing with the diploma and degree programmes of Project 2000, which now include more theory. The necessity for nurses to acquire this knowledge is not limited just to issues related to the causation of mental illness. Nurses need to understand the biological bases of mental illness to appreciate the pathology of psychiatric disorders, how medications work and how the benefits and side-effects of such substances arise. Furthermore, it has become clear that the biological abnormalities found in some mental illnesses can have a direct impact on the planning of patient care. For example, we now know that some of the brain abnormalities in schizophrenia can lead to significant problems with attention and memory (Bilder, 1996); some patients can only concentrate for short periods and will take much longer than average to memorize information. The nurse needs to understand how such situations arise and to assess how much of a problem is experienced by the patient. In this the nurse may be able to draw upon the expertise of the clinical psychologist in the team, who has special training in assessment of cognitive functioning. When assessment of attention and memory is complete the nurse is better able to plan care that takes account of particular limitations of the patient. In another area, nurses will need to appreciate advances in biological knowledge to be effective communicators with patients and their families. The general public is becoming much more aware of research findings in medicine. It is therefore likely that, in the future, many more patients and their families increasingly will want and need comprehensive information regarding the nature of mental illnesses. Indeed, in areas such as schizophrenia and Alzheimer's disease educational programmes delivered by nurses have now been running for some years. (Brooker et al., 1994). One obvious benefit of providing information is that increased understanding of the nature of an illness is likely to lead to greater compliance with treatments. As we know (Bebbington, 1995), non-compliance with treatment is a problem in up to 50% of those prescribed neuroleptic medication.

This chapter sets out to help the nurse obtain a general working knowledge of the normal structure and function of the brain and to appreciate the current state of research in brain imaging and the genetics of mental illness. Four groups of mental illnesses will then be examined to appreciate how each of them is influenced by biological factors and to demonstrate the diverse nature of biological influences.

ANATOMY OF THE BRAIN

A sound knowledge of the anatomy of the brain, particularly in the light of some of the research findings which are discussed in this chapter, is essential. The student should review anatomy and physiology textbooks; a brief review of basic structure and function of the brain is shown in Table 7.1.

The brain weighs slightly less than 1.5 kg in the adult and is composed of trillions of cells. In the developing fetus, the brain starts as a simple tube. During pregnancy, this tube folds up, expands and develops. As Table 7.1 shows, different parts of the brain are responsible for different functions. However, one of the biggest mysteries, which has yet to be unravelled, is the precise way that all of the interconnections between various parts work. Networks of nerve cells that connect parts of the brain, function by a process called neurotransmission. Put simply, this transmission process is effected by chemical messengers which initiate, maintain and, at some point, stop our physical and mental functions. These chemical messengers are called neurotransmitters. As Table 7.1 shows, various parts of the brain are particularly relevant to mental disorders, and the principal areas are:

- The cerebral cortex, which is critical in decision making and higher order thinking, such as abstract reasoning.
- The limbic system, which is involved in regulating emotional behaviour, memory and learning.
- The basal ganglia, some of which coordinate movement.
- The hypothalamus, which regulates hormones throughout the body and controls behaviours such as eating, drinking and sex.
- The locus ceruleus, which manufactures the hormone noradrenaline that is centrally involved in the body's response to stress.
- The raphe nuclei, which are made up of serotonin neurones that regulate sleep and are involved in the regulation of behaviour and mood.
- The substantia nigra, which is a collection of dopamine-producing cells involving the control of complex movements, thinking and emotional responses.

NEURO-IMAGING

One of the major problems of research into the causation of mental illness has been the difficulty of studying the brain in life. Until 20 years ago, much of the major research was carried out by post-mortem studies that relied on studying microscopic sections of brain tissue. Some indirect evidence of how the brain functions was gleaned from neurosurgical exploration and from observation of patients after accidental brain injury. One of the classic examples of how observation led to treatment was the case of Phineas Gage, a US railway worker in the 19th Century who suffered a dramatic personality change after he survived a piece of metal being driven into the front of his brain in an accident. This observation, among others, led to a Portuguese psychiatrist, Moniz, introducing the prefrontal lobotomy in 1935. This operation was an attempt to produce 'personality change' in sufferers of mental illness. An account of how brain surgery for mental illness has developed is out of place here but the above illustrates how hit and miss the development of treatments has been. The development of methods that enable the visual study of the brain in life has therefore been of great importance in the expansion of knowledge of the nature of mental illness.

The first major advance in the detailed X-ray examination of the brain was computerized axial tomography (CT or CAT) scanning. Essentially, CT scans are a series of X-ray pictures of different levels of the brain and eventually a number of 'slices' are put together on a computer to give a three-dimensional picture. CT scanning, however, provides a picture of structure only and early scans were often of very poor quality. Further, each scan involves bombarding the patient with a high dose of X-rays (400 times that of a chest X-ray). Newer techniques include magnetic resonance imaging (MRI). In this procedure the patient is placed within a cylindrical machine that generates a magnetic field. Radio waves, which are induced in brain tissues by this field, can be detected and computerized and a clear picture is generated. A great advantage of this procedure is that it avoids the use of radiation. However, MRI scans still provide only a picture of brain

TABLE 7.1 Structure and function of the brain (part 1)

CEREBRUM	Largest portion of the brain. Responsible for conscious perception, thought and motor activity. Governs muscle coordination and the learning of rote movements. Can override most other systems. Divided into two hemispheres, each of which is divided into four lobes.
Dominant hemisphere	Left side is dominant in most people (95% of right handed and more than 50% of left handed people). Responsible for the production and comprehension of language, mathematical ability and the ability to solve problems in a sequential, logical fashion.
Non-dominant hemisphere	Right side is non-dominant in most people. Responsible for musical skills and recognition of faces and tasks requiring comprehension of spatial relationships.
Corpus callosum	Largest fibre bundle in the brain. Connects the two cerebral hemispheres and passes information from one to the other, welding the two hemispheres together into a unitary consciousness, allowing the 'right hand to know what the left hand is doing'.
Cerebral cortex	A few mm thick and about 0.25 m^2 in area . Sheet of grey matter containing 30 billion neurons interconnected by almost 110 x 10^3 m of axons and dendrites. Forms the corrugated surface of the four lobes of the cerebral hemispheres. Connected to various structures of the brain and has a great deal to do with the abilities we think of as uniquely human, such as language and abstract thinking, as well as basic aspects of perception, movement and adaptive response to the outside world. Damage to certain cortical areas usually results in predictable deficits, depending on the area affected.
Frontal lobes	Aid in planning for the future, motivation, control of voluntary motor function and production of speech. Play an important part in emotional experience and expression of mood.
Parietal lobes	Reception and evaluation of most sensory information (excluding smell, hearing and vision).
Central sulcus	Groove or fissure on the surface of the brain that divides the frontal and parietal lobes.
Temporal lobes	Receive and evaluate olfactory and auditory input and play an important role in memory. Associated with brain functions such as abstract thought and judgement.
Lateral fissure	Separates the temporal lobe from the rest of the cerebrum.
Occipital lobes *Clinical Example:*	Reception and integration of visual input. Aphasia, absent or defective speech or comprehension, results from a lesion in the language areas of the cortex. The several types of aphasia correspond to different lesion sites. Damage to Broca's area, which contains the motor programmes for the generation of language, results in expressive, motor aphasia, with difficulty producing either written or spoken words but no difficulty comprehending language. Damage to Wernicke's area, which contains the mechanisms for the formulation of language, results in receptive, or sensory aphasia, where words are produced but their sequence is defective in linguistic content, resulting in paraphasia (word substitution). neologisms (insertion of new and meaningless words) or jargon (fluent but unintelligible speech) and there is a general deficiency in the comprehension of language. If the lesions occurs in the connection between the two areas, conduction aphasia results, in which a person has poor repetition but relatively good comprehension.
DIENCEPHALON	Consists only 2% of the CNS by weight. However, it has extremely widespread and important connections and the great majority of sensory, motor and limbic pathways involve the diencephalon.
Thalamus	Comprises 80% of the diencephalon. All sensory pathways and many other anatomical loops relay in the thalamus. Takes sensory information and relays it to areas throughout the cortex. Influences prefrontal cortical functions such as affect and foresight. Influences mood and general body movements associated with strong emotions, such as fear or rage.

TABLE 7.1 Structure and function of the brain (part 2)

Pineal gland	Endocrine gland involved in reproductive cycles. During darkness it secretes an antigonadotropic hormone called melatonin, which decreases during light, thus increasing gonadal function. Important in mammals with seasonal sexual cycles; its effects in humans are not yet clear, although tumours of the pineal gland affect human sexual development. May also be involved in the sleep–wake cycle.
Hypothalamus	Weighs only 4 g. Major control centre for the pituitary gland, for maintaining homoeostasis and regulating autonomic, endocrine, emotional and somatic functions. Controls various visceral functions and activities involved in basic drives and is very important in a number of functions that have emotional and mood relationships. Directly involved in stress-related and psychosomatic illnesses and with feeding and drinking behaviour, temperature regulation, cardiac function, gut motility and sexual activity. Coordinates sleep–wake cycle responses to other areas of the body. Contains the mamilliary bodies, which are involved in olfactory reflexes and emotional responses to smells.
BRAIN STEM	Connects the spinal cord to the brain. Location of cranial nerve nuclei. Controls automatic body functions such as breathing and cardiovascular activity.
Midbrain	Contains ascending and descending nerve tracks. Visual cortex centre. Part of auditory pathway. Regulates the reflexive movement of the eyes and head. Aids in the unconscious regulation and coordination of motor activities. Contains the part of the basal ganglia, the substantia nigra, that manufactures dopamine.
Pons	Contains ascending and descending nerve tracks. Relay between cerebrum and cerebellum. Reflex centre. Contains the locus ceruleus, which manufactures most of the brain's noradrenaline.
Medulla oblongata	Conduction pathway for ascending and descending nerve tracks. Conscious control of skeletal muscles. Involved in functions such as balance, coordination and modulation of sound impulses from the inner ear centre for several important reflexes: heart rate, breathing, swallowing, vomiting. coughing, sneezing.
Reticular formation	Central core of the brainstem. Controls cyclic activities such as the sleep–wake cycle (called the reticular activating system, or RAS). Plays an important role in arousing and maintaining consciousness, alertness and attention. Contributes to the motor system, respiration, cardiac rhythms and other vital body functions.
Clinical Example:	Damage to the RAS can result in coma. General anaesthetics function by suppressing this system. It may also be the target of many tranquillizers. Ammonia (smelling salts) stimulates the RAS, resulting in an increase in arousal.
BASAL GANGLIA	Several deep, grey matter structures that are related functionally and are located bilaterally in the cerebrum, diencephalon and midbrain. Control muscle tone, activity and posture. Coordinate large muscle movements. Major effect is to inhibit unwanted muscular activity. Cause extrapyramidal syndromes when dysfunctional.
Clinical Example:	Parkinson's disease, characterized by muscular rigidity, a slow shuffling gait and a general lack of movement, is associated with a dysfunction of the basal ganglia, probably a destruction of the dopamine-producing neurone of the substantia nigra (part of the ganglia but located in the midbrain).

TABLE 7.1 Structure and function of the brain (part 3)

· ·

LIMBIC SYSTEM	Forms the limbus, or border of the temporal lobes, and is intimately connected to many other structures of the brain. Concerned both with subjective emotional experiences and with changes in bodily functions associated with emotional states. Particularly involved in aggressive, submissive and sexual behaviour and with pleasure, memory and learning. Associated with mood, motivation and sensations central to preservation.
Clinical Example:	Klüver–Bucy syndrome develops when the entire limbic system is removed or destroyed. Symptoms include fearlessness and placidity (absence of emotional reactions), an inordinate degree of attention to sensory stimuli (ceaseless and instructive curiosity) and visual agnosia (the inability to recognize anything).
Hippocampus	Consolidates recently acquired information about facts and events, somehow turning short-term memory into long-term. Contains large amounts of neurotransmitters.
Clinical Example:	Surgical removal of the hippocampus results in the inability to form new memories of facts and events (names of new acquaintances, day-to-day events, why a task was begun) although long-term memory, intelligence and the ability to learn new skills are unaffected. A similar memory problem is Korsakoff's syndrome in which patients have relatively intact intelligence but cannot form new memories. Patients typically confabulate (make up answers to questions). This syndrome occurs in chronic alcoholism. This is also found in Alzheimer's disease in which the memory loss is profound and there is extensive cellular degeneration in the hippocampus .
Amygdala	Generates emotions from perceptions and thoughts (presumably through its interactions with the hypothalamus and prefrontal cortex). Contains many opiate receptors.
Clinical Example:	Electrical stimulation of the amygdala in animals causes responses of defence, raging aggression or fleeing. In humans, the most common response is fear and its related autonomic responses (dilation of the pupils, increased heart rate and release of adrenaline). Conversely, bilateral destruction of the amygdala causes a great decrease in aggression and animals become tame and placid. This is in effect another kind of memory dysfunction: there is impairment of ability to learn or remember the appropriate emotional and automatic responses to stimuli.
Fornix	Two-way fibre system that connects the hippocampus to the hypothalamus.
CEREBELLUM	'Little brain'. Full range of sensory inputs finds its way here and in turn projects to various sites in the brainstem and thalamus. Although it is extensively involved with the processing of sensory information, it is also part of the motor system and is involved in maintenance of equilibrium and muscle tone and in postural control and coordination of voluntary movements. It is now thought that, because of connections to other brain regions, the cerebellum may be involved in cognitive, behavioural and affective functions.
Clinical Example:	The malnutrition often accompanying chronic alcoholism causes a degeneration of the cerebellar cortex, resulting in the anterior lobe syndrome, in which the legs are primarily affected and the most prominent symptom is a broad-based, staggering gait and a general incoordination, or ataxia, of leg movements.
VENTRICLES	Each cerebral hemisphere contains a relatively large cavity, the lateral ventricle. A smaller midline cavity, the third ventricle, is located in the centre of the diencephalon, between the two halves of the thalamus. The fourth ventricle is in the region of the pons and medulla oblongata and connects with the central canal of the spinal cord, which extends nearly the full length of the spinal cord.
Clinical Example:	Although the clinical significance of these findings is uncertain, imaging techniques have shown enlargement of the ventricles in many psychiatric disorders (e.g. schizophrenia), suggesting an atrophy of many critical structures in the brain.
SPINAL FLUID	Cerebral spinal fluid (CSF) comes from blood choroid plexuses, located in the ventricles and fills the ventricles, subarachnoid space (between the brain and the skull) and the spinal cord. CSF bathes the brain with nutrients, cushions the brain within the skull and exits through the bloodstream. Within the central nervous system, approximately 140 ml of spinal fluid travels from its point of origin to the bloodstream at approximately 1.4 ml per minute.
Clinical Example:	Neurotransmitters and their metabolites can be measured in the CSF, plasma and urine and give an approximation of neurotransmitter production and metabolism in the brain. This provides clues to abnormal neurotransmission in some mental illnesses.
BLOOD–BRAIN AND BLOOD–CSF BARRIERS	Neuronal function requires a microenvironment that is protected from changes elsewhere in the body that may have adverse effects. Blood–brain and blood–CSF barriers protect the CNS in several ways. 1. Large molecules, for example, plasma proteins, present in the blood are excluded from the CSF and nervous tissue. 2. The brain and spinal cord are protected from neurotransmitters in the blood, for example, adrenaline produced by the adrenal gland. 3. Neurotransmitters produced in the CNS are prevented from precipitously leaking into the general circulation. 4. Toxins are excluded either because of their molecular size (too big) or because of their solubility (only substances soluble in water and cell-membrane lipids can pass these barriers) — therefore many drugs are not able to enter the brain and spinal cord.

structure at a specific moment and cannot show blood flow or metabolic patterns. Newer techniques, however, have allowed scientists to study the brain while the person carries out physical and mental tasks. Two of these, positron emission tomography (PET) and single photon-emission tomography (SPET) have been used extensively in research in mental illness. In these techniques, a radioactive isotope is injected into the patient who is then scanned. The scans allow researchers to study blood flow patterns through various parts of the brain, the metabolism of glucose and the activity of various brain chemicals. Much research is now being conducted with these techniques, including study of the brain during tasks such as mental arithmetic calculation and comparing brain activity of patients with mental illnesses with that of normal people.

Brain imaging techniques (Table 7.2) are now being used in conjunction with older methods such as electroencephalography (EEG). Brain electrical activity is recorded while scanning and pictures of function are obtained. Specialized psychological tests (Frith *et al.*, 1991) have also been conducted while imaging takes place. Using these methods in combination with other research techniques obviously provides a more comprehensive picture and allows us to see how thinking processes and symptoms such as delusions and hallucinations relate to both brain structure and brain chemistry. The advances of imaging in studying the working brain are now helping us understand how gross brain structures and their abnormalities relate and thus provide us with a much more integrated picture of structure and function in various illnesses.

ELECTROENCEPHALOGRAPHY

Electroencephalography involves the study of electrical activity in the brain recorded by electrodes placed on various sites over the scalp. Its main application has been in epilepsy to detect the abnormal bursts of electrical activity that can lead to changes in consciousness or to abnormal movements or behaviour. It has also been used to study sleep and other altered states of consciousness. However, its usefulness in research into the common mental illnesses has been very limited.

NEUROTRANSMITTERS

The process of neurotransmission concerns the way in which nerve cells communicate. An understanding of this process is essential for mental health nurses and aids appreciation of the way in which neurotransmission can be disordered in various mental illnesses. Such knowledge will assist the nurse to understand how drug therapies work and how side-effects of such treatments might arise. Neurotransmitter substances are chemical messengers, manufactured in the neurone and released from the axon at the presynaptic cell membrane into the space between the nerve cells (the synapse). The neurotransmitters are then received by the post-synaptic membrane of the dendrite of the next nerve cell at specific receptor sites. This either causes stimulation of the receiving nerve cell (called excitation) or the neurotransmitter preventing the receiving nerve cell from further action (inhibition). Whether

TABLE 7.2 Brain imaging techniques

Technique	How it works	What it images	Advantages/disadvantages
Computed tomography (CT)	Series of X-rays computer constructed into 'slices' of the brain that can be stacked by the computer, giving a three dimensional view.	Brain structure.	Provides clearer pictures of the brain than X-rays alone.
Magnetic resonance imaging (MRI)	A magnetic field surrounding the head induces brain tissues to emit radio waves that are computerized for clear and detailed construction of sectional images of the brain.	Brain structure (newer MRI techniques show brain activity).	Avoids the use of harmful radiation, although MRI can be adapted to use radioactive materials also.
Positron emission tomography (PET)	An injected radioactive substance travels to the brain and shows up as a bright spot on the scan; different substances are taken up by the brain in different amounts depending on the type of tissue and the level of activity.	Brain activity and function.	Allows the injection of labelled drugs for the study of neurotransmitter receptor activity or concentration in the brain.
Single photon emission computer tomography (SPECT)	Similar to PET but uses more stable substances and different detectors to visualize blood flow patterns.	Brain activity and function.	Useful in diagnosing cerebrovascular accidents and brain tumours.

there is excitation or inhibition depends on the original stimulation. Once the process is complete, the neurotransmitters are transported back into the synapse and re-absorbed across the membranes in a process known as re-uptake. The axons are covered by a myelin sheath which insulates the nerve cell. This sheath also acts as a filtering and stabilizing system in its own right, by providing nourishment to the nerve cells in the form of glucose and oxygen. At the same time, it acts as a regulator for neurotransmitters and other important chemicals such as sodium and potassium.

Neurotransmitters are important substances and the discussion below shows that abnormality in amount or action of neurotransmitters is a central feature of many mental illnesses. As Table 7.3 shows, there is an overall understanding of what these substances are, where they are produced and what their function is. Nevertheless, the precise details of their nature and action is still unclear. There are still many possible combinations of these neurotransmitter substances to be researched and therefore there are numerous mysteries yet to be explored and resolved.

GENETICS AND MENTAL ILLNESS

A revolution in the thinking about this subject and human nature itself has occurred in recent years. Currently, world-wide research efforts are in progress to provide a total genetic profile of the human being. In this endeavour, known as the Human Genome Project, researchers in every research-active country in the world are linked in a common effort to define and map every single unit of genetic structure. In theory, this will enable scientists to see how every human characteristic is produced and passed on to the next generation. It is hoped that this understanding will lead to an ability to eradicate many diseases and protect us from processes such as malignancy and infection. There is the probability that genetic treatments will emerge in the next few years and diseases such as cystic fibrosis and muscular dystrophy may soon be treatable with genetic technologies. There is also promising research in developing treatments for various types of cancer and researchers have isolated genes that are responsible for a whole array of conditions. A number of tests are now available that will diagnose genetic disorders in the unborn child (for example, muscular dystrophy). All of this knowledge stems from our ability to work with genes at a molecular level. Research has also been greatly assisted by new computer techniques. Researchers in neuroscience have made substantial progress with disorders such as Alzheimer's disease and Huntington's chorea. However, the picture with schizophrenia, mood disorders and other psychiatric conditions, although optimistic and exciting, is still far from clear (McGuffin *et al.*, 1994). What is emerging is, that, for mental health professionals to understand the nature of mental illness, they need to have a greater appreciation of the science of genetics. However, the education of mental health professionals also needs to integrate this knowledge with findings from different areas. Results of multiple research methods targeting specific questions in genetics, anatomy, biochemistry and psychology, will eventually be drawn together to help in the understanding of how mental illnesses are caused, evolve and are maintained.

Each group of mental illnesses discussed below is the focus for considerable research effort and it may be that the findings in genetics provide the basis for completely new classification systems for mental illness. In these systems, illnesses will probably be classified not only according to their clinical presentation (as is the current case) but also their aetiology. In turn this may involve labelling an illness by the name of the specific gene or group of genes that are involved in causation.

The probability must be considered that, with the isolation of genetic causes for some mental illnesses, mental health nurses may eventually be called upon to provide genetic counselling. In general medicine, nurses are now beginning to assume this role and nurses are working as genetic counsellors in centres where prenatal testing for disorders such as muscular dystrophy is carried out. These nurses work alongside their medical colleagues to supply information and counselling to women and their families who may be faced with distressing dilemmas when considering the risks of giving birth to a child who may have a genetic disorder that may give rise to a lifetime of problems.

OTHER METHODS OF STUDYING HUMAN INHERITANCE

There are a number of ways researchers have studied human inheritance.

TWIN REGISTERS

For many years, several centres in the world have meticulously collected detailed information on twins, both genetically identical and non-identical. Obviously this research provides strong indirect evidence for the genetic causation of various illnesses.

ADOPTION STUDIES

A number of centres have studied biological and adoptive family members to examine the relative importance of developmental and environmental factors in the causation of mental illness. Several high profile studies have examined groups of identical and non-identical twins reared in different family environments. A combination of twin studies and adoption studies provides the strongest indirect evidence for causation.

FAMILY STUDIES

For more than a century, medical researchers have examined family trees to see if some diseases occur more often than expected in families, and data from a variety of sources have been used in studies on familial mental illness. However, such

TABLE 7.3 Neurotransmitters and neuromadulators in the brain

AMINES

Amine neurotransmitters are synthesized from amino molecules such as tyrosine and histidine. Found in various regions of the brain, amines affect learning, emotions, motor control and other activities.

Substance	Location	Effect	Function
Monoamines Noradrenaline (NA)	Derived from tyrosine, a dietary amino acid. Located in the brainstem (particularly the locus ceruleus).	Can be excitatory or inhibitory.	Levels fluctuate with sleep and wakefulness. Plays a role in changes in level of attention and vigilance. Involved in attributing a rewarding value to a stimulus and in the regulation of mood. Plays a role in affective and anxiety disorders. Antidepressants block the re-uptake of NA into the presynaptic cell or inhibit monoamine oxidase from metabolizing it.
Dopamine (DA)	Derived from tyrosine, a dietary amino acid. Located mostly in the brainstem (particularly the substantia nigra).	Generally excitatory.	Involved in the control of complex movements, motivation, cognition and regulating emotional responses. Many drugs of abuse (such as cocaine and amphetamines) cause DA release, suggesting a role in whatever makes things pleasurable. Involved in the movement disorders seen in Parkinson's disease and in many of the deficits seen in schizophrenia and other forms of psychosis. Antipsychotic drugs block dopamine receptors in the post-synaptic cell.
Serotonin (hydroxytryptamine or 5-HT)	Derived from tryptophan, a dietary amino acid. Located only in the brain (particularly in the raphe nuclei of the brainstem).	Mostly inhibitory.	Levels fluctuate with sleep and wakefulness, suggesting a role in arousal and modulation of the general activity levels of the CNS, particularly the onset of sleep. Plays a role in mood and probably in the delusions, hallucinations and withdrawal of schizophrenia. Involved in temperature regulation and the pain control system of the body. LSD (the hallucinogenic drug) acts at 5-HT receptor sites. Plays a role in affective and anxiety disorders. Antidepressants block its reuptake into the presynaptic cell.
Acetylcholine	Synthesized from choline. Located in the brain and spinal cord but is more widespread in the peripheral nervous system, particularly the neuromuscular junction of skeletal muscle.	Can have an excitatory or inhibitory effect.	Plays a role in the sleep–cycle. Signals muscles to become active. Alzheimer's disease is associated with a decrease in acetylcholine-secreting neurons. Myasthenia gravis (weakness of skeletal muscles) results from a reduction in acetylcholine receptors.
Amino acids Glutamate	Found in cells of the body where they are used to synthesize structural and functional proteins. Also found in the CNS where they are stored in synaptic vesicles and used as a neuro-transmitter.	Excitatory.	Overexposure to glutamate can be toxic to neurons and may play a role in brain damage caused by stroke and in some degenerative diseases such as Huntington's disease. Drugs that block glutamate (which are under development) might prevent seizures and neural degeneration from over-excitation.
Gamma-aminobutyric acid (GABA)	A glutamate derivative, most neurons of the CNS have receptors.	Major transmitter for postsynaptic inhibition on the CNS.	Drugs that increase GABA function, such as the benzodiazepines, are used to treat anxiety and to induce sleep.

Peptides

Peptides are chains of amino acids found throughout the body. About 50 have been identified to date but their role as neurotransmitters is not well understood. Although they appear in very low concentrations in the CNS, they are very potent. They also appear to play a 'second messenger' role in neurotransmission; that is, they modulate the message of the nonpeptide neurotransmitters.

Substance	Location	Effect	Function
Endorphins and enkephalins	Widely distributed in the CNS.	Generally inhibitory.	Can reduce pain. The opiates morphine and heroin, bind to endorphin and enkephalin receptors on presynaptic neurons, blocking the release of neurotransmitters and thus reducing pain.
Substance P	Spinal cord, brain and sensory neurons associated with pain.	Generally excitatory.	Found in transmission pathways. Blocking the release of substance P by morphine reduces pain.

studies are difficult to carry out and researchers have often, been forced to to rely on death certificates and medical records, which are often grossly inaccurate.

COMBINATIONS

The above methods are still used in genetic research but are now often combined with molecular genetic technology. These combined efforts are beginning to provide some fascinating findings.

SCHIZOPHRENIA

Schizophrenia is the major consumer of mental health care resources in this and other countries. Many mental health nurses trained when it was fashionable to regard schizophrenia as a manifestation of sociopolitical processes, and views of antipsychiatrists such as Thomas Szasz and R D Laing exerted great influence not only on other psychiatrists but also on a generation of mental health nurses. There are still a few mental health professionals, though decreasing in numbers who argue that schizophrenia is not a biological disorder. Nonetheless, the overwhelming evidence, some of which will be reviewed here, is that schizophrenia is probably a group of brain diseases that have their origins in processes occurring before birth (Gournay, 1996). However, this is not to say that social and psychological factors are unimportant. Indeed, there is also a large amount of evidence that shows that social and psychological factors are major determinants of long-term outcome.

What follows is a summary of knowledge in various areas of biology; some of this is well-proven, some more tentative. While the developments of research in each area are clearly exciting, the major challenge is to draw together all of this new knowledge and provide a comprehensive picture of causation. What seems to be agreed is that schizophrenia is not one but probably a group of disorders, though there may be some common core characteristics in the majority of individual disorders or subtypes. However, this is speculation at present.

IMAGING RESEARCH IN SCHIZOPHRENIA

Earlier studies of imaging research concentrated on clearly identifiable factors such as ventricular size. Van Horne and MacManus (1992) reviewed 39 studies that agreed that ventricular enlargement was a major though not universal finding in schizophrenia research. Since then, more sophisticated scanning techniques have shown abnormalities in many parts of the brain including the temporal lobes, frontal lobes, basal ganglia, thalamus, corpus callosum and hippocampal formation. Research using positron emission tomography (PET) scans has compared people with schizophrenia with 'normal' populations. A number of studies using PET have shown a reduction in glucose metabolism in the frontal area of the brain. Such patients show the so-called negative symptoms such as withdrawal and the blunting of mood and emotion. Imaging research has been taken further by some researchers

who have examined various structural abnormalities in patients and related these to their long-term outcome. At the Hillside Hospital, New York, researchers are studying people with schizophrenia over a number of years from their very first presentation (Lieberman *et al.*, 1993). In a study such as this, research teams can observe a number of different variables such as brain structure, neuropsychological function and symptomatology before and during the months and years of treatment. These researchers have already shown that patients who have obvious structural abnormalities (demonstrated at initial assessment before treatment has commenced) have poorer treatment outcome. Importantly, the findings from this research show clearly that structural and psychological abnormalities are not entirely related to treatment. Previous claims that drug therapy was totally responsible for such abnormal findings were obviously incorrect.

NEUROPSYCHOLOGICAL FINDINGS

Research showing brain structure to be connected with various mental functions is of great importance to mental health nurses. There has been considerable research that has examined the various processes of memory, attention, problem solving and other aspects of thinking by the use of specialized neuropsychological tests. In recent years these neuropsychological examinations have been used in combination with research into the structural problems referred to above. It seems that many people with schizophrenia have marked abnormalities in their thinking processes and that these abnormalities are linked to certain symptom types. For example, the psychologist Chris Frith and his colleagues in London have shown that general problems with memory are linked to negative symptoms and thought disorder (Frith *et al.*, 1991). Other researchers in different parts of the world have shown that small numbers of people with schizophrenia gradually deteriorate in intellectual ability, regardless of whether they receive treatment. Recent research in the USA (Heinrichs and Awad, 1993) has attempted to separate people with schizophrenia into subtypes according to their psychological functioning. These subtypes range from a general dementia, to highly specific defects of problem solving, to no problems whatsoever. This division may be helpful for nurses in care planning (Heinrichs and Awad, 1993). Using this classification, it becomes possible to develop very specific care plans for patients with the severer forms of illness (who have the most widespread problems of thinking, memory and attention). For example, such plans will take into account that these individuals are probably only able to concentrate for a few minutes at a time. Interviews and treatment sessions should be planned to accommodate these difficulties. When information is given to people who suffer these cognitive deficits, it will need to be given repeatedly and in different forms (e.g. verbally and in writing).

GENETIC EVIDENCE FOR SCHIZOPHRENIA

The risk of someone in the general population developing schizophrenia during their lifetime is 1 in 100 (Gottesman, 1991). It has been known for many years that this risk increases to about 1 in 10 for a sibling of someone with schizophrenia and to nearly 1 in 2 for an identical twin. This latter figure obviously points to other, as yet unidentified, factors which are implicated in causation, for if the illness was entirely genetically determined *all* identical twins would be affected. What is also beginning to emerge clearly from genetic research is that some types of schizophrenia run in families and therefore a family tree of such cases will reveal a large number of members affected (Sharma and Murray, 1993). However, in other cases, schizophrenia seems to arise as an isolated phenomenon, thus suggesting, if nothing else, that there are genetically different varieties of this group of illnesses. Recent studies have attempted to localize probable genetic abnormalities to specific chromosomes and work carried out in the UK and Iceland shows that, in some cases at least, chromosome 5 is a likely candidate (Sherington *et al.,* 1988). However, other studies have failed to replicate these findings. This again points to the probability that schizophrenia is a group of disorders and that causative genes may be located in various chromosomes or that there may be combined genetic influences at work (Sasaki and Kennedy, 1995).

Most genetics researchers believe that the basis of schizophrenia lies in faulty development of the brain during pregnancy (i.e. that schizophrenia is a neurodevelopmental disease) and that this developmental problem is caused by an abnormal gene or genes. It also seems likely that in some people this group of genetic factors may combine with others to produce schizophrenia in later life. Another possibility is that genetic factors render the fetus susceptible to problems that may occur at birth (such as cerebral anoxia) or at other periods of pregnancy and that the symptoms result from the neurological damage so produced.

VIRUSES AND SCHIZOPHRENIA

It has been known for some years that there is a greater incidence of schizophrenia in people born in the late winter and early spring. This pattern seems to relate to outbreaks of viral disease, particularly influenza, occurring during the third to sixth month of pregnancy, infection being likely to lead to problems in the development of the central nervous system (Eagles, 1992). Research has shown that, for some as yet unknown reason, female fetuses seem to be vulnerable. This, taken with the evidence that there is likely to be an increased genetic loading in females who develop schizophrenia, indicates a complex relationship between problems with the development of the central nervous system and other factors.

MATERNAL UNDERNUTRITION AND BIRTH INJURY

It is also likely that maternal undernutrition may be important in vulnerability to schizophrenia and, again, research shows that female fetuses are more susceptible. The key time for vulnerability to undernutrition is apparently in the first three months of pregnancy (Susser and Lin, 1992). Other research has shown that birth injury may also be a factor in causation as several studies have shown a statistical link between this and the development of schizophrenia. There are still a number of theories regarding how birth injury may affect the developing brain but one fascinating hypothesis (as stated above) is that birth injuries occur because the fetus is already susceptible in some way and that a period of oxygen starvation, for example, merely enhances an underlying process.

MOOD DISORDERS

Much is known of the biological factors associated with mood disorders, however, one major difficulty is to define what a mood disorder is and how this differs from normal mood variation. There is also a need to distinguish between those mood disorders that are probably predominantly biological in their causation and those that are predominantly produced by psychological or social factors. This is further complicated by theories that suggest that there is already an underlying biological susceptibility in cases where social factors seem to be important contributory causes.

BRAIN IMAGING IN MOOD DISORDERS

Research using brain imaging techniques in mood disorders is not as well developed as similar research on schizophrenia. Various studies have suggested that patients with major mood disorders may have larger ventricles than control populations and that there may be a smaller cortical mass in depressed individuals than in normal controls. Recent studies involving the functional imaging of the brain during various tasks have shown that there are reduced areas of glucose metabolism in the prefrontal cortex during the depressive illness but that these manifestations revert to normal after successful treatment with drugs. In obsessive–compulsive disorders, psychological treatment involving behaviour therapy reverses abnormal findings (Lucey *et al.,* 1995). It would therefore be interesting to examine whether patients with depression receiving cognitive therapy also show these biological changes and whether these changes are similar to those that occur with drug therapy. This goes to the core of some key philosophical issues in psychiatry. Specifically, findings that show that psychological treatment affects brain function open the debate about the reciprocal relationship between thinking processes and biological function. In turn, we need to consider whether we should continue to think of mind and body as separate.

GENETIC AND MOOD DISORDERS

The genetic evidence for bipolar disorder is much stronger than that for schizophrenia. While the lifetime risk of developing bipolar illnesses in the general population is about 0.5%, the risk rises to 1 in 4 for non-identical twins. In virtually all cases, both identical twins will be affected (Slater and Cowie, 1971).

Chromosome research in bipolar illness is more advanced than in schizophrenia. We have known for some years of the strong evidence of single chromosomes being involved in causation. Knowledge comes from epidemiological studies of religious groups in the USA (the Hutterites and Amish). These groups have remained separate from the rest of US society and have tended to intermarry.

A number of groups of research workers from various countries are sharing their data on genetic linkage studies. It is becoming clear that different types of major depressive illness are very different genetically. The so-called schizo-affective disorders have very different causation from the two types of bipolar illness which, in turn, differ from each other. The National Institute of Mental Health Genetics Initiative, in the USA, has developed a sophisticated diagnostic interview to assist with diagnosis and categorization. This sets out to standardize the procedure for classifying patients who enter genetic studies. However, it appears that the clinical picture alone is not a very good reflection of underlying genetic causes. It will undoubtedly be several years before it is fully understand how mood disorders are caused and exactly how the chemical processes of neurotransmission are affected in depression. Only when there is accurate information available about the precise basis of neurotransmission will we be able to confidently develop more sophisticated drug treatments for affective illnesses.

BIOLOGICAL MARKERS OF DEPRESSION

Some years ago, the finding that the adrenal hormone, cortisol, was present in abnormally high levels in depressed patients led some researchers to believe that a simple biological test could be developed to diagnose the condition accurately. In fact such a test was developed (the dexamethasone suppression test). This involves giving the patient a small does of the steroid, dexamethasone. This acts on the pituitary and reduces the production of the adrenocorticotropic hormone which, in turn, reduces adrenalin production for 24 hours. In some depressed patients, this reduction of cortisol production does not occur, reflecting an underlying disturbance of neurotransmitters. The problem with this test is that probably only 50–60% of patients with depression will show a positive result and it cannot therefore be used as a reliable diagnostic tool. Other researchers have tried to identify other biological markers. Thyroid hormone and growth hormone responses have been studied in detail with, as yet, promising but inconclusive outcomes.

NEUROTRANSMITTERS IN DEPRESSION

The accidental discovery of antidepressant drugs nearly 50 years ago led to a number of findings concerning the biochemical abnormalities present in depression. Until just a few years ago, the monoamine oxidase inhibitors and the tricyclic anti-depressants were the mainstay of treatments for depression. The simple central theory underpinning their use was that depression was caused by a shortage of noradrenaline (Gelder *et al.*, 1994). However, in recent years, the vast amount of research undertaken has led to more complex biochemical theories. The general view seems to be that, in depression, there is a problem with the regulation of the overall system of neurotransmitters. Many studies now support the theory that concentrations of serotonin are below normal in mood disorders. The new generation of drugs act by preserving serotonin concentration at normal levels. These are the selective serotonin re-uptake inhibitors of which Prozac (fluoxetine) is the best known example. However, the researchers who developed these drugs were also interested to examine the relationships of serotonin to other neurotransmitter substances and the various salts that form the basic medium of nerve cells. As a result, for example, it has been long known that lithium carbonate can regulate and stabilize mood. Lithium compounds have been used for many years, not only to treat mood disorders but also, prevent episodes of severe mood swing. Overall, there are encouraging results from this simple treatment approach. Many patients who have suffered years of distress from mood swings have found stability by taking small daily doses of a lithium compound. For reasons that are not entirely clear, not all patients benefit from this approach, which demonstrates that depression, like schizophrenia, is a group of illnesses rather than a single entity.

SEASONAL AFFECTIVE DISORDER

In 1984, Rosenthal and his colleagues in the USA published an important paper that defined Seasonal Affective Disorder (Rosenthal *et al.*, 1984). The description of this newly discovered syndrome was based on research stemming from previous observations that some patients developed recurrent depressive disorders at a particular time of the year (usually in autumn or winter). These patients also underwent a change from depression to their normal state, or indeed an upswing of mood into mania or hypomania, at a specific time of year (usually spring). To make a diagnosis of Seasonal Affective Disorder, the clinician needs to ensure that there are no other obvious influences (for example, depression that occurs in workers who may be regularly unemployed during the winter). The original research into this disorder was also supported by the observation that suicide rates were higher in northern countries when winter days were short. Early in the investigation of this condition there was considerable enthusiasm for the belief that artificial light therapy would correct an underlying abnormality of the circadian rhythm. However, as studies have become more rigorous, it has become clear that light therapies are largely ineffective in treatment.

ANXIETY STATES

Although the last Mental Health Nursing Review recommended that mental health nurses refocus their efforts on those with serious and enduring mental health problems, there is still an important continuing need for nurses to be cognisant of both the nature and treatment of anxiety disorders. The UK has led the world in training nurse behaviour therapists. The first course to train nurses as autonomous therapists began at the Maudsley Hospital in 1972. Since then, 200 nurse behaviour therapists have been trained in centres around the UK and it is likely that training in behaviour therapy for nurses and others will expand rapidly over the next few years. It is now recognized that, although there is an obvious need to focus on disorders such as schizophrenia, mental health nurses have a valuable role to play in dealing with the various forms of anxiety states. In future, it may be that specialist mental health nurses have a role as supervisors of practice nurses, other health professionals and non-professionals delivering brief behavioural or cognitive behavioural intervention for anxiety states.

Anxiety states have been thought of as caused by life stresses or acquired by conditioning. We are now beginning to see that anxiety states may indeed be associated with both structural and biochemical abnormalities, and genetic factors may be much more important than was previously assumed. The main anxiety states are as follows:
• Panic disorder.
• Panic disorder with agoraphobia.
• Specific phobias.
• Social phobias.
• Obsessive–compulsive disorder.
• Post-traumatic stress disorder.
• General anxiety disorder.

Detailed discussion of each of these conditions is impossible here. However, what is described below is an account of how biological influences contribute towards the causation and maintenance of various anxiety states and how these biological variables may be important in determining the optimal treatment approach.

IMAGING RESEARCH IN ANXIETY DISORDERS

There are now several studies that show structual and functional abnormalities in imaging of the brains of patients with panic disorder. Some of the earliest studies using CAT or MRI scans showed underdevelopment of the frontal and temporal lobes of people with panic disorder. More recent work has confirmed the presence of abnormalities and studies using functional imaging with single photon-emission computed tomography (SPET) have shown decreased blood flow in the frontal lobes of patients with panic disorder.

In obsessive–compulsive disorders (OCD) the same functional imaging techniques have shown that cortical and sub-cortical regional cerebral blood flow patterns differ between patients with OCD and healthy controls. It is also known that patients with OCD generally have a smaller caudate nucleus than normal controls (Robinson *et al.*, 1995). Although these structural and functional abnormalities have been reported in many studies, researchers are still trying to determine just how they link with the types of symptom that are presented. In the groups

of patients studied, there is a wide variation in measurements of various brain structures with some patients being within a normal range, while others have very abnormal measurements. This is similar to the case with schizophrenia and perhaps indicates that, in terms of brain anatomy, anxiety states may be much more heterogeneous than we have hitherto imagined. As with other research in mental health the results of brain imaging studies must be linked with other research. It is probably safe to say that it may be many years before imaging plays an important part in the diagnosis of these or other psychiatric conditions.

THE GENETICS OF ANXIETY DISORDERS

Familial studies of anxiety disorders have been undertaken for many years. This research consistently shows higher than expected levels of anxiety in relatives of anxiety sufferers. Twin studies show a rate of concordance of up to 50% in anxiety disorders in general. Regarding specific syndromes, evidence is gradually beginning to suggest that panic disorder and agoraphobia share the same genetic causation but are different aetiologically from general anxiety disorders. However, it is also clear from other research that psychosocial factors are important in both the causation and maintenance of these conditions. The contribution of genetic factors is thus very difficult to determine.

There have been several studies examining a possible genetic contribution in obsessive–compulsive disorder. The picture again is one where genetics is not the sole causative factor. Researchers seem to be agreed that obsessive-compulsive disorder may result from the combined affect of both the specific inherited tendency to obsessive–compulsive symptoms and a more general inherited tendency to the broader characteristic of neuroticism (McGuffin *et al.*, 1994).

Despite the very wide prevalence of specific phobias the genetics of these conditions have not been widely researched. However, there are at least two twin studies, one from the register kept at the Maudsley Hospital and one from the National Norwegian twin register (Gottesman, 1991; Shields, 1982), which show higher concordance rates in identical twins compared with non-identical twins. These data, with other familial studies, indicate that there is a genetic contribution to specific fears and phobias although it is also clear that social and psychological factors are involved.

BIOLOGICAL CHANGES IN PANIC DISORDER

For many years it has been known that patients experiencing panic attacks can develop states of hyperventilation which are so severe that they lead to the state of intense muscular spasm known as tetany. When one breathes in excess of bodily requirements the body becomes depleted of carbon dioxide. In turn this leads to an increase in the level of alkalinity of body fluids, which eventually produces a range of physical symptoms including pins and needles, numbness, yawning and sighing and other frightening but essentially harmless symptoms. Eventually the body attempts to deal with the physiological abnormalities produced by over-breathing by suspending respiration, which allows the conservation of carbon dioxide. Thus, the old method of stopping people panicking by having them rebreathe their own air using a paper bag makes physiological sense. Some researchers have shown that patients with high levels of anxiety are in a constant state of mild hyperventilation and suffer symptoms such as pins and needles virtually continuously. However, it now clear that not all patients who panic show this pattern of hyperventilation and some people are more susceptible than others.

DEMENTIAS

There are many varieties of dementia, with many causes, and this discussion will focus on two common types–a comprehensive explanation of all the biological factors associated with all the different types is outwith the scope of this book. Some research findings are discussed and it should be noted that knowledge of these conditions is changing all the time. Mental health nurses must appreciate that biological concepts in dementia frequently need revising.

For many years it has been known that dementias are caused by different underlying processes. Generally, it is considered by researchers that 50% of cases arise from Alzheimer's disease, with about a further 20% attributable to vascular disease and so-called multi-infarct dementia. A further 20% of cases have been assumed to be a mixture of Alzheimer's disease and multi-infarct dementia with the remaining 10% or so of cases arising from a variety of causes including trauma and sundry affects of other physical illness. However, it is now known that approximately 20% of cases of dementia are caused by a newly defined condition called Lewy Body Disease (LBD). This is characterized by the presence of abnormal areas (called Lewy bodies) within the subcortical neurones, which are similar to those found in Parkinson's disease. McKeith and his colleagues (McKeith *et al.*, 1995) have defined the condition, based on the presenting clinical signs and symptoms. They have shown that patients with this disorder have a fluctuating confusion and one or more of the following symptoms:

1. Visual hallucinations.
2. Parkinsonism.
3. Syncopal falls.

These patients are also extremely sensitive to neuroleptic drugs and often develop very severe reactions to traditional tranquillizing medications. These reactions include severe rigidity, postural hypertension, an increase in confusion and on occasion, sudden collapse and a rapid deterioration leading to death. Unlike Alzheimer's disease, where more women than men present with the disorder, LBD is a condition where men present approximately 1.5 times more frequently than women. The survival times of patients suffering LBD are much shorter than in Alzheimer's disease. Patients with Alzheimer's disease will generally live about 5 years from diagnosis, compared with average survival times of only 26 months in LBD.

The discovery of LBD as the second most common cause of dementia has practical implications for treatment. For example, the Committee on the Safety of Medicines now suggests that all patients with a diagnosis of dementia be prescribed neuroleptics with caution and that those with LBD should probably not be prescribed traditional neuroleptics, unless they are given in very low doses. There is some evidence that patients with LBD may respond to the newer atypical anti-psychotics such as risperidone and clozapine. Furthermore, drugs like chlormethiazole may be helpful for the relief of nocturnal symptoms (McKeith *et al.*, 1995)

IMAGING IN ALZHEIMER'S DISEASE

There is now evidence that in the early stages of Alzheimer's disease there are clear abnormalities in ventricular size and that these can be seen clearly on MRI scans. However, during the later stages of the illness, patients show a classic, gross shrinking of the brain tissue. Examination of the brain after death shows that there is an excessive deposit of amyloid protein. These deposits eventually develop, with the result that the brain becomes enmeshed in plaques and tangles. The consequence is extensive changes in the function of the nervous system, as these deposits reduce the function of the synapse. Eventually there is a progressive breakdown of the connections between the various parts of the brain as these neurofibrillary tangles increase. There is also a gradual reduction in the ability to use higher thinking and reasoning and eventually all aspects of memory, judgement and language fail. In the later stages of the disease process, physical immobility occurs because of the involvement of sensory and motor areas of the brain. The disease therefore causes a gross devastation of all psychological and physical functioning and in the worst cases deterioration progresses to the point where the patient exists in a little more than persistent vegetative state.

NEUROTRANSMITTERS IN ALZHEIMER'S DISEASE AND LEWY BODY DEMENTIA

It has been known for some time that patients with Alzheimer's disease have reduced levels of acetylcholine in the brain (Eagger and Harvey, 1995). Over the years research has focused on neurotransmitters, many of which have been implicated in either the causation or the maintenance of the disease. In LBD, research has shown very similar results. Researchers are now beginning to show differences between the two disorders. For example, the sensitivity to neuroleptic medication in LBD may be caused by the loss of neurones in the substantia nigra, in turn leading to a reduction of dopamine. This reduction in dopamine is not enough in itself to be the cause of the physical symptoms of parkinsonism seen in LBD. Neuroleptic drugs given to LBD sufferers cause the D2 receptors to become blocked and dopamine falls to even lower levels. This in turn causes the symptoms of acute rigidity and then the rapid deterioration described above.

PHYSICAL AND MENTAL ASPECTS OF NURSING IN DEMENTIA

Dementias obviously cause profound changes in psychological functioning. Patients also often show severe physical deterioration and loss of basic physical functions. Because of this, the need for physical nursing care is very important. Therefore the mental health nurse who deals with the elderly should be appropriately trained in the nursing care of the physical illnesses which so often accompany these conditions and such nurses need to keep abreast of developments in both the general and mental health areas.

The Mental Health Nursing Review (Department of Health, 1994) suggests that nurses focus on patients with serious and enduring illness but also recognized that there is a clear role for mental health nurses working with the elderly. However, these roles are substantially different to those in illnesses such as schizophrenia. Recent research has shown that mental health nurses can be effectively trained in diagnosing various states of dementia (Spear and Herzberg, 1995). It can therefore be argued that a nurse suitably trained in diagnostic skills could be used in a cost-effective way to assist the screening processes currently carried out by general practitioners. Other research suggests that mental health nurses can have valuable roles assisting the carers of people with dementia by providing them with information to increase their coping skills and thus reduce psychological distress. In general there seems little reason why community mental health nurses should not be trained in similar psychosocial interventions to those of nurses working with the serious mentally ill. However, nurses working with the elderly need to have skills in physical care and the combination of physical and psychological care skills obviously needs very specific attention in nurse educational programmes.

SUMMARY

It is becoming apparent that many psychiatric disorders are caused in part at least by biological variables and it seems clear that the next few years will reveal precise genetic causes or at least partial causes for many common disorders. In addition, it is likely that increasingly sophisticated brain imaging techniques will show structural abnormalities not only in disorders such as Alzheimer's disease and schizophrenia but also in others that for many years have been considered to be primarily psychological.

Various research methods including biochemical investigation and neuropsychological testing will together produce definitive pictures of brain function and thus demonstrate just how mental illnesses are caused and maintained. Gradually therefore, the respective roles of biological, psychological and social processes in causation and maintenance of mental illnesses will become defined. It is likely that the classification of mental illnesses will change in the light of this research. Certainly, the future holds a great deal of promise for the development of drug treatments. In the longer term it is also likely that genetic research will provide treatments for some of the mental illnesses. It is also entirely probable that genetic testing may lead to screening programmes for some of the more devastating illnesses. However, such programmes raise obvious ethical and philosophical problems. For example, how much would the knowledge that one is likely to produce a child who will develop Alzheimer's disease in their 70s influence parents in deciding whether or not to proceed with pregnancy? How does one weigh this knowledge alongside the possibility of many years of happy and productive life before the onset of the disease?

The biological aspects of mental health nursing education have been inadequately addressed in the past. The new knowledge discussed above forms the basis for changes in training that will better inform all therapist–patient contacts.

KEY CONCEPTS

- Mental health nurses need to have a sound knowledge of the anatomy of the brain.
- New techniques in neuro-imaging have allowed scientists to study the brain over a period of time while the patient carries out physical and mental tasks.
- An understanding of neurotransmission is essential to mental health nurses. It enables a better understanding of drug therapies and the side-effects of such treatments.
- The isolation of genetic causes for some mental illnesses means that mental health nurses may well have a future role in genetic counselling.
- There is overwhelming evidence to show that schizophrenia is probably a group of brain diseases which have their origins in processes occurring before birth.
- There is a need to distinguish between those mood disorders that are predominantly biological in their cause and those that are mainly produced by psychological or social factors.
- There is an important continuing need for nurses to be cognisant of both the nature and treatment of anxiety disorders.
- Mental health nurses working with the elderly should be appropriately trained in the nursing care of physical illnesses that often accompany dementias.

REFERENCES

Bebbington PE: The content and context of compliance. *Int Clin Psychopharmacol* 9(5):41–50, 1995.

Bilder R: Neuropsychology and neurophysiology in schizophrenia. *Curr Opin Psychiatry* 9(1):57–62, 1996.

Brooker C, Falloon I, Butterworth A, *et al.*: The outcome of training community psychiatric nurses to deliver psychosocial intervention. *Br J Psychiatry* 165(2):222–230, 1994.

Department of Health: *Working in partnership. The report of mental health nursing review.* London, 1994, HMSO.

Eagger S, Harvey R: Tacrine and other anticholinesterase drugs in dementia. *Curr Opin Psychiatry* 8(4),264–267, 1995.

Eagles JM: Are polio viruses a cause of schizophrenia. *Br J Psychiatry* 160(5): 598–600, 1992.

Frith C, Leary J, Cahill C, *et al.*: Performance on psychological tests: demographic and clinical correlates of the results of these tests. *Br J Psychiatry* 159(13):26–29, 1991.

Gelder M, Gath D, Mayou R: *Concise Oxford textbook of psychiatry.* Oxford, 1994, Oxford Universtity Press.

Gottesman I: *Schizophrenia genesis.* New York, 1991, Genesis.

Gournay K: Schizophrenia: a review of the contemporary literature and implications for mental health nursing theory, practice and education. *J Psychiatr Ment Health Nurs* 3(1):7–12, 1996.

Heinrichs R, Awad A: Neurocognitive subtypes of chronic schizophrenia. *Schizophr Res* 9(1):49–58, 1993.

Lieberman J, Jody D, Geisler S: Time course and biological correlates of treatment response in first episode schizophrenia. *Arch Gen Psychiatry* 50(3):369–376, 1993.

Lucey J, Costa D, Blanes T, *et al.*: Differential correlates with obsessive compulsive and anxious–avoidant dimensions. *Br J Psychiatry* 167(5):629–634, 1995.

McGuffin P, Owen M, O'Donavan M: *Psychiatric genetics.* London, 1994, Gaskell.

McKeith I, Galasko D, Wilcock G, *et al.*: Lewy Body dementia—diagnosis and treatment. *Br J Psychiatry* 167(6):709–717, 1995.

Robinson D, Wu H, Munne R, *et al.*: Reduced candidate nucleus volume in obsessive compulsive disorder. *Archi Gen Psychiatry* 152:393–398, 1995.

Rosenthal N, Sack D, Gillin J: Seasonal affective disorder: A description of the syndrome and preliminary findings with light therapy. *Archi Gen Psychiatry* 41:72–80, 1984.

Sasaki T, Kennedy J: Genetics of psychosis. *Curr Opini Psychiatry* 8(1):25–28, 1995.

Sharma T, Murray R.M: Etiological theories in schizophrenia. *Curr Opini Psychiatry* 7(1):39–423, 1993.

Sherrington R, Brynjolfsson J, Peturrson H: Localization of a susceptibility. Locus for schizophrenia on chromosome 5. *Nature* 336:164–167, 1988.

Shields, J: *Schizophrenia, the epigenetic puzzle.* Cambridge, 1982, Cambridge University Press.

Slater E, Cowie V: *The genetics of mental disorder.* Oxford, 1971, Oxford University Press.

Spear J, Herzberg J: The community psychiatric nurse in the dementia service. *Curr Opini Psychiatry* 8(4):237–239, 1995.

Susser E, Lin S: Schizophrenia after pre-natal exposure to the Dutch hunger winter of 1944–1945, *Arch Gen Psychiatry* 49(7):983–988, 1992.

van Horne J, MacManus I: Ventricular enlargement in schizophrenia. *Br J Psychiatry* 16(5):687–697, 1992.

FURTHER READING

Deakin JFW: Neurobiology of schizophrenia. *Curr Opin Psychiatry* 9(1):50–56, 1996.

> *An excellent overview of brain structure, neurochemistry and brain function in schizophrenia with an wide selection of contemporary research references. It is also helpful as important papers are summarized in an annotated bibliography.*

Fraser A, Molinoff P, Winokur K: *Biological basis of brain function and disease.* New York, 1994, Raven Press.

> *This reference text covers the traditional textbook topics such as neuropsychiatric diseases, neuroimaging and neurosciences but also covers the biological aspects of the majority of psychiatric disorders. Also included are important topics such as the neurobiology of sleep and other areas of interest to nurses. Heavy going in some places, but also stimulating and informative.*

Hollander E, Zohar J, Olivier B: *Current insights in obsessive compulsive disorder.* Chichester, 1994, John Wiley.

> *This book contains a number of important sections concerning biological and pharmacological aspects of obsessive compulsive disorder but is particularly recommended as it integrates an array of different perspectives thereby putting the biological into context.*

McGuffin P, Owen M, O'Donovan N, et al.: *Seminars in Psychiatric Genetics.* London, 1994, Royal College of Psychiatrists.

> *This paperback gives readers from various backgrounds an excellent overview of the current state of molecular genetics. Introductory chapters give anatomical and physiological background and the jargon of genetics is explained. Following chapters cover: schizophrenia affective disorders, neurotic disorders, mental retardation, dementia and other areas.*

Maier, M: Invivo magnetic resonance spectroscopy: applications in psychiatry. *Br J Psychiatry* 167(3):299–305, 1995.

> *This review, although rather technical in places , gives an up-to-date account of nuclear magnetic resonance technology, plus a very helpful reference list.*

Watson S: *Biology of schizophrenia and affective disease.* Washington, 1995, American Psychiatric Press.

> *A truly definitive text which covers all of the major aspects of the biological bases of these two diseases. It is best viewed as a reference text and is certainly not light bedtime reading!*

• Chapter •
8

The Legal and Ethical Context of Mental Health Nursing

Learning Outcomes

After studying this chapter you should be able to:

- Demonstrate an awareness and understanding of the legislative processes that directly affect psychiatric nursing practice.

- Acquire a working knowledge of current mental health law as applicable in England and Wales.

- Examine the implications for practice of the relationship between psychiatry, the law and morality.

- Assist in the development of ethical awareness among mental health nurses by an examination of some of the ethical issues pertaining to practice.

*P*sychiatric nurses work within an increasingly competitive health care environment in which the law has an increasing effect upon the delivery and outcome of mental health practice. Psychiatry and law are inextricably linked. The development of contemporary approaches to the care, treatment and management of mentally disordered individuals is paralleled by developments in civil and criminal legislation. Both psychiatric and legal interventions may be claimed to exist in order to fulfil a societal requirement for authority and control over those who are unable, or decline, to accord with its essential regulations and limitations. Contemporary psychiatric care demands an awareness and appreciation of the manner in which legal issues affect all aspects of practice.

Nurses are increasingly being required to assess the morality of their practice, both by an examination of the potential ethical dilemmas of practice that may arise and, importantly, by maintaining a considered view of the moral context in which mental health care is delivered. Such an 'ethical awareness' is fundamental to effective nursing practice. Most importantly, to be able to ethically justify all aspects of care delivery is essential in a health care setting where potential for allegations of paternalistic and coercive practice is heightened by the nature of clinical contact.

The relationship between the law and morality shows the intrinsic relationship between legal and psychiatric approaches. Although they should not be regarded as mutually constitutive, i.e. 'legal' does not always equate with 'moral', the legal and ethical arenas offer scope for many related issues to be addressed.

The mentally disordered and their families are now using the law to express legitimate grievances and to fight for needed changes in the way psychiatric care is provided. This emphasizes the need for psychiatric nurses to be aware of, and understand, the legal provisions and ethical approaches that relate to their practice. An analysis of legal and ethical issues pertaining to psychiatric nursing practice enables a considered response to perhaps inevitable accusations of psychiatry being coincident with custodial and punitive approaches to care. Furthermore, such awareness enhances the freedom of both nurse and patient and ultimately results in better care for all psychiatric patients.

This chapter will address both legal and ethical aspects of psychiatric nursing. Although law and ethics are covered separately, the inevitable overlap between the two will be evident.

The law, as stated, refers to current legislation in England and Wales. An outline of the relationship between the law and morality, together with a brief examination of a number of potential 'ethical dilemmas', is offered.

PSYCHIATRIC NURSING AND THE LAW

'Nurses are becoming increasingly concerned at the effect of the law on their work' (Young, 1991).

THE NURSE'S STATUTORY ROLE

The Nurses, Midwives and Health Visitors Acts of 1979 and 1992 empowered the United Kingdom Central Council for Nursing, Midwifery and Health Visiting (UKCC) to regulate the nursing, midwifery and health visiting professions. The UKCC maintains the professional register, which contains the names of all those who meet the requirements for registration, and determines the standard for entry to professional education and training. It also investigates allegations of professional misconduct to determine when the right to practise should be removed. The statutory duties of a nurse are established in the UKCC's Code of Conduct (UKCC, 1992) and elaborated and enhanced in a number of UKCC advisory papers.

LITIGATION AND THE NURSE

Working within a consumer-focused health care environment in which the rights of the patient are accorded an increasingly high regard, nurses must be attentive to the legal right of patients to take action against those in whom they have entrusted their care and treatment, when this care and treatment has been perceived to have been harmful.

NEGLIGENCE

The law in England with regard to a *doctor's* duty of care has been clearly established by a number of judgments. The most notable of these is Bolam v Friern Hospital Management Committee (1957) in which a judicial sanction for a 'medical standard' of care was established: 'The Bolam principle may be formulated as a rule that a doctor is not negligent if he acts in accordance with a practice accepted at the time as proper by a responsible body of medical opinion even though other doctors adopt a different practice. In short the law imposes the duty of care; but the standard of care is a matter of medical judgement' (Kennedy and Grubb, 1994).

In contemporary mental health practice with the increasing range of nursing roles and accordant responsibilities, the legal position of a nurse must be regarded like that of a doctor: 'Nurses, as well as doctors, may sometimes make mistakes. All that has been said in relation to doctors applies equally to them. A nurse will be judged in accordance with the standard of skill and carefulness to be expected of a nurse in this position and speciality with this seniority' (Brazier, 1992).

The basis for a claim made in negligence is that (1) the defendant owed a duty of care to the plaintiff and (2) the defendant was in breach of that duty. The onus is then on the plaintiff 'to prove that the defendant's negligence caused his injury' (Mason and McCall–Smith, 1994). Most claims for negligence made against health care staff for what is termed 'medical injury' are brought in tort (a civil wrong). It may be that the patient who makes such a claim will be unable to clearly identify the individual whom they regard as responsible for their injury. In such a case, the patient may have to decide who is responsible from a large number of health care staff from a variety of professional disciplines.

In most cases (in non-contractual NHS settings) the patient will proceed against the employing authority, which has a vicarious liability for any negligence committed by its employees. Claims against staff within non-NHS settings may be different, as the patient directly contracts for the delivery of care and may take direct legal action against either an individual or the hospital or clinic for failure to supply the care contracted for: 'The private nurse should therefore be aware of her contractual position' (Young, 1994). The case of Wilsher v Essex Area Health Authority (1987) focused on the vicarious liability of the health authority.

Nurses have, perhaps, traditionally been perceived as unlikely defendants of accusations of negligence. This accords with the conventional view of the nurse acting under the authority of their employer (or even the doctor) but, within a financially conscious health service in which 'value for money' and an assurance of 'quality' are demanded, nursing can no longer regard itself as being beyond the reach of potentially litigious 'consumers' of their services.

BATTERY AND ASSAULT

'An action in battery arises when the plaintiff has been touched in some way by the defendant and when there has been no consent, express or implied' (Mason and McCall Smith, 1994). The plaintiff does not have to prove that any harm or injury has resulted from the contact. The possibility of an action in battery being taken against a nurse may be regarded as unlikely; it is rarely successful when taken against a doctor. (See Devi v West Midlands Regional Health Authority 1981 for an example of a successful action in battery against a doctor).

Accusations of assault being made against a nurse may be viewed as far likelier. The case of Pountney v Griffiths (1975) offers an example of a judicial response to a private prosecution taken by a patient within Broadmoor Hospital against a male nurse who, the patient claimed, had punched him (the patient) on the shoulder while escorting him from a visit by his family. The case eventually reached the House of Lords where Lord Edmund Davies quoted with approval the words of Lord Widgery CJ in his judgment in the divisional court:

In my judgment where a male nurse is on duty and exercising his function of controlling patients in the hospital, acts done in pursuance of such control or purportedly in pursuance of such control are acts within the scope of Section 141 [Mental Health Act 1959] and are thus protected by the section'.

Following this decision it is difficult to think of any action done in relation to a detained patient which will not be caught by this wide interpretation.

(Dimond and Barker, 1995)

The powers of nurses and other authorized health care staff with regard to conveying or detaining patients under the Mental Health Act 1983 are addressed in Section 137 (2) of the Act which states:

> A constable or any other person required or authorised by or by virtue of this Act to take any person into custody, or to convey or detain any person shall ... have all the powers, authorities, protection and privileges which a constable has within the area for which he acts as a constable.

The implications of Section 137 (2) are perhaps not as far-reaching as might at first appear and do not offer sanction to staff acting in an overtly controlling manner: 'It would be surprising if the intention behind Section 137 (2) of the Mental Health Act 1983 was to provide the full range of police powers to hospital staff' (Gunn, 1992).

Potential accusations of negligence or assault or the (less likely) potential for accusations of battery should not imply that nurses need adopt defensive practice strategies, but rather, an awareness of nurses' legal responsibilities and the legal position of the patient must inform their practice. The circumstances in which a psychiatric nurse may face accusations of negligence and the precautions that can be taken to ensure that such accusations are unfounded, should be appreciated.

THE LAW

'The law provides an essential framework for the care of those with a mental disorder – probably more than in any other area of health and social care' (Department of Health and Welsh Office (DoH & WO), 1993).

THE COURTS

If an offence is alleged to have been committed, following a decision to prosecute (usually taken by the Crown Prosecution Service) the case will initially be decided within one of two courts of law.

Magistrates' Court

There are two types of magistrates. The commonest is the lay person who has been accepted as a Justice of the Peace, to sit (generally with two others) in a magistrates' court. Their task is to hear the evidence, in the case of summary offences, decide the question of guilt and sentence the offender when found guilty. The other sort of magistrate is the paid professional lawyer who may sit alone and is

known as the stipendiary magistrate. Stipendiary magistrates are only employed in metropolitan areas.

(Faulk, 1994).

Much of the legislative work required of current mental health law may be dealt with by the magistrates' court. In the case of an indictable offence (i.e. one which renders the individual committing it liable to be charged with a crime) the magistrate, after hearing the evidence, must decide whether to deal with the case (within the magistrate's powers) or to commit the defendant to a Crown Court.

Crown Court

In a Crown Court, the case (both for the prosecution and defence) is argued by barristers and guilt is decided by a jury. A judge presides over the court and ensures that the proceedings adhere to the law. Certain Sections of the Mental Health Act can only be applied by a Crown Court (see below).

MENTAL HEALTH LEGISLATION

All clinical practice may be regarded as having concomitant legal requirements. An understanding of both previous and contemporary legislation will assist nurses' awareness and application of practices governed and influenced by legal processes.

HISTORY

Legislation on admission to mental hospitals and the treatment of the mentally ill within them was established by the Lunacy Act of 1890. Patients entered mental hospitals via the court process with its associated bureaucracy and the stigma of being seen publicly as a 'mental patient'.

The Mental Treatment Act 1930 permitted the admission of some patients to psychiatric hospitals without the requirement that they first be 'certified'. The delivery of mental health care in England and Wales was radically reformed by the Mental Health Act 1959. The principal aim of this Act was to reduce the numbers of mentally ill patients in institutions and to introduce the concept of 'informal' (voluntary) admissions to mental health care. The Act reflected a recognition of the unfortunate position to which historical and socially pejorative policies had condemned many mentally ill patients and was regarded as a major advancement in mental health care: 'The impetus of the Act was doubtlessly economic, but it also took account of and embodied the dissatisfaction which had been mounting for years amongst those concerned with the plight of the mentally ill' (Nolan, 1993).

The Mental Health Act 1959 referred to four main groups of mental disorders:
1. Mental illness.
2. Subnormality.
3. Severe subnormality.
4. Psychopathic disorder.

The Act reflected a contemporary medical approach to mental illness and its management rather than the social and legal perception of the needs of the mentally ill that had been the basis of previous legislation. Nonetheless, it maintained the requirement for legal intervention in the care and management of some mentally disordered patients. English and Welsh mental health law received a thorough revision with the emergence of the 1983 Mental Health Act which repealed all existing mental health legislation.

The reader now should be in a position to assess the impact of mental health legislation on the care and management of mentally disordered individuals.

THE MENTAL HEALTH ACT 1983

The information that follows is derived from:
1. The 1983 Act itself.
2. The *Code of Practice: Mental Health Act 1983* (DoH & WO, 1993).
3. The *Mental Health Act 1983 Guidelines* (Bethlem and Maudsley NHS Trust, 1994).

The Mental Health Act 1983 (hereafter referred to as the 'Act') is the legislation governing the formal detention and care of mentally disordered people in hospital. An accurate under-standing of the Act is essential for complying with its associated legal responsibilities. A sound knowledge of the most commonly used detention orders, patient rights and the Code of Practice is essential for high standards of care and good professional practice. (The 1959 Mental Health Act was repealed in 1983 and the current Act came into force on the 30th of September, 1983).

CONTENTS OF THE ACT
The Act identifies four categories of mental disorder.

Mental illness
The Act does not define 'mental illness' and leaves this as 'a matter for clinical judgement'. The mental illness should be of a nature or degree to warrant the detention of the patient in the interests of his or her health or safety or for the protection of others.

Mental impairment
Mental impairment means 'a state of arrested or incomplete development of mind (not amounting to severe mental impair-ment) which includes significant impairment of intelligence and social functioning and is associated with abnormally aggressive or seriously irresponsible conduct'.

Severe mental impairment
Severe mental impairment means' a state of arrested or incom-plete development of mind which includes severe impairment of intelligence and social functioning and is associated with abnormally aggressive or seriously irresponsible conduct'.

Psychopathic disorder
Psychopathic disorder means 'a persistent disorder or disability of mind (whether or not including significant impairment of intelligence) which results in abnormally or seriously irresponsible conduct'.

A person may not be dealt with under the Act as suffering from mental disorder by reason only of promiscuity or other immoral conduct, sexual deviancy or dependence on alcohol or drugs.

The Act is divided into 10 parts, the principal parts being: Part II—Compulsory Admission to Hospital, Part III–Patients Concerned with Criminal Proceedings and Part IV–Consent to treatment. Each part of the Act is further split into numbered paragraphs or groups of paragraphs. These paragraphs have become known as 'sections'. Patients held under the Act are compulsorily detained.

PART II – COMPULSORY ADMISSION TO HOSPITAL
The legal implications of nursing the mentally disordered patient are most clearly demonstrated when the patient is compulsorily admitted and detained under the provisions of the Act. 'Psychiatry is the only medical discipline which has special legal powers to detain and treat people against their will' (Cope, 1995). The process of psychiatric detention may originate in a court of law, in the community or in a hospital setting.
A patient may (DoH & WO, 1993) be compulsorily admitted under the Act where this is necessary:
• in the interests of his or her own health, or
• in the interests of his or her own safety, or
• for the protection of other people.

Section 2—Admission for Assessment
This allows for compulsory admission and detention for up to 28 days for assessment or assessment followed by treatment for mental disorder. The period of detention is not renewable and if continued detention is required it may be followed by a Section 3 application (see below).

Grounds for admission or detention
These apply where the patient is suffering from a mental disorder of a nature or degree that warrants detention in hospital for assessment for at least a limited period and he or she should be detained in hospital in the interests of his or her own health or safety or with a view to the protection of other persons.

Application
The applicant (nearest relative or Approved Social Worker) must have seen the patient personally within the past 14 days. The application must also be supported by two registered medical practitioners, one of whom must be qualified in psychiatry and be approved for this purpose under Section 12 (2). One of the doctors should (if practicable) have had previous acquaintance with the patient. The applicant is

responsible for ensuring the patient gets to hospital although this responsibility may be delegated to others (for example, ambulance staff). Patients must be informed of their legal position and rights and may apply to have their case reviewed by a Mental Health Review Tribunal (see below) during the first 14 days of detention.

Treatment

The patient's consent to treatment should be obtained whenever possible. However, under the Act doctors may treat mentally disordered patients with medication for mental disorder for 3 months with or without consent. (See Part IV of the Act below.)

Applications for discharge

The patient may be discharged from detention by the responsible medical officer (RMO), the nearest relative, the Managers (see below) and the Mental Health Review Tribunal.

Appeals by patients

A patient detained under Section 2 can apply to the Managers or to the Mental Health Review Tribunal for discharge. If the patient applies to the Mental Health Review Tribunal he or she must do so within the first 14 days of detention.

Section 3 — Admission for Treatment

Allows compulsory detention for up to 6 months for treatment and is renewable in the first instance for 6 months, then subsequently for periods of 1 year.

Grounds for admission or detention

The patient is suffering from mental illness, mental impairment, severe mental impairment or psychopathic disorder (a patient who is suffering from any other disorder or disability of mind cannot be detained for treatment under this order) *and* the mental disorder is of a nature or degree that makes it appropriate for the patient to receive such treatment in hospital *and* it is necessary in the interests of the patient's health or safety or for the protection of others that he or she should receive such treatment and it cannot be provided unless he or she is detained *and*, for a patient suffering from psychopathic disorder or mental impairment, there is an additional condition that medical treatment is likely to alleviate, or prevent a deterioration in, his or her condition.

Application

The applicant (nearest relative or Approved Social Worker) must have seen the patient within 14 days. If the applicant is an Approved Social Worker, every effort must be made to contact the nearest relative before completing the application. If the nearest relative objects to the detention the Approved Social Worker cannot proceed. However, any unreasonable objection by the relative may be grounds for the County Court to transfer the powers of the nearest relative to another person, who becomes 'acting nearest relative'. Two medical recommendations are required (see Section 2).

Treatment

Medication for mental disorder can be given to a patient on Section 3 for 3 months with or without their consent. (See Part IV of the Act below.)

Applications for discharge

The patient may be discharged from detention by the RMO, the nearest relative, the Managers or the Mental Health Review Tribunal.

Appeals by patients

A patient under Section 3 can make an application to the Managers as often as he or she likes in every period of detention. The patient can apply to the Mental Health Review Tribunal once in every period of detention–in the first 6 months and again in the second 6 months if renewed.

It is often the case that a patient will apply to both the Managers and the Mental Health Review Tribunal for discharge from detention. The Managers and the Tribunal will each hear the patient's appeal. If the Managers hear an appeal and refuse to discharge, the patient will automatically be reminded of the right of appeal to a Mental Health Review Tribunal, if he or she has not already done so.

Section 4 – Emergency Admission for Assessment

This allows for compulsory admission and detention for up to 72 hours for assessment. It is designed for emergencies in the community when those involved cannot cope with the mental state of the patient and need to admit him or her to hospital. The order is used under urgent necessity with the clear intention that an immediate Section 2 will be arranged once the patient is in hospital. It is not to be used for patients already detained in hospital. (See Section 5(2) below.)

Grounds for admission or detention

There is urgent necessity for the admission of a person to hospital for assessment. It should only be used where the delay in waiting for a second opinion for a Section 2 would be undesirable because of the serious nature of the patient's current illness and ability to cope in the community setting.

Application

The applicant (nearest relative or Approved Social Worker) must state that it is of urgent necessity that the patient is admitted for assessment and that compliance with normal procedure would involve unreasonable delay. The applicant must have seen the patient in the previous 24 hours. One medical recommendation is required by a doctor, who must have seen the patient within the previous 24 hours. It is preferable that the doctor making the recommendation has had previous acquaintance with the patient.

Treatment

Section 4 patients are, for the purposes of Consent to Treatment (see below) in the same position as informal patients and Common Law rules apply. Therefore treatment can only be given with the patient's consent or under a Common Law emergency situation.

Applications for discharge

Only the patient's RMO can discharge the patient. There are no rights of appeal by the patient or the nearest relative against an order of such short duration.

Appeals by patients

There are no appeal rights. For the sake of good practice it should be noted that Section 4 should only be used if there is *serious intent* for the patient to be placed on a Section 2 order. Arrangements for obtaining the second medical opinion should be initiated immediately.

Section 5 (2) — Doctor's Holding Power (Report on a Hospital In-patient)

This section permits the detention of an informal in-patient for up to 72 hours to allow a doctor to make an application for admission under Section 2 or 3.

Grounds for admission or detention

A mentally disordered patient is already receiving treatment in hospital as an informal patient and wishes to leave the hospital before there is time to complete a Section 2 or Section 3 assessment.

Application

The doctor in charge of the patient's care completes a Form 12. One medical recommendation is required, which does not have to be made by a Section 12 (2) approved doctor.

Treatment

The patient is not subject to Consent to Treatment provisions and therefore retains his Common Law right to refuse treatment.

Applications for discharge

Only the patient's RMO can discharge the patient. Any patient detained under Section 5 (2) should be discharged immediately if:

1. An assessment for Section 2 or 3 is carried out and the decision is made not to make an application.
2. The decision is taken that no assessment for Section 2 or 3 is needed.

Appeals by patients

No appeals are possible. It is considered to be bad medical practice to use Section 5 (2) more than once on the same patient within a short space of time. The intentions should be to place the patient on a Section 2 or 3 order.

Section 5 (4) — The Nurse's Holding Power

This allows a Registered Nurse (see Box 8.1) to detain an informal patient, who is already being treated for mental disorder, for up to 6 hours. When reading the following, you should consider the circumstances when Section 5 (4) might be invoked, whether it is an appropriate nursing intervention and how applying it might affect the nurse–patient relationship.

Grounds for detention

These apply where the patient is suffering from a mental disorder to a degree that makes it necessary for his health or safety, or for the protection of others, for him or her to be immediately restrained from leaving hospital. It can only be used if the patient is indicating either verbally or otherwise that he or she wishes to leave the hospital *and* it is not practicable to obtain a doctor to furnish a report under Section 5 (2).

Application

The holding power begins after the nurse has recorded his or her opinion on Form 13 and ends either 6 hours later or on the arrival of a doctor to make a report under Section 5 (2). The nurse must be on the professional register of the UKCC in:

Box 8.1

Using Section 5(4)

Before using the powers of Section 5(4) the nurse should assess:

- The likely arrival time of the doctor as against the likely intention of the patient to leave. Most patients who express a wish to leave hospital can be persuaded to wait until a doctor arrives to discuss it further. Where this is not possible the nurse must try to predict the impact of any delay upon the patient.

- The consequences of a patient leaving hospital immediately and the harm that might occur to the patient or other, taking into account:
  – what the patient says he or she will do;
  – the likelihood of the patient committing suicide;
  – the patient's current behaviour and in particular any changes in usual behaviour;
  – the likelihood of the patient behaving in a violent manner;
  – any recently received messages from relatives or friends;
  – any recent disturbance on the ward (which may or may not involve the patient);
  – any relevant involvement of other patients.

- The patient's known unpredictability and any other relevant information from other members of the multidisciplinary team.

(Bethlem and Maudsley NHS Trust, 1994)

- Part 3–First level nurse trained in the nursing of persons suffering from mental illness.
- Part 5–First level nurse trained in the nursing of persons suffering from mental handicap.
- Part 13–First level nurse trained in mental health nursing.
- Part 14–First level nurse trained in mental handicap nursing.

Treatment
Treatment can take place only with the patient's consent or under Common Law

Application for discharge
Not applicable.

Appeals by patients
Not applicable. From Code of Practice, Mental Health Act 1983:

PART III–PATIENTS CONCERNED WITH CRIMINAL PROCEEDINGS
Part III of the Act describes the application of mental health legislation to those who have involvement with the criminal justice process. Such individuals are commonly termed 'Mentally disordered offenders' and their care management is frequently the responsibility of Forensic Mental Health Services.

Section 35–Remand to Hospital for Report on Mental Condition
This provides for detention for a maximum period of 28 days and for further periods of 28 days to 12 weeks maximum.

Grounds for detention
These are, to prepare a report on the person's mental condition. The order is an alternative to remanding a person in custody for a medical report in circumstances where it would not be practicable to obtain the report if he or she were remanded on bail.

Application
In the Crown Court this can apply to any person awaiting trial for an offence punishable with imprisonment or who is at any stage of such a trial prior to sentence. In the Magistrates' Court, it applies to any person convicted of an offence punishable on summary conviction with imprisonment but before sentencing *or* charged with such an offence (if the court is satisfied that he or she did the act or made the omission charged) *or* if he or she has consented to the exercise of the power. The court must be satisfied on the written or oral evidence of a registered medical practitioner (Section 12 approved) that there is reason to suspect that the accused person is suffering from mental illness, mental impairment, severe mental impairment or psychopathic disorder. The patient must be admitted to hospital within 7 days of the date of remand.

Treatment
The patient is not subject to Consent to Treatment provisions and therefore retains the Common Law right to refuse treatment. The outcome of an assessment under Section 35 will be either (1) the person is suffering from a mental disorder that makes it appropriate for him or her to be detained in hospital for medical treatment or (2) the person is not so suffering. In the case of (1) the medical reports should be accompanied by two medical recommendations to enable a Section 37 order to be imposed (see below). In the case of (2) the person can be dealt with under normal court powers.

Applications for discharge
The court may terminate the remand at any time.

Appeals by patients
A patient detained under Section 35 can commission an independent psychiatric report at their own expense and apply to the court for their remand to be terminated.

Extension of Section 35
Further periods of remand (after the first 28 days) may only take place if it appears to the court on the oral or written evidence of the registered medical practitioner that this is necessary for completion of the assessment.

Section 36—Remand to Hospital for Treatment
This provides for the detention of an individual in hospital for a maximum of 28 days, with further periods of 28 days for not more than 12 weeks in all.

Grounds for detention
To remand to hospital for medical treatment. This is an alternative to the Home Secretary's power under Section 48 (see below) to transfer unsentenced prisoners to hospital in an emergency. It is not necessary to establish a link between the person's assessed mental disorder and the alleged offence.

Application
In the Crown Court, this applies to any person who is in custody, awaiting trial before the court for an offence punishable with imprisonment or who is in custody at any stage of such a trial prior to sentence. The court must be satisfied on the written or oral evidence of two registered medical practitioners (one of whom must be Section 12 approved) that the person is suffering from mental illness or severe mental impairment of a nature or degree that makes it appropriate for him or her to be detained in hospital for medical treatment.

Treatment
The patient is subject to the Consent to Treatment provisions of the Act (see below).

Applications for discharge
The court may terminate the order at any time.

Appeals by patients
A patient detained under Section 36 can commission an independent psychiatric report at their own expense and can apply to the court for the remand to be terminated on the basis of the report.

Extension of Section 36
Further periods of remand depend simply on the written or oral evidence from the registered medical practitioner to the court that such a further remand is warranted.

Section 37—Hospital Order
Directs the admission of a patient to a named hospital, that has consented to admit the patient, for an initial period of up to 6 months with a first renewal period of 6 months and subsequent renewal periods of 1 year.

Grounds for detention
The offender is suffering from mental illness, mental impairment, severe mental impairment or psychopathic disorder *and* the disorder is of a nature that makes it appropriate for him or her to be detained in hospital for treatment *and* in the case of a patient suffering from psychopathic disorder, or mental impairment, such treatment is likely to alleviate or prevent deterioration of his or her condition. The court must be satisfied that, having regard to all the circumstances, a Hospital Order is the most suitable method for dealing with the case.

Application
This can be applied by a Crown Court or a Magistrates' Court. Section 37 is an alternative to a penal disposal for offenders who are found to be suffering from mental disorder when sentenced. No causal relationship has to be established between the offender's mental disorder and their criminal activities. The court must be satisfied on the written or oral evidence of two registered medical practitioners (one of whom must be Section 12 approved and one of whom must be from the admitting hospital). The patient does not have to be at court when the order is made but their legal representative must be present. The court must be satisfied that the patient will be admitted to the hospital within 28 days of the date of the order.

Treatment
The treatment rules are the same as for Section 3. The 3-month treatment period begins from the date when the patient is admitted to hospital and not from the date of the Court Order itself as courts and prisons are not covered by the Consent to Treatment rules of the Act.

Applications for discharge
The patient may be discharged from detention by the RMO, the Managers or a Mental Health Review Tribunal. Mental Health Review Tribunal appeals can only be accepted during the second 6 months of detention since the case will have been examined at the outset by the courts. The nearest relative can apply to the Mental Health Review Tribunal, but only during the second 6 months of detention. The nearest relative does not have the power to order discharge.

Appeals by patients
A patient detained under Section 37 can appeal to the Managers as often as he or she likes. An appeal can also be made to the Mental Health Review Tribunal. The patient can appeal against the order to a court within 21 days of the order being made. The appeal would be to a Crown Court if a Magistrates' Court made the original order and to the Court of Appeal if the Crown Court made the order.

Section 38—Interim Hospital Order
This order provides for the detention of an individual for an initial period of 12 weeks maximum, with further periods of 28 days at a time, but no more than 6 months in all. When a person is convicted by a court, but not yet sentenced, the court may make this order to assess the patient for mental disorder. This is done to determine whether the patient should be sentenced to hospital. Section 38 is used to evaluate the person's response to hospital treatment, without any irrevocable commitment (on either side) to this method of dealing with the person should it prove unsuitable.

Grounds for detention
The grounds for detention are that the person is suffering from mental illness, mental impairment, severe mental impairment or psychopathic disorder *and* there is reason to suppose that the mental disorder is such that it may be appropriate for a Section 37 to be made *and* the court is satisfied on the evidence of the registered medical practitioner who would be in charge of the person's treatment that the patient will be admitted to hospital within 28 days of the order.

Application
As with Section 37; however, a Magistrates' Court cannot make an interim hospital order in respect of an unconvicted person. The court must be satisfied on the written or oral evidence of two registered medical practitioners (one of whom must be Section 12 approved and one of whom must be from the admitting hospital).

Treatment
The patient may be treated for mental disorder with or without his or her consent and is therefore subject to the Consent to Treatment provisions (see below).

Applications for discharge
Only the court can discharge.

Appeals by patients

As a Section 38 order is a form of sentence the patient can appeal against it to the Crown Court or Court of Appeal (not to Managers or the Mental Health Review Tribunal).

Section 41—Order Restricting Discharge

When a Hospital Order (Section 37) is made, an order restricting discharge may be made under Section 41. Therefore, a Hospital Order with an accompanying 'Restriction Order' will be recorded as Section 37/41. Restriction Orders are applied for for more serious persistent offenders; the Home Office is responsible for granting leave and allowing discharge (except for discharge via a Mental Health Review Tribunal).

Grounds for restriction

The court must be satisfied, having regard to the nature of the offence, past record of the offender and the risk of further offences, that a Restriction Order is necessary for the protection of the public.

Application

Only Crown Courts can make a Restriction Order. A Magistrates' Court may commit an offender to the Crown Court with a view to a Restriction Order being made. Section 41 directs the admission of a patient to a named hospital (which has consented to the patient's admission) on specific restrictions, which may be without limit of time or for a specific period. Admission must take place within 28 days of the court order. The court requires that at least one of the registered medical practitioners gives evidence to the court verbally.

Treatment

As with Section 37, the 3-month treatment period begins when the patient is admitted to hospital.

Leave

The restrictions do not allow the RMO to grant leave or transfer the patient without the consent of the Home Secretary. Requests for leave of absence, transfer or discharge must be made to the Home Office by the RMO.

The granting of leave within the hospital grounds does not require the Home Secretary's consent. Any leave beyond the hospital grounds requires the prior consent of the Home Secretary.

Applications for discharge

The nearest relative cannot order the patient's discharge, nor can they apply to a Mental Health Review Tribunal.

Appeals by patients

A patient can apply to a Mental Health Review Tribunal during the second 6-month period of detention and, subsequently, on a yearly basis. A patient cannot be discharged from the Restriction Order by the RMO or the Managers without the consent of the Home Secretary.

Conditionally discharged patients

Most Section 37/41 patients who are discharged by the Home Office or Mental Health Review Tribunal are 'conditionally discharged', which means that the Section 41 remains in place. Such patients normally have discharge conditions set by the Home Office (such as seeing their consultant psychiatrist or social supervisor regularly). If these conditions are broken the Section 41 enables the patient to be recalled by the Home Office to hospital, where the patient then reverts to detention under the Section 37/41 order.

Conditionally discharged restricted patients (Section 41 only) may apply to a Mental Health Review Tribunal 12 months after their conditional discharge, and every 2 years thereafter, for an absolute discharge. Patients under Section 41 can be admitted informally to hospital for psychiatric treatment without the need for recall being required.

Section 47–Transfer to Hospital of Prisoners (Transfer Direction)

The Home Secretary directs the transfer of a prisoner suffering from mental disorder to a named hospital which has consented to take the prisoner. The Home Secretary normally applies special restrictions (Section 49; see below) to the Direction and the following Section 47/49 details relate to such orders. The Home Secretary can at any time order the person back to prison.

Grounds for detention

The Home Secretary must be satisfied that:
1. the prisoner is suffering from mental illness, psychopathic disorder, mental impairment or severe mental impairment *and*
2. the nature or degree of that disorder makes it appropriate for the prisoner to be detained in a hospital for treatment and, in the case of psychopathic disorder or mental impairment, that such treatment is likely to alleviate or prevent deterioration of the prisoners' condition.

Admission to the specified hospital must be within 14 days of the transfer direction. The order ceases after this period if admission to hospital does not take place. Section 47 requires two recommendations from registered medical practitioners (one of whom must be Section 12 approved).

Treatment

Consent to Treatment rules apply.

Applications for discharge

The nearest relative cannot order the patient's discharge or apply to a Mental Health Review Tribunal.

Appeals by patients

The patient can apply to the Mental Health Review Tribunal the Transfer Direction is made and subsequently at yearly intervals.

Section 48–Removal to Hospital of Other Prisoners (Unsentenced Prisoners)

The criteria used by the Home Secretary for transfers of unsentenced prisoners to hospital are the same as for Section 47 except that 'The prisoner is in urgent need of such treatment'.

Grounds for detention
The Home Secretary must be satisfied that:
1. the person is suffering from mental illness or severe mental impairment (only) *and*
2. the mental disorder is of a nature or degree appropriate for the person to be detained in hospital for treatment *and*
3. the person is in urgent need of such treatment.

A Restriction Direction (Section 48 plus Section 49 Restriction; see below) must be made by the Home Secretary for people detained in a prison or remand centre.

On return to court for final sentencing the order will cease to have effect and would be replaced by a Section 37 or 37/41 if appropriate or another decision, such as sentencing to prison.

Section 49–Restriction on Discharge of Prisoners Removed to Hospital (Restriction Direction)

This section has the same effect as a Restriction Order given under Section 41. If the patient is subject to a fixed term sentence and is still in hospital at the time the sentence would have ended, the detaining order changes from Section 47/49 to a 'notional' Section 37 which begins on the expiry of the Restriction Direction.

Restriction may be terminated at any time by the Home Secretary. The patient may also be discharged from hospital with the consent of the Home Secretary.

Leave of Absence for Restricted Patients–Sections 37/41, 47/49 and 48/49

The RMO must decide on the degree of supervision of the restricted patient within the hospital grounds. Any leave outside the hospital, transfer to another hospital or transfer to another unit within the same hospital requires the Home Secretary's consent. If the patient needs to go to another hospital for urgent medical treatment the Home Secretary's consent can be assumed on the understanding that the patient is escorted to and from the hospital and that adequate steps are taken to minimize the risk of absconding. The Home Office should be notified of such movements to other hospitals and when the patient returns. In the event of the patient's escape from hospital or failure to return from leave, the local police and the Home Office should be informed immediately.

Section 136—The Police Power to Remove to a Place of Safety

This section authorizes a police officer who finds a person who appears to be suffering from a mental disorder in a place to which the public has access, to remove him or her to a place of safety. The police officer may do so if:
1. the person appears to be in immediate need of care and control *and*
2. the police officer thinks it is necessary to do so in the person's interest or for the protection of other persons.

A person removed to a place of safety under this order may be detained there for a period not exceeding 72 hours for him or her to be examined by a registered medical practitioner and to be interviewed by an Approved Social Worker and for arrangements to be made for care and treatment. The Consent to Treatment provisions do not apply to this part of the Act.

PART IV—CONSENT TO TREATMENT

As a general rule, patients on long-term detention orders can be treated for mental disorder for 3 months with or without their consent. This means treatment for mental disorder only. Treatment for physical illness is completely excluded from this and comes under Common Law provisions (for example, anaesthetic for a brain scan is a 'physical investigation' and so if a patient does not consent, the administration of the anaesthetic does not come under the Act but under Common Law). The issue of the patient's 'capacity' to make decisions about medical treatment is essential to any examination of consent to treatment (see below).

Section 57—Treatment that Requires the Patient's Consent and a Second Opinion

Psychosurgery and sexual implantation of hormone treatments cannot be given to any patient, whether formal or informal, without the consent of the patient *and* a second opinion. If at any time a previously consenting patient withdraws that consent, treatment must not be given.

Section 58—Treatment Requiring Consent *or* a Second Opinion

Section 58 covers the prescription and administration of medication for mental disorder, after the expiry of 3 months of a detaining order, and the administration of electroconvulsive therapy. Electroconvulsive therapy may be administered if the patient consents; if not, a second opinion must be obtained. If the patient consents to treatment with medication for mental disorder after the 3-month period, the responsible medical officer must so certify (using Form 38). If the patient does not consent, or cannot give consent, to the continuation of medication for mental disorder after the 3-month period, the Mental Health Act Commission (MHAC, see below) must be contacted. The MHAC will send a doctor, who will consider the case. If the MHAC doctor feels that the treatment is likely to alleviate or prevent a deterioration in the patient's condition and the patient is not capable of understanding the nature, purpose and effect of the treatment, or will not consent, the doctor will so certify (using Form 39). Once this form has been completed the treatment may proceed.

When an MHAC doctor comes to give a second opinion for treatment that the patient does not consent to or cannot give valid consent to, the doctor will examine the patient and will require to speak to each of the following:
1. A Registered Nurse.
2. A doctor.
3. Another professional (for example, a psychologist) who knows the patient.

PATIENTS' RIGHTS UNDER THE MENTAL HEALTH ACT 1983

The responsibility for giving information, in the form of leaflets, about the patient's rights and about procedures relating to appeals etc., rests with the Managers via their authorized agents. However, information also needs to be given to the patient orally. Nurses should ensure that patients understand their rights and that this is noted in the nursing records. The explanation of rights should be a process that continues throughout the patient's period of detention. Information on the Act should be freely available to all patients, both informally and formally. Section 132 of the Act requires hospitals to ensure that all detained patients are informed of their rights and understand them as clearly as possible. The key areas on patient rights under the Act are:
1. Consent to treatment.
2. Rights of appeal to the Mental Health Review Tribunal and the Hospital Managers.
3. The Mental Health Act Commission and its role in visiting patients and investigating complaints.

THE ROLE OF 'THE MANAGERS' UNDER THE MENTAL HEALTH ACT 1983

'Managers' are defined under Section 145 of the Act as:

- a. In relation to a purpose vested in the Secretary of State for the purpose of his functions ..., and in relation to any accommodation provided by a local authority and used as a hospital by or on behalf of the Secretary of State ..., the district health authority or special health authority responsible for the administration of the hospital.

- b. In relation to a special hospital, the special health authority established to carry out the functions of the Secretary of State.

- c. In relation to a mental nursing home registered in pursuance of the Registered Homes Act 1984, the person or persons registered in respect of that home.

- d. In relation to a hospital vested in a National Health Service trust, the directors of the trust.

Under the provisions of the Act, Managers may appoint 'Officers' to act on their behalf. Managers have statutory powers, responsibilities and duties concerning the admission of patients, transfer of patients, scrutiny and receipt of documents, detention, review of detention and discharge, the giving of information and access to Mental Health Review Tribunals.

NURSES AND THE ADMINISTRATION OF MEDICATION

The following is based on *The Mental Health Act Commission, practice note 2: Nurses, the administration of medicine for mental disorder and the Mental Health Act* (Mental Health Act Commission, 1994). Nurses administering medication to detained patients who are subject to the provisions of Section 58 of the Act must ensure that they are entitled to do so by meeting all necessary legal requirements, that is, that Form 38 or 39 is completed. A copy should be kept with the medical card and reference should be made to it at the time any medication for mental disorder is administered.

ACCESS TO HEALTH RECORDS ACT 1990

'Psychiatric records are regarded as particularly sensitive because of the recording of opinions as well as facts, the nature of the diagnosis, the possible adverse response of the patient to disclosure, and the frequent inclusion of third party information' (Cope and Chiswick, 1995).

Traditionally, psychiatric patients have been able to gain access to written reports about themselves in certain circumstances, for example, reports written for Mental Health Review Tribunals. The opportunity for patients to gain formal access to the majority of their written records was not made available until the Access to Health Records Act, which came into force on the 1st of November 1991. This Act applies only to records written after this date. Formal limitations to access are summarized in Box 8.2.

A patient may request to see their records and, if he or she believes them to be inaccurate, ask that they be amended. The person responsible for writing the record may either make the requested amendment or make a note within the record of the part(s) that the patient believes to be inaccurate. Nurses are guided in the completion and maintenance of records by the UKCC's *Standards for Records and Record Keeping* (UKCC, 1993), which outlines the legal status of records. An important aspect of record keeping of which nurses must remain aware is that:

> Any document which records any aspect of the care of a patient or client can be required as evidence before a court of law or before the Preliminary Proceedings Committee of the Council (UKCC) or other similar regulatory bodies for the health care professions including the General Medical Council, the comparable body to the UKCC for the medical profession.
>
> *(UKCC, 1993)*

For nurses, a major implication of the Act and the UKCC's Standards is that they emphasize the requirement to maintain accurate written records and to ensure that the highest standards of record keeping and report writing are upheld. Furthermore, the Act and Standards promote, wherever possible, the maintenance of a nurse–patient relationship that is as open and truthful as possible.

Box 8.2 — *Limitations to access to health records*

Information can be withheld if:

1. Disclosure is 'likely to cause serious harm to the physical or mental health of the patient or any other individual'; or
2. The information is 'relating to, or provided by, an individual other than the patient who could be identified by that information, unless the third party has consented'.

(Access to Health Records Act, 1990)

Box 8.3 — *The role of the Mental Health Act Commission*

1. Reviews the operation of the Act and the way in which powers of detention are exercised.
2. Monitors the consent to treatment provisions of the Act to ensure that patients' rights are maintained and protected.
3. Carries out official visits to hospitals, social services and boroughs and elsewhere to talk to patients and professionals and to inspect documentation.
4. Produces and monitors the Code of Practice.
5. Issues Practice Notes on special issues related to the Act.
6. Reports biennially to Parliament.
7. Provides second opinion approved doctors for Consent of Treatment.
8. Receives complaints in regard to any matter relating to the detention and treatment of patients under the Act.

Box 8.4 — *Functions of the Mental Health Review Tribunal*

The Mental Health Review Tribunal can:

1. Discharge patients from hospital.
2. Recommend a leave of absence.
3. Decide on a delayed discharge, conditional discharge or transfer to another hospital.
4. Reconvene if their recommendation is not complied with.

THE MENTAL HEALTH ACT COMMISSION

The MHAC is answerable to, and complies with directions from, the Secretary of State but it is otherwise independent in its functions. Membership of the Commission includes lawyers, nurses, social workers, psychologists, doctors and sundry lay persons. Any person authorized by the MHAC has the right of access to detained patients and their records. Members of the Commission, although generally giving notice of their intention to visit, can make unannounced visits and it is an offence under Section 129 of the Act to refuse such an authorized person access to either patients or their records. The relationship between all health care professionals and the MHAC should be regarded as both positive and mutually beneficial. The role of the Commission (Box 8.3) is to achieve the highest quality of care and management of patients. For members of a clinical service where high standards are maintained, a visit from the MHAC should not provoke anxiety. Nurses should welcome its involvement and the endorsement of practice that results from a positive MHAC report. It is essential, of course, that the high standards that the MHAC ordinarily sees are continually maintained and evident.

MENTAL HEALTH REVIEW TRIBUNALS

The Mental Health Review Tribunal is the statutory body responsible for hearing patient appeals against detention (Box 8.4). It is an independent organization, much like a 'mobile court'. Members of the Tribunal are drawn from the legal profession, medicine and lay people. and are appointed by the Lord Chancellor. At a Tribunal hearing there will be at least one lawyer, doctor and lay person present. The legal member will be the chairman. Tribunal hearings are held with all participants (doctor, social worker and patient) present.

Nurses are increasingly being required to play a significant role in the tribunal process, both prior to the tribunal and in the review itself.

The nurse must ensure the following:

- that the patient has the appropriate knowledge about the application and an application form,
- that arrangements are being made for him (her) to receive legal aid (or other) representation should he (she) so wish,
- that, if requested, she (he) prepares a report for the hearing, deciding which parts (if any) have to be excluded from disclosure to the patient, and
- that she (he) is prepared to give evidence before the tribunal should this be requested.

(Dimond and Barker, 1995)

LEGAL ASPECTS OF COMMUNITY MENTAL HEALTH NURSING

Developments in the practice of caring for the mentally disordered have led to a rapid increase in the number and range of community mental health services. Such developments have required the provision of new legislation and the revision of existing laws. A demand for further legal authority with regard to those who are cared for beyond the hospital environment is frequently supported or condemned depending upon the commentator's origin and perspective.

MENTAL HEALTH ACT 1983, SECTION 117

Section 117 of the Mental Health Act 1983 requires the provision of after-care services for discharged in-patients who have been detained under Sections 3, 37, 47 or 48 'until such time as the District Health Authority and the local services are satisfied that the person concerned is no longer in need of such services'. Nurses will be involved in '117 meetings' at which all members of the multidisciplinary clinical team plan the after-care of patients due for discharge from hospital. The reduction in in-patient mental health facilities experienced in recent years has led to a concomitant increase in the number of mentally disordered individuals being cared for and treated in community settings. The need to match the increase in numbers of 'community patients' with a coincident increase in appropriate resources has not perhaps been successfully met (Eastman, 1995). Demands for an increase in the level of supervision of discharged psychiatric patients followed a number of highly publicized catastrophic events in which mentally disordered individuals committed grievous harm to themselves or others, following discharge from an in-patient setting (e.g. Ritchie *et al.*, 1994). There was wide-ranging public concern that such events could have been minimized if not prevented altogether if the mentally disordered individual had received an appropriate level of supervision following discharge.

THE CARE PROGRAMME APPROACH

The Care Programme Approach (CPA) is concerned to ensure that all patients accepted by the specialist psychiatric services receive the optimum care and supervision following their discharge into the community. The CPA applies to all patients whether or not they have been, or are, subject to the provisions of the Mental Health Act. The CPA ensures that the principles central to Section 117 of the Act are adhered to for both formal and informal patients. Personalized care packages are developed for each patient and a key worker is appointed to ensure that the care package is implemented (DoH, 1990). The care package should include a Care Plan, a nominated key worker and a process for regular review of the individual's care.

The provisions of the CPA apply also to patients who have not been admitted to hospital but who have been under the care of a community mental health team. The development of the CPA has led to the extension of the role of the Community Psychiatric Nurse (CPN), who often required to act as key worker to individual patients. Although the key worker may belong to any discipline, it has been noted that 'CPNs (given their origins) will be identified to occupy many of these positions' (White and Brooker, 1990).

SUPERVISION REGISTERS

To assist in providing a comprehensive and safe community care package for discharged in-patients, providers of mental health care have been required to establish registers of individuals requiring a high level of supervision following discharge from hospital. This was perceived as particularly important with regard to the potential for catastrophe if the severely mentally disordered individual was not closely supervised following discharge. The report of the inquiry into the care of Christopher Clunis, who had a significant background of mental health care and who attacked and killed a man at a London Underground station, advocated that a register of such individuals should be established to improve communication between all agencies and persons involved in an individual patient's care (Ritchie *et al.*, 1994).

NHS Management Executive Guidelines on the introduction of supervision registers state:

> The Secretary of State for Health announced in December 1993 a requirement on all health authorities to ensure that mental health service providers establish and maintain supervision registers which identify those people with a severe mental illness who may be a significant risk to themselves or others

> *(NHS Management Executive, 1994)*

Supervision registers are established alongside the provisions of the CPA (see above) and have been described as forming 'a subset of those suitable for CPA The aim of supervision registers was to target patients with the most serious forms of illness and to ensure that they receive appropriate treatment' (Coffey, 1995).

The required contents (NHS Management Executive, 1994) of supervision registers are as follows:

Part 1 Identification
- i Patient's full name, including known aliases, home address including postcode (or 'no fixed address'), sex, and date of birth.
- ii Patient's current legal status in respect of the Mental Health Act.

Part 2 Nature of Risk
- i Category of risk and nature of specific warning indicators.
- ii Evidence of specific episodes of violent or self-destructive behaviour (including relevant criminal convictions) or severe self-neglect.

Part 3 Key Worker and Relevant Professionals
- i Name and contact details of patient's key worker.

- ii Name and contact details of other professionals involved in the care of the patient including the consultant responsible for the care of the patient.

Part 4 Care Programme
- i Date of registration.
- ii Date of last review.
- iii Date of next programmed review.
- iv Domponents of care programme.

The ethical implications of placing patients on supervision registers have been addressed. Among the principal objections are that supervision registers may infringe the civil liberties of the individual and will operate in a discriminatory way in that they will reflect the 'discriminatory manner of mental health care in which women and ethnic minorities are over represented' (Harrison, 1994).

MENTAL HEALTH (PATIENTS IN THE COMMUNITY) ACT 1995

In 1993, the Department of Health conducted an internal review of the care of the mentally ill in the community (DoH, 1993) largely in response to growing concerns that 'community mental health care' was neither fully effective nor reliable. Section 7 of the Mental Health Act 1983 allowed patients to be 'received into guardianship' (Mental Health Act 1983) but 'the actual authority of the guardian is very weak' and 'guardianship orders are rarely used' (Crichton, 1994).

The Mental Health (Patients in the Community) Act (1995) came into force on 1st April 1996 and is an amendment to Section 25 of the Mental Health Act 1983. The Act has potentially far-reaching legal and ethical implications for mental health practice. The principal purpose of the Act is to ensure a system of supervision of care in the community for patients who have been detained in hospital in England and Wales under the Mental Health Act 1983 or in Scotland under the Mental Health (Scotland) Act 1984. The Act extends the period during which, under the 1983 Mental Health Act, certain patients who are absent without leave may be taken into custody and returned to hospital. It also removes the previous 6-month time limit on the period for which patients detained in hospital in England and Wales may be given leave of absence. In Scotland, it restricts the total period for which leave of absence may be granted to 1 year.

The RMO must make the application for supervision to the Health Authority that is to be responsible for providing the patient's after-care services. The RMO must be satisfied that supervision is justified by the risk of harm to the patient or others and must consult the patient and others before making the application. The process of supervision is as follows.

Following discharge, the patient will have a nominated supervisor and may be required to reside at a specified place or to attend for medical treatment, occupation, education or training. Access to the patient at any place where he or she may be residing must be given to the patient's supervisor, any registered medical practitioner, any approved social worker or any other person authorized by the supervisor.

The patient cannot be required to receive medication against his or her will. Supervision will last initially for 6 months, after which it may be renewed, if the stated conditions are satisfied, for a further 6 months and subsequently for periods of 1 year at a time.

If the patient refuses the services provided, or fails to comply with any of the requirements, there will be a review, which may consider whether the patient's condition is such that he or she needs to be readmitted to hospital under the provisions of the Mental Health Act 1983.

Patients can apply to a Mental Health Review Tribunal for their supervision to be terminated. A Tribunal considering the application of a patient currently detained in hospital may recommend that the patient's RMO considers applying for supervision.

For nurses, this Act has most impact on those working in the community who may be nominated as supervisors under the Act. 'It will give Community Psychiatric Nurses (CPNs), doctors and social workers unprecedented scope to intervene in their clients' lives if they breach contracts hammered out prior to leaving hospital' (McMillan, 1995). The significance of the supervisor's role suggests a move towards action being taken against nurses, who may find themselves at 'risk' because of the nature of the role: 'The more independent the nurse's function, the greater the risk of a finding of liability' (Brazier, 1992).

It will assist the reader's understanding to give thought to the reasons behind the development of legislation for mentally disordered patients in the community and how far that legislation is enforceable by nurses.

COURT DIVERSION SCHEMES

'Mentally disordered homeless defendants charged with minor offences are more likely to be remanded into custody than others charged with similar offences' (Joseph, 1992). To address this situation, attempts are being made to divert the mentally disordered individual away from custody. Nurses can play a significant role in 'court diversion' and are frequently involved in an assessment of individuals brought into custody prior to their appearance before a court of law. The results of such assessments can play an essential role in informing the court's decision on disposal of an individual. The emergence of this aspect of the psychiatric nurse's role has assisted in raising the profile of nursing within the multidisciplinary team. Nurses, possibly with medical colleagues, see individuals prior to their appearance in court and endeavour to make an assessment of their mental state and behaviour (and other contributory factors) to make effective and considered recommendations to the court about an individual's mental health requirements.

'A pivotal role can be played by CPNs in diversion, thereby alleviating the tremendous personal distress experienced by mentally ill people who become caught up in the criminal justice system' (Hillis, 1993).

ETHICS

From the formulation of the Hippocratic Oath in Ancient Greece to the present day, doctors have debated among themselves the codes of conduct which should govern the art of healing. These days philosophers, theologians, lawyers and journalists insist on joining the debate.

(Brazier, 1992)

Ethics is a branch of philosophy that, in its simplest definition, informs us what is right and wrong about our thoughts, intentions and actions. Such an apparently advantageous philosophical tool may appear to offer a simple method of defining what is right and wrong with a variety of nursing practices and therefore a subsequent means of rectifying any perceived 'wrongs' to adhere to the most 'right' (and, therefore, presumably, the most 'ethical') course.

Unfortunately, ethics does not always allow for such a simplistic approach, hence the ever growing ethical discourse in health care and elsewhere. An awareness of ethics and ethical thinking, however, assists in the essential assessment and understanding of the morality of practice.

There is, inevitably, some common ground occupied by the moral and legal requirements of a society and much of what is perceived as 'moral' within Western society is reflected by the laws governing individual and societal activity. The delivery of care and treatment to those who suffer from mental disorders presents psychiatric nurses with various issues that require ethical consideration. Concern for questions about the patient's dignity, autonomy, potential de-humanization and 'labelling', and justice and paternalism, may all be heightened within the area of mental health care. The relationship between patient and health care professional, although perhaps 'one-sided' in respect of knowledge and skill, is generally acknowledged as being most effective when both parties are equally involved in striving for the same aim, i.e. the well-being of the patient. The mentally disordered individual may be either unable or unwilling to take part in such an 'equal' relationship due to an incapacity to fully perceive the disabling effects of his or her disorder.

According to the nature and severity of the mental disorder, the patient may be in a particularly vulnerable position when receiving health care. A mental disorder may prevent him or her from exercising those rights which, for the majority of recipients of health care, are perhaps taken somewhat for granted. For nurses, to maintain an adherence to morality in delivery of care (both with regard to professional codes and, perhaps, personal ideology) may be viewed as of particular significance in the field of mental health. The resolution of ethical dilemmas requires the application of ethical awareness, a skill that all psychiatric nurses should strive to develop.

MORALITY AND THE LAW

Morality is not reducible to established laws, i.e. to examine what is legal, or what the law says on a particular matter, is not necessarily to discover what is morally right or wrong. On occasion, doing what is perceived to be right may require breaking the law. Therefore it is not possible simply to resolve moral dilemmas by resolving legal ones. The law itself may be subjected to moral scrutiny and criticism and the question of whether one is morally bound to obey an established law is always an open one. 'Many acts are immoral but not illegal; many acts are illegal but not immoral' (Bavidge, 1989).

The somewhat sparse literature on psychiatric nursing and ethics focuses primarily on the various practical issues that are a frequent cause of concern and on ethical debate. Such dilemmas of practice are the most easily perceptible and frequently raised ethical issues within mental health practice. These 'practice-based' dilemmas, which arise from the nature of clinical work, provide the potential for clearly identifiable moral predicaments.

INFORMED CONSENT

Central to the concept of informed consent is consideration of the degree and quality of information that must be exchanged between a health care professional and a patient so that the patient may make an informed decision about his or her health care. The right of a competent individual to give or withhold consent to any form of treatment is generally acknowledged.

Giving appropriate information is central to a demonstration of respect for the patient's right to self-determination (autonomy). The completion of a consent-to-treatment form is not, in itself, evidence of valid informed consent: 'Informed consent is an autonomous authorization by individuals of a medical intervention' (Beauchamp and Childress, 1994). Such authorization cannot be offered without a clear explanation and understanding of the information and issues involved. The question whether a mentally disordered individual may be deemed competent (or incompetent) to give or withhold consent has been addressed. 'The fact that a person is suffering from a mental disorder, as defined in the Mental Health Act (1983) does not in itself preclude that person from giving a legally effective consent' (Skegg, 1984).

CONFIDENTIALITY

Nurses caring for mentally disordered individuals receive, generate and generally have access to a wide range of confidential material concerning their patients. This information may range from a minor verbal exchange told 'in confidence' by a patient or relative (in response to which, of course, an assurance of confidentiality cannot be given) to the highly sensitive recordings of an individual's physical, psychological, sexual and social history etc. contained in a patient's case notes or within a report for a Mental Health Review Tribunal.

A responsibility to ensure that such information remains confidential is both implicit and explicit in professional and ethical codes of practice. Disclosure of confidential material may be (legally) permissible in specific instances. Doctors are given guidance on the disclosure of confidential information by the General Medical Council which, in its 'Blue book', offers exceptions to the duty of confidentiality (see Box 8.4).

The case of W v Egdell (1990) highlights a judicial view in favour of disclosure in the public interest. The case concerned the communication of information by Dr Egdell. W was detained in a secure hospital and the information disclosed was an independent psychiatric report that the doctor had prepared about him for a forthcoming Mental Health Review Tribunal. The report opposed W's transfer from the secure hospital to a medium secure facility and stated that, in the doctor's opinion, W remained a danger. W's solicitors decided not to forward the report to the Tribunal (and withdrew the application for W's transfer). To ensure that the findings of the report were not repressed, Dr Egdell sent it to W's hospital (plus a copy to the Home Secretary). W subsequently sued Dr Egdell, claiming damages for the breach of the duty of confidence. W's claim was dismissed as was his subsequent appeal.

What concerns might arise when information, which one knows to be confidential, has been (in the reader's view) inappropriately communicated?

PATIENTS' RIGHTS

In contemporary practice, nurses should be able to demonstrate an active respect for the rights of their patients. An awareness of the rights of mentally disordered patients must also form part of the repertoire of psychiatric nursing skills.

Nurses should ensure that they (and their patient) are fully informed, for example, of their right to appeal against detention, to refuse treatment and to complain about any element of their care management. Not least among the ever growing number of rights accorded to the psychiatric patient, and possibly the most important, are the rights to be treated with respect and for dignity to be maintained at all times. Of course, patients also have the right to legal representation, the right to suitable health care and the right to receive appropriate and accurate information.

As part of the reader's development plan, summarize the

legal and moral rights of a patient detained under the Mental Health Act 1983.

RESPECT FOR AUTONOMY

Autonomy has been defined as 'Personal rule of the self that is free from both controlling interferences by others and from personal limitations that prevent meaningful choice, such as inadequate understanding' (Beauchamp and Childress, 1994). Nurses are required to ensure that their patient's autonomy is respected despite the powerful position of privilege that the nurse frequently enjoys. A sick individual in need of treatment places him- or herself at the 'mercy' of their carer's discretion and their capability of acting in accordance with the patient's best interests with an overriding respect for patient autonomy. A mental disorder, according to its severity, may diminish an individual's capacity to exercise autonomy. A mentally disordered individual may not be allowed to act autonomously because of incapacitation or because it is decided by others that 'autonomous' action would not be in that individual's best interests.

The reader should at this point think of situations in mental health practice where an individual's autonomy may be overridden in their 'best interests' What ethical and legal considerations must be taken into account?.

The care and management of mentally disordered individuals offers many examples of potential 'ethical dilemmas' of practice. For example, the concept of power and coercion within the nurse–patient relationship (power issues may be claimed to permeate both traditional and contemporary mental health practice) and the many concerns regarding the application of physical and social control of patients.

TABLE 8.1 Table of statutes and cases.

Table of Statutes

Access to Health Records Act 1990
Lunacy Act 1890
Mental Health Act 1959
Mental Health Act 1983
Mental Health (Patients in the Community) Act 1995
Nurses, Midwives and Health Visitors Act 1979
Nurses, Midwives and Health Visitors Act 1982

Cases

Bolam v Friern Hospital Management Committee (1957)
Devi v West Midlands Regional Health Authority (1981)
Pountney v Griffiths (1975)
W v Egdell (1990)
Wilsher v Essex Area Health Authority (1987)

 Box 8.5

Guidelines on the disclosure of confidential information

1. The patient or his legal adviser gives written consent.
2. Information is shared with other doctors, nurses or health professionals participating in caring for the patient.
3. Where, in particular circumstances, on medical grounds it is undesirable to seek the patient's consent, information regarding the patient's health may sometimes be given in confidence to a close relative.
4. When, in the doctor's opinion, disclosure of information to some third party other than a relative would be in the best interests of the patient, the doctor must make every effort to get the patient's consent. Only in exceptional circumstances may the doctor go ahead and impart that information without the patient's consent.
5. Information may be disclosed to comply with a statutory requirement, for example notification of an infectious disease.
6. Information may be disclosed when it is so ordered by the court.
7. Rarely, disclosure may be justified on the grounds that it is in the public's best interest which, in certain circumstances such as, for example, investigation by the police of a grave or very serious crime, might override the doctor's duty to maintain the patient's confidence.
8. Information may also be disclosed if necessary for the purpose of a medical research project approved by a recognized ethical committee.

(General Medical Council, 1993)

KEY CONCEPTS

- Effective psychiatric nursing demands an awareness and understanding of the legal and ethical implications of practice and how each may influence and inform nursing activity.
- Psychiatric nurses must ensure that their practice adheres to legal requirements and be aware that, within an increasingly litigious health care environment, the potential for allegations of malpractice must always be considered.
- A thorough knowledge of relevant mental health legislation must be acquired in order that nursing practice is fully informed and nurses are able to assist their patients in experiencing the psychiatric 'system'.
- Legislation aimed specifically at ensuring safe and effective community psychiatric nursing practice is increasing.
- The ability of identify ethical problems and to offer them considered analysis are skills which may be developed by knowledge of ethical theory and its practical application.
- The rights of mentally disordered individuals, whilst receiving care and treatment, must be acknowledged in accordance with an ongoing respect for individual autonomy.

SUMMARY

This chapter has attempted to highlight the essential requirement for psychiatric nurses to develop and maintain a comprehensive awareness and understanding of the legal and ethical issues which influence their practice.

Delivering care and treatment to mentally disordered individuals in whatever clinical setting is a role which carries significant responsibilities. It is hoped that this chapter has assisted in explaining the legal and moral responsibilities of psychiatric nursing and the effect upon practice.

The reader is directed towards further reading in relation to ethics and law; the study and comprehension of both is a beneficial and worthwhile task.

REFERENCES

Bavidge M: *Mad or bad?* Bristol, 1989, Classical Press.

Beauchamp T, Childress J: *Principles of biomedical ethics.* Oxford, 1994, Oxford University Press.

Bethlem and Maudsley NHS Trust: *Mental Health Act 1983 Guidelines.* London, 1994, Maudsley Hospital.

Brazier M: *Medicine, patients and the law.* London, 1992, Penguin Books.

Coffey M: Supervision registers and mental health problems. *Nurs Times* 91(28):36–37, 1995.

Cope R, Chiswick D: Ethical issues in forensic psychiatry. In: Chiswick D, Cope R: *Seminars in practical forensic psychiatry.* London, 1995, Royal College of Psychiatrists.

Cope R: Mental health legislation. In: Chiswick D, Cope R: *Seminars in practical forensic psychiatry.* London, 1995, Royal College of Psychiatrists.

Crichton J: Supervised discharge. *Med Sci Law* 34(4):319–320, 1994.

Department of Health: *The care programme approach for people with a mental illness referred to the specialist psychiatric services.* London, 1990, Department of Health.

Department of Health: *Legal powers on the care of mentally ill people in the community: Report of the internal review.* London, 1993, Department of Health.

Department of Health and Welsh Office: *Code of practice: Mental Health Act 1983.* London, 1993, HMSO.

Dimond BC, Barker FH: *Mental health law for nurses.* Oxford, 1995, Blackwell Science.

Eastman N: Anti-therapeutic community mental health law. *BMJ* 310:1081–1082, 1995.

Faulk M: *Basic forensic psychiatry.* London, 1994, Blackwell Scientific Publications

General Medical Council. *Professional conduct and discipline: Fitness to practice.* London, 1993, General Medical Council.

Gunn MJ: Personal searches of psychiatric patients. *Crim Law Rev* 767–777:1992.

Harrison K: Supervision registers: unethical, illegal and unenforceable. *Ment Health Nurs* 14(5):6–8,1994.

Hillis G: Diverting tactics. *Nurs Times* 89(1):24–27, 1993.

Joseph P: *Psychiatric assessment at the Magistrates' Court.* London, 1992, Home Office and Department of Health.

Kennedy I, Grubb A: *Medical law texts with materials.* London, 1994, Butterworths.

McMillan I: Threatening treatment. *Nurs Times* 91(11):17, 1995.

Mason JK, McCall–Smith RA: *Law and medical ethics.* London, 1994, Butterworths.

NHS Management Executive: *Introduction of supervision registers for mentally ill people from 1 April 1994.* London, 1994, Department of Health.

Nolan P: *A history of mental health nursing.* London, 1993, Chapman & Hall.

Ritchie J, Dick D, Lingham R: *The report of the inquiry into the care and treatment of Christopher Clunis.* London, 1994, HMSO.

Skegg PDG: *Law, ethics and medicine.* Oxford, 1984, Clarendon Press.

United Kingdom Central Council for Nursing, Midwifery and Health Visiting: *Code of professional conduct.* London, 1992, UKCC.

United Kingdom Central Council for Nursing, Midwifery and Health Visiting: *Standards for records and record keeping.* London, 1993, UKCC.

White E, Brooker C: The future of community psychiatric nursing: What might 'The Care Programme Approach' mean for practice and education? *CPNJ* December 27–28, 1990.

Young A: *Law and professional conduct in nursing.* London, 1991, Scutari Press.

FURTHER READING

Bloch S, Chodoff P: *Psychiatric ethics*. Oxford, 1991, Oxford University Press.
Offers an overview of aspects of law relevant to mental health practice. It deals with admission to hospital, civil commitment, hospital orders, treatment and management and issues arising beyond hospitalization.

Dimond BC, Barker FH: *Mental health law for nurses*. Oxford, 1995, Blackwell Science.
This very useful text offers a clear exposition of the relationship between contemporary mental health legislation and nursing practice.

Fletcher N, Holt J, editors: *Ethics, law and nursing*. Manchester, 1995, Manchester University Press.
A contemporary approach to the relationship between the three areas of professional knowledge. Examines the nurse's position within a legal and ethical context and provides the reader with an easily readable yet comprehensive account of the relationship between nursing and legal and ethical considerations.

Hoggett B: *Mental health law*. London, 1990, Sweet and Maxwell.
Provides an in-depth and comprehensive account of medical law, with wide-ranging use of statute and case law.

Mason JK, McCall–Smith RA: *Law and medical ethics*. London, 1994, Butterworths.
An excellent and highly accessible account of medical law and its relationship with ethical decision making. Utilizes statute and case law to expose all aspects of its subject matter.

Quality and Standards in Nursing Practice

Learning Outcomes

After studying this chapter, you should be able to:

- Identify the origins of quality and standards in nursing.

- Define the concepts of quality, audit and standard.

- Discuss the impact of political policy making on quality issues within the mental health services.

- Describe the quality assurance cycle.

- Compare and contrast a variety of quality assurance programmes.

*T*here is much confusion and disagreement among nurses about quality and its meaning in the mental health care setting. This chapter offers an overview of the conflicts and difficulties surrounding the issues of quality in mental health. The evolution of the concept of quality in health care is outlined, following both political and professional developments. Management approaches to quality assurance are explained and clinical approaches discussed. At present there are no common views of what quality means or how it can best be monitored. It is hoped that nurses will develop their own ideas and, within their work environment, come to a common view of what quality means and of ways to demonstrate the level of service they provide. The future development of quality assurance in health care is uncertain because of the political influences on it. For robust quality assurance initiatives to be developed, it is suggested that there is a need for them to be clinically rather than politically led.

WHERE HAS THE IDEA OF QUALITY ASSURANCE COME FROM?

The National Health Service (NHS) was set up by Government in 1948. It was the first health care system in Western society to offer free medical care to all. The service was built by nationalizing all voluntary and local authority hospitals and extending the previously limited insurance scheme to the whole population. Overnight everyone became entitled to free health care, provided either by a general practitioner or hospital, funded by the state. The move was not popular within the medical profession, as, prior to nationalization successful doctors were able to build up their case loads and thus their earnings. However, it was popular with the general public because they could now expect to be treated at no cost, whenever they were in need.

The NHS was launched amid claims that it would separate the best health advice and treatment from the ability to pay and universalize the best care. People's expectations of health care were raised. They had been told to expect the best. However, this expression of the level of quality was ill thought out and certainly not backed by methods to monitor its delivery. The numbers using the service have risen steadily since its inception, perhaps assisted by the technological advances in medicine and increased life expectancy. This has, however, resulted in rising costs and lengthening waits for treatment. Advances in medical technology and the lengthening waits could be considered marks of success: people are using the service, recovering, and returning to use the service when they are next in need. People were told to expect excellence; they have instead experienced disappointments, complaints and dissatisfaction with the NHS. In addition, the Black Report (Department of Health and Social Security (DHSS), 1980) commissioned by the Labour Government but not published until after the Conservatives won the 1979 General Election, reported that there were still major inequalities in health care provision. The promise to universalize 'best care' had been broken.

POLITICS AND SOCIAL POLICY

The Conservative Government was elected in 1979, marking a change in political philosophy and subsequently in social policy. The move was away from a mixed economy and towards the New Right. Thus there was a move towards a free market economy and individualism. This philosophical change first affected the health service when the Government commissioned an independent inquiry into management of the NHS. The inquiry panel was headed by Roy Griffiths, then managing director of Sainsbury's. Recommendations from the inquiry (DHSS, 1983) included a change in the management structure, and the introduction of accountability for and quality assurance to services. This was the first time that monitoring the quality of health care had been mentioned explicitly.

Professionals were concerned by the shift in social policy. The move away from consensus management and the introduction of general management was regarded with grave suspicion. How could managers, with no experience of the health service, really take charge of something as complex as a hospital? However, there was little organized protest and the changes took place.

THE MARKET PLACE AND VALUE FOR MONEY

Working for Patients (DHSS, 1989) introduced the concept of an internal market to the NHS. Again, professionals' concerns at the introduction of competition were not heeded. This move to introduce a market economy led to the establishment of purchasing authorities and Trusts. They were responsible and accountable to the Department of Health (DoH) for purchasing high quality health care for their local populations, within a fixed budget. Thus the concept of value for money was introduced. Purchasing authorities drew up contracts with Trusts stating the amount and quality of services they wished to purchase. For the first time, hospitals were asked to account for the way their money was spent. In order to monitor the services, both purchasing authorities and Trusts established quality departments. This led to increasing amounts of money being spent on the monitoring of services and reduced the money available for actually providing patient care. It is arguable whether any improvement to services has been noticed by the patients themselves.

STANDARDS FOR CARE

The Government established its Citizens Charter initiative and, as part of this, the *Patient's Charter* (DoH, 1991). This set out for the first time standards of care for the NHS. Monitoring of Patient's Charter standards was introduced and league tables of results were published by the National Health Service Executive (NHSE). Comparisons between the Trusts do not, however, take in to account the fact that they have vastly different catchment populations, with vastly different needs. The establishment of the league tables has again required spending on staff to monitor achievements at Trust Purchaser and NHSE levels and further deflected funds away from direct patient care. A revised charter *The Patient's Charter and You* was published in 1995 (DoH, 1995). This Charter goes further than the first, setting rights and standards for different services in the NHS and new expectations of services. These include standards for appointment waiting times and the length of wait for certain operations, rights to information about treatment and the type of ward you will be admitted to for a planned admission and expectations that every hospital will display information on how well they are achieving the Charter standards. However, waiting lists remain, as does discontent with services.

Private sector initiatives in quality, such as those of retailers Marks and Spencers and Sainsbury's, are made up of three parts: a reliable product, value for money and a no-questions-asked refund if you are dissatisfied. The health service, despite spending ever increasing amounts on quality assurance departments, at all levels from the NHSE to Trusts, is far from achieving this guarantee of quality. Perhaps it is time to stop and ask if it actually possible to achieve this within health care provision and if, in fact, it is what patients want.

QUALITY IN NURSING

Alongside this government thrust towards quality assurance in health care, the moves to professionalize nursing and to define quality nursing practice have continued. The movement to professionalize nursing reportedly started as early as the 1860s (Dingwall *et al.*, 1988) when the idea of paying and training nurses to work in the workhouses was introduced. It has continued ever since with almost continual debates over how nurses should be trained, levels of registration and what should be expected from regulatory bodies. A number of reports have been commissioned both by Government and the Royal College of Nursing (RCN). The United Kingdom Central Council for Nurses, Midwives and Health Visitors (UKCC), the National Boards and a generic register for all nurses were introduced as part of the *Nurses, Midwives and Health Visitors Act* (DHSS, 1979). Following this, perhaps the most major change in nurse education occurred with the introduction of Project 2000 (UKCC, 1986). The focus of training moved away from wards and into institutes of higher education.

The struggle to define quality in nursing leapt forward with the establishment of the RCN Standards of Care Project in 1985, the introduction of the Code of Professional Conduct (UKCC, 1992) and the UKCC's publication of standards for the administration of medicines (UKCC, 1992) and for record keeping (UKCC, 1993).

With the advent of diploma level graduates, nursing no longer seemed satisfied with traditional methods of nursing care or methods of monitoring it. Of course the moves to introduce research into practice to define quality of nursing care began earlier than the mid-1980s but the impetus was increased. Nursing was no longer considered a vocation but a career.

It is unclear how much of the move towards professionalism has been driven from within nursing and how much has been encouraged from outside the profession. What is clear is the constant battle for power between managers and the medical profession since the Griffiths Report (DHSS, 1983).

POWER STRUGGLE

The introduction of general management brought corporate decision making with it. Doctors, who up until 1983 had made decisions based on clinical judgements alone, now had to account to the general manager and became only a part of the corporate management process. The introduction of general management was only partially successful in reducing medical dominance of health care (Strong and Robinson, 1990). It was reported that nurses showed no initiative and lacked any developed sense of professional identity and that even senior nurses could be easily bullied by members of the medical profession (Strong and Robinson, 1990). If this was the case, how could managers rely on nurses to be their allies when tackling a difficult doctor? Management's idea was to try to increase professional identity among nurses by flattening the nursing hierarchy and reducing bureaucracy in the profession.

The power struggle between managers and the medical profession was further fuelled by the introduction of the purchaser–provider split. Contracts stated the levels of activity required for payments made by the purchaser. Thus cost implications of clinical decisions had to be considered. *Working for Patients* (DHSS, 1989) also included a requirement for medical audit. Doctors were told for the first time to demonstrate the effectiveness of treatments.

Medical audit and, subsequently, clinical audit also had implications for the move to professionalize nursing. Clinical audit demands a demonstration of the effectiveness of services. Purchasers may decide whether or not to purchase a service based on its effectiveness, both in terms of quality and cost. Part of the process of clinical audit is to examine the effectiveness of the nursing component of the service. This can only be achieved if the nursing component is measurable. Doctors need nurses to be able to demonstrate the effectiveness of nursing for the overall service to be considered effective.

Thus the move to professionalize nursing has not come from within the profession alone. It has also been encouraged by management, as a tool to assist in controlling the power of the medical profession and by the medical profession, in an attempt to demonstrate the effectiveness of the services they lead.

Perhaps the confusion around the issue of quality assurance in nursing is now easier to understand. Perhaps also the pressure to demonstrate quality nursing practice is also clearer.

What is obvious is that it is no longer considered adequate for the quality of nursing care to be monitored by counting boxes of chocolates received from grateful patients.

WHAT DO QUALITY AND QUALITY ASSURANCE MEAN?

If nurses must demonstrate quality nursing care it is essential to understand what the term 'quality' means and how the quality assurance process can be used to monitor care.

QUALITY

Quality is defined in the Concise Oxford Dictionary (Allen, 1990) as the degree of excellence of something. Ellis and Whittington (1993) suggest that the word can also be used as a neutral term, referring just to the nature or characteristics of something. There are difficulties in defining the concept of quality because it is a combination of an abstract idea and the expression of desirability or level of excellence to be attained (Green *et al.*, 1991). This difficulty is apparent in health care, where it can be seen that individuals have different views on what good care is and how it should be provided. Ellis (1988) defines quality as that which gives complete customer satisfaction. This definition has limitations within health care provision. Who are the customers? Are they the local purchasing authority, general practitioners or the service users?

Quality in mental health presents a unique challenge because some users are receiving care against their will. If service users are the customers, can services ever offer complete satisfaction to those compulsorily detained under sections of the Mental Health Act or to those community service users placed on the Supervision Register (NHSME, 1994 (HSG(94)5))? Ovretveit (1992) states that quality health care gives people what they need, as well as what they want, at the lowest cost. This definition also has limitations in the field of mental health as it may be difficult to gain agreement between individual service users and professionals on what the service users' needs are.

When considering mental health service provision at a national level there is marked controversy between service users, user groups, professionals, the general public and Government over service users' needs. Among questions being asked in the press are, 'Should people with long-term disabling mental health problems be cared for in the community or should they be in hospital?' 'How can professionals guarantee public safety when planning care for someone with a history of violence?' 'Do user groups really represent the views of service users?'

QUALITY ASSURANCE

The concept of quality assurance comes from industry. Originally, quality control was introduced as a simple way to ensure that goods met requirements. Goods were checked against a set standard and any not meeting it were rejected. Monitoring can take place at any stage of production, from raw materials to the finished product. As frequent rejection of goods not meeting the standard is expensive, action to identify reasons for substandard products and to rectify processes has been introduced. Ellis and Whittington (1993) suggest that managers usually see the introduction of analysis, feedback and rectification of processes as the origin of quality assurance.

Quality assurance is the process by which quality is defined, monitored and evaluated. Once evaluation has occurred the process begins again. It is therefore often referred to as the quality assurance cycle (see Figure 9.1). Each stage of the cycle is crucial to the development of the goods or service.

Quality assurance has its own vocabulary, and terms used can cause confusion. 'Standard' and 'audit' are perhaps those used the most frequently. An understanding of these concepts is needed to participate fully in the quality assurance process or cycle. A standard is an agreed, measurable level of attainment. Standards can be agreed anywhere from individual service through to national level. They may relate to a single discipline or be multidisciplinary (Hooper *et al.*, 1995). Audit is the process of measuring performance against a standard with the aim of identifying both good and bad practice (Hooper *et al.*, 1995).

Quality assurance is a simple idea. However, implementation of the process is complex and fraught with potential for disagreement. For example: Who should participate in the process? What is the acceptable standard and who should lead initiatives? First a decision must be made on what service or part of the service is to be examined, then an acceptable level or standard for the service must be agreed. Once agreement is reached it is necessary to consider how monitoring or audit can be best undertaken, to ensure reliable and valid results that give an accurate view of the service. The results of any audit must then be examined to evaluate the service. When evaluating the service, questions must be asked, such as:

- Has the standard been reached or not?
- If it has could the service be further improved?
- If not, was the standard realistic or does it need to be altered?
- If the standard was right but not met, how should the service be changed to ensure an improvement?

Once any necessary changes to standards or service have been introduced, the quality assurance cycle begins again.

The first cycle may take several months to complete. Agreement on the service to be examined and the standard acceptable must be gained from all involved. Some may be wary of the process, concerned about repercussions should services not meet the standard. These concerns must be addressed by those leading the initiative. A high level of commitment and motivation is needed for the process to maintain momentum and thus ensure service development. Once initial differences of opinion have been discussed, agreements reached and the fears of repercussions allayed, subsequent cycles may be speedier.

APPROACHES TO QUALITY ASSURANCE

Quality assurance is the basis for any quality programme. The boom in interest in quality has, however, led to the development of a number of different approaches. Some have been management-led while others have been led by the medical or nursing professions. All approaches have their roots in industry. The development of different approaches has, however, added to the confusion surrounding quality.

There are two contrasting philosophical bases for quality programmes; the initiative can use a bottom-up or a top-down approach.

In a bottom-up approach, the quality programme is developed at a local level. In a top-down programme it is decided at a higher level and imposed locally. A bottom-up approach is frequently favoured, as it encourages ownership of initiatives, reduces suspicion and increases motivation. This approach, however, is rarely initiated at the most local level. Often senior ward staff or a whole clinical directorate decide on a quality assurance programme. Thus what is intended as a bottom-up approach may appear as a top-down approach to junior or untrained ward staff. Individuals' perceptions of the quality assurance programme are, therefore, dependent on position in the hierarchy. Most quality assurance programmes will therefore be seen by some as a bottom-up and by others as a top-down approach. A programme that encourages ownership and motivation and leads to a minimum of suspicion will be one that has clear relevance and benefits to the area.

There is no one right way of approaching quality assurance. Kitson (1990) suggests it is not so much the method selected but the way in which it is introduced and implemented that makes a programme a success. There is no reason why a programme must only contain a single approach. It may be that a combination of approaches is more effective.

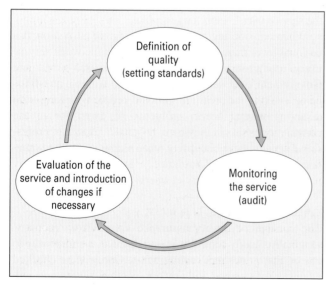

Figure 9.1 The quality assurance cycle

When implementing a quality assurance programme consideration must be given to:
- The complex dynamics surrounding quality assurance in health care.
- What is required to be achieved.
- Who is required to be involved.
- How others will be interested and motivated.
- How much time there is to devote to the programme.

QUALITY ASSURANCE PROGRAMMES

Total Quality Management
As the name suggests, this is an organization-wide approach that seeks to involve staff at every level. The process is management-led and attempts to develop a culture of quality improvement.

There are five core values of Total Quality Management (TQM):
1. Putting the customer first.
2. Meeting and exceeding customer expectations.
3. Getting the service right first time.
4. Reducing the costs of poor quality.
5. Empowering staff and recognizing staff value.

The difficulties of implementing a TQM approach within a mental health setting are, perhaps, twofold.

When earlier the development of quality in the health setting was considered, two agendas were highlighted: that of management and that of the professionals. It was noted that the values of managers may differ from those of professionals, yet to implement TQM effectively requires a common agenda. Sensitive negotiation is needed to define common ground. Unless this is undertaken the TQM programme will fail.

The second difficulty is in putting the customer first. The question 'who is the customer?' was raised when considering definitions of quality. This type of programme not only demands a definition of the customer but also that the customer is put first. However, what is not made clear is whether the customer's needs and wishes are put first. When considering a person with a mental health problem these needs and wishes may not correspond, as in the example of some-one detained against their will under a section of the Mental Health Act.

Continuous Quality Improvement
This is an organization-wide approach, often developed from Total Quality Management. Continuous Quality Improvement requires continuing quality improvement across the whole organization. It is a progressive initiative, so when standards have been achieved, new higher standards are set and implemented. This type of initiative needs a consistent management philosophy for quality that is shared and acted on by staff and managers at all levels.

A difficulty with implementing this approach in the mental health setting is in gaining agreement on the philosophy for quality. This can only be achieved through sensitive negotiation and may be very time consuming.

The Adult Learning Model of Quality Assurance
This model was developed within the Canadian health services (Wilson, 1987). It is unusual, as it is one of few programmes developed specifically for use in health care. The programme's development was management-led.

The programme involves a six-step process:
1. Documentation of existing quality monitors.
2. Recording of established practices.
3. Development of strategies for audit.
4. Comparison of practice against standards.
5. Development of an audit programme.
6. Endorsement of departmental programme by the Director of Quality.

One of the benefits of this programme is that existing quality initiatives are recognized and can be incorporated. It is a management method for quality assurance, thus it could be seen as a top-down approach. There is a need to gain commitment and cooperation from all members of the team for the programme to be effective.

Quality Circles
The idea of quality circles was developed in Japanese industry in the 1960s. Benefits from quality circles in industry have been found to be:
1. Improvement in the quality of products.
2. Cost reduction.
3. Improved staff attitudes.
4. Development of staff supervision.

Quality circles were introduced into the health service in the early 1980s as a management initiative. They consist of small groups of people who volunteer to meet together, usually weekly, to identify, analyse and solve job-related problems. Having developed a solution they then have a responsibility to convince the manager and, if successful, to implement the solution and monitor the results.

Quality circles are a bottom-up approach to quality, though their introduction may be management-led and therefore they may be perceived as imposed. The fact that they rely on voluntary commitment means that participants are likely to be motivated. However, within a nursing team it may be difficult for volunteers to arrange to meet regularly, because of shift patterns and commitments to patient care. An additional difficulty may be that the multidisciplinary team is not equally represented, e.g. volunteers may all come from the nursing team or from the medical team. Therefore, there must be a team agreement that the quality circle's decision is accepted, even by those who have not volunteered as members. This may lead to biased decisions on service and care provision.

Benchmarking

Benchmarking is a process in which standards for a service are established, applied and evaluated. Standards are identified from the best or most appropriate performance known to be achievable in that field. This is a management framework for quality monitoring. Links may be made with other organizations with a similar service, so that practices can be compared, in the search for the best or most appropriate performance.

The approaches to quality assurance described above are all management-led initiatives. This list is not exhaustive. There are many other management approaches that you may come across within your organization. The principles of the approaches are similar in that they usually address issues across the whole of a service or organization. For such an approach to succeed a common understanding of and philosophy for quality is essential. It is difficult to achieve this in a large organization because of the size of the workforce and the different priorities of different professionals. Although there is a need to understand the difficulties, they should not be seen as insurmountable problems and they can be overcome with time and sensitive negotiation.

STANDARDS SETTING

Much has been written in the nursing press about standards and standards setting. The concept of standards setting in nursing developed rapidly between the mid-1980s and early 1990s. The leaders in this could be considered to be the RCN, who established their Standards of Care project in 1985.

How and where standards should be set and their benefits to care have been debated. The motivation for standards setting is the subsequent benefit to care. Unless standards positively influence care, they are pointless. The result of the debate on how and where standards should be set seems to be that each service or organization must find the way that works best for them. It may be appropriate to use standards set in a similar area, rather than 'reinventing the wheel'. It may be the necessary or preferred option, however, to set individual standards for a specific clinical area or service.

Defining, identifying and quantifying care is complex. The model recommended by the RCN to facilitate this process (Kitson, 1986) is Donabedian's structure, process and outcome model.

PROCESS

When setting standards the initial step is to agree and document the philosophy or value system. It is then necessary to focus on the service provided and its component parts. Focusing on the parts of the service assists in the identification of specific standards. The service may have been commissioned to provide in-patient care to adults suffering from acute mental health problems. This gives an overview of the service but it does not say exactly what the nursing staff do. An element of the service may be to provide care to people who are actively suicidal. This says a little more but what does

it involve? What assessment should the nurses be undertaking and how often? What interventions should be carried out and by whom? These decisions will be guided by statements from professional bodies, organizational policies, local guidelines and current research. Once the elements of the service have been identified and the level of good practice has been agreed, a standard exists.

Donabedian's framework is used to scrutinize the standard, breaking down the steps needed to achieve it into three parts: the structure, the process and the outcome. The structure refers to the ward environment, resources and staffing levels. The process is how the standards are achieved, e.g. a standardized assessment is completed, the nursing system and therapeutic interventions prescribed. The outcome is the observable, measurable results, e.g. the completed assessment and the implementation of the prescribed intervention. Box 9.1 gives an example of a standard statement and how it is broken down into structure, process and outcome.

 Box 9.1

An example of a standard for care plans, scrutinized using the Donabedian framework

Problem identification, objective setting and a problem solving approach to meeting the needs of patients are used in developing nursing care plans.

Structure:
- There are professional standards on records and record keeping.
- There is a Trust policy on the requirements for nursing records.
- Each patient is assigned a named nurse, responsible for the coordination and delivery of care.

Process:
- Each nurse will undergo a local education programme with regard to the nursing process.
- The nurse writes a statement of objectives designed to resolve the problem identified.
- The nurse and patient write their perceptions of the problem as patient centred.
- What the nurse will do is written down.
- What the patient will do is written down.
- The nurse and patient sign the care plan. If this is not possible, reasons are recorded.

Outcome:
- The problem is identified in terms of the patient.
- The objective is realistic and relates to the identified problem.
- The objective is measurable and contains a time element.
- The signature of the named nurse is on the care plan.
- The signature of the patient or a reason for no patient signature is on the care plan.
- The patient has a copy of the care plan.

(Bethlem and Maudsley Trust: Mental Health Nursing Practice Standards and Audit, compiled by David Russell, 1992.)

Kitson (1986) states that a major difficulty in discussing standards is being able to distinguish between the philosophy or value statements and statements of standards, which need to be broken down into discrete, understandable, measurable units. It is essential to be able to do this to audit the standard. The outcomes identified in Box 9.1 are discrete and measurable. The auditor can examine nursing documentation to see if the care plan is signed and dated by both the nurse and the patient. Feedback on the level at which the standard is being achieved can then be offered.

Standards may be set for the nursing component of services or they can be set as multidisciplinary standards. Multi-disciplinary standards should identify, where necessary, the professional responsible for carrying out a particular component of the standard; e.g. if the standard set covers medication, it may be necessary to specify that the medication is prescribed by the doctor or nurse, as legally it cannot be prescribed by the psychologist or social worker.

Once standards are set they must be audited so that an evaluation of the service can be made. Again audit may be carried out by one discipline or may be multidisciplinary. If the standards are for nursing practice it is usual that they are audited by nurses. When the standards cover a multidisciplinary service they may be audited by any of the disciplines or a team made up of members from different disciplines.

AUDIT TOOLS

Several audit tools have been developed for use in evaluating nursing practice. Examples are Qualpacs (Wandalt and Ager, 1974), Psychiatric Monitor (Goldstone and Doggett, 1990) and the Nottingham Audit (Howard and Hurst, 1987).

These tools avoid the need to set individual standards, as the standard of care required is documented. However, when used to evaluate a service, they may not be as flexible as is required nor examine all the areas considered important. Balogh *et al.* (1992) suggest that although an 'off the shelf' audit may appear attractive managers do not often consider the cost of staff time and training needed to use it.

CLINICAL PROTOCOLS AND GUIDELINES

A service already may have established clinical protocols or guidelines for aspects of care provision. If they are specific, they can be used to audit actual care delivery rather than establishing new standards. This is a method frequently preferred by doctors. It can be adopted by nurses or, perhaps more profitably and in line with government guidance (NHS, Management Executive, 1993) as a multidisciplinary clinical audit initiative.

QUALITY OF LIFE—AN OUTCOME MEASURE IN MENTAL HEALTH CARE

Quality assurance programmes have little relevance to people using mental health services unless the outcome, as well as the structure and process of mental health services, is addressed. An outcome measure that is increasingly used to evaluate the effectiveness of many mental health services is Quality of Life (QoL). We will consider the rationale for using QoL as an outcome measure, QoL indicators for those with mental health problems and QoL measures and uses.

RATIONALE

Goodinson and Singleton (1989) define QoL as 'freedom of action, a sense of purpose, achievement in one's work or family life, self esteem, integrity and the fulfilment of some fundamental aspects of biological and physiological function'. A mental health problem is likely to encroach upon the quality of a person's life. Institutional care to help with this com-pounds the encroachment. Detention for involuntary treatment under a section of the Mental Health Act may severely restrict an individual's QoL. Therefore, concern with a client's QoL should be of key interest to mental health nurses. While improving the QoL of patients, researching QoL provides nurses with an opportunity to evaluate the efficacy of different treatments and interventions, to identify the point at which to make specific intervention in an illness and it provides means to allocate nursing resources cost-effectively.

Seeking cures for mental illness remains an important objective of many researchers. However, the absence of such cures is focusing attention on identifying the psychosocial factors that sustain the debilitating effects of disorders. Developing effective interventions and appropriate outcomes against which to measure the effects of these interventions is crucial. QoL research offers this promise.

Quality of Life is an important outcome measure of the usefulness of health services (Vetter *et al.*, 1988). The use of QoL is gaining ground among many purchasers of mental health services in the UK (Simmons, 1993). Assessing, pro-moting and monitoring the QoL of people with mental health problems is crucial. It is a major target of the DoH drive to improve the health of the nation (DoH, 1992). To be used successfully as an outcome measure, it is important for mental health service providers to be aware of QoL indicators while planning services.

QUALITY OF LIFE INDICATORS

Indicators of QoL are concerned with mental and physical well-being, having mutually enhancing relations with other people, engaging in social, community and civic activities, and having a sense of reasonable self-actualization, so-called higher order needs (Flanagan, 1978). Indicators for those with mental health problems, whether living in institutional settings or not, commonly focus on different aspects. These include their living situation, family and social relations; leisure activities; work; finances; personal safety; and health issues. These are the so-called lower order needs (Lehman *et al.*, 1982). Such people are motivated more by lower order than higher order needs, unlike those living without severe or enduring mental health problems.

Callaghan (1993) and Callaghan and Adams (1994) suggest conditions that may improve the QoL of those living in mental health settings. These include:

• More contact with relatives.
• Improved finances.
• Protection against harm from others.
• Greater privacy.
• Opportunities to engage in work-related activities.
• Easier and more access to staff.
• More homely surroundings furnished with personal possessions.
• A degree of choice on whom to share living space with.
• Maintenance of confidentiality, even from relatives if necessary.
• Acknowledgement of clients' needs to master increasingly complex social and cognitive skills with provision of opportunities to engage in work-related activities.
• Unified treatment programmes, presenting no contradictions and comprehensive enough to allow clients to internalize and integrate values and ways of behaving.
• Care to ensure that the setting does not resemble 'cold storage' for the client, i.e. isolated activities should not occupy the client intermittently but a unified lifestyle should be encouraged, incorporating therapy and activities cohesively.
• Reduction of the potentially harmful effects of institutionalization. These include (i) loss of contact with the outside world, (ii) enforced idleness through lack of interesting activities, (iii) loss of friends and personal possessions and (iv) a poor ward atmosphere and the loss of prospects.

MEASURING QUALITY OF LIFE

While QoL may be useful to evaluate the effect of mental health services on users, how to measure it is often debated by researchers. There are many and varied measures of QoL. These include indexes (Karnofsky and Burchenal, 1949), interviews, which may be structured (Lehman *et al.*, 1982), semi-structured (Heinrichs *et al.*, 1984) or unstructured (Norman and Parker, 1990), visual analogue scales (Padilla and Grant, 1985) and Quality Adjusted Life Years (QALYs) (Williams, 1985). However, many of these measures may be inadequate (Goodinson and Singleton, 1989).

First used in the late 1940s, indexes are rating scales developed for use by health care staff to assess the QoL of patients. Indexes are limited because they ignore the important, subjective indicators of QoL. They also place staff in the paternalistic position of deciding the QoL of patients whose views did not contribute to the ratings of their QoL. Their use is limited nowadays.

Semi-structured interviews are the commonest measures in use and potentially the most valuable. These usually develop from interviews with the people whose QoL they assess.

Unlike indexes, they include subjective indicators. More recently, Norman and Parker (1990) used unstructured interviews to assess the effect of transferring previously hospitalized persons with long-term mental illness to a community setting.

The QoL Questionnaire (Bigelow *et al.*, 1991) offers a comprehensive and relevant measure of QoL and appears sensitive enough to capture the vicissitudes of QoL domains.

Perhaps the most contentious QoL measures developed recently are QALYs. QALYs offer economic, QoL and life expectancy measures to decide how best to allocate increasingly scarce health resources equitably. Aside from the moral issues of utilizing such an approach especially in a mental health setting, QALYs were not validated in such settings. They would have limited value here because life expectancy has less relevance. Box 9.2 identifies some recently published QoL measures used in research with mentally ill people and describes the dimensions of QoL assessed by each measure. Bowling (1991) provides a review of QoL measurement scales; not all are relevant to mental health care.

Quality of life measures and dimensions

Quality of Life Interview (Bigelow *et al.*, 1990)
• Housing; self and home maintenance; finances; employment; psychiatric medication; physical health; meaningful use of time; psychological well-being; interpersonal functioning.

Quality of Life Questionnaire (Bigelow *et al.*, 1991)
• Psychological distress; well-being; ability to cope with stress; basic need satisfaction; independence; interpersonal interaction; spouse role; social support; work at home; work in a job; employability; meaningful use of leisure time; negative consequences of alcohol; negative consequences of drug use.

Quality of Life Profile (Oliver, 1992)
• Work or education; leisure and social participation; religion; finances; living situation; legal and safety issues; family relations; social relations; health.

Client's Quality of Life Instrument (Pinkney *et al.*, 1991)
• Leisure and recreation; employment; education; finances; living arrangements; social activity; involvement with family, friends and community; ability to cope.

Quality of Life Self-Report (Skantz *et al.*, 1990)
• Housing; physical environment; household and personal care; public service; knowledge and education; contacts; dependence; finances; inner experiences; religion; mental health; physical health; work; leisure.

(Simmons, 1993)

USING QUALITY OF LIFE AS AN OUTCOME MEASURE

The last 15 years has seen a resurgence in evaluative research in mental health that has used QoL as an outcome measure. In general, this research is problematic: over-reliance on objective and often inadequate measures, few attempts to relate processes to outcomes in care delivery and, importantly, a poor understanding of the link between the objective conditions of life and a person's perception of the conditions (Holmes, 1989).

Two recently published reviews (Simmons 1993; Callaghan and Adams, 1994) suggest ways that QoL may be used effectively as an outcome measure. These include:

- Assessment of both subjective and objective indicators of QoL
- Researchers' awareness of social response bias, idiosyncratic reports and interpretation of feelings when assessing subjective indicators of QoL.
- Assessment based on self-reports, which include some element of satisfaction with life in general and specific features.
- The method of assessment should provide some guidance through a semi-structured interview but not constrain the respondents' opportunities to talk about areas important or of concern to them.
- Some assessment of the person's welfare (as opposed to satisfaction with life) that takes the form of more objective measures.

THE FUTURE

POLITICAL INFLUENCES

The political influences of quality on health are uncertain. Current Government policy is clear; it is aimed at improving effectiveness. There is a strong link between improving both the clinical and the cost effectiveness of services, with guidance on specific target areas yet to be agreed (NHSE, 1995). It is unclear whether this policy will continue if there is a change in Government.

MANAGEMENT INFLUENCES

Management initiatives have up to now been influenced by Government policy and guidance. They are likely to continue to be influenced in this way. Uncertainty, caused by the potential for a change in Government to affect policy development, will inevitably be reflected in management quality assurance initiatives.

CLINICAL INFLUENCES

Clinically-led quality assurance initiatives, although influenced by Government policy, have the potential to develop independently. Such initiatives began before the reforms following the Griffiths Report (DHSS, 1983) formally put quality assurance on to the agenda for the NHS. Nurses and other health care professionals have recognized the importance of quality of care to patients for many years. This will not alter with change in Government. It is in this area that there is a chance to develop independent quality assurance programmes and projects. To keep quality assurance on the agenda for patients in the future, it may be necessary for health care professionals to work together to develop programmes that are robust enough to continue, despite changes in Government. It is only in this way we can make sure that quality services for patients continue to develop.

SUMMARY

Improving the QoL of people with mental health problems has been placed on the national health care agenda. QoL is used in many countries as an outcome measure against which to evaluate the quality of both hospital and community based mental health services. QoL measures are available, many of which are reliable and valid and can be used with relative ease by any mental health professional. The method selected to assess QoL must be that which allows service users the opportunity to discuss areas important to them and of concern to their quality of life. QoL fits neatly into quality assurance programmes of service providers in the mental health field.

Quality assurance has developed rapidly over the past 15 years and it is likely that it will continue to do so. The direction in which it will develop is less clear, though involvement of nurses in clinically-led initiatives will ensure that patients' needs maintain a high profile irrespective of other influences.

KEY CONCEPTS

- The development of quality assurance in nursing care has been influenced by two distinct agendas: political and professional.
- An understanding of quality assurance terminology is essential for nurses to be able to develop programmes with other health care professionals, based on a common philosophy.
- There are many different approaches to quality assurance, some management-led, others led by professionals. There is no one right way to monitor quality of care. There is a need to develop a system that works for the particular area of practice.
- Clinical protocols, guidelines and standards may be used as the basis of clinically-led quality assurance programmes.
- Management-led quality assurance programmes have a requirement to examine both cost and clinical effectiveness.
- The future development of quality assurance in health care is uncertain if it continues to be politically driven. Changes in Government may lead to alteration in policy. Only clinically-led quality initiatives can overcome this uncertainty.

REFERENCES

Allen RE: *The concise Oxford dictionary of current English.* Oxford, 1990, Clarendon Press.

Balogh R, Bond S, Parker K: Off-the-shelf audit: is it feasible? *Nurs Stand* 7(4):35–38, 1992.

Bigelow D, Gareau M, Young D: A quality of life interview. *Psychosoc Rehab* 14(2):94–98, 1990.

Bigelow D, McFarland B, Olson M: Quality of life of community mental health program clients. *Community Ment Health J* 27(1):43–55, 1991.

Bowling A: *Measuring health: a review of quality of life measurement scales.* Milton Keynes, 1991, Open University Press.

Callaghan P: *Quality of life: the importance of theory to practice in English Special Hospitals.* Paper presented at the 5th International Congress of Mental Health Nursing, September 1993, University of Manchester.

Callaghan P, Adams R: The contribution of quality of life to developing therapeutic nursing in Special Hospitals. *J Psychiatr Ment Health Nurs* 1(2):109–114, 1994.

Department of Health: *The Patient's Charter.* London, 1991, HMSO.

Department of Health: *The Health of the Nation.* London, 1992, HMSO.

Department of Health: *The Patient's Charter and you.* London, 1995, HMSO.

Department of Health and Social Security: *The Nurses, Midwives and Health Visitors Act.* London, 1979, HMSO.

Department of Health and Social Security: *Inequalities in health: report of a Research Working Group (Chairman: Sir Douglas Black).* London, 1980, DHSS.

Department of Health and Social Security: NHS Management Enquiry Team: *National health service management enquiry: the Griffiths Report.* London, 1983, HMSO.

Department of Health and Social Security: *Working for patients.* London, 1989, HMSO.

Dingwall R, Rafferty AM, Webster C: *An introduction to the social history of nursing.* London, 1988, Routledge.

Ellis R, editor: *Professional competence and quality assurance in the caring professions.* London, 1988, Croom Helm.

Ellis R, Whittington D: *Quality assurance in health care.* London, 1993, Edward Arnold.

Flanagan J: A research approach to improving out quality of life. *Am Psychol* 12(3):138–147, 1978.

Goldstone LA, Doggett T: *Psychiatric monitor.* Newcastle-upon-Tyne, 1990, Polytechnic Products Ltd.

Goodinson SM, Singleton J: Quality of life: a critical review of current concepts, measures and their clinical implications. *Int J Nurs Stud* 26(4):327–341, 1989.

Green W, Hinchliff S, Fordham J, Schober J: *Quality assurance.* London, 1991, HMSO.

Heinrichs DW, Hanlon TE, Williams T, Carpenter J: The Quality of Life Scale: an instrument for rating the schizophrenic deficit syndrome. *Schizophr Bull* 10(3):388–396, 1984.

Holmes CA: Health care and the quality of life: a review. *J Adv Nurs* 14(10):833–839, 1989.

Hooper A, Grover R, Gawith L: A glossary of terms encountered in quality assurance and related work. *Q-Net, The Mental Health Quality Assurance Network.* Issue 2, London, 1995, Sainsbury Centre.

Howard D, Hurst K: *The central Nottinghamshire psychiatric nursing audit.* Nottingham, 1987, Central Nottinghamshire Health Authority.

Karnofsky D, Burchenal J: The clinical evaluation of chemotherapeutic agents in cancer. In: McCleod CM, editor: *Evaluation of chemotherapeutic agents.* New York, 1949, Columbia Press.

Kitson A: Standards of care in psychiatric nursing. *Nurs Times* 82(52):51–54, 1986.

Kitson A: Editorial (quality assurance supplement). *Nurs Stand* 5(9):3, 1990.

Lehman AF, Ward NC, Linn LS: Chronic mental patients: the quality of life issue. *Am J Psychiatry* 139(10):1271–1276, 1982.

National Health Service Executive: *Improving the effectiveness of clinical services.* EL(95)105, Leeds, 1995, NHSE.

National Health Service Management Executive: *Meeting and improving standards in healthcare.* EL(93)59, Leeds, 1993, NHSME.

National Health Service Management Executive: HSG(94)5 *Introduction of the Supervision Register for mentally ill people from 1st April 1995.* Leeds, 1995, NHSE.

Norman I, Parker F: Psychiatric patients' views of their lives before and after moving to a hostel: a qualitative review. *J Adv Nurs* 15(9):1036–1044, 1990.

Oliver J: The social care directive: development of a quality of life profile for use in community services for the mentally ill. *Soc Work Soc Serv Rev* 3(4):5–45, 1992.

Ovretveit J: *Health Service quality: an introduction to quality methods for health services.* Oxford, 1992, Blackwell.

Padilla GV, Grant MM: Quality of life as a cancer nursing outcome variable. *Adv Nurs Sci* 8(1):45–58, 1985.

Pinkney AA, Gerber G, Lefave H: Quality of life after psychiatric rehabilitation: the client's perspective. *Acta Psychiatr Scand* 83(2):86–91, 1991.

Simmons S: Quality of life in community mental health care: a review. *Int J Nurs Stud* 31(2):183–193, 1993.

Skantz K, Malm U, Dencker S, May P: Quality of life in schizophrenia. *Nord Psykiatrica Tiddsker* 44(3):71–75, 1990.

Strong P, Robinson J: *The NHS under new management.* Milton Keynes, 1990, Open University Press.

United Kingdom Central Council for Nursing, Midwifery and Health Visiting: *Project 2000: a new preparation for practice.* London, 1986, UKCC.

United Kingdom Central Council for Nursing, Midwifery and Health Visiting: *Code of professional conduct.* London, 1992, UKCC.

United Kingdom Central Council for Nursing, Midwifery and Health Visiting: *Standards for the administration of medicines.* London, 1992, UKCC.

United Kingdom Central Council for Nursing, Midwifery and Health Visiting: *Standards for records and record keeping.* London, 1993, UKCC.

Vetter N, Jones D, Victor C: The quality of life of the over 70s in the community. *Health Visitor* 61(1):10–13, 1988.

Wandalt D, Ager G: *Qualpacs, quality patient care scale.* New York, 1974, Appleton-Century Crofts.

Williams A: *Quality adjusted life years and coronary artery bypass grafting.* London, 1985, HMSO.

Wilson CRM: *Hospital-wide quality assurance.* Ontario, 1987, WB Saunders

FURTHER READING

Ellis R, Whittington D: *Quality assurance in health care: a handbook.* London, 1993, Edward Arnold.
> *Provides an inventory of quality assurance techniques, guidance on selecting a technique, and setting up a quality assurance system.*

Firth-Cozens J: *Audit in mental health services.* Hove, UK, 1993, Lawrence Earlbaum Associates.
> *Offers advice on selecting topics for audit and methods for monitoring practice.*

Kemp N, Richardson E: *Quality assurance in nursing practice.* London, 1990, Butterworth Heinemann.
> *Discusses how standard setting can be effective in monitoring and evaluating professional practice.*

Mishra R: *The Welfare State in crisis; social thought and social change.* Hemel Hempstead, 1984, Harvester Wheatsheaf.
> *Examines the arguments underlying theories of welfare provision.*

Nolan P: *A history of mental health nursing.* London, 1993, Chapman & Hall.
> *A historical perspective on the development of mental health nursing.*

Rogers A, Pilgrim D, Lacey R: *Experiencing psychiatry: users' views of services.* London, 1993, MIND.
> *Describes patients eye-views of mental health services.*

Royal College of Nursing Standards of Care Project: *Quality patient care: the dynamic standard setting system.* London, 1990, RCN.
> *Offers a framework for standard setting and evaluation of nursing care.*

Smith R, editor: *Audit in action.* London, 1992, BMJ.
> *A compendium of articles on audit originally published in the BMJ.*

Strong P, Robinson J: *The NHS under new management.* Milton Keynes, 1990, Open University Press.
> *Reports a research study of seven health authorities and the effects of the implementation of recommendations from the Griffiths management inquiry (DHSS 1983). Offers first-hand accounts of the dynamics of management and professionals within the NHS.*

Thornicroft G, Brewin CR, Wing J, editors: *Measuring mental health needs.* London, 1992, Gaskell.
> *Offers the perspective of managers, purchasers, clinicians and researchers.*

• *Chapter* •
10

Supervision and Professional Practice

Learning Outcomes

....

After studying this chapter, you should be able to:

• Describe the different approaches to supervision taken from the literature.

• Explore the various forms clinical supervision takes.

• Analyse components of the supervisory relationship.

• Identify areas of responsibility between participants in the supervisory relationship.

• Explore elements of a working model suitable to particular clinical areas.

• Discuss research methods suitable for evaluating the effectiveness of supervision.

*C*linical supervision has been known in certain mental* health settings for several years but has only recently become the focus of interest across the branches of nursing. Added impetus has come from the Department of Health's Mental Health Nursing Review Team who consider it an integral part of mental health nursing practice. The Review Team's *Working in Partnership* (Department of Health, 1994) recommends supervision as an important developmental target for all nursing staff, yet it is still not considered an integral part of a majority of clinical settings. Within mental health nursing clinical supervision is a recognized element of practice and an ethical and professional necessity. It not only offers the opportunity to consider and address the high levels of emotional and physical contact nurses experience in their work with patients but helps clinicians develop their own personal and specialist skills.

The United Kingdom Central Council for Nurses, Midwives and Health Visitors (UKCC) suggest that clinical supervision will play an increasingly important part in clinical care (UKCC, 1995). Recent interest in clinical supervision is characterized by concern over maintaining high clinical standards of care and an emphasis on the professional development of nurses.

In the National Health Service, 'supervision' is often equated with managerial activity. Clinical work is seen to be scrutinized critically by a domineering overseer concerned with punitively monitoring performance, such as time-keeping, rates of work and rigidly applied standards of practice. Such an image may be reinforced by the reality of having a supervisor who is responsible for individual performance review and who may have an influence over promotional prospects. The UKCC (1995) has attempted to allay these fears by stating that supervision is not:

1. The exercise of managerial responsibility and managerial supervision.
2. A system of formal individual performance review procedures.
3. Intended to be hierarchical in nature.

Supervision, as a separate entity related to nursing practice is discussed here, drawing from the literature and the authors' own experiences. The supervision of clinical practice is increasingly advocated throughout nursing as a means of enhancing professional development. The theoretical background and the application of supervision is explored and a working example is presented. Clinical supervision needs a high level of perseverance and commitment both from the individuals involved and at an organizational level. It is an area of nursing practice that can provide recognition of the effects of caring, not only for individuals but for teams of nurses. It is also an example of a professional activity that nurses can promote in other disciplines as a model of good practice.

DEFINITIONS

The emergence of supervision in mental health nursing (coming from counselling and psychotherapy, where it is an established prerequisite for practice) reflects an acknowledgement of the complexities of interpersonal relationships involved in working closely with troubled individuals.

This concern, primarily with practitioner–patient casework, is reflected in Hess' (1980) view of supervision as 'essentially a dyadic human interaction with a focus on modifying the behaviour of the supervisee, so he or she may provide a better service to a third person'. Here, the emphasis of the supervisory relationship is on making sure that supervisees are adequately prepared for their work with patients. This view is supported by Taylor (1994) who sees supervision as 'an intensive interpersonally focused, one-to-one relationship in which one person is designated to facilitate the development of therapeutic competence in the other person'. This perspective places importance on the nature of the relationship between participants, while acknowledging that the primary purpose is to develop the supervisee's competence in casework. Such a position suggests that supervision is an educational process, where the supervisee is enabled to develop competence through the guidance of a senior colleague.

Ironbar and Hooper (1989) support this view, suggesting that the supervisor should be someone with extensive clinical experience and training, who can provide expert support and guidance and who is trusted and respected by the supervisee. They propose eight objectives for supervision. It should:

1. Discuss in detail specific aspects of the practitioner's casework.
2. Focus on the skills base of the interventions, the goals of therapy and the nature of the practitioner's relationships with clients.
3. Encourage self-evaluation of the practitioner's approach.
4. Give guidance and advice on professional practice.
5. Offer support and validation for professional decisions.
6. Give feedback to individuals on their performance.
7. Promote professional self-development.
8. Help the practitioner cope with personal and professional stress.

According to these objectives the educational aspect of supervision is clear. By focusing on goals, interventions and relationships the supervisor encourages self-evaluation and development, while providing feedback, advice and guidance. However, a supportive dimension to supervision is also proposed. The supervisor helps the practitioner to cope with professional stress and provides validation and support for professional decisions.

This supportive dimension is emphasized by Farkas–Cameron (1995) who conceptualizes supervision as a 'self-actualizing' process of 'engaging in a potentially supportive, trusting and respectful relationship with a colleague to advance one's level of clinical practice'. This aspect of supervision is crucial. For a practitioner to subject their practice freely to scrutiny they must trust that it will be received and treated in a respectful and supportive way. However, in attempting to introduce a system of clinical supervision, Farkas–Cameron encountered fear among some nurses that it was synonymous with personal therapy. They questioned whether or not it would help them cope with professional challenges or develop therapeutic relationships with their patients. Farkas–Cameron, in common with Hess (1980) and Taylor (1994) , focuses the supervision on the supervisee's clinical practice. This is important if the supportive element is not to be experienced as intrusive or irrelevant.

A third aspect of supervision is emphasized by Holloway and Neufeldt (1995), who suggest that 'supervision plays a critical role in maintaining the standards of the profession'. This implies that the supervisor has a quality assurance role in relation to the clinical work of the supervisee although the UKCC (1995) draw a clear distinction between supervision and appraisal. The supervisor may also have a managerial or evaluative role for the practitioner but this must remain distinct from the supervisory 'quality assurance' role, which is primarily concerned with helping to achieve and maintain high ethical and professional standards. Greenburg (1980) describes a potential conflict between these roles. A practitioner will wish to appear competent to a supervisor who can influence their future career development. This may lead to a less open supervisory relationship, where the supervisee glosses over or disguises difficulties with which they need assistance and guidance, resulting in poor performance of their practice role. Shohet and Wilmot (1991) recommend that the management of these power discrepancies should be discussed and negotiated between the participants.

These aspects of the supervisory process correspond to those described by Proctor (1988), who characterized three functions of supervision:

1. Formative, which refers to the supervisee's learning process and is concerned with acquiring competence in the application of skills and with the development of the practitioner's professional identity. This occurs mainly through reflection on casework guided by the supervisor's training and experience.
2. Restorative, which refers to the attention and validation that is paid to the emotional effects of the therapeutic work on the practitioner. This occurs mainly through debriefing and enables the supervisee to recognize and manage stress and avoid burn-out.
3. Normative, which refers to the aspect of supervision that is concerned with professional and ethical standards of the

supervisee's practice, where the supervisor provides a quality control role.

The definitions discussed here reflect the origins of supervision in counselling and psychotherapy by focusing primarily on the practitioner's casework (McLeod, 1993). However, psychiatric nursing is an increasingly diverse profession, with practitioners working in a wide variety of settings with a broad range of responsibilities in addition to their casework. Burrow (1995) points out that nurses are subject to contractual obligations, not only to their patients but also to their employers and to their professional body. These factors combine to make nursing a complex and stressful occupation where the practitioner has to balance a number of sometimes conflicting demands in a safe and reasonable manner. Supervision in psychiatric nursing cannot be restricted to the casework but must also concern itself with the practitioner's ability to discharge these broader obligations and responsibilities. In view of this, the authors suggest that supervision in psychiatric nursing is:

> a trusting and respectful relationship between two or more practitioners, which serves formative, restorative and normative functions with regard to all aspects of the professional work of one or more participants.

THEORETICAL MODELS OF SUPERVISION

Here the authors present and offer a critique of theoretical models with regard to their practicality in the workplace. Using the definition of supervision above, several questions immediately arise, which include:

- How is the task achieved?
- What activities occur in the context of the relationship?
- What kind of conceptual framework is used to organize an understanding of what takes place?

Answers are important, to give the participant guidance about their roles and because the supervisee may be reluctant (consciously or unconsciously) to expose certain aspects of their work to scrutiny. Reasons for this reluctance include feelings of inadequacy, guilt and shame or the fear of being thought negligent or incompetent. These feelings are commonplace and closely related to the nature of therapeutic work they are invariably evident when under stress or close to burn-out.) They are also a direct result of deficits in the practitioner's theory or skills repertoire.

It is therefore a crucial part of the supervisor's role to help the practitioner recognize and manage these difficulties while taking appropriate action. Without some clear 'map', guidance or model to assist in making choices about supervisory style, the supervisor can be drawn into colluding with the supervisee's avoidances, thus neglecting formative, restorative or normative responsibility. According to Page and Wosket (1994) a supervision model should enable the participants to locate themselves by providing such a map. It should also

articulate both the process and methodology of supervision and be practical and adaptable to different situational demands.

Developmental, process and cyclical models have been proposed and will be looked at in detail. The cyclical model provides a structure in which the supervisor and supervisee can locate themselves (both within individual sessions and across the period of their relationship) by relating their concerns to the appropriate stage of the process. This can also be informed by reference to the developmental model, which indicates, in particular, the developmental stage of the supervisee in their career as a practitioner. The process model gives a comprehensive guide to the possible methods available to the supervisor. These methods are placed clearly in the context of the supervision process by the cyclical model. In combination they offer a practical and flexible framework which is adaptable to differing situational demands.

DEVELOPMENTAL MODEL

Stoltenberg and Delworth (1987) describe an approach to supervision that refers to the developmental stage of the supervisee. Their model identifies the supervisor as the one who needs to modify both the style and focus of the supervision as the practitioner gains in experience and confidence. Hawkins and Shohet (1989, 1991) characterize this developmental model in four stages based on the practitioner's development.

Stage 1: Novice

Supervisees are inexperienced and anxious about their role and ability. They are often highly motivated but are dependent on the supervisor for guidance and to assess their work. They tend to focus on particular aspects of their role, lacking the insight and experience to form a broad overview of their clinical and managerial work. The supervisor needs at this stage to provide a well-structured environment for novices, including positive feedback, encouragement about their performance and clear guidance on areas for improvement.

Stage 2: Apprentice

Supervisees have progressed beyond the initial anxieties and are beginning to develop a more sophisticated understanding of their role. They function more autonomously, though there may be episodes of over-confidence or reverting to a state of dependence with corresponding periods of despondency. This may result in disillusionment with the supervisor who is seen as incompetent and inadequate. The supervisee will need to feel well-supported by the supervisor, who should provide less structure than in the novice phase of development while maintaining the safe boundaries of the relationship, as the supervisee may begin to test out their supervisor's authority through cancelling or arriving late for appointments or by more outright verbal challenges.

Stage 3: Journeyman

Supervisees are less dependent on the supervisor, showing increased self-confidence and more stable motivation. They develop a working overview of their role and are able to prioritize more effectively, adapting to varied professional demands. The supervision becomes more of a professional conversation between colleagues, with periodic confrontation.

Stage 4: Master

Supervisees have mastered their role and achieved personal autonomy, insightful awareness, stable motivation and recognizes the need to confront professional problems. Supervision at this stage primarily serves to help consolidate professional development.

This formulation of the developmental stages of practitioner development may provide a useful model for assessing the corresponding demands of supervision in practice. However, it is not a fixed blueprint and each practitioner will develop at their own pace and with their own particular strengths and weaknesses. It has also been criticized for failing to take account of the developmental stage of the supervisor and, in particular, it provides little guidance on the actual focus of the activity or methodology that takes place in the supervision session.

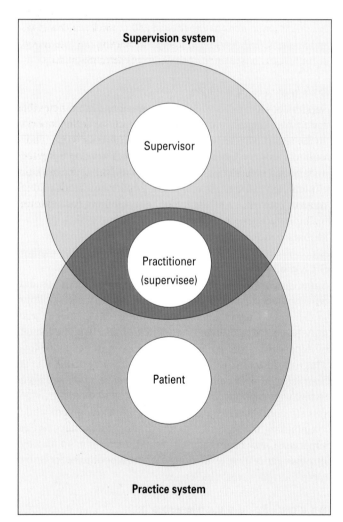

Figure 10.1 Process model of supervision (Hawkins and Shohet, 1989)

PROCESS MODEL: STYLES AND MODES

Hawkins and Shohet (1989) propose a model of supervision, which focuses mainly on the process that occurs in the supervisory session (Figure 10.1); it is designed for counselling and psychotherapy supervision but can be adapted to a broader arena such as nursing. They aim to distinguish between different supervisory styles by looking at the range of options open to the supervisor. According to Hawkins (1985) the supervisory context has three elements:

1. The practitioner.
2. Their practice.
3. The supervisor.

These elements constitute two interconnecting dyadic or interactive systems: first the practice system, which connects the practitioner and their practice; and second the supervision system, between practitioner (supervisee) and supervisor. The supervisory system interacts with and guides the practice system, supervisory being generated in this way. Hawkins and Shohet (1991) describe six options, or 'modes', for approaching the supervision task and it is the way these modes are combined that defines the supervisor's style.

The six modes are divided into two categories: those concerned with the supervision system and those concerned with the practice system.

The Practice System

Three modes focus on the practitioner's clinical work as it is reported in the supervision session.

1. Content

The emphasis here is on exploring the factual content of the supervisee's working life. Interest is focused on how the practitioner spends their time, the size of their caseload, the demands of paperwork and any other particular aspects of their role, and on the content of their patient contact.

2. Strategies and interventions

This mode is concerned with the choices of intervention made by the supervisee and when and why such choices were made. This relates both to the supervisee's work with patients and to other performance aspects of his or her role, such as decision making and resource management. It is concerned with exploring alternatives and developing strategies.

3. Process

Here the supervisor pays particular attention to the supervisee's approach to work, and to their confidence and enthusiasm, stage of development and learning needs. Attention is also paid to the dynamic processes that occur in relationships with patients, as well as between supervisee and colleagues.

The Supervision System

The final three modes focus on the way the practitioner's clinical work is reflected in the supervision session.

4. Practitioner countertransference

Here the emphasis is on the way the supervisee is affected by the clinical work. Certain patients may provoke emotional reactions, positive or negative, which make therapeutic work difficult for the practitioner. The work may also be experienced as either very exciting and stimulating or very exhausting and draining. The supervisor concentrates on helping the supervisee to manage these emotions and to explore their roots in the clinical work.

(Countertransference has been succinctly defined as the feelings evoked in the therapist or nurse by the patient. See: Winnicott, 1949; Money-Kyrle, 1958; Brown and Pedder, 1991.)

5. Mirror or parallel process

The emphasis here is on the way the supervisory relationship reflects the supervisee's experience of their clinical work. If a particular patient or staff member has been acting in a passive or aggressive way towards the supervisee, for example, the supervisee may behave in a similar way towards the supervisor. This phenomenon has been well documented by Mattinson (1975), who suggests that it can be recognized by behaviour that is out of character with the supervisee's personality and previous experience.

6. Supervisor countertransference

Here the supervisor concentrates on their own 'here and now' experiences of the supervision session, using the thoughts, feelings and images that emerge in response to the supervisee's description of their clinical work to help illuminate interpersonal or other processes that may be taking place.

Supervisory Style

According to Hawkins and Shohet (1989), supervisors tend to have their own style, which depends on the particular combinations of these modes they use. The style will usually reflect the supervisor's theoretical orientation. Most supervisors, for example, will be interested in the content of the supervisee's work (mode 1) but a supervisor working from a predominantly behavioural perspective will also take a close interest in mode 2 (strategies and interventions) and mode 3 (concerned with process) (Linehan, 1980). A supervisor whose orientation is mainly psychodynamic will also be interested in mode 3 but will place a stronger emphasis on modes 4 and 6 (practitioner and supervisor countertransference) as well as on mode 5 (mirror or parallel processes) (Moldawsky, 1980). A supervisor whose orientation is client-centred or humanistic will also emphasize mode 5 (Wilmot and Shohet, 1985) as well as showing concern for modes 2 and 3 (Rice, 1980).

It is useful to identify these different modes of supervision to help supervisors become aware of their own supervisory style. Overreliance on a certain combination of modes can restrict the scope of the supervision. For example, if excessive emphasis is placed on mode 2 (strategies and interventions), the supervision may serve as an intellectual discussion of techniques at the expense of more contextual issues surrounding the supervisee in their working

circumstances. Similarly, supervision that concentrates exclusively on modes 4, 5 and 6 (practitioner and supervisor countertransference and the mirror process), can resemble personal therapy for the supervisee, which does not take sufficient account of their clinical responsibilities and may be experienced as intrusive. This model can also be useful for the supervisee in considering and negotiating their supervisory needs, though it does not specifically address the negotiation of a contract nor is it a means of structured evaluation.

This process model is a useful guide through individual supervision sessions but does not provide a perspective on the supervisee's or supervisor's development or their relationship over time. Hawkins and Shohet (1989) have suggested that this can be achieved by integrating it with a developmental approach. For example, an inexperienced practitioner will need to focus mainly on activities undertaken and on the methods employed, requiring the supervisor to use modes 1 (content) and 2 (strategies and interventions). As the supervisor becomes more experienced, however, the emphasis of concern will shift towards their own approach to and feelings about the work, and their own learning needs. Here the supervisor's emphasis will be on the use of modes 3 (process) and 4 (practitioner countertransference). An experienced practitioner may be more preoccupied with subtle aspects of their professional life and it may be appropriate for the supervisor to respond by focusing more on modes 5 (mirror process) and 6 (supervisor countertransference).

CYCLICAL MODEL

Page and Wosket (1994) have attempted to design a flexible framework that both offers a clear map of the entire supervision process and suggests a workable methodology, incorporating a range of different approaches. They conceptualize supervision as a cyclical process (Figure 10.2). This process is considered seamless and takes place both in individual sessions and throughout the life of a supervisory relationship. There are five stages in the model.

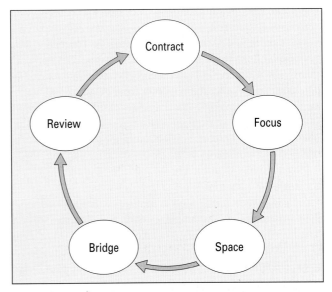

Figure 10.2 Cyclical model of supervision (Page and Wosket, 1994)

Stage 1: Contract

The parties negotiate the task and structure at the outset. Ground rules and boundaries are agreed, including the timing, frequency and duration of the sessions as well as the nature and focus of the relationship. Supervision is not a managerial relationship but the supervisor may sometimes also have a managerial role for the supervisee. It is important to clarify where the boundary falls between supervision and management and to decide how material discussed in a supervision session is to be handled outside, when it comes to appraisal for instance, or if evidence of malpractice emerges. Equally, supervision is not personal therapy for the supervisee, so some agreement should be reached about the content of sessions and the responsibilities of each party. The contract agreed at the outset may be revisited and revised many times throughout a healthy supervisory relationship.

A contracting stage will also occur at the beginning of a supervision session, when some agreement is reached about, for example, the duration and content of the session.

Stage 2: Focus

The focus is the work under consideration at the time. Usually this involves the practitioner presenting some aspect of work for exploration, as will happen in an individual session but it may also be that some themes emerge across sessions that represent the supervisee's longer-term preoccupations in relation to their practice. These might be issues concerning patient work, such as therapeutic interventions and techniques or organizational aspects of the supervisee's working life or more personal issues, such as stress. The issue is clarified until each participant has an understanding of the concern and some sense of how it might be explored in supervision. This develops the supervisee's responsibility for making the best use of supervision and ensures that the content and method are relevant to their needs and practice.

Stage 3: Space

The major collaborative work of supervision takes place at this stage. The issue is reflected upon extensively and investigated both through questioning and challenging and also by attending to transference issues and parallel process. This takes place both on a micro level within supervision sessions and on a macro level, in relation to the supervisee's main practice concerns that emerge thematically from the sessions, across the supervision process. The emphasis of this stage is not on finding solutions but on generating ideas and insights into questions. This is where reflection and exploration can be pursued and where insight and understanding can develop.

Stage 4: Bridge

Ideas and insights generated in the 'space' are applied to on the work situation. This might involve, for example, solving a work difficulty using insights gained or deciding on a course of action to address an identified deficit in skills, knowledge or experience. On the macro level this may be manifest by the practitioner deciding to move into a new clinical area to gain some specific experience. Some sort of planning and goal

setting will usually be involved, ensuring that the supervision process has a tangible impact on the supervisee's practice.

Stage 5: Review

The final stage is concerned with reviewing and evaluating the quality of the supervisory relationship and the effectiveness of the work done in supervision. This may occur at any time during the supervision process, certainly after an agreed period and usually in some form towards the end of each session. It involves each party providing feedback to the other on the quality and usefulness of the supervision. This is important for the practitioner as their professional and practical development depends to a large extent on the quality of the supervision they receive. Likewise, it is equally important that a good supervisor will always be concerned to improve the quality of the supervision provided. This is particularly so where the supervisor has some formal assessment role for the supervisee, who should be made aware of any doubts about the quality of their work and given every opportunity and assistance to improve. Recontracting follows seamlessly from review, at which stage participants renegotiate their agreement in the light of their evaluation and feedback.

TYPES OF SUPERVISION

Methods of supervision can take many guises. These will depend on the type of supervision required, the resources available to carry it out and the emphasis placed on its importance to and influence on practice.

FORMAL AND INFORMAL SUPERVISION

Formal supervision occurs when two or more practitioners make a contract to meet together regularly at a certain time for supervision. Informal supervision takes place when one practitioner approaches another without any predetermined format, to discuss aspects of their work. These approaches are not mutually exclusive. Indeed, informal supervision can be a valuable source of new ideas and support and should be encouraged. However, this cannot replace formal supervision, which provides a clear structure for detailed discussion of issues that may not arise informally, and ensures difficult issues are not avoided. A system of formal supervision makes sure that practitioners receive the supervision they require, rather than leaving this to chance encounters in the staff room.

INDIVIDUAL SUPERVISION

Individual supervision takes place between two practitioners, one of whom is usually more senior and experienced. It allows the supervisee the undivided attention of an important resource for a time, providing invaluable opportunities for learning, support and nurturing. The supervisee can put aside competitive concerns about colleagues and enter freely into detailed discussions of their own working lives, allowing the supervisor to make a full assessment of their capabilities and competence. The clinical possibilities and developments that emerge, however, may reflect the experience, theoretical approach and competence of the supervisor. This can be restrictive for some supervisees who incline to a different approach or whose learning needs cannot be met by a particular person. Individual supervision is probably the form most frequently practised and the supervisor is often someone who has specific skills and expertise in the particular clinical field. Considerable emphasis is being given to allow the supervisor to be chosen rather than allocated. With the introduction of PREP and the preceptorship role for newly qualified staff, recognition is being given to the developmental and mutual learning possibilities of supervision in addition to formal instruction.

GROUP SUPERVISION

Group supervision takes place when two or more practitioners from various practice areas come together with a supervisor to discuss their work. This provides a broad range of clinical and life experiences, so the practitioner benefits from the experience of the supervisor and of fellow supervisees, as well as from witnessing and participating in the supervision offered to other members. Possibilities for exploration through methods such as role-play are also enhanced, although the time allocated for supervision of each member's work will be reduced. The focus of supervision also needs to be more clearly defined in the contracting stage, to clarify how formative, restorative and normative functions are to be undertaken, as it may be inappropriate to address individual issues in a group setting. Whole wards, units or a clinical team may invite an expert to come to the ward on a regular basis to offer group supervision on specific areas of practice. For example, group therapy sessions held on the unit could be written up and presented at a group supervision session or team development issues could be addressed with the help of an outsider.

PEER SUPERVISION

Peer supervision takes place between colleagues of the same grade and depends on mutual respect developed over a period of working together. It may take place individually, or in a group or whole-team format. The equality of grades would usually preclude a managerial role but participants may be required to provide feedback on each other's work as part of the supervision and learning experience. Some may find this difficult, leading to an emphasis on support rather than challenge, and thus collusion. This may be increased where colleagues with similar clinical experience at similar career points may have little skills development to offer each other. However, it can be a good way of introducing some quality control into a service and can help to improve communication between staff and develop team cohesiveness. Care planning meetings would be an example, where staff meet regularly to discuss their patient work and help each other to plan and evaluate effective clinical interventions.

TEAM SUPERVISION

Team supervision is similar to group supervision but involves practitioners who work together. This can save time and produce a range of perspectives on work situations. It can lead to the swift implementation of practice changes that come out of supervision and help to improve communication. It can also enhance feelings of team support and cohesiveness and reduce the isolation of staff whose individual caseload is not known to other team members. However, it can also be threatening for staff to expose their practice in front of juniors or colleagues. Some units offer peer review, where staff meet as a group and discuss issues as colleagues who aim to continually evaluate and review current practice and who take turns to facilitate sessions.

Most clinical units are involved in practising a debriefing system following serious incidents, where staff meet to discuss the situation and identify areas of good practice and areas in need of improvement. This practice has become necessary in acute clinical areas, as nurses are involved increasingly in violent and disturbing incidents. However, these responsive meetings are only the beginning of the debriefing process, helping to contain the anxiety and stress of an incident there and then. The effects of violence have been shown to take many months to surface, through emotional and physical symptoms (Whittington and Wykes, 1991). The need for continuing support and debriefing has been taken up in some clinical areas, with ward or clinical team sessions often being held at the end of each shift or working day. The overall aim is to evaluate and complete the day's work, while still at work rather than allowing situations and feelings to overspill into the next day or be ruminated over outside work.

LIVE OR ON-LINE SUPERVISION

Such supervision takes place during work being supervised. The supervisee may initially observe the supervisor performing a task before trying themselves, first with assistance, then with guidance and eventually unaided. This can also be used to supervise casework as it takes place, and is useful in helping translate theory into practice and in developing skills. Any supervisee editing of reports is omitted as the supervisor observes the work first hand, but it provides only 'snapshots' of the supervisee's working life and can be a valuable addition to formal supervision sessions.

THE SETTING, PURPOSE AND FUNCTION

Supervision should be part of the working life of a nurse and not something squeezed in or tagged on after-hours. Standards for the frequency and minimum amount of time supervision requires to prove worthwhile are suggested.

Any professional helper should have at their disposal technical skills and abilities to bring to the helping relationship, grounded in sound theoretical and academic roots. However, relating to another person brings with it all the complexities and subtleties of human interaction. The practitioner delivers a service to the patient, to the best of their ability, and aims to help the patient understand the meaning and rationale behind the advice and actions offered. At the same time, to gain greater understanding of the patient, they have to appreciate the effects that their actions have. In other words, the professional has to self-evaluate their own work and expose it to scrutiny by the patient and by other colleagues. Only when the professional becomes aware of their personal frame of reference can they begin to explore and work with the effects this has on the patient and vice versa. This awareness brings with it a wider range of options to choose to work from (i.e. the patient's, practitioner's and the supervisor's perspectives). Whether the practitioner uses supervision or has a systematic, self-taught method of reflection, they come to the relationship not as the 'expert' but as an equal partner in the learning experience.

Schon (1983) describes the professional–patient relationship as bound by the professional's responsibility to understand their actions and behaviours not only from their own perspective but, more importantly, from the patient's.

Wright (1991) considers the unconscious processes that develop within nursing that prevent this insight and closeness developing between nurse and patient. Routine activities are used by nurses to safeguard themselves from the emotional and psychological stress evoked by working closely with disturbed patients. Where primary nursing is working properly and nurses are allowed to work closely with patients there is an acceptance of these stresses and mechanisms, as an integral part of the therapeutic process. Wright describes the Cassel Hospital (Richmond, Surrey) where the system of supervision has operated since the 1950s. Daily meetings between nurses and other members of the clinical team focus on the patient and their relationship with the community at large, while also including the patient's important contact with their nurse. Considerable emphasis is placed on how this relationship develops and the feelings it evokes in the nurse.

The Bethlem and Maudsley NHS Trust has worked with clinical supervision since the late 1980s, with many of the principal components originating from the work of an in-patient psychotherapy ward (Jackson and Cawley, 1992; Jackson and Williams, 1994). The ward was established in the late 1970s to treat a range of acute psychiatric illnesses using a psychoanalytical approach and has been compared to the Menninger clinic program in the USA. The work on this ward initiated a network of clinical supervision throughout the hospital and a training course, developed by the Revd John Foskett, was established in 1979. The course, which continues to run successfully, is aimed at all health professionals from different backgrounds. Clinical supervision has been an inherent part of student nurse training at the Maudsley and has led to emphasis on its relevance, in the current Project 2000 branch programme. Through the use of role-play, group dynamics and critical incident analysis students are encouraged to learn how to take personal responsibility for their learning. With this comes increased self-awareness and an environment where they can examine their own as well as other people's individual differences through attitudes, values, beliefs and prejudices that all influence patient care. The development of listening skills and being able to attend to other people's emotions as well as one's own, help to generate the skills necessary for providing feedback and constructive criticism to promote change and personal growth within the supervisory relationship. Through offering the space to reflect on such issues students of all levels can begin to explore how they solve problems, deal with difficult situations and, perhaps most importantly, how they identify and begin to confront feelings that may emerge when providing therapeutic patient care. Supervision can be viewed then as integral to many aspects of nurse training and practice, as laid out in Box 10.1.

Minardi (1994) views clinical supervision as a collaborative exchange between two or more practitioners concerning their clinical practice and any issues surrounding that work. The purpose is essentially threefold:
1. To support the practitioner by providing time and space to discuss important clinical practice issues
2. To facilitate learning through reflection
3. To aid the monitoring of practitioners' competency.

Supervision sessions are planned and negotiated between the supervisor and supervisee and are usually carried out in a one-to-one situation once every 10 working days, for an hour at a time. Some clinical areas are developing practice standards for supervision as part of their quality assurance initiatives and state minimum contact times ranging from monthly to once a fortnight.

Box 10.1 *Supervision of professional practice*

Supervision of professional practice involves:
- Being an integral part of any practitioner's daily practice.
- Monitoring the effectiveness of the practitioner in the helping relationship.
- Proividing the opportunity for continued learning and a greater understanding of the therapeutic relationship in all its complexities.
- Recognition of the effects of unconscious aspects of professional caring, both on the practitioner and the help they offer.

THE SUPERVISORY RELATIONSHIP

The supervisory relationship is regarded as central to the effectiveness of supervision. Here we consider blocks that might prevent the relationship forming or being used adequately and offer practical assistance to overcome them. How to negotiate a learning contract for both students and qualified staff members is presented and reference is made to discussing and promoting career development and enhancing professional practice. The supervisory relationship is shown as a safe place where feedback and learning can take place.

Any survey on clinical supervision soon reveals that each clinical area approaches supervision in a slightly different way. In recent publications, papers give variations in the components of supervision and how to implement it. (See for example, Coleman and Rafferty, 1995; Devine and Baxter, 1995; Leach, 1995). However a strong, common theme is the value placed upon a constructive working relationship between the supervisor and supervisee. The quality of this relationship is uppermost; it does not seem so important to have close connection with line management. To develop such a relationship, conditions of trust, non-collusiveness, warmth and genuineness need to be in place (see Box 10.2).

Nurses do not automatically become effective supervisors virtue of their experience, education or personality (Clarkson and Gilbert, 1991). There is need for high levels of awareness of the supervisee's own thoughts and experiences and the supervisor's influential thoughts, feelings and behaviour. Formal training is one route to achieving this. Experience of effective supervision is another. What is most beneficial, perhaps, is an amalgamation of the two. Only through continuing the learning cycle can the future skills and knowledge of more experienced nurses be passed on and adapted for future practice.

It is easy for the relationship to develop into a question and answer session, with the supervisor under the misapprehension that they are there to provide all the answers and the supervisee looking to find answers to all their clinical difficulties. This is not the case. The relationship is one of mutual learning and development.

Fear and anxiety within the relationship has been identified by Shohet and Wilmot (1991) as a prime influence on establishing it successfully. Fear and anxiety on both sides can be an effective screen to prevent issues being identified and explored, rather than being used to help understand the processes that are occurring between the supervisor and supervisee and in the supervisee's client relationships.

Box 10.2 *Student nurses' perceived qualities of a supervisor*

A supervisor should be able to provide the following:
- A relevant, sound knowledge base with appropriate clinical skills and experience.
- Be able to negotiate objectives and assess learning needs.
- Demonstrate an interest and recognition of the supervisee's current situation and work pressures.
- Be capable of forming a supportive and professional relationship.

(Fowler, 1995)

PRACTICAL ISSUES

Some practical problems can be encountered in the supervisory relationship. These include: how and whether to change supervisor; developing the professional profile; presenting oneself to a supervisor; choosing a supervisor in the first place, and what characteristics the practitioner should look for. Here, a multidisciplinary approach to supervision is presented, which draws on the expertise of other professionals as supervisors and supervisees.

BLOCKS TO SUPERVISION

One element involved in providing effective supervision is to recognize potential limitations and blocks to the supervisory relationship and to find ways of overcoming them. Hawkins and Shohet (1989) identify the following areas as a useful framework for considering the practical implementation of clinical supervision for practising nurses.

Previous Experience of Supervision

A person's prior experience of supervision, whether good or bad, can influence both the supervisor and the supervisee and their approach to the new relationship. It is suggested that these experiences, good or bad, should be shared at the beginning of a new supervisory relationship and that the elements each party wishes to repeat or avoid are discussed.

Personal Inhibitions

Often a one-to-one relationship brings up past experiences and memories re-emerge that can stimulate painful and negative feelings. Being put on the spot and recognizing any such painful memories is a useful mechanism to help practitioners assess how their patients might be feeling. These unconscious processes are an important element of the learning experience through supervision. Therefore the supervisor and supervisee have to be able to recognize emotional blocks and to work through them, so that insight can be enhanced and learning take place.

Difficulties in the Supervisory Relationship

Some of these issues have been looked at earlier, with the main stumbling block to the development of a satisfactory relationship being anxiety and fear on both sides. Previous bad experience of a supervisor will affect how the supervisee and supervisor approach the new relationship. Setting the scene early in the relationship and negotiating what is expected of both parties will help allay some of the fears but it is largely up to the supervisor to recognize and deal with the subtleties that will arise from the relationship. Other difficulties emerge if expectations are unrealistic for either party. Some supervisees expect their supervisor to offer sound advice and solutions to all clinical difficulties. It is difficult for experienced clinicians to say that they do not know the answer, so supervisors may feel they ought to know and therefore avoid contact with a supervisee who is demanding such wisdom. Supervision is a mutual learning experience and therefore an explorative and developmental relationship. This means that both sides need to be able to admit that they do not know the answer but are willing to explore the issues and develop new ways of tackling problems.

Organizational Blocks

Often supervision is considered a luxury rather than a necessity in a busy psychiatric setting. Nurses see themselves as the last stage in the caring set-up, needing time and attention devoted solely to them and to discussion of their work and therapeutic relationships. Indeed, some clinical areas have given specific and regular commitment to structured supervision. Nurses meet during the working week for regular clinical evaluation and reflection. Some people have seen this as a way of avoiding contact with patients and more as a time for nurses to 'sit around and moan to each other'. Supervision has been described as 'not proper work' or 'not the best use of a nurse's time'. The organization (in this instance an NHS Trust, hospital or community setting) needs to recognize the value and usefulness of supervision sessions for the maintenance of high quality and professionally directed practice. This is where the importance of research and monitoring the effects of supervision on nurses' work becomes paramount. For too long nurses have assumed that what they do is the best or correct way, without participating in systematic evaluation. The authors will discuss later some ideas on how to monitor the effects of supervision and what is hoped will be an inspiration for all clinicians to become their own private investigators.

Practical Blocks

Areas that can lead to blocks in the development of supervision on a ward or department or even the fulfilment of supervisory contracts can be manifold. One such block is the senior staff's commitment to supervision and whether they are able to obtain supervision for themselves. Often senior staff are expected to be the ones responsible for the supervision of staff but get little or no support to carry this out. It is recommended, therefore, that all staff expected to act as supervisors receive supervision themselves. The provision of appropriate supervisors for senior nursing staff can be a block in itself. Looking outside the nursing discipline to other professionals within the clinical team for supervision can provoke anxiety. It also requires additional time and effort in the negotiation, and sometimes, explanation, of what is required. It should not, however, be overlooked as a means of finding highly expert clinicians to act as willing nurse supervisors.

Cultural Blocks

Progressive change in nursing often happens in such a way that no real change in the organizational defences occurs and the real need for therapeutic closeness to patients remains inhibited (Fabricius, 1991). Cultural blocks to supervision are one way that prevents nurses from working closely and therapeutically with patients. Keeping busy with the day-to-day

activities of clinical work is far less emotionally and mentally demanding than having to consider one's personal influence on the developments of a therapeutic relationship.

BENEFITS OF SUPERVISION

Five areas of benefit from clinical supervision, as outlined below, have been identified by nursing staff at the Bethlem and Maudsley Hospital.

Support

There is a risk of overusing this word, which reduces its potency. Nurses have seen supervision as offering them support through the allocation of time to discuss, openly and without fear of recrimination, personal thoughts and feelings associated with their working lives. These thoughts and feelings can then be explored and worked with to provide a more positive outcome. Through offering a safe environment to explore such issues, supervision can offer a setting where the nurse is able to be vulnerable, like their patients. This allows them greater freedom to consider the therapeutic situation and gather insight and regain confidence, and identify options available to them and appropriate to their own personal capabilities.

Team Building

Through supervision, clinical leaders are able to understand and recognize in their staff areas of strength and ability that could otherwise be overlooked or disregarded. Supervision can be a motivational experience and an area where new ideas and skills can be safely examined. The shared environment of caring has a cumulative effect on patient care. If staff are being adequately looked after and supported at work, patients will ultimately benefit.

Monitoring Performance

Within the supervisory relationship, staff are able to recognize areas in need of development and those areas they excel in and can share with others. This also allows the supervisor to observe for signs of stress and help the supervisors deal with them effectively. A system of appraisal can also be fuelled by supervision and the wider context of the nurse's performance evaluated.

Improving and Developing Skills

Through being able to examine their role in supervision, nurses can look at areas in need of change. Through being supervised, the supervisee can use the experience to enhance not only the delivery of patient care but also feedback and a culture of sharing among staff.

Information Sharing

Supervision promotes a productive relationship that develops sharing of direct information and case management issues.

POTENTIAL DIFFICULTIES IN THE SYSTEM

Formal Training

Nurses cannot be expected to become natural supervisors or supervisees. It is often a difficult transition from being the carer to the cared for. Also, nurses should not and need not be treated as patients. Supervision is not a form of free private therapy.

What is Expected of Me?

Neither supervisor nor supervisee know what is expected of them or what is required for their specific relationship. (This is one way of experiencing first-hand how a patient feels when given a named nurse and not told how to deal with the nurse.)

Patient Turnover

A high turnover of acutely disturbed patients has emphasized safety in acute clinical areas. This often means that time for staff to meet for supervision is considered a low priority.

Night Supervision

Often nurses on nights receive less allocated time for supervision. Time outside normal working hours has often to be used to meet supervisors.

Working Closely with Those Who Can Affect My Career

Disquiet remains around the issues of developing close working relationships with senior or influential staff. Questions of confidentiality and safe practice have to be negotiated at the outset. Nurses still shy away from working in such an open forum with other professional disciplines.

Choice

Little consideration is given to the element of choice of supervisor.

MONITORING EFFECTS THROUGH RESEARCH

Past and current research into supervision, and research methods which could be easily adopted in wards and departments, prove the worth of supervision and its effect on patient care.

There are many anecdotal instances of how and why clinical supervision is useful and improves practice. However, systematic measurement and evaluation of the effects of supervision have remained elusive and sparse. Currently the University of Manchester in collaboration with the Department of Health is carrying out a nationwide evaluation of the effects of implementing supervision through measurements of stress, job satisfaction and emotional burn-out. Such a widespread study has not been carried out previously and the results are awaited with considerable interest. It is not possible of course for individual nurses or teams to carry out such a large study but smaller projects should be encouraged.

Bergin and Strupp (1972) carried out a survey of psychologists and psychiatrists, which revealed growing dissatisfaction with the traditional experimental designs and statistical procedures, which were considered inappropriate for the subject of therapeutic change. Garfield (1983) concludes that this is largely responsible for the lack of outcome studies and that being able to show systematic change rather than statistical significance is more revealing and can contribute to uncovering the active processes that take place within therapy.

Single case studies have been used for educational purposes, with benefit to the individual effort and to the effect supervision has had on patients and their families and (Vidoni, 1975; Leach, 1986; Graham, 1994).

Reflective journals are appearing in greater numbers as a means of exploring clinical competence of student nurses and of structuring what is discussed in supervision sessions (Cameron and Mitchell, 1993).

Retrospective examination of related issues such as staff sickness levels, turnover and morale has also suggested that clinical supervision has an effect on these areas. It is always difficult with these measures, however, to exclude the effect of other issues such as patient turnover and dependency levels, and other extraneous circumstances.

Barlow *et al.* (1984) review the progression of research in behavioural change and look both at traditional and alternative research methods. Some methods that might be considered appropriate for monitoring the supervision process follow.

The term *developmental research* was first used by Thomas (1978) in social work where observations are made and data collected at various stages throughout a treatment programmes. The programme is analysed to check whether it needs fine tuning or changing in any way. The final result is a programme that can then be compared with another in a similar clinical situation.

The main difference between *quasi experimental designs* and the more traditional experimental design is that random allocation of sample groups is not used. Conclusions are drawn from the effect of the research intervention rather than comparing the differences between the two groups. Another way of overcoming this non-equivalence among the groups is to use a time series method for example, taking measurements at the beginning, middle and end of therapy sessions.

Individual case analysis. Traditional research methods have concentrated on sample groups, while practitioners are encouraged to see patients as individuals. Individual differences (otherwise described as intersubjective variability) in patients' responses to interventions continue to engage practitioners and provide a substantial amount of unexplored terrain as far as research strategies are concerned. The effect supervision has on the practitioner and the patient can readily be applied to individual case analysis and has been touched upon earlier.

Personal knowledge is essential for ethical choices in clinical practice and presupposes personal maturity and freedom. Every solution to a problem requires new methods of enquiry and different conceptual structures. These will all affect the shape and patterns of knowing, and identify the patterns through which connection modifies the whole (Carper, 1978).

Supervision of professional practice provides a specific time in clinical work to evaluate and reflect on current practice. This in itself demands considerable personal and organizational commitment. This commitment helps to produce nurses who are both willing and able to work closely with patients in a therapeutic relationship that is characterized by consideration, sensitivity and understanding. Through dialectical reconstruction between two or more people additional insights into the art and science of nursing can be formed. Without such consideration nurses can be left feeling impotent to act, to change, to develop and to grow (Vaughan, 1992).

The lack of research in nursing, particularly on the effect of supervision on practice, could be significantly countered if nurses were to consider clinically relevant methods rather than see research as a hurdle for academic or career developments. Research is vital to nursing to avoid the need to rely on other disciplines for new knowledge and as a means of evaluating objective evidence for therapeutic interventions more effectively.

SUMMARY

The supervision of clinical practice can take many guises and will largely depend on the philosophy of the practitioner and/or their working environment. The theories presented in this chapter will help practitioners decide how they wish to pursue clinical supervision for themselves and their colleagues. There are (as in any interpersonal process) areas which will prove difficult and challenging. Supervision needs the commitment and support of all involved, which takes time and energy, but once in place pracitioners will not want to work without it!

The authors have undergone their own supervision and have experienced stimulating and devastating supervisors. It is a two way process and much can be learnt from all experience when explored safely and sensitively.

Nursing is about caring and supervision is one mechanism through which nurses can learn to care for themselves whilst at the same time analyzing and improving ways in which they care for patients.

KEY CONCEPTS

• Clinical supervision is an important part of all clinical nursing activity.
• There are a number of different methods that have been developed from which to choose a system of supervision best suited to the individual's or clinical team's philosophy of care.
• Clinical supervision covers aspects of educational, supportive and professional standards of nursing.
• Theoretical background can influence the style and delivery that supervision takes.
• Clinical supervision should be an integral part of any nurse's day-to-day clinical activity.
• The relationship between supervisor and supervisee is important and sets the scene in which supervision will work or falter.
• Research into clinical supervision is a potential source of new knowledge and of considerable importance for nurses to use as an exemplar to other professions.
• The implementation of clinical supervision has a direct influence on the quality of patient care.

REFERENCES

Barlow DH, Hayes SC, Nelson RO: *The scientist practitioner. Research and accountability in clinical and educational settings.* Massachusetts, 1984, Allyn & Bacon.

Bergin A, Strupp HH: *Changing frontiers in the science of psychotherapy.* Chicago, 1972, Aldine.

Brown D, Pedder J: *Introduction to psychotherapy*, 2 ed. London, 1991, Tavistock/Routledge Publications.

Burrow S: Supervision: clinical development of management control? *Br J Nurs* 4(15)879–882, 1995.

Cameron BL, Mitchell AM: Reflective peer journals: developing authentic nurses. *J Adv Nurs* 18(2):290–297, 1993.

Carper BA: Fundamental patterns of knowing in nursing. *Adv Nurs Sci* 1(1):13–23, 1978.

Clarkson P, Gilbert M: The training of counsellor trainees and supervisors. In: Dryden W, Throne B, editors: *Training and supervision for counselling in action.* London, 1991, Sage.

Coleman M, Rafferty: Using workshops to implement supervision. *Nurs Stand* 9(50):27–30, 1995.

Department of Health, Mental Health Review Team: *Working in partnership: A collaborative approach to care.* London, 1994, HMSO.

Devine A, Baxter TD: Introducing clinical supervision: a guide. *Nurs Stand* 28(40):32–34, 1995.

Fabricius J: Running on the spot or can nursing really change? *Psychoanal Psychother* 5(2):97–108, 1991.

Farkas–Cameron M: Clinical supervision in psychiatric nursing, a self actualising process. *J Psychosoc Nurs* 33(2):31–7, 1995.

Fowler J: Nurses' perception of the elements of good supervision. *Nurs Times* 91(22):33–37, 1995.

Garfield SL: Effectiveness of psychotherapy: the perennial controversy. *Prof Psych Res Prac* 14(1)35–43, 1983.

Graham IW: Reflective practice: using the action learning group mechanism. *Nurs Educ Today* 15(1):28–32, 1994.

Greenburg L: Supervision from perspective of the supervisee. In: Hess A, editor: *Psychotherapy supervision: Theory research and practice*. New York, 1980, Wiley.

Hawkins P: Humanistic psychotherapy supervision. *Self Soc: Eur J Humanist Psychol* XIII(2) March/April, 1985.

Hawkins P, Shohet R: *Supervision in the helping professions*. Buckingham, 1989, Open University Press.

Hawkins P, Shohet R: Approaches to the supervision of counsellors. In: Dryden W, Thorne B, editors: *Training and supervision for counselling in action*. London, 1991, Sage.

Hess A: Training models and the nature of psychotherapy supervision. In: Hess A, editor: *Psychotherapy supervision: Theory research and practice*. New York, 1980, Wiley-Interscience.

Holloway E, Nerfeldt SA: Supervision. Its contribution to treatment efficacy. *J Consult Clin Psychol* 63(2)207–213, 1995.

Ironbar N, Hooper A: *Self instruction in mental health nursing*. London, 1989, Bailliere Tindall.

Jackson M, Cawley R: Psychodynamics and psychotherapy on an acute psychiatric ward. *Brit J Psychiat* 160:41–50, 1992.

Jackson M, Williams P: *Unimaginable storms*. London, 1994, Karnac.

Leach G: Nurse/therapist supervision as an impetus to change. In: Kennedy R, Heymans A, Lischler L, editors: *The family as in-patient*. London, 1986, FAB.

Leach L: Doing it for themselves. *Nurs Stand* 29(45):22, 1995.

Linehan M: Supervision of behaviour therapy. In: Hess A, editor: *Psychotherapy supervision: Theory, research and practice*. New York, 1980, Wiley-Interscience.

Mattinson J: *The reflection process in casework supervision*. London, 1975, Tavistock.

McLeod J: *Introduction to counselling*. Milton Keynes, 1993, Open University Press.

Minardi HA: *Clinical supervision in nursing* 2nd International Conference on Nurse Practitioner Practice. Unpublished.London, 6th August, 1994.

Moldawsky S: Psychoanalytic psychotherapy supervision. In: Hess A, editor: *Psychotherapy supervision: Theory, research and practice*. New York, 1980, Wiley-Interscience.

Money-Kyrle R: Normal countertransference and some deviations. In: Moras K, Scrupp HH: Pretherapy interpersonal relations, patients alliance and the outcome on brief therapy. *Arch Gen Psychiatry* 405–409, 1982.

Page S, Wosket V: *Supervising the counsellor: a cyclical model*. London, 1994, Routledge.

Proctor B: *Supervision: a working alliance*. East Sussex, 1988, Alexia, [Video].

Rice L: A client-centred approach to the supervision of psychotherapy. In: Hess A, editor: *Psychotherapy supervision: Theory, research and practice*. New York, 1980, Wiley-Interscience.

Schon DA: *The reflective practitioner*. 1983, Basic Books Inc.

Shohet R, Wilmot J: The key issue in the supervision of counsellors: the supervisory relationship. In: Dryden W, Throne B, editors: *Training and supervision for counselling in action*. London, 1991, Sage.

Stoltenberg C, Delworth U: *Supervising counsellors and therapists*. San Francisco, 1987, Josey Bass.

Taylor M: Gender and power in counselling supervision. *Br J Guid Counsel* 22(3)319–326, 1994.

Thomas EJ: Research and service in single case experimentation: conflicts and choices. *Soc Work Res Abstr* 14(1):20–31, 1978.

UKCC for Nursing, Midwifery and Health Visiting: *Clinical Supervision for Nursing and Health Visiting. Registrar's Letter*. London, 1995, UKCC.

Vaughan B: Exploring the knowledge of nursing practice. *J Clin Nurs* 1(3):161–166, 1992.

Vidoni C: The development of intense positive countertransference feelings in the therapist toward a patient. *Am J Nurs* 75(3):407–409, 1975.

Whittington R, Wykes T,: Coping strategies used by staff following assault by a patient: an exploratory study. *Work Stress* 5(1)37–48, 1991.

Wilmot J, Shohet R: Paralleling in the supervision process. *Self Soc: Eur J Humanist Psychol* XIII(2) March/April, 1985.

Winnicot DW: Hate in the countertransference. In: *Through paediatrics and psychoanalysis*. London, 1978, Hogarth Press.

Wright H: The patient, the nurse, his life and her mother: psychodynamic influences in nurse education and practice. *Psychoanaly psychother* 5(2):139–149, 1991.

FURTHER READING

Atkins S, Murphy K: Reflection: a review of the literature. *J Adv Nurs* 18(8):1188–1192, 1993.
   A comprehensive review of the literature, offering a useful start for any nurse wishing to know more of the theory behind the practice.

Bishop V: Clinical supervision questionnaire results. *Nurs Times* 90(48)40–42, 1994.
   Some interesting assumptions and practical problems encountered with nurses and supervision.

Boyd E, Fales A: Reflective learning: Key to learning from experience. *J Humanist Psychol* 23(1):99–117, 1983.
   An interesting article; provides some thought provoking information, although a little heavy going.

Butterworth T, Faugier J: *Clinical supervision and mentorship in nursing*. London, 1992, Chapman & Hall.
   A good introduction to clinical supervision written specifically for nurses by nurses.

Houston G: *Supervision and counselling*. Norfolk, 1990, MF Barnwell.
   Although based around counselling and therapy, this book gives useful information on the process of supervising clinical practice.

Reising G, Daniels M: A study of Hogan's model of counsellor development and supervision. *J Counsel Psychol* 30(2):235–244, 1983.
   An overview of Hogan's model which, although being written by and for psychologists, is relevant to nurses.

Schon DA: *The reflective practitioner*. 1983, Basic Books Inc.
   A very important text that gives valuable and research based information on the whole aspect of reflective practice, of which clinical supervision is an offshoot.

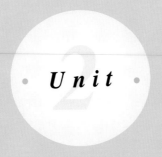

Unit 2

Principles of
Organizing Care

11

Community Care

*T*he mental health system is part of a rapidly changing health care environment. For the past four decades, concerted efforts have been made to move mental health care out of the institution and into the community. Key historical developments in community mental health nursing from 1954 to 1985 are outlined here. Later we will discuss developments since 1985 in greater detail.

ORIGINS OF COMMUNITY MENTAL HEALTH NURSING SERVICES

The decade 1950 to 1960 saw the beginning of a more liberal era in psychiatry. Before this, mental health care had been largely custodial, with patients detained for lengthy periods, sometimes a lifetime. People with mental illness were removed from their communities and placed in large institutions away from public view. Often these hospitals were self-sufficient communities, with work provided on asylum farms and in asylum workshops. Policies were decided locally, nurse training was poorly coordinated at a national level and staff were often as institutionalized as the patients (Ministry of Health, 1945).

THE COMMUNITY PSYCHIATRIC NURSE

Treatment of people with mental health problems in the community was partly facilitated by antipsychotic medication introduced in the 1950s. The 1959 Mental Health Act made admission and discharge easier, with less formal admissions and the provision of sheltered accommodation and work schemes outside the large asylums. The first 'out-patient' nurses in Britain were appointed at Warlingham Park Hospital, Surrey in 1954 (Moore, 1960, 1964). The role of the community psychiatric nurse (CPN) then was similar to that of the psychiatric social worker and involved monitoring out-patients, setting up therapeutic groups and assisting with accommodation issues. In 1957, the role of in-patient nurses at Moorhaven Hospital, Devon, was extended to include supervision of clients outside hospital. From this point, the number of CPNs rapidly increased and the in-patient population began to decline. By 1966, 225 CPNs were employed by 42 hospitals. The CPN:population ratio grew from 1:50 000 in 1980 to 1:23 800 in 1985 (Community Psychiatric Nurses Association, 1985) although this does not match the 1:7500 recommended by the Royal College of Psychiatrists (1980). Despite this rapid increase, there were vast regional variations, both in ratio of CPNs to local population and in the amount of training that nurses working in the community received.

Until the 1970s, CPNs remained largely hospital based and their key duties included: monitoring medication, assessing mental state, supervising out-patient clinics and group work. The majority of referrals were made by hospital consultants, clients tended to have diagnoses of schizophrenia and major depression and the nursing service was delivered within the model of medical care. Throughout the 1970s, CPNs moved away from the hospital setting and were often attached to GP surgeries, accepting referrals from a wider range of sources and caring for clients with a variety of mental health problems. As a result, CPNs became largely autonomous practitioners, assessing care needs independently of secondary psychiatric services and planning and implementing care. CPNs began to specialize in certain areas, such as behavioural psychotherapy and elderly care (CPNA, 1985).

EVALUATION OF COMMUNITY MENTAL HEALTH NURSING SERVICES

Because of the lack of evaluative studies conducted in the field, the effectiveness of the growing numbers of CPNs was not widely addressed. One GP (Shaw, 1977) examined the work of CPNs over a 6-month period with clients he had referred to a community psychiatric nursing service. When compared to hypothetical care without the CPN service, he found that his clients received fewer prescriptions for psychotropic medication and more rapid assessment. Corrigan and Soni (1977) and Pullen (1980) proposed that decreased admission rates indicated successful community psychiatric nursing intervention. However, decreased admission rates are not necessarily an indicator of quality service provision and their findings may have suggested that some clients were neglected, when admission may have been indicated (Hunter, 1980). A large scale, 5- year study of community psychiatric nursing care of clients with schizophrenia (Hunter, 1978) found that clients cared for by CPNs spent more time in hospital and attending day-care facilities, while the most disturbed clients were not receiving adequate amounts of community psychiatric nursing care. A comparison of routine out-patient follow-up and CPN follow-up (Paykel *et al.,* 1982) found no difference in the effectiveness of either type of care on symptom reduction but clients who were seen by a CPN reported greater satisfaction with their care.

These studies went some way to evaluate community mental health nursing services but there was no adequate large scale study carried out during this period, when the government was increasingly suggesting that community care should be developed.

TRAINING OF COMMUNITY MENTAL HEALTH NURSES

Training in community mental health nursing was not established until 1970, when a short course was introduced in London, which was later expanded to a 1-year course in community psychiatric nursing (Rawlings, 1970). Further courses were developed in a piecemeal fashion during the 1970s. The United Kingdom Consultative Council for Nursing, Midwifery and Health Visiting (UKCC) and National Boards, created in 1982, established three ENB courses — ENB 810, 811, 812 — specializing in community mental health nursing. However, health authorities found secondment of nurses difficult and places on these courses were limited. In 1985, only 22% of mental health nurses in the community had received specialist training (CPNA, 1985). The UKCC recognized that community mental health nursing skills were a priority for basic training and the focus of the Project 2000 syllabus (UKCC, 1987) was divided between institutional and non-institutional settings.

GOVERNMENT INVOLVEMENT IN MENTAL HEALTH SERVICE DEVELOPMENT

The increase in community mental health nursing has largely resulted from Government involvement in promoting movement of mental health care provision from institutional settings into the community (Table 11.1). Governments have been increasingly interested in defining aspects of community care, resulting in the 1990 NHS and Community Care Act (House of Commons, 1990). Tooth and Brooke (1961) predicted that the decline in number of long stay hospital patients would result in such beds being discontinued after 16 years. The then Minister of Health, Enoch Powell, declared that the psychiatric in-patient population should be halved by 1975 and the process of de-institutionalization began, spurred on by such as Goffman (1961) and Wolfensberger (1970). Other Western countries adopted similar philosophies, with Sweden, in particular, providing psychiatric out-patient care in primary health care settings and Italy introducing rapid policy changes in hospital closures (Tansella *et al.,* 1987).

In 1975, a Government White Paper set a target of 47 900 in-patient beds (from 104 400) after the closure of large psychiatric institutions (Department of Health and Social Security (DHSS), 1975). Further legislation in the 1980s continued the trend of bed closures and relocation of services to the community. In 1981, the Government produced a consultative document discussing resources in the move towards community care. There appeared to be conflict between the motivation of hospitals to discharge patients and the reluctance of Local Authorities to accept responsibility for providing post-discharge facilities (DHSS, 1981). Proposals to rectify this began to be made. A House of Commons Social Service Committee Report (House of Commons, 1985) and an Audit Commission Report (Audit Commission, 1986) reviewed progress of community care provision and criticized the unclarified resource issue. These two reports noted that clients had been discharged from psychiatric hospitals without adequate community facilities or resources to support them. The concern over the health service–local authority divide was highlighted and it was suggested that budgets should be given to local services to purchase effective care, provided by multi-disciplinary teams, with cooperation between statutory and voluntary agencies.

As a result of these findings, a review of the funding situation was commissioned by Government. The Griffiths Report was published in 1988 (Griffiths, 1988) and recommended that responsibility for community care should be clarified both nationally and locally, yet with funding to remain unchanged in general structure. Large scale closures of hospital beds would be achieved with special funds and should be jointly planned by health and social services, with 'care-managers' appointed for long stay patients. Griffiths also proposed that GPs should become more involved in the care of the mentally ill and should liaise with social services regarding care needs of individual clients.

Each of these reports acknowledged the important role of the CPN in delivery of community care but the Griffiths Report proposed that management of community services should be the responsibility of local authority social service departments and care largely provided by mental health social workers, with only the acutely mentally ill remaining under health authorities. The Royal College of Psychiatrists (1988) criticized this separation of services and advocated that health authorities should be responsible for all clients with mental health problems.

In 1989 two Government White Papers — Caring for People (Department of Health (DoH), 1989a) and Working for Patients (DoH, 1989b) — were published, which set the scene for the NHS and Community Care Act 1990. Their key points included:

TABLE 11.1 Summary of Government involvement in the development of community mental health care

1961	Predictions of decrease in hospital beds	The 1950s and 1960s saw the beginning of the community care movement in Britain and bed closures were proposed.
1975	Better Services for the Mentally III	The Government began to consider the resource implications of transferring services from hospitals into the community.
1981	Care in the Community	The health–social services divide was identified as an issue in the move towards community care provision.
1985	Social Services Committee Report	The Report further examined the difficulties of funding health and social service departments separately.
1986	Audit Commission Report	Rationalization of funding was identified as a critical area for development, with short-term funding suggested to enable the development of community services.
1988	Griffiths Report	The Report recommended that special funds should be made available for the closure of large psychiatric hospitals. More emphasis on primary care involvement. Health authorities were to be responsible only for those with acute illness; social services to assume responsibility for those with long-term mental health needs.
1989	Caring for People; Working for Patients (White Paper)	The proposed a single budget to cover care costs, with local authorities having a budget for residential placement costs. Hospital discharges were to be coordinated by health and social services.
1990	NHS and Community Care Act	The Act divided purchasing and provider units, with GPs allowed to become fund-holders. Made allowances for hospitals to become trusts. Local authorities were given responsibility for care provision, with local care plans to be jointly agreed by health and social services. Encouraged liaison between statutory and voluntary agencies.
1991	Care Programme Approach introduced	All clients accepted by specialist psychiatric services had to be registered on the CPA, with particular attention given to those with severe mental health needs. Key Workers to be appointed to coordinate care, maintain contact with the client and review care on a regular basis.
1993	Supervised Discharge proposed	Psychiatric services would be able to extend leave periods under the 1983 Mental Health Act and recall clients to hospital.
1994	Supervision Registers introduced	Provision of registers for those clients deemed vulnerable or dangerous.

- Commitment to the principles of community care.
- A single budget to cover the cost of care.
- Local authorities to be given a budget for placement of all new applicants for residential care.
- Hospital discharges to occur only when adequate health and social care were provided, with individual care plans for all discharged clients.
- The introduction of capital charges on all NHS hospitals, resulting in higher costs of in-patient beds.

The NHS and Community Care Act 1990 marked the culmination of years of development and has radically restructured health care provision in the UK. The purchaser–provider divide was made explicit, with fund-holding GPs able to purchase specialist services from health authorities and to directly employ CPNs. Hospitals became able to apply for Trust status and thus regulate their own finances. Local authorities were given responsibility for the provision of community care, with local social services and health authorities required to draw up jointly agreed care plans based on local implementation of needs-led care for vulnerable psychiatric clients. Enabling people to live in their own homes, supporting carers and working with voluntary agencies to provide care were to be emphasized. Much of the NHS and Community Care Act was implemented in April 1993.

In 1990, the Government also produced a circular on the Care Programme Approach (CPA) for people with a mental illness referred to specialist psychiatric services (DoH, 1990). This circular particularly emphasized the need for services to be provided for those clients deemed vulnerable, with long-term mental health needs. The circular said that each client should be allocated a Key Worker, often a CPN, who would have responsibility for the coordination of assessment of health and social care needs, delivery of care, maintenance of contact with clients and their carers and regular review of care plans. The CPA was implemented in April 1991.

Following concerns regarding incidents of inadequate care provision, particularly lack of follow-up care, the Government required health service provider units to establish supervision registers, an extension of CPA registers, which identify those clients at risk of committing acts of serious violence, suicide or serious self-neglect (NHS Management Executive, 1994). This development was based largely on the conclusions of the Ritchie Report (Ritchie *et al*., 1994), which indicated that Supervision Registers would improve communication between those agencies involved in caring for particularly vulnerable or dangerous clients. In addition, the Government also planned to introduce a programme of supervised discharge from April 1996, which would allow psychiatric services powers of recall to hospital (DoH, 1993).

IMPACT OF GOVERNMENT POLICY ON THE ROLE OF THE COMMUNITY MENTAL HEALTH NURSE

This legislation has not been implemented without difficulty. Much of it has had direct implications for mental health nurses working in the community and the ambiguity of many policy documents has resulted in nurses feeling confused and uncertain of their role, faced with increasing demands. The organization of CPN services has developed into two distinct areas: those working in primary care, mainly attached to GP practices, and those working in a multidisciplinary team from a statutory specialist service base, for example a psychiatric hospital or day care base. The 1985 CPNA survey found that the trend towards providing care from primary health care centres was growing, although 37% of CPNs were still working from psychiatric hospitals. It found that many CPNs and GPs were in favour of basing nurses in primary care settings. With GPs providing at least part-treatment for more than 90% of people with mental health problems, it seemed appropriate for CPNs to work alongside the primary care-giver. However, those most in need of intensive community care are the severely mentally ill, discharged early from hospital or not admitted at all. Follow-up of these people requires a multidisciplinary approach in conjunction with primary care services.

Community psychiatric nursing has been subject to the same social policy trends as the rest of the health service but has had to adapt to a changing and often conflicting role. The Social Services Committee Report of 1985 (House of Commons, 1985) acknowledged the important role of the CPN in delivering community care and highlighted the difficulties of role development of generic mental health workers, advocating that mental health social workers should be employed to work cooperatively with other community professionals. A Community Nursing Review (DHSS, 1986) proposed a model that would assist in combining the two major strands of community mental health nursing. Neighbourhood nursing services were proposed with responsibility for coordinating nursing in primary care settings, alongside specialist multidisciplinary psychiatric teams. The two services would operate in tandem, with close liaison expected. Implementation, however, was left to the discretion of local health authorities and has not been widely adopted.

The Griffiths Report acknowledged that CPNs have 'an invaluable role in meeting the needs of both clients and informal carers' but advocated that the management of community services should be the responsibility of local authority social service departments, with CPNs working primarily with the acutely ill, rather than with clients with long-term health care needs. This is in contrast to the more recent Government philosophy of prioritizing vulnerable clients with severe, enduring mental health needs, in both health and social service care planning.

THE MENTAL HEALTH NURSE WORKING IN A PRIMARY HEALTH CARE SETTING

The 1990 NHS and Community Care Act further widened the gap between primary and secondary care services with the introduction of GP fundholding. Although GPs have historically been the gatekeeper to specialist mental health services, studies have shown that they are often inadequately trained to screen for psychiatric illness and do not refer to specialist services with consistency (Goldberg *et al.*, 1982; Hoeper *et al.*, 1984). The Royal College of Psychiatrists noted in 1980 that the GP should be the coordinator of services for clients with psychiatric illness, if not the principal service provider, yet emphasis on the role of the GP as service planner does not take into account the limitations of demands-led primary care services. A more pro-active, assertive service is required to provide care to the most vulnerable. Local initiatives to improve liaison between specialist services and GPs (Strathdee and Williams, 1984; Tyrer, 1984) have been successful but the Government did not address the national need for improvements in joint working between primary and secondary health care until 1992 (NHS Management Executive (NHSME), 1992). Those GPs who have access to specialist community mental health teams generally develop systems of liaison, yet this may not change the GP's ability to detect mental health problems (Warner *et al.*, 1993). The development of fundholding practices denotes a shift in power between primary and secondary health care services. The GP is now in a position to buy specific services, including the direct employment of CPNs. CPNs working apart from multidisciplinary teams, including those working in primary health care settings, are often isolated and inadequately supported and supervised (Wooff *et al.*, 1986; Wooff and Goldberg, 1988). They have tended to concentrate traditionally on working with clients with neurosis — the 'worried well' — while clients with more chronic conditions have been referred to secondary services. A major survey of CPNs in 1990 (White, 1990) found that 80% of people with schizophrenia did not receive care from a CPN. Those clients with less severe mental health problems tend to respond quickly to interventions and provide the CPN with greater job satisfaction than those clients for whom 'cure' is not an option (White and Brooker, 1990). However, the work of CPNs with clients with minor mental health problems may actually be ineffective and costly (Gournay and Brooking, 1994). GPs still continue to see large numbers of people with severe mental health problems, who are not in contact with specialist psychiatric services (Kendrick *et al.*, 1991). The opportunity exists for primary health care to use its community mental health nursing services to provide care to those who are unwilling to use traditional psychiatric care systems.

THE CARE PROGRAMME APPROACH AND COMMUNITY MENTAL HEALTH NURSING

The CPA (DoH, 1990) refocused community mental health nursing on those clients with severe, long-term mental health problems. The CPA applies to all clients accepted by specialist psychiatric services and all patients considered for discharge from hospital. Many health providers have focused particularly on those deemed vulnerable, those with long-term mental health needs and patients subject to Section 117 of the 1983 Mental Health Act (patients who have been on Sections 3, 37, 37/41, 47/49 and 48/49). The CPA requires:

- Systematic assessment of health care needs of clients in the community and of patients in hospital who are being considered for discharge.
- Systematic assessment of social care needs by health and social workers.
- Regular (at least 6-monthly) review of vulnerable clients and their care plans.
- A system of recording care provided and feedback to the relevant authorities when resources are not available to meet needs.

To coordinate these functions, a Key Worker is appointed. The Government recommended that the role of the Key Worker is most appropriately assumed by community mental health nurses and mental health social workers. The role of the Key Worker is central in the delivery of care and may involve coordination of a number of agencies, dependent on the complexity of the individual's care needs. The primary responsibilities of the Key Worker include: developing a care plan with the client, carers and other professionals; providing a point of contact for the client, carers and professionals; convening and participating in regular reviews; convening urgent reviews and mobilising emergency services when necessary; and maintaining a close therapeutic relationship with the client.

Although the CPA emphasizes the importance of multidisciplinary team working and liaison with primary health care, the Government has failed to recognize that the traditional functions of the CPN working in primary health care are not always suitable to fulfil the responsibilities of the Key Worker role. A study of CPNs training in 1990 clearly demonstrated that they viewed their role as one of primary prevention, receiving referrals mainly from GPs and treating clients with anxiety-related problems using counselling techniques and behavioural and cognitive therapies (Brooker, 1990). The introduction of the CPA challenged these beliefs and appropriate retraining was advocated (White and Brooker, 1990). CPNs did not feel skilled in the care of clients with severe, long-term mental health problems. In order to provide CPNs with the skills to function in the complex role of Key Worker, appropriate training must be provided. The Government has recently committed itself to better training for Key Workers, with a 10-point plan focusing on service implications of prioritizing clients with severe mental health problems (DoH, 1993). However, it is not clear what this training will involve, how it will be resourced or how its effectiveness will be monitored.

GOVERNMENT LEGISLATION AND COLLABORATIVE WORKING

The 1989 Government White Papers heralded a range of changes including the CPA (DoH, 1990). CPA in particular emphasizes the integration of primary and specialist health care with social services:

> Although all patients concerned will be patients of a Consultant Psychiatrist, modern psychiatric practice calls for effective inter-professional collaboration between psychiatrists, nurses, psychologists, occupational therapists and other health service professional staff:- social workers employed by Social Service authorities and general practitioners, the primary health care team and proper consultation with patients and their carers.

This would seem a positive step in developing community care, yet further action has since been necessary to attend to loopholes and target the most vulnerable mentally ill patients (i.e. the *Health of the Nation* (DoH, 1992), a review of the Mental Health Act (DoH and Welsh Office, 1983) with Community Supervision Registers (DoH, 1994a) included). These have been reactions to public and professional concerns, with changes in social perceptions pressuring the Government to respond piecemeal.

Raftery (1991) states that:

> Policy in practice resembles a mosaic, parts of which make sense to different groups but whose overall message may be less than completely coherent.

The timing of the introduction of the CPA followed several tragedies involving health and social care. Following the recommendations of the Spokes enquiry into the killing by a client of hospital social worker Isabel Schwartz, clarification was sought on responsibility for after-care. Individual pre-discharge plans were to be specified and a register of designated patients kept. This was of particular importance to homeless individuals with mental health problems. In October 1991 The Royal College of Psychiatrists, on the recommendation of the Spokes enquiry, published good medical practice in after-care of potentially violent or vulnerable patients discharged from in-patient psychiatric treatment; by then the CPA had been launched. The implementation of CPA was left to the discretion of local districts but should have been completed by October 1995.

Care Management versus Care Programming

The CPA implemented by health authorities and care management, in which local Social Service departments are to take the lead, are variants of the 'case management' interventions which appeared in the USA in the mid-1970s as a response to the perceived future of the then existing community support programmes (Shepherd, 1990). The essential difference is the extent to which they include purchasing as well as service provision.

Care programming essentially consists of direct service provision and generally does not include purchasing. Care management has purchasing as its central role together with a smaller amount of direct service provision in terms of needs assessments and brokerage with providers.

Care management emphasizes the need for social services to adopt a more flexible needs-led, as opposed to a service level, approach to care. Although packages of care are intended to be needs-led (after carefully assessing individual needs), availability both of resources and care managers suggests that distinguishing what is social care as opposed to health care may not be easily done, resulting in unmet needs. Resources available for the changes in procedures necessitated by the CPA were not made available specifically (Hudson, 1992). However, the mental illness specific grant was identified as a potential source of funding which could be complementary to the introduction of care programming.

Practical Implementation Issues Surrounding the Care Programme Approach

Today's pattern of local comprehensive mental health services providing fewer beds, shorter admissions and emphasis on care in the community, results in patients spending large periods of time at risk of committing offences or at increased risk of harming themselves and others.

Community care in response to legislation has embraced the functional equivalents of occupation, social networks and medical treatments. Generally, health and social care providers have adopted this principle with increased vigour. However, providing the functional equivalent of public protection, control and containment is an unresolved challenge and has far-reaching implications for the clinician and provider.

Mass media attention and clinical inquiries into scandals in mental hospitals that revealed cruel, dehumanizing aspects of custodial care (Martin, 1984) have given way to inquiries into scandals in the community. The scandals of in-patient services have been replaced by community care deaths (e.g. the Report on Christoper Clunis, (Ritchie *et al.*, 1994)). Further guidelines from the Department of Health (1994a) provide a framework for providers in the care and treatment of patients with specific and severe mental health disorders on discharge from hospital .

Supervision Registers and Supervised Discharge

The introduction of Supervision Registers and plans for providing supervised discharge (DoH, 1993; NHSME, 1994) further involves the Community Mental Health Nurse (CMHN) as Key Worker for the care of most vulnerable clients. The purpose of Supervision Registers is to identify those clients at most risk of harming themselves or others and, in service planning, to prioritize care for those most in need of intensive support and monitoring. Concerns about the role of the Key Worker in operation of the Supervision Register were raised by the Royal College of Psychiatrists in 1994 (Caldicott, 1994). These concerns are pertinent to CMHNs working as Key Workers and include:

- Lack of clarity regarding the accountability of Key Workers and the legal implications for Key Workers when care breaks down and an incident occurs.
- The potential risk of harm to the therapeutic relationship caused by Key Workers having to impose care regimes on clients, in order to meet their responsibilities as Key Workers.
- The issue of confidentiality and civil liberties.

Tension is likely within progressive units when they are seeking to maximize autonomy of patients by providing care in a less restrictive way but also have to ensure that worries and demands for the public safety are addressed. For the practitioner, concerns arise over professional accountability and the consequences that a public inquiry may have.

Ensuring Effective Working — Key Workers
All clients referred to specialist psychiatric services are required by the CPA to have a Key Worker appointed to coordinate care. Key Workers cannot be responsible for all the care of any individual but they can ensure that if problems arise, they are brought to the attention of others caring for the person (Kingdon, 1994).

Key Workers can come from various disciplines and can include psychologists, social workers, occupational therapists and psychiatrists. Their major responsibilities are to be specific contacts for the user and carer, GPs and others. It is the responsibility of Key Workers to ensure that reviews of the client occur regularly according to need. Key Workers need not necessarily come automatically from the statutory sector, though the relationship between the agency and the client must be emphasized. Importance should be given to the client's choice regarding gender and ethnic background to facilitate a trusting relationship between client and Key Worker. The client should also be given the right to request a change of Key Worker.

The responsibilities and accountability of Key Workers' roles and function require clear, agreed guidelines and adequate and professional training to be available within the provider units.

Needs Assessment
Individuals accessing mental health services should receive assessment for health and social care needs. Where specific needs are identified, the appropriate discipline should be engaged in the client's care for further detailed specialist assessment. Closer inter-disciplinary collaborative working should not result in excessive documentation if a full multi-disciplinary attendance is available for the client reviews.

Collaborative Working
Audrey Leathard (1991) described the effectiveness of inter-disciplinary approaches as a need to overcome the barriers to inter-disciplinary team functioning. These barriers include role ambiguity, status inequality, conflicting authority and power structures, leadership styles and pay differentials between the professional groups.

The organization of continuing care and supervision for severely mentally ill people outside hospital is best undertaken by a combination of team members, that is: a nurse, social worker, psychiatrist and occupational therapist or psychologist. This will ensure a planned system in which all disciplines appropriate to the patient's care can work together to provide consistent, patient, high quality cooperation with the family or carer and thus facilitate empowerment of the patient him- or herself. This view is endorsed further by Kingdon (1992).

CONTINUITY OF CARE AND THE COMMUNITY MENTAL HEALTH NURSE
The potential for fragmentation of care is an issue that CPNs must address, particularly those nurses fulfilling the role of Key Worker under the CPA and Supervision Registers. The NHS and Community Care Act encouraged the CPN to work in primary health care by introducing GP fundholding, yet the CPA and the Supervision Register increase the responsibility of the CMHN to become involved with those clients with severe mental illness, largely cared for by multidisciplinary teams. CMHNs are in a strong position to bridge this gap and encourage liaison between primary and specialist health care. With their range of responsibilities and skills, CPNs have to work across agencies, liaising and disseminating information, both clinical and educational. Goldie (1977) examined the division of labour in mental health work, looking at ways in which non-medical personnel secure professional status. Three models of working were suggested: a role ancillary to the psychiatrist but under psychiatrist leadership; role overlap, with doctors assigned a coordinating, rather than a directive role; an anti-psychiatry position, denying all hierarchy. CMHNs are in a prime position to adopt the middle line, blurring their role somewhat and acting as intermediary between primary and specialist health care services. This requires a commitment, not only from CMHNs but also from primary and specialist health care services to enable effective inter-agency working. The CPN attached to primary health care teams will have to develop links with multidisciplinary teams and the multidisciplinary community mental health nurse must develop good working relationships with primary care. Quality leadership, supervision and training are essential but a national directive to coordinate such an approach is currently lacking.

COMMUNITY MENTAL HEALTH IN THE 1990S

MODELS OF COMMUNITY CARE

Intensive Home-based Care
Comprehensive models of community care treatment have successfully demonstrated examples of good practice. A study, conducted in Montreal in 1979, examined comprehensive multidisciplinary care for clients suffering mainly from schizophrenia or depression (Fenton *et al.*, 1979). The

provision of community care compared to hospital treatment proved effective for some clients and a general reduction in disruption to families was noted.

A study of 130 clients needing admission in Madison, Wisconsin clearly demonstrated the benefits of a comprehensive multidisciplinary team approach to community care (Stein and Test, 1980). Clients cared for in the community received an intensive care package for 14 months, consisting of 24-hour crisis support, counselling, family education and interventions to improve basic living and social skills. Compared to a hospitalized control group, clients receiving community care had fewer and shorter hospital admissions, reported less symptomatology and greater satisfaction with care and were more socially integrated. The Madison study was replicated in Sydney, Australia (Hoult *et al.*, 1981; Hoult, 1986) with similar results. Both studies reported a rapid deterioration in mental state when intensive community care ceased.

The first comprehensive trial of intensive home based care in Britain, the Daily Living Programme, was conducted in south Southwark, London (Muijen *et al.*, 1992). The Daily Living Programme team consisted mainly of psychiatric nurses who worked with a consultant psychiatrist, senior registrar, social worker and occupational therapist. Clients presenting for admission were randomized into a home based care group and a control group. Clients in the treatment group who required hospitalization were admitted for short periods of crisis intervention only, with responsibility for care remaining with the Daily Living Programme staff. Home based care consisted of intensive 24-hour support for clients and their carers across a wide range of areas including psychiatric treatment, housing, finance and work. As a result, admission rates in the treatment group dropped dramatically compared to the control group and clients and their carers reported greater satisfaction with home based care. This model of working requires an extension of the CPN role into areas of care usually provided by other multidisciplinary team members, such as support with housing and financial issues. CPNs working as case managers in an intensive service need to become adept at making those decisions usually made by a psychiatrist, such as mental state assessment, admission and discharge and the use of medication. Although the extended role is stimulating, nurses also need adequate training and support from other multidisciplinary team members in view of the intensive relationships built up with clients throughout treatment (McNamee, 1993).

The model of intensive community support has since been replicated and adapted throughout Britain (Burns *et al.*, 1993; Dean *et al.*, 1993) and further study has demonstrated that CMHNs can be effective practitioners in the area of community support, although community resourcing and training of staff remain important considerations (Muijen *et al.*, 1994).

Key Components of Effective Community Based Services

To provide an appropriate community service for a range of individuals with mental health needs, a variety of interventions, treatment settings and facilities must be available. These include acute care and crisis intervention, continuing care and outreach, day care, respite facilities, rehabilitation services, social care liaison and advocacy (e.g. housing and financial support) family and carer support, consultation and liaison and access to work schemes.

Crisis intervention is discussed in depth in Chapter 13. Ideally, services that provide acute care and crisis response should be available on a 24-hour basis and information regarding such services should be made available to clients, carers, health care professionals and the local community. Crisis arrangements should provide immediate psychiatric assessment and have access to a range of further facilities including continuing care teams and in-patient facilities. Comprehensive mental health services provide both crisis response and continuing care for clients (Stein and Test, 1980).

Day care facilities vary widely in their functions and philosophies, providing an alternative to hospital admission, support and monitoring for clients living at home, long-term structure and support for clients with long-term mental health needs, intensive therapy and a central point for information, training and resources (Holloway, 1988). An innovative approach to day care services is the 'clubhouse' model, developed in New York (Beard *et al.*, 1982) and adapted by services in the UK (Shepherd *et al.*, 1993). In this model, service users become members of the clubhouse and assume responsibility for its functions and activities, which promotes the acquisition of skills and fosters a sense of ownership and positive social status.

THE CYCLE OF CARE PROVISION

Continuity in the provision of care can be viewed as a cyclical process with different professionals stepping in and out of the arena to meet the clients' needs as they arise. All professionals are seen as having important roles to play at different stages of health and illness. The importance of the role played by relatives or significant others is also discussed, as is their need for support throughout. Continuity of care will be discussed below as we explore a typical cycle of care.

REFERRAL

Psychiatric referrals have various origins, for example:
- General practitioners.
- Social services departments.
- Probation service, courts, etc.
- Other agencies, e.g. schools.
- General hospitals (particularly Accident and Emergency Departments).
- Other psychiatric teams.
- Self.
- Family or friends.

There are many reasons for referral being sought including, for example:
- Stress.
- Life crises.
- Lack of support network or its inability to cope.
- Concern by relatives or carers.
- Psychiatric assessment.
- Advice and information.
- Previous mental health problems recurring.

Most referrals to most psychiatric teams are made by GPs but presumably these have often arisen because of:
- An initial self-referral to the surgery,
- A referral by a significant other to the GP. ('Significant other' refers to a person with whom the client has a meaningful relationship, i.e. relative, friend, carer etc).
- Concern expressed by a another member of the primary health care team (i.e. practice nurse, district nurse, health visitor etc).

Initial referral to the GP may occur for a variety of reasons, some of which are listed below:
- Accessibility and availability.
- Previous relationship with GP.
- Privacy.
- Less stigma attached.

Accessibility and Availability

What is meant by these terms? Moak (1990) on reviewing the quality of psychogeriatric services, provides the following:

> Availability depends upon a process for heightening awareness of the need to provide specialised services for assuring responsible allocation of resources for such services access is a function of the location of services....

It is generally acknowledged that GPs and primary health care teams provide far better access for people by being based within the local community they serve. Sharp and Morell (1989) state that:

> the General Practitioner plays a major role in the management of the mentally ill and is often the first point of access for the client...

— a point worthy of note, in terms not only of access and referral but of community care in general. For many, the GP is the family doctor. The GP may have known the client and his or her family for many years and have a valuable understanding of their life circumstances as a whole. In 1983 the Health Education Council and Consumers' Association conducted a general household survey in respect of health information. They found that 95% of respondents claimed to trust their GP. There would appear to be a good channel of communication between client and GP (or other primary health care professionals). This could well arise from a previous relationship with the professional concerned or a general feeling, reported by many, that the barrier to care is often slight.

Just as there is a stigma to being diagnosed mentally ill, there is a potential stigma to attending the out-patient department of a psychiatric hospital or attending a community mental health team base. Moak (1990), in exploring issues of accessibility, argues that those 'seeking primary care services are usually amenable to psychiatric referral within the same clinic'. A psychiatrist or other mental health professional, visiting a client at a primary health care team base, brings less stigma and helps to keep the privacy and dignity of the client intact.

The role of the GP in developing mental health care was first established by Shepherd *et al.* (1966). A large study involving London GPs found that 15 000 people were at risk in any 12-month period and 14% consulted at least once for a condition diagnosed as being largely psychiatric in nature. Further studies since have validated these findings (Goldberg and Blackwell, 1970; Regier *et al.*, 1985).

Potential clients, while residing in the community, will nearly always make their GP the first point of contact, whether or not they have contact with the secondary services. In the case of the homeless, they will often attend a clinic or hostel aimed primarily at their needs and from there make contact with a GP.

McDonald (1993) describes primary health care as being 'the first level of contact of individuals, the family and community with the national health system, bringing health care as close as possible to where people live and work and thus [primary health care] constitutes the first element of a continuing health care process'.

Kendrick *et al.* (1991) in a major survey of 500 GPs in the South West Thames Region found that 90% of them were happy to undertake the physical care of patients with long-term mental health needs but were reluctant to take on complete responsibility for their mental health care. Three-quarters wanted the psychiatric services to maintain primary responsibility and four-fifths believed that the CMHN should be the Key Worker. However, from the survey all GPs were happy to undertake care shared with the secondary services.

The GP is often best placed to identify and assess psychiatric morbidity in Great Britain. Almost all (98%) of the population is registered with a GP; 60–70% of the registered population consult a GP each year and only 10% fail to do so over a three year period (Sharp and Morell, 1989).

ASSESSMENT

Assessment can be defined as the systematic collection and analysis of information from which the client's needs for care are identified. This information will continue to be gathered while interventions are made and the programme of care is evaluated.

After receiving the referral, usually by letter but sometimes by telephone, the psychiatric team must consider how to proceed, what action is to be taken and by whom. Most of these decisions can be made through discussion of the referral at a team meeting, when representatives from other disciplines will be present. The choice of professional to complete the assessment may well result from a number of factors, for example:

- Professional expertise or skills.
- Continuity (i.e. which professional is most likely to become the Key Worker for the client).
- Other demographic factors, e.g. gender, ethnicity and age.
- Previous knowledge or relationship with client.
- Safety factors.
- Whether the crisis outlined in referral is likely to lead to hospital admission.

Other factors for consideration in planning an assessment are:
- Whether the referring person is willing to be involved.
- Where the assessment is to take place (this should ideally be client centred and should take into account their wishes as far as possible).
- Whether or not the client knows the referral has been made. (If not, then who is to inform them should be decided prior to the assessment.)
- Whether or not the client would like non-professional support during the assessment (e.g. family, friend, carer, befriender, advocate).

Ideally all the above questions should be answered before the assessment begins, as to some extent the answers will provide pertinent information to the psychiatric team. In a crisis where immediate action is required, there is not often time to ask such questions, although the venue of the assessment is often pre-ordained. Even after the assessment has begun, steps can be taken to involve others at the client's request. If an assessment leads to section procedures under the Mental Health Act (DoH and Welsh Office, 1983) then the approved social worker present has a duty to inform the nearest relative and to exchange some information with them.

In *Caring for People: Community Care in the Next Decade and Beyond* (DoH, 1989a) the Government states that:

assessment should take account of the wishes of the individual and his or her carer and of the carer's ability to continue to provide care and where possible, should include their active participation. Effort should be made to offer flexible services which enable individuals and carers to make choices.

The process of assessment is an ideal opportunity for professionals, carers and the client to share information and in most circumstances decisions about treatment and interventions can be made jointly.

Slade (1994) argues that:

by taking account of the viewpoints of both the client and the team, neither of which is 'right' in itself, a more balanced consideration of the person's needs can be made.

He illustrates this through the use of the following diagram (Figure 11.1), which illustrates the factors he feels influence differing perceptions of need.

All assessments should be needs-led as opposed to service-led, i.e. professionals should not get into the habit of prescribing programmes of care based upon the service available. Through the process of care management, social service departments, as purchasers, may have funds available for alternatives based upon the client's actual need.

So what information is to be gathered during the assessment itself and how is it to be done? The means most often used is the medically trained staff, involving psychiatric and medical histories and culminating in an examination of the mental state of the individual, whatever form of assessment is

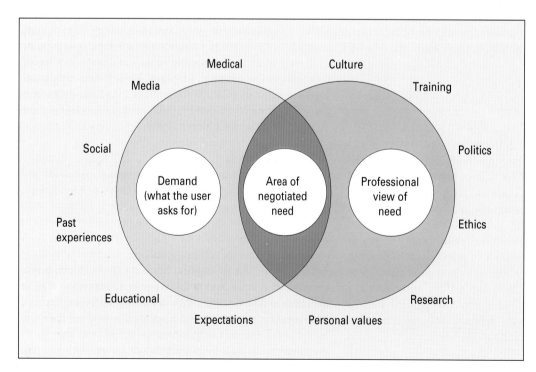

Figure 11.1 Factors that influence perceptions of need (courtesy of Slade, 1994)

used. Whether the assessment is to lead to a specific diagnosis or not, the factors shown in Box 11.1 are important.

After the overall psychiatric assessment and consideration of arguments about the assessment of need, the next step would be to further question the client about what he or she feels would be of use to them at this time i.e. what do they want? This is a good starting point for planning and negotiating interventions and an overall package of care. Of course there are exceptions to this, including:

- Where a decision for the client to be formally detained in hospital is made.
- Where the client being assessed is felt by the professional(s) to be mentally unwell (although not to an extent where formal detention in hospital is required) but the client differs and feels that he or she is not unwell (termed 'lack of insight').

In the first instance, professionals can start to address issues and enter into negotiation once the client has been admitted. In the latter example it is necessary to adopt flexible working strategies with the client and their family, working hard towards building relationships and completing further assessments of need.

TREATMENT — PACKAGES OF CARE

Interventions, in terms of the treatment plan, are obviously linked directly to the assessment and its outcomes. It is always good practice to discuss the information gleaned during an assessment interview with the multidisciplinary team as a whole. Often colleagues, whether from another discipline or not, can offer different perceptions and ideas to the case

material presented. Again, decisions regarding interventions, if any, can be made within such a multidisciplinary meeting.

Typical outcomes following discussions of assessment material and potential interventions can include:

- Referral back to the GP with advice and information regarding resources available.
- Offer of a package of short-term treatment to be negotiated with the client (and significant others, if appropriate). Such a package might include:
  - counselling
  - medication
  - psychological interventions
  - involvement in activities (e.g. day care, group therapy, training)
  - social interventions (e.g. housing, finances, child care etc.)
- Intensive community support of both client and family or carers.
- Admission to hospital (either on a voluntary basis or under a section of the Mental Health Act 1983).

Treatment is discussed in a general sense here, as many of the issues are similar in different situations. Whether hospitalized or community based, all clients should be offered the opportunity to participate in discussions and decisions regarding their care. Wilson–Barnett (1989) also reminds us of the importance of supplying clients with adequate information. This should include their treatment and care, medication and education about their illness. Some information and a rationale for the care to be given will be contained in the written programme of care, which may take the form of an action plan or care plan. All patients should receive a copy of this plan, which, ideally, should have been negotiated with them and can form the basis of a contract between client and professional. Organizations such as MIND, National Schizophrenia Fellowship (NSF) and the Manic Depressive Society produce leaflets on different illnesses. These are designed specifically to be understood by lay people. Some hospitals now provide drug information services that produce leaflets explaining psychiatric medication, what it does and any side-effects etc. In addition to Pharmacy Departments, this information is easily obtained from MIND. Holdsworth *et al.* (1994) in an article directed predominantly towards primary care, discuss the use of such materials. They argue that:

> self help materials present the user with therapeutic procedures in written, audio and audio-visual form and in Great Britain have been found to be particularly effective against anxiety and alcohol misuse.

This raises questions as to why the range has not so far been broadened to include psychological interventions. Whatever information and advice given to the client, sharing such knowledge with relatives and carers, where appropriate, must also be remembered. The NSF in a recent survey into the needs of carers (Hogman and Pearson, 1995) stated that 'the need for information is of primary concern for carers... it enables people to adjust to the situation and cope with it'. They

Box 11.1

Important factors to consider during the process of assessment.

1. Demographic details (gender, ethnic origin, mental status, occupation, living circumstances).
2. Reason for referral and referring agency.
3. Presenting problems (e.g. history, duration, severity, treatment received so far). Should incorporate views of client, carers and relatives.
4. Past psychotic history.
5. Pre-morbid personality (may provide a valuable baseline for interventions and information received should take into account views of significant others where possible).
6. Appearance and behaviour of client (includes a literal description).
7. Client's speech (rate, volume and content in addition to any signs of formal thought disorder).
8. Client's mood (e.g. clinical variation reported, constancy, appropriateness, ideas of self harm or suicide).
9. Thought content.
10. Abnormal beliefs and preoccupations (e.g. delusions, hallucinations, passivity phenomena, e.g. thought insertion, depersonalization).
11. Cognitive state (includes orientation, attention, concentration, memory etc).
12. Insight (i.e. client's view of illness and attitudes about this).
13. Assessment of potential risk (e.g. risk of harm to self or others, previous history of such).

found that lack of information and understanding results in further distress to families attempting to come to terms with a member being diagnosed as having severe mental illness.

In line with the *Patient's Charter* (DoH, 1992) every client has the right to a named worker, either a Key Worker or primary nurse. This professional will help to ensure continuity of care throughout the client's contact with the mental health service. By the very nature of allocating a professional to co-ordinate a client's care, all others involved with that person's care, including relatives and carers, will know to whom to relay information and where to receive it from. This reduces confusion and avoids information being missed or not adequately recorded, a criticism made in the recent inquiry into Christopher Clunis (Ritchie, 1994). These ideas support the CPA and Supervision Registers.

The Key Worker is often identified at the point of assessment. If the client is subsequently admitted to hospital for treatment, the Key Worker will hand over information needed by the allocated primary nurse to ensure that the therapeutic work progresses. As a result, treatment will be less disruptive for the client and the relatives and carers. A primary nurse has similar responsibilities to a Key Worker but, generally, this only spans the duration of the stay in hospital. A Key Worker, on the other hand, provides a longer-term commitment to the client's care. Bebbington and Kuipers (1994) argue that a Key Worker should be allocated to a client 'for a minimum of one or two years'. They follow this by stating that although every client has a Key Worker 'it is important that other members of the team know patients well enough to pick up the case when the Key Worker is not available'.

When treatment has taken place in hospital, this raises specific issues of planning for discharge. The use of a tool such as the CPA register is certainly one element of good practice in psychiatry. It formalizes the planning of the discharge process and thus after-care prior to the client returning to the community. As said earlier, any client thought vulnerable can be placed on the register as it does not apply only to clients detained under treatment orders.

> The Care Programme Approach was designed to build on existing good practice by systematising procedures, clarifying responsibilities and improving the continuity of care
>
> *(Shepherd et al., 1995)*

The allocated primary nurse is responsible for ensuring that a planning meeting takes place prior to discharge and that all interested parties attend. This, of course, includes relatives and carers (if the client is agreeable) and the primary health care team. A formal treatment package for after-care will be agreed by all concerned and specific tasks will be allocated to named people, professionals or otherwise. This document will then be circulated by the Key Worker (under the CPA) ensuring that everyone, including the client, knows exactly what is planned in terms of after-care and what role each person is expected to play. The Key Worker will then take over the responsibility for the coordination of the client's care, in the continuity cycle.

AFTER-CARE

The continuity of care provision highlighted through referral, assessment and treatment phases is consolidated, to some extent, in the after-care phase. After-care usually follows an admission to hospital but can also follow a period of intensive support in the community.

During after-care, treatment, support and monitoring are still live issues but the needs of the client can often change slightly or take on slightly different meanings. To illustrate this point, the Department of Health Social Services Inspectorate (1991) defines needs in terms of the NHS Community Care Act 1990. Needs are 'the requirements of individuals to enable them to achieve, maintain and restore an acceptable level of social independence of quality of life'.

While we can argue that the idea of needs applies throughout the cycle, it is particularly relevant to a time of less intensive professional support and applies mainly to rehabilitation. Bridges *et al.* (1994) define rehabilitation as:

> a process which aims to minimise the negative effects of the dynamic relationships between biological, psychological, functional and environmental factors and maximise the person's latent abilities and strengths. Its long term goal is to help a person travel through an illness career at minimum personal cost and maximal personal benefit particularly in terms of achieving an optimal level of functioning and well-being — even if the illness has a deteriorating course'.

They too conclude that 'continuity of care is an essential element'. After-care, as a follow-on to and a consolidation of treatment, has many functions, of which the most important is the prevention of further relapse or at the very least the minimization of such an event. The prevention of relapse involves the following:

* Treatment compliance.
* Continuing education of the client.
* Ongoing education of family and carers about the client's illness.
* An understanding of expectations.
* A detailed history of the client's illness.
* An acknowledgment of coping strategies, warning signs, critical or difficult periods etc.
* An understanding of other factors that may exacerbate relapse (e.g. substance misuse).
* Regular reviews and monitoring of client progress.
* Ensuring that client needs are met and that services are provided.
* Effective interprofessional working with open channels of communication maintained.
* Crises being quickly and effectively dealt with as they arise.

A large proportion of these items will be covered directly by the CPA and should be dealt with through effective discharge and after-care planning. Some, however, are worthy of more consideration here.

Keefler and Kaitar (1994) examine the use of family psychoeducation in the after-care of clients with a diagnosis of schizophrenia. They state, from a review of the literature, that family psychoeducation programmes are seen to be valuable in prevention of relapse. Such programmes involve establishing a collaborative and cooperative style of working with the family, through education regarding the illness. This helps the family gain better understanding, in addition to exploring how they could respond to the client, when unwell, in a more appropriate manner. This idea fits very well with the findings of the NSF survey mentioned earlier.

Two terms have been highlighted here—'cooperation' and 'collaboration'—but what do these mean exactly? Cooperation is being 'prepared to help another organization or individual meet their objectives and work together on them' (Payne, 1993). Collaboration is slightly different in that it is working together in a planned way to ensure consistency and continuity.

Interprofessional working, although a necessity, often presents problems in terms of effectiveness. Leathard (1991) discusses its effectiveness in terms of barriers that often appear. Among these barriers, she includes role ambiguity, status inequality, conflicting authority and power structures, different leadership styles and pay differentials between professional groups. For example, a CPN may find it difficult to confront a consultant psychiatrist over the completion of a task. However, these barriers must be addressed and overcome for the care provided and indeed the service as a whole to be of value to clients.

Grave (1994), in considering the changing perceptions towards mental illness since the mid-1980s, argues that because of a move away from an illness model 'the psychiatrist becomes only one expert among many'. He follows this by stating 'The medical profession is not necessarily in a leadership role but [is] rather one of a number of professional groups who provide timely specialised intervention'. This idea refers back to the view given earlier of continuity of care being coordinated by one professional with others stepping in and out of the arena.

The aim of after-care, whether in the short or the long term and dependent mainly on the needs and wishes of the client, is to conclude the continuity of care cycle by returning the focus of care to the referring agency (if possible) or ideally the primary health care team and GP. GPs appear to hold a variety of views regarding accepting responsibility for coordinating mental health care. In a study of 58 GPs, Strathdee (1987) found that linking GP practices directly with psychiatrists could more easily result in consultations and the provision of expert advice when needed and that GPs were happy, on that basis, to maintain personal responsibility. Kendrick *et al.* (1991) found that many GPs favoured shared responsibility.

> The critical question is not how the General Practitioner can fit into the mental health services but rather how the psychiatrist can collaborate most effectively with the primary care medical services and reinforce the effectiveness of the primary physician as a member of the mental health team.
>
> *(WHO, 1973).*

Harder (1988) found from looking at issues related to working with GPs that 'in clinical work, GPs value quick support, prompt case summaries when patients are discharged and the possibility of case discussion on the telephone'.

All this should happen as a matter of course. After all, it is widely recognized that GPs act in the role of goal keeper to psychiatric services (Lazarus, 1994) and, in fact, deal with a multitude of mental health problems that never actually reach psychiatry (Walters *et al.*, 1994). Malcolm (1994) argues that primary health care is 'care which can be generalist, holistic, continuing and comprehensive'. He contrasts this with secondary care, which he argues is 'specialist, dealing with only one aspect of the person's needs and is episodic'.

In an era of purchasers and providers of health care, GP fundholders are in a prime position to be able to access specialist mental health care when needed. Malcolm follows this idea, stating 'As an organised entity primary health care could become the budget holder for referral to secondary care and thus become a practical strategy for shifting the balance of care from secondary to primary'. Such a primary health care service may take us further towards achieving better health care for everyone (Malcolm, 1994).

Having already introduced the notion of stigma and a stated preference by some health professionals towards primary health care, referral back to the GP does appear to be an ideal situation. However, this should be accompanied by:

• Back-up if needed from the psychiatric team.
• A completed care package with needs addressed.
• A client who is engaged with the GP and complying with medication.
• A client subject to the CPA or Supervision Registers.

So, in conclusion, continuity of care can be seen as a cyclical process over time, whereby clients are able to move uninterrupted through the care system. The idea of a cycle fits well here as it recognizes and takes into account the different

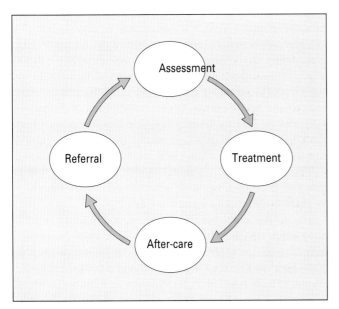

Figure 11.2 The continuity of care cycle

needs of clients, the involvement of various professionals and the often cyclical nature of mental illness itself (Figure 11.2).

THE ROLE OF THE COMMUNITY MENTAL HEALTH NURSE

Although the goal of the legislation could be viewed as admirable, implementation may be fraught with difficulties; most predictably lack of resources will be cited. It is widely felt that there will never be enough resources to satisfy all demands.

The Mental Health Nursing Review (DoH, 1994b) recommends that the essential focus for the work of mental health nurses lies in working with people with serious or enduring mental illness. Given that, there is a lack of available resources and, as Naish (1994) suggests, 'fears are rife that its cost implications have fated it to become another departmental dust gathering'. However, the Mental Health Nursing Review has made 42 recommendations that require mental health nurses to reshape their role and develop services for the future, both in the short and the long term.

The Mental Health Nursing Review (DoH, 1994b) responds to the CPA with the following recommendation:

> We recommend that action is taken to ensure that mental health nurses play a central role in services made available under the Care Programme Approach and in the provision of supervised discharge.

Service providers have to ensure that available resources are used efficiently, decide on the priorities and target vulnerable client groups, that is the severely mentally ill. The Health Committee Report (DoH, 1994a) identifies a number of 'gaps' in current provision including the allocation and usage of beds, both acute and long-term, and secure bed placements for mentally disordered offenders in community based services. With minimum use of compulsory powers and lack of available inpatient beds, nurses are placed under enormous pressure in providing assertive follow-up and closer supervision, aimed at preventing harmful acts by people with mental disorders.

The current structure and ethos of community services places limitations on the professionals' knowledge about risk and assessment. It has to be recognized that no legislation will predict disasters and prevent their occurrence. The authority and accountability of the Key Worker role is little comfort to practitioners at times of public inquiry and the ensuing burden of responsibility.

Jayne Zito, whose husband Jonathan died after being attacked by a man with a history of mental health problems, states:

> Community care is not a given or natural resource. It is a policy that needs careful planning, adequate resourcing and effective monitoring.

(Zito Trust, 1995)

Nurses working alongside those from other disciplines are developing a range of specific techniques, interventions and treatment options. This can be viewed as a valuable contribution to the development of mental health nursing and nursing clinical expertise. There are too few studies available that focus on people with schizophrenia. (See, as an example Brooker *et al.*, 1993 on the training of community nurses undertaking psychological interventions with families caring for a sufferer of schizophrenia.) A further development, the Thorn Nursing Initiative, aims to enhance mental health nurses' clinical skills and knowledge of people experiencing severe and enduring mental health problems (Gamble, 1995).

Enhancing the therapeutic role of mental health nurses through such a range of specific techniques and interventions will give them the opportunity to explore multiple interventions with people with acute and enduring mental health needs. This can form part of a holistic approach to identified needs, taking account of the clients' and carers' perspectives and the informed views mental health nurses can provide. However, as Holloway (1994) acknowledges, balancing the need to make decisions with the importance of promoting individual choice and autonomy is a dilemma inherent in psychiatry.

TRAINING AND DEVELOPMENT

The Key Worker role carries greater individual responsibility. It is imperative that adequate initial and continuing training on community care developments and the changing role of Key Workers takes place.

Mental health nursing students need to be equipped with relevant knowledge about severe mental health problems if they are to educate patients and families experiencing mental illness. Nursing theories, such as those of Peplau (1990), Orem (1985) and Roy (1976), still followed in many in-patient and community settings, need revision to include multidisciplinary care systems where all disciplines have an input. This is essential to working collaboratively across disciplines.

Individual assessment of clients also has to be carried out with an awareness of relevant research knowledge. An example of this is literature concerning the nature of risk assessment and decision making (Monahan, 1988; Pollock *et al.*, 1989). Training programmes need to include an overview of Government policy, implications for practice, risk assessment, needs led assessment, monitoring and supervision, Mental Health Act training, role and function of Key Workers, problem solving and cognitive behavioural approaches, and inter-agency and inter professional working.

The Secretary of State's 10-point plan (DoH, 1993) commits itself to developing a framework for training Key Workers in their duties under the CPA.

The proposed amendments to the Mental Health Act Code of Practice (DoH and Welsh Office, 1983) due for implementation in April 1996 will have a direct impact on the role of the Key Worker. The Order requires that a person, following discharge from hospital, will reside at a fixed address, attend day care provision and take appropriate prescribed treatments. If the individual terminates these agreements, he or she will be recalled to hospital. This Act does not provide for the housing or accommodation required. It merely acts as a tagging system, ensuring that community health teams know the whereabouts of the individual 24 hours a day. This amendment is aimed at individuals, well known to community mental health teams, with severe and enduring mental health problems. These individuals are sometimes referred to as the 'revolving door', a metaphor for the problematic situation where a patient who has been released on voluntary medication decides they are well enough and stops receiving treatment, resulting in a relapse of the illness.

The responses to this proposal have been varied. The central issue, clearly stated by MIND and the Mental Health Act Commission document, is that personal liberty is not to be taken lightly.

The Mental Health Act Commission also proposes that community treatment orders be introduced in the form of special guardianship. However, guardians cannot enforce medication and little research has been done on the role of guardianship. Further examination of these legal matters is needed.

The recent report of the inquiry into Christopher Clunis (Ritchie, 1994) gave detailed comments on appropriate supervision of the patient and the value of measures to ensure that seriously mentally ill people receive close supervision and support.

Mental health legislation, in its efforts to attain satisfactory supervision of those clients coming into contact with mental health services, is still in its early stages of evaluation. However, research evaluating the CPA by Pierides *et al.* (1994) confirms its effectiveness in improving the delivery of care to people suffering from severe mental illness.

In this case analysis of the report, Ritchie (1994) suggests that providing good quality, effective care in the community is dependent on available resources, the quality of facilities, and quality staff, effectively supported and trained. Provider units that fail to deliver adequate care and control for the vulnerable and difficult group of severely mentally ill people will continue to pose unacceptable risks, both to the public and clinicians themselves.

FACTORS AFFECTING CONTINUITY OF CARE

Carson and Bartlett (1993) looked at particular stresses facing CMHNs. Stress levels from 250 nurses working in community teams were analyzed. The results indicated that 4 out of 10 nurses were experiencing high levels of psychological distress. The study concludes that while major changes are occurring in the psychiatric area for both in-patient and community nurses, stress is exacting its toll on mental health nurses in terms of higher absence rates, lower self-esteem and personal unfulfilment. Carson and Bartlett suggest that further studies will need to concentrate on effective stress reduction strategies, which will enable professionals to cope with increasing workloads and expectations. The Sainsbury Centre for Mental Health also looked at job satisfaction and burn-out in community teams. The Report identified role ambiguity

relating to an individual's discipline and the team in which he or she belongs. Placing practitioners into teams poses special difficulties that can lead to conflicting team aims (Onyett *et al.* 1995).

From the studies cited, it is clear that major changes in legislation and working practices can result in stress and poor job satisfaction.

PROVIDING SUPPORT AND CONTINUITY

Community mental health teams need to be clear about their aims and overall philosophy. Most teams provide a mixture of extended support, that is (for people with neurotic disorders) treatment of acute crises and provision of alternatives to in-patient hospitalization where feasible and intensive support for a more disabled population where individual needs may require a more social rather than medical input.

Mental health teams need to have clear priorities and to monitor workload to ensure that targets in respect of purchaser requirements are met. The need to measure the workload of nurses has been acknowledged. Bridel (1993) suggests that efficient rostering and determining the right mix of skills will affect the cost of the service both in the short run and in terms of future staffing levels.

Gournay (1995) states that case management will be the main mechanism for providing community care in the future and that individuals with severe and enduring mental health problems should be named in caseloads of no more than six or eight. The appropriate balance between professional and non-professional staff requires careful thought according to the range of functions the team is undertaking.

The Ritchie Report (1994) highlights effective communication and accountability within teams. This requires clear and decisive leadership. Rafferty (1993) proposes a definition of leadership as the ability to identify a goal, to determine a strategy for achieving that goal and to inspire one's team to join in putting that strategy into action. Therefore leaders ideally should have vision and the ability to support, strengthen and inspire their teams.

Clear operational management is required for all team members. Individual team members remain responsible for their own actions within their professional boundaries.

It is important that team members do not feel personally responsible for decisions taken in response to their roles as Key Workers. Responsibilities need to be shared and varied between members of the team and the team has to be accountable for transmitting information and for the performance of central actions. Striking a balance between the need to preserve confidentiality between clinicians and patients and involving other professionals or agencies is important. Clinicians' failure to pass on information to workers in voluntary agencies was another finding of the Ritchie Report (1994).

The shortage of resources means that teams will have to use every resource available to them and involve the carers and general practitioners as part of an effective and integrated community mental health team.

SUMMARY

The first out-patient nurses in Britain were appointed in Warlingham Park Hospital in 1954. Their role involved monitoring out-patients, setting up therapeutic groups and facilitating accommodation issues. Community psychiatric nurses remained largely hospital based until the 1970s when they began to work from GP surgeries and became more autonomous, specializing in areas such as behavioural psychotherapy. More recently, community mental health nurses have become part of multidisciplinary teams working from a statutory specialist base.

Community mental health nurses increasingly face conflicting demands from local and national policies, creating role strain and ambiguity. The introduction of the CPA (DoH, 1990) has re-focused community mental health nursing to those clients with severe and enduring mental health problems, and community mental health nurses have extended their role as Key Workers. However, conflict has arisen as GP fundholders may demand that the needs of other priority groups are met. The organization of community mental health care is best undertaken by a multidisciplinary team, to ensure a planned system of needs assessment and care delivery. A range of acute, day, respite, rehabilitation, and social care needs to be available, alongside advocacy and carer support. Users of services emphasize the need for choice, flexibility and alternatives to hospital care. Community mental health nurses must assess these needs in a manner which accommodates both choice and risk.

KEY CONCEPTS

- Community mental health nursing has developed rapidly since the 1950s.
- Legislation has had a great impact on community service development and the role of the community mental health nurse.
- Multidisciplinary working and interagency planning are essential components of an effective community mental health service.
- Training and development are important considerations in the provision of community mental health services.
- Primary health services have an important role in the delivery of community mental health care.

REFERENCES

Audit Commission: *Making a reality of community care.* London, 1986, HMSO.

Beard J, Propst RN, Malamud TJ: The Fountain House model of psychiatric rehabilitation. *Psychosoc Rehab J* 5:47, 1982.

Bebbington PE, Kuipers L: The social management of long-standing schizophrenia (i): the deployment of clinical techniques. *Clinician* 12:1738, 1994.

Bridel JE: Why measure workload? *Prof Nurs* 362, 1993.

Bridges K, Huxley P, Oliver J: Psychiatric rehabilitation: redefined for the 1990s, *Int J Soc Psychiatry* 40:1, 1994.

Brooker C: A description of clients nursed by community psychiatric nurses whilst attending English National Board clinical course no. 811: clarification of current role. *J Adv Nurs* 15:155, 1990.

Brooker C et al: Skills for CPNs working with seriously ill people. In: Brooker C, White E, editors: *Community psychiatry,* vol 2. London, 1993, Chapman & Hall.

Burns T et al: A controlled trial of home-based acute psychiatric services (i): clinical and social outcome. *Br J Psychiatry* 163:49, 1993.

Caldicott F: Letter to the Secretary of State for Health, *Psychiatry Bull* 18:385, 1994.

Carson J, Bartlett H: Stress and the psychiatric nurse. *Nurs Times* 89:38, 1993.

Community Psychiatric Nurses Association: *National survey update.* Bristol, 1985, CPNA Publications.

Corrigan J, Soni DS: Community psychiatric nursing: an appraisal of its impact on community psychiatry in Manchester, England. *J Adv Nurs* 2:247, 1977.

Dean C et al: Comparison of community based service with hospital based service for people with acute, severe psychiatric illness, *BMJ* 307:473, 1993.

Department of Health: *Caring for people: community care in the next decade and beyond.* London, 1989a, HMSO.

Department of Health: *Working for patients. Presented to the Parliament by the Secretaries of State for Health, Social Security.* London, 1989b, HMSO.

Department of Health: *The Care Programme Approach for people with a mental illness referred to the specialist psychiatric services.* London, 1990, DOH.

Department of Health: *Care management and assessment — summary of practice guidance.* London, 1991, HMSO.

Department of Health: *Health of the Nation key area handbook, mental illness,* London. 1992, HMSO.

Department of Health: *Legislation planned to provide supervised discharge of psychiatric patients.* London, 1993, DOH.

Department of Health: *Draft guidelines to arrangements for inter-agency working for the care and protection of severely mentally ill people.* 1994a, HMSO.

Department of Health: *Working in partnership: a collaborative approach to care— report of the Mental Health Nursing Review Team.* London, 1994b, HMSO.

Department of Health and Social Security: *Better services for the mentally ill.* London, 1975, HMSO.

Department of Health and Social Security: *Care in the community: a consultative document on moving resources for care in England.* London, 1981, HMSO.

Department of Health and Social Security: *Neighbourhood nursing — a focus for care.* London, 1986, HMSO.

Department of Health and Welsh Office: *Mental Health Act Code of Practice,* ed 2. London, 1983, HMSO.

Department of Health Social Services Inspectorate: *Care management and assessment: practitioners guide.* London, 1991, HMSO.

Fenton F, Tessier L, Streuning E: A comprehensive trial of home and hospital psychiatric care. *Arch Gen Psychiatry* 36:1073, 1979.

Gamble C: The Thorn nurse initiative. *Nurs Stand* 9(15):31, 1995.

Goffman E: *Asylums.* New York, 1961, Anchor Books/Doubleday.

Goldberg D, Blackwell B: Psychiatric illness in general practice: a detailed study using a new method of case identification. *BMJ* 11:439, 1970.

Goldberg D, Steele JJ, Johnson A and Smith C: Ability of primary care physicians to make accurate rates of psychiatric symptoms. *Arch Gen Psychiatry* 39:829, 1982.

Goldie N: The division of labour among mental health professionals — a negotiated or imposed order? In: Stacey M *et al.,* editors: *Health and the division of labour.* London, 1977, Croom Helm.

Gournay K: Changing patterns on mental health care. Implications for evaluation and training. *Psychiatric Care* 2(3):93, 1995.

Gournay K, Brooking J: Community psychiatric nurses in primary health care. *Br J Psychiatry* 164:231, 1994.

Grave B: Reform of mental health care in Europe — progress and change in the last decade. *Br J Psychiatry* 165:431, 1994.

Griffiths R: *Community care: agenda for action. A report to the Secretary of State for Social Services.* London, 1988, HMSO.

Harder J: Working with general practitioners. *Br J Psychiatry* 153: 513, 1988.

Hoeper EW *et al.:* The usefulness of screening for mental illness. *Lancet* 1:33, 1984.

Hogman G, Pearson G: *The silent partners: the needs and experiences of people who provide informal care to people with a severe mental illness.* Surbiton, Surrey, 1995, National Schizophrenia Fellowship.

Holdsworth N, Paxton R, Seidal S, Thanson D, Shrubb S: Improving the effectiveness of self help materials for mental health problems common in primary care. *J Ment Health* 3:413, 1994.

Holloway F: Day care and community support. In: Lavender A, Holloway F, editors: *Community care in practice.* Chichester, 1988, Wiley.

Holloway F: Need in community psychiatry, a consensus is required. *Psychiatr Bull* 18:321, 1994.

Hoult J *et al.:* Psychiatric hospital versus community treatment: the results of a randomized trial. *Aust NZ J Psychiatry* 17:160, 1981.

Hoult J: Community care for the acutely mentally ill. *B J Psychiatry* 149:137, 1986.

House of Commons second report from the Social Service Committee Session 1984/5 on community care. London, 1985, HMSO.

House of Commons: *National Health Service and Community Care Act.* London, 1990, HMSO.

Hudson B: Coming up roses. *Health Service J* 3:20, 1992.

Hunter P: *Schizophrenia and community psychiatric nursing.* Surbiton, Surrey, 1978, The National Schizophrenic Fellowship.

Hunter P: Social work and community psychiatric nursing—a review. *Int J Nurs Stud* 17:131, 1980.

Keefler J, Kaitar E: Essential elements of a family psychoeducational programme in the aftercare of schizophrenia. *J Ment Fam Ther* 20(4):369, 1994.

Kendrick T *et al.:* Provision of care to general practice patients with disabling long-term mental illness: a survey in 16 practices. *Br J Gen Practice* 44:301, 1991.

Kingdon D: Interprofessional collaboration in Mental Health. *J Inter-Prof Care* 2:141, 1992.

Kingdon D: Making care programming work. *Adv Psychiatr Treat* 1:41, 1994.

Lazarus A: A proposal for psychiatric collaboration in managed care. *Am J Psychother* 48(4):600, 1994.

Leathard A: Going inter-disciplinary. *Nursing* 4:33, 1991.

McDonald J: *Primary health care—medicine in its place.* London, 1993, Earthscan.

McNamee G: A changing profession: the role of nursing in home care. In: Weller MPI, Muijen M, editors: *Dimensions of community mental health care.* London, 1993, WB Saunders.

Malcolm L: Primary health care and the hospital: incompatible organisational concepts? *Soc Sci Med* 39(4):455, 1994.

Martin JP: *Hospitals in trouble.* Oxford, 1984, Blackwell.

Ministry of Health: *Report of sub-committee on mental nursing and the nursing of the mentally defective.* London, 1945, HMSO.

Moak GS: Improving quality in psychogeriatric treatment. *Psychiatr Clin N Am* 13:99, 1990.

Monahan J: Risk assessment of violence among the mentally disordered: generating useful knowledge. *Int J Law Psychiatry* 11:249, 1988.

Moore S: A psychiatric outpatient nursing service. *Mental Health* 20:51, 1960.

Moore S: Mental nursing in the community. *Nurs Times* 467, 1964.

Muijen M *et al.:* Community psychiatric nursing teams: intensive support versus generic care. *Br J Psychiatry* 164:211, 1994.

Muijen M *et al.:* Home based care and standard hospital care for patients with severe mental illness: a randomized controlled trial. *BMJ* 304:749, 1992.

Naish J: Professions unite on nurse leadership plans. 1,1,4, Nursing Manual, 1994.

NHS Management Executive: *Introduction of supervision registers for mentally ill people from 1 April 1994.* London, 1994, HMSO.

NHS Management Executive: *The health of the nation: first steps for the NHS.* London, 1992, HMSO.

Onyett S, Pillinger T, Muijen M: *Making community mental health teams work.* London, 1995, The Sainsbury Centre for Mental Health.

Orem D: *Concepts of practice.* New York, 1985, McGren Hill.

Paykel ES, Mangen SP, Griffith JH, Burns TP: Community psychiatric nursing for neurotic patients: a controlled trial. *Br J Psychiatry* 140:573, 1982.

Payne M: *Linkages, effective networking in social care.* London, 1993, Whiting & Birch Ltd.

Peplau HE: Interpersonal relations model :principles and general applications. In: Reynolds W, Cormack D, editors: *Psychiatric and mental health nursing in London.* London, 1990, Chapman & Hall.

Pierides M, Roy D, Craig T: The Care Programme Approach, preliminary results one year after implementation in an inner city. *Psychiatr Bull* 18:249, 1994.

Pollock N, McBain I, Webster CD: Clinical decision making and the assessment of dangerous patients. In: Howells K, Hollin CR, editors: *Clinical approaches to violence.* Oxford, 1989, John Wiley.

Pullen I: Description of an extramural service for psychiatric emergencies. *Health Bull* 38:163, 1980.

Rafferty AM: *Teaching questions.* London, 1993, Kings Fund.

Raftery J: Social policy and community psychiatry. In: Bennett DH, Freeman HL, editors: *Community psychiatry.* Edinburgh, 1991, Churchill Livingstone.

Rawlings JA: Course in community psychiatry. *Nurs Mirror* 130:20, 1970.

Regier DA *et al.:* The chronically mentally ill in primary care. *Psychol Med* 15:265, 1985.

Ritchie JH, Dick D, Lingham R: *The report of the inquiry into the care and treatment of Christopher Clunis.* London, 1994, HMSO.

Roy C: *Introduction to nursing: an adaptation model.* New Jersey, 1976, Prentice Hall.

Royal College of Psychiatrists: Comments on the Griffiths report. *Bull R Coll Psychiatrists* 12:385, 1988.

Royal College of Psychiatrists: Community psychiatric nursing: a discussion document for the working party of the section for social and community psychiatry. *Bull R Coll Psychiatrists* 4:114, 1980.

Sharp D, Morell D: The psychiatry of general practice. In: Williams P, Wilkinson G, Rawnsley K, editors: *Scientific approaches in epidemiological and social psychiatry.* London, 1989, Routledge.

Shaw A: CPN attachment in a group practice. *Nurs Times* 73(12):9, 1977.

Shepherd G: Case management. *Health Trends* 2:59, 1990.

Shepherd G, Singh K, Mills N: Community services for the long-term mentally ill: a case example — the Cambridge Health District. In: Weller MPI, Muijen M, editors: *Dimensions of community mental health care.* London, 1993, WB Saunders.

Shepherd G *et al.:* Implementing the Care Programme Approach. *J Ment Health* 4:261, 1995.

Shepherd M *et al.: Psychiatric illness in general practice.* Oxford, 1966, Oxford University Press.

Slade M: Needs assessment: involvement of staff and users will help to meet needs. *Br J Psychiatry* 165:293, 1994.

Stein L, Test MA: Alternative to mental hospital treatment. 1. Conceptual model, treatment program and clinical evaluation. *Arch Gen Psychiatry* 37:392, 1980.

Strathdee G: Primary care psychiatric interaction: a British perspective. *Gen Hosp Psychiatry* 9:69, 1987.

Strathdee G, Williams P: A survey of psychiatrists in primary care: the silent growth of a new service. *J R Coll GPs* 34:615, 1984.

Tansella M, de Silva D, Williams P: The Italian psychiatric reform: some quantitative evidence. *Soc Psychiatry* 22:37, 1987.

Tooth GC, Brooke EM: Trends in the mental hospital population and their effect on future planning. *Lancet* 1:710, 1961.

Tyrer P: Psychiatric clinics in general practice: an extension of community care. *Br J Psychiatry* 145:9, 1984.

United Kingdom Consultative Council for Nursing, Midwifery and Health Visiting: *Project 2000 paper 9.* London, 1987, UKCC.

Walters L, Gannan M, Murphy D: Attitudes of General Practitioners to the psychiatric services. *Int J Psychol Med* 11:44, 1994.

Warner R, Gater R, Jackson M, Goldberg D: Effects of a community mental health service on the practice and attitudes of general practitioners. *Br J Gen Pract* 43:507, 1993.

White E, Brooker C: The future of community psychiatric nursing: what might 'the Care Programme Approach' mean for practice and education? *CPNJ* 10(6):27, 1990.

White E: *The third quinquennial survey of community psychiatric nursing.* London, 1990, CPNA Publications.

Wilson–Barnett J: Limited autonomy and partnership: professional techniques in health care. *J Med Ethics* 15:12, 1989.

Wolfensberger W: The principle of normalisation and its implications to psychiatric services. *Am J Psychiatry* 127:291, 1970.

Wooff K, Goldberg D: Further observations on the practice of community care in Salford: differences between community psychiatric nurses and mental health social workers. *Br J Psychiatry* 153:30, 1988.

Wooff K, Goldberg D, Fryers T: Patients in receipt of community psychiatric nursing care in Salford 1976–1982. *Psychol Med* 16:407, 1986.

World Health Organization: *Psychiatric and primary medical care.* Copenhagen, 1973, WHO.

Zito Trust: *Learning the lessons.* London, 1995, Zito Trust.

FURTHER READING

Wolff G et al: Public education of community care. A new approach. *Br J Psychiatry* 168:441–447, 1996.
> *The findings from a controlled study of the effect of a public education campaign and community attitudes to mentally ill people.*

Thomas P, Greenwood M, Kearney G, Murray L: The first twelve months of a community support bed unit. *Psychiatr Bull* 20:455–458, 1996.
> *This study acknowledges that traditional in-patient care is not essential for everybody, with evidence that people suffering from acute and severe mental health problems can successfully be managed in the home setting.*

Department of Health: *Building bridges: a guide to arrangements for interagency working for the care and protection of severely mentally ill people.* London, 1995, Department of Health.
> *An excellent resource document for health and social care purchasers and providers.*

Marriott S, Hassiotis A, Ray J, Tyer P: From inter-agency to multi-disciplinary work in a sector generic mental health team. *Psychiatr Bull* 20: 345–347, 1996.
> *This study suggests how the changes associated with implementing a multi-disciplinary model within a sector team can enhance the effectiveness of the service provided.*

Brooker C, Repper J, Booth A: Examining effectiveness of community mental health nursing. *Ment Health Nurs* 16(3):12–15, 1996.
> *This paper reviews research evidence currently available, suggesting other alternative types of research with the potential to inform practice.*

Dean C, Freeman H: *Community mental health care: international perspectives on making it happen.* London, 1996, Gaskell/Royal College of Psychiatrists.
> *A comprehensive list of contributions from an international perspective, on the developments of community mental health services.*

Health Promotion:
Its Application to Mental Health

Learning Outcomes

After studying this chapter you should be able to:

- Discuss the concepts of health in relation to mental health.

- Compare and contrast different perspectives arising from the definition of health.

- Identify the main concepts of health promotion.

- Use the concepts of health promotion to discuss how they can be applied to mental health promotion.

- Discuss the approaches used in health education that the mental health nurse may employ when assessing clients.

- Compare and contrast different models of health promotion and give examples of how these may be integrated into a plan of care for a client or group of clients.

- Offer examples of how values may direct the outcome of health promotion when dealing with a client or group of clients.

CHAPTER OUTLINE

- *Health*

- *Health promotion*

- *Health education*

- *Values in health promotion*

- *Models of health promotion*

---

*T**he traditional view of mental health has been** to focus care and treatment on illness and disease, usually within an institution. However, the establishment of specific mental health targets in *The Health of the Nation* (Department of Health, 1992) and the introduction of *Caring in the Community* (Department of Health, 1990) which endeavours to provide more care and treatment in the patient's own environment, mean that the mental health practitioner must draw on alternative bodies of knowledge and skills to meet the needs of the individual.

From a variety of sources (commercial, academic and governmental), individuals are being asked to consider healthy living and the development of a 'healthy lifestyle' (see Figure 12.2). The term that has been used to encompass these ideas is 'health promotion'. Many publications have clearly identified that health promotion is not only central but integral to modern day nursing practice (Delaney, 1994). However, the various definitions and interpretations of the term have often resulted in confusion, misapplication by nurses or lack of action.

This chapter will examine the theories of health promotion that have developed from disciplines such as psychology, education, epidemiology and sociology and identify their application to the mental health field. Health promotion is integral to the work of nurses and health care professionals in the modern health care system. The discussions in this chapter will assist the student to challenge the traditional medicalization of health and to begin to consider developing interventions in health promotion that do not rely on the traditional approach of medical care.

The chapter identifies various aspects of health promotion and explores each discrete area independently. These are then brought together to discuss a number of current models of health promotion that are used when designing and delivering a health promotion programme. The discussions are not intended to provide a definitive theoretical approach to the subject but are designed to provoke thought within the student to develop skills that enhance health gain and a positive approach to health.

HEALTH

Focus on health promotion has increased since the 1980s. It is rapidly establishing itself as an important force in public health and as such is being incorporated into contemporary approaches to health and health care (Bunton and Macdonald, 1992). Health promotion can now be seen to be challenging the traditional views of health in the medical model. It is taking a wider view by considering social and economic aspects and identifying health as an issue central to human life (Downie *et al.*, 1990). However, to promote health it is first necessary to understand and explore the term 'health'.

In ancient Greece the main function of a physician was to treat disease and to restore the health of the individual. This was achieved by treating any imperfections caused by accidents during birth or arising from everyday life (Dubos, 1960). Views about health have changed much since the ancient Greeks: the World Health Organization (WHO, 1946) have defined health as a state of complete physical, mental and social well-being and not merely the absence of disease or infirmity.

Health can be seen as both a negative and positive attribute. The disease model of health, for example, can be considered as a negative model. In this model, health is seen as the opposite of disease or illness. Health is perceived as made up of a number of predetermined factors, based upon the culture within which it is defined. The factors considered to constitute health are compared statistically to those that have been determined as the norm or ideal state (Sim, 1990). However, this view of health can only be considered in relation to disease and does not allow the individual to determine their own perspective of health. It relies entirely on the views of the health professionals.

In 1984 the WHO reviewed their definition of health and suggested that the extent to which an individual or group is able to realize aspirations and satisfy needs is important (WHO, 1984) (see Box 12.1). This suggests that health is a continuum, health and ill health being at opposite ends and that the definition of health is the subjective view of the individual in relation to the way he or she perceives the symptomatology. This more encompassing view can be considered as an example of positive health.

Downie *et al.* (1990) suggest that an important aspect of positive health is well-being. Well-being is the *feeling* of health that the individual has. It can be experienced by the person who is not strictly in positive health. An example of this might be the individual who has contracted a flu virus but is unaware of it in the absence of symptoms.

Closely associated with well-being is the concept of fitness. Downie (1990) believes that if individuals can carry out normal, everyday activities without any undue physical discomfort then they would probably consider themselves to be fit. Strength, stamina, suppleness and skills need to be considered to determine one's level of fitness (Downie, 1990). However, this again must be seen as a subjective assessment as individuals' levels of fitness relate specifically to their lifestyle and the activities they need and want to undertake and will change throughout their lives, according to age and personal circumstances.

Smith and Jacobson (1988) suggested from their research that there is a close link between fitness and mental health. In their findings they suggest that exercise not only assists individuals in moving towards physical fitness but that it also makes them feel good mentally. This link between physical and mental health is again identified in a study by Clarke and Lowe (1989). Their study considered the positive aspects of health and being healthy and the findings suggested that a prerequisite for health was a positive mental attitude, which could be achieved mainly in the pursuit of enjoyable activities in enjoyable company. This again demonstrates that the definition of health is subjective and rarely consistent. Farrell (1991) believes the mentally healthy are those who are able to solve problems in a mature way and deal with crises, possibly within a supportive network of family and friends. Being mentally healthy also involves getting to know oneself, understanding one's own needs, being able to achieve the possible and accepting why certain things cannot be achieved, while recognizing what causes personal stress and learning how to deal with it successfully (Farrell, 1991).

Unfortunately there is a dearth of research-based literature that attempts to define mental health. However, two useful studies from the USA, although both quite old, do attempt to explore this area. Bush *et al.* (1975) used an ethnoscientific approach in an effort to offer a definition of mental health. The study was performed using participant observation and repeated interview techniques. Throughout the contact with respondents, researchers identified frameworks and terms within those frameworks, which the subject placed in a hierarchy to identify their feelings about mental health. Findings from this study suggested that different groups of people perceived mental health as having different meanings. A clear gender difference was identified by the use of different terminology to describe beliefs. Males felt that to be mentally healthy it was necessary to be in control and to have material wealth. Females, however, considered that to be mentally healthy it was necessary to have inner strength and luck and to use prayer and to have a sound genetic background.

The second study that attempts to define mental health was

Box 12.1 *A definition of health promotion*

The definition of health promotion offered by the Ottawa Charter for Health Promotion (WHO, 1986) states that health promotion is a process that enables people to increase control over, and to improve, their own health.

undertaken by Kjervik and Palta (1978). This study aimed to determine beliefs about the meaning of mental health by establishing the differences in characterizing healthy males and healthy females. A random sample of 150 mental health nurses was used. The sample was divided into three equal groups, each group having a separate set of instructions: to consider what they thought an ideal, normal, healthy male was like, to consider what an ideal, normal, healthy female was like and finally to consider what they thought an ideal, normal, healthy adult was like. The findings of the study suggested that there was a close relationship between social acceptability of traits (those aspects that society in general perceived as desirable and necessary) and perceptions of health. They also suggested that the conceptions of healthy males differ little from those of healthy adults but conceptions of healthy females differ significantly from those of healthy adults. This implies that there is a significant gender difference when attempting to define mental health. Males and females may not hold the same definitions of mental health and there may be several paradigms of mental health within the same society.

Although dated, the findings from both these studies suggest that it is difficult to establish a conclusive definition of mental health. Mental health is not only difficult to define but the studies suggest that different views of mental health can coexist in the same society. In present day society, with its multi-ethnic and cultural mix, it is suggested that this is only to be expected.

Mental health has often been considered as a modern day euphemism for mental illness. This frequently results in confusion, not least because such a definition of mental health is grounded firmly in a disease model of health with negative connotations. Evans (1992) supposes that, as with our physical health, our mental health is an ever changing state and reflects our responses to both our internal and external environments. Evans suggests that our mental health is intrinsically connected to our physical, emotional and social health and as such cannot and should not be considered in isolation. A model of mental health needs to consider factors such as self-image, a sense of mastery and autonomy, a sense of security, relationships, emotional expression, reality based behaviour and how these relate to the individual's view of the self. The combination of these ideas suggests that health is a complex concept and that its definition has progressed far from simply including being free from ascertainable disease. Definitions of health (Figure 12.1), both physical and mental, must consider the social, economic, environmental, political, psychological and spiritual aspects of the person in relation to meeting their own needs and wants. This suggests that we should employ the concept of holism when considering health.

HEALTH PROMOTION

As exploration of the term 'health' has demonstrated, emphasis traditionally has been placed upon illness and disability. The approach to health has always appeared to be reactive as opposed to proactive. However, since the realization that a reactive approach towards health has proved ever more costly, interest in a more proactive approach has increased, namely that of health promotion. Indeed, with the launch of *The Health of the Nation* (Department of Health, 1992) providers of health care have been requested by Government to ensure that a health promotional approach is taken and a number of specific targets have been identified, towards which health care providers need to work.

The increased interest in a proactive approach to health care, focusing on the prevention of illness and disease and the development of healthy lifestyles, has facilitated a unifying concept. That is, health promotion has brought together a number of separate fields of study under one umbrella (Bunton and Macdonald, 1992) and as such more than adequately complements the developing definitions of modern day health. Dines and Cribb (1993) suggest that health workers are being asked to become more aware of how policies and practice affect health and suggest that health promotion therefore does not belong to any one institutional setting or professional role. The broad range of theory drawn into health promotion facilitates a multidisciplinary knowledge base, suggesting that the changes in the discipline make it multidisciplinary and, therefore, an integral part of the public health movement.

Health promotion represents those strategies that actively and positively promote the health of whole populations (Bunton and Macdonald, 1992) and can, therefore, be seen to have no obvious boundaries (Dines and Cribb, 1993). However, while medicine has its part to play, it is clear from this view that health promotion has freed itself from a medically dominated approach to health care; indeed it takes little impetus from medicine or the medical model.

Although this definition widens the scope of health promotion rather than focusing on components and strategies, it could prove problematic in its implementation as it suggests that health promotion, along with the public health movement,

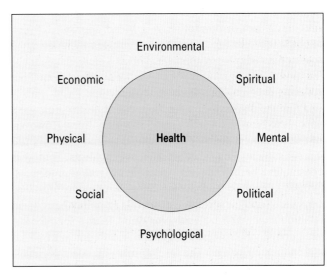

Figure 12.1 Definitions of health

is one of the few true interdisciplinary approaches to health care (Green and Raeburn, 1988).

Downie *et al.* (1990) believe that the overall goal of health promotion is to achieve a balance of physical, mental and social facets of positive health coupled with the prevention of physical, mental and social ill health. However, it would seem difficult, if not impossible, for the individual to achieve this in isolation and thus health promotion needs to function on two distinct levels. These are the individual or lifestyle approach and the structural or fiscal–ecological approach (Bunton and Macdonald, 1992), both of which play equally critical parts in the success of health promotion.

THE LIFESTYLE APPROACH

The lifestyle approach to health promotion focuses predominantly on the individual. It identifies the behaviours of the individual that may put them at risk of ill health and those associated with increased morbidity or premature death, and aims to reduce them. Such an approach includes ensuring that the individual is given appropriate information about their behaviours and that the health promoter transfers the knowledge and skills at a level the individual can understand. The rationale behind such an approach is that, with increased knowledge about their behaviours, the person will undergo an attitude shift and the result will be a change in behaviour. Examples of areas that would be included in the lifestyle approach are ceasing smoking, reducing alcohol consumption, use of non-prescribed drugs and assertiveness training.

THE STRUCTURAL APPROACH

The structural approach in health promotion, however, is not always under the control of the individual. Structural approaches consider the way in which society is controlled to promote and maintain a healthy population. Examples of this approach are housing policy, taxation on tobacco and alcohol, legislation regarding the driving of vehicles and the use of seat belts. When considering the structural approach in health promotion the importance of policy making and policy changing is evident. Draper (1986) suggests that policy making in health promotion is a broad approach, which attempts to recognize, assess and then change health-damaging features of today's environment. This is a clear statement of the importance of health promotion, not disease oriented but reducing everyday environmental risk factors.

From the discussion so far, the focus of health promotion appears to be on the development of healthy lives. However, health promoters enable the individual to lead a healthy life it is not sufficient to give information to individuals about what constitutes a healthy life and expect them to follow guidelines. Social, economic and ecological environments must be considered and the influence of sociology cannot be ignored (Bunton *et al.*, 1995). Health promotion, from a sociological perspective, is considered within the wider context of social and cultural influences. The development of modern societies, with increasing focus on the body, lifestyle, effective use of leisure time, personal development and the consumer culture,

must be considered when establishing an understanding of the discipline of health promotion (Bunton *et al.*, 1995).

The need for policy making and change in health promotion can be seen as far removed from the individual approach. Donati (1988) however, identifies the link between these two approaches and states clearly that policy change needs to develop from a 'bottom up' approach, involving the individual's perspective, suggesting that policy introduction conceived as purely a 'top down' approach will have limited effect on health promotion. This can be explained by considering the imposition of rigorous policy upon individuals, without consultation, which ultimately limits choice. It does not facilitate behaviour and attitude change by means of education or the development of awareness of social, economic, political and environmental influences.

The apparent gap between these two approaches to health promotion is bridged by the health protection methods used. Health protection measures can be seen as those activities that combine both policy approaches and individual, educational approaches. Examples of such approaches are breast screening, cervical smears and immunization programmes.

The broad remit of health promotion, which has two principal themes, has been considered above. However, within each of those themes there are a number of sub-themes, all of which are ultimately directed at the reduction of ill health and premature death. Maben and Macleod–Clark (1995) believe, when considering health promotion, that there are a number of concepts that relate to its meaning. These include well-being, empowerment, health education, collaboration, participation, equity and holism. It is clear, as with the definition of health, that the definition of health promotion has different emphases. Many definitions of health promotion exist (Tones, 1981; Tannahill, 1985), all slightly different but with interconnecting themes. It would not seem possible to establish a universal definition and it would appear more beneficial to define health promotion in the context in which it is employed. Maben and Macleod–Clark (1995) support this view and suggest that the definition of health promotion will depend upon who is asked and what the agenda is. Thus, definitions of health promotion will vary according to the organizations that use them and the political, social and theoretical considerations these organizations use in their daily functioning, which determine the approach they take. This allows the definition of health promotion to cover the issues associated with identified health promotional goals and target populations, as well as the type and focus of the interventions (Rootman, 1985).

MENTAL HEALTH PROMOTION

Mental health promotion proves just as difficult to define. This may be because there is a dearth of literature about mental health promotion, which is matched by a reluctance to address the subject or to debate whether mental health promotion should be considered as a separate concept (Hancock and Hancock, 1993). Ideally, health should be viewed holistically; therefore to separate mental health from physical or social health raises false divisions. This is particularly true when considering health promotion and is borne out in a study of community psychiatric nurses that focuses on perceptions of mental health promotion (Childs, 1995).

Health promotion is all too frequently based on ill health and the prevention of ill health, suggesting that the individual can only ever be well or ill. However, by considering prevention alone, mental health promotion falls into the medical model in that limited goals dictate levels of achievement. Rakusen (1990) believes that promotion allows mental health to be considered as a process and as such prevention will occur naturally. Mental health promotion cannot be easily defined or limited to one area. It focuses on joy rather than pleasure, truth rather than techniques and thriving rather than surviving (Rakusen, 1990). This approach considers mental health to be a continuum which the individual moves along, striving to achieve a level of functioning that is pleasing.

Stark (1986) considers the concept of primary prevention in mental health and believes that current health care systems are oriented towards curative care. In contrast primary prevention seeks to reduce the increase in rate of psychopathology and therefore the use of mental health services. It can be considered as an opportunity to enhance the social and emotional well-being of the individual. Prevention, therefore, should not be based on the assumption that it deals with an individual who has, or will develop, a mental illness but that the ultimate aim should be that psychological disorders do not occur. Mental health promotion should not be focused on

groups experiencing emotional disorders or behavioural deviance but on the needs and strengths of a community. In this context health professionals need to accept that the members of the community are experts in their own social environment and therefore able to identify the important issues relating to the promotion of their mental health.

Mental health promotion has proved difficult to define. It is an area that has been poorly researched and much of the literature explores the issues from an anecdotal position. However, mental health promotion should not be seen as an individual intervention. It is a process that incorporates aspects of prevention. Mental health promotion focuses predominantly on psychological health but is an integral part of working with an individual and as such should not be separated from the wider approach of health promotion. The individual must be viewed holistically. Perhaps the most important aspect of mental health promotion is the need for it to be directed to the population at large. It is not an approach that should be geared only towards those who experience mental ill health. It is something everyone can benefit from.

MENTAL HEALTH PROMOTION AND THE NURSE

Health promotion is gradually becoming an important aspect of nursing. Nurses are being encouraged to develop their roles to incorporate the major elements of health promotion (Maben and Macleod–Clark, 1995). Traditionally, nursing has viewed health promotion in the medical model and sought to promote

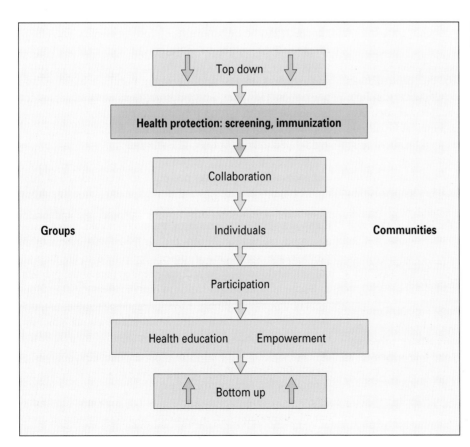

Figure 12.2 Health promotion through policy change

health through disease prevention. However, as the definition of health has progressed, so has the need to review nursing, its contribution to health care and the way in which health promotion is incorporated. Delaney (1994) suggests that, although integral to nursing, it has proved difficult to identify the distinct health promotional activities that are integral to nursing practice. However, it is far easier to identify the part that health education plays in the nurse's role. The focus is directed towards patient, carer and colleague education. As identified earlier, health education is only one aspect of health promotion. Nurses, therefore, must work towards establishing clear health promotional activities within their practice and continue to develop nurse education to ensure that this much wider view is included.

HEALTH EDUCATION

In exploring a definition of health promotion the need to develop knowledge and skills in achieving a healthy lifestyle has been identified. The common term for this is health education (see Box 12.2). Most definitions of health promotion include an element of health education. However, as Speller (1985) asserts, the terms 'health promotion' and 'health education' are not interchangeable.

There is frequently confusion between the terms. On reviewing the literature, health promotion appears to be the dominant concept, which incorporates health education (Saan, 1986; Tannahill, 1985).

APPROACHES TO HEALTH EDUCATION

The first approach to health education, proposed by Tones (1981) was the educational approach. In this, information about health is given to individuals to promote understanding. In giving the information no attempt is made to change attitudes or look for healthy behavioural outcomes. An example of this approach is offering information to a group about drug abuse; role-plays may be used to demonstrate how to refuse drugs if they are offered. Tones suggests that this approach is often used where the health educator believes it unethical to use persuasion or coercion to change health-related behaviour or attitudes. This approach provides the individual with

complete choice about whether or not to use the information to enhance lifestyle.

However, over recent years the approach to health care has altered dramatically. Much more consideration is now being placed on the maintenance of a healthy population and not just on the treatment of illness, and as such the approaches to health education have been modified. Tones and Tilford (1994) now suggest three approaches to health education:
1. The preventive approach.
2. The radical approach.
3. The self-empowerment approach.

The Preventive Approach

The preventive approach to health education is based on assumptions that prevention of illness is better than cure and that the behaviour of an individual plays a significant part in the aetiology of illness and disease. Forster (1992) believes this approach can be considered in three areas: primary, secondary and tertiary prevention.

Primary prevention encourages individuals to behave in a way that will assist in the avoidance of developing disease or illness. Activities undertaken here are genetic counselling, in relation to diseases such as Huntington's chorea. This type of education focuses on such issues as the effect of stress and how to reduce it, using techniques such as relaxation exercises, becoming involved in leisure activities, taking adequate rest and establishing effective social networks.

Welch *et al.* (1987) considered health education in mental health and suggested that knowledge and skills acquisition were essential in implementing a primary prevention approach. To be of benefit, they also believe it is essential for health educators to identify ethical, legal and value concerns as there is a need to distinguish between individual and societal rights and between public education and persuasion. However, a common problem using this approach in mental health is that it is difficult to identify illness or disease patterns, as mental ill health may be of a learned nature and related to complex social influences.

Much of this activity occurs in schools or in health clinics and focuses on the younger person. Topics considered in these environments are the normal development processes, body image, adequate nutritional intake and the avoidance of disorders such as anorexia or bulimia nervosa. Successful outcomes rely heavily on the skills of the educator in presenting a convincing argument that relates to the individual's lifestyle without introducing fear as part of the process.

Secondary prevention aims to halt or reverse the development of diseases or illness. Physical health screening for such diseases as cancer play a major part in this approach. However, halting or reversing disease development in mental health proves far more difficult. The predominant approach here is to promote education both of health care professionals and the general public in recognizing early warning signs of mental illness, to limit the development of severely incapacitating disorders. An example of this would be providing education about the signs of stress. By ensuring that individuals understand the

Box 12.2 *A definition of health education*

Health education focuses on enabling and supporting individuals to set their own agendas for health. This means that the individual can decide on what health means and the ways achieve it. Health education, therefore, is implemented in ways relevant to the individual or group of individuals. French (1990) identifies the differences in terms of approach and suggests that health education is practically based and is rooted in educational activity. It is not about behavioural change or political action.

signs and symptoms of stress and how to manage it, they are far less likely to develop stress-related mental illnesses such as anxiety states.

Tertiary prevention is aimed at preventing further complications once disease or illness is already in existence. Health educators need to focus on identifying ways in which individuals can adopt that lifestyle which minimize their limitations and provide maximum fulfilment. Examples of this approach would be to assist individuals or their families to deal with the stress and management of an already established illness. Brooker's research (1993) offers an excellent example of this approach. Brooker studied families who were caring for schizophrenics at home. His findings suggest that educating relatives is a crucial component of psychosocial interventions in the care and treatment of individuals suffering from schizophrenic illness. This type of approach is a strategy that seeks to prevent further exacerbation of mental illness and has an overall purpose of enabling families to cope with the stress of caring for severely disabled individuals, by relieving them of some of their anxieties.

The Radical Approach

The radical approach moves away from the individual approach and attempts to look further ahead than merely providing information regarding illness and disease. In fact Tones and Tilford (1994) suggest that it attempts to reject the medicalization of health and the 'victim blaming' that is associated with it. This approach to health education focuses on the social, political and economic factors that promote unhealthy lifestyles and tackles the determinants of health and disease at a social level.

The radical approach aims to develop public awareness of the different ways in which commercial interest does not always promote health and healthy lifestyles. Pike and Forster (1995) suggest that, when following an approach that seeks to deal with the roots of ill health and disease, it is frequently more beneficial to deal with topics such as poverty rather than attempting to persuade the disadvantaged to alter their lifestyle.

A clear example of this approach can be seen when considering the relationship between unemployment and mental illness. The research study performed by Banks and Jackson (1982) used the general health questionnaire to assess young people moving from employment to unemployment and vice versa. They were able to test young people before they left school and at intervals afterwards. Their findings suggest that symptoms of mental ill health increased significantly in those who left school and became unemployed and decreased in those who found work. Banks and Jackson believe this to be a significant indicator in the relationship between ill health and unemployment, as there was no significant difference in mental health between the two groups while they were still at school.

This example identifies the need for such an approach to health education. That is, it would be more beneficial to address the issue of unemployment to reduce the incidence of mental illness than to encourage the unemployed to focus on the maintenance of mental health. However, Pike and Forster (1995) suggest that knowledge alone is not enough to ensure the radical approach is actioned as with the preventative approach. There is a persisting need to use persuasion if community action is to result.

The Self-Empowerment Approach

The self-empowerment approach is characterized by the individual's ability to choose and determine the type of lifestyle desired. This is an important part both of physical and psychological well-being. The underlying goal of health promotion can be described as the achievement of equity, that is, the equal distribution of both power and resource. To this end Tones and Tilford (1994) state that an empowered community is able to facilitate the development of individual or self-empowerment and is dependent upon a reciprocal relationship between individuals and their environment.

To achieve this, health educators need to support and guide individuals not only in providing information to enable informed choices to be made but also in identifying the skills needed to determine health and lifestyle. In Tone's (1981) earlier work he identifies four strategies that are aimed at achieving self-empowerment:

1. Promote beliefs and attitudes that are favourable to deferring immediate rewards for more substantial future benefits.
2. Increase the internal locus of control, that is, challenge the beliefs that both health and lifestyle are controlled by fate or powerful people.
3. Endeavour to enhance self-esteem.
4. Encourage the development of certain social skills, for example, by assertiveness training.

The combination of these strategies aims to help individuals, either alone or with a group, to influence local and national policies that are believed to inhibit, or limit, individuals in achieving the health and lifestyle that they themselves have determined.

Much of the discussion surrounding health education has focused on ill health or its prevention. However, Rakusen (1990) considers that health education incorporates emotional education. This removes it from the arena of sickness and makes it potentially available to anyone, regardless of how the person defines him or herself. Emotional education, in the widest context, enables mental health to be considered as a continuum that allows each individual to intervene to develop ways of dealing with his or her emotions. This concept of health education in mental health suggests that everyone has a right to emotional education, just as everyone has a right to intellectual education, and in the final analysis enables mental health education to be seen as developing 'mental fitness, just as most health education can be seen as developing physical fitness (Rakusen, 1990).

Health education and health promotion are often considered to be one and the same thing. However, it is evident from this discussion that health education is only part, albeit a significant one, of health promotion. It is offered predominantly at two levels. First, on an individual one that focuses on different approaches to preventing ill health and empowering the individual to choose and determine the type of lifestyle required. Secondly, health education is approached from a wider perspective that attempts to tackle the causes of health and disease at a societal level.

VALUES IN HEALTH PROMOTION

It is not possible to examine health promotion in any depth without considering the influence that values have on the implementation of a programme. Health promotion, in its simplest form, is about preventing the onset of disease and illness and providing support for those conditions that are chronic or long term, while helping individuals to achieve their highest functional level and promoting the concept of health. All of these activities provoke different responses in people and therefore some form of controversy is bound to arise. Controversy derives from the different values people place on various aspects of health and health promotion (see Box 12.3 for the range of factors which impact upon health promotion).

Burnard and Chapman (1988) state that holding values, or valuing something, is concerned with prizing one's own beliefs. Values are concerned with choosing one's beliefs and then acting upon them. Most values are based on the individual's previous experience and personal beliefs and the beliefs of his or her cultural background, and these values allow the individual to perform, or refuse to perform, certain actions. However, this is not always done at a conscious level and many individuals are unaware of their own value system. This may often be reflected in an individual not knowing how to make decisions or how to act in given situations.

O'Keefe (1995) states simplistically that values in health promotion are expressed in terms of how people should and should not act in given circumstances. This explanation, however, does not recognize the complexity of values and their relationship to the individual.

Downie *et al.* (1990) offer a more encompassing view of values and distinguish between liking values and moral values. Liking values can be described as those values the individual holds in preference to others. This suggests that these values are offered in comparison to others; one value is worth more

to the individual than another. An example of this is perhaps the individual who enjoys live music and would therefore value going to a live musical performance rather than watching something on television and would forgo a favourite television programme to attend a live musical performance. Moral values, however, are those which the individual values for their own sake. Downie *et al.* (1990) offer the example of an elderly gentlemen living on his own who forgoes a number of other things to maintain his independence and continue to live alone. This value cannot be compared with any others as there is no demonstrable gain, purely the gentleman's independence.

Health promotion programmes are clearly linked with changing the attitudes and behaviour of individuals, attempting to alter behaviour so that it minimizes the risk of ill health or further damaging health in chronic conditions. Downie *et al.* (1990) believe that attitudes and values are closely linked. They suggest that attitudes are constructed from cognitive, affective and conative components and as such reflect the major components of values; these are beliefs, feelings and behaviour. Values, therefore, can be said to be more than how people should or should not act. Both moral and liking values identify preferences, which express and affect attitudes.

Society itself can be said to hold a number of values. However, different societies hold different values and even within one society smaller groups often hold values that are not necessarily reflective of the whole society. For any society to continue to function and develop there must be some values that are widely held, those held by the majority. These are known as consensus values and reflect, in general, the society from which they come. It is not possible to state categorically that all members of the society will hold these values, but the majority of the population will. These values are also dynamic in that they are adapted and modified in relation to changing circumstances of the society; they are sometimes reflected by being part of the society's legal system.

However, consensus values are not the only ones that affect the individual's beliefs, behaviour and feelings. For a person to maintain a sense of individuality, personal values, as discussed above, combine with consensus values to form the individual's overall values. Personal values provide the individual with a sense of personal development and forward movement.

Downie *et al.* (1990) believe that this combination of values is essential for individuals to flourish. The values are a reflection of the individual's physical and psychological beliefs about human beings and the limits placed upon them in the process of living.

Within health promotion it is essential to recognize the important influence that an individual's values has upon the holder. When working with a group or individual, the development of any health promotional activity must acknowledge the values of that group or individual to ensure that the activity is understood and is relevant. Without this acknowledgement, the activity will have little significance and be of no value in altering lifestyle.

One of the difficulties working with culturally based values is that it is not appropriate to identify values held by an

---

Box 12.3

Values affecting health promotion

1. Personal experiences
2. Personal beliefs
3. Cultural background
4. Ability to make decisions based on information
5. Unconscious influences

individual as right or wrong, or better or worse than anybody else's. In health promotion it is essential that the individual's values are recognized and accepted, as condemning another's values will immediately inhibit the relationship between health promoter and client. Values are frequently demonstrated in the way people behave but, perhaps more importantly, can be reflected in the way things are said. When promoting health with anyone, values are arguably one of the most important things to consider. Without careful consideration, regardless of effort, health promotion will not occur.

MODELS OF HEALTH PROMOTION

We have already established that the term 'health promotion' is best defined within the area that it is used and that the definition should represent the issues associated with health promotional goals and target populations, as well as with the type and focus of the interventions (Rootman, 1985). To this extent, it is not possible to identify models of health promotion that consider mental health alone. The models of health promotion explored below must be adapted to the client population, to the type of interventions the health promoter is employing and to the goals one is aiming for.

THE HEALTH BELIEFS MODEL

The Health Beliefs model of health promotion has established itself as a framework that attempts to explain and predict behaviours related to health. The model was originally designed to predict preventive behaviours, those behaviours that are actively encouraged to prevent the onset or further exacerbation of illness, but it has also been used to predict the behaviour of both the chronically and acutely ill (Bunton and Macdonald, 1992).

The model attempts to account for the individual's readiness to take an active role in changing behaviour in relation to aspects of health. However, although this appears to be a simple approach, a number of factors need to be considered for any movement towards identified goals. The earlier exploration of definitions of health plays an important part in this model. For this approach to be successful it is essential for the individual to place some value on their health in comparison to other aspects of their life. For example, if individuals are keen on sports the use of tobacco may reduce their ability to participate. They would therefore place a value on that aspect of their health and be more encouraged to change their behaviour in terms of tobacco usage. However, if individuals were experiencing a severe depressive illness they may not consider their health, or the ability to participate in sports activities, to be of any value and such an approach to change their health-related behaviours would not be of particular value.

Other issues that need to be considered when using this model are the individual's susceptibility to the illness and how serious the possible health problem is perceived by the individual to be. It is necessary also to assess the extent to which

the individual considers possible consequences of the health problem to be detrimental to their lifestyle and whether the effort in changing behaviour, to minimize the risk from a potential health problem, is worth the disruption to the current lifestyle. The extent to which the individual believes in the diagnosis and possible treatment of the health problem is particularly relevant when working with someone who has mental health problems. This can be especially difficult when working with individuals who have psychotic type illness or who have feelings of worthlessness. They may consider that the health problem is insignificant or that they are not worthy of the input necessary to change their behaviour.

For this model of health promotion to be effective it is essential that the approach taken is always from the client's point of view. The foundations of this model are the beliefs held by the individual. Pike and Forster (1995) believe that cues to action are useful tools to help motivate or maintain the individual's behavioural change. They suggest that health warnings on tobacco products or displays of fat content on food products can be of particular benefit.

TANNAHILL'S MODEL OF HEALTH PROMOTION

Tannahill (1985) proposes a model of health promotion that he believes enables the health professional to define, plan and actually promote health. In this model three spheres of activity are identified: health education, health protection and prevention. These spheres of activity overlap and thereby produce what Tannahill calls the seven domains, which he suggests are all integral to health promotion. These are:

1. Preventive Services: This domain considers the prevention of illness. Activities included in this domain are immunization programmes, screening for congenital disorders, cervical screening and developmental surveillance.

2. Preventive Health Education: Within this domain efforts are made through education to influence the lifestyles of individuals to prevent ill health. Individuals are encouraged to use available preventive services. An essential element in this domain is to ensure that adequate communication channels are available so that the individual knows that appropriate preventive services are both provided and accessible.

3. Preventive Health Protection: This domain functions on a macro level and considers legal controls. It focuses on ensuring that laws, regulations and policies are in place to prevent ill health and promote good health. Areas that would be included are the fluoridation of water supplies and driving and waste disposal laws.

4. Health Education for Preventive Health Protection: The social environment is the main focus of this domain. Efforts are made to stimulate the social environment to ensure that it can support preventive health protection methods and guarantee their success. Such efforts would consider the relationship between poverty and unemployment and poor mental health (Banks and Jackson, 1982), ensuring that it was recognized and that the issues were

taken into account when developing national policy.

5. Positive Health Education: In this domain health education is aimed at influencing behaviour on positive health grounds, for example, the use of leisure time directed towards the achievement of fitness and well-being. Positive health education also encompasses working with groups and communities to develop positive health attributes. These attributes, such as a high level of self-esteem, Tannahill (1985) believes to be central to the enhancement of true well-being.

6. Positive Health Protection: This domain, again, moves away from the individual and focuses on such things as the introduction of a smoking policy within the workplace to facilitate the provision of clean air for the majority of employees. It works too at a macro level by encouraging the commitment of public funds to schemes such as the provision of accessible leisure facilities.

7. Health Education Aimed at Positive Health Protection: Within this domain efforts are made to raise awareness and ensure support is obtained to exert influence on policy - makers. This ensures that positive health protection measures are considered when new policies are being developed.

This model of health promotion clearly demonstrates the wide range of activities that can be incorporated into health promotion. Although the model identifies seven domains, each domain should not be seen in isolation. It is a model that encourages the incorporation of aspects of one domain into another. An activity in a single domain cannot be undertaken in a rigid fashion or without considering how others may impact on the way in which it is implemented.

Tannahill (1985) suggests that the major principle of the model is empowerment. It is not of great significance whether the approach is for an individual, a group or a community. What is of importance is that the individual or individuals are in control of how health promotional activities move forward and that the activities can be adapted to be more relevant to them. External forces outside their influence must not dictate how the individual relates to health promotion.

SETTINGS APPROACHES TO HEALTH PROMOTION

Health promotion and health education both address health problems caused by, or dependent upon, the interaction between external and personal factors. These factors influence the pathways of health and disease (Baric, 1990). Baric suggests that, to accommodate these factors, there is a need for a multisectoral intervention within the framework of health promotion and this must incorporate participation of the community in primary care (see Figure 12.2).

Health promotion can be considered in terms of healthy cities, healthy communities and healthy enterprises. Each of these can be viewed as a community in its own right. To develop an effective health promotion programme, the community must base the concepts of such a programme on self-reliance and self-determination. The health activities in the programme are expected to be incorporated into the everyday life of the community and not seen as 'special' activities. These health activities are geared towards dealing with the community's problems and represent a support system for the community endeavouring to improve its own health and management of disease.

In this approach to health promotion much of the work is done by the defined community. The roles of community members, who do the work, are also clearly defined. Outside help may be requested, but help that is mainly focused on raising the competence of community members to deal with their own problems.

This approach to health promotion is characterized by two types of activity: external and community forces.

External forces: this area functions predominantly at a regional or local level. An appropriate agency develops a movement popularizing the concept of a healthy city, community or enterprise, using the help of mass media and the support of political representatives. These methods are used to create and popularize training facilities and workshops for community members. At these locations they acquire the skills necessary to carry out health promotion programmes in their community. The content of this training is based in the health promotion framework and includes such matters as dealing with different community problems, one of which is health.

Community forces: this area focuses on the shift of activities from the centre to the identified community. First and foremost it is essential that the community makes a commitment to being 'healthy'. A multisectoral approach is used to assess the community resource and identify the needs of its population. These needs are then translated into a plan of action that is directed to achieving specific solutions to identified problems. The plan, which is developed in terms of interventions, consists of both short- and long-term aims and objectives that form the basis for evaluating the programme. In this approach evaluation is considered as part of the intervention and feedback mechanisms are included as part of the programme so that adjustments can be made once the programme is running.

This type of settings approach has been used to establish health promotion programmes in cities, schools and hospitals. Healthy Sheffield (Halliday and Adams, 1992) is a good example of such an approach, which considered the health challenges presented to the population of the city, and, using the Health For All targets (WHO, 1985), identified seven guiding principles that were used to establish seven key objectives to meet the overall aim of a healthy Sheffield.

SUMMARY

This chapter has broadly considered the subject of health promotion and tried to identify the literature that covers the multiplicity of factors contributing to the subject. Health promotion is developing into an activity of great importance, both at a national and local level. It has been clearly shown that health promotion is an essential part of modern day health care delivery. To date much of the activity has been based on existing data, adapting them to meet the perceived need of the local population or individual. However, with the launch of *The Health of the Nation* (Department of Health, 1992) there has been an increase in emphasis on health promotion. The specific targets within it show the need to establish new data that directly reflect the needs of the population. As has been suggested, health promotion is more effective when directed towards the needs of the local population. It is essential, therefore, that there is a move towards developing more meaningful local profiles that can demonstrate trends in both health and illness.

Mental health promotion is difficult to explore from the literature alone. Mental health only begins to raise its profile and become significant when the individual becomes mentally ill. This, however, defeats the overall aim of mental health promotion, which needs to be directed towards the population in general. As Rakusen (1990) suggests, everyone is entitled to emotional education and therefore to limit the activities of mental health promotion to only a few specialists will prove ineffective and will result in mental health promotion being directed only towards the mentally ill. Mental health promotion is not about developing specific programmes for the mentally ill but more about ensuring that the promotion of mental health is incorporated into the everyday activities of those involved in health care.

To separate mental health promotion from health promotion in general also proves difficult. When considering physical health, it is not possible to completely divorce it from mental health. Likewise, mental health cannot be separated entirely from physical health. It would therefore appear impractical to attempt to separate the two when developing ways of promoting health (Childs, 1995). As an example of this, if someone needs a special diet and if their finances are such that they can ill afford this, it is likely that they will become anxious about the situation. Therefore, to focus purely on the physical issues of taking the recommended diet ignores both the psychological issues of anxiety and the sociological issues of inadequate income to support the necessary lifestyle.

The development of health promotion has implications for nurses. Fundamentally, nurses need to consider whether or not their views and philosophies about health and health care are broad enough to integrate health promotion into their nursing care. Traditionally nurses have, on the whole, considered nursing to be about caring for the sick. Moreover, health education and health promotion have been considered the remit of the health visitor alone (Macleod–Clark, 1993).

Macleod–Clark (1993) suggests that attempts to incorporate a health perspective into practice have been seen as 'add ons' and not integral to practice. The health model of nursing focuses on patients being involved in decisions about, and actively participating in, their care. It enhances individuals' knowledge, enables them to become more autonomous and empowers them to take responsibility for their own health (Macleod–Clark, 1993). This is a significant shift in the way nurses practice but it is essential for the effective inclusion of health promotion in care provision.

KEY CONCEPTS

- Definitions of health, both physical and mental, must consider the social, economic, environmental, political, psychological and spiritual aspects of the individual.
- Health promotion is not only central but integral to contemporary nursing practice.
- Ideally, health should be seen from a holistic point of view. To separate mental health from physical or social health raises artificial divisions.
- Health education is only one component of health education. The two terms should not be used interchangeably.
- Health promotion is more effective when directed towards the needs of the local population.
- Nurses must consider whether their views and philosophies about health and health care are broad enough to allow them to integrate health promotion into their nursing care.

REFERENCES

Banks MH, Jackson PR: Unemployment and the risk of minor psychiatric disorder in young people: cross-sectional and longitudinal evidence. *Psychol Med* 12(7):789–798, 1982.

Baric L: A new approach to community participation. *J Inst Health Educ* 28(2):41–52, 1990.

Brooker C: Evaluating the impact of training community psychiatric nurses to educate relatives about schizophrenia: implications for health promotion at a secondary level. In: Wilson–Barnett J, Macleod Clark J, editors: *Research in health promotion and nursing*. Basingstoke, 1993, Macmillan.

Bunton R, Macdonald G: *Health promotion, disciplines and diversity*. London, 1992, Routledge.

Bunton R, Nettleton S, Burrows R: *The sociology of health promotion–critical analyses of consumption, lifestyle and risk*. London, 1995, Routledge.

Burnard P, Chapman C: *Professional and ethical issues in nursing, the code of professional conduct*. Chichester, 1988, John Wiley.

Bush MT, Ullom JA, Osborne OH: The meaning of mental health: a report of two ethnoscientific studies. *Nurs Res* 24(2):130–138, 1975.

Childs A: Perceptions of mental health promotion: a study of community psychiatric nurses. In: Trent D, Reed C, editors: *Promotion of mental health*, Vol 4. Aldershot, 1995, Avebury.

Clarke R, Lowe F: Positive health — some key perspectives. *Health Promot* 3(2):401–406, 1989.

Delaney F: Nursing and health promotion: conceptual concerns. *J Adv Nurs* 20(5):828–835, 1994.

Department of Health: *Caring in the community*. London, 1990, HMSO.

Department of Health: *The health of the nation–A strategy for health in England*. London, 1992, HMSO.

Dines A, Crabb A, editors: Health promotion: concepts and practice. Oxford, 1993, Blackwell Scientific Publications.

Donati P: The need for new social policy perspectives in health behaviour research. In: Anderson R, Davis J, Kickbusch D, *et al.*, editors: *Health behaviour research and health promotion*. Oxford, 1988, Oxford University Press.

Downie RS: Ethics in health education: an introduction. In: Doxiadis S, editor: *Ethics in health education*. Chichester, 1990, Wiley.

Downie RS, Fyfe C, Tannahill A: *Health promotion: models and values*. Oxford, 1990, Oxford Medical Publications.

Draper P: Nancy Milio's work and its importance for the development of health promotion. *Health Promotion* 1(1):101–106, 1986.

Dubos R: *Mirage and health*. London, 1960, Allen & Unwin.

Evans JA: Model of mental health. *Nurs Times* 88(16):55–56, 1992.

Farrell E: *The mental health survival guide*. London, 1991, MacDonald Optima.

Forster D: Promoting health. In: Kenworthy N, Snowley G, Gilling C, editors: *Common foundation studies in nursing*. Edinburgh, 1992, Churchill Livingstone.

French J: Boundaries and horizons, the role of health education within health promotion. *Health Educ J* 49(1):7–10, 1990.

Green LW, Raeburn JM: What is it? What will it become? *Health Promot* 3(2):151–159, 1988.

Halliday M, Adams L: Healthy Sheffield: the consultation experiment. *Health Educ J* 51(1):43–46, 1992.

Hancock D, Hancock B: Mastery of the environment. *Elder Care* 5(6):22–23, 1993.

Kjervik DK, Palta M: Sex-role stereotyping in assessments of mental health made by psychiatric–mental health nurses. *Nurs Res* 27(3):166–171, 1978.

Maben J, Macleod-Clark J: Health promotion: a concept analysis. *J Adv Nurs* 22(10):1158–1165, 1995.

Macleod–Clark J: From sick nursing to health nursing. In: Wilson–Barnett J, Macleod–Clark J, editors: *Research in health promotion and nursing*. Basingstoke, 1993, Macmillan.

O'Keefe E: Values and ethical issues. In: Pike S, Forster D, editors: *Health promotion for all*. Edinburgh, 1995, Churchill Livingstone.

Pike S, Forster D: *Health promotion for all*. Edinburgh, 1995, Churchill Livingstone.

Rakusen J: Emotional education. *Openmind* 46(4):10–11, 1990.

Rootman I: Using health promotion to reduce alcohol problems. In: Grant M, editor: *Alcohol policies*. Copenhagen, 1985, World Health Organization.

Saan H: Health promotion and health education, living with a dominant concept. *Health Promot* 1(3):253–255, 1986.

Sim J: The concept of health. *Physiotherapy* 76(7):423–428, 1990.

Smith A, Jacobson B: *The nation's health: a strategy for the 1990s*. London, 1988, King Edward's Hospital Fund.

Speller V: Defining health promotion service implications. *Health Educ J* 44(2):34–35, 1985.

Stark W: The politics of primary prevention in mental health: the need for a theoretical basis. *Health Promot* 1(2):179–185, 1986.

Tannahill A: What is health promotion? *Health Educ J* 44(4):167–168, 1985.

Tones BK: Health education: prevention or subversion? *R Soc Health J* 101 (3):114–115, 1981.

Tones BK: Health education and health promotion: new directions. *J Inst Health Educ* 23(4):37–40, 1983.

Tones K, Tilford S: *Health education: effectiveness, efficiency and equity*, 2 ed. London, 1994, Chapman & Hall.

Welch MJ, Boyd MA, Bell D: Education in primary prevention in psychiatric-mental health nursing for baccalaureate students. *Inter Nurs Rev* 34(5):126–130, 1987.

World Health Organization: *Constitution*. Geneva, 1946, World Health Organization.

World Health Organization: *Report of the working party on concepts and principles of health promotion*. Copenhagen, 1984, World Health Organization.

World Health Organization: *Targets for health for all: Targets in support of European regional strategy for health for all by the year 2000*. Copenhagen, 1985, World Health Organization.

World Health Organization: *Ottawa charter for health promotion*. *Health Promot* 1(4):iii–iv, 1986.

FURTHER READING

Beck E, Lonsdale S, Newman S, Patterson D: *In the best of health: the status and future of health care in the UK*. London, 1992, Chapman & Hall.
> The Government seems convinced that shifting the balance of the NHS in favour of disease prevention and health promotion will improve the nation's health. This book addresses how health care systems have to adapt to such changes and examines the wider financial implications and professional issues.

Doyal L: *The political economy of health*. London, 1981, Pluto Press.
> This classic text demonstrates that ill health in both developed and under developed countries is largely a product of the social and economic organization of society. The role of health promotion is therefore significant.

Thornicroft G, Brewin C R, Wing J: *Measuring mental health needs*. London, 1992, Gaskell.
> This book describes the different approaches that can be taken to identify the mental health needs of individuals and of the population and how mental health needs can be measured.

Trent DR, editor: Promotion of mental health, Vol 1. Aldershot, 1992, Avebury.
> This book presents 34 contributions from the first national conference on mental health promotion in the UK.

Wilson–Barnett J, Macleod–Clark J: Research in health promotion and nursing. Basingstoke, 1993, Macmillan.
> This book demonstrates the importance of research in this vital area and its relationship to nursing practice. As such it seeks to develop and enhance the health-promotion role of all nurses.

Crisis Theory and Intervention

Learning Outcomes

After studying this chapter you should be able to:

- Define crisis.

- Discuss the development of crisis theory.

- State what occurs in a crisis.

- Describe the phases of a crisis.

- Discuss the three types of crisis.

- Describe the factors that influence the outcome of crisis.

- Define crisis intervention, and give its aims and general principles.

- Describe four types of crisis intervention.

- Apply the nursing process to crisis intervention.

A crisis occurs when an individual's customary coping mechanisms are inadequate to deal with a perceived threat. Disequilibrium can occur, during which time the individual must find some new way of coping; failure to do so will result in the development of a chronic maladaptive state. Crisis theory provides a framework for preventive, supportive and therapeutic intervention with the individual at risk and his or her family. It is a systematic process of problem resolution and has been found to reduce greatly the incidence and severity of mental illness.

A crisis can occur for anyone and any references here to gender in specific terms are not of significance but are intended as generic references only. The individual involved in crisis intervention is also referred to as a client, unless reference is specifically made to other studies.

Crisis is determined from the Greek words for 'decision' or 'turning point'. The Chinese ideogram or character for crisis is interpreted both as a *danger* and as an *opportunity*. In times of crisis an individual is uncertain what to do. The usual homoeostatic, direct problem solving mechanisms do not work or are not currently possible. The anxiety and distress that is experienced enables the client to try new and different ways of solving problems. Within this willingness to try new methods lies the opportunity for growth and resolution. Crisis intervention is designed to help with the immediate effects of a stressful event on a person.

DEVELOPMENT OF CRISIS THEORY

Historically, crisis theory is derived from psychoanalytical theory, which proposes that there are unconscious links to behaviour arising from present threats and those of the past.

Crisis theory's emphasis on an individual's coping mechanism has a direct parallel in ego psychology, which emphasizes the adaptive function of the ego. The origins of crisis theory lie in Lindemann's (1944) classic study of grief reactions, which followed his intensive work with ulcerative colitis patients.

Lindemann reported on the evaluation and treatment of 101 persons, all of whom had experienced the death of a close relative. A large number were victims or close relatives of victims from the fire at Coconut Grove, Boston, in 1942, which claimed the lives of 491 people. Lindemann observed that acute grief was 'a normal reaction to a distressing situation' and that such reaction presented a commonality of experience. Lindemann suggested that normal grief reactions were generally acute, had a definable onset and lasted for a relatively brief period. They followed a pattern of identifiable stages and were not ordinarily pathological although they might appear so. Finally, Lindemann believed that the likelihood of psychopathological sequelae could be minimized by timely intervention.

Lindemann's colleague, Gerald Caplan, developed the theory of crisis. As described by Caplan (1964):

> A crisis is provoked when a person faces an obstacle to important goals that is, for a time, insurmountable through the utilisation of customary methods of problem-solving. A period of disorganisation ensues, a period of upset, during which many different abortive attempts at solution are made. Eventually some kind of adaptation is achieved, which may or may not be in the best interests of that person and his fellows.

Caplan's crisis theory is based on the concept of emotional homoeostasis: all people are constantly faced with 'hazards' that are usually surmountable. Occasionally, the hazards will be too large or the individual particularly susceptible and crisis will occur. This presents opportunities for the internal boundary realignment that is potentially constructive, especially if the individual is aware, from past experience, that mastery is forthcoming.

Once mastery of the distressing situation has occurred, through use of habitual methods, the individual is said to have successfully 'coped with the problem'. Occasionally the problem is so severe that it cannot be mastered by the usual methods and it is then that the individual is entering 'crisis', says Caplan.

Others have expanded and modified Caplan's crisis model. Klein and Lindemann (1961) stated that crisis does not occur in a social vacuum and that an individual's crisis is often reflective of what is occurring in his or her social group. This was expanded upon in the work of Parad and Caplan (1960), in which it was noted that families can equally experience crisis.

Rapoport (1962) viewed crisis as not only a response to a current threat but one that might be partially rooted in previously threatening situations. Furthermore, she felt these situations were potentially likely to 'reactivate unresolved or partially resolved unconscious conflicts'.

Crisis theory was identified at a time of increased social awareness in America. In 1963 President Kennedy passionately addressed the Congress and the Nation on the need for a national health program with new approaches to mental health. Congress appointed a Joint Commission on Mental Illness and Health, which funded a nationwide network of centres whose emphasis was the prevention of emotional disorders.

WHAT OCCURS IN A CRISIS

In a crisis there is heightened confusion and anxiety but also greater susceptibility to suggestion and desire for help.

If an individual's existing repertoire is not sufficient they will try all manner of new methods and eventually may find some coping method. They will adapt to the situation and return to the previous state of mental health, having developed increased constructive coping methods. This is why a crisis does not usually last for longer than 4 to 6 weeks. Conversely, if maladaptive coping mechanisms are developed the individual will reach a lower level of functioning, resulting in the decreased possibility of resolving future crises successfully.

Crisis is any transient situation that requires the individual to reorganize his or her psychological structure and behaviour.

PHASES OF A CRISIS

1. Initial impact or shock phase lasting a few hours to a few days with an increase in anxiety.
2. Defensive retreat.
   The individual tries previously successful ways of problem solving and adjusting. If these coping mechanisms are successful, they will resolve the crisis. However, if they are unsuccessful then.
3. Recoil and adjustment will occur when the increase in anxiety produces a 'reaching out' for assistance.
4. Resolution or adaptation and change.

If the individual is unable to find new methods of coping or is emotionally isolated, then it is usually impossible to prevent a major crisis. This is typified by exhaustion, digestive symptoms, a sense of unreality and distance from others, feelings of guilt, irritability and anger and rumination over how the event could have been avoided. The individual's behaviour becomes increasingly impulsive and unproductive. He or she may have a feeling 'going crazy' and relationships may suffer.

According to Burgess and Baldwin (1982), the characteristics of an individual in crisis are:

1. Decreased ability to maintain perspective because of parallel changes in emotional and cognitive states.
2. Decreased ability to mobilize resources, because of confusion, with the result that alternative solutions cannot be conceived or evaluated.
3. Decreased ability to solve problems.

If the crisis is only partially resolved it tends to return. Earlier crises may affect the character of later ones. This can occur in two ways: either the crisis effect is addictive, with the result that later ones are more intense or there can be growing desensitization and less intensive crisis reaction.

TYPES OF CRISIS

Crisis can be divided into three types: Developmental, Situational and Traumatic. Occasionally more than one type of crisis can occur at the same time.

DEVELOPMENTAL CRISES (MATURATIONAL)

Developmental crises occur at transition points, the periods that everyone experiences in the process of biopsychological growth and development. They are accompanied by changes in thought, feelings and abilities. Erikson (1963, 1968) identified specific periods in normal development when a developmental crisis could occur, precipitated by a rise in anxiety. Such events as birth, starting school, puberty, moving away from home, marriage, ageing and retirement fall into this category.

As each stage of development is dependent on the mastery of the previous one, unsuccessful mastery of one stage is likely to affect subsequent ones. Some conflicts related to role change are found in Case study: Developmental crisis.

SITUATIONAL CRISES

These are external traumatic events or situations that are outside the normal pattern of living. They are often sudden, unexpected and uncomfortable. Situational crises often follow on from the loss of an established support; the most usual response to such loss is depression. These crises can develop from the loss of a role and consequently alter the individual's perception of self. Examples are redundancy, bereavement, illness or divorce. Some of the stresses related to redundancy are shown in Case study: Situational crisis.

TRAUMATIC CRISES (ADVENTITIOUS)

These are crises that are accidental, rare and unexpected. They call upon coping methods not required previously. Traumatic crises can expose individuals to life threatening situations, e.g. earthquakes, fires, accidents, terrorist action and rape.

There are two broad categories of victim level in such crises. Primary victims directly experience physical, material and personal losses from the traumatic event (Bolin, 1982). Secondary victims witness trauma and suffer vicariously. They may have friends or family killed in a disaster but not feel themselves eligible for help because they are not true victims. Case study: Traumatic crisis, outlines some of these features.

FACTORS INFLUENCING THE OUTCOME OF A STRESSFUL EVENT

1. The person's perception of the event.
2. The physical and emotional status of the person.
3. The coping techniques or mechanisms and the level of maturity.
4. Previous experience with similar situations.

Case study: Developmental crisis

Mrs G was a 31-year-old woman who attended a mental health clinic 6 months after the birth of her first child. She reported symptoms of anxiety, difficulty in sleeping, poor concentration and excessive worry about her daughter. Mrs G had returned to work a month previously and her daughter was being looked after by a local childminder. Mrs G and her husband had planned her return to work during her pregnancy, as they required her income and Mr G was happy with the situation.

Mrs G felt that she was able neither to concentrate on her work nor to look after her daughter adequately and this was reinforced by comments from Mrs G's mother who felt it was negligent for a small child to be away from its mother.

Mrs G had tried to discuss the subject with her husband, who failed to understand why she had 'changed her mind about returning to work' and only praised the competence of the childminder.

In summary, here was a young mother struggling with her change in role, feeling unsupported by her family and having to meet the dependency needs of an infant and be a wage earner. This precipitated a crisis for her.

Case study: Situational crisis

Mr D was a 52-year-old married man with two teenage children. He had worked for the same firm as Supplies Manager for 16 years when the company made him redundant.

After breaking the news to his wife, he refused to discuss it with anyone else. Each day he would leave the house at the time he had usually set off for work, dressed in a suit, sit in the public library all day and return home at his usual time.

This continued daily for 3 weeks until his wife persuaded him to attend his family doctor's surgery.

Mr D was able to express for the first time that he felt overwhelming guilt and viewed himself as a failure to his family and did not want anyone else to know about his redundancy, especially his children who were currently taking examinations.

Case study: Traumatic crisis

Ms W was brought to an Accident and Emergency Department by a friend who had visited her unexpectedly that evening. When the friend arrived at Ms W's flat the front door was found battered with the lock was hanging off. Ms W was sitting calmly in a chair and refused to say what had happened. Her friend believed that Ms W had been attacked and after reporting the break-in to the police, drove her friend to hospital.

On arrival Ms W remained calm and continued to deny that anything had happened. When the casualty staff attempted to take her pulse and blood pressure Ms W became distressed, agitated and started screaming and cowering in a corner. A female doctor was called, who had considerable experience with victims of assault. Ms W confided in her that she had been raped by the intruder but had been too embarrassed and humiliated to admit this.

A rape crisis centre was contacted, which gave information about police and legal procedures and offered counselling to Ms W.

5. The objectively realistic aspects of the situation.
6. Cultural aspects.
7. The availability of family and friends to help and their response.

At each phase, previous experience moulds what occurs but does not completely determine it. Every crisis outcome is determined by choices, which are made partly actively and partly by chance, and by other aspects of the situation. These include:

- The bodily state of the individual at the time, the purely chance aspects of the development of the external stress and the availability of external social resources and the communication system, as well as the personality of the individual.

Among personal factors the following should be assessed:

- Does the present situation link symbolically to any similar problems of the past and if so how adequately were they resolved?
- What previous experiences have had an impact on the present problematic situation?

Aguilera and Messick (1990) devised a paradigm which sets out the difference in outcome of a stressful event, depending on the presence or absence of balancing factors (Figure 13.1).

CRISIS INTERVENTION

Crisis intervention is a model for the treatment of acute states of psychological decompensation, including some formal psychiatric disorders. In addition to crisis resolution the intervention maximizes the related potential for psychic growth and maturation, and so represents an important tool in preventative psychiatry.

(Hobbs 1984)

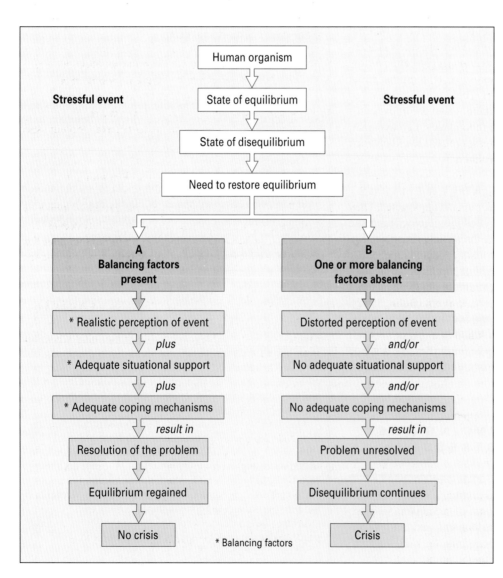

Figure 13.1 Paradigm: the effect of balancing factors in a stressful event (reproduced courtesy of Aguilera DC: *Crisis intervention: theory and methodology*, 7 ed. St Louis, 1994, Mosby-Year Book Inc.)

AIMS OF CRISIS INTERVENTION

1. To relieve present distress, notably anxiety, confusion and hopelessness.
2. To restore the individual's previous functional capacity.
3. To help the individual, the family and significant others learn what personal actions are possible and what resources exist.
4. To understand the relationship of the present crisis with past experiences and persistent psychological problems.
5. To develop new attitudes, behaviours and coping techniques.
6. To emphasize the healthy aspects of an individual's personality, strengths, potentials and ability to solve problems.

Crisis intervention is based on the theory that aid during a crisis will help the person to adapt in a healthy manner. The immediate aim is a resolution of the crisis and a return to a state of equilibrium. A minimum aim is to restore the person to the level of competence prior to the crisis. In the disequilibrium of crisis periods it has been found that minimal intervention produces maximal lasting benefit. Individuals are more susceptible to influence at these times.

The role of the intervenor is active participation with the individual. Together they collaborate to resolve the crisis. The intervenor enables the individual to resolve the problem him- or herself, thus promoting opportunities for growth.

FACTORS INFLUENCING THE OUTCOME OF CRISIS INTERVENTION

1. Attitude of therapist and value placed on crisis work.
2. Use of time in that assessment is done as quickly as possible.
3. Use of non-traditional practices for such matters as appointment times and location of service.
4. Similarities between the value systems of therapist and the individual. The therapist must be open to what constitutes a problem for the individual.

GENERAL PRINCIPLES

Ewing (1978) clarified the commonalities of crisis intervention and regarded the following as general principles.

Crisis Intervention is Accessible and Brief

Caplan believed that crises are self-limiting and last no longer than 6 weeks, regardless of adaptive resolution. With this in mind crisis intervention, if it is to be effective, needs to be readily and rapidly available (Chowdhury *et al.,* 1973; Johnson and Thornicroft, 1991).

The provision of acceptable and effective crisis intervention is regarded by service users (Rogers *et al.,* 1993) and GPs (Strathdee, 1990) as crucial. Box 13.1 summarizes some of the important elements of a crisis service. Parad and Parad (1968) concluded that 'in the midst of crisis having to wait for help the crisis may subside with some crippling and sometimes tragic results. A little bit of help at the right time may be more effective than a long period of help after the crisis has subsided'.

Crisis Intervention is Offered to the Individual, the Family and Social Network

The family is important to the mental health requirements of its members because it satisfies their needs and in a crisis situation it supports the individual. Crises are rarely experienced by the individual alone but have effects on family and social networks.

Crisis Intervention Addresses Itself to Any Form of Crisis

While clinicians may argue what constitutes a crisis, it would appear to be more helpful that the client defines what situations are crises. In recent years the general public have begun to demand urgent help at times of emotional distress.

Crisis Intervention is Focused on the Client's Present Problem

In crisis intervention the therapist helps the individual analyse the stressful event and assists in resolving the immediate problem. Crises often 'stir up' issues from the past that have not been resolved. These however are not dealt with until the crisis is resolved.

Crisis Intervention Aims Both to Resolve Present Crises and to Develop More Adaptive Coping Mechanisms for the Future

Crises offer the potential for constructive growth and resolution of old conflicts.

Crisis Intervention is Reality Orientated

Bancroft (1979) noted that, among the principal types of coping behaviours following a stressful event, denial was prominent. The client distorts reality to the degree that the problem no longer exists. The therapist takes active measures to focus on the realities of the present situation.

In Crisis Intervention Therapists Take Non-Traditional Roles

Therapists have an extended role in helping the client with all aspects of daily living.

Box 13.1 *Elements of a crisis service*

1. Accessible 24 hours a day, 7 days per week.
2. Crisis outreach.
3. Experienced, trained professionals.
4. Community crisis beds.
5. Respite beds.
6. Relapse prevention by psycho-educational interventions.

CRISIS INTERVENTION AND THE NURSING PROCESS

Brammer (1979) describes a logical, problem-solving approach as a framework for effective crisis intervention. The first step involves an appraisal or assessment of the situation. Such an assessment may be based upon the expected behaviour patterns specific to the crisis event. During the next step, the nurse must decide on the type of help that is required. Thus a plan of action is formulated, through utilization of the information gained. The third step is one of action or intervention. In this instance, intervention is based upon the application of skills designed to promote adaptation and regain equilibrium.

Finally, the client is near a state of crisis resolution. At this time the nurse evaluates and reinforces those techniques which have been successfully employed in achieving ego equilibrium. Because of the close similarity of this framework to the nursing process the steps of crisis intervention are described in terms of the nursing process. Psychiatric nurses base their pattern of care on the nursing process, which is a problem-solving approach. It involves collection of data, formulation of needs, planning of interventions and implementation and evaluation of the process.

ASSESSMENT

To make any intervention effective a full assessment of the problem needs to be done. The first question that needs to be addressed is 'Is this individual really in crisis?' Someone may be angry, crying and upset but not overwhelmed and in a state of crisis. The nurse, through talking to the individual, who as we know is susceptible to help at this point, asks the client to describe his or her feelings. This is done in a manner that is non-judgemental and appreciative of the distress the person feels. By the nurse's acceptance of these feelings a rapport is built, which will not only aid future work together but also allows the individual to start to acknowledge that feelings are valid.

As seen in Aguilera and Messick's (1990) paradigm (Figure 13.1) there are balancing effects that are important in the development and resolution of a crisis. A full assessment of these balancing factors needs to be done.

Identify the Precipitants of the Event

There is a need to identify the precipitating events. The nurse should explore what event occurred to threaten the client and what particular needs of the individual were threatened. Knowledge of when the event occurred is necessary together with some time framework of when symptoms appeared. When did he start to feel anxious? When did the client start to find that he or she was unable to make decisions?

Individual's Perception of the Event

This is vital because it forms the cornerstone of intervention. What constitutes a crisis for one person may be unnoticeable for another. Without value judgement or criticism the nurse needs to explore why the individual feels that the event was so disastrous. What basic needs are threatened?

The manner in which a client describes an event can often give clues to precipitating events. The present crisis may be symbolically or actually connected to events in the past. For example a woman talking about abusive events that occurred in childhood may later reveal that she has been raped.

Support Networks

The extent or absence of social support networks must be assessed. Does the individual live alone? Does he or she have close friends? Who could the client talk to openly and feel understood by?

Once a tree of support has been drawn, it can be used for the individual to decide what help and support to request from different people. For the nurse, it also guides what interventions may be necessary, and for whom. When a support network is absent or minimal then other forms of intervention may be indicated. Isolation, estrangement or alienation from others are important social correlates of suicide, as are adverse life events particularly in the form of losses.

Coping Skills

The nurse assesses the strengths and weaknesses of the client's coping skills by questioning. How has he or she handled previous crises, what has worked or failed before and what has been tried since the event occurred? These all need to be described as specifically as possible. Then some degree of assessment can be made on the adaptiveness of these methods. It is also necessary to know the level of effect that has occurred. Is the client still working, able to go out, eating, sleeping, abusing alcohol etc?

PLANNING

The second step of crisis intervention is planning, which is a collaborative problem-centred approach. It involves the active participation of the client, with ownership of the problem being the client's.

Alternative solutions are discussed, with the nurse emphasizing that options are available outside the familiar repertoire of coping methods. The nurse assesses the need for environmental intervention by eliciting the client's view on what coping mechanisms need to be strengthened and which new ones practised. The basic philosophy is to enable the individual to use coping mechanisms with support, education and encouragement from the nurse. While the individual may feel helpless and out of control, with the assistance of the nurse he or she can resolve the chaos.

During the planning phase, goals of intervention are set. These should include:
- Establishment of therapeutic relationship between nurse and client, with clearly defined boundaries.
- Definition of the problem.
- Re-establishment of a realistic interpretation of the event.
- Improved self-esteem.

- Involvement of social support networks and provision of support for them.
- Recognition of healthy coping methods.
- Belief that the client can master the problem.

IMPLEMENTATION

The third phase of crisis intervention is implementation. Implementation may take place at a variety of levels. Jacobson (1979) has described four crisis-orientated therapies:

1. Non-specific crisis treatment.
2. Environmental intervention.
3. Generic crisis-orientated intervention.
4. Individual crisis-orientated treatment.

Non-Specific Crisis Treatment

General support includes nurturing, caring, listening and willingness to help. The nurse's belief in the client's ability to solve problems and potential for growth are powerful reinforcers for mastery of the situation.

Environmental Interventions

Environmental interventions directly change the individual's physical or interpersonal situation. They may include removing the client from a stressful situation, for example suggesting some time off work if he or she is having work-related stresses. A client living alone who experiences the death of a parent may receive comfort from staying with a relative or friend for a period. It may be that a young couple could be relieved of stress in coping with the arrival of a new baby if a grandparent or other relative came to stay and took over looking after the child temporarily.

Generic Crisis-Orientated Intervention

The generic approach is designed to reach high risk groups as quickly as possible. It is designed to reach individuals who have experienced similar types of crisis. Cohen and Ahearn (1980) take account of the emotional reactions to disasters and have designed disaster-specific interventions to assist victims.

The uniform symptomatology of grief reaction is well defined by Lindemann (1979). Proper management of grief reaction can prevent prolonged and serious consequences. Bereavement counselling is regarded as the classic model of this type of crisis intervention.

Individual Crisis-Orientated Treatment

These are interventions designed to meet an individual's specific problem. The nurse must have a good understanding of the client's psychodynamics to interpret what led to the current crisis. While individual focused intervention can be applied to all crises, it is most usually used for developmental crises, crises in which the individual response endangers the client's safety or where generic intervention has been insufficient.

EVALUATION

The final phase of crisis intervention, with the nurse and client jointly evaluating if the problem, has been resolved. Has equilibrium been restored? What techniques worked, which did not and why? To expand the client's potential for future problem solving in crises, appraisal of what took place is needed.

After working through the crisis, some clients may wish to seek therapy for the resolution of old conflicts and the nurse will then refer them to the appropriate service.

WORKING WITH CRISIS

The purpose of crisis intervention is resolution of the immediate crisis and restoration to the previous level of functioning. Burgess and Baldwin (1982) propose three essential qualities for those working with crisis:

1. Active: requires being actively involved, being direct: 'quickly create an optimistic therapeutic ambience while developing a therapeutic alliance in which the client accepts responsibility for change'.
2. Accurate: need to assess the situation quickly, to screen relevant from irrelevant information.
3. Accountable: need to be prepared to put personal therapeutic expertise and skills into practice.

REQUIRED SKILLS

Nurses are often the first health care professionals in contact with the individual in crisis; therefore they are uniquely positioned to intervene in crisis. As has already been mentioned the nurse needs to have a wide range of expert skills available for intervention. (See Chapter 3 for further information on forming a therapeutic relationship.)

Communication

Interpersonal communication is affected by the sensitivity of the participants and consists of both verbal and non-verbal aspects.

The nurse can assist communication by re-arrangement of the environment. Some individuals may find it easier to communicate in their home rather than in a health care setting, that some might find the support from a relative being present helps them to talk.

As communication is a fundamental requirement for intervention, whatever the nurse can do to optimize it should be done.

Listening is the foundation of therapeutic communication and involves energy and concentration. Distractions, such as telephone calls, messages and excessive noise, must be minimized. Maintaining eye contact, being close (not threatening the client) and speaking in a normal, audible tone encourages the client to talk. The nurse conveys objectivity by neither agreeing nor disagreeing at this stage. Listening requires decoding both the content and the feelings expressed in the message. Real listening is difficult. The nurse needs to suspend their judgement, personal thinking and experience. Listening is a sign of respect and re-enforces verbalization by the individual in crisis.

Holistic Care

Individuals in crisis are often behaviourally chaotic and need assistance to undertake some functions of everyday living. The nurse involved in crisis intervention needs to have a wide definition of their role and be prepared to be flexible in what they offer, including practical support if required, e.g. assisting a client with shopping, making arrangements for children to be collected from school.

Team Working

Interdisciplinary interaction is a basic tenet of community health care. Teamwork is an approach both to providing services and determining ways in which members can work together. Communication between members of the team and a collaborative approach to distribution of case load enhances the ability of any team member to offer intervention to individuals in crisis. The ability to work in a team and have open, honest relationships enable nurses to accept support and supervision.

By discussing the individual work they are undertaking, objectivity can be maintained, together with confidence of their ability to offer intervention. Where there is an absence of team working, individual nurses may take unrealistic therapeutic risks, experience excessive stress and blur the boundaries of their relationships with clients. Team discussions and individual supervision enable the details and goals of the intervention to be communicated and, as importantly, the nurse's feelings about the situation to be aired. Feedback and suggestions can give directional guidance and help a reflective approach to practice.

SETTINGS FOR CRISIS WORK

Nurses work in many settings in which they encounter individuals in crisis. Nurses working in obstetric, paediatric, adolescent or geriatric settings are constantly observing developmental crises.

Situational crises are readily observable in general hospitals where death, loss of role or health, and changes in body image have a serious impact on individuals and their families, bringing many to crisis point.

Community health nurses can observe people in their own environments and recognize families or individuals in crisis, e.g. the child who has a new sibling and who refuses to go to school, the elderly man who has been recently mugged becoming withdrawn and refusing to leave the house. Crises can be identified from many sources.

TYPES OF CRISIS INTERVENTION

The form of crisis intervention offered will depend on both the type of crisis and the specific needs of the individual. Some specific forms of crisis intervention have developed in response to commonly encountered crises.

FAMILY WORK

A person seldom lives in total isolation. Usually, when a crisis occurs for an individual, the family and social network are affected. It is not uncommon for parents to be retiring or recovering from bereavement of a spouse at the time their children are struggling with the challenges of parenthood.

When working with families in crisis the nurse needs to determine which members of the family are most affected and why. Who is the scapegoat? Who has symptoms? Who is the identified client? The family is viewed as a system, with each member affecting and being affected by the others. For example, when a child has been caught stealing from the local sweet shop, the crisis is not just the child's but the family's. The nurse is very directive in bringing all members of the family together. Everyone is given the opportunity to verbalize what their analysis of the problem is, what they feel, and say how they are affected.

The available resources and possible solutions are discussed. The nurse assists them in forming a plan of joint action, who is doing what and when. The nurse arranges a follow-up meeting so that they can report back to each other. In some families the intervention may be to help the members to strengthen diffuse boundaries, by fostering the cessation of inappropriate action between generations. In other families the nurse may support the relaxation of overly rigid boundaries by improving communication between members who are isolated.

MARITAL CRISIS INTERVENTION

In some situations, short-term marital crisis intervention is a useful alternative to marriage counselling, especially if long-term commitment to engagement in counselling is doubtful.

SPECIAL CLIENT POPULATIONS

There is growing emphasis on crisis intervention with a number of special client groups such as rape victims, juvenile offenders, drug abusers, families of the critically ill and disaster victims.

CRISIS GROUPS

The goals for group crisis intervention are the same as for individual work. The advantage for some people is that the individual members feel less isolated and often make social contacts. The feeling that one is not alone offers support and encourages more open expression of feelings. The best known example of a group crisis intevention organisation is Alcoholics Anonymous.

PREVENTIVE WORK

Crisis intervention is a major technique of preventive psychiatry. Crises can be avoided by identifying what factors lead to a crisis and offering rapid intervention. Working with high risk groups such as victims of violence, newly diagnosed terminally ill and families of people with AIDS can greatly contribute to their ability to adapt and cope with their stresses.

EDUCATION OF INDIVIDUALS

Educating individuals about the preventive aspects of crisis and early adaptive responses is vital and is often part of the evaluative stage of intervention work.

For all health care professionals involved with clients, there is a role for preventive education, from teaching coping strategies, to information on how to access help. Likewise nurses have a responsibility to themselves and their colleagues in enabling supportive strategies and social networks to be created, which allow them to discharge the stresses inherent in their work. This underpins adaptive responses and ensures an uninterrupted flow of work.

TELEPHONE CONTACT

Crisis intervention is sometimes offered by telephone rather than face to face contact, for example by organizations such as Saneline, Childline and The Samaritans.

The Samaritans answer 2 million calls every year, half a million from first time callers. Their purpose is to 'offer appropriate support. It is being acceptable to those in crisis. It is being easily accessible and it is being available when needed ... every day, every night' (Armson, 1994).

See Boxes 13.2 and 13.3 for examples of crisis intervention services.

Box 13.2 *Examples of crisis intervention services*

The Daily Living Programme

A 3-year, randomized controlled study began at the Maudsley Hospital in October 1987, funded by the Department of Health. Its aim was to compare home based intervention versus standard hospital care for seriously mentally ill patients facing emergency admission. During the trial period the two groups were evaluated on clinical outcome, social functioning, family burden and cost of treatment.

The groups assigned to the Daily Living Programme (DLP) and to standard in-patient care were all from south Southwark, London and 80% were first presentations.

The principles of the DLP were to offer:

a) Continuity of care: patients entering the DLP received treatment and support until the end of the 3-year project.

b) Care coordinated by a Key Worker who also organized local resources.

c) Crisis intervention offered wherever the patient lived.

d) Rehabilitation and skill training as required.

e) Support for relatives and other members of the social network.

f) 24-hour care, 7 days a week.

g) Advocacy for patients as individuals and as a group.

The type and intensity of care were tailored to the individual's needs and offered a comprehensive range of services including financial.

Assertive outreach was implemented for all DLP patients.

Findings

Often DLP patients required a very brief admission at the start of the study, when they continued to be cared for the DLP. They used 20% of hospital bed days compared to the control group.

During the first 20 months, three patients committed suicide (two in the control group) and one was charged with homicide.

The cost of supporting the DLP sample was significantly lower than for hospital based services in both the short and medium term. The DLP did not shift costs to the other agencies, the patient or his or her relatives.

Satisfaction was greaterfor DLP patients, and their relatives, even for those experiencing severe crisis.

DLP patients had a greater degree of social adjustment.

Muigen et al., 1992

East Barnet crisis intervention services

The crisis services in east Barnet have been established for over 20 years and offer many lessons applicable in crisis intervention work as an effective tool in the management and prevention of psychiatric disorders.

They have set up many specific crisis intervention services for distinct client groups, including a crisis approach to schizophrenia.

In the crisis approach to schizophrenia drugs are used at dosages below the threshold for side-effects. This treatment is combined with social interventions that deal with the human problems resulting from this illness.

As crisis theory is mainly concerned with the individual and his social context, the intervention strives to maximize the resources of the individual and family in solving the problems that beset them. While the Barnet services recognize that drugs and hospitalization are an important service, their overall aim is to understand and treat the problem in its personal, family, social and human context.

When an individual becomes mentally ill there is a great deal of shame and guilt. The Barnet team recognize the family's need to be absolved from guilt and blame that is often offered by a medical model of understanding schizophrenia but believe that the family is an integrated part of the problem and that guilt and blame need to be addressed to support the family in their crisis.

cont.

Box 13.2 — *Examples of crisis intervention services (cont)*

The Barnet mode for crisis intervention addresses the family through three levels of analysis:
1. The parental level.
2. The identified client.
3. The sibling level.

Parental level – the age at which schizophrenia is diagnosed in males peaks at 21 years and then declines; for females there is a diagnostic plateau up to the late 30s. These ages often coincide with parents' own crises. Mothers often struggle to give up the role of mothering and find themselves faced with limited or unsatisfying outside contacts. Fathers, too, often experience mid-life crises. Their expectations of life have been unfulfilled, their jobs may be insecure or boring, their marriage unsatisfying and or may feel that they have fewer options than when younger.

In some families the relationship of the parents is a constant battle, in others there is cold avoidance.

The crisis of the child's illness throws these and any other problems into focus and 'blaming each other' often follows.

The identified client – a growth into adulthood involves forming a family context and assuming a work role. When individuals fail to make this transition and remain in a state of arrested development they tend to be called schizophrenic, when they present symptoms. This is an example of developmental crisis. Schizophrenia can be viewed as a means to lay claim to many of the rights of childhood, such as unconditional love and lack of responsibility, while still having many of the freedoms of adulthood. Research has shown that there is an increase in crisis events in the 6 weeks prior to the admission to hospital of individuals with schizophrenia.

The sibling level — siblings can often be placed in the role of the forgotten child, with emotional deprivation and deep resentment. The 'parental child' is one thrown into the role of an adult through family crisis and often has deep seated emotional immaturity. The final role given to siblings can be called the 'shadow child', who carries a secret phobia of madnes; the 'shadow child' scans his or her own children for signs of these and if they occur, feels secretly relieved as the problems can then be faced and dealt with.

The Barnet team have reviewed the management of schizophrenia with these concepts in mind and formulated the following strategies that address the human context of the behaviours:
- Humanize, normalize.
- Open the channels of communication and relatedness.
- Work on family relationships.
- Develop modes of communication.
- Develop modes of relationship.
- Devlop conflict management.
- Work on extra-familial relationships.
- Develop follow-up, support and crisis intervention.

Box 13.3 — *High risk factors for suicide*

- Males.
- Older age group – 45 years plus.
- Divorced, separated or widowed.
- Living alone.
- Socially isolated.
- Unemployed or retired.
- Past psychiatric history, depression, delusions or hallucinations.
- Family history of affective illness.
- Previous suicide attempt.
- Recent event – bereavement, separation, loss of job.
- Poor physical health – chronically or terminally ill.
- Evidence of depressive illness.
- Abuse of alcohol.

SUMMARY

This chapter examines how individuals, their families and social networks respond when faced with overwhelming stresses; through examination of crisis theory it looks at the stages and interventions that form a therapeutic approach to crisis and how individuals either avoid or grow from their crisis.

KEY CONCEPTS

- Crisis can be viewed as a decision or turning point. Crisis theory evolved from the study of grief reaction and bereavement. All crises have some elements of commonality. The phases of a crisis are mainly predictable and the characteristics of the individual experiencing the crisis form a pattern of response.
- Crises can be developmental, situational or traumatic. Developmental crises are transition points in the maturational process when psychological equilibrium is upset. Situational crises occur in response to a traumatic event or situation outside the normal pattern of living.
- Traumatic crises are accidental, rare and unexpected, often with multiple losses and gross environmental changes.
- There are definable factors that influence the outcome of a stressful event.
- Crisis intervention is a brief, active, directive, problem-solving approach that focuses on the individual's immediate problems, with the goal of re-establishing psychological equilibrium or the pre-crisis level of functioning. It also aims to make links between previous experiences and current crises, with the development of enhanced coping mechanisms.
- Accessible, appropriate and adequate resources are necessary for crisis intervention. Intervention is based on current problems only and is offered to include the client, the family and social network.
- The methodology of crisis intervention includes assessment, planning, implementation and evaluation. On assessment the precipitants of the crisis are identified, together with the individual's perception of the event. The client's support networks and coping skills are assessed. The planning stage involves collaborative definition of the problem through formation of a therapeutic relationship.
- Implementation may take a variety of forms: non-specific, environmental, generic or individual approaches. Non-specific includes interventions that provide the individual with the feeling that the nurse is caring, concerned and willing to help. Environmental interventions directly change the individual's physical or interpreted situation.
- Generic approaches are aimed at high risk, homogeneous groups. The individual approach includes interventions that aid a particular individual to achieve an adaptive resolution and are based on a clear understanding of the person's psychodynamics.
- Evaluation is a joint activity and reviews what has been achieved or resolved and how. Further work may be indicated and referrals to suitable services follow.
- Fundamentals of crisis intervention include formation of therapeutic relationships, communication, holistic care and team working.
- The work of the crisis intervenor is possible only through supervision, communication and support and an emphasis on reflective practice.

REFERENCES

Aguilera DC, Messick JM: *Crisis intervention: theory and methodology*. St Louis, 1990, Mosby Year Book Inc.

Armson S: *The Samaritans*. In: Jenkins R, Griffiths S, Wylie I *et al*, editors: *The prevention of suicide*. London, 1994, HMSO.

Bancroft J: Crisis intervention. In: Bloch S, editor: *An introduction to the psycho-therapists*. Oxford, 1979, Oxford University Press.

Bolin R: *Long-term family recovery from disaster*. Boulder, 1982, Institute of Behavioural Science.

Brammer LM: *The helping relationship process and skills*. New Jersey, 1979, Prentice Hall.

Burgess AW, Baldwin BA: *Crisis intervention — Theory and practice*. 1982, Prentice Hall.

Caplan G: *An approach to community mental health*. Tavistock/London, 1964, Grune & Stratton.

Chowdhury N, Hicks RC, Kreitman N: Evaluation of an aftercare service for para-suicidal patients. *Soc Psychiatry* 36:67, 1973.

Cohen RE, Ahearn F Jr: *The handbook for mental health care of disaster victims*. Baltimore, 1980, Johns Hopkins University Press.

Erikson EH: *Childhood and society*. New York, 1963, WW Norton.

Erikson EH: *Identity, youth and crisis*. New York, 1968, WW Norton.

Ewing CP: *Crisis intervention as psychotherapy*. Oxford, 1978, Oxford University Press.

Family Service Association of America: *Crisis intervention: selected readings*. New York, 1962, Family Service Association of America.

Hobbs M: Crisis intervention in theory and practice: a selective review. *Br J Med Psychol* 57(23):1984.

Jacobson GF: Crisis-orientated therapy. *Psychiatr Clin N Am* 2(1):39, 1979.

Johnson S, Thornicroft G: *Emergency services in England and Wales: report of study commissioned by the Department of Health*. London, 1991, HMSO.

Klein DC, Lindemann E: Preventative intervention in individual and family crisis situations. In: Caplan G, editor: *The prevention of mental disorders in children*. New York, 1961, Basic Books.

Knapp M, Beecham J, *et al.*: Service use and cost of home-based versus hospital-based care for people with serious mental illness. *Br J Psychiatry* 165:195,1994.

Lindemann E: Symptomatology and management of acute grief. *Am J Psychiatry* 101:141, 1944.

Lindemann E: *Beyond grief*. New York, 1979, Jason Aronson.

Marks I, Connolly J, Muijein I, *et al.*: Home-based versus hospital-based care for people with serious mental illness. *Br J Psychiatry* 165:179, 1994.

Muigen I, Marks I, Connolly J, *et al.*: The daily living programme. *Br J Psychiatry* 160:379, 1992.

Parad HJ, Caplan G: A framework for studying families in crisis. *J Soc Work* 5:3015, 1960.

Parad HJ, Parad LG: A study of crisis-orientated planned short term treatment, Part 2. *Soc Casework* 49:418. 1968.

Rapoport L: The state of considerations. Social Services Review 36. In: Parad H, editor: *Crisis intervention: selected readings*. New York, 1965, Family Service Association of America.

Rogers A, Pilgrim D, Lacey R: *Experiencing psychiatry: Users' views of services*. 1993, MIND.

Strathdee G: The delivery of psychiatric care. *J Royal Soc Med* 83:222, 1990.

FURTHER READING

Bengelsdorf H, Alden DC: A mobile crisis unit in the psychiatric emergency room. *Hosp Community Psychiatry* 38:662–665, 1987.

Brown GW, Andrews B, Bifulco A, Adler Z, Bridge L: Social support, self esteem and development. *Psychol Med* 16:813–832 1986.

Caplan G: *Principles of preventative psychiatry*. New York, 1964, Basic Books.

Falloon RH, Fadden G: *Integrated mental health care*. Cambridge, 1993, Cambridge University Press.

Marmar J: Crisis intervention and short term dynamic psychotherapy. In: Daranloo H, editor: *Short term psychotherapy*. New York, 1980, Jason Aronson.

Murgatroyd S, Woolfe R: *Coping with crisis*. London, 1982, Harper & Row.

Newton J: *Preventing mental illness in practice*. 1992, Routledge.

Roberts CA: *Primary prevention of psychiatric disorders*. 1967, Ontario Mental Health Foundation.

Sifneos PE: *Short term psychotherapy and emotional crisis*. 1970, Harvard University Press.

Tyrer P, Higg R, Strathdee G: *Mental health and primary care –A challenging agenda*. 1993, Mental Health Foundation.

Woolley N: Crisis theory: a paradigm of effective intervention with families of critically ill people. *J Ad Nurs* 15:1402–1408, December, 1990.

In-Patient Mental Health Nursing Care

Learning Outcomes

After studying this chapter you should be able to:

- Describe recent changes in in-patient psychiatric care.

- Identify the components of the clinical environment and the day-to-day organization of patient care.

- Discuss the scope of nursing within in-patient psychiatric settings.

- Evaluate outcomes related to in-patient mental health nursing practice.

*T*his chapter examines the organization of in-patient care on adult acute admission wards. For a number of years there has been a gradual shift in the focus of mental health care from psychiatric hospitals to the community. There has been a marked drop in the psychiatric in-patient population. However, there remains a need for continued access to in-patient facilities for a number of people with severe mental illness. The chapter emphasizes the changing nature of nursing care within the in-patient environment and the need to make the best use of the available resources. It acknowledges the challenge of delivering sensitive and responsive services under current pressures and that the development of the nurse–patient relationship is crucial to this work. The need for in-patient care as a vital part of a range of contemporary mental health services remains and with it the requirement to monitor and evaluate the nature and quality of such provision.

RECENT CHANGES IN IN-PATIENT CARE

Although 26% of the UK population have symptoms of mental illness in any given year, only about 1 in 10 of these people (576 000) receive specialist mental health services. According to Goldberg (1990) only about four admissions will occur for every 250 people under psychiatric care in the community. The total number of psychiatric in-patients has been declining steadily over a number of years. For the past 10 years, there has been an average annual decrease of 6%. A number of influences are changing the delivery of in-patient care and shifting traditional treatment from the hospital to other less restrictive and cheaper settings. Most people with mental health problems can be cared for much of the time in the community. Indeed, most people prefer to be looked after in their own homes. Purchasers of mental health services are mindful of expensive hospital beds and are keen to monitor length of stay, occupancy rates and other factors that may demonstrate inefficiency and waste of in-patient facilities.

Despite the provision of a variety of community facilities and treatment, some people suffer relapses from time-to-time that necessitate admission to hospital. Other precipitating factors include the risk of harm to self or others, crisis, and a first episode of serious mental illness. Although in-patient care has declined, even among the most developed community programmes there continues to be a need for some hospital places for short-term and long-term care. Preferably such care should not take place in old, remote institutions but in purpose-built local facilities. Acute care is required for patients who are disturbed or suicidal. A ward's protective environment assists in stabilization, treatment and re-establishment in the community. Acute units can also be places of sanctuary for vulnerable patients and provide respite for relatives.

Approximately £1.8 billion is spent annually on adult mental health services in England and Wales. Currently, 66% of resources on mental health are spent on in-patient care (Figure 14.1). The greater expenditure on in-patient beds compared to community services has been of concern, since resources to develop alternative services are already limited.

Nevertheless, the number of psychiatric beds has declined markedly since the 1950s. In 1995 there were 47 296 psychiatric in-patients in England. A new pattern of services for acute care is developing and shorter lengths of stay have become common. Guze and Unutzer (1993) predict that this trend will continue and that eventually in-patient units will be small and intensively staffed. Units will function as intensive care facilities for only the most severely disturbed. When acute patients are admitted,

they will be stabilized and transferred to lower levels of care as rapidly as possible.

RECEIVING PSYCHIATRIC IN-PATIENT CARE

So who does receive psychiatric in-patient care? Table 14.1 gives the major diagnosis of patients admitted to NHS Hospitals, England, 1989-1990. The need for mental health care, including hospital admission, varies widely with local circumstances. Hospital admission rates for different populations can vary by a factor of 5 and are associated with social deprivation including poverty and isolation. Certainly this is the case across most large cities in England where wards contain high numbers of disturbed young patients detained under the Mental Health Act 1983. The Audit Commission, responsible for examining economy, efficiency and effectiveness in use of NHS resources, suggest that if a service is well managed and targeted, only the most severely ill people, such as those diagnosed as psychotic will be admitted to hospital. Everyone else will receive care in the community. The cost of hospital care and the distress caused by admission certainly brings into question the appropriate use of in-patient care (Figure 14.2).

Caldicott *et al.* (1994) report discrepancy between actual and ideal numbers of psychiatric admission beds in London, where the true bed occupancy has been as high as 130%. Recent research continues to show that patients are admitted to hospitals mainly for good reasons. A series of articles comparing bed occupancy levels, reasons for admission and use of the Mental Health Act 1983, among London health districts, shows that, most patients were diagnosed as psychotic or suffering from affective disorders (Flannigan *et al.*, 1994a,b; Bebbington *et al.*, 1994). Eighty-five per cent were urgent unplanned admissions and 26% were admitted compulsorily under a section of the Mental Health Act 1983. Thomas (1995) reports that patients admitted to the Bethlem Royal and Maudsley Hospital Community Directorate have severe mental illness and are

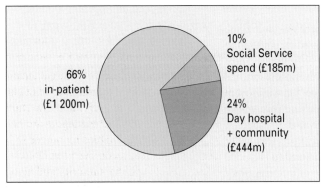

Figure 14.1 Expenditure on mental health services (Adapted from DoH, Welsh Office Health and Social Services Statistics, CIPFA data for England and Wales, 1992–93; reproduced courtesy of DoH.)

TABLE 14.1 Major diagnoses of patients admitted to NHS hospitals, England, 1989 - 1990

Main diagnosis	Total ordinary admissions	Duration of stay (days) Median	Mean
Mental disorders	303 378	14	255.7
Senile & presenile organic psychotic	47 423	20	197.7
Schizophrenic psychoses	33 585	31	723.3
Affective psychoses	30 949	29	92.9
Other psychoses	33 960	15	71.7
Neurotic & personality disorders	31 382	14	49.3
Alcohol dependence syndrome	20 530	9	16.4
Drug dependence	2 967	9	18.7
Physiological malfunction from mental factors	698	2	6.6
Mental retardation	56 047	4	620.3

Source: Department of Health, 1993, Hospital Episode Statistics, Volume 1, Finished consultant episodes by diagnosis, England, Financial Year 1989-90, HMSO

usually in crises. The decisions to admit patients are taken very seriously and usually involve senior nurses, doctors and managers.

THE CLINICAL ENVIRONMENT

The NHS has a public image of shabby and austere buildings. Nowhere is this more evident than in the field of mental health. It is known that nothing touches the lives of mentally ill people more than the setting where they are cared for (Gostin, 1986) yet most psychiatric hospitals are daunting, if not dangerous, places. The size and complexity of the building itself can increase patients' anxiety. In the late 1950s Osmond (1957) suggests that since mentally ill people have been studied closely, intensively and in more ways than almost any other group, their needs should be able to defined very exactly. He believes that requirements for mentally ill people are well able to be defined and that from this architects can be employed to devise efficient structures. Unfortunately there is little published research on the link between design of buildings and health outcomes or ideal therapeutic environments for the mentally ill. Exceptions include Dix and Williams (1996) who describe the design of a psychiatric special care unit for a small group of highly disturbed mentally ill people.

Sayce (1995) suggests that patients' disturbed behaviour may well result from the environment rather than mental distress. A recent report by MIND found that users were deeply dissatisfied with care on acute psychiatric units in general hospitals. They complained of lack of safety, lack of privacy, an over-clinical atmosphere and not enough opportunity to talk about problems (Sayce *et al.*, 1995).

Recently, more attention has been paid to the surroundings where patients are treated. The MILMIS (Monitoring Inner London Mental Illness Services) indicators relating to ward conditions identify environments that may well be detrimental, distressing and arousing (MILMIS, 1995). The Report of the Mental Health Nursing Review Team highlighted serious deficiencies of mental health services sited at district general hospitals, which were found unsuitable environments for people with mental health problems (HMSO, 1994). Although no one wants see a return to large remote institutions, there were some advantages from the size of old type psychiatric hospitals. First, some degree of specialization of function for individual in-patient units was possible. Secondly, they could provide a range of facilities and specialized staff, not readily available to smaller, dispersed units (such as occupational therapy services). Ward staff were able to use these services selectively to complement ward facilities.

Most people agree that in-patient facilities must provide the least restrictive conditions that meet the needs of patients. Nevertheless, staff who care for the mentally ill may, from time-to-time, have to exercise some degree of physical management and control. The level of security needs careful consideration since this will influence the philosophy of care, staffing levels, nursing skills and training, and the facilities required. For example, the use of seclusion, rapid tranquillization, control and restraint procedures and breakaway techniques, all require a different approach and exert different demands on staff.

The main response to violence and disturbed behaviour on in-patient units has been a coercive and sometimes punitive approach. Rather than use this, staff require training that focuses on prevention and minimization of violence, such as identifying triggers to anger. Powell *et al.* (1994) found that one of the three commonest antecedents to violent incidents at the Maudsley Hospital was the restrictions on patients associated with routine hospital regime. The identification of these triggers may assist staff prevent further occurrences of violence.

Most acute in-patient services are now expected to cope with patients with disturbed behaviour and those with management difficulties. Some psychiatric hospitals and mental health units have intensive care areas or units that cater for patients whose behavioural disturbance cannot adequately be contained on an open ward. Intensive care areas provide a locked facility with a high patient: nursing staff ratio and often contain a seclusion room. For further discussion on the prevention and management of violence see Chapter 19.

DAY-TO-DAY ORGANIZATION OF NURSING CARE

Organization of the patients' day and care in the in-patient unit varies with local needs and resources. The introduction of clinical directorates and decentralized management structures means that many charge nurses or ward managers are held accountable for ward budgets. This enables resources to be used in the best way. Not only have resources been devolved but clinical staff at ward level have the authority and autonomy to develop their own philosophy of care that complements the treatment ideology. Since the mid-1980s many mental health nurses have adopted a person-centred philosophy, under which the range and focus of nursing care is determined by individual patients' needs and preferences. The nursing workforce is organized to reflect this philosophy, which aims to enhance the patient's autonomy and recognize individuality. Many in-patient units operate either primary nursing or team nursing. Under primary nursing a patient is allocated to a named nurse (the primary nurse) who has associate, identified nurses when unavailable. Alternatively, the patient can be allocated to a team, with one member of the team as the named nurse. Only nurses in that team will be directly involved in caring for the patient. To provide a more individual approach to patient care the traditional hierarchical form of nursing establishment has been replaced by a flatter and more flexible structure. Such flexibility enables a greater number of qualified nurses to spend time in direct patient contact and be more clinically focused.

However, to ensure safety, security and effective use of resources most in-patient units operate a combination of flexibility and routine. In-patients follow a daily sequence of washing, dressing, eating and participating in whatever therapeutic and recreational activities staff offer. Routine enables some continuity and allows people to know in advance what is likely to happen at various times, for example, meals and meetings. Nevertheless, it is important that the patient's day is not organized around a set of ward routines. As far as practicable patients should be consulted over how they like to spend the day and the timing of events, for example, when they usually wake up or go to bed. Many people with mental health problems have difficulties with daily activities; for example some patients have day–night reversal. Late rising in the day leads to patients being active late at night or in the small hours. They may want to stay up late watching television or playing music, which can disturb others, resulting in resentment and feelings of hostility. Part of the patient's care plan may be

directed at trying to improve their level of social integration into the ward and their level of social functioning. The following specimen care plan (Table 14.2) is for a patient who has had three episodes of schizophrenia. AB is a 25-year-old man who has been unemployed since the first episode of his illness. He normally lives at home with his parents but was admitted to hospital following failure to take medication, expressing persecutory delusions and becoming socially withdrawn.

Since the ward or unit is probably part of a larger organization, staff and patients will be expected to conform to hospital or health service protocol, for example, a no-smoking regime. In addition to local regulations and procedures, an

TABLE 14.2 A specimen care plan

Needs and problems	Goal	Action
AB says that he feels tired all the time; this leads him to spend most of the day in bed.	For AB to be able to stay up during the daytime once during the next 3 days.	Find out what AB might enjoy doing and structure a programme of daily activities that suit his abilities and provide him with the opportunity to achieve success.
		Negotiate a reasonable time to get up.
		Explore with AB what makes it difficult to stay awake during the day.
		Negotiate a reasonable bedtime and provide social time markers such as a bath, hot drink and quiet environment from 10 p.m.
		If AB awakes in the night, offer him a milky drink and an opportunity to talk; encourage him to return to bed.
		If AB cannot sleep ask him to restrict his movement to the ward area away from other sleeping people and to keep as quiet as possible.
AB avoids contact with other people because he says that they are trying to 'read my mind' and that he feels frightened and annoyed about this.	For AB to explore his feelings of fear and annoyance with one person over the next 4 days, in an attempt to plan strategies to cope effectively with them.	AB's primary named nurse will work to establish a relationship with him, based on reliability, acceptance, warmth and mutual trust.
		A regular time will be set when AB and his nurse will spend an agreed amount of time together in an activity of his choice.
		Once a relationship is established, AB can be encouraged to keep a journal, noting down his thoughts and feelings as they occur so that any pattern to the circumstances in which he feels frightened or annoyed can be identified.
		This journal may then be used as a basis for discussion during meetings with his nurse.
		When and if any triggers to AB's fear and annoyance have been identified, this care plan needs to be reviewed and reformulated to move on to an appropriate following stage.

operational policy that specifies the purpose, structure and day-to-day functioning of the ward is needed. This ensures it runs efficiently and smoothly.

THE THERAPEUTIC MILIEU

It has long been known that the dynamics of in-patient psychiatric wards can be put to direct therapeutic or anti-therapeutic use. Maxwell Jones (1952) described the in-patient environment as a therapeutic community, with cultural norms for behaviours, values and activity. He saw patients' social interactions among peers and health care workers as treatment opportunities. For example, he suggested that interpersonal difficulties between patients provided fertile material for psychodynamic intervention. He believed that clinical staff should share in the community governance with the patient group, on an equal basis. He further emphasized the benefit of mutual participation of patients in each other's treatment, predominantly through sharing of intimate information and feedback in group settings such as the community meeting.

In 1969 Abroms introduced the concept of the therapeutic milieu. He suggested that it served the two main purposes of setting limits on disturbing and maladaptive behaviour and teaching psychosocial skills. In 1978 Gunderson, in a seminal paper, further elaborated the concept of the therapeutic milieu. He described three features of the therapeutic community: distribution of responsibility and decision making; clarity of the role and leadership of programmes; and high levels of interaction between patients and staff. He also described five functional components: containment, support, structure, involvement and validation.

CONTAINMENT

The function of containment is to keep the patient safe and to sustain his or her physical well-being. Containment includes the provision of food, shelter and medical attention, as well as the steps necessary to prevent the patient from harming self or others. Therefore it includes a continuum of interventions, with seclusion and restraint being the most extreme. Containment is intended to reinforce temporarily the internal controls of patients. It allows them to test reality, particularly their omnipotent beliefs concerning their own destructiveness.

Containment is necessary to provide safety and foster trust. Therapeutic use of containment communicates to patients that the nurse will impose external controls as necessary to keep patients and the environment safe. Appropriate and consistent limit setting is essential to meeting this goal. Nursing examples of therapeutic containment include the use of observational levels, time-out and seclusion.

SUPPORT

Support is about staff's conscious efforts to help patients feel cared for and enhance their self-esteem. It is the unconditional acceptance of the patient, whatever their given circumstances. (See Chapter 3 for an exploration of acceptance.) The function of support is to help patients feel comfortable and secure and to reduce their anxiety. Support may take many forms on the in-patient unit, under the general description of paying attention to the patient.

Support can be communicated through empathy and by being available, appropriately offering encouragement and reassurance, giving helpful direction, taking the patient out of the hospital for various activities, offering food or drinks and engaging patients in activities that they are reluctant to get involved in. Other nursing examples include giving information, advising and teaching, promoting reality testing and modelling healthy relationships and interactions. To provide support, nursing staff activity must be coordinated, cohesive and consistent with the patient's treatment goals. Supportive nurturing enhances self-esteem. Those milieux that offer support also provide nurturing and permit, encourage and direct patients to become engaged in other therapeutic efforts on the ward.

STRUCTURE

Structure refers to all aspects of a milieu that provide predictable organization of time, place and person. This dependability in activity, staff and environment helps the patient feel safe. Having a routine including a timetable of meetings, groups, social events and other ward activities is one feature of structure. Other nursing examples include setting limits within the ward and the use of negotiation and contracts. The more these uses of structure are planned with the patient according to shared ideas of what is adaptive and maladaptive, the more the structure becomes therapeutic in itself. The patient can then begin to accept responsibility for behaviour and its consequences.

Providing structure helps the patient to control inappropriate behaviours. The nurse invokes appropriate consequences if the patient is unable, for whatever reason, to either impose or honour effective limits. As consequences are consistently applied, the patient learns to delay impulsive and inappropriate responses through consistent expectations and behavioural responses.

INVOLVEMENT

Involvement is part of the ward structure that goes beyond compliance with rules and activities. It refers to those processes that help patients to become awareness of their social environment and to interact with people. Its purpose is to strengthen the patient's sense of self and to modify behaviour that is anti-social or inappropriate. Interpersonal communication and group activities provide patients with opportunities to interact with others in their immediate environment.

Nursing examples of involvement include the use of open doors and open rounds and facilitating patient-led groups, community activities and self-assertive experiences. Wards that emphasize involvement encourage the use of cooperation, compromise and confrontation. Through this involvement, patients learn appropriate interaction patterns and experience the consequences of unacceptable behaviours. For example, a patient who displays anger or offensive behaviour that distances others can be encouraged to participate in activities that will assist in talking about his or her feelings, working out differences and receiving feedback. This supportive experience strengthens the patient's sense of self, behavioural control and social interaction skills. Therefore, encouraging involvement provides corrective experiences for the patient.

VALIDATION

Validation means that the individuality of each patient is recognized. It is the act of affirming a person's unique view of the world. Validation can help patients develop a greater capacity for closeness and a more consolidated identity. The mental health nurse displays validation through individual attention, empathy and non-judgmental acceptance of the patient's thoughts, feelings and perspectives. Other nursing examples of validation include individualized treatment planning, showing respect for the patient's rights and providing opportunities for the patient to succeed. Therapeutic listening and acknowledging the feelings underlying the patient's personal experience reinforce individuality. Clarification of these feelings assists the patient in understanding and accepting their unique experience. This strengthens the patient's sense of individuality and encourages the integration of pleasant and unpleasant aspects of personal experience.

The appropriateness of these functions in short-term inpatient settings is being re-evaluated in light of the nature of contemporary in-patient psychiatric care. While not disputing their importance and usefulness, Gutheil (1985) suggests that, since its development over 40 years ago, the therapeutic milieu has undergone significant alteration and corruption by emphasis on community care, increased use of psychopharmacology, high staff turnover and lack of psychoanalytically trained staff.

Evaluation of the functional components of support, structure, involvement and validation is sparse. Jackson and Cawley (1992) describe the effects of a psychodynamic approach in an acute admission ward over a 13-year period. Influenced by the therapeutic community movement, they suggest that psychoanalytic ideas offer a way of understanding psychotic thinking and inexplicable or bizarre behaviour. These ideas amplify the psychotherapeutic component of management and sometimes set the scene for more intensive psychotherapy. The authors suggest that the best setting for such work is an inpatient milieu, staffed by a multidisciplinary team. Although nurses are not trained psychotherapists their work is often effectively psychotherapeutic. The traditional pattern of 'nurses care and doctors treat' no longer applies and the treatment of severely disturbed patients was strengthened by listening closely to them and by attempting to understand their experience using psychoanalytic concepts.

Though the ward referred to by Jackson and Cawley no longer exists, some of the fundamental principles of the therapeutic milieu remain in many modern in-patient settings. These include patients' participation in decision making, multidisciplinary staff and a belief in the rehabilitative potential of the environment. It must be emphasized that these aspects of care do not just happen but are brought about by staff who aim to provide high quality, clinically effective care. It is important that in-patient mental health nurses know what factors contribute to providing a safe, structured and supportive environment and how they can positively influence patient outcome.

PATIENTS' PARTICIPATION IN DECISION MAKING

Most modern mental health services embrace the idea of user-involvement. It is widely accepted that service users have a right to be involved not only in decisions about their own care but more generally about service delivery and development. Users' participation often means attending meetings. At ward level a variety of meetings take place. These range from ward business meetings to therapy groups (see Chapter 30). Outside the ward environment there are often user group meetings and hospital-based, user-run advocacy schemes that have input into management meetings. Although slower to develop than in the USA and some European countries, most British mental health services now support various advocacy models. These models usually take the form of patients' councils and mental health forums. In addition, Glazier and May (1995) describe the involvement of users in training professionals. While acknowledging the benefits of such involvement, the authors highlight the difficulties encountered both by professionals and the service users acting as trainers in changing cultural norms. This topic is discussed in more detail in Chapter 3.

MULTIDISCIPLINARY STAFF

Multidisciplinary working is accepted practice on in-patient units. The complex nature of people's mental health problems requires contribution from different professions. However, the bringing together of different professionals poses problems and suitable methods of coordination are required if an effective and efficient team is to result. On many in-patient units there is often dissatisfaction about the way teams operate. Work is sometimes hampered by rivalry, power struggles and by, conflict and disagreements about decision making, the division of labour and leadership. Such conflict often gives rise to the secondary effects of poor communication, goal ambiguity and low morale. Where multidisciplinary staff try to be egalitarian, there is often confusion over leadership, responsibility, authority and accountability. Doyle (1977) describes a mental health centre where all team members were treated as equal. All staff including the psychiatrist, psychologist, social workers, nurses and attendants were expected to rotate shifts and interchange jobs. After a few months, staff became so preoccupied with defining their philosophical and therapeutic positions that patients' needs were not met. Ambiguity over leadership and responsibility finally resulted in considerable stress and conflict among the staff. This was reduced when the approach was reversed and clear role definition and leadership were restored.

Most in-patient units produce information booklets detailing the members of the multidisciplinary team and their functions. Ranger (1986) suggests that patients have a very traditional view; they regard doctors as being in charge and see nurses and doctors as being most involved in assessment and treatment. Patients in the study were unclear about the role of psychologists. Ranger suggests that this is hardly surprising since many of the other disciplines were also unsure of the psychologists' role. Social workers ranked low on involvement with patients but patients saw themselves as being less involved than any of the professionals in all areas except occupational therapy.

Communication between members of the team is a top priority for those involved in care of the mentally ill. Nurses and other disciplines are involved in a variety of multidisciplinary meetings. Pollock (1986) suggests that ward rounds exemplify how the multidisciplinary team functions. One observational study in which the content of ward rounds was analysed for ten neurotic and ten psychotic patients demonstrated that most of the time was taken up by discussions on diagnostic and medical matters (Sanson–Fisher *et al.*, 1979). Doctors spoke almost eight times as much as non-medical staff, including nurses. Occupational therapists spoke the least. Fewtrell and Toms (1985), in an experimental study compared a new ward round format with traditional ward round procedures. The new model included Key Workers; each qualified member of staff was allocated responsibilities for a particular patient that included participating in the assessment interview. In the new format patients were encouraged to ask questions and give their opinions both among themselves and with staff. This produced a swing away from discussing purely medical aspects of care to more social and domestic ones. Primary nurses now attend ward rounds instead of the senior nurse on duty. The responsibility for supporting the patient during the ward round and communicating with other members of the multidisciplinary team is devolved to each patients primary or associate nurse. The organization of care using primary nursing has improved communication by reducing repetition and thereby eliminating misunderstanding.

To resolve the main difficulties that arise through multidisciplinary team work it is essential that nurses develop a number of coping strategies. These can include maintaining regular contact, up-dating and involvement in decision making. Most importantly it is essential that nurses do not become isolated or alienated and that they try to avoid stress and burn-out. Mechanisms to help prevent these negative reactions include attending staff support groups, variability of work, building-in time away from the clinical area to carry out project work or research, attending study days and courses, visiting other departments or units, clinical supervision and proper appraisal.

REHABILITATIVE POTENTIAL OF THE ENVIRONMENT

The forming of relationships is considered to be a therapeutic tool provided by an in-patient environment. In-patients must have the opportunity to form beneficial relationships both among themselves and with hospital staff. Mental health nursing is based on the one-to-one therapeutic relationship. However, constraints of working on busy, acute psychiatric wards would seem to make it impossible for nurses to meet up regularly with the number of patients who might benefit from forming such relationships. Many nurses complain that, because of the fast turnover of patients and reduced length of stay, they are unable to form therapeutic relationships and have therefore slipped back into a more custodial role. This is particularly true where psychopharmacology is the main treatment regime. In such settings, the main purpose of the milieu is to provide a safe environment where medication can take effect and the patient's condition can be stabilized sufficiently for discharge. Prior (1993) suggests that under such circumstances the object of focus centres on improving patient behaviour. However, a hospital milieu is not compatible with such a focus on behaviour since, by definition, the latter necessitates the patient's contact with society, to test behavioural competence. According to Prior, in-patient units are therefore rendered 'functionless'.

Although such arguments are popular, there is nevertheless a consensus that hospital care cannot be dispensed with altogether at the present time. Current Government policy is that priority should be given to people with serious or long-term problems who are at high risk of repeated admissions. Such a policy is not without its problems. Guthiel (1985) suggests that staff on in-patient units dealing with the seriously mentally ill are vulnerable to low morale and it is important that staff feel they are doing constructive work.

It seems unlikely that these conflicts and dilemmas will be resolved unless traditional ways of working are challenged. Prior's study (1993), comparing the social worlds of a number of psychiatric hospital in-patients with those of patients who had left hospital 5 years previously, points out that in one hospital, patients were often allocated to wards as much on the basis of nursing interests as on the basis of patient need. The patient population had been divided into groups according to various nursing and administrative interests, for example, disturbed patients and 'rehab' patients.

Handy (1991), studying psychiatric nurses on an admission ward, found that they spent most of their time carrying out ward routines such as serving meals and administering medication, while the personal problems that caused patients to be admitted received relatively little attention. The seniority of nursing staff related inversely to the amount of time they spent with patients and related positively to that spent on administration or with other disciplines. There was a tendency for patients to be dealt with by the most inexperienced and least qualified staff, while decisions concerning them were taken by senior staff with less knowledge of them. Robinson (1995), in measuring nursing interactions in delivery of care on three wards at Rampton Hospital, found that nurses spend almost twice as much time away from direct contact with patients as they do in direct care. The high levels of indirect care and the heavy burden of administration call for more innovative use of nursing skills.

It is clear that there is pressure for mental health nurses to concentrate only on those patients who require detailed and intensive interventions. Other patients, who are deemed less severely ill, may require some nursing input but, in the main, therapeutic services and care will be sought elsewhere. Nurses working on in-patient units need to examine the values and assumptions underlying their work if they are going to find ways of providing appropriate and effective methods of delivering care.

SENSITIVE AND RESPONSIVE SERVICES

There is increasing concern about the way in which mental health services have failed to respond to the needs of certain groups, particularly women and people from ethnic minority groups. Services are often inappropriate, insensitive and in some cases discriminatory.

RESPONDING TO WOMEN'S NEEDS

Official statistics from the Department of Health suggest that more women than men are admitted to psychiatric hospitals every year. This being the case, to give special attention to the needs of women as if they were in the minority seems a curious undertaking. However, the harrowing experiences many women suffer as a result of their encounters with mental health services makes attention necessary. Reports suggest an alarming incidence of attacks on women who use mental health services (Copperman and Burrows, 1992). Nilberts and Crossmaster (1989) reported that 71% of women had been threatened by physical violence, 38% had been sexually assaulted. These findings resulted in a number of actions In April 1995 the Department of Health provided additional rights under the new Patient's Charter. These include informing patients prior to admission whether it is planned for them to be cared for in a ward for men and women. If so, in all cases, patients can expect single-sex washing and toilet facilities. If patients prefer to be cared for in single-sex accommodation their wishes are to be respected, wherever possible.

Identifying concerns and raising awareness has stimulated wider initiatives. Many psychiatric hospitals have produced local policies and guidelines to help staff provide safety and privacy in mental health settings. These include policies relating to allegations of sexual assault, abuse and rape. Other initiatives include the introduction of women-only wards, women-only areas on some in-patient units and the choice of same-sex named nurse or Key Worker. The therapeutic benefits of women-only wards are:

1. Less threatening environment, particularly for women who have suffered violence or abuse.
2. Opportunities to share concerns with staff and other patients without being inhibited by the presence of men, e.g. sexual or marital issues, diet, children.
3. Shared experience of mental illness with other women.
4. Staff having higher awareness of issues affecting women that could affect mental health problems and progress of recovery.

5. Less embarrassment in supervision from women staff.
6. Counselling and group work, enabling sharing of womens' issues.
7. Ability to offer women-centred support, interpreters and advocacy, and specific occupational therapy activities.

While such endeavours are essential, they are not enough on their own. Batcup and Thomas (1994) argue for stronger and more radical measures to provide a safer modern mental health service in ways that are more acceptable to patients. These include challenging the processes that perpetuate abuse and inequality in the context in which they occur, and scrutinizing knowledge, employment structures, training and policies for explicit and implicit oppressive and sexist assumptions. Additionally there should be continual assessment and evaluation of ward space and nurses' time to provide optimal conditions of safety and privacy.

RESPONDING TO THE NEEDS OF ETHNIC MINORITY GROUPS

People from different ethnic minority groups often experience difficulties when using mainstream mental health services. Indeed, it is often suggested that black and other ethnic groups are disadvantaged by the psychiatric system. One simple explanation for this problem is the lack of cross-cultural understanding by professionals. African–Caribbeans in Britain have higher admission rates to psychiatric hospitals and are diagnosed as schizophrenic more often than the white population (London, .1986). Asian people appear to experience delayed entry into mental health services until a crisis point is reached, possibly because they are more reluctant than others to reveal their symptoms to GPs. Pilgrim and Rogers (1993) suggest two reasons to explain the apparent over-representation of Afro-Caribbeans with schizophrenia and the under-representation of Asians. The first looks at cultural differences; the second suggests a vulnerability to distress caused by adverse environmental factors, including social deprivation and unfavourable conditions such as racial harassment, discrimination, poor housing, unemployment, and lack of educational opportunities. Certainly, transcultural research demonstrates that the high admission of Caribbeans is to be explained by factors operating in the UK rather than the country of origin (Hickling, 1991).

To improve the effective delivery of mental health services for black and other ethnic groups many NHS Trusts are trying to recruit staff who reflect the local population of the communities they serve. Although there has been much progress in some areas, for example the development of better understanding and closer links with black communities, there continue to be difficulties recruiting nurses from black and other ethnic groups. Many service providers now have policies or guidelines for good practice when working with black or other ethnic mental health service users. The implementation of such policies, particularly in relation to equal opportunities, is essential if patients from ethnic groups are to have confidence that racism and discrimination is being eliminated. Such policies will also help ensure that services are appropriate, adequate and accessible and that they are monitored regularly. Staff should receive training and guidance relating to good practice, including an awareness of cultural differences and their effect on health patterns and patients' needs. Staff must ensure that they understand the implications of the various policies, particularly with regard to legal requirements.

THE SCOPE OF NURSING

Mental health nurses have continually extended the caring and treatment aspects of their role. In in-patient settings, the increased workload resulting from higher admission rates, faster turnover, shorter lengths of stay and the intensity and severity of symptoms calls for radical changes in the way care is organized. Unfortunately, established ways of working die hard and the culture on many psychiatric hospital wards proves difficult to change and then sustain. This is not to deny that some traditional nursing interventions may still prove useful. However, many of the problems facing contemporary nurses require different approaches and a wider range of solutions. These include brief in-patient admissions, crisis management, rapid stabilization, psycho-educative approaches and the use of cognitive behavioural interventions.

When patients are admitted to hospital, it must be made very clear what the purpose of that admission is and what can and cannot be achieved. Lamb (1988) suggests that it is important to help the patient (and their relatives) to understand why admission to hospital is necessary. The admission should be seen as part of a continuum of care, not as a discrete episode. From the beginning the emphasis is, therefore, on how the admission can be used to improve and maintain future adaptation in the community. The assessment of the patient should not only be directed at the resolution of the patient's mental health problems but at the knowledge, behaviour and coping mechanisms that he or she requires to adapt to life in the community. Once these have been identified, a planned programme can be developed with the patient and implemented.

Where appropriate family members, friends and significant others should be included in the care planning process. There is now considerable evidence that suggests that it is possible to provide effective support for families and that this can significantly reduce the patient's risk of symptomatic relapse (Tarrier *et al.*, 1988). Interventions shown to be effective include a psycho-educative approach and improving the communication and problem solving abilities of families. Combined with the emotional support offered in 'family therapy' as described by Leff *et al.* (1989), skills training in these interventions now forms the basis of the Thorn nursing initiative as described in Chapter 32.

Structured activities run by nurses in the ward environment are often an important part of a patient's individualized care plan. These include stress management and relaxation, therapeutic groups and social skills training. In addition to providing opportunities for social interaction and learning new skills, such groups and programmes provide a cost-effective way to implement mental health nursing care. For example a recent study by Thomas and Smedley (1995) showed that out of 1231 recent hospital admissions 23% were re-admitted following relapse resulting from non-compliance with medication. One of the factors contributing to non-compliance is that patients do not understand the importance of the medication; nor are they informed adequately about side-effects. It is also known that most patients will retain only a small amount of any information given about drugs. Therefore, a once-only teaching or information session will not be adequate. Education groups relating to medication and other health teaching activities, where continual contact, reinforcing and clarification can take place, seem much better ways to address these problems

MAKING THE BEST USE OF RESOURCES

In England, there are approximately 30 000 qualified mental health nurses working in in-patient units. Mental health nurses are the largest single occupational group in psychiatric organizations. In the constant search for cost-effectiveness in health care, the organization and management of nursing is continually scrutinized. Reforms in the NHS, such as introduction of general management, resource management and the internal market, have created interesting challenges both for those managing the services and those working within them. One of the most important challenges is how to ensure that the NHS can deploy professional staff to greatest effect. Nursing staff costs are usually a major part of a service's operational costs. Attention to effective use of nursing staff and other resources is an important part of the mental health nurse's role in prudent management of in-patient care. The right people must be in the right place at the right time. This means more than just making sure there are adequate numbers of nurses on duty to carry out the work. It means getting the right grade and skill mix to provide the care. This in turn is dependent on the identified needs of the patients.

Qualified mental health nurses are becoming scarcer and what are acceptable, safe levels of nurse staffing on in-patient units is now a critical issue. Unfortunately, this situation has not received sufficient attention. Various methods have been developed to try to quantify nursing care delivery in in-patient units; however, most of these lack sophistication and flexibility. This has resulted in most wards and units continuing to base their nursing establishments on tradition, general principles and non-systematic methods, for example, by the ratio of nurses to bed numbers, traditional rostering and deployment of nurses. It is usually the ward manager who ensures that the ward is adequately staffed, with a trained nurse in charge of each shift and a balance of grades.

This traditional method of allocating resources has given way in some areas to more systematic methods including workforce planning, workload measurement, patient dependency and classification systems and skill mix reviews. In their own way all of these approaches try to address the issues of how much nursing time is needed and which grades of nurses are required. Workload is often described in terms of its component parts, which are

1. Direct patient care, e.g. discussing self-care with a patient.
2. Indirect patient care, e.g. answering relatives' queries.
3. Other activities, e.g. ordering supplies.

Martin (1992) provides an example of this type of analysis by detailed examination of patient activities in five in-patient areas using work sampling observation. Martin found that patients spend on average 56.8% of their waking time apparently doing nothing. Time spent in direct patient interaction, including all one-to-one and group encounters on the ward regardless of purpose, by qualified and unqualified nurses, accounts for 21.8% of work time. By far the highest proportion of time spent on one activity was communicating with other staff (35.6%). The results of this study led Martin to ask the searching question 'What do qualified psychiatric nurses do?'

In general nursing, there are a number of methods to assess workforce requirements. Most existing systems use measures of patient dependency as a basis of assessing workload, and relate them to nursing activity. Some systems categorize nursing care into basic and technical care; others are based upon individual care plans (Rhys-Hearn and Potts, 1978). American psychiatric nurses have a tradition of using patient classification systems (Sovie, 1988; Treanor and Cotch, 1990). Queen (1995) suggests that the patients' need for nursing care is typically grouped into four or five categories (see Table 14.3). Each higher level of grouping represents more intense needs for nursing care than the previous one. A value (usually number of hours) is then assigned to each category representing the amount of nursing care required in a specific period (usually an 8-hour shift). This number is then multiplied by the number of patients on the ward who require each category of nursing care. These values are summated and the final figure represents the number of nursing care hours required for all of the patients on that ward for the specified time.

Although this example shows how a patient classification system can be used as framework for determining resource, as yet there has been little similar work carried out among British mental health nurses. A number of British research studies, while not directly addressing issues related to workload, patient classification or skills mix, have provided rich data on the use of nursing time, the types of interventions used and nurses' involvement in other activities (Altschul, 1972; Cormack, 1983).

EVALUATING PRACTICE AND IMPROVING CARE

The increasing pressures on the resources available for mental health care mean that nurses are expected constantly to evaluate their practice and seek methods to improve effectiveness and efficiency. Not only must nurses demonstrate that what

they do, they do well, but they must also produce benefits. These pressures have given rise to a number of nursing initiatives aimed at improving clinical decision making and changing practice and the delivery of services. In the main, these endeavours are welcomed and have resulted in improvements, but it must also be remembered that they are means to an end and that they are often costly and time-consuming to carry out and sometimes result in nurses spending less time on direct patient care.

QUALITY ASSURANCE

Quality assurance is a clinical and managerial framework that ensures a systematic and continual monitoring and evaluation of agreed levels of service and care provision. The activities involved in quality assurance and standard setting are described in full in Chapter 9. Most psychiatric hospitals employ a quality assurance nurse, with special responsibility to take a lead on quality initiatives. In addition, in-patient nurses are involved in some type of quality-related activity, such as quality circles or audit meetings. Audit packages directly targeted at mental health services have been slow to develop. Recently, however, increased numbers of off-the-shelf audit packages have become available. Examples include the Central Nottinghamshire Psychiatric Nursing Audit (CNPNA) (Howard and Hurst, 1987) and Psychiatric Monitor (Goldstone and Doggett, 1989). There seems to be a lack of enthusiasm for the widespread use of these systems. Nevertheless, the importance accorded to improving the quality of mental health services is evident by the number of NHS Trusts that have a Director of Quality on their management team. In many cases this role is combined with that of Director of Nursing.

CLINICAL AUDIT

Clinical audit is a systematic and critical analysis of the quality of professional care. The term 'clinical audit' includes nursing audit but covers audit by other professionals usually working together. The Department of Health recently commissioned an evaluation of the development, progress and impact of audit in health services in England (Willmot *et al*, 1995). Among its findings the evaluative study found that audit activities range diversely, covering all aspects of health care. These activities include discharge planning, record keeping, development of collaborative care plans and management of pain, suicide and deliberate self-harm. The results from audit activities have led to changes in practice, service management and on culture and attitudes and generally have had a lasting effect within provider units. There was diversity in profession and status of those leading audit activities although most were led by board-level directors or by service managers.

EVIDENCE-BASED PRACTICE

The term 'evidence-based' practice reflects the aspiration that nurses should deliver care and therapy based on procedures that are known, through research evidence, to be effective.

TABLE 14.3 Nursing care categories

Category	Nursing services needed
Category I (1 nursing care hour per 8-hour shift)	The patient: • Is able to perform activities of daily living with no or minimal supervision and assistance • Actively participates in treatment programme • Independently attends activities and appointments on or off grounds • Sleeps restfully during the night
Category II (5 nursing care hours per 8-hour shift)	The patient: • Requires supervision or some assistance in performing activities of daily living • Requires nursing supervision at all times while outside the in-patient unit • Participates in treatment programme with individual nursing intervention to complete activities of daily living • May or may not sleep restfully during the night, requiring some nursing intervention
Category III (8 nursing care hours per 8-hour shift)	The patient: • Requires intermittent, individual nursing intervention to complete activities of daily living • Requires full visual observation by nurses at all times • Demonstrates disruptive perceptual, cognitive or affective disturbance • Is at risk of harm to self or others • Requires redirection, orientation, or externally imposed limit setting • Does not sleep restfully through the night, requiring ongoing individual nursing intervention
Category IV (8 nursing care hours per 8-hour shift)	The patient: • Is totally dependent in all activities of daily living • In unable to understand or is resistant to treatment programme • Demonstrates severe and persistent perceptual, cognitive and/or affective disturbance • Is at risk of harm to self or others • Has a profound chronic sleep disturbance

Patient category	Nursing care hours required per shift	Patient census
I	1 x 6	= 6
II	3 x 7	= 21
III	5 x 4	= 20
IV	8 x 1	= 8
	TOTAL 18	= 55 hours nursing care required
	55	= 6.875 or 7 staff needed per 8-hour shift

Whereas there are over one million randomized, controlled trials in medicine, there are few such studies in mental health nursing. Indeed many areas of mental health nursing are not amenable to research methods such as randomized controlled trials. Therefore, there must be a place for the consideration of other types of research findings such as by qualitative methods. Nevertheless, research findings derived from other disciplines are often used in nursing practice and nurses need to keep up to date with these developments as they emerge. One way of doing this is through making use of clinical practice guidelines. These support clinicians by making them aware of advances in research, through systematically collecting and appraising available experimental evidence and helping them to build it into their routine clinical practice.

Following the American Psychiatric Association the Royal College of Psychiatrists has taken the lead in developing clinical practice guidelines to support and improve clinical care through informed decision making. The College has adopted the definition used by the American Agency for Health Care Policy and Research:

> A clinical practice guideline is a systematically developed statement which assists practitioner and patient decisions about appropriate health care for specific clinical circumstances.

Many mental health nurses are involved in the development of clinical practice guidelines. However, the Royal College's programme only commenced in January 1995, so it will be sometime before individual guidelines are available. The adoption of evidence-based nursing practice requires a shift in thinking, attitudes and behaviour of many nurses. Even if evaluations of nursing practice are carried out successfully, the results need to be disseminated and, most importantly, acted upon. There may be professional opposition because of new ways of working, adapting to change and retraining. Despite these obstacles, the move towards evidence-based nursing is worthwhile since it is likely to have major impact on clinical practice, which could result in real and lasting improvements in patient care.

RISK MANAGEMENT

Mental health care is a risk activity. In-patient units exist to assess and treat people with mental illness and, to keep them safe, as well as to relieve symptoms. Every effort must be made to ensure that people who are admitted to in-patient wards, staff and members of the public come to no harm as a result of their contacts with the service. Evaluation of an in-patient setting also involves the assessment of risk. Risks are usually related to situations that could result in legal action involving patients, families, the hospital or the health care provider. Issues related to involuntary admission. refusal of treatment, informed consent, confidentiality, access to health records, security, least restrictive environment, seclusion and restraint are confronted daily by the in-patient nurse (see Chapter 8). It is recommended that all nurses become aware of the law governing the mentally ill and related legislation.

Risk management has become an essential part of the clinical and management process of in-patient care and complements overall aims to improve the quality of services and the working environment. The aim of risk management is to

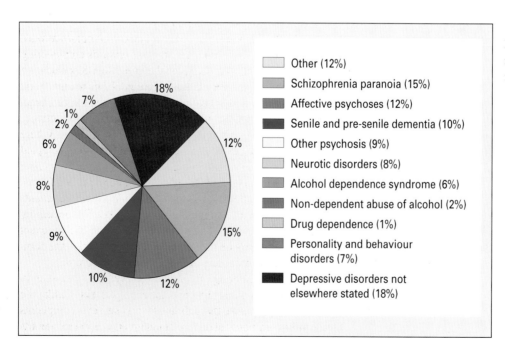

Figure 14.2 Distribution by diagnosis of all admissions to mental illness hospitals, England, 1986

ensure that risk is identified, analyzed and controlled and, where possible, eliminated; or, at the least, to reduce the effect of risk that cannot be eliminated. The four stages in risk management are summarized in Figure 14.3.

MEASUREMENT OF OUTCOMES

Mental health nurses in the in-patient setting must be able to articulate the value of nursing care and prove their worth. In a modern mental health service with a strong emphasis on effectiveness and outcomes, nurses must be able to show what happens to people as a result of nursing interventions. In mental health nursing the measurement of outcomes is particularly difficult. In the absence of data on effectiveness, interventions should be used that are based on consensus or the best indications available. So far there are very few areas where the relationship between patient outcomes and nursing interventions is clearly understood. Nevertheless, there are a number of outcome measures that are used when evaluating nursing care. The views of service users has become one such outcome and measures for it are regarded as central to any evaluation of in-patient mental health nursing.

Users' Views

In addition to the involvement of users in planning services, mental health professionals are increasingly seeking out and acting upon the views of service users. User input can be solicited through meetings, questionnaires, consultation with

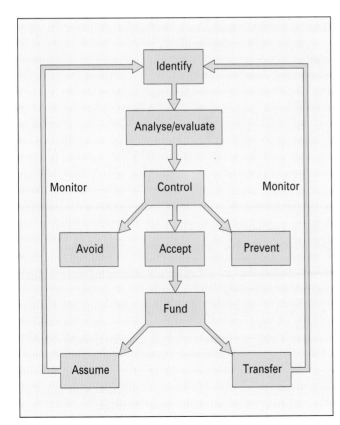

Figure 14.3 Stages of risk management

user representative groups, mechanisms such as suggestion boxes and complaints procedures. Most mental health nurses directly involved in providing care are ideally placed to explore the views of service users about the care and treatment they receive.

Although there is no single recommended method for obtaining users' views, there is a tradition of using anonymously answered self-completion satisfaction questionnaires. This tradition seems to have emanated from the pioneering work of Raphael (1972). To date much of the user feedback gathered through satisfaction surveys has related to hotel and service aspects of care, for example the cleanliness of the environment and the quality of the food. Not denying the importance of these, research and audit show that there are many aspects of treatment and the behaviour of professionals that are of even greater importance to users. These include communication, information about treatments and choice. McIver (1991), while acknowledging the strengths of the Raphael questionnaire for psychiatric patients, points out that exploratory work, to find out which subject areas and issues were considered by users to be important, is not mentioned. Examples of such an approach do exist. For example Camden Consortium with Good Practices in Mental Health (GPMH) have produced information from views of users. This is given under six main headings:

1. Hospital admission.
2. Safety.
3. Physical surroundings.
4. Hospital staff.
5. Treatment.
6. Rights.

Similar work has been carried out at the Bethlem and Maudsley Trust, where a number of discussion groups with service users has led to the production of two questionnaires to survey the views of in-patients.

Patients' Complaints

Complaints are most likely to be initiated with nurses at ward level. Recently there has been progress towards empowering nurses to deal with complaints on the spot. Most hospitals have a local complaints policy that provides guidance to nurses and other front-line staff in dealing with complaints. Current practice is that nurses to whom a complaint is made actively attempt to resolve matters informally, there and then. Where this cannot be achieved because the explanation is not accepted or involves a multiplicity of issues or warrants a fuller investigation, complainants are encouraged to make a formal complaint. An offer is made to refer details to the Complaints Officer, who will instigate an investigation. On becoming aware of a complaint, nursing staff are trained to elicit relevant information, reassure on confidentiality and advise the complainant of the procedure, aided by publicity material.

Regular monitoring of complaints reveals a cross-section of types of complaints by psychiatric in-patients. Unlike the information gathered through satisfaction surveys, complaints are most commonly about the standards and appropriateness of medical and nursing care in relation to assessment, diagnosis and treatment. Complaints about nurses' behaviour also feature highly, especially that nurses' are disrespectful or ignore patients' wishes.

SUMMARY

This chapter has described the changes that have occurred on psychiatric wards and the role of the in-patient mental health nurse. It is time to shift the discussion from community versus institutional care and concentrate instead on transforming services so that they are responsive, coordinated and offer real choice to users. There appears to be a place for in-patient care; in fact it seems that in many cases good community care depends on adequate in-patient facilities. Scott (1995) suggests that mental health services should not regard hospital and community services as opposites but see the role of in-patient care as part of the range of services. Admission to in-patient units is usually needed by those who are acutely or severely ill (particularly if they or their families are unable to cope with community support alone), those who may be a danger to themselves or others and those who need respite.

The polarities of opinion regarding community and institutional care are often of little use to service users. Fortunately, this divide is being bridged by a number of initiatives, often nursing led, which are beginning to address the community care–hospital interface. Many of these initiatives adopt the philosophy of patient-centred care, not just of health but of social care too, where a range of services ensures appropriate care for people at different stages of illness and disability. These include the Key Worker approach where the patient is clearly assigned to one professional with continuing responsibility for that patient, whether in hospital or the community. Rainsford and Cann (1994) describe the use of 'bridging therapy' on a mental health unit dealing with people with acute psychosis. The nursing staff have developed a system of follow-up and outreach as a means of bridging the gap between hospital and community care. Other initiatives include the rotation of ward nurses and community nurses and the use of models of psychiatric, consultation, liaison nursing (Tunmore and Thomas, 1992).

It is expected that in-patient wards will progressively decrease in size and will focus exclusively on brief admissions, stabilization through rapid neuroleptic medication and early discharge. The nurse's role in caring for concentrated numbers of very disturbed patients needs to be reviewed and new models of care needed to be developed. These models must encompass some of the fundamental principles upon which previous care was based. Regardless of how severely disturbed today's in-patients may be, they still need to be listened to and, where possible, understood. More than ever, they need help with problem solving and require social and emotional support.

KEY CONCEPTS

- The total number of psychiatric in-patient beds has been declining steadily over a number of years.
- In many cases good community care depends on adequate in-patient facilities.
- The dynamics of in-patient wards can be used to direct therapeutic or anti-therapeutic use.
- Forming relationships is considered to be a therapeutic tool provided by an in-patient environment.
- In-patient wards will focus on brief admissions, rapid stabilization and early discharge.
- Most acute in-patient services are now expected to cope with patients with disturbed behaviour and those who present with management difficulties.

REFERENCES

Abroms G: Defining milieu therapy. *Arch Gen Psychiatry* 21:553, 1969.

Altschul A: *Patient–nurse interaction: a study of interactive patterns in acute psychiatric wards.* Edinburgh, 1972, Churchill Livingstone.

Batcup D, Thomas B: Mixing the genders, an ethical dilemma: how nursing theory has dealt with sexuality and gender. *Nurs Ethics: Int J Health Care Prof* 1(1):43,1994.

Bebbington POE *et al.*: Inner London collaborative audit of admissions in two health districts (ii): ethnicity and the use of the Mental Health Act. *Br J Psychiatry* 165 (6):743, 1994.

Caldicott F, Lelliott P, Thompson C: *Monitoring Inner London mental illness service.* London, 1994, Royal College of Psychiatrists.

Copperman J, Burrows F: Reducing the risk of sexual assault. *Nurs Times* 88(26):64, 1992

Cormack D: *Psychiatric nursing described.* Edinburgh, 1983, Churchill Livingstone.

Dix R, Williams K: Psychiatric intensive care units, a design for living. *Psychiatr*

Bull 20(9)527-529, 1996.

Doyle MC: Egalitarianism in a mental health centre: an experiment that failed. *Hosp Community Psychiatry* 28:521, 1977.

Fewtrell GW, Toms DA: Patterns of discussion in traditional and novel ward-round procedures. *Br J Med Psychol* 58(1):57, 1985.

Flannigan CB *et al.*: Inner London collaborative audit of admissions in two health districts (i): introduction, methods and preliminary findings. *Br J Psychiatry* 166(6):734, 1994a.

Flannigan CB *et al.*: Inner London collaborative audit of admissions in two health districts (iii): reasons for admission to psychiatric wards. *Br J Psychiatry* 165(6):750, 1994b.

Glazier S, May P: Changing cultural norms. *IHSM Network* 2(25):6, 1995.

Goldberg D: Filters to care: a model. In: Jenkins R, Griffiths S, editors: *Indicators for mental health in the population.* London, 1990, HMSO.

Goldstone LA, Doggett DP: *Psychiatric nursing monitor: an audit of the quality of nursing care in psychiatric wards.* Leeds, 1989, Poly Enterprises.

Gostin L: *Institutions observed: towards a new concept of secure provision in mental health*. London, 1986, King's Fund.

Gunderson J: Defining the therapeutic process in therapeutic milieus. *Psychiatry* 41:327, 1978.

Gutheil TG: The therapeutic milieu: changing themes and theories. *Hosp Community Psychiatry* 36(12):1279, 1985

Guze BH, Unutzer J: Studies of psychiatric inpatients. In: Freeman HL, Kupfer DJ, editors: *Curr Opin Psychiatry* 6(2):233, 1993.

Handy J: Stress and contradiction in psychiatric nursing. *Hum Relat* 44(1):39, 1991.

Hickling FW: Psychiatric hospital admission rates in Jamaica, 1971 and 1988. *Br J Psychiatry* 159:817, 1991.

HMSO: *Finding a place: a review of mental health services for adults*. Audit Commission, London, 1994, HMSO.

Howard D, Hurst K: *The Central Nottinghamshire psychiatric nursing audit*. Nottingham, 1987, Central Nottinghamshire Health Authority.

Jackson M, Cawley R: Psychodynamics and psychotherapy on an acute psychiatric ward: the story of an experimental unit. *Br J Psychiatry* 160:41, 1992.

Jones M: *Social Psychiatry in practice. A study of therapeutic communities*, Tavistock, 1952, London.

Lamb HR: When the chronically mentally ill need acute hospitalisation: maximising its benefits. *Psychiatr Ann* 18:426, 1988.

Leff J *et al.*: A trial of family therapy v a relatives' group for schizophrenia. *Br J Psychiatry* 154(1):58, 1989.

London M: Mental illness among immigrant minorities in the United Kingdom. *Br J Psychiatry* 149(34-36):265, 1986.

Martin T: Psychiatric nurses' use of working time. *Nurs Stand* 6(37):3436, 1992.

McIver S: *Obtaining the views of users of mental health services*. London, 1991, King's Fund Centre for Health Services Development.

MILMIS Project Group: Monitoring Inner London mental illness services. *Psychiatr Bull* 19(5):276, 1995.

Nilberts D, Crossmaster M: Assaults against residents of a psychiatric institution: residents' history of abuse. *J Interpers Violence* 4:342, 1989.

Osmond H: *Function as the basis of psychiatric ward design*.

Pilgrim D, Rogers A: *A sociology of mental health and illness*. Buckingham, 1993, Open University Press.

Pollock L: The multidisciplinary team. In: Hume C, Pullen I, editors: *Rehabilitation in psychiatry*. Edinburgh, 1986, Churchill Livingstone.

Powell G, Caan W, Crowe M: What events precede violent incidents in psychiatric hospitals? *Br J Psychiatry* 165(1):107, 1994.

Prior L: Mind, body and behaviour; theorisations of madness and the organisation of therapy. *Sociology* 25(3):403, 1991.

Prior L: *The social organisation of mental illness*. London, 1993, Sage.

Queen VA: Inpatient psychiatric nursing care. In: Stuart GW, Sundeen SJ: *Principles and practice of psychiatric nursing*. St Louis, 1995, Mosby.

Rainsford E, Caan W: Experience of supervising discharges. *J Clin Nurs* 3(3):133, 1994.

Ranger S: *Functioning of the multidisciplinary team: a study of 3 teams in a psychiatric rehabilitation setting [dissertation]*. London, 1986, Institute of Psychiatry.

Raphael W: *Psychiatric hospitals viewed by their patients*. London, 1972, King Edward's Hospital Fund for London.

Rhys–Hearn C, Potts D: The effect of patients' individual characteristics upon activity times for items of nursing. *Int J Nurs Stud* 15(1):23, 1978.

Robinson KD: Are nurses fulfilling their proper role? Measuring cultural trends in mental health nursing care. *Psychiatr Care* 2(1):27, 1995.

Sanson–Fisher RW, Poole AD, Harker J: Behavioural analysis of ward rounds within a general hospital psychiatric unit. *Behav Res Therapy* 17:333, 1979.

Sayce L: Response to violence: a framework for fair treatment. In: Crichton J: *Psychiatric patient violence: risk and response*. London, 1995, Duckworth.

Sayce L *et al.*: Users' perspective on emergency needs. In: Phelan M, Strathdee G, Thornicroft G, editors: *Emergency mental health services in the community*. Cambridge, 1995, Cambridge University Press.

Scott J: Mental health services. In: Merry P, editor: *NHS handbook 1995/96*, ed 10. Tunbridge Wells, Kent, 1995, JMH Publishing.

Sovie M: Variable costs of nursing care in hospitals. *Ann Rev Nurs Res* 6:131, 1988.

Tarrier N *et al.*: The community management of schizophrenia: a controlled trial of behavioural intervention with families to reduce relapse. *Br J Psychiatry* 153(5):532, 1988.

Thomas B: *Rethinking acute in-patient psychiatric care*. Presented at the Australian and New Zealand Psychiatric Nurses 21st International Conference, Canberra, October 1995.

Thomas B, Smedley N: *Reasons for admission to acute psychiatric wards*, Unpublished report, Bethlem and Maudsley NHS Trust, 1995.

Treanor J, Cotch K: Staffing of adult inpatient facilities. *Hosp Community Psychiatry* 41(5):545, 1990.

Tunmore R, Thomas B: Models of psychiatric consultation liaison nursing. *BJN* 1(9):447,1992.

Willmot M *et al.*: *Evaluating audit: a review of audit activity in the nursing and therapy professions: findings of a national survey*. London, 1995, CASPE Research.

FURTHER READING

Beishon S, Virdee S, Hagell A: *Nursing in a multi-ethnic NHS*. London, 1995 Policy Studies Institute.
> *This book describes the racial harassment of ethnic minority staff throughout the NHS and discusses further policy implications.*

Department of Health: *24 hour nursed care for people with severe and enduring mental illness*. London, 1996, Department of Health.
> *This report describes a study aimed at looking at the need for 24-hour staffed accommodation for severely mentally ill patients as an alternative to acute hospital care. It suggests that 24-hour nursing care will release acute beds that are needed for other patients requiring intensive short-term care.*

Hawton K, Cowen P, editors: *Dilemmas and difficulties in the management of psychiatric patients*. Oxford, 1990, Oxford Medical Publications.
> *This book provides a wealth of practical clinical guidance by addressing some of the dilemmas and difficulties that arise in psychiatric practice.*

Hearn J, Sheppard DL, Tancred–Sheriff P, Burrell G: *The sexuality of organization*. London, 1992, Sage publications.
> *A collection of essays that examines sexuality in organizations including the labour process, sexual harassment and men's sexuality. It shows various ways in which the very processes of organizations reflect power relations suffused with dominant forms of sexuality.*

Vincent C, editor: *Clinical risk management*. London, 1995, BMJ Publishing Group.
> *This provides a comprehensive guide to the principles of risk management. It will assist nurses to recognize potential risks in the clinical area and suggests ways of dealing with them.*

Watkins M, Hervey N, Carson J, Ritter S: *Collaborative community mental health care*. London, 1996, Arnold.
> *A particularly useful and up-to-date text describing the multiprofessional team approach to modern mental health services.*

Liaison Mental Health Nursing and Mental Health Consultation

<table>
<tr><td>

Learning Outcomes

....

After studying this chapter, you should be able to:

• Define liaison mental health nursing.

• Identify mental health problems related to the key areas of *The Health of the Nation*, *(Department of Health, 1992)*.

• Describe a model of mental health consultation.

• Outline the process of consultation.

• Compare and contrast consultation with other types of collaborative activity.

• Identify role characteristics of the mental health nurse involved in liaison and consultation activities.

</td><td>

CHAPTER OUTLINE

• *Liaison mental health nursing*

• *Mental health consultation*

• *The consultation process in liaison mental health nursing*

• *Education and training*

</td></tr>
</table>

L*iaison mental health nursing is a component part* of mental health nursing linked closely with liaison psychiatry and other areas of nursing (Box 15.1). It is concerned with assessment, treatment, care, study and prevention of mental health problems among people with physical illness. Often the terms 'liaison' and 'consultation' are used interchangeably to describe a range of activities and processes. Here, consultation is used to describe a specific form of collaborative work between professionals. Interprofessional consultation is one person helping another with a particular problem without taking on the responsibility of the solution.

LIAISON MENTAL HEALTH NURSING

AN OUTLINE OF LIAISON WORK

Liaison mental health nursing usually involves the mental health nurse applying skills and knowledge to the care of patients with physical illnesses and somatic complaints, in a general hospital setting. Liaison mental health nurses (LMHNs) may work with patients who express their emotional distress through somatic disorders and many are skilled in the assessment and care of patients following deliberate self-harm. Liaison mental health nurses also provide support for staff as part of their routine practice, for example, through clinical supervision, and through difficult or stressful situations. This involves close working relationships and collaboration with other professionals. The LMHN may be integrated into a multidisciplinary clinical team, attend multidisciplinary meetings, case conferences and ward rounds and provide education and support for non-psychiatric colleagues in a range of settings.

Liaison refers to acts of communication or cooperation between different groups, units or services, whose work focus is usually different. Liaison psychiatry is an umbrella term used to cover clinical practice in a range of settings and services. Lipowski (1981) defines liaison psychiatry as 'the diagnosis, treatment, study and prevention of psychiatric morbidity in the physically ill, of somatoform and factitious

Box 15.1

The goals of liaison mental health nursing

....

- To promote mental health care in a range of different services and settings.
- To prevent the escalation of mental health problems and reduce psychiatric morbidity among patients with physical health problems.
- To establish the effect of mental health problems on treatment and care in physical illness.
- To enable non-psychiatric colleagues to promote mental health as a routine part of their work.
- To evaluate the effect on patient well-being and hospital resources when mental health problems are recognized and followed with appropriate interventions.
- To identify areas where mental health problems go unrecognized and are unattended.
- To develop collaborative working arrangements with colleagues in other services in a range of different settings.

disorders, and of psychological factors affecting physical conditions'. This gives a broad definition of the scope of practice in the field. Each of the activities and components in the definition are themselves wide ranging and diverse. Such a broad definition is appropriate for clinical practice at the interface of psychiatry and medicine. Lloyd (1980) suggests that liaison psychiatry should remain ill-defined, as it is a style and locus of practice rather than a discrete subspecialty.

HISTORICAL DEVELOPMENT

The origins of liaison psychiatry lie in the 1930s when the term 'psychiatric liaison' was first used in the USA (Lloyd, 1980; Lipowski, 1983). Psychiatric liaison units were established in, and became a key part of, general hospital-based mental health services by the 1980s as psychiatry aligned itself with medicine. Liaison mental health nursing has evolved as a response to psychosocial problems of patients admitted to general hospitals with physical illnesses (Robinson, 1982).

There are many accounts of the role of the LMHN, in various clinical settings, from the USA, where liaison mental health nursing and mental health consultation are a well established component of advanced nursing practice (Robinson, 1982). The American Nurses Association (ANA) Council on Psychiatric and Mental Health Nursing have published standards for psychiatric consultation liaison nursing (ANA, 1990). There is a small but increasing amount of literature from British mental health nurses involved in liaison mental health nursing (Jones, 1989; Tunmore, 1990, 1994; Regel and Davies, 1995).

The incidence of psychiatric morbidity among general hospital patients in Britain is well documented (Torem *et al.*, 1979; Sensky *et al.*, 1985; Brown and Cooper, 1987; House and Jones, 1987). Estimates of psychiatric morbidity among medical in-patients are 30–65% (Gomez, 1987). A review of London's specialist health services (Department of Health (DoH) 1993a) reports mental illness in up to 25% of acute

medical admissions, and alcohol problems in 30% of medical and surgical admissions. As many as 50% of patients in all medical specialties referred for investigation do not have physical disorders to account for their symptoms.

Psychiatric units may provide services in liaison with specialties such as neurosciences, cardiac, cancer and renal services, plastic surgery, orthopaedics, paediatric surgery, and neonatal intensive care. Regel and Davies (1995) identify other areas, including critical care, burns and accident and emergency departments. Psychiatric problems may be associated with post-traumatic stress disorder, somatization disorders, chronic pain, chronic fatigue syndrome, multiple sclerosis, and irritable bowel syndrome.

THE HEALTH OF THE NATION

For the first time, targets for promotion of health and prevention of illness in the United Kingdom have been set out. *The Health of the Nation* (DoH, 1992) addresses priorities for improving health and quality of life and reducing preventable deaths in five key areas:

1. Coronary heart disease and stroke.
2. Cancers.
3. Mental illness.
4. HIV/AIDS and sexual health.
5. Accidents.

These targets present a great challenge to all nurses. Mental health nurses are in a unique position since they can apply their skills and knowledge across each of these areas. While mental illness is one of the key areas, it is not a mutually exclusive category. It coexists with each of the other areas (Figure 15.1). Psychiatric liaison encourages collaboration with colleagues from elsewhere and enables mental health nurses to promote mental health in each of the key areas.

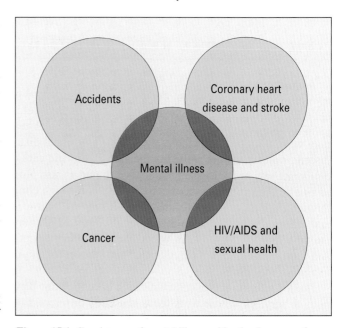

Figure 15.1 Coexistence of mental illness with other key areas from the *Health of the Nation*

There are many psychiatric problems and mental health interventions associated with the key areas. For example, substance misuse involves a range of behaviours with major consequences for the health and well-being of individuals with various physical health problems. It has direct implications for health promotion in all key areas. It is associated with a high proportion of heart conditions, cancers, HIV transmission, unplanned pregnancy, sudden death and suicides (DoH, 1994).

The Health of the Nation and Suicide

The Health of the Nation (DoH, 1992) uses suicide rates as one measure for mental illness targets. Reduction of the overall suicide rate can result from improvements in other key areas identified in. For example, suicide may be related to a diagnosis of AIDS or cancer.

It is inappropriate to generalize from data on suicide from other countries and cultures. Local cultural and religious influences may militate against a verdict of suicide as the cause of death. Definitions of suicide for research purposes may be different from official definitions. Contradictions in statistics may be caused by different criteria being used for selection of patients and classification of information. See Chapter 17 for a more detailed discussion.

Coronary Heart Disease and Stroke

Many studies have investigated the role of psychosocial factors in heart disease (Box 15.2). High levels of anxiety have been identified among patients following their first heart attack (Thompson, 1989). Treatment for hypertension appears to increase reports of psychosomatic symptoms, emotional problems, feelings of depression and unhappiness. Depression and low mood among this group of patients may be attributed to the side-effects of medication (Goldberg *et al.*, 1980).

Psychiatric complications following open heart surgery are reported in 32% of patients (Smith and Dimsdale, 1989). These include disorientation to place and time, perceptual illusions, delirium, hallucinations, paranoid ideation and agitation.

Patel *et al.* (1985) demonstrate the effectiveness of behavioural modification and the cognitive reappraisal techniques of cognitive therapy among patients with hypertension.

Box 15.2 *The health of the nation — coronary heart disease and stroke*

- Over 30% of open heart surgery patients may experience psychiatric disorder (Smith and Dimsdale, 1989).
- 25% of patients experience major depression while 20–40% experience minor depression following a stroke (Robinson *et al.*,1983; Eastwood *et al.*,1989; Morris *et al.* 1990).
- Anxiety disorders have been reported in up to 27% of stroke patients (Castillo *et al.*,1993). Generalized anxiety disorders are a common accompaniment to major depression in stroke patients (Starkstein *et al.*,1990).

Intervention significantly reduced the level of blood pressure over a 4-year period. Wadden (1983) found relaxation training an effective treatment for some patients. Stress management and behavioural techniques, including breathing exercises, relaxation and meditation, appear to reduce heart disease and the complications of hypertension. These may provide the basis for a cost-effective primary prevention programme to reduce risk factors for coronary heart disease.

Mental health promotion is a component of rehabilitation programmes for patients following myocardial infarction. Programmes may address stressful situations, anticipation of chest pain, emotional reactions such as anger, anxiety, depression and irritation and the importance of social networks, work and leisure activities and physical exercise (Fridlund *et al.*, 1992).

Lipowski (1983) identifies the need for liaison psychiatry services for the elderly. He observes how elderly patients with cognitive impairment are often viewed as a nuisance on medical and surgical wards. Goodstein (1983) describes a psychiatric consultation liaison service for elderly patients following cerebrovascular accidents. Stroke patients who fail to show signs of improvement are sometimes viewed as malingerers who desire dependent relationships. Stockwell (1972) suggests that general nurses least enjoy caring for those suffering from illnesses that they consider should be cared for elsewhere. However, she also reports that older, dependent stroke patients are among those that nurses enjoy caring for most.

To most patients, the most distressing aspect of a sudden stroke with its unpredictable rate and extent of recovery, is the loss of control they experience. Anxious preoccupation about having another stroke may lead to patterns of avoidance behaviour.

The patient's response to a stroke is influenced by practical consequences related to loss of function, reaction of others, availability of social support, physical appearance and sexuality, finance and additional illnesses. The nature of the disability may assume significance in relation to earlier life events. Patients may report fears of death, insanity, disfigurement and loss of physical function. They may develop feelings of guilt, experiencing the stroke as punishment, and rationalize previous behaviour to explain the illness. A stroke, just like a diagnosis of cancer or AIDS, may be perceived as life threatening. Severe and distressing psychological reactions usually associated with bereavement, such as denial, bargaining and depression are common consequences (Fedoroff *et al.*, 1991).

Many depressed stroke patients remain untreated. Treatment depends on recognition and acknowledgement of depression. Acceptance of depression as a natural grief reaction and lack of awareness of depression may account for the discrepancy between the numbers of stroke patients with depression and those treated for it (Feibel and Springer, 1982; Finklestein *et al.*, 1987).

Armstrong (1991) argues that emotional distress is the result of cognitive and physiological processes in stroke patients. Inability to relate experience to expression and the dissociation of these gives rise to psychological distress.

However, Castillo *et al.* (1993) link the site of the lesion with the type and severity of psychiatric problem. Anxiety experienced by stroke patients may result from pathophysiological processes occurring after a stroke rather than a psychological reaction either to the stroke or to decreased independence. Their research suggests that right hemisphere lesions are more frequently associated with patients experiencing anxiety alone while anxiety and depression are more likely in patients with left sided lesions. Anxiety appears to be commoner among depressed than non-depressed patients.

Cerebrovascular accidents are associated with prior alcohol abuse among patients (Starkstein *et al.*, 1990; Casteillo *et al.*, 1993). Chick *et al.* (1985) report effective interventions for alcohol related problems among general hospital in-patients in a randomized controlled trial. They recommend routine nursing assessment and screening involving brief counselling interventions for early detection of alcohol problems. This intervention should coincide with recovery from medical illness, when patients are more amenable to advice, support and information.

Box 15.3   *The Health of the Nation — Cancers*

Mortality rates where suicide is established as the cause of death are higher among cancer patients:
- During the first year following diagnosis (Allebeck *et al.*, 1989).
- During the first 2 years following diagnosis (Storm *et al.*, 1992).
- With lung cancer, cancers of the gastro-intestinal system and cancer of the mouth and pharynx (Allebeck and Bolund, 1991).
- With non-localized cancers compared with localized cancers or where the extent of the disease is unknown (Louhivouri and Hakama, 1979; Storm *et al.*, 1992).
- With advanced or rapidly progressing cancer (Bolund, 1985).
- Not having treatment (Louhivouri and Hakama, 1979).

Box 15.4   *The Health of the Nation — HIV and AIDS*

- Severe depressive illness has been reported in 17% of hospitalized AIDS patients (Perry and Tross, 1984).
- Rates of non-opiate substance abuse are significantly higher than those of the general population (Atkinson *et al.*, 1988).
- There is a higher level of suicidal ideation among patients who are HIV positive but who had not developed AIDS than among patients diagnosed with AIDS (McKegney *et al.*, 1992).
- The likelihood of psychiatric problems such as delirium and dementia is high among patients diagnosed with AIDS (McKegney and O'Dowd, 1992)
- Mental illness has been identified among as many as 80–90% of gay men with HIV infection (Perry and Tross, 1984; WHO, 1988).
- HIV dementia is prevalent among 10–15% of people known to be HIV positive (McArther *et al.*, 1994).

Suicide, coronary heart disease and stroke

There appears to be relatively little research to link suicide with cardiac problems (Hacket and Stern, 1987) and strokes. Farberow *et al.* (1966) match characteristics from case records of suicide with non-suicide controls among a sample of patients with respiratory and cardiac disease. An increased risk of suicide seems to be linked to higher levels of agitation, depression and anxiety. High dependency combined with dissatisfaction, complaining behaviour and a lack of support from family and hospital are other risk factors. The importance of a close and supportive relationship in suicide prevention is emphasized (Badger, 1990). In the absence of research into the relationship among heart disease, stroke and suicide, over-inclusion of suicide risk factors may be preferable to under-estimation of risk.

Cancer

A high level of psychiatric disorder is reported among cancer patients. Psychological distress and psychiatric disorders are prevalent during the first 2 years after diagnosis (Derogatis *et al.*, 1983). Specialist cancer centres have encouraged the development of psychological care and liaison mental health nursing (Tunmore, 1989).

Mental illness and psychological distress may be more prominent at particular stages of the disease. Psychiatric morbidity increases following diagnosis and news of recurrent disease (Moorey and Greer, 1989). Links between high anxiety levels and the end of chemotherapy and radiotherapy treatment have been identified and relate to outcome (Peck and Bolland, 1977; Forester *et al.*, 1987). Problems such as delirium, dementia, depression and psychosis affect compliance with treatment (Goldberg, 1983). Attention to coping strategies and proper assessment of cancer patients may prevent or help to reduce non-compliance.

Breast cancer accounts for 22% of all cancer diagnoses. About 20% of women who have had mastectomy for breast cancer develop mental illness following surgery (Morris *et al.*, 1977; Maguire *et al.*, 1978). Higher levels of anxiety and depression have been found among women on chemotherapy (Payne, 1989). The relationship of psychological responses and breast cancer has been linked to attitudes towards cancer. Watson *et al.* (1991) suggest that a fatalistic attitude, characterized by lack of control, is related to a tendency to control emotional responses. Interventions that encourage expression of feeling will help develop coping strategies and may improve the patient's quality of life.

Suicide and cancer

The risk of suicide among cancer patients is greater than for the general population (Storm *et al.*, 1992), clearly indicating the need for preventive psychological support and care (Box 15.3). Poisoning is the commonest means of both suicide and parasuicide among cancer patients. Poisoning and drowning are commoner among women and hanging, jumping from a great height and shooting are common among men with cancer (Allebeck and Bolund, 1991).

Research on differences between the sexes in suicide rates has been inconclusive or contradictory. Allebeck and Bolund (1991) report similar rates, though Fox *et al.* (1982) found an increase among men with cancer but not among women. Louhivouri and Hakama (1979) report a higher risk for men than women. Storm *et al.* (1992) found that men have a higher risk than women during the first year following diagnosis. Allebeck and Bolund (1991) found no statistically significant relationship between age group and suicide rate among cancer patients.

HIV/AIDS and Sexual Health

Liaison mental health nursing and psychiatry services have developed in response to problems associated with psychological adjustment to HIV infection and AIDS and management of neuropsychiatric disorder (Grant, 1988; Fernandez *et al.*, 1989). Mental illness occurs in 80–90% of gay men with HIV infection (Perry and Tross, 1984; WHO, 1988). These high levels follow diagnosis and include anxiety, depression, guilt and despair as part of an adjustment reaction (Box 15.4). Neuropsychiatric problems among patients with HIV infection are wide ranging and include both cognitive and motor impairment. Psychotic symptoms such as elevated mood, ideas of grandeur, delusions, hallucinations and blunted and inappropriate affect may be present (Vogel-Scibilia *et al.*, 1988; Kieburtz *et al.*, 1991).

Testing for HIV infection appears to produce transient mood disturbance; pre and post test counselling may successfully reduce this (Ironson *et al.*, 1990; Perry *et al.*, 1990). Uncertainty about the future course of the illness may lead to a higher level of distress. Chuang *et al.* (1989) argue that earlier stages of the disease involve more threatening stressors than those involved with coping with death and dying, for example, fear of pain, isolation, rejection, and general fear of the unknown.

High rates of depression are common (Law *et al.*, 1993) and severe depressive illness has been reported in 17% of hospitalized AIDS patients (Perry and Tross, 1984). Rates of alcohol abuse in this group vary but rates of other substance abuse, non-opiate, mainly cannabis and psychostimulants, are significantly higher than in the general population (Atkinson *et al.*, 1988). The DoH (1994) call for training on the social, emotional and behavioural issues in sexual health and drug misuse for all staff involved in health care.

The relationship between the presence or absence of physical symptoms of HIV infection and mental state has been investigated (Atkinson *et al.*, 1988; Gorman *et al.*, 1991; Kessler *et al.*, 1991). High levels of self-reported problems appear to be associated with an increased rate of psychiatric illness and mental health problems (Wilkins *et al.*, 1991; Law *et al.*, 1993). Distress associated with uncertainty may be replaced by 'acceptance' following AIDS diagnosis. Alternatively, certainty and awareness of the diagnosis may help some to face fears and achieve a sense of control through the development of different perspectives, new meanings or understanding.

Other psychosocial factors, such as knowing others who have died or are dying of HIV related illnesses and lack of social support may increase the level of distress experienced, for example, lack of a close confidant–someone to talk to about serious problems–may increase the likelihood of depression (Ostrow *et al.*, 1989).

Suicide, HIV and AIDS

Several studies examine the incidence of suicide among people with HIV and AIDS (Seth *et al.*, 1991; McKegney and O'Dowd, 1992). Seth *et al.* (1991) review the psychiatric illnesses among patients referred to a liaison psychiatry team over a 1-year period. Out of a total of 60, 32 were depressed. Suicidal intentions were expressed by 10 of these and 1 committed suicide. Marzuk *et al.* (1988) report that men diagnosed with AIDS and aged 30–39 years are 36 times more likely to commit suicide than those in the general population of the same age but AIDS free. The risk of suicide is highest in the first 6 months following the diagnosis of AIDS. Suicide may be impulsive with little or no prior indication (Chuang *et al.*, 1989).

Charlton *et al.* (1993) link the rise in mortality since 1984 among men aged 15–44 years to suicides, open verdicts and AIDS. While AIDS may not be recorded as a cause of death, HIV infection and AIDS may be involved in the increased rate of suicide and open verdicts. Marzuk *et al.* (1988) suggest that AIDS related suicides are underestimated and that suicide may be 'hidden'. Deaths may be related to intravenous drug use, overdoses of prescribed medication and treatment refusal or non-compliance. The availability of social support, the opportunity to share common experiences with others and the reduction of stigmata related to HIV infection and AIDS may reduce the numbers of AIDS related suicides (Charlton *et al.*, 1993).

Accidents

The Health of the Nation (1992) addresses accidents in a wide context. Here the focus is on the role of the mental health nurse in the accident and emergency department and the level of psychiatric morbidity among patients attending general hospital casualty services.

Deliberate self-harm, depression, schizophrenia, personality disorders and drug and alcohol dependence are among the commonest diagnoses of attenders at accident and emergency departments (Anstee, 1972; Friedman *et al.*, 1983; Hillard *et al.*, 1983). Psychiatric assessment of violent or threatening behaviour in the accident and emergency department may result in referral to appropriate psychiatric services (McNiel *et al.*, 1992).

Salkovskis *et al.* (1990) divide accident and emergency attenders into four main categories depending on the factors influencing their attendance: psychiatric emergencies (overt psychological symptoms), psychiatric problems (e.g. self-poisoning, alcohol ingestion), physical ailments strongly influenced by psychological factors and physical ailments with little or no psychological influence. Their study reports a rate of persistent psychiatric disturbance just under 50% across each of these categories.

Storer *et al.* (1987) show that referral to a community psychiatric nurse linked to the accident and emergency department significantly reduce unnecessary and inappropriate demands on general medical services. They report a decrease in the number of GP visits and an overall reduction in NHS use as a result of community psychiatric nursing intervention. The study identifies a demand for mental health care and demonstrates the feasibility of liaison mental health nursing services in this setting.

Drug misuse is associated with fatal overdose, physical injury and accidental injuries such as road traffic accidents, burns and head injuries (English National Board for Nursing, Midwifery and Health Visiting (ENB), 1995).

Alcohol is a known cause of accidents and often a factor in suicide and attempted suicide (Royal College of Psychiatrists, 1988). Drug and alcohol misusers make heavy demands on the accident and emergency department.

Despite these research findings, what constitutes appropriate use of accident and emergency departments in general hospitals is the focus of some debate. Sheehan (1992) suggests that fear, ignorance and tradition resulted in the rejection of a resolution at the 1991 Royal College of Nursing Congress supporting the employment of psychiatric nurses in casualty departments of all general hospitals. Research suggests that many people visit the casualty department with complaints that could be treated in general practice (Myers, 1982; Davison *et al.*, 1983; Warren, 1989). However, if services are to reflect consumer demand then accident and emergency departments may need to adapt for the groups of patient that attend. Storer *et al.* (1987) cite research findings from the 1960s and 1970s indicating that while the accident and emergency department is an obvious choice for both crisis management and community mental health intervention, liaison psychiatry services have failed to develop as expected in this location. Anstee (1972) argues that psychiatric services should be part of the total service provided through the casualty department. Atha *et al.* (1989) argue that the development of community based mental health services and the reduction of in-patient psychiatric beds may lead to the accident and emergency department being the only medical service open to patients on demand. The community psychiatric nurse may have an increasingly active part to play in provision of mental health services through accident and emergency departments.

Deliberate self-harm

Deliberate self-harm is one of the commonest psychiatric diagnoses reported by accident and emergency services (Anstee, 1972; Friedman *et al.*, 1983; Hillard *et al.*, 1983). Evidence suggests that accident and emergency based psychiatric services may reduce the suicide rate among attenders. Catalan *et al.* (1980) examined the ability of nurses to assess deliberate self-poisoning patients and suggest that such assessment services could be set up easily in most district general hospitals. Hillard *et al.* (1983) compared the suicide rate among the general population with that of the psychiatric emergency service population and found a far higher risk among attenders. The risk appeared particularly high among patients diagnosed with affective disorders, substance misuse and schizophrenia and those who made repeated visits to the emergency service. Psychiatric services linked to accident and emergency departments are an important development in services for those most at risk of suicide.

Liaison psychiatry services are identified in *The Health of the Nation* as cost-effective means of providing a mental health service in different settings. The costs of such high quality services may be offset against the amount of money spent on, for example, inappropriate investigations and unnecessary or extended hospital admissions. The cost-effectiveness of liaison psychiatry services has been demonstrated in a range of settings besides those key areas set out in *The Health of the Nation* (Levitan and Kornfeld, 1981; Mumford *et al.*, 1984; Hammer, 1990; James and Hamilton, 1991; Strain *et al.*, 1991).

MENTAL HEALTH CONSULTATION

Mental health consultation may be incorporated into community programmes for promotion of mental health, prevention of mental disease treatment and rehabilitation of people with mental illness. This preventive approach, operating at primary, secondary and tertiary levels of prevention, is in keeping with mental health promotion programmes (see Chapter 12).

Consultation activities provide a vehicle for promotion of mental health and prevention of mental illness and suicide in a range of non-psychiatric settings including voluntary organizations, housing departments and associations, education services, youth groups, the criminal justice system, employers, trade unions and local media.

An increasing proportion of programmes is delivered by professionals with no specialist preparation in psychiatry, mental health nursing or psychiatric social work. Mental health problems can be managed by the primary care team where staff have received appropriate training. However, the Audit Commission (1994) survey of mental health services in England and Wales suggests that cooperation between mental health care services, social services and primary health care teams needs to be improved. Training in the management of mental health problems is not a routine part of staff education in primary health care settings. For example, less than 20% of practice nurses are qualified mental health nurses and less than 40% of GPs have experience in psychiatry.

The DoH (1994) review of mental health nursing suggests a framework for collaborative work by nurses, midwives and health visitors in preventive mental health care (Table 15.1). The report recommends collaboration between mental health nurses and their non-psychiatric colleagues on the primary health care team, including health visitors, district nurses, school nurses and practice nurses. Interagency working and collaboration will help to equip non-psychiatric professionals with some of the skills they require to manage a range of mental health problems in the community. Mental health consultation is one form of collaborative work that can be included within this framework.

Mental health consultation is a means of improving the professional practice of non-psychiatric professionals and of contributing to the overall standard of mental health care. Consultation benefits the patient as it may enable them to remain under the care of the main professional carer, without unnecessary or inappropriate referral to a specialist mental health service. The non-psychiatric professional benefits through learning how to manage problems they would otherwise consider beyond their capabilities. If others are equipped with the appropriate skills, mental health nurses can focus their attention and services on the needs of people with more severe or serious mental health problems. The reasons for specialist psychiatric referral may become more clearly identified and result in a better and more appropriate use of the services available.

CAPLAN'S MODEL OF MENTAL HEALTH CONSULTATION

Caplan (1964) describes a model of mental health consultation developed as part of a programme of mental health promotion and prevention of mental health problems. The model identifies four types of consultation based on the main emphasis of the consultation:
1. Client-centred case consultation.
2. Programme-centred administrative consultation.
3. Consultee-centred case consultation.
4. Consultee-centred administrative consultation.

For each type of consultation the primary focus is either a case problem or an administrative problem associated with a mental health programme. The route of the consultant's intervention may be direct or indirect. The consultant is responsible for identifying the most appropriate type of consultation for a given situation (Figure 15.2).

Client Centred Case Consultation
The main aim of the consultant is to provide appropriate and effective treatment for the consultee's client following an assessment of the problem. This may involve referral to a specialist or the provision of guidelines for non-specialist management. Education of the consultee is an important secondary function of client-centred consultation.

Programme Centred Administrative Consultation
The consultation focuses on problems of administration of mental health promotion programmes in prevention, treatment or rehabilitation of mental illness. For example, planning and administration of services, policy development and recruitment, training and deployment of staff. The consultant provides a specialist assessment of the programme and recommends a plan of action. Education of the consultee so that they will be better able to deal with similar future problems on their own is a subordinate goal.

Consultee Centred Case Consultation
The main focus for this type of consultation is the consultee and their current work problem. The consultant will talk to the consultee about the client but spend little or no time providing

TABLE 15.1 Areas for consultation and liaison work between nurses, midwives and health visitors and mental health nurses

	Primary prevention	Secondary prevention	Tertiary prevention
Aim	To reduce incidence of mental illness by identifying the vulnerable and at risk	The early detection of mental illness and prompt early intervention	Treatment and active intervention for people with established mental illness
Route			
Mental health nurse involvement	Consultation and liaison	Consultation and liaison casework	Consultation and liaison, treatment, active intervention
Involvement of other professionals	Health visitors, district nurses, school nurses, practice nurses	Health visitors, district nurses, school nurses and practice nurses	Health visitors, district nurses, school nurses and practice nurses
Location of work	Primary health care setting, general hospitals	Primary health care setting, general hospitals	Hospital; residential, day and community care

a specialist assessment. The goal is to improve the consultee's functioning rather than to provide a specialist assessment of the client. The consultant is aware that the consultee is experiencing problems with the client and is therefore likely to hold distorted views and perceptions of the situation. The consultant picks up any internal inconsistencies, omissions and distortions in the consultee's account. The consultant works with the consultee's perceptions to help the consultee resolve the situation. Through this process the consultee increases his or her awareness of the range of issues involved and gains a better understanding of their part in the situation.

Caplan identifies four categories of difficulty experienced by non mental health professionals which interfere with their ability to deal adequately with the mental health problems of their clients. These are a lack of understanding of psychological factors, lack of skill or resources in dealing with the problems, lack of professional objectivity and lack of confidence and self-esteem.

Lack of understanding of psychological factors

The consultee's understanding of psychology and psychopathology is limited or they are at a loss as to how to relate theory to practice in order to understand and address the work problem. The consultant may add to the consultee's knowledge or clarify information about the situation, identifying patterns of psychosocial interaction in a way that is meaningful to the consultee. The type and level of information provided by the consultant must be consistent with that associated with the consultee's profession. This type of consultation aims to educate and develop the consultee without trying to turn him or her into a mental health professional.

Lack of skill

The consultee may lack the necessary skills to deal effectively with the client, for example, the professional use of self in dealing with psychological issues. The consultant assists the consultee to develop a relevant plan of action. The consultant works within the range of action appropriate to the consultee's

level of ability and professional subculture. This activity is similar to supervision in that it focuses on the development of professional skills. The mental health specialist may be able to contribute to training programmes to ensure that appropriate skills are learned effectively in the future.

Lack of objectivity

Even knowledgeable, experienced and skilled professionals may encounter situations where they are unable to function properly through subjective factors. For example, the consultee may identify too closely with a client; something about a case may trigger personal involvement and sensitivity. The consultee's judgement is likely to be distorted and less professionally effective. Caplan refers to this as a 'problem theme' intruding into the professional person's functioning. This may arise from some deep-seated aspect of the consultee's personality or a current personal conflict. The consultee may attribute the discomfort they experience to the client, displacing their own anxiety. The consultant aims to disentangle the consultee's personal life from the work problem. The focus remains on the work problem and the development of a more reality-based set of expectations for the client. The consultation helps the consultee return to professional functioning and re-establish their objectivity.

Lack of confidence and self-esteem

Professional workers without the benefit of adequate supervision and who work alone may be more likely to experience this. The consultee's functioning may be upset by a range of factors including illness, fatigue, infirmity, inexperience or youth. The consultant provides support that promotes a sense of self-esteem and self-confidence, assuming that the consultee is technically competent and able.

Consultee Centred Administrative Consultation

This aims to help the consultee master problems in planning and maintenance of mental health promotion programmes, prevention and control of mental illness and interpersonal dynamics of agency operation.

It is most appropriate for a group of administrators. The consultant acts as a facilitator for the group in addressing interpersonal motivations and interpersonal relations from a group dynamic perspective. Few mental health consultants will have as thorough an understanding of administrative problems as they have of individual psychology. They must exercise caution in limiting the consultation to interpersonal and group dynamic aspects of the administrative situation. The 'theme interference' of consultee-centred consultation also applies to this approach. The consultant needs to be cautious about their role becoming that of the supervisor or group psychotherapist. Mental health consultants need to complement their traditional knowledge of their own profession with further study of administration, human resource management and social sciences, to operate effectively in this area.

Care route \ Level	Case consultation	Administrative consultation
Direct	Client centred	Programme centred
Indirect	Consultee centred	Consultee centred

Figure 15.2 Mental health consultation

THE CONSULTATION PROCESS IN LIAISON MENTAL HEALTH NURSING

Liaison mental health nursing involves both the provision of care directly to the patient (or to the patient and their family) and the provision of care indirectly through another non-psychiatric professional. These two routes of care provision are represented in the model of mental health consultation in Figure 15.2 as consultation activities for direct and indirect care.

CONSULTATION ACTIVITIES FOR DIRECT CARE

As a direct care provider, the mental health nurse is involved in mental health assessment, psychological interventions, and evaluation of care. The nurse may be skilled in a range of interventions including individual, family or group therapy, cognitive and behaviour therapy, crisis intervention, health promotion, staff support, stress management and counselling. The nurse intervenes on an interpersonal level to expand the mental health services available in non-psychiatric settings.

In direct care activities the types of problem that arise are considered to be patient-centred case problems. Most of the nurse's time is spent with the patient and the interaction is primarily supportive and goal directed. The goal may be to:

1. Assess a patient's mental state.
2. Assist the patient and their family or carer through a crisis.
3. Counsel and support the person who has impaired physical functions; has loss of self esteem; is grieving; has suffered family abuse, violence, or rape; is demonstrating impaired mental or emotional functioning; or is needing guidance in coping with a personal life situation that is an actual or perceived threat to their mental health.

In direct care activities the patient and the mental health nurse are the main participants. The mental health nurse uses advanced nursing skills and knowledge to provide direct care that results in measurable changes in the patient's health and is directly responsible for implementing, evaluating and documenting care. The nurse also collaborates with other staff, providing them with information that may contribute to the patient's well-being.

CONSULTATION ACTIVITIES FOR INDIRECT CARE

When the LMHN functions in an indirect manner, the consultee is responsible for resolving the identified problem. The LMHN assists the consultee to improve their problem-solving skills in the specific presenting situation and in handling similar problems in the future. The liaison nurse is acknowledged as an expert in promoting and developing human resources to resolve the current problem and to enhance the consultee's own abilities and efforts.

Indirect activities incorporate education, systems evaluation and programme development into the consultation process. Consultation takes place between the liaison mental health nurse and other non-psychiatric professionals in schools, business and industry, civic and community organizations and voluntary sector organizations. Problems can range from managing aggression in public service organizations to the development of interpersonal and communication skills among employees.

THE PROCESS OF CONSULTATION

Mental health consultation may be represented as a process involving several phases.

Phase 1: Preparation and orientation for consultation.
Phase 2: The Working Phase:

> Assessment
> Planning
> Implementation
> Evaluation.

Phase 3: The Termination Phase.

Phase 1: Preparation and Orientation for Consultation

The entire consultation process is affected by the setting and staff involved in the relationship. The philosophy, organizational structure, policies and procedures, culture and staff expectations will vary. Extensive preparatory work is often necessary to develop appropriate relationships and systems of communication between the consultant and the consultee. The consultant and consultee may work within different areas of the same organization. For example, the consultant mental health nurse may be based in an accident and emergency department and the consultee as staff nurse on a medical ward in the same general hospital. Alternatively, they may work in organizations that are usually quite separate. For example, the consultee may be based in a residential nursing home and the consultant in an NHS Community Mental Health Trust.

A shared perception of mental health problems and role expectations is an essential part of this relationship. It is important that arrangements for consultation are authorized by both the consultee's and the consultant's senior managers. This includes contracts and payments for services, the development of appropriate job descriptions, determination of the boundaries of practice and responsibility for evaluating the consultant's work. Agreement and explicit recognition of these parameters are required as a basis for the development of the consultation process.

Ideally the consultee should have direct access to mental health consultation at the time they experience difficulties. The consultant needs to be visible within the organization, perceived as approachable by potential consultees and credible in mental health nursing.

In the consultation process, the consultant is attentive to the consultee's language, perceptions, cognitions and ways of working to communicate effectively with them. This is particularly important as it is the consultee and not the specialist who provides the client with treatment. Attention to the professional context of the consultee improves both the content and the style of communication between consultant and consultee.

Elements of the consultation contract

- A brief statement of the problem.
- Name, title, position of consultee.
- Expected outcomes or goals.
- Arrangement of meetings to address the problem.
- Key departments and staff involved.
- If appropriate, the compensation arrangements for consultation.

The consultation contract

The consultation activities of the LMHN are best guided and evaluated using a written agreement between the consultee and the consultant (Lehmann, 1995). This consultation contract represents an agreement between the two parties of the particular services to be provided and the nature of the collaborative arrangement. It may help to prevent misunderstandings and clarify roles. The main points to include in the contract are included in Box 15.5.

Phase 2: The Working Phase

This emphasizes the problem-focused nature of consultation and mirrors the problem-solving cycle of the nursing process (Ritter, 1989; Tunmore, 1992) (see Chapter 2). The working phase incorporates stages of assessment, planning, implementation and evaluation and applies to each of the four types of consultation identified in Caplan's model.

Assessment

This begins with the formulation of the consultation contract. It involves data collection and clarification of information in order to frame the consultation relationship and provide a context for future work. Lewis and Levy (1982) suggest that assessment in mental health consultation will focus on a range of interrelated factors. These will vary in emphasis and importance for each type of consultation but may include, for example, assessment of the request for consultation, the consultee, other professionals' involvement, the milieu, the patient's family and carers, the physical health problem and assessment of the patient's notes (Box 15.6).

Planning

The assessment provides the basis for the development of a plan. The LMHN identifies actual and potential problems, including possible sources of conflict, stress or dysfunction, within the health care system. Benefits and strengths, including problem-solving abilities, present coping strategies and other resources identified during the assessment stage, are also incorporated into the plan.

The LMHN frames the problem in a way that gives an objective view of the situation. The key issues addressed have a work focus rather than focusing directly on the consultee's difficulty (see Consultee-Centred Consultation). Theoretical concepts that promote learning and can be generalized to fit other similar situations the consultee may experience, are used

in developing the plan. The language and ideas of the consultee may be incorporated into the proposed interventions. Interventions should be feasible, practical, time limited and in line with the skills and abilities of the consultee who is responsible for their implementation. This means that the consultee is able to retain responsibility for the care plan and its implementation.

Planning involves the identification of expected outcomes for each problem area and their incorporation into a written plan. Outcomes should be realistic and achievable. They must be mutually agreed by the consultee and the consultant and give a clear indication of these professionals' shared expectations. Goals are based on the expected outcome and should provide effective measures of achievement for evaluation.

Implementation

The consultee selects the interventions to be tried and implements them. This stage includes trying out alternative interventions that have resulted from the planning stage. The implementation stage ends either after an agreed period of time or when the interventions result in the desired change. Implementation of the plan by the consultee may take place after the mental health nurse has left the setting.

Evaluation

This stage addresses the effects of planned interventions and the extent to which they met the desired goals. It involves determining whether the problem has been resolved, the degree of success and identifying any additional problems that arose during the process.

Phase 3: The Termination Phase

Termination involves pulling together the threads of the consultation process and psychological and physical closure and withdrawal. The work involved in this phase depends on a variety of factors including the setting, the nature of the consultation contract, the organization, and the relationship between the consultant and consultee. If the LMHN is a staff member of the same organization as the consultee their visibility and availability will continue. If they are an 'outside' consultant, termination will be more formal.

Summary report

A formal written report of the consultation allows all members of the organization to have access to relevant information. The format of the report will vary with the type of consultation, the setting, the level of organization involved, and the issues addressed. Suggestions for areas to be included in the report are shown in Box 15.6. The report should be clear and concise, with detail on the mental health nurse's perspective on the consultation process.

Professional Development

The mental health nurse may use the consultation contract and summary report for self-evaluation of their own performance. Reflection on the consultation process will help identify areas for revision and improvement in the future. Self-evaluation, a necessary part of the consultation process (Box 15.7), should include goal setting, problem solving, communication skills, and application of theory to practice. Peer review and consultee satisfaction are other complementary means of evaluating performance and outcomes.

The consultation process involves an acknowledgement of equality between the consulting professionals. Lehmann (1995) describes a coordinate professional relationship between the consultant and the consultee. The consultative relationship is a coequal one where each party has respect for the other's expertise and professionalism. Steinberg (1989) emphasizes how the consultant is 'working with *other people's* perspectives, assumptions and expertise'. It is these fundamental attributes that distinguish consultation from other forms of interprofessional collaboration. Both parties consult in the process of consultation and both need a shared understanding and specific skills for successful collaboration.

Box 15.6

Assessment

Assessment of the request for consultation
Is the LMHN actively sought by the consultee? Is the consultation request made because the LMHN happened upon the consultee, their presence promoting the consultation? Is the request from an individual or more than one person or is it a team request? The request may be expressed in terms of someone else's problem, for example a ward Sister who states that 'the students have been finding Mr Thomas's behaviour quite strange'. What is the consultee asking of the consultant? They may be seeking clarification about treatment, expressing concern about the level of distress experienced by a patient. They may be asking for advice on a mental health programme for staff, on the patient's psychological care or on the most appropriate way of responding in a difficult situation. They may, through the consultation request, emphasize their own feelings of worry or sense of helplessness about a particular patient or situation.
    The request for consultation may reflect an underlying problem. The consultee may be unaware of the actual problem; they may be aware of it but be unable to clearly articulate the problem.

Assessment of the consultee
What is the consultee's understanding of the psychological factors associated with the problem? Does he or she have the appropriate skills and resources to manage it? Does the consultee seem to be experiencing personal stress? Has the consultee had problems over similar issues before? Does he or she have knowledge of the issue involved but lack experience and confidence in managing the problem? How long has the consultee worked in the unit and does he or she have much experience in the field? Has the consultant worked with the consultee before? What is the consultee;s understanding and expectation of consultation? What is the working relationship like? To what extent are there shared understandings or conflicts?

Assessment of other professional involvement
Are different professionals likely to have very different perspectives and understanding of the problem? Do any differences lead to conflicts within the team that affect the problem? Are there other interprofessional conflicts? Is there any evidence of conflict between the patient and other members of staff? How experienced are others in managing the problem? Is the consultant seen to be encroaching on another's professional territory? Is there a Key Worker or primary carer system in operation?

Assessment of the milieu
What is the clinical setting? It may be a specialist service, an intensive care unit, an accident and emergency department, a medical or surgical ward. What is the general dependency level of patients on the unit? How is the patient's behaviour perceived? Are they seen as appropriately placed? How has the patient found the milieu? Do they have a sense of privacy and personal space? Have they been distressed by events they may have experienced or something they may have overheard? Do staff on the unit have strong leadership or a team spirit? What is the relationship between this unit and the consultant?

Assessment of the patient's family and carers
Are family involved? Who is the main carer? What is their relationship with the patient? Are there conflicts between the carers, family members and staff? What does the family have in terms of support? How do the carers and relatives relate to the doctors, nurses and other clinical staff?

Assessment of the physical health problem
Does the patient have a physical illness, a somatic complaint or physical injury? Is there a common pattern of behaviour, thoughts, and feelings associated with this kind of physical health problem? What perceptions of the physical health problem are held by the patient, by their family and carers, and by the nursing, medical and other clinical staff? Could there be a physiological basis to the behaviour; for example, could it be related to treatment, medication, illness or injury?

Assessment of the patient's notes
What is the history of illness, treatment and care? How has the patient coped and responded on previous occasions? Are any pattern or trends evident, for example, non-attendance at out-patient clinics and frequent attendance at accident and emergency departments? What is the treatment protocol? Have there been recent changes? Do the notes report on the patient's thoughts and feelings and on their moods and behaviour? Who has written the notes? Is there a primary nurse or Key Worker involved? What information is missing?

Key characteristics of consultation have been identified (see Box 15.8) (Steinberg, 1989; Tunmore and Thomas 1992). It is important to be able to differentiate consultation from other collaborative activities such as supervision, teaching and liaison. There are important similarities and differences between these activities.

Box 15.7 *Summary of the consultation process*

Phase 1 Preparation and Orientation for Consultation
Setting ground rules
Identification and definition of roles and relationships
Hopes and expectations of consultation from both parties
Agreeing a contract
Practical arrangements of meetings — when, where, how often and for how long.

Phase 2 The Working Phase
Assessment
Planning
Implementation
Evaluation
Documentation of the consultation — consideration of who keeps what records, what format is appropriate and where any record should be kept.

Phase 3 The Termination Phase
Summary Report
Purpose, dates, time, and consultation activities
Problem statement
Assessment of the problem
Proposed interventions
Alternative approaches
Evaluation criteria and outcomes.

Box 15.8 *Key characteristics of consultation*

- 'To consult' describes the behaviour of both parties in the consultation relationship.
- The consultant works indirectly on the problem or question through the consultee.
- Consultation emphasizes the consultee's perspective of the problem and not the consultant's.
- The consultee retains total responsibility for the work problem.
- The consultee is autonomous. They may accept or reject whatever comes from the consultation.
- The consultee is regarded as a competent professional within their own area of practice.
- Consultation is an educational activity. The consultant facilitates the work and the professional development of the consultee.

Supervision

Different types of supervision are described in Chapter 10 where the important distinction is made between management and clinical supervision. The main differences between consultation and supervision are associated with hierarchical and administrative responsibilities and relationships. The supervisor is more senior, has more experience, holds higher qualifications and has more responsibility for performance and outcomes. The consultant has no administrative authority or powers of coercion over the consultee. They are not in a line management relationship. The consultant has no responsibility for carrying out the recommended plan or programme and the consultee may accept or reject any or all recommendations.

Teaching

Consultation incorporates a learning process for both the consultee and the consultant. However, the aim of consultation is not to impart a specific body of knowledge to the consultee but rather to facilitate their problem-solving skills through support and guidance. The consultant may provide the consultee with new information and knowledge to help with a current work problem and similar situations should they arise in the future.

Liaison

This refers to collaborative work between different agencies whose focus of work is usually quite separate. Different perspectives come together in a particular forum. Liaison work does not necessarily include consultation although these forms of collaborative interagency activity are often related. Liaison work may involve a mental health nurse attending an oncologist's ward round or providing a clinic in an accident and emergency department.

The development of mental health consultation and liaison nursing services is a challenging process. The mental health nurse may find that the liaison service can be abused or used as a last resort for patients who are seen as difficult management problems, rather than the basis of a collaborative and educational approach between psychiatric and medical services. Non-psychiatric staff may simply want to pass on the problem rather than understand how better to manage it themselves (Brooks and Walton, 1981; Thomas, 1983).

Commitment to liaison and consultation activities may be lacking from either or both parties. Mental health consultation may be available but given a low priority by mental health teams and non-psychiatric services. The development of consultation skills is dependent on adequate experience of the consultation process.

Appropriate use of the consultant may be dependent on the ability of the consultee to identify the problem. The consultee has to define the problem and identify the need for mental health consultation before they request it. Non-psychiatric staff may fail to define the problem as one that is amenable to psychiatric intervention. For example, they may perceive a depressed mood as a 'natural' consequence of a cancer diagnosis that cannot be changed.

The mental health nurse may prefer to demonstrate their own worth by providing direct clinical services to patients rather than engage in consultation activities. Professional and territorial issues may override the aim of mental health consultation to promote mental health and reduce the incidence of mental disorder. Consultation may be seen as giving away the skills and knowledge of the mental health nurse to non-mental health professionals and, in turn, as devaluing the expertise of the mental health nurse and undermining their professional status.

EDUCATION AND TRAINING

In the USA, degree programes at Master's level for specialist preparation in psychiatric liaison have been described (Robinson, 1972; Nelson and Schilke Davis, 1979; Lambert and Lambert, 1981). British mental health nurses have no such programmes. However, the need for education has been identified (Tunmore, 1994; Regel and Davies, 1995). Liaison mental health nursing could form part of the general preparation of mental health nurses for registration and be promoted through post-registration education programmes. The English National Board for Nursing, Midwifery and Health Visiting includes concepts of liaison nursing in the indicative content for the specialist community mental health nursing qualification (ENB, 1994).

Education programmes for liaison mental health nursing should cover a range of theoretical perspectives, the relationships between physical and mental health and illness, mental health consultation, different practice settings and skills in psychological therapies.
Relevant theoretical perspectives include:
- Adaptation and stress.
- Crisis intervention.
- Human development.
- Interpersonal and group dynamics.
- Management of change.
- Organizational behaviour.
- Problem-solving approaches.
- Psychosocial factors influencing health.
- Psychological reactions to physical illness.
- Sociocultural variation.
- Staff management.
- Systems theory.

Appropriate areas of clinical preparation should provide the LMHN with an understanding of the relationships between physical and mental health and illness. These may include:
- Substance misuse.
- Alcohol problems among medical patients.

- Assessment and management of mental health problems in people with physical illness.
- Common medical illnesses and their symptoms, treatments and disabilities.
- Deliberate self-harm.
- Management of psychological trauma.
- Organic mental disorders: delirium and dementia.
- Psychosomatic and anxiety disorders.
- Use of psychotropic medication in physical illness.

Programmes need to cover mental health consultation and other forms of interagency collaborative work such as clinical supervision, staff support and debriefing in different practice settings. The settings may include, for example, the intensive care unit, the accident and emergency department and medical and surgical units.

The development of skills in a particular therapeutic approach or type of psychological intervention, e.g. cognitive behaviour therapy, may benefit certain groups of patient or help with particular types of problem. Advanced training in psychological skills is an important part of the LMHN's role.

SUMMARY

This chapter identifies liaison and consultation as collaborative activities where mental health nurses provide services in a range of different settings and for patients with a variety of different problems. The development of psychiatric liaison services and the promotion of mental health consultation in both the primary health care setting and the general hospital are means of promoting mental health and preventing mental illness among people with a range of physical health problems.

Through both direct and indirect care activities the liaison mental health nurse aims to improve coping abilities among patients with a variety of different physical illnesses, provide support to patients and staff in stressful situations and, by working closely with colleagues from other areas of health care, to reduce the stigma associated with mental illness.

Mental health consultation is a form of collaborative interagency work that provides a structured and systematic approach for the application of the skills and knowledge of the mental health nurse across different service settings and clinical areas. Through the continued use of this flexible, transferable and adaptable approach to care, mental health nurses can promote the creative use of a wide range of diverse nursing skills. A coordinated approach to liaison and consultation activities in organizations and across traditional boundaries will extend the benefits of mental health care to a wider population and highlight the contribution of mental health nurses to overall health needs.

KEY CONCEPTS

- Liaison and consultation involve different but related activities.
- Liason and consultation respectively provide means of working with non-psychiatric services, professionals and other groups.
- Liaison and consultation facilitate work across established boundaries.
- Liaison mental health nursing has grown within general hospital settings and accident and emergency departments.
- Mental health consultation provides a model for the development of mental health services in primary care.
- Education programmes incorporating models of consultation and liaison will assist in the future development of appropriate mental health services.

REFERENCES

Allebeck P, Bolund C: Suicides and suicide attempts in cancer patients. *Psychol Med* 21(4):979–984, 1991.

Allebeck P, Bolund C, Ringback G: Increased suicide rate in cancer patients. *J Clin Epidemiol* 42:611–616, 1989.

American Nurses Association: *Standards of psychiatric consultation nursing practice*. Kansas City, Missouri, 1990, ANA Council on Psychiatric and Mental Health Nursing.

Anstee BH: Psychiatry in the casualty department. *Br J Psychiatry* 120:625–629, 1972.

Anstee BH: The pattern of psychiatric referrals in a general hospital. *Br J Psychiatry* 120:631–634, 1972.

Armstrong C: Emotional changes following brain injury: psychological and neurological components of depression, denial and anxiety. *J Rehab* 57(2):15–22, 1991.

Atha C, Salkovskis P, Storer D: Accident and emergency: more questions than answers. *Nurs Times* 85(15):28–31, 1989.

Atkinson JH *et al.*: Prevalence of psychiatric disorders among men infected with human immunodeficiency virus. *Arch Gen Psychiatry* 45(9):859–864, 1988.

Audit Commission: *Finding a place: a review of mental health services for adults.* London, 1994, HMSO.

Badger TA: Men with cardiovascular disease and their spouses: coping, health and marital adjustment. *Arch Psychiatr Nurs* 4(5):319–324, 1990.

Bolund C: Suicide and cancer medical and care factors in suicides by cancer patients in Sweden 1973–1976. *J Psychosoc Oncol* 3:31–53, 1985.

Brooks P, Walton HJ: Liaison psychiatry in Scotland. *Health Bull* 39:218–227, 1981.

Brown A, Cooper AF: The impact of liaison psychiatry service on patterns of referral in a general hospital. *Br J Psychiatry* 150:83–87, 1987.

Caplan G: *Principles of preventive psychiatry.* New York, 1964, Basic Books.

Castillo C *et al.*: Generalised anxiety disorder after stroke. *J Nerv Ment Dis* 181(2):100–106, 1993.

Catalan J *et al.*: Comparison of doctors and nurses in the assessment of deliberate self-poisoning patients. *Psychol Med* 10(3):483–491, 1980.

Charlton J *et al.*: Suicide deaths in England and Wales: trends in factors associated with suicide deaths. *Popul Trends* 71:34–42, 1993.

Chick J, Lloyd G, Crombie E: Counselling problem drinkers in medical wards: a controlled study. *BMJ* 290:865–867, 1985.

Chuang HT *et al.*: Psychosocial distress and well-being among gay and bisexual men with human immunodeficiency virus infection. *Am J Psychiatry* 146(7):876–880, 1989.

Davison AG, Hildrey AC, Floyer MA: Use and misuse of an A&E department in the East End of London. *J R Soc Med* 76(1):37–40,1983.

Department of Health: *The health of the nation — first steps for the NHS.* London, 1992, HMSO.

Department of Health: *The report of the inquiry into London's health service, medical education and research.* London, 1993a, HMSO.

Department of Health: *The health of the nation — mental illness key area handbook.* London, 1993b, HMSO.

Department of Health: *Working in partnership: a collaborative approach to care.* London, 1994, HMSO.

Derogatis L *et al.*: The prevalence of psychiatric disorders among cancer patients. *J Am Med Assoc* 249(6):751–757, 1983.

Eastwood MR *et al.*: Mood disorder following cerebrovascular accident. *Br J Psychiatry* 154:195–200, 1989.

English National Board for Nursing, Midwifery and Health Visiting: Creating life-long learners; partnerships for care. Guidelines for the implementation of the UKCC's standards for education and practice following registration. London, 1995, ENB.

Farberow NL *et al.*: Suicide among patients with cardiorespiratory illness. *J Am Med Assoc* 195(6):422–428, 1966.

Fedoroff JP *et al.*: Are depressive symptoms nonspecific in patients with acute stroke? *Am J Psychiatry* 148(9):1172–1176, 1991.

Feibel J, Springer C: Depression and failure to resume social activities after stroke. *Arch Phys Med Rehab* 63:276–278, 1982.

Fernandez F *et al.*: Consultation–liaison psychiatry and HIV related disorders. *Hosp Community Psychiatry* 40(2):146–153, 1989.

Finklestein S *et al.*: Antidepressant drug treatment for poststroke depression: retrospective study. *Arch Phys Med Rehab* 68:772–776, 1987.

Forester BM, Kornfield DS, Fleiss JL: Psychiatric aspects of radiotherapy. *Am J Psychiatry* 135(8):960–963, 1987.

Fox BH *et al.*: Suicide rates among cancer patients in Connecticut. *J Chronic Disability* 35:89–100, 1982.

Fridlund B, Pihlgren C, Wannestig L: A supportive–educative caring rehabilitation programme; improvements of physical health after myocardial infarction. *J Clin Nurs* 1:141–146, 1992.

Friedman S *et al.*: Predicting psychiatric admission from an emergency room—psychiatric, psychosocial and methodological factors. *J Nerv Ment Dis* 171(3):155–158, 1983.

Goldberg EL, Comstock GW, Graves CG: Psychosocial factors and blood pressure. *Psychol Med* 10:243–255, 1980.

Goldberg RJ: Systematic understanding of cancer patients who refuse treatment. *Psychother Psychosom* 39(3):180–189, 1983.

Gomez J: *Liaison psychiatry: mental health problems in the general hospital.* New York, 1987, Free Press.

Goodstein RK: Overview: cerebrovascular accident and the hospitalised elderly — a multidimensional clinical problem. *Am J Psychiatry* 140(2):141–147,1983.

Gorman JM *et al.*: Glucocorticoid level and neuropsychiatric symptoms in homosexual men with HIV infection. *Am J Psychiatry* 148(1):41–45, 1991.

Grant SM: The hospitalised AIDS patient and the liaison mental health nurse. *Arch Psychiatr Nurs* 2(1):35–39,1988.

Hacket TP, Stern T: Suicide and other disruptive states. In: Hacket TP, Cassem NH: *Massachusetts general hospital handbook of general hospital psychiatry.* Massachusetts, 1987, PSG.

Hammer JS: The cost–benefit of psychiatric consultation/liaison services in the medical setting. *Curr Opin Psychiatry* 3(5):687–691,1990.

Hillard JR *et al.*: Suicide in a psychiatric emergency room population. *Am J Psychiatry* 140(4):459–462, 1983.

House AO, Jones SJ: The effects of establishing a psychiatric consultation–liaison service: changes in patterns of referral and care. *Health Trends* 19:10–12, 1987.

Ironson G *et al.*: Changes in immune function and psychological measures as a function of anticipation and reaction to news of HIV-1 antibody status. *Psychosom Med* 52(3):247–270, 1990.

James DV, Hamilton LW: The Clerkenwell scheme: assessing efficiency and cost of a psychiatric liaison service to a magistrates' court. *BMJ* 303:282–285, 1991.

Jones A: Liaison consultation psychiatry—the CPN as clinical nurse specialist. *Community Psychiatr Nurs J* April:7–18, 1989.

Kessler RC *et al.*: Stressful life events and symptom onset in HIV infection. *Am J Psychiatry* 148(6):733–738, 1991.

Kieburtz K *et al.*: Manic syndrome in AIDS. *Am J Psychiatry* 148(8):1068–1070, 1991.

Lambert CL, Lambert VA: Nursing students and a mental health consultation programme. *Psychiatr Mental Health Services* March:29–35, 1981.

Law WA *et al.*: Symptoms of depression in HIV-infected individuals: etiological considerations. *Neuropsychiatry Neuropsychol Behav Neurol* 6(3):181–186, 1993.

Lehmann FG: Consultation liaison psychiatric nursing care. In: Stuart G, Sundeen S, editors: *Principles and practice of psychiatric nursing*, ed 5. London, 1995, Mosby.

Levitan SJ, Kornfeld DS: Clinical cost and benefits of liaison psychiatry. *Am J Psychiatry* 136(6):790–793, 1981.

Lewis A, Levy J: *Psychiatric liaison nursing: the theory and clinical practice.* Reston, Virginia, 1982, Reston Publishing Co., Inc.

Lipowski ZJ: Liaison psychiatry, liaison nursing and behavioural medicine. *Compr Psychiatry* 22(6):554–561, 1981.

Lipowski ZJ: The need to integrate liaison psychiatry and geopsychiatry. *Am J Psychiatry* 140(8):1003–1005, 1983a.

Lipowski ZJ: Current trends in consultation liaison psychiatry. *Can J Psychiatry* 28(5):329–338, 1983b.

Lloyd GG: Whence and whither liaison psychiatry? *Psychol Med* 10:11–14, 1980.

Louhivouri KA, Hakama M: Risk of suicide among cancer patients. *Am J Epidemiol* 109:59–65, 1979.

Maguire GP *et al.*: Psychiatric problems in the first year after mastectomy. *BMJ* 1:963–965, 1978.

Marzuk PM *et al.*: Increased risk of suicide in persons with AIDS. *J Am Med Assoc* 259(9):1333–1337, 1988.

McArther JC *et al.*: Dementia in AIDS patients: incidence and risk factors. *Neurology* 43(11):2245–2252, 1994.

McKegney FP, O'Dowd MA: Suicidality and HIV status. *Am J Psychiatry* 149(3):396–389, 1992.

McNiel DE *et al.*: The role of violence in decisions about hospitalization from the psychiatric emergency room. *Am J Psychiatry* 149(2):207–212, 1992.

Moorey S, Greer S: *Psychological therapy for patients with cancer — a new approach.* Oxford, 1989, Heinemann Medical Books.

Morris PLP, Robinson RG, Raphael B: The prevalence course and selected correlates of depressive disorder in hospitalised stroke patients. *Int J Psychiatry Med* 20:327–342, 1990.

Morris T, Greer S, White P: Psychological and social adjustment to mastectomy. *Cancer* 40:2381–2387, 1977.

Mumford E, Schlesinger HJ, Glass GV *et al.*: A new look at evidence about reduced cost of medical utilization following mental health treatment. *Am J Psychiatry* 141(10):1145–1158, 1984.

Myers P: Management of minor medical problems and trauma: general practice or hospital? *J Royal Soc Med* 75:879–883, 1982.

Nelson JKN, Schilke Davis D: Educating the liaison mental health nurse. *J Nurs Educ* 18(8):14–20, 1979.

Ostrow DG *et al.*: HIV related symptoms and psychological functioning in a cohort of homosexual men. *Am J Psychiatry* 146(6):737–742, 1989.

Patel C *et al.*: Trial of relaxation in reducing coronary risk: four year follow up. *BMJ* 290:1103–1106, 1985.

Payne S: Anxiety and depression in women with advanced cancer: implications for counselling. *Counsel Psychol Q* 2(3):337–344, 1989.

Peck A, Bolland J: Emotional reactions to radiation treatment. *Cancer* 40:180–184, 1977.

Perry SW, Jacobsberg L, Fishman B: Psychological responses to serological testing for HIV *AIDS* 4:145–152, 1990.

Perry SW, Tross S: Psychiatric problems of AIDS inpatients at the New York

hospital: preliminary report. *Public Health Rep* 99:200–205, 1984.

Regel S, Davies J: The future of mental health nurses in liaison psychiatry. *BJN* 4(18):1052–1056, 1995.

Ritter S: *Bethlem Royal and Maudsley Hospital manual of clinical psychiatric nursing principles and procedures.* London, 1989, Harper & Row.

Robinson L: A psychiatric nursing liaison programme. *Nurs Outlook* 20(7):454–457, 1972.

Robinson L: Liaison mental health nursing 1962–1982: a review and update of the literature. *Gen Hosp Psychiatry* 4:139–145, 1982.

Robinson RG *et al.*: A two year longitudinal study of post-stroke mood disorders: findings during the initial evaluation. *Stroke* 14:736–741, 1983.

Royal College of Psychiatrists: Guidelines for training in liaison psychiatry. *Bull R Coll Psychiatrists* 12(9):389, 1988.

Salkovskis PM *et al.*: Psychiatric morbidity in an accident and emergency department: characteristics of patients at presentation and one month follow-up. *Br J Psychiatry* 156:483–487, 1990.

Sensky T *et al.*: Referrals to psychiatrists in a general hospital — comparison of two methods of liaison psychiatry: preliminary communication. *J R Soc Med* 78(6):463–468, 1985.

Seth R *et al.*: Psychiatric illness in patients with HIV infection and AIDS referred to the liaison psychiatrist. *Br J Psychiatry* 159:347–350, 1991.

Sheehan A: Mental health nurses needed in acute general settings. *BJN* 1(14):696, 1992.

Smith LW, Dimsdale JE: Postcardiotomy delirium: conclusions after 25 years? *Am J Psychiatry* 146(4):452–458, 1989.

Starkstein SE *et al.*: Relationship between anxiety disorders and depressive disorders in patients with cerebrovascular injury. *Arch Gen Psychiatry* 47(3):246–251, 1990.

Steinberg D: *Interprofessional consultation.* Oxford, 1989, Blackwell Scientific.

Stockwell F: *The unpopular patient.* RCN Research Project Series 1 (no. 2). London, 1972, Royal College of Nursing.

Storer D *et al.*: Community psychiatric nursing intervention in an accident and emergency department: a clinical pilot study. *J Adv Nurs* 12(2):215–222, 1987.

Storm HH, Christensen N, Jensen OM: Suicides among Danish patients with cancer: 1971–1986. *Cancer* 69(6):1507–1512, 1992.

Strain JJ, Llyons JS, Hammer JS *et al.*: Cost offset from a psychiatric consultation liaison intervention with elderly hip fracture patients. *Am J Psychiatry* 148(8):1044–1049, 1991.

Thomas CJ: Referrals to a British liaison psychiatry service. *Health Trends* 15:61–64, 1983.

Thompson DR: A randomized controlled trial of in-hospital nursing support for first time myocardial infarction patients and their partners: effects on anxiety and depression. *Adv J Nurs* 14:291–297, 1989.

Torem M, Saravay SM, Steinberg H: Psychiatric liaison: benefits of an active approach. *Psychosomatics* 20:598–611, 1979.

Tunmore R: Liaison psychiatric nursing in oncology. *Nurs Times* 85(33):54–56, 1989.

Tunmore R: Liaison psychiatry–setting the pace. *Nurs Times* 186(34):29–32, 1990.

Tunmore R: Nursing care planning. In: Brooking J, Ritter S, Thomas B, editors: *A textbook of psychiatric and mental health nursing.* Edinburgh, 1992, Churchill Livingstone.

Tunmore R: Encouraging collaboration—liaison mental health nursing, *Nurs Times* 90(20):66,1994.

Tunmore R, Thomas B: Models of psychiatric consultation liaison nursing. *BJN* 1(9):447–451, 1992.

Vogel Scibilia SE, Mulsant BH, Keshavan–Matcheri S: HIV infection presenting as psychosis: a critique. *Acta Psychiatr Scand* 78(5):652–656, 1988.

Wadden T : Predicting treatment response to relaxation therapy for essential hypertension. *J Nerv Ment Dis* 171(11):683–689, 1983.

Warren R: The other 99 per cent. *Health Serv J* 99(5139):232–233, 1989.

Watson M *et al.*: Relationships between emotional control, adjustment to cancer and depression and anxiety in breast cancer patients. *Psychol Med* 21(1):51–57, 1991.

Wilkins JW *et al.*: Implications of self-reported cognitive and motor dysfunction in HIV positive patients. *Am J Psychiatry* 148(5):641–643, 1991.

World Health Organization: *Global programme on AIDS: report of the consultation on the neuropsychiatric aspects of HIV infection.* Geneva, 1988, WHO.

FURTHER READING

Baldwin S, Godfrey C, Propper C, editors: *Quality of Life: Perspectives and policies*. London, 1990, Routledge.
> *This book addresses the philosophical and policy issues around this increasingly important topic through detailed studies of what constitutes a good quality of life for particular client groups.*

Bowling A: *Measuring health: A review of quality of life measurement scales*. Buckingham, 1991, Open University Press.
> *This book reviews a wide range of popular measures of functional disability and health status, especially those concerned with psychological well-being, including morale, anxiety and depression.*

Critchley DL, Maurin JT, editors: *The clinical specialist in psychiatric mental health nursing*. New York, 1985, John Wiley & Sons.
> *This remains one of the few contributions to nursing literature that specifically addresses theoretical, research and practice issues at the advanced level appropriate for the clinical nurse specialist.*

Hodes M, Moorey S, editors: *Psychological treatments in disease and illness*. Tavistock, 1993, The Dorset Press.

Lloyd GG: *Textbook of general hospital psychiatry*. London, 1991, Churchill Livingstone.

McDowell I, Newell C: *Measuring health: a guide to rating scales and questionnaires*. Oxford, 1987, Oxford University Press.
> *This is a useful reference book that brings together information on different health measurement techniques. The chapter on psychological well-being will be of particular interest to nurses who wish to evaluate the progress of patients.*

Wilson–Barnet J, Batehup L: *Patient problems: a research base for nursing care*. Scutari Press, London, 1988.
> *The authors address some of the major challenges in patient care through describing the research that explores the social, psychological and physical aspects of health and illness.*

Wilson-Barnet J, MacLeod Clark J, editors: *Research in health promotion and nursing*. London, 1993, Macmillan.
> *This book presents a research based perspective of the relationship between health promotion and nursing practice. It examines the impact of nursing interventions on the lifestyles of patients', including those with coronary heart disease, HIV/AIDS and the mentally ill.*

Nursing Interventions with Long-Term Clients

Learning Outcomes

After studying this chapter, you should be able to:

- Describe and discuss the development of care in the community.

- Demonstrate an awareness of the assessment tools available for use with this patient group.

- Outline the importance of pharmacological interventions in treating resistant schizophrenia

- Have an awareness of the use of psychosocial interventions to complement drug treatment.

- Demonstrate the use of a case management approach to delivering mental health care.

*O*ne person in every hundred will experience an episode of schizophrenia during their lives. However, not everyone with schizophrenia will have enduring problems. Some (around 15%) may have only one episode and others may have frequent episodes; the remainder are chronically ill.

People with enduring mental health problems can be subdivided into three groups:
1. Old long-stay.
2. New long-stay.
3. New long-term.

Old long-stay patients are those who have spent most of their adult lives in hospital. New long-stay patients are often referred to as 'revolving-door' patients because they continual move unsuccessfully between hospital, home and the community, until there are no options left but long-stay wards. New long-term patients are those who are repeatedly using in-patient and community services (Perkins and Repper, 1996).

Most people with enduring mental illness will have a diagnosis of schizophrenia (Ford *et al.*, 1995). However, it is important to note that other illnesses, such as affective, personality and anxiety disorders, can also result in an enduring illness.

THE HISTORICAL CONTEXT

The care of, and provision of services for, the mentally ill has changed dramatically in the last 100 years. In this section these changes are briefly outlined.

ASYLUMS
During the early 19th Century the mentally ill were placed in asylums. These were places of refuge, shelter and sanctuary, designed to protect vulnerable people from exploitation, cruelty and distress. Care focused on providing a humane environment in which to look after the mentally ill.

Asylums began to decline in use because of overcrowding and inadequate staffing. Changes in public attitudes to mental illness and the development of psychiatry as a specialized branch of medicine contributed further to their demise. Psychiatry became an accepted branch of medicine and new medical methods for managing mental disorder were gradually adopted. Nursing during this era had largely custodial responsibilities.

TREATMENT MODALITIES

New medical treatments including electroconvulsive therapy (ECT), leucotomy (brain surgery) and insulin coma treatment were used in continental Europe and were imported to the UK in the early 1930s. This period saw the idea develop that mental disorder could be treated with medical intervention and would require less continuous long-term care in hospital.

The 1950s saw the introduction of antipsychotic drugs such as chlorpromazine, which had a significant impact on the treatment of people with schizophrenia. This was reflected in the Mental Treatment Act of 1959 which recognized that people could be treated voluntarily and not as detained patients.

SOCIAL POLICY–COMMUNITY CARE ACT

In 1983 the Department of Health and Social Services (DHSS) launched the Care in the Community Programme, which marked a radical change in care philosophies and practices. Community Care was to support quality of life, rights and status of those who needed it in their home environment. The design of community care services was based upon a needs-led, consumer-oriented model and promoted self-advocacy as the mechanism for determining service provision at local level.

Community Care is a partnership among an informal community network, the individual and statutory services. The introduction of joint finance in the mid-1980s by the DHSS was an attempt to encourage integrated planning and service delivery. Emphasis was placed on joint funding for joint initiatives with the NHS.

Lack of coordination and effective communication among departments on bureaucratic issues, differences in managerial culture and absence of a system for joint monitoring between the two services led to the failure of the system.

This failure was addressed by the Social Service Select Committee in the House of Commons in the mid-1980s. They recommended that a joint plan and the resources to meet expected needs should be available for everyone leaving psychiatric hospitals.

While the Community Care policy was being implemented, the 1983 Mental Health Act was enacted by Parliament. This provides a framework for deciding whether compulsory admission to hospital is justified. It also sets conditions under which a legally detained patient can be forcibly treated. The Act allows compulsory admission in the interests of the individual's health and of the safety of others.

The 1983 Mental Health Act was formulated at a time when most treatment and care was provided in hospitals. It did not take account of development of community services, the growing practices of treating people at home and the maintenance of people with long-term mental disorder in the community.

Since the 1980s there has been a progressive move from institutionalized care to individually tailored care. The shift has been accompanied by closure of many of the large Victorian asylums and a shift in emphasis to treatment from custodial care.

The development of services for the long-term mentally ill in the UK is dominated by hospital closure programmes, resulting in changes in the management of patients with severe and enduring mental illness.

Services for people with mental health problems must be effectively coordinated. Patient needs are often complex and extensive (Challis and Davies, 1986) and may require a range of different interventions over long periods. Significantly, people with serious mental illness tend not to seek help when their condition is deteriorating and may lose contact with services, requiring that steps are taken to avoid this. Experience of organizational problems has led to demands that systems for deliver the range of services required are actually provided.

CARE PROGRAMME APPROACH

The Care Programme Approach (CPA) was introduced by the UK Government as part of its drive towards care in the community, The CPA aims to improve delivery of services to people with severe mental illness and minimize the risk of them losing contact with services. Its essential elements are the assessment of health and social need, a written care plan, the nomination of Key Workers and regular reviews of patients' progress.

Although the principles behind the introduction of the CPA have been welcomed, its implementation has had problems. Some psychiatrists consider the criteria for inclusion too broad and services too under-resourced to cope with the added workload. Some local services have adopted criteria for including patients on the CPA that suit their local needs.

CRITERIA FOR INCLUSION ON CPA REGISTER

The criteria are:
1. A diagnosis of severe and persistent mental illness and any of the following: history of repeated relapse, severe social disability, refusal of multiagency involvement and coordination, history of serious suicidal risk or self-harm, severe self-neglect, violence or danger to others.
2. All patients who fulfil criteria for Section 117 after-care; that is, patients admitted under Sections 3, 37, 41, 47 and 48 of the Mental Health Act 1983.

The CPA ensures that anyone discharged from specialized psychiatric services requiring after-care programmes will have their have their needs met as part of a planned and reviewed care plan. The care plan will be devised by a multidisciplinary team including the responsible medical officer, a social worker, GP, patient's carer or relative, the patient, community psychiatric nurse and a ward nurse prior to discharge.

The care plan covers the following areas:

1. Where the patient will live.
2. Their finances.
3. Relationships with friends and family.
4. Employment prospects.
5. Any psychological or psychotic difficulties.
6. Any predictors of relapse.
7. Known risk factors.
8. Any other relevant information.

A Key Worker is nominated at the pre-discharge meeting and is a member of the team, with mental health experience. In most cases the community psychiatric nurse or social worker is deemed the most appropriate. The role of the Key Worker includes:

- Keeping close contact with the patient.
- Monitoring that the agreed programme of care is delivered.
- Taking immediate action if care is not being delivered.
- Liaising with all those involved in the patient's care and organizing review meetings.

SUPERVISION REGISTER

This is a revised part of the CPA, introduced on 1st April 1995. It states that all individuals who are under the care of a hospital unit or trust and known to be at significant risk of being violent, committing suicide or self-neglect as a result of mental illness should be registered. This particular group can then be flagged up promptly should any difficulties arise. This also highlights the nature of the needs of patients on the register and ensures prompt and well coordinated working practices.

The following criteria for inclusion on the Supervision Register have been proposed:

1. Diagnosis of a major mental illness.
2. Documented history of relapse following non-compliance.
3. History of serious violence or serious danger to others resulting from the illness.
4. History of having been detained in hospital under a section of Mental Health Act 1983.

NURSING CARE OF THE LONG-TERM MENTALLY ILL

Most long-term patients can be maintained for most of the time in the community. However, even in the best community services some patients suffer relapses that will necessitate admission to hospital. Care of the long-term mentally ill should be a shared responsibility between in-patient and community services. Because of the nature of presentation of the long-term mentally ill (i.e. disengagement with services, non-compliance with medication, vulnerability to stress), there may be periods when they relapse and experience acute symptoms.

One of the aims of care in an in-patient setting is to control acute symptoms, i.e. provide crisis resolution, to assist the patient's return to his or her optimum level of functioning prior to relapse.

To achieve a minimal use of in-patient care requires assertive outreach work by a highly flexible and well organized staff team and also very close cooperation from the in-patient unit itself.

The in-patient nurse caring for the long-term mentally ill in crisis must understand the theory of crisis intervention and be skilful in applying this to practice. The nurse must complete a nursing assessment, identify areas of need and plan nursing interventions to address them.

Tyrer (1985) suggests that a hospital base should be sited within easy reach of a well defined catchment area with sub-units (day centres, community mental health centres etc.) actually located within it. In this way there is continued access to a wide range of treatment options, from individual counselling to hospital admission. Hospitals can become a back-up for community services rather than the other way round. The continuity of clinical responsibility, across community and in-patient settings, is the key organizational factor in ensuring the success of this approach.

ASSESSMENT AND OUTCOME MEASUREMENT

Accurate assessment is an essential part of designing and implementing any nursing interventions. However, many assessment tools used by nurses fail to demonstrate that they are valid and reliable (see Chapter 18). Mental health nurses must ensure that the assessment tools that they use have these qualities. A variety of instruments have been developed for use with the long-term acutely ill. However, few measures have been developed specifically for use with people with long standing illnesses (Hemsley, 1994). A sample of those frequently used in clinical practice will be outlined (see also Chapter 18). The reader should consult the source reference for further information.

THE REHAB SCALE

The REHAB is a 23-item scale that examines both general and deviant behaviour. It includes quality of speech, quality of relationships and antisocial behaviours. This scale has been demonstrated to be both valid and reliable. An extensive database of norms for the long-term mentally ill are available and are useful in determining the severity of an individual's illness.

THE SOCIAL BEHAVIOUR SCHEDULE

This measures challenging and bizarre behaviour (Wykes and Sturt, 1986). A carer is interviewed using a structured interview techique to determine frequency and severity of behaviours.

TREATMENT AND REHABILITATION

In this section a wide range of treatment interventions will be discussed, ranging from pharmacological therapy to social skills training.

PHARMACOLOGICAL INTERVENTIONS

The use of antipsychotic drugs such as chlorpromazine and haloperidol is highly effective in treating, predominantly, the positive symptoms (hallucinations, delusions, thought disorder) of schizophrenia (see for example, Barnes and Kane, 1996). However, they often have little impact on the negative and affective symptoms of the illness. Further, antipsychotic drugs have been shown to produce a range of distressing side-effects that are strongly associated with non-compliance. Although most people with schizophrenia will respond to treatment with these drugs, between 20% and 30% will not show a clinically significant response (Rotrosen, 1995). It is these treatment-resistant individuals who make up the majority of the long-term mentally ill. For a more detailed discussion about antipsychotic drugs refer to Chapter 27.

Atypical Antipsychotics

Clozapine, the first atypical antipsychotic drug of superior efficacy and low risk of extrapyramidal side-effects (EPS) was reintroduced in 1990. A number of controlled studies (see for example, Kane *et al.*, 1988) and uncontrolled ones (Clozapine Study Group, 1993) have demonstrated that clozapine is not only effective in treating the positive symptoms of schizophrenia but also the negative and affective symptoms of the illness (Tugrul, 1995). However, clozapine can cause neutropenia in approximately 1% of people treated and therefore requires regular blood monitoring (Pickar, 1995). Because of this potentially fatal effect, clozapine is only licensed for use in treating people with resistant schizophrenia (see Chapters 18 and 27 for more information about clozapine).

Research into the receptor-binding profile of clozapine has led to the development of a new generation of antipsychotic drugs that will be introduced gradually during the late 1990s. The only other new antipsychotic drug that is commercially available at present is risperidone. Risperidone does not require haematological monitoring, carries a low risk of EPS and some studies have demonstrated that it can be as effective as clozapine in treating resistant schizophrenia (Heinrich *et al.*, 1991).

However, Barnes and Kane (1996) raise important questions about comparing novel and traditional antipsychotic drugs. They highlight that both clozapine and risperidone have been closely monitored in controlled trials and therefore the optimum dose range has been determined. This may account, in part, for the lower incidence of side-effects. Mental health nurses have a useful role to play in evaluating the risks and benefits of treatment options with patients. Further, they must also be involved in monitoring their patients' individual responses to different medications. Antipsychotic drugs can only be considered to be one part of treatment. People with long-term illnesses need to develop a range of skills to help them to live more independently.

Medication Management

It is important that patients are educated about all aspects of their treatment, specifically medication (for a review of educational interventions see Chapter 18). Patients should be informed of their diagnosis and the treatment options that are available. They should then be informed of both the positive and negative effects of these interventions and be helped to weigh up the risks and benefits. They can then negotiate and evaluate their treatment options with mental health care professionals.

Mental health nurses must monitor the side-effects from antipsychotic drugs closely. This is most efficiently and accurately done using validated assessment tools such as the Extrapyramidal Side Effect Rating Scale (Simpson and Angus, 1970). Nurses can also help reduce the distress caused by other side-effects such as weight gain, drowsiness and constipation. Table 16.1 shows effective interventions for management of common side-effects from antipsychotic drugs. Nurses must be aware of the irreversible and potentially fatal side-effects caused by antipsychotic drugs.

Preventing Irreversible Side Effects

Permanent abnormal involuntary movements, known as tardive dyskinesia (TD), are observed in approximately 20% of people treated with antipsychotic drugs (Kane and Smith, 1982). Possible risk factors for developing TD are:

1. Increasing age.
2. Increasing duration of illness and drug therapy.
3. Female gender (Jeste and Caliguiri, 1993).
4. Persistent negative symptoms (Liddle *et al.*, 1993).
5. The presence of an affective disorder.
6. Concurrent diabetes.
7. A possible genetic predisposition.

TD is known to occur when approximately 80% of striatal dopamine D_2 receptors are blocked, which occurs with fairly low doses of traditional antipsychotics (Gerlach and Peacock, 1995). Glazer *et al.* (1993) demonstrated that as many as two-thirds of patients on antipsychotic medication for 25 years will develop TD at some stage. Several effective preventive interventions have been suggested. First, mental health nurses need to take all the probable risk factors into account when assessing the risk of TD. Gerlach (1994) has suggested that the idea of giving the 'lowest possible dose' needs to be considered and that patients would benefit from the 'shortest possible treatment period'. However, other authors are wary of the efficacy of this approach (Barnes and Kane, 1996). It is also indicated that low-level D_2 receptor blockers (i.e. clozapine or risperidone) be used if the risk of TD is high.

Treatment of TD has been shown to be ineffective (Feltner and Hertzman, 1993). Studies have investigated the use of benzodiazepines, lithium, carbamazepine, beta-blockers (Gerlach and Peacock, 1995), ECT (Kaplan *et al*., 1991) and vitamin E (Adler *et al*., 1993); all these approaches were found to elicit a limited response.

THE USE OF ELECTROCONVULSIVE THERAPY IN THE LONG-TERM MENTALLY ILL

Enns and Reiss (1992) defined electroconvulsive therapy (ECT) as:

> a medical procedure in which a brief electrical stimulus is used to induce a cerebral seizure under controlled conditions.

ECT was introduced in 1938 by Cerletti and Bini (Cerletti, 1940) to treat severe psychosis and soon became the treatment of choice for the maintenance of chronic schizophrenia. After the development of antipsychotic medication, ECT was mainly used to alleviate severe affective disorders (Enns and Reiss, 1992). Although there is a large body of literature from early studies, serious methodological flaws have been found (Christison *et al*., 1991). It was advocated that schizophrenic patients with catatonia, affective symptoms (Folstein *et al*., 1973) or acute episodes (Small, 1985) would most benefit from ECT; however, its role in the treatment of chronic schizophrenia remained unclear.

Early experiments using genuine ECT and 'sham ECT' as a control showed no benefits of using ECT in chronic schizophrenics (Miller *et al*., 1953; Heath *et al*., 1964). However, there has recently been renewed interest in this area for 'treatment-resistant' patients. Studies have suggested that some of these previously unresponsive people may benefit from ECT (Friedel, 1986). Sajatovic and Meltzer (1993) cite a number of studies that indicate that a combination of ECT and antipsychotics may be useful for treatment-resistant individuals, although it is unclear whether any positive effects are maintained at follow-up (Brandon *et al*., 1985).

Recently, several case studies have again suggested that ECT is an effective maintenance treatment in chronic patients to prevent relapse (Lohr *et al*., 1994; Hoflich *et al*., 1995, Stiebel, 1995). It is clear that there is a need for methodologically sound, controlled studies of the use of ECT for treatment-resistant schizophrenia before any strong conclusions can be drawn. This has been hindered, perhaps, by the many important legal and ethical issues surrounding this treatment.

NEGATIVE SYMPTOMS

Negative symptoms can affect cognition, emotion, speech and motivation (Hogg, 1996). Typical distressing negative symptoms include apathy, social withdrawal, impaired ability to establish and maintain self in the community, poor self-care and self-management of illness, difficulty in engaging in recreational or occupational activities and trouble managing finances and negotiating social relationships (see Chapter 18). Negative symptoms can be less responsive to antipsychotic medication than other aspects of severe mental illness. Further, between 40% and 50% of patients relapse while on regular medication or suffer significant negative symptoms (Carpenter

TABLE 16.1 Management of side-effects

Side effect	Nursing interventions
EPS (parkinsonism, akathisia, dystonia, dyskinesia)*	First instance, use p.r.n. (as required) anticholinergic; consider prophylactic use if persistent. If patient is distressed consider other treatment options or reduce dose.
Weight gain	Dietary advice and exercise.
Sedation	Give smaller dose in the morning, single dose at night or reduce dose.
Anxiety	Consider using p.r.n. benzodiazepines.
Nausea	Consider an anti-emetic. Advise patient that these effects are usually transient.
Constipation	Dietary advice (bran cereal, increase fibre intake). Consider bulk-forming laxatives.
Seizures	Consider using anti-convulsants or reduce dosage.
Sexual dysfunction	Evaluate the impact on the patient's life, then consider treatment options.

* *may be irreversible.*

et al., 1988). For these reasons behavioural approaches together with pharmacological interventions are often used to alleviate these problems.

Liberman *et al.* (1994) propose that, to understand why behavioural models are effective, the vulnerability–stress model needs to be taken into account. The basic principle of this model is that psychological and social stressors and mediators can influence the course of a schizophrenic illness (Nuechterlein, 1987). Coping and social skills training can help to buffer stress, medication is used for the underlying vulnerability (Liberman and Kopelowicz, 1994) and the provision of supportive services can act as a protective factor (Liberman *et al.*, 1994). The most commonly used behavioural approaches will be outlined and discussed.

Token Economies

The use of interventions to increase motivation, based on giving rewards when tasks are performed, have been well documented. The best known example of this type of intervention is the token economy regime. In this model the performance of a pre-specified target behaviour is immediately followed by a tangible reinforcement (Kazdin, 1982).

In a randomized controlled trial by Li and Wang (1994), a token economy was used as part of the rehabilitation of 52 chronic schizophrenic patients. A reinforcement schedule was administered on a daily basis by trained mental health nurses. Results demonstrated significant improvements in the psychosocial function of the experimental group compared to controls.

A study by Dickerson *et al.* (1994) examined the effect of a token economy on patients' performance and the level of violence. In this study, patients earned points for hygiene, attendance at unit activities and medication compliance. Points could be exchanged for tangible reinforcers such as soft drinks and snacks. Dickerson *et al.* (1994) demonstrated, over a 5-year period, that such interventions could reduce levels of violence and improve psychosocial functioning.

Such interventions have been criticized because improvements are not sustained when the token economy stops. Further, the ethics of such interventions have also been questioned. However, token economies have been shown to consistently improve the level of social functioning in people with chronic schizophrenia.

Social Skills Training

Social skills training can be defined as:

> behavioural techniques or learning activities that enable people to establish or restore instrumental/affiliate skills in domains required to meet the interpersonal, self care and coping demands of community living.

> *(Liberman et al., 1994)*

Deficits in social and role functioning are key factors in schizophrenia (American Psychiatric Association (APA), 1987). The inability to cope with the environment and social isolation can lead to stress and poor community functioning, which is associated with relapse.

There is evidence in the large body of literature (Liberman, 1992) to suggest that social skills training, when carefully designed and delivered, can increase patients' knowledge and skill levels (Wallace and Liberman, 1985) and halve relapse rates.

In 1990, Benton and Schroeder conducted a meta-analysis of 27 controlled studies of social skills training (SST) in schizophrenia. They assessed:

1. The magnitude of the treatment effects.
2. Whether positive effects could be generalized and maintained.
3. The impact of differences in diagnosis and training.

They found that in contrast with controls, SST is significantly more effective in improving social skills acquisition, durability and generalization as well as leading to earlier discharge from hospital and reduced relapse rates. However, these improvements were independent of differences in diagnosis or method of training.

The process is designed to help the psychiatrically disabled person function at an optimal level in as normal a social context as possible (Bennett, 1978). Social skills training is aimed at solving problems concerned with activities of daily living, such as personal hygiene, dressing and grooming, as well as other broader aspects such as medication management, family relationships, job finding, occupation and friendship (Liberman *et al.*, 1994). Deficits in social and independent living skills are prevalent among the long-term mentally ill. These include deficiencies in non-verbal communication skills such as eye contact, posture and facial expression as well as inadequate problem-solving abilities (Liberman, 1992). Programmes from manuals, 'in vivo' and homework tasks are emphasized, to spur generalization.

To promote the clinical application of social skills training, these techniques have been made 'user friendly' by packing them in modules, e.g. trainer's manuals, patient workbooks and demonstration video cassettes. Each module is goal-specific and targeted on areas of community living. Examples from the medication management module (Liberman *et al.*, 1994) include:

- Understanding the benefits of medication.
- Having knowledge of self-administration.
- Recognizing side-effects of medication.
- Negotiating with health care professionals.
- Understanding the benefits of long-acting injectable medication.

Sessions include role-play scenes, modelling and rehearsal, to improve skills. At times, sessions are video-taped to aid feedback.

In addition to the highly structured modular format (Wallace *et al.*, 1992), there are also moderately structured approaches to delivering social skills training such as problem-solving groups (Hierholzer and Liberman, 1986). Participants are taught the problem-solving skills that they need for daily living. This problem-solving method involves:

1. Deciding that a problem exists and defining it clearly.
2. Identifying the alternative solutions to the problem.
3. Evaluating the advantages and disadvantages of each solution.
4. choosing the best option or options.
5. identifying the necessary resources to carry out the chosen solution.
6. picking a time and carrying out the solution.

FAMILY INTERVENTIONS IN RELAPSE PREVENTION

In people with a history of repeated relapse, or in those at high risk of treatment non-compliance, living alone or in a family environment that has a high level of expressed emotion, relapse prevention is an important aspect of care.

Effective interventions that prevent relapse rely on close cooperation between the patient, their carer or relative and mental health professionals. An ethos of trust and informed partnership between these groups must be developed (Smith and Birchwood, 1990). Education about early intervention strategies also needs to be provided emphasizing that the patient and carer are invaluable in recognizing the potential for relapse and need to initiate treatment (National Schizophrenia Fellowship, 1995). Treatment compliance will be enhanced when the suffer and carers have a stable, trusting relationship with mental health professionals.

Patient-specific signs of relapse can be obtained by careful interviewing of patients and relatives about any changes in thinking and behaviour prior to a recent relapse. The interview should identify the date of onset of symptoms, time between admissions and dates when changes in behaviour and thinking were observed. These baseline data will help predict an impending relapse and enable appropriate steps to be taken.

FAMILY INTERVENTIONS FOR PEOPLE WITH ENDURING MENTAL HEALTH PROBLEMS.

Family interventions are often implemented to help patients and carers cope more effectively (Liberman *et al.*, 1994). It is most often the families of the long-term mentally ill who provide the care and support in the community (National Schizophrenia Fellowship, 1995). Most intervention for families follows a similar format:

1. Behavioural assessment.
2. Education about schizophrenia and care.
3. Communication skills training.
4. Problem-solving.
5. Coping with special problems.

When comparing family interventions with intensive individual therapy for discharged patients at 2-year follow-up (Strachan, 1992), the family interventions significantly reduced the number and length of admissions, reduced incidence of acute exacerbation of symptoms and lowered the number of emergency crisis sessions needed. Social and vocational adjustment were also increased and the effective doses of medication needed to maintain patients were lower. In 1990, Brenner *et al.*, showed that a family treatment programme that addressed cognitive and behaviour deficits led to improvements in social adjustment and cognitive functioning and was effective in lowering psychopathology.

It is also appropriate to work with the family as a whole in efforts to prevent or resolve crisis. There is now a considerable body of research that emphasizes the importance of family interaction in schizophrenia (Leff and Vaughn, 1985). Families in which relationships are critical, hostile, dominant, over-involved and with high levels of face-to-face contact were designated High Expressed Emotion (Brown *et al.*, 1972). It has been demonstrated that lowering the amount of expressed emotion (EE), encouraging warmth and positive remarks and using maintenance medication can significantly reduce relapse rates in vulnerable families and improve community outcomes (Gamble, 1993).

This can be achieved through education, relative groups and family work or simply reducing the amount of face-to-face contact within vulnerable families (Leff *et al*, 1982, 1984; Liberman *et al*, 1994). An outline family work of this kind includes:

- Identification of difficulties within the family.
- Modelling of skills by therapist.
- Rehearsal of skills learnt using role-play etc.
- Constructive feedback and reinforcement.
- The use of homework assignments.
  (See Chapter 23 for a more in-depth examination of Expressed Emotion studies and family interventions.)

It is important to note that the most effective psychosocial treatments, whether in in-patient or community settings, contain elements of:

1. Practicality.
2. Problem-solving of everyday challenges.
3. Socialization.
4. Vocational activities.

However, psychosocial treatment has been shown to be effective with this client group only if it is long-term (Hoggarty *et al.*, 1991).

COGNITIVE REMEDIATION

Clear cognitive deficits in people with schizophrenia have been demonstrated. All nursing interventions must take note of these deficits. Mental health nurses should spend short periods of time (no more than 20–30 minutes) with patients. Any information given should be presented in a clear, concise way and may often need to be repeated.

Interest has focused recently on whether these cognitive deficits can be restored (Green, 1993). Although cognitive remediation has been extensively examined in brain injury patients, such interventions have been largely overlooked for people with schizophrenia. However, neuropsychological models for rehabilitation do exist and may be applicable to psychiatric patients (see, for example, Powell, 1981).

The substitution transfer approach offers the patient alternative strategies for achieving goals (Wilson, 1989). This approach aims to get an intact part of the brain to take over the functions of the damaged part. Green (1993) cites the example of memory rehabilitation. Patients with defective verbal memory could be trained to use aids such as checklists or to use visual imagery as a mnemonic device. Such interventions may be of importance in improving the quality of life of people with schizophrenia. Mental health nurses should be actively involved in the design and development of such interventions.

PSYCHOLOGICAL MANAGEMENT OF SYMPTOMS

As previously discussed, a high proportion of people with schizophrenia do not respond to treatment with antipsychotic medication or are left with distressing residual symptoms. This section describes some of the psychological treatments that have recently been developed to complement drug therapy.

WORKING WITH DELUSIONS

Evidence from research into the formation and maintenance of delusional beliefs suggests that nursing interventions that inform the patient that their beliefs are not real will not be effective. Further, if, as Kaney and Bentall (1989) suggest, delusions are a mechanism to protect an individual's self-esteem, such interventions may be very distressing. Patients need to be helped to develop ways of testing out their delusional beliefs for themselves. Beliefs that are less tenaciously held should be examined first. The nurse can gently support and encourage the patient to compare their beliefs with reality. Gradually more strongly held and persistent beliefs can then be examined. Interventions should also be graded according to cognitive effort. Those requiring the least effort should be examined first. Only with this type of graded intervention have significant improvements in delusional thinking been demonstrated (Tarrier *et al.*, 1993; Bentall *et al.*, 1994).

WORKING WITH HALLUCINATIONS

A variety of approaches for working with hallucinations have been proposed, such as thought -stopping (Allen *et al.*, 1985), distraction, and verbal suppression procedures (such as listening to music or covert counting). However, Bentall *et al.* (1994) argue that, using their theoretical model of hallucinations, focusing treatment may reduce the frequency of the voices or the distress caused by them, by helping the patient gradually to re-attribute the voices to the self.

In this study, patients were helped to identify the physical characteristics of the voices, the content of the voices and any related thoughts and assumptions about voices (Bentall *et al.*, 1994). The formulation of the meaning and function of the voices often involved the patients accepting the voices as self-generated. Bentall *et al.* report that some patients became aware that the voices themselves were not distressing but that their thoughts about them had caused great distress. Such interventions may be of considerable use to mental health nurses, although training and supervision in these techniques would be required.

CRISIS INTERVENTIONS

The psychological reaction to loss of well-being, and the possibility that this may herald a relapse, places a strain both on the patient and relative, which can accelerate relapse. The availability of support and quick access to the mental health team will help reduce these effects.

There are certain individuals who implement strategies of their own when recognizing loss of well-being. This may include changing their behaviour, engaging in other social activities, seeking professional help or recommencing medication. Achieving these ends may require some changes in service provision. Services need to be flexible and responsive to the needs of individuals and their carers (in other words, proactive rather than reactive) for crisis interventions to be effective.

The earlier a crisis is identified, the better the chances for effective intervention. This involves working with service users to predict those situations that are most likely to create an intolerable threat to their equilibrium and then helping them develop preventive strategies.

When a crisis occurs, support can be offered using a problem-solving approach. By their very nature, crises are unpredictable and emotive. For this reason it is important that case managers (mental health professionals) do not work alone. Debriefing and winding down after dealing with a crisis is important.

CASE MANAGEMENT

Case management was developed to overcome patients' difficulties in finding and accessing mental health services. It involves having a single person responsible for monitoring a long-term supportive relationship with the client, regardless of where the client is or the number of agencies involved. This involves planning for the long-term and liaison with other services (Harris and Bergman, 1987). In brief, the case manager coordinates the delivery of individual 'packages of care'. The role of the case manager therefore contains elements of social work, nursing, occupational therapy and administrative skills. Intagliata (1982) lists six main elements of case management:

1. Comprehensive assessment of individual needs.
2. The development of an individualized 'package of care' to meet those needs.
3. Ensuring that the service is accessible, continuous, coordinated and flexible.
4. Monitoring the quality of services provided and liaison with service providers.
5. Adjusting levels of support according to fluctuating levels of functioning.
6. Providing long-term commitment.

ASSERTIVE COMMUNITY MANAGEMENT

This approach uses a multidisciplinary team, rather than a single person, to provide services directly to patients' homes or community locations, to stabilize patients in the community (Witheridge, 1990). This is because those in need of services often find it most difficult to attend out-patients' appointments or to contact services to ask for help. Studies have shown that assertive case management can be effective in improving communication and continuity of care (Witheridge, 1990), and can improve economic efficiency and provision of services and clarify accountability (Wasylenki *et al.*, 1993). One of the benefits of assertive case management can be attributed to a small team of staff working together on a daily basis (Hoge *et al.*, 1994). One of its most important functions is to avert hospitalizations, through close monitoring of the patient's illness and medication and by using aggressive crisis intervention (Stein and Test, 1980).

WORKING WITH INFORMAL CARERS

This should be routine practice, rather than something that only occurs where carers are problematic (Smith and Birchwood, 1990). Case managers should involve carers in identifying needs and in the planning and implementation of care.

The burden of caring for people with long-term mental illness is well documented. Fadden *et al.* (1987) specifically identified the following detrimental effects on carers' lives:
1. Reduced social and leisure activities.
2. Increased financial burden.

Fadden and co-workers also highlighted the fact that carers found it difficult to understand and accept the illness.

Winefield and Harvey (1994) suggested that some of this burden could be alleviated through support and regular contact with mental health services. They carried out a survey of 121 carers and identified the following needs:
1. Support.
2. Less social isolation.
3. To know that there are others in the same or similar situation.
4. Information about illness and treatment.
5. Advice about coping strategies.
6. To gain familiarity with mental health resources.

Holden and Lewine (1982) demonstrated that carers felt left out of treatment and would like help to develop more realistic expectations about the course and outcome of the illness. Further, Shapiro *et al.*, (1983) state that carers want to increase their understanding of serious mental illness and its impact on the family. A recent survey into carers' needs and experiences by the National Schizophrenia Fellowship (1995) pro-

duced similar results but also highlighted that 71% of carers experienced physical or mental health problems as a direct result of their caring role.

Mental health nurses can provide invaluable advice and support to their patients' carers through case management. This can be achieved by giving information about illness, treatment and local resources and trying to increase carers' understanding and awareness of long-term mental illness.

MAINTAINING AND EXPANDING SOCIAL NETWORKS

Poor social networks contribute to the vulnerability of the long-term mentally ill. The case manager should help the patient to exercise choice and develop a social network.

LIAISON WITH HOSPITALS

The role of effective case management in hospital settings is more specialized. Stein and Test (1980) argued that with adequate community programmes, hospitals would only be used for patients who are in imminent danger, pose a threat to others or have significant medical problems. However, people who persistently experience psychotic symptoms may require structure and care that can only be provided in a hospital.

SUMMARY

Working with people with enduring mental illness presents significant challenges for mental health nurses. Progress may often be slow and patients may have little motivation to take part in day-to-day activities. However, important developments in psychopharmacology, specifically the introduction of clozapine, may make a significant impact on this patient group. A range of psychosocial interventions including social skills training and the psychological management of symptoms provide the framework for mental health nurses to impact dramatically on the quality of life for this patient group. Such interventions are relevant both to ward based nurses and to those working in the community.

The success of new drug treatments and psychosocial interventions may often mean that patients who have been hospitalized for long periods of time may wish to lead more independent lives or return home. Such changes will have an impact on their carers and family. Mental health nurses play an important role in supporting and educating carers.

The use of case management as a method of organizing care will expand the role of nurses working in the community. The will have to develop a variety of skills and perform a variety of different and contrasting roles.

KEY CONCEPTS

- Community care is an informal partnership between an informal community network, the individual and statutory services.
- People with serious mental illness often tend not to seek help when their condition is deteriorating.
- Behavioural family management is often implemented to help patients and carers cope more effectively.
- Case management involves having a single person responsible for monitoring a long-term supportive relationship with a client, regardless of the number of agencies involved.
- Mental health nurses have an important role to play in supporting and educating carers.
- New drug treatment and psychosocial interventions may often mean that patients previously hospitalized for long periods can lead more independent lives in the community.

REFERENCES

Adler LA, Peselow E, Duncan E, Rosenthall M *et al.*: Vitamin E and tardive dyskinesia: time course of effect after placebo substitution. *Psychopharmacol Bull* 29(3):371–374, 1993.

Allen H, Halperin J, Friend R: Removal and diversion tactics and the control of auditory hallucinations. *Behav Res Ther* 23:601–605, 1985.

American Psychiatric Association: *Diagnostic and statistical manual of mental disorders,* 3 edi (revised) Washington DC, 1987, American Psychiatric Association.

Barnes TRE, Kane JM: Choosing between old and new antipsychotics. *Curr Opin Psychiatry* 9:41–44, 1996.

Bennett DH: Social forms of psychiatric treatment. In: Wing JK, editor: *Schizophrenia–towards a new synthesis.* London, 1978, Academic Press.

Bentall RP, Haddock G, Slade PD: Cognitive behaviour therapy for persistent auditory hallucinations: from theory to therapy. 25:51–66, 1994.

Benton MK, Schroeder HE: Social skills training with schizophrenics: A meta analytic evaluation. *J Consult Clin Psychol* 58(6):741–747, 1990.

Brandon S, Cowley P, Macdonald C, Neville P, Palmer R, Wellstood–Eason S: Leicester ECT trial: Results in schizophrenia. *Br J Psychiatry* 146:177–183, 1985.

Brenner HD, Kraemer S, Hermanutz M, Hodel B: Cognitive treatment in schizophrenia. In: Straube ER, Hahlweg K, editors: *Schizophrenia: concepts, vulnerability, and intervention.* New York, 1990, Springer-Verlag.

Brown GW, Birley JLT, Wing JK: Influence of family life on the course of schizophrenic disorders: A replication. *Br J Psychiatry* 121:241–263, 1972.

Carpenter WT, Heinrichs DW, Wagman AMI: Deficit and non-deficit forms of schizophrenia: the concept. *Am J Psychiatry* 145:578–583, 1988.

Cerletti U: L'electroshock. *Revista Sperimentale di Freniatria* 64:209–310, 1940.

Challis DJ, Davies BP: *Case management in community care.* Aldershot, 1986, Gower.

Christison GW, Kirch DG, Wyatt RJ: When symptoms persist: choosing among alternative somatic treatments for schizophrenia. *Schizophr Bull* 17(2):217–245, 1991.

Clozapine Study Group: The safety and efficacy of clozapine in severe treatment resistant schizophrenic patients in the UK. *Br J Psychiatry* 163:150–154, 1994.

Dickerson F, Ringel N, Frederick P, Boronow J: Seclusion and restraint, assaultiveness and patient performance in a token economy. *Hosp Community Psychiatry* 45(2):168–170, 1994.

Enns MW, Reiss JP: Electroconvulsive therapy. *Can J Psychiatry* 37(10):671–678, 1992.

Fadden G, Bebbington P, Kuipers L: The burden of care: the impact of functional psychiatric illness on the patient's family. *Br J Psychiatry* 150:285–289, 1987.

Falloon IR, Boyd JL, McGill CW: *Family care of schizophrenia.* London, 1984, Guilford Press.

Folstein M, Folstein S, McHugh PR: Clinical predictors of improvement after electroconvulsive therapy of patients with schizophrenia, neurotic reactions and affective disorders. *Biol Psychiatry* 7:147–152, 1973.

Ford R, Beadsmoore A, Ryan P, *et al.*: Providing the safety net: case management for people with a serious mental illness. *J Men Healt,* 1:91–99, 1995.

Friedel RO: The combined use of neuroleptics and ECT in drug resistant schizophrenic patients. *Psychopharmacol Bull* 22: 928–930, 1986.

Gamble C: Working with schizophrenic clients and their families. *Br J Nurs* 2(17):856–859, 1993.

Gerlach J: Oral vs. depot administration of neuroleptic in relapse prevention. *Acta Psychiatr Scand* 89(supplement 382):28–32, 1994.

Gerlach J, Peacock L: Intolerance to neuroleptic drugs: the art of avoiding extrapyramidal side effects. *Eur Psychiatry* 10(supplement 1):27s–31s, 1995.

Glazer WM, Morgenstern H, Doucette JT: Predicting the long term risk of tardive dyskinesia in outpatients maintained on neuroleptic medication. *J Clin Psychiatry* 54(4):133–139, 1993.

Green MF: Cognitive remediation in schizophrenia: Is it time yet? *Am J Psychiatry* 150(2):178–187, 1993.

Harris M, Bergman HC: Case management with the chronically mentally ill: a clinical perspective. *Am J Orthopsychiatry* 57:296–302, 1987.

Heath ES, Adams A, Wakeling PLG: Short courses of ECT and simulated ECT in chronic schizophrenia. *Br J Psychiatry* 110:800–807, 1964.

Heinrich K, Klieser E, Lehmann E, Kinzler E: Experimental comparison of the efficacy and compatibility of risperidone and clozapine in acute schizophrenia. In: Kane JM, editor: *Risperidone: major progress in antipsychotic treatment.* Oxford, 1991, Oxford Clinical Communications.

Hemsley D: Schizophrenia investigation. In: Lindsay SJE, Powell GE, editors: *The handbook of clinical adult psychology.* London, 1994, Routledge.

Hierholzer RW, Liberman RP: Successful living: a social skills and problem solving group for chronic mentally ill. *Hosp Community Psychiatry* 37:913–919, 1986.

Hoflich G, Kasper S, Burghof KW, Scholl HP *et al.*: Maintenance ECT for the treatment of therapy resistant paranoid schizophrenia and Parkinson's disease. *Biol Psychiatry* 37(12):892–894, 1995.

Hoge MA, Davison H, Griffith EEH, Sledge WH, Howenstine RA: Defining managed care in public sector psychiatry. *Hosp Community Psychiatry* 45(11): 1085–1089, 1994.

Hogg L: Psychological treatments for negative symptoms. In: Haddock G, Slade P D, editors: *Cognitive behavioural interventions in psychotic disorders.* London, 1996, Routledge.

Hoggarty GE, Anderson CM, Reiss DJ, Kornblith S, *et al.*: Family psychoeducation, social skills training, and maintenance chemotherapy, in the aftercare treatment of schizophrenia: II Two year effects of a controlled study on relapse and adjustment. *Arch Gen Psychiatr,* 48(4):340–347, 1991.

Holden DF, Lewine RRJ: How families evaluate mental health professionals, resources, and effects of illness. *Schizophr Bull* 8(4):626–633, 1982.

Intagliata J: Improving the quality of community care for the chronically mentally disabled: the role of case management. *Schizophr Bull* 8(4):655–674, 1982.

Jeste DV, Caliguiri MP: Tardive Dyskinesia. *Schizophr Bull* 19:303–315, 1993.

Kane J, Honigfeld G, Singer J, *et al.*: Clozapine for the treatment resistant schizophrenic. *Arch Gen Psychiatr,* 45:789–796, 1988.

Kane JM, Smith J: Tardive dyskinesia: Prevalence and risk factors. *Arch Gen Psychiatry* 39:473–481, 1982.

Kaney S, Bentall RP: Persecutory delusions and the self serving bias: Evidence from a contingency judgement task. *J Nerv Ment Dis* 180:773–780, 1989.

Kaplan Z, Benjamin J, Zohar J: Remission of tardive dystonia with ECT. *Convuls Ther* 7(4):280–283, 1991.

Kazdin AE: The token economy: a decade later. *J Appli Behav Anal* 15:431–455, 1982.

Leff J, Kuipers L, Berkowitz R, Eberlein-Vries R, Sturgeon D: A controlled trial of social intervention in families of schizophrenic patients. *Br J Psychiatry* 141:121–134, 1982.

Leff J, Vaughn C: *Expressed emotion in families: its significance for mental illness.* New York, 1985, Guilford.

Li F, Wang M: A behavioural training programme for chronic schizophrenic patients. *Br J Psychiatry* 165(supplement 24):32–37, 1994.

Liberman RP: *Handbook of psychiatric rehabilitation.* New York, 1992, Macmillan.

Liberman RP, Koploeicz A: Basic elements in biobehavioural treatment and rehabilitation of schizophrenia. *Int Clin Psychopharmacol* 9(5): 51–58, 1995.

Liberman RP, Kopelowicz A, Young AS: Biobehavioural treatments and rehabilitation of schizophrenia. *Behav Ther* 25(1):89–107, 1994.

Liddle PF, Barnes TRE, Speller J, Kibel D: Negative symptoms as a risk factor for tardive dyskinesia in schizophrenia. *Br J Psychiatry* 163:776–780, 1993.

Lohr WD, Figiel GS, Hudziak JJ, Zorumski CF *et al.*: Maintenance electroconvulsive therapy in schizophrenia. *J Clin Psychiatry* 55(5):217–218, 1994.

Miller DH, Clancey J, Cumming E: A comparison between unidirectional current nonconvulsive electrical stimulation given with Reiter's machine, standard alternating current electroshock (Cerletti method), and pentothal in chronic schizophrenia. *Am J Psychiatry* 109:617–620, 1953.

National Schizophrenia Fellowship: *The silent partners: the needs of people who provide care for people with a severe mental illness.* Kingston upon Thames, 1995, NSF.

Nuechterlein KH: Vulnerability models: state of the art. In: Haffner H, Gattaz W, Jangerik W, editors: *Searches for the cause of schizophrenia.* Berlin, 1987, Springer-Verlag.

Perkins RE, Repper JM: *Working alongside people with long term mental health problems.* London, 1996, Chapman & Hall.

Pickar D: Current concepts in schizophrenia: international symposia report new standards for assessment and treatment, part 2. Treatment issues and broadening options. *J Clin Psychiatry* 56(6):269–280, 1995.

Powell GE: *Brain function therapy.* Aldershot, 1981, Gower Press.

Rotrosen JP: Current concepts in schizophrenia: international symposia report new standards for assessment and treatment part, 2. Treatment issues and broadening options. *J Clin Psychiatry* 56(6):269–280, 1995.

Sajatovic M, Meltzer HY: The effect of short term electroconvulsive treatment plus neuroleptics in treatment resistant schizophrenia and schizoaffective disorder. *Convuls Ther* 9(3):167–175, 1993.

Shapiro RM, Possidente RN, Plum KC, Lehman AF: The evaluation of a support group for families of the chronically mentally ill. *Psychiatr Q* 55(4):236–241, 1983.

Simpson GM, Angus JWS: A rating scale for extrapyramidal side-effects. *Acta Psychiatr Scand* 212(supplement 44):11–19, 1970.

Small JG: Efficacy of electroconvulsive therapy in schizophrenia, mania, and other disorders. I. Schizophrenia. *Convuls ther* 1:263–270, 1985.

Smith J, Birchwood M: Relatives and patients as partners in the management of schizophrenia. *Br J Psychiatry* 156:654–660, 1990.

Stein L, Test MA: Alternative to mental hospital treatment I: Conceptual Model, treatment program, and clinician evaluation. *Arch Gen Psychiatry* 37:392–393, 1980.

Stiebel VG: Maintenance electroconvulsive therapy for chronically mentally ill patients: A case series. *Psychiatr Serv* 46(3):265–268, 1995.

Strachan A: Family management. In: Liberman RP, editor: *Handbook of psychiatric rehabilitation.* New York, 1992, Academic Press.

Tarrier N, Beckett R, Harwood S, Baker A, Yusupoff L, Ugartebru I: A trial of two cognitive–behavioural methods of treating drug-resistant residual psychotic symptoms in schizophrenic patients. *Br JPsychiatry* 162:524–532, 1993.

Tugrul KC: Current concepts in schizophrenia: international symposia report new standards for assessment and treatment, part 2. Treatment issues and broadening options. *J Clin Psychiatry* 56(6)269–280, 1995.

Wallace CJ, Liberman RP: Social skills training for schizophrenics: A controlled clinical trial. *Psychiatry Res* 15:239–247, 1985.

Wallace CJ, Liberman RP, Mackain SJ, Blackwell G, Eckman TA: Effectiveness replicability of modules for teaching social instrumental skills to the severely mentally ill. *Am J Psychiatry* 149:654–658, 1992.

Wasylenki DA, Goering RN, Lemire MS, Lindsey S, Lancee W: The Hostel Outreach Program: Assertive Case Management for homeless mentally ill persons. *Hosp Community Psychiatry* 44(9):849–853, 1993.

Wilson B: Models of cognitive rehabilitation. In: Wood RL, Eames P, editors: *Models of brain injury rehabilitation.* Baltimore, 1989, Johns Hopkins University Press.

Winefield HR, Harvey EJ: Determinants of psychological distress in relatives of people with chronic schizophrenia. *Schizophr Bull* 19(3):619–625, 1994.

Witheridge TF: Assertive community treatment: a strategy for helping persons with severe mental illness to avoid rehospitalization. In: Cohen NL, editor: *Psychiatry takes to the streets: outreach and crisis intervention for the mentally ill.* New York, 1990, Guilford Press.

Wykes T, Sturt E: The measurement of social behaviour in psychiatric patients: an assessment of the reliability and validity of the SBS. *Br J Psychiatry* 148:1–11, 1986.

FURTHER READING

Haddock G, Slade PD, editors: *Cognitive behavioural interventions in psychotic disorders.* London, 1995, Routledge. *Reviews the use of psychosocial interventions in schizophrenia, including a medication management programme.*

Phelan M, Strathdee G, Thornicroft G: *Emergency mental health services in the community.* Cambridge, 1995, Cambridge University Press.
This book provides a comprehensive overview of research findings and theoretical models, describing emergency mental health services in the community.

Watkins M, Harvey N, Carson J, Ritter S: *Collaborative community mental health care.* London, 1996, Arnold.
This book provides a multiprofessional team approach to dealing with the challenges of community-centred mental health care.

Weller MPI, Muijen M: *Dimensions of community mental health care.* London, 1993, WB Saunders.
Written by a team of leading professionals, this text provides an in depth examination of diverse approaches to community care for people who are mentally ill

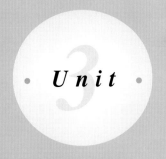

·*Unit*·

3

Applying Principles in Nursing Practice

17

Understanding Suicidal Behaviour

Learning Outcomes

After studying this chapter you should be able to:

- Explore the nature of depression in depth.

- Describe the epidemiology of suicidal behaviour.

- Understand depression and suicidal behaviour from the point of view of the service user or patient.

- Analyse predisposing factors leading to depression and deliberate self-harm.

- Discuss the processes involved in undertaking an assessment of the risk of suicidal behaviour.

- Identify a range of nursing interventions in working with people who are depressed and suicidal.

CHAPTER OUTLINE

- *Depression*

- *Suicide and suicidal behaviour*

- *Other kinds of self-harm*

- *Nursing interventions in the hospital setting*

- *Nursing interventions in the community*

- *Managing one's own feelings*

Working with people who are depressed and suicidal is both difficult and challenging. The critical issues for mental health nurses include:

- understanding and supporting someone who feels that they and their life are worthless.
- assessing suicidal risk
- managing suicidal behaviour.
- confronting the possibility of suicide.
- coping with the effects of suicidal behaviour on others.

At the centre of all of this is the person who presents with depressed and suicidal feelings and behaviour. The relationship between this person and the Key Worker or nurse is crucial to the development of the therapeutic work that can take place. Both parties come with their own knowledge and experiences; however, it is the nurse's role to apply this knowledge and skills base in the duty of care to the individual being nursed. This body of knowledge and skills adds a third dimension to the nurse–patient relationship (Figure 17.1). The chapter will focus, therefore, on the three aspects of caring for a suicidal patient. These are: the person who is

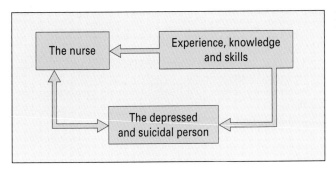

Figure 17.1 The three-dimensional aspects of caring for a suicidal and depressed person.

depressed and suicidal; the nurse offering the care; and the experience, knowledge and skills brought to the therapeutic relationship.

To illustrate this model, the chapter includes the real-life experiences of service users and professionals, as well as relevant literature. The overall aim is to promote greater understanding of the complex and intricate mechanisms involved in caring for someone who has turned their back on life itself.

DEPRESSION

WHAT IS DEPRESSION?

Depression is something that most people feel at some time in their lives, as an experience of feeling 'down', 'blue', 'low'. Clinical depression differs from this both qualitatively and in duration; it is usually characterized by a profound, persistent and all-pervasive depressive mood. It is, however, difficult to describe and classify. In reviewing what he considered to be the 'confusion' surrounding the classification of depression, Kendall (1976) noted that 'the boundaries between depression and sadness, between depressive illnesses and anxiety states, between affective psychosis and schizophrenia, and between recurrent depression and personality disorder are all arbitrary and ill-defined'. There appear to be standard features, but as Hamilton (1989) pointed out, depressed people found in clinical practice often differ in their symptoms from those found in classical descriptions. Hamilton is among many who have found a high prevalence of anxiety with depression, expressed both psychically and physically. It is generally agreed, however, that there is a common core of a prevailing mood of sadness, helplessness and hopelessness, and self-esteem is low. The following Case study gives a literary example of depression.

In *The Bell Jar*, Esther experiences apathy and poor self-esteem. She cannot be bothered to wash herself or her clothes and she does not care enough about herself to be concerned with appearance or hygiene. She has not been sleeping. The future stretches ahead of her in apparent futility—she describes it as 'desolate'. Significantly, she seeks safety. She feels safe in the familiarity of the clothes she is wearing and she also feels safe in the room because there are no windows, presumably a reference to her self-destructive wishes (which she indeed enacts throughout the book). There is also an air of detachment in this passage; Esther expresses herself in a very matter-of-fact way. There are no words that express emotion at all.

Depression is expressed differently in different cultures. Helman (1990) notes, for example, that somatization (experiencing psychological distress as physical symptoms) is a major feature of depression in some cultures, especially Far Eastern ones. Instead of complaining of depressed mood, people seek medical attention for physical symptoms such as feeling 'tired all the time', headaches, palpitations, vague pains and dizziness. Depression is experienced as physical pain, instead of emotional pain. There is therefore the risk of depression

remaining unrecognized because of the façade of physical symptoms.

The problems of identifying and classifying depression make it difficult to ascertain its incidence. One study of depression in primary care found that 1 in 20 people in the community are likely to be depressed (Blacker and Clare, 1987). Wright (1994) points out that, while figures vary, there is likely to be at least one depressed patient seen at any given GP surgery session. However, only 1 in 400 people get referred to a psychiatrist for depression and only 1 in 1000 is admitted to hospital for depression. Most people with depression, then, are encountered in community settings.

Women are more likely than men to be diagnosed as depressed. There are several possible explanations for this, including medical diagnostic habits as well as the fact that women may suffer from depression post-natally, although social factors may be more important (Tennant, 1985).

WHAT CAUSES DEPRESSION?

There are a number of theories that attempt to understand the causation of depression. The causes proposed include: biological causes or genetic predisposition; childhood experiences leading to increased vulnerability in the face of stressful events in adulthood (Brown and Harris, 1978); social and relationship factors: and fundamentally distorted thought processes (Beck, 1967). Whatever the theoretical bases for understanding the causes, it is usually possible to identify one or more life events that may have triggered the depression, such as divorce, unemployment or bereavement. In our second

---

Case study: **An example of depression from literature**

In her semi-autobiographical novel, *The Bell Jar*, Sylvia Plath provides a revealing account of depression through the central character, Esther:

- 'At first I wondered why the room felt so safe. Then I realised it was because there were no windows.
- The air conditioning made me shiver.
- I was still wearing Betsy's white blouse and dirndl skirt. They drooped a bit now, as I hadn't washed them in my three weeks at home. The sweaty cotton gave off a sour but friendly smell.
- I hadn't washed my hair for three weeks, either.
- I hadn't slept for seven nights.
- My mother told me I must have slept, it was impossible not to sleep in all that time, but if I slept it was with my eyes wide open, for I had followed the green, limnous course of the second hand and the minute hand and the hour hand of the bedside clock through their circles and semi-circles, every night for seven nights, without missing a second, or a minute or an hour.
- The reason I hadn't washed my clothes or my hair was because it seemed so silly....
- I could see day after day glaring ahead of me like a white, broad, infinitely desolate avenue.
- It seemed silly to wash one day when I would only have to wash again the next.
- It made me tired just to think of it'.

(Plath, 1963)

---

case study, 'Winston's' experiences show clear long-standing problems and critical events that are likely to have contributed to his depression.

It is important to recognize the individual's own experience, help them understand what their problems and needs are and to work from that. Theories of causation only help practitioners when they provide pointers and guidelines that can be implemented effectively in practice. In most cases, individuals are offered a range of interventions based on an eclectic view of causation; for example, the person may find antidepressants helpful (suggesting a biological factor in depression) along with a period of cognitive–behavioural treatment (suggesting distorted thinking).

SERVICE USER PERSPECTIVES

How do people who have become depressed experience their depression? One woman described her feelings, as follows:

> Nothing seems worth it. Any good feelings of pleasure or warmth seem to have gone for good. I try and imagine how I could ever have felt happy, and I can't.

(quoted in Rosenthall and Greally, 1988)

Lewis (1995) argued that scant attention has been paid to the question of individuals' experience of depression. Through a qualitative analysis of in-depth interviews with depressed people, she uncovered a number of themes. The first theme related to the identification of a problem as 'depression'. People varied in their reaction to the diagnosis, ranging from relief to rejection. For example, 'Angie' said:

> The sense of relief, that I knew I wasn't going round the bend and that I wouldn't have to put up with this forever.... It never occurred to me that I could be depressed, I just thought that I was a nasty person.

Other themes included trying to understand and explain the depression. Some people explained their depression in terms of individualized explanations, such as 'Penny':

> I am bad with my monthlies and things like that. And get really depressed and, you know, and really down then, and I don't want to go anywhere.

Others saw social circumstances as causing their depression. 'Frank' saw his unemployment as crucial:

> They said to me, 'It's up to you to pull out now'. I say, 'I can't'. I said, 'If I got a job tomorrow—this'd all go, in a week, or a fortnight; it'd go'.

SUICIDE AND SUICIDAL BEHAVIOUR

Suicide figures are unreliable and likely to be underestimated through problems of definition and dependence on coroners' verdicts. The most recent Government figures show that there were 3299 recorded verdicts of suicide in England in 1993 (Department of Health, 1995). This adds up to more than 60 suicides a week in England alone. Of these, most were men (2534, compared with 765 women). There has been a consistently greater prevalence in male suicides, with the highest number of suicides among men in their 30s (Charlton *et al.*, 1993).

INCIDENCE OF SUICIDE

Reporting on the suicide rates in England and Wales between 1975 and 1984, McClure (1987) found an overall increase of 30% in male suicides, most apparent in the 25–54 years age group. McClure suggested that corresponding increases in unemployment, wine and spirit consumption and divorce rates could give some indication as to the causes of the increase in suicide among younger men. Among even younger men, suicide rates have increased dramatically. Health Education Authority figures suggest that rates of suicide among 15 to 24-year-old males have increased by 71% since 1982 (Aggleton, 1995).

Unemployment also appears to be a factor in suicide. It is thought to provide a trigger to depression, demoralization and social isolation, summarized as adding stress to an already vulnerable state and one enhanced by an economic recession (Pritchard, 1992). At the same time, professional people are also at high risk of suicide, e.g. vets, pharmacists, dentists and doctors. This may be because of ready access to means of suicide, such as lethal drugs (Kingdon and Jenkins, 1995).

Studies have shown that a large proportion (approximately 70%) of suicides will have had contact with psychiatric services (Busteed and Johnston, 1983; Crammer, 1984). An associated diagnosis or history of mental illness is a principal

---

> ### Case study: **Factors leading up to depression**
>
> Winston was a 52-year-old married man living with his wife and three daughters. They lived in a flat on a housing estate that was described as becoming ever smaller as the daughters began to bring friends and boyfriends home with them. Winston was born in Jamaica where his twin brother remained with their grandmother, who had brought them up. Winston had not seen his grandmother since he left Jamaica, 20 years earlier. He had returned to Jamaica only once, a year earlier, for his grandmother's funeral.
>
> He worked as a boiler maintenance man in the city, working shift hours (mainly the night shift as this brought in more money for the family). Winston's wife Beverley worked part-time in an office for a small haulage company. Money was short and there was often friction in the house over financial difficulties, the daughters' behaviour and the whole family's dislike of the area in which they lived. The flat had been burgled twice in the last 6 months and during the second burglary, racist graffiti were daubed on the living room walls. Shortly afterwards, Winston came home to an empty flat and a note from his wife, saying she had left him. He consulted his GP 3 weeks later, complaining of sleeplessness, lack of appetite and feeling that life was not worth living. He had continued to go to work and nobody at work knew what had happened.

feature (accounting for 93%) of which depression, alcoholism, schizophrenia, anxiety states, barbiturate dependence and psychotic states have been identified. Alcoholism and depression are associated with the majority of suicides (Barraclough, 1974).

CULTURAL FACTORS IN SUICIDE

Suicide is seen across the world in different cultures and races, leading Crammer (1984) to describe it as part of human nature. In Britain, concern has recently been raised about the relatively high number of suicides among young women of Asian ethnicity, especially when compared with rates in other ethnic minority groups (Soni-Raleigh and Balajaran, 1992).

Sociologists are keen to point out the marked differences in the rates of suicide by country and among groups of countries (Kelleher and Daly, 1990). Cross-cultural comparisons should be made with caution, since differences in meaning and attitudes associated with suicide result in some countries being very open with statistics and information, while others refrain from releasing true figures (Charlton *et al.*, 1993).

Kelleher and Daly (1990) discussed the increased rates of suicide in Cork, Ireland, where coroners have traditionally been reluctant to deliver verdicts of suicide. Significantly there appeared to be no evidence to support the hypothesis that mental illness had contributed to the increase in suicide, which led Kelleher and Daly to propose the increase was probably the result of social changes, especially those concerning traditional values and behaviour. In his study, unemployment appeared to be a factor in 60% of suicides.

In Canada, statistics show a recent increase in the number of suicides in newly retired pensioners (Delisle, 1992). Central American literature concentrates on the high proportion of youth suicides traced to the possession of firearms (Dudley *et al.*, 1992) and an increased use of crack (Marzuk *et al.*, 1992). Crack, a particularly addictive derivative of cocaine, is increasingly evident in major cities throughout England and therefore a subject needing further investigation.

DEFINING SUICIDAL BEHAVIOUR

The literature concerning suicide and suicidal behaviour is vast and a topic of considerable debate in its own right. Taiminen (1992) argued that most research has concentrated on macro studies (using large case numbers, even whole population studies) in the hope of finding areas of commonality. These large studies, he claimed, have distilled the useful information but also diluted the complex.

Attempts to define suicide and suicidal behaviour present problems. Many people will admit to having thought of ending their lives but have never really had the intention of carrying it out. Fairbairn (1995) argued that our understanding of the motive and intentions of suicide is contained in the labels chosen to describe it. It is therefore essential to have clear terminology.

Alvarez claimed that research has made suicide more respectable but has done little to improve society's acceptance of its existence. 'The real motives which impel a man to take his own life are elsewhere, they belong to the internal world,

devious, contradictory, labyrinthine and mostly out of sight'. (Alvarez, 1971).

In his seminal work on suicide, Stengel argued against the use of intention to commit suicide as a criterion for defining suicidal behaviour. He recognized the complex nature of an individual's motivation as an essential factor in acts of self-harm: 'suicide means the fatal, and suicide attempt means the non fatal act of self-injury, undertaken with more or less conscious self-destructive intent, however vague and ambiguous'. (Stengel, 1970).

OTHER KINDS OF SELF-HARM

There are a number of terms for non-fatal self-harming behaviour including parasuicide (Kreitman and Dyer, 1980) pseudocide, and deliberate self-harm (Morgan, 1979). Some terms, such as attempted suicide and suicidal behaviour, imply an intention to commit suicide but, as already argued, such an intention is neither always present nor easy to ascertain (even when death occurs).

DIFFERENTIATING BETWEEN NON-FATAL SUICIDAL BEHAVIOUR AND OTHER KINDS OF SELF-HARM

Here we suggest three distinct but overlapping kinds of non-fatal self-harming behaviour:

1 Self-harm without any suicidal intent, such as repetitive cutting, burning or injuring the body.

> I saw my brother's razor on the bathroom sink one night and I just thought to myself, if I cut myself I'll be alright. So I cut my wrist. As I watched the blood flow I felt no pain. I just felt clean, released, almost detached from what I had just done.

> *(Pembroke, 1994).*

2 Self-harm where the feelings of suicidal intent are ambivalent, such as taking an overdose of paracetamol without fully knowing the consequences and then seeking medical help. Rosalind's experience is presented here:

> For the first time I really wanted to die. I locked myself in the bathroom and started to scrape... but it all felt too much. In tears I went and showed the staff my distress, all I longed for was to be heard, acknowledged, cared for and loved .

> *(Pembroke, 1994)*

3 Self-harm where the intention and wish is to die, such as described by Anne Jennings:

> I had attempted to commit suicide and had been convinced that I would succeed, only to my horror, three days later, to find I had failed.... Death for me would have been final, the end to the unbearable torture and turmoil.

> *(Jennings, 1989).*

The term 'parasuicide' means the deliberate taking of a substance above the recommended prescribed dose or deliberate self-injury. This covers all three aspects given above because it carries no implications of the degree of actual suicidal intent. However, in practice it is more likely to be used to refer to the last two. The first, self-mutilation (such as superficial cutting) may be a distinct phenomenon, motivated by the need to alleviate tension and without suicidal intent or an inherent risk of suicide (Hawton and Catalan, 1987). Unless explicitly stated otherwise, parasuicide will be used in this chapter for the sort of self-harm that may include suicidal motivation.

INCIDENCE OF PARASUICIDE AND NON-FATAL SELF-HARM

It is even more difficult to get clear and concise information about self-harm from official sources than it is about suicide. National figures have not been released since 1981. At that time, official statistics showed that at least 100 000 people attend hospital following an overdose or deliberate self-harm each year (Office of Health Economics, 1981). Again, this is likely to be an underestimation of the total number of parasuicides, since many people will consult their GPs rather than attend hospital (Kennedy and Kreitman, 1973) or may only contact the Samaritans or other non-statutory helping agencies or do nothing.

During the 1960s and 1970s there was an enormous increase in the incidence of parasuicide in adults throughout Britain (Alderson, 1974) and the Western world (Wexler *et al.*, 1978). Many British cities reported increasing rates, for example Edinburgh (Holding *et al.*, 1977) and Oxford (Bancroft *et al.*, 1979). Jones (1977) predicted that adult self-poisoners would fill all available emergency medical beds by 1984. In 1980, it was reported that parasuicide was the commonest reason for emergency medical admission for women and second (to myocardial infarction) for men (Kreitman and Dyer, 1980). However, nationally there was a recorded decline in the 1980s (Brewer and Farmer, 1985). Hence by 1989 it was reported that parasuicide accounted for only 11% of all acute adult admissions to a general hospital (Fuller *et al.*, 1989).

METHODS OF SELF-HARM

Self-poisoning

The commonest method of deliberate self-harm is self-poisoning. This accounts for around 90% of reported parasuicides (Goldberg and Sakinofsky, 1988). Substances used in overdoses range from prescribed sedatives and psychotropic drugs to non-prescription analgesics through to substances not intended for ingestion, for example domestic bleach or petrol (Hawton and Catalan, 1987). Analgesics, such as aspirin and paracetamol, are the most commonly used non-prescribed drugs. This has been a source of concern as many people do not realize the potentially fatal consequences of taking overdoses, especially of paracetamol with its effect on the liver and there have been calls for urgent attention to address this problem.

Hawton and Blackstock (1976) found that where prescription medicines were used, especially psychotropic drugs, usually these had only recently been prescribed. This is not as surprising as it first sounds. Over a third of people who commit a parasuicide seek help from their GP within 2 weeks of an admission. Morgan (1979) claimed that one of the most important risk factors for determined self-harm consists in visiting the doctor in order to obtain the drugs. However, many people use medication prescribed for someone else (Jones, 1977).

Alcohol is often used to enhance the effect of medication taken and also to numb the experience or for 'Dutch courage'. Studies report the use of alcohol in 25–40% cases, with men twice as likely to use alcohol in this way as women (Platt *et al.*, 1988; Owens and Jones, 1988).

Self-injury

Self-injury is less likely to be reported than self-poisoning and may not come to the attention of medical or mental health services. Cutting of wrists and arms is most usual, although sometimes other parts of the body may be cut. Other methods may be more violent and include attempted hanging, jumping from high buildings and jumping in front of trains. Violent methods such as these are invariably associated with high suicidal intent (Michel, 1987).

DEMOGRAPHIC FACTORS IN PARASUICIDE

Unlike suicide, parasuicide is more prevalent in young women aged 15–19 years. In the 1970s it was estimated that 1 in 100 young girls referred to a general hospital were referred following a parasuicide (Hawton and Catalan, 1987). The rates have decreased in this group but it has been reported that women are more likely to harm themselves when under the age of 35 (Dyck *et al.*, 1988). While women in general are more likely than men to harm themselves through parasuicide, the sex difference appears to be diminishing. (See, for example, Fuller *et al.*, 1989).

The incidence of self-harm among children is unclear and likely to be under-reported. In a US study of 175 children, 13 (7%) had made a suicide attempt, as reported by either the mother or the child. Eight of the 13 children reported attempts that were not reported by their mothers (Walker *et al.*, 1990).

Self-harm in elderly people is a major problem because it is more likely to be fatal and they are more at risk of subsequent suicide. Frierson's (1991) study of 95 people between the ages of 60 and 90 who had attempted suicide showed that there was a high degree of premeditation and serious suicidal intent in this group. They were significantly different from younger people who had attempted suicide and were more likely to be depressed and to use potentially fatal methods.

SOCIAL AND ECONOMIC FACTORS

Various social problems are common among people who commit parasuicide. Some mentioned by researchers are low socio-economic class, social deprivation, poor housing, poverty, social isolation (Bancroft *et al.*, 1979; Kreitman and Dyer, 1980; Morgan, 1979; Michel, 1987; Keinhorst *et al.*, 1991). There also appears to be a strong relationship between male unemployment and parasuicide; Hawton and Rose (1986) found that rates of parasuicide were up to 15 times higher for unemployed than for employed men. It is difficult to associate parasuicide with unemployment in women mainly because of the research problem of defining women's unemployment (Hawton and Rose, 1986).

The association between attempted suicide and marital status is complicated and seems to vary with age and between the sexes. Among married people, a suicide attempt is more likely to occur where the relationship has been disrupted through separation. Marital difficulties, including so-called domestic violence, are common (Buglass and McCulloch, 1970; Hawton and Catalan, 1987). Bancroft *et al.* (1979) reported that 50% of married men and more than 10% of married women in their sample had had extramarital relationships during the previous year. Divorced people of both sexes have higher rates of parasuicide than single or married people (Holding *et al.*, 1977; Platt *et al.*, 1988).

MENTAL HEALTH PROBLEMS AND PARASUICIDE

Psychiatric disorder has been identified in a number of parasuicide samples at rates of 25–50% of the population. For example, using the Present State Examination, Newson-Smith and Hirsch (1980) identified psychiatric disorder in 31% of a series of people who had taken overdoses. However, the number in this category declined over time, with the result that 3 months after the overdose only 8% were identified as having a definite psychiatric disorder; many people's 'illnesses' had resolved within a week.

A US study of more than 650 people attending psychiatric out-patient clinics found that over half had a history of suicidal ideation and 25% reported at least one suicide attempt (Asnis *et al.*, 1993). Suicidal behaviour was prevalent in most diagnostic groups, although people with mood disorders such as depression were significantly more likely to have suicidal ideation.

The commonest psychiatric disorder associated with parasuicide is depression. Morgan (1979) found that as many as 39% of men and 59% of women in his sample were affected by a reactive depression, although estimates from other studies are lower. The concept of hopelessness in depression has been emphasized in the work around suicide risk. For example, one study of elderly people who had attempted suicide found that they had significantly higher hopelessness scores than similarly depressed people who had not attempted suicide (Rifai *et al.*, 1994). In addition, higher levels of hopelessness correlated with a high drop-out rate from treatment. Beck *et al.* (1975) proposed that hopelessness might be the main symptom preceding suicide.

Although it is clear that most people who have deliberately harmed themselves were not suffering from a formal mental illness at the time of the act, many have psychiatric symptoms, especially those associated with depression. Michel (1987) found that people identified as having low suicide intent after parasuicide showed sleeplessness (23%) and depressed mood (26%). With those who had higher suicidal intent, a higher proportion of *symptoms* were reported — delayed sleep (36%), worrying (67%), depressed mood (75%), irritability (55%), feelings of hopelessness (61%) and poor concentration.

LIFE EVENTS AND LONG-TERM PROBLEMS

Hawton and Catalan (1987) suggested that parasuicide problems can be divided into those that occur shortly beforehand (which often act as precipitants) and long-term or chronic problems, in the context of which acute problems have arisen. Paykel (1980) identified a number of life events including serious physical illness of self or close family members and serious arguments with spouse. People who had harmed themselves had experienced such life events at four times the rate of the comparable population.

Bancroft *et al.* (1979) found that crisis events involving a key person (e.g spouse, family member, partner) were the commonest that occured during the week prior to parasuicide. A major quarrel with the key person was the most likely precipitant. Long-standing problems identified in this study included sexual problems, problems with children and physical ill health.

A PSYCHODYNAMIC PERSPECTIVE ON SUICIDAL BEHAVIOUR

It is possible that sociomedical theories of suicide and self-harm detract from an understanding of the inner world of the person involved. It could also be argued that social pressures bring to the surface inner negative feelings and a sense of hopelessness (Alvarez, 1971). Psychoanalytical approaches have much to offer in this respect.

In April 1910, the Vienna Psycho-Analytical Society held its first symposium on suicide. Adler and Stekel presented different approaches. Adler spoke of an inferiority complex and revenge, while Stekel related the act to masturbation and its associated guilt. He also presented the principle that no one kills themselves who has not wanted to kill another. Freud refused to take sides and wanted to know more about the relationship between melancholia and mourning. He was concerned with how to reconcile the impulses of self-preservation and self-destruction.

In *Mourning and Melancholia*, Freud (1917) first discussed the idea of the ego trying to restore to life whatever has been lost from identification with the lost object. The normal mourning process concludes successfully by the gradual realization that the loved or lost object does not exist in the outside world, but is slowly compensated for by establishing an internal object replacement. In melancholia, or depression, this process produces so much guilt and hostility that it becomes too much for the sufferer. It is as if the melancholic person believes they have somehow destroyed or murdered the lost object themselves. This manifests itself in an internal persecutor who is punishing and seeks revenge. In essence, Freud was attempting to describe the struggle in the internal world of the mind that led to his later writings on what he called the death instinct.

Melanie Klein developed Freud's work and introduced the term 'projective identification' (Klein, 1921). Her explanations help our understanding of the suicidal patient. She suggests that while, in attempting suicide, the ego intends to murder its bad object, the intention at the same time is always to defend the loved object. Projective identification is the mechanism where the good or loved object is always protected (Klein, 1946). Elizabeth Bott–Spillus (1983) described succinctly how the work of Klein evolved its present clinical use and offered her own explanation of projective identification. The patient, according to Bott–Spillus (1983) gets the external object (i.e. therapist or nurse) to understand what they are feeling, by subjecting them to the same experience. On the basis of this theory it is not surprising that caring for a suicidal patient is extremely uncomfortable and emotionally highly charged. The person projects part of him or herself into the nurse. This can prompt the nurse to think, feel and even behave in a manner similar to the patient. If the nurse can recognize these influences, he or she will be able to process them in a healthy frame of mind and then help the patient to understand the patient's own feelings, allowing for a process of re-internalization (Ogden, 1979).

Treating a person who has attempted suicide brings further elements of confusion and dilemma. McGinley and Rimmer (1992) described this confusion as arising from having to care for both the victim and the perpetrator of the suicide act. If seen in this way, it is not surprising that staff are left with similar contradictory and confusing feelings, such as ambivalence, resentment and anger.

NURSING INTERVENTIONS IN THE HOSPITAL SETTING

Nurses are often those health professionals in the forefront of caring for someone who is suicidal. Often the patient's first contact with a nurse is in the Accident and Emergency Department (A&E). Rarely are nurses in A&E trained in mental health skills. They, especially younger and less experienced nurses, often appear to have negative attitudes to people who harm themselves (McLaughlin, 1994). Nevertheless, they have to deal with many people aftre parasuicide. In one busy inner London department, there are as many as 800–1000 attendances after parasuicide each year (Minghella, 1989). Even in suburban departments the numbers are high; for example, a survey in Guildford found nearly 2000 attendances after overdoses over a 5-year study period (Boyes, 1994). Following assessment in casualty, the person may be admitted to a general hospital ward and again encounter negative attitudes. One survey found that most parasuicide patients felt isolated and ignored while in hospital. A young woman described her experience in casualty as harsh.

> They scare you so you don't do it again. They say, "We don't know why you've taken it, you're going to die". They should be more kind and caring.(quoted by Strong, 1995)

However, Davenport (1993) talked of the need for nurses to adopt a calm and supportive approach to people who have overdosed on paracetamol and who are brought to casualty for what is usually unpleasant and stressful treatment.

Someone who is considered to be severely depressed and at high risk of suicide is likely to be admitted to a psychiatric unit, at least for a short while. Unfortunately, it has been argued that traditional psychiatric treatments are ineffective and more often enhance the negative aspects of feelings in someone who is suicidal (Giovacchini, 1978). In hospital, a standard nursing approach aimed at preventing suicide attempts is to assign the suicidal person to a single room, furnished sparsely and under close surveillance. The patient's personal possessions are often removed, especially any objects that might be used to inflict further self-harm. Restrictions are also made to the person's movements, including limiting access to other areas of the ward and a ban on leaving the ward.

Although precautions vary from hospital to hospital the ultimate aim is to maintain the patient's life in a safe environment. Nursing interventions in such settings have been described as offering little or nothing to help rectify the person's state of mind, except perhaps to reassure them that something is being done. Yet it has been suggested that such procedures can lead to mistrust and resentment (Bydlon––Brown and Billman, 1988). The following case study illustrates how people may feel on being admitted to psychiatric hospital following a suicide attempt.

Case study: **The experience of being admitted to hospital after a suicide attempt**

Anne Jennings took a medically serious overdose and had intended to kill herself. Following medical treatment she was admitted to a psychiatric hospital.

'The worst ordeal of that first day on the psychiatric ward, was that there was no privacy at all, even though I had my own room. Any idea that I had had of being alone and quiet was dispelled within the first half hour of arriving. Apart from having a nurse allocated to watch me, there were numerous forms to be filled in, possessions to be accounted for and, more disturbing, a barrage of interviews with various members of the staff, as well as students.... The effect on me was that although I was clearly receiving a lot of attention and time, I felt "uncontained" and invaded'.

(Jennings, 1989)

NURSING OBSERVATION IN PRACTICE

Observation of patients is a common means of intervention and prevention used by hospital nurses. Guidelines and policies concerning the degree of observation required must be simple to follow, easily carried out with clear instructions and agreed by medical and nursing staff, according to Goh *et al.* (1989). However, the authors do not mention the relevance of discussing these levels of observation with the patient themselves. This clearly must happen at an individual level (with the suicidal person involved) but it has also been argued that service users should be consulted at a service level, for example when formulating hospital policies on self-harm (Pembroke, 1994).

Providing a safe environment within an institution may contradict an anti-custodial psychiatric philosophy, aimed at enhancing the person's ability to live and function more effectively outside hospital. Often when patients are placed under close observation or scrutiny (i.e. the nurse is not to let the patient out of sight or to keep the patient at arm's length distance at all times) their freedom is limited or restricted. Decision making is removed and the patient's environment is completely controlled by the nurse. Within this setting there is a risk of patients becoming increasingly devoid of any control over their actions. Indeed, it has been noted that individuals are more likely to harm themselves under this regime, leaving staff feeling increasingly anxious and on edge about the patient's level of safety (Pauker and Cooper, 1990). A cycle of anxiety and concern ensues, leaving the nurse unable to assess the situation objectively. These feelings of inadequacy can be relayed to the patient, who feels unsafe and uncared for. In one study, while nurses perceived close observation as the most effective method of preventing further self-harm in suicidal patients, nurses also expressed the view that such special supervision was non-therapeutic (Reid and Long, 1993). The problem is often exacerbated when procedures are not properly thought through; for example, when agency nurses are deployed to observe a suicidal person they do not know and will not meet again or when suicidal women are closely observed by male nurses. 'Pearl described her experience as 'embarrassing and humiliating' when talking about having to use the toilet with the door not fully shut and a male nurse outside'.

Good interpersonal skills are essential when undertaking special observation with suicidal people. An interpersonal approach encourages staff and patients to consider their working relationship and gives patients an element of choice and control over how to work through internal conflicts in a structured way. It means treating the suicidal person with dignity and respect, one of the items on the Mental Health Task Force User's Charter (1994) along with providing the least restrictive treatments. This approach also brings with it the stress of working closely with a suicidal person and all the anxieties and concerns associated with allowing that person to remain in control of their behaviour and be responsible for it.

Reid and Long (1993) suggest that there should be a planned therapeutic programme of care throughout special supervision and that nurses especially need to be able to convey empathy to patients during this time. It may be that initially the nurse can do nothing but sit with the patient and convey the message of protection through non-verbal and verbal communication. Verbally, the nurse needs to explain that he or she is there to keep the person safe and prevent them from coming to any further harm. Non-verbally, this is reinforced through careful observation that is not over-intrusive and punitive but supportive and containing.

Often this constant care is still not enough and can leave nurses feeling hopeless and useless themselves. Carrying out one-to-one observations can be very demoralizing and draining. The nurse is also under scrutiny so it is important to remain calm and confident. On completing the observation the nurse should be able to pass on and evaluate the experience so he or she can leave the patient in the care of the next nurse. This handover may be done in the presence of the patient, encouraging the patient to participate to reinforce their responsibility and involvement in the plan of care.

ASSESSMENT OF SUICIDE RISK

Psychiatrists have been described as poor assessors of suicide risk (Rabiner *et al.*, 1982; Salmons, 1984) but this is clearly an area where most mental health professionals need to be able to apply specific knowledge and skills effectively. For people who are admitted to psychiatric hospital, there are particular times when the risk of suicide or self-harm is increased. The start of treatment (usually during the first week) is considered to be the most likely time for a suicide or attempt (Copas and Ashley, 1982). Other times identified as higher risk are near to discharge or other major alterations in the patient's situation (Ashton, 1986). The patient's safety is a priority in the nurse's role for assessing the risk of self-harm and should be incorporated into any plan of care. This assessment should include consideration of those factors known to represent an increased potential for suicide, identified in the literature as considerable risk factors (see Table 17.1).

Hradeck (1988) suggested that there are additional elements that need to be assessed. These are:

1 Factors leading up to the crisis.
2 The patient's strengths and abilities to cope and use of coping mechanisms.
3 The nature and strength of the patient's support systems, such as family and friends.

Assessment scales have been used successfully in the clinical field and are gradually finding a place providing mental health professionals with a framework for assessing suicidal risk. One such scale is Beck's suicidal intent scale (Beck *et al.*, 1974). This consists of a series of questions, scored according to the circumstances surrounding the parasuicide and the act itself, which the patient answers. Pierce (1981) carried out a study in an attempt to check the accuracy of an adapted version of this scale and found that it was short, easy to use and useful in assessing suicide risk.

Kienhorst *et al.* (1991) suggested that a simple questionnaire to assess suicide risk could be helpful but that a scale's ability to predict suicide will depend largely on the specific person and his or her situation. Although suicide is the most obvious outcome measure for validating such a scale, the drawbacks and implications of using this as a validation method are considerable. In-patient suicides are few each year, so only a few unrecorded incidents would invalidate the scale. (Pallis *et al.*, 1984).

Snaith *et al.* (1978) claimed that scales used in the clinical setting need to be constructed from the responses of patients. Patients' behaviour was reported to be different in the psychiatric interview from that when with family members or at home. Assessment therefore needs to be backed up or supplemented by the reports of others such as relatives, friends and colleagues, as well as by the patient's self-report.

TABLE 17.1 Identifying suicide risk factors

	High risk
Social and economic factors	
	Male
	Older
	Separated, divorced
	Living alone
	Middle class professional
	Unemployed
Psychological and psychiatric factors	
	Depression
	Schizophrenia
	Previous parasuicide (especially violent methods)
	Hopelessness
	Alcohol dependence
	Drug dependence
	Recent bereavement (especially loss of spouse)
	Family history of suicide
Physical health	
	Long-term illness
	Epilepsy
Circumstances of parasuicide	
	Planned, well-prepared
	Timed so that intervention unlikely
	Precautions against discovery
	Did not seek help afterwards
	Suicide note
Motivation	
	Wanted to die or still wants to die
	Expected to die

Clinical scales, then, seem to have some value in gathering information to help make decisions about how best to help the patient, yet no one tool is sufficient to cover the many facets of suicidal behaviour. Even a comprehensive list of suicidal characteristics does not leave the clinician wholly confident. A number of factors can hamper recognition of the underlying risk. It is apparent that some people will talk openly about their plans and thoughts while others deny any intent (Morgan and Priest, 1984).

Gathering as much information as possible from many different sources is therefore recommended, as suggested in Table 17.2. The nurse can obtain a self-report questionnaire from the patient and may also wish to make their own assessment through other suicidal intent scales (see for example Snaith *et al.*, 1978; Pallis *et al.*, 1984).

Bydlon-Brown and Billman (1988) reported a nursing-led study observing how nurses cared for suicidal patients. They found that there were numerous factors that influenced and complicated decision making. Some issues identified were staff and patient transference, biased attitudes towards psychiatric diagnosis, reliance on intuition, and variability of experience, education and the patient's contact with staff. The authors developed a suicide assessment tool, aimed at helping nurses assess subsequent observation levels, based on the nurses' judgements and the patient's behaviour. A senior nurse member and the patient's primary nurse score the tool and decide the final outcome together. However, the article does not discuss how the scale was validated, whether there was discussion with other disciplines or whether the suicidal person was involved. It does highlight the fact that assessment is often based upon intuition and non-verbal communication rather than on any systematic form of measurement and collaboration.

During an assessment interview it may prove difficult to listen and be attentive to a person whose problems appear to be either trivial or serious and insurmountable, or whose suicide attempt might appear to lack intent, or on the other hand when someone seems determined to kill themselves. Professionals can erect barriers to prevent a rapport from developing in order to protect themselves from the strong emotional, cultural, moral and spiritual dilemmas they are facing. Improvement in communication between care givers and the care receivers is identified as a necessary improvement area in this situation (Gibbs, 1990). See Table 17.2 for a guide to assessment strategies to use in clinical practice.

A Qualitative Study of How Registered Mental Health Nurses Determine Suicide Risk

Semi-structured interviews were carried out with a range of qualified mental health nurses at a psychiatric hospital in London (Hardy, 1993). The purpose of the study was to establish how these nurses ascertained suicide risk for psychiatric in-patients. Emphasis was placed on describing current ward practice and factors that might influence the nurses' decisions. In addition the subsequent effects of caring for the suicidal patient were identified.

All twelve interviews were tape recorded, transcribed and analyzed using the grounded theory approach (Glaser and Strauss, 1967). Each individual response was analyzed for key words, repeated phrases and emerging patterns. Category generation continued until saturation point was achieved, where nothing new was being discovered from the data.

The respondents varied in clinical grade and experience, from senior clinical nurse specialists to staff nurses. All were trained nurses with at least 3 years' experience in acute and specialist ward areas (e.g. deliberate self-harm, challenging behaviour, substance abuse, forensic, and eating disorders). None of the respondents had previously been asked to consider their own thoughts and feelings about suicidal patients. However, most were able to talk at length about their approaches to assessment.

When collating the results, extensive information emerged about current ward practice. This provided substantial evidence from which to offer a summary of experienced nursing practice. The nurses were all from one NHS Trust and therefore generalizations cannot be made but the study does offer an insight into how nurses perceive their own methods of assessing the suicide risk of psychiatric in-patients.

Originally, ten categories emerged from the data, which were then redefined into four major categories. These were:

1 Questioning: Carrying out a formal or an informal interview with the patient. Using open-ended questions to elicit information. 'I'd keep asking until I'd satisfied my need to know'.

2 Observation: Observing the patient, looking for signs, non-verbal communication, any previous scars or wounds, how they respond to the nurse and to others.

3 Interaction: Developing a relationship, being open and honest and encouraging the patient to do the same. Negotiating what is best for the patient.

4 Utilizing existing knowledge: Gathering and using information from many different sources to inform care provision and aid understanding.

The nurses interviewed in this study utilized knowledge gained from their assessment of the patient and their situation to help decide the best plan of care. Part of this process was concerned with distinguishing those patients who had previous attempts, those with a specific plan or method and those who were more impulsive and unwilling or unable to cooperate with staff. The main decisions about emergency responses to patients were made by the nurse, particularly in crisis situations, which invariably occurred outside of normal working hours when access to other disciplines was limited.

Negotiating a Plan of Care Within a Safe Environment

The nurse's first task is to establish a relationship with the patient that is based on open and honest communication. The nurse needs to keep the patient informed of treatment decisions and always discuss them with the patient, to keep the patient involved and convey a sense of the patient remaining in control of the situation. The following case study describes how this might work in practice.

The Exploration of Feelings

As soon as the acute crisis is over, understanding the underlying problems can help the patient begin to make changes. Using Cawley's 'levels of psychotherapy', it is possible to regard this stage of the nurse–patient relationship as somewhere between the 'supportive' (first) level and the 'intermediate level' (Cawley, 1977). The first level involves unburdening of problems, non-judgmental help and listening, and opportunity to vent feelings. Once a relationship has been established the nurse can begin to offer time to explore the predisposing and precipitating factors leading to the patient's present situation, tending towards the intermediate level of psychotherapy. Some of the potential work at this level (such as interpretation of unconscious motives) is not appropriate without specialist training and supervision, however.

Regular scheduled meeting times will help present the patient with a structured approach to what might feel like a very unstructured and uncontrollable situation. The nurse should ensure the meetings start and finish on time, to provide the boundaries needed for the containment of strong emotions. For the patient to explore such feelings, the nurse has to provide an environment that will encourage exploration. The room should be reasonably free from interruptions, furnished comfortably with chairs of comparable height, emphasizing the equality of the relationship. The same room should be used

---

TABLE 17.2 Methods for making a nursing assessment of suicide risk

Personal interview and discussion with the patient:
    For the purpose of getting to know the patient and their present risk of self-harm and to negotiate levels of intervention required to keep the patient feeling safe.

Self-rating scale or questionnaire:
    Completed by the patient.

Suicidal Intent or Global rating scales:
    Completed by the nurse, relatives or friends in discussion with the patient.

Discussion with friends and relatives:
    Can be carried out by the nurse to pick up any additional information or discrepancies in the patient's personal account.

Discussion within the clinical team:
    All members of the multidisciplinary team should be allowed to express their opinions so that decisions are verified and action carried out consistently.

for each session but the time, frequency and duration of the session is most important. This conveys the message that the nurse recognizes the sensitivity and importance of the situation and will help to foster a relationship based on trust. The aim is for the patient to come to see and use the sessions as their own (Brown and Pedder, 1991).

The essence of the nurse–patient relationship is to use the interpersonal dynamic as a tool for understanding. How the nurse feels toward the patient is often dismissed yet, through the psychodynamic approach, projective identification offers a way of understanding the therapeutic potential that is being overlooked. The nurse is able to use valuable material that the patient is constantly communicating at a subconscious or unconscious level. The process of therapy is about helping patients to live more comfortably with parts of themselves that were previously ignored and so caused much suffering.

In-patient nursing interventions also need to work towards the patient's discharge and the ending of the relationship. This is a high risk time for patients. Often, ending therapeutic relationship can rekindle feelings from other losses. There are practical strategies that may help, such as working together with the patient's partner and liaising with community nurses.

NURSING INTERVENTIONS IN THE COMMUNITY

Depressed and suicidal clients are referred to community nurses from a variety of sources, although most often from GPs or in-patient units. It is important to recognize that the risk of suicide is raised after hospital discharge, especially within the first month when the person can feel unsupported and is often unsupervised (Goldacre *et al.*, 1993).

Case study: **Negotiation between nurse and patient**

'Sarah', who took an overdose of tablets, was placed on one-to-one observation. Whenever the one-to-one observation ceased, Sarah would leave the ward or take more tablets while still on the ward. Eventually the nurse working with her — Nasrin — expressed her concern to Sarah, discussing with her how they could help her move forward. Sarah and Nasrin eventually agreed that Nasrin would come and check Sarah's safety every 5 minutes. This went on well for a couple of hours: Sarah did not attempt to harm herself. During the next hour they discussed it again. This time they decided that Nasrin would come every 10 minutes and in-between times Sarah would come and find the nurse. This meant that Sarah was still being observed every 5 minutes but that she was taking responsibility for keeping herself safe and seeking help when feeling vulnerable and in need of staff input. Eventually the system was reduced to every half an hour, with Nasrin and Sarah each taking responsibility for alternate half hours.

Some people have argued that suicide prevention in the community is hampered by unhelpful attitudes and popular misconceptions about suicide, such as 'those who talk about it never do it' (Kingdon and Jenkins, 1995). General practitioners often do not recognize suicide risk or signs of depression and fail to ask patients about suicide plans or previous attempts. Studies have revealed that GPs themselves feel they have little knowledge or skills to apply when dealing with depressed and suicidal patients (Michel and Valach, 1992). However, there are a number of strategies both at primary and secondary care levels that can be deployed effectively.

The mental health nurse's role in working with depressed and suicidal people in the community may be divided into four main areas.

ASSESSMENT

The community nurse needs to be especially careful to assess depression and suicide risk accurately, since there are often no other mental health professionals working with the client. When seeing a client for the first time, assessment should include taking a thorough history, including current mood and feelings of self-worth, previous experiences of depression or self-harm, noting attitudes towards depression and recording a family history, since depression or suicide in close relatives increases the client's own risk (Perry and Anderson, 1992). Self-report questionnaires to assess depression may also help, the Beck Depression Inventory (BDI) being most widely used. (Beck, 1978). Asking the client during the assessment about any suicidal feelings is essential. Some nurses worry that by mentioning suicide they may be 'putting ideas into the client's head'. Experience suggests that it is highly unlikely that if a person has not thought of suicide, they will suddenly consider it because it has been mentioned by a nurse. If a person is feeling suicidal, it may help them to share their feelings with someone else and the fact that the nurse has asked about and is aware of the possibility of suicide may encourage a feeling of safety. A checklist of suicidal risk factors could be useful, with particular attention paid to social factors, such as whether the person lives alone. If a person is referred following parasuicide, the sorts of suicidal intent scales mentioned earlier are also useful for assessment.

THERAPEUTIC INTERVENTIONS

The community nurse may use similar therapeutic interventions to those used by hospital based nurses. However, the lack of physical containment in the community means that special care must be taken to ensure the client's safety. If suicidal ideas or threats are present, they must be taken seriously and actively explored. If necessary, a crisis response may be initiated. Crisis responses include arranging for a psychiatrist's assessment, with the possibility of hospital admission, providing intensive support such as staying with the client at home for an extended period, and offering temporary respite from the home situation. Asking if he or she feels safe often helps in making a decision with the client about how best to proceed. Bancroft (1986) presented a behavioural, problem-solving approach to working with crisis:

- Explain the principles of problem-solving to the client.
- Help the person to define the problem appropriately and realistically.
- Try to think creatively.
- Use assessment of the person's previous coping resources to help him or her reflect on strengths and weaknesses.
- Together, consider the practical consequences and implications of each option.
- Encourage the person to make a choice, after due consideration and when it 'feels right'.
- Break down the chosen method of coping into manageable steps.
- Negotiate a contract with the person in which a commitment is made to carry out each step.
- Help the person to evaluate the effectiveness of these steps.

However, Fine and Sansone (1990) have argued that there is a difference between working with someone in a crisis and working with someone who has long-standing self-harming behaviours or threats. Similarly, Porritt (1990) talked of 'taking over responsibility' in a crisis as a short-term measure only. A person's autonomy is sacrificed to prevent suicide when crisis measures are taken. Fine and Sansone suggested that this may be acceptable and indeed necessary in a real crisis but some individuals relate by engaging others into assuming responsibility for their own suicidal behaviour, and consistently avoid taking personal responsibility. Ironically, this can result in reduced self-esteem and confirmation that they are not able to take control of their own life. Fine and Sansone proposed a number of strategies, such as exploring the behaviour with the client, emphasizing the client's own responsibility and autonomy, setting and enforcing clear and explicit limits and taking crisis action only if there really is a crisis. They stress that the practitioner must make a clear assessment to be able to differentiate accurately between acute and what they call 'chronic' suicidal behaviour. They also emphasize the need to keep full records of interactions and strategies agreed with clients and to keep other professionals informed. A form of intervention for prevention of further parasuicide among people who have deliberately harmed themselves has been described by Morgan *et al.* (1993) and has seen parallels in self-help organizations. A 'green card' was given to people who attended casualty after parasuicide, inviting them to seek help at any time provided there had been no further self-harm. This seemed to have an effect in reducing repetition. A similar approach could be used by community nurses, perhaps using a nurse–client contract approach.

Buckman (1992) suggested the following principles when dealing with any threat, including suicidal threats:

- Stay calm.
- Identify the objective of the threat and acknowledge it. This means letting the person know you understand what he or she is saying, and acknowledging the feelings behind the threat.
- Ask the person to suspend the threat in favour of discussion.

PRACTICAL HELP AND SUPPORT

The community nurse is in a position to give practical help to clients with their day-to-day lives. For example, if a person is socially isolated and has had a long period of unemployment (both risk factors in suicide) the community nurse can offer support, information and even resources to help the client change the situation. It may be impractical to seek a job; it may be important to encourage the setting of realistic goals about needs such as employment or a satisfying relationship. However, the nurse can often help the client regain control of his or her life by assisting with, say, finding voluntary work, providing information about where to get benefits advice, and looking for alternative accommodation. Practical steps such as these are often overlooked by nurses and yet they may provide concrete examples of progress for someone who is in a vicious circle of low self-esteem leading to apathy, hopelessness and inaction.

LIAISON

Communicating with other professionals in community settings is an essential aspect of the community nurse's role. With the primary health care team, liaison may include providing information or training sessions about depression and suicidal behaviour and ensuring clients' GPs are fully informed about interventions and progress.

Liaison with other agencies, statutory and non-statutory, will provide access for the client to a range of resources that might be helpful, such as social clubs, self-help support groups, alcohol counselling services and training schemes. Assertiveness training may be beneficial for a depressed woman, for example, to help her feel in control of herself and her environment, although as Smith (1987) pointed out, such changes have consequences and women may well need the nurse's continued support to appreciate the context and effects of proposed life changes.

Liaison can also involve family and friends, working with the client's own 'natural' resources. Falloon *et al.* (1992) have found that working with families at the earliest stages of depression may help prevent major depressive episodes.

MANAGING ONE'S OWN FEELINGS

Peplau (1952/1988) described the concept of psychodynamic nursing as being able to understand one's own behaviour to help others identify personal difficulties and to apply the principles of human relations to problems that arise at all levels of experience. Landeen *et al.* (1992) proposed that establishing a therapeutic relationship in the psychiatric setting is something that cannot be taught easily but which comes with increased personal exposure to, and contact with, patients. Yet involvement with suicidal people can be stressful and emotionally draining. These ideas fit with the model of the three-dimensional aspects of caring depicted in Figure 17.1. The nurse and the depressed person bring their own experiences and knowledge to the relationship, which need to be understood alongside the tangible facts of precipitants, behaviours, assessment and treatment.

The culture of health care delivery tends to be centred on assisting patients to regain or improve their health. When working with the suicidal patient, strong feelings are generated such as frustration and anger, in particular, in nurses who are unprepared for the psychological affects of trying to establish a relationship with someone who does not want that care. This inevitably leaves the nurse with additional feelings of guilt and frustration (Braverman, 1990).

Nurses have been shown to remove themselves from stressful situations, by elaborate means, to avoid conflict (Menzies, 1960; Fabricius, 1991; Dartington, 1993; Shur, 1994). Such avoidance of personal thoughts and feelings towards death and dying is commonplace in our society. Kubler–Ross (1969) describes this as an internal struggle that leaves people with overwhelming feelings of fear, denial and avoidance when coming to terms with a sudden death. Despite Kubler–Ross's work being largely concerned with death through terminal illness, it is relevant to suicide. By inhibiting any involvement in activities associated with death and dying, people are prevented from being able to ask questions and prepare themselves adequately.

Nurses therefore need to have the opportunity of exploring their own personal feelings towards suicidal patients. Allowing the nurse to explore personal emotions and attitudes will help prepare them to offer greater empathy and a non-judgemental approach to the patient. The nurse may experience feelings of anger, frustration, sadness, guilt, fear and loss, all of which may be very similar to the patient's feelings. Once nurses are able to identify emotions within themselves, they may be more able to help patients explore and identify their own feelings.

DEALING WITH SUICIDE

Some people will still choose death in spite of all the efforts of nurses, doctors, family and friends. Mental health professionals need to prepare themselves for this possibility. Through the rejection of life itself, the patient may have rejected all of their own responsibility and any offers of help.

Suicide has a profound effect for family, friends and mental health professionals. Any bereavement brings with it the probability of a myriad of difficult feelings, such as ambivalence, shock and disbelief, but with suicide these feelings are complicated by the nature of the death and may cause complicated grief reactions in those left behind (Worden, 1987). This mother whose son killed himself said:

> It is incredibly hard for me to talk about it. If I say my son is dead there is a shut-down at that point. But this is what I want more than anything else. I want someone to give me licence to talk more about it. I want to say he was my son. He was important. He did die and he did take his own life. All these are facts I want you to know.

(Quoted by Strong, 1995)

Parkes (1975) noted that with death of any sort:

> Pain is inevitable.... It stems from the awareness of both parties that neither can give the other what he wants. The helper cannot bring back the person who's dead, and the bereaved person cannot gratify the helper by seeming helped.

Sudden death by suicide, in most cases, is seen as a violation of those left behind but also a violation of the belief in life itself (Wright, 1991). The following quotes are taken from the sample of nurses interviewed about suicide (Hardy, 1993).

> I had the experience where the patient I was primary nurse to committed suicide. I remember thinking, I'm glad she did it when I wasn't on duty and that was partly because I didn't want to take the blame and responsibility. I realize that is a bit like I'm covering my back, but suicide often does turn into a bit of a witch hunt. ('Maria')

> The other factor is that we've got a registration number and the fact that if a person commits suicide on your ward there seems to be a swoop of administrators and doctors all pointing the finger at you. That person could lose you your job. ('Raj')

> I've seen nurses leave after dealing with all that. I've seen nurses ignore people who are genuinely upset about someone I know who recently jumped.... People get fed up, nurses can detach themselves in an attempt to deal with it all. I think the whole business of working with someone who is suicidal is very painful... it needs an awful lot of skill and insight and self-understanding. ('Sue')

> I think it's a rejection of you, isn't it, and what you stand for and can offer, ultimately as a nurse, being there all the time and that's just not good enough. You need to have skills, instinct, experience. It's all so useful. ('Mike')

A SHORT NOTE ON ETHICAL ISSUES

There are probably two main ethical considerations in working with someone who is suicidal and depressed. Firstly, there is the issue of confidentiality. Is it possible or advisable for the nurse to keep confidential someone's plans to commit suicide? It would seem not; the nurse has a duty of care to the patient and must inform the responsible medical officer if there is a real threat of suicide. In our view it is probably best never to promise complete confidentiality to the patient, as there are always potentially difficult disclosures that the nurse may have to share with other professionals. Mental health service users consider it essential to be fully informed of the confidentiality policy, which they expect should serve to preserve confidentiality to the maximum extent that is compatible with offering an effective service. (Mental Health Task Force User Group, 1994).

The second, related, consideration concerns so-called 'rational' suicide. Are there some circumstances in which the suicidal person has a right to commit suicide and the nurse has no right to intervene? Again, professional ethics would suggest otherwise but this is a vexed question. Certainly, Szasz (1986) argued strongly against suicide prevention. Fairburn (1995) contended that suicide nearly always hurts or harms other people and that, even if it does not, it could still be regarded as morally wrong because the possibility of harm to others will always exist. He was thus able to argue that intervention to try to prevent suicide is morally justifiable.

Autonomy is important. However, I think it can be overridden where its exercise involves harming others. So, to my mind, intervention in another person's suicide can be justified on the grounds that if one does not, one will be harmed; by the feelings or nightmares one might have afterwards, or by the effects on one's career if one works in one of the caring or other public services.... This does not mean, however, that I believe that we are morally obliged to intervene, only that we may intervene in order to prevent harm.

SUMMARY

This chapter set out to enable the reader to gain an understanding of the complex nature of depression and suicidal behaviour. Proposing a three-dimensional model of care, emphasis has been placed not only on knowledge and skills but also on the experiences and feelings of nurses and service users as essential parts of the therapeutic process. The nature, incidence and associated factors of depression, suicide and non-fatal suicidal behaviour have been presented, demonstrating the enormous impact of these conditions and their importance for mental health nursing. Nursing interventions in both hospital and the community have been suggested, with special reference to the assessment of suicidal risk. The emotional effects of working with people who are depressed and suicidal, and who may indeed commit suicide, have also been discussed together with brief ethical considerations.

KEY CONCEPTS

- Nurses are often the health professionals in the forefront of caring for someone who is suicidal.
- Clinical depression is usually characterized by a profound, persistent and all-pervasive depressive mood.
- The relationship between the suicidal person and the nurse is crucial to the development of therapeutic work.
- People with depression are offered a range of interventions based on an eclectic view of causation.
- Observation of patients is a common means of intervention and prevention used by hospital nurses.
- Nurses need to have the opportunity to explore their own personal feelings towards suicidal patients.

REFERENCES

Aggleton P: *Young Men Speaking Out*. London, 1995, Health Education Authority.

Alderson MR: Self-poisoning: what is the future? *Lancet* 1:1040–1043, 1974.

Asnis GM, Friedman TA, Sanderson WC et al.: Suicidal behaviors in adult psychiatric outpatients. *Am J Psychiatry* 150(1):108–112, 1993.

Alvarez A: The savage god—a study of suicide. London, 1971, Penguin Books.

Ashton J: Preventing suicide in hospital. *Nurs Times* 82(52):36–37, 1986.

Bancroft J: Crisis intervention. In: Bloch S: *An introduction to the psychotherapies*. Oxford, 1986, Oxford University Press.

Bancroft J, Hawton K, Simkin S et al.: The reasons people give for taking overdoses: a further enquiry. *Br J Med Psychol* 52(4):353–365, 1979.

Barraclough B, Bunch J, Sainsbury P: A hundred cases of suicide. Clinical Aspects. *Br J Psychiatry* 125:355–373, 1974.

Beck AT: *Depression: clinical, experimental and theoretical aspects*. London, 1967, Staples Press.

Beck AT: *Beck Depression Inventory (revised edition)*. Philadelphia, 1978, Center for Cognitive Therapy.

Beck AT, Kovacs M, Weissman A: Hopelessness and suicidal behaviour: an overview. *JAMA* 234:1146–1149, 1975.

Beck AT, Schuyler D, Herman J: Development of suicidal intent scales. In: Beck AT, Resnick HLP, Lettieri DJ: *The prediction of suicide*. Maryland, 1974, Charles Press.

Blacker CVR, Clare AW: Depressive disorder in primary care. *Br J Psychiatry* 150:737–751, 1987.

Bott Spillius E: Some developments from the work of Melanie Klein. *Int J Psychoanal* 64:321, 1983.

Boyes AP: Repetition of overdose: a retrospective 5-year study. *J Adv Nurs* 20(3):462–468, 1994.

Braverman BG: Eliciting assessment data from the patient who is difficult to interview. *Nurs Clin N Am* 25(4):743–749, 1990.

Brewer C, Farmer R: Self-poisoning in 1984: a prediction that didn't come true. *BMJ* 290:391, 1985.

Brown GW, Harris T: *Social origins of depression*. London, 1978, Tavistock.

Brown D, Pedder J: *Introduction to psychotherapy: an outline of psychdynamic principles and practice*. London, 1991, Tavistock.

Buckman R: *How to break bad news*. London, 1992, Papermac.

Buglass D, McCulloch SW: Further suicidal behaviour: the development and validation of predictive scales. *Br J Psychiatry* 116:483–491, 1970.

Busteed EL, Johnston C: The development of suicide precautions for an inpatient psychiatric setting. *J Psychosoc Nurs Ment Health Serv* 21(5):15–19, 1983.

Bydlon–Brown B, Billman RR: At risk of suicide... . *Am J Nurs* 88(10):1358–1361, 1988.

Cawley RH: The teaching of psychotherapy. *Association of University Teachers of Psychiatry Newsletter*, 1977.

Charlton J, Kelly S, Dunnell K et al.: Suicide deaths in England and Wales: Trends in factors associated with suicide deaths. *Popul Trends* 71(**Issue**):34–42, 1993.

Copas JB, Ashley R: Suicide in psychiatric inpatients. *British Journal of Psychiatry* 141 November:503–511, 1982.

Crammer JL: The special characteristics of suicide in hospital inpatients. *Br J Psychiatry* 145 February:460–476, 1984.

Dartington A: Where angels fear to tread. Idealism, despondency and inhibitions in thought in hospital nursing. *Winnicott Studies* 7:21–41, 1993.

Davenport D: Structured support at a time of crisis. Treatment of paracetamol overdose. *Prof Nurse* 8(9):558, 560–562, 1993.

Delisle I: Le Suicide a l'arge de la retraite [Suicide at the age of retirement]. *Can Nurse* 55:39–41, 1992.

Department of Health: *Health and personal social statistics for England, 1995 edition*. London, 1995, HMSO.

Dudley M, Waters B, Kelk N et al: *Youth suicides in New South Wales: urban–rural trends*. Med J Australia 156(2):83–88, 1992.

Dyck RJ, Bland RC, Newman SC, et al: Suicide attempts and psychiatric disorders. *Acta Psychiatrica Scand* 338(supplement):64–71, 1988.

Fabricius J: Running on the spot or can nursing really change? *Psychoanal Psychotherapy* 5(2):97–108, 1991.

Fairburn: *Contemplating suicide: The language and ethics of self-harm*. London, 1995, Routledge.

Falloon IRH, Shanahan W, Laporta M: Prevention of major depressive episodes: early intervention with family-based stress management. *J Ment Health* 1(1): 53–60, 1992.

Fine MA, Sansone RA: Dilemmas in the management of suicidal behaviour in individuals with borderline personality disorder. *Am J Psychother* XLIV(2):160–169, 1990.

Freud S: *Mourning and melancholia*. London, 1917, Hogarth Press.

Frierson RL: Suicide attempts by the old and very old. *Arch Int Med* 151(1):141–144, 1991.

Fuller GN, Rea AJ, Payne JF et al.: Parasuicide in central London 1984–1988. *J R Soc Med* 82(2): 653–656, 1989.

Gibbs A: Aspects of communication with people who have attempted suicide. *J Adv Nurs* 15(2):1245–1249, 1990.

Giovacchini P: *New perspectives on psychotherapy of the borderline adult*. New York, 1978, Masterson.

Glaser B, Strauss A: *Strategies for qualitative research*. New York, 1967, Aldine Publishing.

Goh SE, Salmons PH, Whittington RM: Hospital suicides: Are there preventable factors? *Br J Psychiatry* 154 February: 247–249, 1989.

Goldacre M, Seagroatt V, Hawton K: Suicide after discharge from psychiatric inpatient care. *Lancet* 342(1):283–286, 1993.

Goldberg J, Sakinofsky I: Introprimitiveness and parasuicide: prediction of interview response. *Br J Psychiatry* 153: 801–804, 1988.

Hamilton M: Frequency of symptoms in melancholia (depressive illness). *Br J Psychiatry* 154 February:201–206, 1989.

Hardy S: *A qualitative study of how registered mental health nurses assess suicide risk [Dissertation]*. University of East London, Stratford,1993, unpublished.

Hawton K, Blackstock E: General practice aspects of self-poisoning and self-injury. *Psychol Medicine* 6:571–575, 1976.

Hawton K, Catalan J: *Attempted suicide: A practical guide to its nature and management*, 2 ed. Oxford, 1987, Oxford University Press.

Hawton K, Rose N: Unemployment and attempted suicide among men in Oxford. *Health Trends* 18(1):29–32, 1986.

Helman CG: *Culture, health and illness*, 2 ed. London, 1990, Wright.

Holding TA, Buglass D, Duffy JC et al.: Parasuicide in Edinburgh—A seven year review 1968–74. *Br J Psychiatry* 130 June:534–543, 1977.

Hradeck EA: Crisis intervention and suicide. *J Psychosoc Nurs* 26(5):24–27, 1988.

Jennings A: Going into hospital. *Openmind* 17(1):12–13, 1989.

Jones DJR: Self-poisoning with drugs: the past 20 years in Sheffield. *BMJ* I:28–29, 1977.

Kelleher MJ, Daly M: Suicide in Cork and Ireland. *Br J Psychiatry* 157 October: 533–538, 1990.

Kendall RE: The classification of depression: A review of contemporary confusion. *Br J Psychiatry* 129 May:15–28, 1976.

Kennedy P, Kreitman N: Epidemiological survey of parasuicide in general practice. *Br J Psychiatry* 123:23–24, 1973.

Kienhorst CWM, De Wilde EJ, Diekstra RKW et al.: Construction of an index for predicting suicide attempts in depressed adolescents. *Br J Psychiatry* 159 July:676–682, 1991.

Kingdon D, Jenkins R: Suicide prevention. In: Phelan M, Strathdee G, Thornicroft G, editors: *Emergency mental health services in the community*. Cambridge, 1995, Cambridge University Press.

Klein M: *Love, guilt and reparation and other works*. London, 1921, Virago.

Klein M: *Envy and gratitude and other works*. London, 1946, Virago.

Kreitman N, Dyer JAT: Suicide in relation to parasuicide. *Medicine* 36:1827–1830, 1980.

Kubler–Ross E: *On death and dying*. London, 1969, Tavistock.

Landeen J, Byrne C, Brown B: Journal keeping as an educational strategy in teaching psychiatric nursing. *J Adv Nurs* 17(2):347–355, 1992.

Lewis S: A search for meaning: Making sense of depression. *J Ment Health*

4:369–382, 1995.

Marzuk PM, Tardiff K, Smyth D *et al.*: Cocaine use, risk taking and fatal Russian roulette. *JAMA* 267(19):2635–2637, 1992.

McClure GM: Suicide in England and Wales 1975–1984. *Br J Psychiatry* 150 March:309–314, 1987.

McGinley E, Rimmer J: The trauma of attempted suicide. *Psychoanal Psychother* 7(1):53–68, 1992.

McLaughlin C: Casualty nurses' attitudes to attempted suicide. *J Adv Nurs* 20(6): 1111–1118, 1994.

Mental Health Task Force User Group: *Guidelines for a local charter for users of Mental Health Services*. NHS Executive. BAPS, 1994, Heywood.

Menzies IEP: A case study in the functioning of social systems as a defence against anxiety. *Hum Relat* 13:95–121, 1960.

Michel K: Suicide risk factors: a comparison of suicide attempters with suicide completers. *Br J Psychiatry* 130: 78–82, 1987.

Michel K, Valach L: Suicide prevention: Spreading the gospel to general practitioners. *Br J Psychiatry* 160:757–760, 1992.

Minghella E: Managing parasuicide: The nurse's role. In Wilson–Barnett J, Robinson S: *Directions in nursing research*. London, 1989, Scutari Press.

Morgan HG: *Death wishes? The understanding and management of deliberate self-harm*. Chichester,1979, John Wiley.

Morgan HG, Priest P: Assessment of suicide risk in psychiatric in-patients. *Br J Psychiatry* 145 February:467–469, 1984.

Morgan HG, Jones EM, Owen JH: Secondary prevention of non-fatal deliberate self-harm: The Green Card study. *Br J Psychiatry* 163 July:111–112, 1993.

Newson–Smith JGB, Hirsch SR: Psychiatric symptoms in self-poisoning patients. *Psychol Med* 9(1):493–500, 1979.

Office Of Health and Economics: *Suicide and deliberate self harm*. London, 1981, White Crescent Press Ltd.

Ogden T: On projective identification. *Int J Psychoanal* 60(**issue**):357–373, 1979.

Owens DW, Jones SJ: The Accident & Emergency department management of deliberate self-poisoning. *Br J Psychiatry* 152 December:830–833, 1988.

Pallis DJ, Gibbons JS, Pierce DW: Estimating suicide risk among attempted suicides.II Efficiency of predictive scales after the attempt. *Br J Psychiatry* 144 February: 139–148, 1984.

Parkes CM: *Bereavement*. Harmondsworth, 1975, Penguin.

Pauker SL, Cooper AM: Paradoxical patient reactions to psychiatric life support: Clinical and ethical considerations. *Am J Psychiatry* 147(4): 488–490, 1990.

Paykel, ES: Recent life events and attempted suicide. In: Farmer R, Hirsch S, editors: *The suicide syndrome*. London, 1980, Croam-Helms.

Pembroke LR: *Self-harm: Perspectives from personal experience. Survivors Speak Out*. London, 1994.

Peplau HE: *Interpersonal relations in nursing*. New York, 1952, Putnam's Sons.

Perry MV, Anderson GL: Assessment and treatment strategies for depressive disorders commonly encountered in primary care settings. *Nurse Practit* 17(6):25–36, 1992.

Pierce DW: The prediction validation of a suicide intent scale: A five year follow-up. *Br J Psychiatry* 139 November: 391–396, 1981.

Plath S: *The Bell Jar*. London, 1963, Faber & Faber.

Platt SD, Hawton K, Kreitman N *et al.*: Recent clinical and epidemiological trends in parasuicide in Edinburgh and Oxford: a tale of two cities. *Psychol Med* 18:405–418, 1988.

Porritt L: *Interaction strategies: an introduction for health professionals*. Edinburgh, 1990, Churchill Livingstone,

Pritchard C: Is there a link between suicide in young men and unemployment? A comparison of the UK with other European Community countries. *Br J Psychiatry* 160 January:750–756, 1992.

Rabiner CJ, Weigner JT, Kane JN: Suicide in a psychiatric population. *Psychiatr Hosp* 13(2):55–59, 1982.

Reid W, Long A: The role of the nurse providing therapeutic care for the suicidal patient. *J Adv Nursing* 18(9):1369 –1376, 1993.

Rifai AH, George CJ, Stack JA *et al.*: Hopelessness in suicide attempters after acute treatment of major depression in later life. *Am J Psychiatry* 151(11):1687–1690, 1994.

Rosenthall J, Greally B: *Women and depression*. London, 1988, Islington Women and Mental Health.

Salmons PH: Suicide in high buildings. *Br J Psychiatry* 145: 469–472, 1984.

Shur R: *Countertransference enactment. How institutions and therapists actualise primitive internal worlds*. Northvale, New Jersey, 1994, Jason Aronson Inc.

Smith L: Women and mental health. In: Orr J: *Women's health in the community*. Chichester, 1987, J Wiley & Sons.

Snaith RP, Constantinopoulos AA, Jardine MJ *et al.*: A clinical scale for self-assessment of irritability. *Br J Psychiatry* 132:164–171, 1978.

Soni-Raleigh V, Balajaran R: *Suicide and self-burning among Indians and West Indians in England and Wales*. *Br J Psychiatry* 11:365–368, 1992.

Stengel E: *Suicide and attempted suicide*. Harmondsworth, 1970, Penguin.

Strong S: Thoughts of suicide. *Community Care* (1):16–17, 1995.

Szasz T: The case against suicide prevention. *Am Psychol* 41:806–812, 1986.

Taiminen TJ: Projective identification and suicide contagion. *Acta Psychiatr Scand* 85 December:449–452, 1992.

Tennant C: Female vulnerability to depression. *Psychol Med* 15:733–737, 1985.

Walker M, Moreau D, Weissman MM: Parents' awareness of children's suicide attempts. *Am J Psychiatry* 147(10):1364–1366, 1990.

Wexler L *et al*: Suicide attempts 1970–1975: updating a United States study and comparison with international trends. *Br J Psychiatry* 131:108–185, 1978.

Worden WJ: *Grief counselling and grief therapy*, 2 ed. London, 1987, Tavistock.

Wright A: Depression. In: Pullen I, Wilkinson G, Wright A *et al.*: *Psychiatry and general practice today*. London, 1994, Royal College of Psychiatrists and the Royal College of General Practitioners.

Wright B: *Sudden death. Intervention skills for the caring professions*. London, 1991, Churchill Livingstone.

FURTHER READING

Douglas J: *The social meaning of suicide*. New Jersey, 1976, Princetown.
  A book that looks at suicide's taboo image within society.

Durkheim E: *Suicide: A study in sociology*. London, 1952, Routledge.
  A classic study, referred to as the first study of suicide and turning point in people's conception of suicide.

Morgan HG: *Suicide prevention. The assessment and management of suicidal risk. An NHS advisory service Thematic Initiative*. London, 1994, HMSO.
  A report written in response to the Health of the Nation targets.

Palmer S: Parasuicide: a cause for nursing concern. *Nurs Stand* 7(19):37–39, 1993.
  A useful attitude on the attitudes of nurses towards patients who have taken overdoses.

Richardson R: *Death, dissection and the destitute*. London, 1988, Penguin.
  A historical look at suicide and its implications throughout Europe.

Taylor S: *Durkheim and the study of suicide*. London, 1982, Macmillan.
  Durkheim's classic work given another overhaul.

Varah C: *The Samaritans in the 70s. To befriend the suicidal and despairing*. London, 1973, Constable

MIND: How to help someone who is suicidal. Available from MIND, Granta House, 15–19 Broadway, Stratford, London E15 4BQ.

Chapter 18

Nursing Interventions with Acutely Ill Clients

Learning Outcomes

After studying this chapter you should be able to:

- Describe the signs and symptoms of schizophrenia.

- Discuss the factors that may lead to the development of schizophrenia.

- Show an awareness of the range of assessment tools available and demonstrate the need for their use in mental health nursing.

- Demonstrate an understanding of the developments in pharmacology and how this research will affect mental health nursing.

- Use research to design relevant and effective interventions to reduce the distress caused by different symptoms.

- Design, implement and evaluate educational interventions for patients about aspects of their illness and treatment.

- Demonstrate an awareness of factors that made lead to relapse.

CHAPTER OUTLINE

- *Signs and symptoms of schizophrenia*

- *Aetiology and causes of schizophrenia*

- *The epidemiology of schizophrenia*

- *Assessment and outcome measures in schizophrenia*

- *Treatment*

- *Psychological interventions*

- *Relapse prevention*

- *A personal account of schizophrenia*

The majority of patients admitted to psychiatric wards have psychotic disorders. In this chapter the signs and symptoms of schizophrenia will be outlined, and our understanding of the causes and treatment of schizophrenia will be presented and applied to nursing practice.

SIGNS AND SYMPTOMS OF SCHIZOPHRENIA

Schizophrenia is the commonest of the disorders grouped under the heading of psychoses. Psychoses form a group of mental disorders characterized by distortions of thinking and perception and inappropriate or blunted affect. The most frequently observed psychotic illnesses are:
- Schizophrenia.
- Schizoaffective disorder.
- Schizotypal disorder.
- Delusional disorder.

Since its definition by Kraeplin and Bleuler almost 100 years ago, our understanding of schizophrenia has been gradually refined. There are two main manuals currently in use for classifying mental disorders. They are:
1. The International Classification of Mental and Behavioural Disorders (ICD 10) (World Health Organisation, 1992).
2. Diagnostic and Statistical Manual of Mental Disorders (DSM IV) (American Psychiatric Association, 1994).

ICD 10 is the diagnostic manual most frequently used in Britain, and is currently in its tenth revision.

SYMPTOMS OF SCHIZOPHRENIA

Schizophrenia is characterized by a variety of features. However, it is not necessary to experience all of these symptoms to receive a diagnosis of schizophrenia (Jones and Tallis, 1994). Six symptom groups have been reported in schizophrenia, typically divided into positive (1–3) and negative (4–6) symptoms (World Health Organisation, 1992) :

1. Hallucinations

Hallucinations (auditory, visual, tactile, olfactory, and gustatory hallucinations) can occur in any of the five senses. However, auditory hallucinations are the commonest. Patients often describe voices making derogatory comments, giving commands or a running commentary. There may be one person talking alone or several people speaking at the same time. Voices may be in the first person (e.g. I am evil), or the second person (e.g. you are evil). or the third person (e.g. he or she is evil). It is important to note that auditory hallucinations are not specific to schizophrenia and have been found to occur in the general population (Posey, 1986).

2. Delusions

A delusion is a belief that is incongruent with reality, strongly held and persistent (Winters and Neal 1983). Common types include delusions of grandeur, delusions of persecution and paranoia and delusions of passivity.

Grandiose delusions include a belief in superhuman powers, social or religious importance and the ability to control environmental conditions. Patients who experience persecutory or paranoid delusions may believe that there is a conspiracy against them or that they are going to be harmed or killed. Patients who experience delusions of passivity may experience feelings of being controlled by an external force, for example a belief that their actions are being controlled via transmitters in their brain.

Significantly, delusions are strongly influenced by an individual's cultural background, age and gender.

3. Thought Disorder

Thought disorder manifests itself in two different ways, disorders of thought process and disruption of communication. Disorders of thought process include:
• Thought withdrawal.
• Thought broadcast.
• Thought echo.
• Thought insertion.

Examples of disruption in communication include:
• Thought blocking.
• Flight of ideas.
• Derailment.
• Neologisms (making up words that do not exist).
• Word salad.

• Echolalia (repetition of the last word said to them).
• Incoherent speech.

4. Negative Symptoms

Negative symptoms include:
• Withdrawal.
• Lack of volition.
• Lack of motivation.
• Inertia (lack of energy).
• Lack of social skills.
• Inappropriate social behaviour.
• Poor self-care.

5. Catatonia

Catatonia is when an individual is observed adopting unusual postures or can be sculpted into positions by another person. Patients may often be mute or appear stuporous.

6. Mood

People with schizophrenia often experience changes in their mood such as blunted or incongruous emotions and lability that cannot be attributed to depression or medication.

AETIOLOGY AND CAUSES OF SCHIZOPHRENIA

In this section research relating to the aetiology and causes of schizophrenia will be examined. The role of genetics, obstetric complications and life events in the development of a schizophrenic illness will be discussed.

GENETICS

It has long been suggested that there is a genetic component to the aetiology of schizophrenia (Boyle, 1990). Indeed Kraeplin in 1899 suggested that approximately 70% of people with a psychiatric disturbance were predisposed to develop such a disorder. Bleuler (1950) shared the belief that heredity plays a part in the development of schizophrenia. However, early studies were seriously methodologically flawed. During the early post-war years little genetic research was conducted, as early genetic theories had been adopted by the Eugenics movement (who were committed supporters of Nazism). Recently there has been renewed interest in the role genetics plays in the development of schizophrenia.

Family Studies

To assess the influence of genes in the development of schizophrenia, the degree to which the illness runs (or aggregates) in families must first be determined. Initial studies (summarized by Zerbin–Rudin, 1967) clearly supported the hypothesis that schizophrenia consistently and substantially aggregates in families. However, these early studies have serious methodological difficulties including unclear operational definitions of schizophrenia. It is also difficult to establish how diagnoses were made (e.g. face-to-face interview or from hospital notes).

Pope *et al.* (1982) suggested that any evidence of family aggregation in schizophrenia could be attributed to methodological deficiencies.

More recent genetic studies (see for example, Coryell and Zimmerman, 1988; Gershon *et al.*, 1988; Maier *et al.*, 1990) have proved to have a more thorough methodological grounding. (Kendley, 1993) state that the second generation of family studies have common methodological features. They are:

1. A normal control group.
2. Structured psychiatric measurement and operationalized diagnostic criteria.
3. Blind assessment and diagnosis.

Results from these studies strongly suggests that first degree relatives carry an approximately 4.8% risk of developing schizophrenia.

Twin Studies

Twin studies aim to investigate the prevalence of a schizophrenia in both monozygotic (identical) and dizygotic (fraternal) twins. These studies use similar methodological approaches to the family studies and are reviewed in detail by Gotesman *et al.* (1987); since this review only one major twin study has been undertaken (Onstad *et al.*, 1991). Onstad *et al.* reported that in 15 of 31 sets of monozygotic twins both members had a diagnosis of schizophrenia. They also indicated that in 1 of 28 sets of dizygotic twins both members were diagnosed with schizophrenia. These results are broadly similar to those of previous twin studies (Gotesman *et al.*, 1987) and suggest that genetic factors play a significant role in the development of schizophrenia. This also supports the hypothesis that family environment makes little contribution to the risk of developing schizophrenia.

However, Boyle (1990), in a wide ranging review of twin studies, identifies inconsistencies in their findings. She suggests that discrepancies may be the result of methodological problems such as sample selection (for example, exclusive use of in-patients, which skews the sample) and using different diagnostic criteria for schizophrenia across different studies. Difficulties in determining whether twins are monozygotic or dizygotic are also discussed. Arguably the most significant criticism of twin studies is that they are based on the assumption that the environment of monozygotic twins is not very different from that of dizygotic twins. It is this criticism that led to the development of adoption studies by Kety *et al.* (1976).

Adoption Studies

Kety *et al.* (1976) suggest that studies of adopted individuals and their biological and adoptive families offer a means of

disentangling the genetic and environmental contributions to schizophrenia and permit the examination of one type of influence while the other is randomised or controlled.

There are three main type of adoption studies:
1. The examination of the biological and adoptive relatives of adopted schizophrenics.
2. The examination of adopted-away offspring of mothers with schizophrenia.
3. The study of adopted children of healthy mothers by parents with schizophrenia.

In a study of biological and adoptive relatives (Kety *et al.*, 1987) it was reported that both chronic schizophrenia and latent or uncertain schizophrenia were found to be significantly commoner in the biological relatives of index adoptees than in the biological relatives of control adoptees.

In a study of adopted-away offspring by Tienari (1991) it was demonstrated that the adopted offspring of schizophrenic mothers are significantly more likely to develop schizophrenia than the offspring of controls. These results are broadly in line with previous studies (see, for example, Rosenthall 1972).

Research by Wender *et al.* (1974) found no significant differences in the prevalence of schizophrenia in individuals adopted by parents with schizophrenia compared with people who were adopted by healthy parents or raised by their biological parents.

Adoption studies have been criticized for the use of unclear diagnostic criteria, unreliable methodology and questionable methods of analysis (Boyle, 1990).

It seems likely that there is an important genetic component to the development of schizophrenia. However, it is clear that schizophrenia is not solely a genetic disorder and environmental factors have a role to play. Table 18.1 shows the percentage of affected individuals according to their family relationship.

Obstetric Complications

It has been demonstrated that there is evidence of a genetic aetiology in schizophrenia. However, twin studies have also indicated that there is an environmental component in its

TABLE 18.1 Percentage of schizophrenic individuals according to their family relationship

Familial relationship	Percentage affected
Offspring of parents both with schizophrenia	36.6
Monozygotic twins	44.3
Dizygotic twins	12.1
Offspring of one schizophrenic parents	9.4
Siblings	7.3
Spouses	1.0

(adapted from Gotesman et al., 1987)

development. The most likely time of action for environmental factors is at or before birth (Rifkin *et al*., 1994; O'Callaghan *et al*., 1994).

Controlled studies have consistently indicated an increased likelihood of obstetric complications in people with schizophrenia (McNeil, 1988; Lewis, 1989) and it has been clearly shown that people with schizophrenia have lower birth weights than control subjects (McNeil *et al*., 1993). In a prospective follow-up study of low birth weight babies (cited in Rifkin *et al*., 1994) a higher than expected incidence of psychosis was identified.

Studies have clearly demonstrated that, when compared to controls, people with schizophrenia are more likely to have been born in the winter and early spring (Hare, 1988; O'Callaghan *et al*., 1991). Hare (1988) suggests that there may be a seasonal factor, or factors, occurring before or at the time of birth that increases the risk of developing schizophrenia. Various studies have hypothesized that exposure to epidemic strains of influenza during pregnancy is a risk factor for developing schizophrenia (Sham *et al*., 1992; Takei *et al*., 1994).

It has been suggested that there may be significant differences in psychopathology between people with schizophrenia born in the winter and in the summer. Kendell and Kemp (1987) found, in a sample of 222 subjects, that a diagnosis of paranoid schizophrenia or schizoaffective disorder was more likely in people born in the winter months. However, in a larger study these results were not replicated (Kendell and Kemp, 1987).

LIFE EVENTS

It has long been suggested that life events (for example, death of family member, or the loss of a job) are associated with the development of a psychotic illness (for example, Drake and Sederer, 1986). There is clear empirical evidence that life events are associated with the onset of depressive illnesses (Brown and Harris, 1978; Lloyd, 1980). However, while some studies support the hypothesis that such events are related to the development of psychosis, results have not been consistently replicated (Bebbington, 1987; Day *et al*., 1987).

In a recent project by Bebbington *et al*. (1993), data from the Camberwell Collaborative Psychosis study were used to examine the hypothesis that there is an excess of life events prior to the onset of a psychotic illness. The results demonstrated a clear association between life events experienced and the development of psychosis.

CLINICAL IMPLICATIONS

Implications of this research for mental health nurses are that their actions should include:

- Providing support, information and advice about the risks to people with schizophrenia who may be considering having children.
- Offering information, advice and support to carers of people with schizophrenia, about the risks involved in having children.
- Helping to explain to patients some of the factors that may have contributed to their schizophrenia.

Awareness of the contribution genetic factors make to the development of schizophrenia informs interventions with patients and carers and helps dispel the myth that schizophrenia is caused by bad parenting or dysfunctional families.

THE EPIDEMIOLOGY OF SCHIZOPHRENIA

It has been widely reported that 1% of the population experience an episode of schizophrenia at some time in their lives, with no differences arising from gender or ethnicity. It has also been stated that the incidence of schizophrenia is consistent over time. However, a variety of studies suggest that there may have been a decline in the incidence of first admission rates of schizophrenia over the last 20–30 years (Eagles and Whalley 1985; Der *et al*., 1990). Research by Nicole *et al*. (1992) reports that there is a higher incidence of schizophrenia in men than in women and also suggests that men experience a more severe form of the illness. However, there are serious methodological difficulties in conducting epidemiological research in schizophrenia.

THE INFLUENCE OF PSYCHOSOCIAL FACTORS

It has been well documented that people from lower socioeconomic groupings and socially deprived areas are more likely to receive a diagnosis of schizophrenia (Jarman, 1983; Thornicroft, 1991). Research by Castle *et al*. (1994) found that the incidence of schizophrenia in Camberwell increased in the period 1965–1984. They suggest that this is associated with the influx of individuals of Afro-Caribbean origin and note that the incidence of schizophrenia was 4–8 times greater in this ethnic group than in the general population.

Research by Eagles (1991) upholds the hypothesis that there is a link between schizophrenia and migration to socially deprived areas. However, it is unclear whether this link is because of the fact that people with schizophrenia may be drawn to socially isolated areas (such as bedsits in large cities) because they feel socially inept, or whether social status is an important contributory factor in the development of schizophrenia (Flannigan *et al*., 1994).

It is also important to note that people with schizophrenia are more likely to be single and living on their own (Thornicroft, 1991; Smedley and Thomas, 1995).

RACE AND ETHNICITY

There is substantial evidence that people from ethnic minorities are more likely to receive a diagnosis of schizophrenia than the endogenous population (Fabrega *et al*., 1993). It is not clear whether this is associated with increased incidence of schizophrenia in these ethnic groups or if other factors apply. The following reasons for this apparent anomaly have been proposed (Snowden and Cheung, 1990):

1. Ethnic differences in socio-economic status.
2. Clinician bias in assigning diagnostic labels.
3. A poor understanding of cultural issues by clinicians.
4. Differences in cultures about how mental illness is perceived and managed.

AGE OF ONSET

It has been widely reported that the onset of schizophrenia is generally observed between the ages of 18 and 24 years. It has also been demonstrated in well replicated studies (Loranger, 1984; Angermeyer and Kuhn, 1988; Hambrecht *et al.*, 1992) that men develop schizophrenia at an earlier age than women. It has also been well documented that in women there is a second peak in the onset of schizophrenia after the age of 40 (Hambrecht *et al.*, 1992). It has been suggested that oestrogens may have antidopaminergic properties that protect women from psychotic disorders (Salokangas, 1993).

It has also been speculated that because psychotic symptoms such as hallucinations and delusions rarely occur before adolescence, the period of endocrine change during puberty may be the trigger for the development of psychotic symptoms. A study by Galdos *et al.*, (1993) identified a dramatic rise in psychotic symptomatology around puberty and found that onset of schizophrenia takes place earlier in females than in males.

CLINICAL IMPLICATIONS

Research has the following implications for mental health nurses:

1. Nurses must examine their attitudes towards race and ethnicity and demonstrate an understanding of the way schizophrenia may be coped with and interpreted in different cultures.
2. Mental health nurses may need to help people with schizophrenia develop social networks.
3. Nurses may need to educate patients about how to get all the benefits to which they are entitled.

ASSESSMENT AND OUTCOME MEASURES IN SCHIZOPHRENIA

The ability to measure the effect of nursing interventions is essential in enabling nurses to demonstrate the value of their work. Accurate assessment of an individual's physical and psychological health as well as their social situation will provide information that will help nurses to design interventions that meet individual needs. Unlike the case with a doctor, the nurse's role in the assessment of people with schizophrenia is unclear and poorly defined. However, a variety of models (see for example Peplau, 1990) have been proposed to help nurses formulate an assessment procedure and guide nursing practice. These models have received growing criticism and fail to reflect developments in schizophrenia research (Gournay, 1996).

A wide variety of assessment procedures are available for use by mental health nurses. However, before a nurse decides on which instrument to use, he or she must consider whether:

1. When used again, it will indicate if a change has occurred.
2. It measures what it intends to.

These concepts are referred to as reliability and validity.

The reliability of an instrument is concerned with the consistency of measurement with repeated testing. A measure can be said to be reliable if the same results are consistently produced (Hammond, 1995). Reliability is measured using correlational coefficients to measure internal consistency (e.g. Cronbach's alpha), equivalence (e.g. inter-rating reliability) and stability (e.g. test–retest reliability).

The validity of an instrument is determined by its ability to measure what it claims to measure. An instrument can be reliable without being valid but an unreliable instrument can not be valid (Oppenheim, 1984). Determining whether an instrument is valid is complex. Four main types of validity have been described, face validity, content validity, criterion validity and construct validity.

1. Face validity is the weakest type of validity. It relies on the opinion of the person using the tool to decide whether it is valid (Gibbon, 1995).
2. Content validity is concerned with the items in the instrument. It is concerned with whether all areas are adequately covered. One way of ensuring content validity is to review the relevant literature (Gibbon, 1995).
3. Criterion validity is concerned with the accuracy of each item in an instrument. It can be demonstrated by correlating items with those from an instrument whose validity has already been established (Hammond, 1995).
4. Construct validity examines the internal structure of the instrument. It involves testing hypotheses about its structure using sophisticated data analysis methods (Hammond, 1995).

When mental health nurses are deciding which instrument to use to assess their patient, it is essential they ensure that it is both reliable and valid. A variety of instruments, that have been clearly demonstrated to be both reliable and valid, will be outlined as a guide for designing nursing interventions.

ASSESSMENT OF GENERAL PSYCHOPATHOLOGY

Mental health nurses are often required to assess psychopathology. This is especially true in community settings when subtle changes in psychopathology may provide the first indications of a deteriorating mental state. Given community mental health nurses' increased responsibilities under the revised Mental Health Act, the importance of accurate assessment cannot be over-emphasized.

Brief Psychiatric Rating Scale (BPRS)

The BPRS (Overall and Gorham, 1962) is the most commonly used rating scale for schizophrenia. The scale contains 16 symptom constructs, which are rated by the interviewer on a 7-point scale from 'not present' to 'extremely severe'. The ratings are based on a 20-minute interview. While a high degree of reliability has been demonstrated (Overall and Gorham, 1962) there is little evidence of construct validity. Although the BPRS is easy to use, it relies heavily on the interpersonal skills and judgement of the interviewer.

The Nurses Observation Scale for In-Patient Evaluation (NOSIE)

The NOSIE (Honigfeld and Klett, 1965) is a scale used in assessing in-patients with chronic schizophrenia. Ratings are based on continual observation of behaviour by staff and take approximately 10 minutes to complete. The instrument has 23 items. Each item is rated on a 5-point scale ranging from 'never' to 'always'. While the NOSIE has demonstrated strong validity and reliability (Tress and Paton, 1994), its focus is on behaviour rather than psychopathology. However, this may be useful when assessing patients who are difficult to interview (for example, those who are hyperactive, mute or withdrawn).

Positive and Negative Syndrome Scale (PANNS)

The PANNS (Kay *et al.*, 1988, 1989) is used increasingly to rate the positive and negative features of schizophrenia. It has demonstrated strong validity and reliability. It includes 30 clearly defined items (7 positive symptoms, 7 negative symptoms and 16 general psychopathology items) rated on a 7-point scale ranging from 'absent' to 'extremely severe'. Ratings are based on a 40-minute structured interview.

Individual Assessment of Symptoms

While instruments such as the BPRS, NOSIE and PANNS provide an overall picture of psychopathology in schizophrenia, research suggests that psychological interventions may be more effective when specific symptoms are targeted.

Dimensions of Delusional Experience Scale (DDES)

This instrument is designed to rate five dimensions of delusional experience (Kendler *et al.*, 1983). These are conviction, extension (into other areas of their life), bizarreness, disorganization and pressure (preoccupation and concern). Ratings are based on a semi-structured interview lasting approximately 45 minutes. While this instrument has proved to be generally reliable, its validity has yet to be demonstrated.

Personal Questionnaire Rapid Scaling Technique (PQRST)

Despite the profusion of research into the formation and treatment of auditory hallucinations (Slade and Bentall, 1988), measurement scales that aim to quantify these experiences are scarce and very few have demonstrated validity and reliability (Garety and Wessley, 1994).

The PQRST (Mulhall, 1978) measures the frequency, distress, disruption to life and patients' attributions of voices over a 1-week period.

Assessment of Social Functioning

Social functioning, including social withdrawal and inappropriate behaviour, is commonly impaired in people with schizophrenia (Pantelis and Curson, 1994). Even after an acute episode has passed, functioning may continue to be impaired. Nursing care is often focused on alleviating these deficits and accurate assessment is therefore essential.

The Life Skills Profile (LSP)

This instrument (Rosen *et al.*, 1989) has 39 items, rated on a 4-point scale, with assessment of these dimensions: self-care, non-turbulence (for example, violence and abuse of alcohol and drugs), social contact, communication and responsibility. The scale is designed to measure the individual's functioning over the previous 6 months. This instrument is can be used in both in-patient and community settings and has been shown to be reliable. However, validity has not been determined.

Assessment of Side-Effects

Mental health nurses are in an ideal position to monitor side-effects that may be experienced. Careful monitoring is not only essential to ensure safety but also because unpleasant side-effects may be a major reason for non-compliance (Fleischhacker *et al.*, 1994). Accurate assessment and effective interventions may also greatly increase patient satisfaction with medication. Therefore, careful assessment and intervention by mental health nurses should increase compliance with medication and consequently reduce relapse rates. This hypothesis has not, however, been empirically tested.

The Liverpool University neuroleptic side-effect rating scale (LUNSERS)

The LUNSERS (Day *et al.*, 1995) is a 51-item, self-report questionnaire covering psychological, neurological, autonomic, hormonal and miscellaneous side-effects. The questionnaire also includes 10 'red herring' items. Each item is rated by the patient on a 0–4 rating scale ranging from 'not at all' to 'very much'. In a study by Day *et al.* (1995) the LUNSERS was demonstrated to have good reliability and validity.

Extrapyramidal side-effect rating scale

This scale (Simpson and Angus, 1970) was originally designed to measure drug-induced parkinsonism. Ten items are rated on a 0–4 rating scale based on a physical examination. The instrument has been shown to have a reasonable degree of inter-rating reliability.

Clinical Implications

It is clear that mental health nurses must use assessment tools that are valid and reliable so that they can design effective and appropriate interventions and accurately determine their effect. Assessment tools should be used on a regular basis, not just on admission and at discharge. Careful use will produce an accurate picture of the course of an individual's illness and may make it possible to identify antecedents to relapse and to design preventive interventions. The assessment tools described here also make communication with other disciplines more efficient and minimize repetition.

TREATMENT

In this section pharmacological and psychological treatments of schizophrenia are examined. The new generation of atypical antipsychotics and research into the formation and maintenance of psychotic symptoms are discussed. Implications for nursing practice are presented.

PHARMACOLOGICAL INTERVENTIONS

Pharmacological interventions are an important aspect of caring for people with schizophrenia. Mental health nurses in both in-patient and community settings have important roles to play in pharmacological interventions and it is essential that they have a good understanding of how drugs used to treat schizophrenia work and the side-effects that can be produced.

The Dopamine Hypothesis of Schizophrenia

Chlorpromazine was introduced in the early 1950s and was the first drug to be used to treat schizophrenia. Since that time a wide range of antipsychotic drugs have been developed. The most frequently used include chlorpromazine, haloperidol, droperidol, sulpiride, thioridazine, trifluoperazine and flupenthixol decanoate.

Controlled trials have demonstrated the effectiveness of these drugs in treating predominantly the positive symptoms of schizophrenia (McKay and McKenna, 1993). Carlsson and Lindquist (1963) first proposed that antipsychotic drugs work by blocking dopamine receptors in the brain. (For a description of how antipsychotic drugs work see Chapter 27). Since then it has been found that antipsychotic drugs not only block dopamine receptors but also, for example, noradrenaline (1), serotonin (5-HT) and histamine receptors (McKay and McKenna, 1993).

Hyttel *et al.* (1985), in a review of the receptor-binding profiles of a variety of antipsychotic medication, noted that certain drugs (such as chlorpromazine and thioridazine, for example) have broad-spectrum effects blocking D1 and D2, 1, 5-HT2 and histamine (H1) receptors. Other antipsychotics such as haloperidol and trifluoperazine have a narrower band of action, while sulpiride is effectively specific only to D2 receptors. As the only pharmacological action shared by these drugs is dopamine receptor blockade, it suggests that this is the action that makes antipsychotics effective.

There are, however, two exceptions to this rule. The first is promazine, which had a weak affinity for dopamine receptors and an equally weak antipsychotic action. The second is clozapine.

Positron emission tomography (PET) is an imaging technique that allows visualization of the receptor-binding sites in the brain, making it possible to determine to what extent different receptors are occupied (Waddington, 1989). Farde *et al.* (1992) have demonstrated that near-maximum occupancy (70–89%) of available D2 receptors can be achieved in patients responding to treatment at relatively modest doses of antipsychotics. It can therefore be suggested that high doses of typical antipsychotics do not appear to be any more effective than considerably lower doses (Farde *et al.*, 1992).

It is generally accepted that the full benefit from treatment with antipsychotic medication is not seen for 2–3 weeks after commencing treatment. However, PET studies (Nordstrom *et al.*, 1992) have indicated that maximal occupancy (73–91%) of D2 receptors occurs within a few hours of treatment being commenced. This evidence supports the hypothesis that primary D2 receptor blockade by typical antipsychotics initiates a series of slow adaptive changes in dopaminergic neurones and possible subsequent changes in others. It is these secondary effects that are responsible for the reduction in psychotic symptoms.

Research by Nyberg *et al.* (1995) described D2 receptor occupancy in treatment with low dose haloperidol decanoate. It was reported that after 1 week of treatment the mean occupancy was 73%. However, despite a fall in occupancy over time to 52%, at week 4 psychotic symptoms did not re-emerge. Nyberg *et al.* (1995) suggest that continuously high D2 receptor blockade may not be necessary to prevent relapse.

It can clearly be demonstrated that antipsychotic drugs are effective in treating predominantly the positive symptoms of schizophrenia. It is also evident that the reason for their effectiveness is their ability to block dopamine D2 receptors. However, between 20% and 40% of people with schizophrenia either derive little benefit from these drugs or experience severe side-effects.

TABLE 18.2 Common side-effects from conventional neuroleptic drugs such as chlorpromazine

Symptom	Percentage experiencing symptom during treatment period *
Parkinsonism	20
Oversedation	18
Akathisia	13
Acute dystonia	9

* from Bollini *et al.*, 1994

Side-effects

The four main categories of extrapyramidal side-effects (EPSE) induced by antipsychotic drugs are akathisia, dystonia, dyskinesia and parkinsonism. It is possible that in some patients EPSE may progress into potentially irreversible forms, tardive dyskinesia for example (Gerlach and Peacock, 1995). It is suggested that these side-effects are caused by dopamine blockade in the nigrostriatal system (Johnstone *et al.*, 1978). Effective prevention of such EPSE may involve the use of the lowest effective dose and close monitoring of side-effects. Table 18.2 describes the side-effects that are commonly reported in people taking conventional neuroleptic drugs such as chlorpromazine.

Clozapine

It has been suggested that the introduction of clozapine is probably the most important development in antipsychotic medication since the advent of chlorpromazine (Liberman *et al.*, 1994). In a seminal multicentre collaborative study by Kane *et al.* (1988) clozapine was demonstrated to be superior to traditional antipsychotics in treatment-resistant schizophrenia. Several

TABLE 18.3 Side-effects from clozapine

Side effect	% affected during treatment*
Hypersalivation	54
Drowsiness	46
Constipation	44
Dizziness	41
Nausea	35
Sweating	28
Dry mouth	24
Headache	22
Seizures	9
Hypotension	6
Benign hyperpyrexia	6
Neutropenia	3
Agranulocytosis	3
Tachycardia	2

* from Clozapine Study Group, 1993

controlled (Claghorn *et al.*, 1987) and uncontrolled studies (Meltzer *et al.*, 1989; Mattes, 1989; Owen *et al.*, 1989; Clozapine Study Group, 1993) have made a variety of claims about the superiority of clozapine in treating the positive symptoms of schizophrenia (hallucinations, delusions, thought disorder). However, the proportion of people with treatment-resistant schizophrenia who respond to clozapine is inconsistent. Claims of between 30% and 61% have been reported (Liberman *et al.*, 1994).

Studies have also reported that clozapine is effective in treating the negative symptoms of schizophrenia (Liberman *et al.*, 1994) and improving patient neurocognitive deficits and functional capacities (Meltzer *et al.*, 1989).

Studies have reported that, when compared to traditional antipsychotic drugs, clozapine produces very little or no parkinsonism and dystonia and less liability to tardive dyskinesia. In a review of eight studies by Liberman *et al.* (1991) approximately 43% of people with tardive dyskinesia improved after treatment with clozapine.

A unique range of side-effects has been reported in patients taking clozapine. Table 18.3 describes side-effects reported by patients in a study by the Clozapine Study Group (1993). Significantly, because of the risk of neutropenia, patients undergoing treatment with clozapine will require regular blood tests for the duration of their treatment.

A variety of explanations have been suggested as to why clozapine is effective in treating atypical and treatment-resistant schizophrenia (Farde *et al.*, 1994; Kerwin *et al.*, 1994; Meltzer, 1994; Curtis *et al.*, 1995). Serotonergic receptors; 5-HT2C and 5-HT2, have been cited as possible candidates for clozapine atypicality (Altar *et al.*, 1988; Canton *et al.*, 1990; Curtis *et al.*, 1995). Research by Duinkerke *et al.* (1993) has demonstrated that 5-HT2 antagonists in open clinical trials are effective in treating the negative symptoms of schizophrenia. It is the research into clozapine that has led to development of a new generation of antipsychotic medication.

Risperidone

Risperidone is the first of the new generation of drugs to be commercially available. Recent PET studies (Nyberg *et al.*, 1993) show it is a 5-HT2 antagonist with approximately 25-fold less D2 antagonist activity than found with other antipsychotics (Megens *et al.*, 1992). In controlled clinical trials, risperidone has been demonstrated to be effective in treating the positive, negative and affective symptoms of schizophrenia with a low incidence of EPSE (Megens *et al.*, 1992). Significantly, although risperidone does not appear to be any more efficacious than haloperidol in randomized control studies, there is evidence that it is more effective in treating negative symptoms (Borison *et al.*, 1992).

The side-effects that have been reported for risperidone are insomnia (25.6%), agitation (21.9%), anxiety (12.3%), EPSE (16.7%), headache (14.2%), constipation (6.8%) and nausea (6.2%).

THE ROLE OF MENTAL HEALTH NURSES IN PHARMACOLOGICAL INTERVENTIONS

Mental health nurses have an important role to play regarding medication. For example, the day-to-day administration of medication on wards and in out-patient clinics, the education of patients about their medications (ensuring that they understand possible improvements in symptoms and any side-effects that might occur), decisions to administer PRN or *pro re nata* medication (given as required) and the assessment of side-effects.

There is evidence that mental health nurses do not effectively monitor side-effects. In a study by Bennett *et al.* (1995) it was demonstrated that, although a group of community psychiatric nurses (CPNs) believed that they were able to assess all the side-effects of medication, in practice they only assessed a few. It was also reported that, generally, these CPNs had a negative attitude towards their involvement in medication.

MENTAL HEALTH NURSES' USE OF PRN MEDICATION

The administration of PRN medication by mental health nurses is a frequently used and yet poorly explored aspect of mental health care. A review of the literature identified no studies that investigated whether nurses believe that they are adequately prepared to administer PRN medication (Gray *et al.*, 1996). When used appropriately, PRN can be an effective intervention that can help minimize distress or reduce side-effects.

A study by Gray *et al.* (1996) described the administration of PRN medication by mental health nurses in acute psychiatric units. They found that the three main categories of drugs administered PRN were benzodiazepines, antipsychotics and analgesics. However, the most frequently administered drug was procyclidine (16.4% of all administrations), which was given to reduce the side-effects of antipsychotic drugs.

The most frequent reason for administering PRN medication was because patients had 'requested' it (19.8% of all administrations). PRN medication was also frequently given because patients were 'agitated' (11.9% of administrations) and 'to aid sleep' (9.7% of administrations).

Given that a high proportion of all PRN medication that is administered is used to reduce the extrapyramidal side-effects of conventional antipsychotics, it is essential that nurses make an informed decision to use this intervention.

The study by Gray *et al.* (1996) finds that use of PRN medication for the purposes of rapid tranquillization is common. However, developments in our understanding of psychotropic medication suggest that use of PRN must be based on careful assessment and understanding of pharmacology.

CLINICAL IMPLICATIONS

1. Mental health nurses should have a good understanding of the side-effects that antipsychotic and other drugs used in schizophrenia can produce.
2. Side-effects should be assessed using valid and reliable tools (for example LUNSER and EPSE rating scale described earlier).
3. Mental health nurses should regularly discuss the severity of the side-effects that the patient is experiencing with the multidisciplinary team and review the type and dose of medication prescribed.
4. Mental health nurses should help patients and their carers to minimize the distress caused by side-effects (such as weight gain, dribbling and sedation).
5. The use of PRN medication should be based on a careful assessment using valid and reliable techniques.
6. Nurses should have a good understanding of pharmacology to inform decisions about the administration of PRN.
7. Alternative coping strategies should be considered before administering PRN.
8. The reason for administering PRN must be carefully documented in the nurse's notes.
9. The effect of the administration of PRN must be careful documented in the nurse's notes.

PSYCHOLOGICAL INTERVENTIONS

SCHIZOPHRENIA AS A HETEROGENEOUS ENTITY

The traditional view of schizophrenia being a homogeneous entity has recently been questioned. A variety of different ways of subdividing schizophrenia have been proposed. While symptomatic subtypes including paranoid versus non-paranoid symptoms (Goldstein and Tsuang, 1988) and positive versus negative symptoms (Crow, 1985) remain in use, their empirical validity is questionable.

Recently, research (see for example, Lyon *et al.*, 1994) has focused on the symptoms of psychopathology, in addition to broader classifications. Research has demonstrated the effects of cognitive behavioural interventions in the treatment of specific symptoms of schizophrenia and a variety of models have been proposed to explain the development of these symptoms (Bentall *et al.*, 1990; Tarrier *et al.*, 1990; Parris and Skagerlind, 1994; Morrison *et al.*, 1995).

RESEARCH INTO DELUSIONS

Much contemporary research has focused on delusions and delusion-like beliefs (Hemsley and Garety, 1986; Garety *et al.*, 1991; Kaney and Bentall, 1992; Lyon *et al.*, 1994; Young and Bentall, 1995). This work may have considerable impact on the design and implementation of educational interventions. Peters *et al.* (1995) measured delusional beliefs in psychotic and normal subjects using a Delusion Inventory that included measures of distress, preoccupation and conviction. It was demonstrated that there was an overlap between the ranges of scores produced by the two groups, suggesting that psychotic symptoms are the extreme end of a normal–pathological continuum.

Two main explanations have been proposed to explain

delusional experiences (Lyon *et al.*, 1994). The first suggests that delusional experiences are the rational attempt to explain abnormal experiences (hallucinations, for example). However, as Chapman and Chapman (1988) note, some people with delusions do not have any perceptual abnormalities and many people with perceptual abnormalities do not have delusions.

Hemsley and Garety (1986) propose that delusional thinking may be the result of 'an inability to evaluate novel information and adjust beliefs accordingly', therefore individuals develop a heightened awareness of irrelevant stimuli that form their delusional beliefs.

Hemsley (1993) proposes that schizophrenic symptoms are associated with weakening influence of past experience on current perceptions. Among the most significant features of delusional thinking is an abnormal view of the relationship between events. He suggests that abnormalities in the hippocampal region play an important role in the emergence of psychotic symptoms. This is the region of the brain that is involved in linking and comparing events.

Clearly, if this hypothesis can be empirically validated it will have considerable impact on the design of an educational strategy. Hemsley (1993) suggests that schizophrenics may experience sensory overload, if they are unaware of information that is redundant and can be discarded (also associated with the hippocampus). This hypothesis concurred with well documented attentional and memory deficits in schizophrenia (Hemsley, 1993).

Research by Young and Bentall (1995) examined hypothesis testing in patients with persecutory delusions. Subjects were given visual discrimination problems and were given feedback from the examiner so that they could formulate correct solutions to the task. Subjects with delusions were less able to respond to feedback and found it more difficult than control subjects to focus on a correct hypothesis. Young and Bentall (1995) concluded that deluded subjects were less responsive to positive feedback than were controls. Conversely, when deluded subjects were given negative feedback they were less likely to change their beliefs than were controls.

Kaney and Bentall (1992) used the Attributional Style Questionnaire (ASQ) (Peterson *et al.*, 1982) to demonstrate that depressed and delusional subjects were more likely than controls to rate negative items as global (affecting all areas of life) and stable (unchangeable). However, depressed subjects significantly rated items more frequently as internal (caused by self) while delusional subjects significantly rated items more frequently as external (caused by others). Deluded subjects were also more likely to rate positive items as internal, global and stable. These results have since been replicated (Candido and Romney 1990; Lyon *et al.*, 1994) and suggest that delusions may be a defence mechanism that protects an individual's self-esteem.

Attribution theory suggests that interventions with deluded patients that enhance self-esteem may be more effective than interventions that directly challenge patients' defences.

RESEARCH INTO HALLUCINATIONS AND THOUGHT DISORDER

Bentall *et al.* (1990) define hallucinations as:

> a percept-like experience that occurs in the absence of an appropriate stimulus, that has the full force and impact of a corresponding real perception, and that is not amenable to direct and voluntary control by the experience.

Frith (1979) suggests that hallucinations result from a disorder of the selection processes involved in perception–that is to say, a failure to filter out hypotheses until the correct one is selected. Bentall (1990) argues that individuals who experience hallucinations tend to misattribute internal stimuli to an external source.

Metacognition forms the basis for many of these theories. It is a term that is used to describe psychological processes such as introspection and the ability to control one's thinking. According to this view, internal cognitive events are attributed to external sources. Research by Bentall *et al.* (1991) suggests that in experimental conditions, hallucinating subjects misattribute words to an external source more frequently than normal controls, especially when tasks require high cognitive effort. This theory also accounts for why hallucinations increase in stressful circumstances and sometimes also occur in normal subjects (Posey, 1986).

Thought disorder is a disorder of the way in which communication is perceived by an individual (Howe, 1986). Thought disorder may therefore result in bizarre and incoherent attempts to communicate with others. Research suggests that metacognitive processes are important in regulating speech (Bentall *et al.*, 1990). Harrow and Prosen (1979) postulate that thought disordered patients have a form of impaired perception that prevents them from deciding whether their speech is appropriate to the circumstances. Harvey (1985) suggests that thought disorder is associated with deficits in reality monitoring tasks, that is to say, an inability to discriminate speech that has already been said from what remains to be stated.

COGNITIVE FUNCTIONING IN SCHIZOPHRENIA

Deficits in the cognitive functioning of people with schizophrenia are well documented and have been observed in almost every cognitive measure (Green, 1993). Perceptual, attentional and memory abnormalities have been identified (Neuchterlein, 1995). These have been found to be present even during remissions and may be part of enduring vulnerability (a disproportionate number of biological relatives also have these abnormalities). Other deficits such as working memory, failures in self-monitoring systems and rapid and biased decision-making can be attributed to acute psychotic experiences.

CLINICAL IMPLICATIONS

Many of the findings from recent psychological research will radically affect the way in which nurses work with people with schizophrenia. Significantly, the validity of interventions such as those described by Peplau (1990) must be re-examined in the light of recent research. While results of controlled studies have yet to be produced that demonstrate the effectiveness of such interventions when used by mental health nurses, it is useful to consider the possible applications for nursing practice:

- It may be advantageous for mental health nurses to adopt a symptom-based approach to interventions.
- One-to-one interventions should be short, lasting for 20–30 minutes.
- Nurses should use interpersonal skills to sustain concentration, such as
  - Eye contact.
  - Clear voice tone.
  - Listening skills.
  - Environmental factors (a quiet room, no interruptions).
- Nursing interventions that simply challenge a patient's belief (for example 'You are not the devil') are not effective.
- Patients will need to be encouraged to develop ways of testing their beliefs in a graded and supportive way.
- Nursing interventions should try to enhance an individual's self-esteem.

FAMILY INTERVENTIONS

Although it is widely accepted that families are not a causactvie factor in schizophrenia, there is evidence to suggest that the course of the illness may be affected by the way families interact. It has been consistently demonstrated that interventions aimed at lowering expressed emotion in families are effective in reducing relapse rates in people with schizophrenia (Barraclough and Tarrier, 1992; Kuipers *et al.*, 1992; Falloon *et al.*, 1993). Such interventions aim to reduce the amount of face-to-face contact, critical comments, hostility and over-involvement and examine relatives' attributions of the cause of schizophrenia and behaviour. Family interventions are discussed in detail in Chapter 31.

Recently, interest has focused on applying these ideas to design interventions for use in community settings such as hostels. Preliminary research by Moore *et al.* (1992) identified varying levels of expressed emotion in a group of hostel workers. Interventions by mental health nurses to lower expressed emotion in this group may be effective in reducing relapse rates and may provide information and support to help individuals cope with the illness.

RELAPSE PREVENTION

Relapse is frequently observed in people with schizophrenia. In this section strategies to enhance treatment compliance and minimise the risk of relapse are presented.

COMPLIANCE

Controlled trials have demonstrated that antipsychotic drugs are the most effective method of treating the symptoms of schizophrenia. However non-compliance with antipsychotic

medication is common. Reported rates of non-compliance range from 10–75%, depending on the patient sample and the operational definition of compliance used (Talbot *et al.*, 1986; Young *et al.*, 1986). Kent and Yellowlees (1994) found that non-compliance with medication was the main reason for admission to psychiatric hospital in 43–62% of cases. It is clear that non-compliance with medication is a serious problem, which mental health nurses are in an ideal position to address. However, it is necessary to first identify why patients are non-compliant.

A 2-year prospective study of treatment compliance (Buchanan, 1992) highlighted the following variables affecting compliance: socio-demographic factors, patients' insight into illness, patients' attitude towards treatment, illness variables, treatment variables, previous compliance and compulsory detention. Sellwood and Tarrier (1994) also examined factors affecting non-compliance and highlight that side-effects from medication and service delivery could also be contributing factors. It has also been suggested that people with schizophrenia who use cannabis and other non-prescription drugs are also less compliant (Cuffel *et al.*, 1993).

Non-Prescription Drug Use

A survey by the Royal College of Nursing (Sandford, 1995) highlights the use of illicit drugs by users of mental health services. Of mental health nurses who responded to the survey, 68% claimed that they had had incidents of illicit drug use in their clinical area. The level of non-prescription drug use that exists is unclear. However, there is substantive evidence that the use of substances such as cannabis, alcohol, cocaine, amphetamines, heroin, ecstasy and benzodiazepines has a significant effect on the mental health of people with schizophrenia.

Several studies have described patterns of non-prescription drug use in people with schizophrenia (Brady *et al.*, 1991; Cuffel *et al.*, 1993; DeQuardo *et al.*, 1994). Cuffel *et al.* (1993) identified three patterns of substance abuse: no substance abuse (54%), abuse of alcohol and cannabis (31%) and polysubstance abuse (14%). It was suggested that while both of the substance-abusing groups experienced more affective disturbance, there was no increase in the amount of psychotic symptoms experienced.

Cuffel *et al.* (1993) state that people with schizophrenia who abuse non-prescription drugs tend to be young, male and of low socio-economic status. It is also suggested that there is an increased likelihood of substance abuse in their family history (Tsuang *et al.*, 1982) and they have better premorbid social functioning (Dixon *et al.*, 1991).

Several studies have suggested that people with schizophrenia may use a variety of non-prescription drugs to 'self-medicate'. Lehman *et al.* (1989) identified two types of self-medication. The first suggests that factors such as a negative affective state, impaired cognition and poor self-esteem, predispose people with schizophrenia to abuse non-prescription drugs (Ram *et al.*, 1992; Soni *et al.*, 1994). The second theory suggests a relationship between the pharmacological effect of specific substances and the symptoms presented by the individual. It has been suggested that cannabis use alleviates the negative symptoms of schizophrenia and reduces the extrapyramidal side-effects. Correlational analysis has been used to support this hypothesis. However, poly-substance abuse is common and as a consequence it is difficult to determine the effect of a single substance.

Research by Cuffel *et al.* (1993) examined the patterns of substance abuse among people with schizophrenia. No patterns of substance abuse were identified based on the pharma-cological effects of the drug. A study by Dixon *et al.* (1991) indicated that people with schizophrenia predominately use drugs that induce psychotic symptoms. DeQuardo *et al.* (1994) reported that heavy substance abusers believed their cannabis use to be self-medicating; however, ward staff reported an increase in psychopathology.

There is clear evidence that the use of non-prescription drugs can have a negative effect on the symptoms of schizo-phrenia. Knudsen and Vilmer (1984) also suggest that cannabis can reduce the effectiveness of neuroleptic drugs. Negrete *et al.* (1986) suggest that there is a strong link between cannabis use and the severity of symptoms experienced. They demons-trated that active users of cannabis had more hallucinations and delusions than 'past users' and 'never users'. Active users also had more frequent visits to hospital.

While it is difficult accurately to measure the level of non-prescription drug use in people with schizophrenia, it is clear that it is a significant problem, especially in inner-city areas. There is also strong evidence that non-prescription drug use will affect the severity and course of the illness. However, there is little research that can be used to design interventions to tackle this growing problem.

SIDE-EFFECTS

It has been frequently observed that individuals who experi-ence side-effects from antipsychotic medication are less compliant (Falloon 1984; Diamond 1985). However, in a study by Kelly *et al.* (1987), only 10% of non-compliance was associated with side-effects.

DEMOGRAPHIC VARIABLES

There is clear evidence that individuals with family support are more compliant (Piatowska and Farnill, 1992). However, evi-dence of other demographic factors influencing compliance is less clear. It has been suggested that variables such as low socio-economic status (Young *et al.*, 1986), gender (Tunnicliffe *et al.*, 1992), age (Tunnicliffe *et al.*, 1992) and ethnicity (Buchanan, 1992) can affect compliance. However, the empirical data are unclear and consistent results have not been produced.

SYMPTOM VARIABLES

It has been suggested that people with schizophrenia who experience delusional beliefs are less compliant, as are those who generally experience more severe positive symptoms (Sellwood and Tarrier, 1994). However, research by Buchanan (1992) demonstrated that the level of psychopathology expe-rienced was not significantly correlated with compliance.

PREVIOUS COMPLIANCE

One of the most frequently reported results in research examining compliance in people with schizophrenia is that past behaviour predicts future behaviour (Buchanan, 1992). Therefore, if indi-viduals were compliant in the past they will tend to be so in the future. However, this leaves a substantial group of patients who will continue to be persistently non-compliant.

INSIGHT INTO ILLNESS AND ATTITUDE TOWARDS TREATMENT

David (1990) suggests that insight is constituted by three over-lapping areas:
1. Insight itself–awareness by the patient that they have an illness.
2. The ability of the patient to relabel psychotic experiences as pathological.
3. A willingness to accept treatment.

Various studies have examined relationships between insight and compliance (for example, Ghaemi and Pope, 1994; Kemp and David, 1995) and there is clear evidence that poor insight is an accurate predictor of non-compliance. However, Kemp and David (1995) suggest that the relationship between insight and compliance is shaped by context, cultural influences, prior experience of treatment and the relationship with health care professionals.

David *et al.* (1992) find that neuropsychological factors such as low IQ (intelligence quotient) and poor cognitive func-tioning may predispose people with schizophrenia to lack of insight.

A study by Amador *et al.* (1994) using the Subjective Awareness of Mental Disorder scale reported that, in a sample of 412 subjects with a DSM-IIIR diagnosis of schizophrenia, 40% were completely unaware and 57% were either partially or completely unaware that they had a mental illness.

Compliance research has been earmarked as a priority by the Department of Health, which emphasizes that ensuring compliance is an essential task in working with people with schizophrenia. Mental health nurses have a critical role to play in enhancing compliance and increasing satisfaction with treatment.

CLINICAL IMPLICATIONS

Gerlach (1994) argues that depot antipsychotics can be effectively used to ensure compliance; this should lead to fewer relapses and less frequent hospitalizations. It is also argued that side-effects can be minimized because it is easier to determine the lowest effective dose. However, there are sig-nificant disadvantages with depot administration. These include the delay in the disappearance of side-effects when depot administration is stopped and a feeling of being con-trolled (Gerlach, 1994). Significantly, the new generation of antipsychotics such as clozapine, risperidone and ziprasidone are not available as depot preparations. As the drugs become used more frequently, it will not be possible to ensure compliance by depot injection.

If compliance is to be effectively enhanced, mental health nurses will need to:
• examine their own attitudes towards non-prescription drug use, to work effectively with drug-using patients.
• use educational interventions to reduce the use of non-prescription drugs.
• assess patients' attitudes towards treatment and insight into their own illness.
• address patients beliefs about their illness and treatment.

A PERSONAL ACCOUNT OF SCHIZOPHRENIA

My experience of schizophrenia is the cognitive equivalent of staring into bright sunshine or listening to very loud road traffic for a long period of time. In my history I have had few episodes of voice hearing. When I did hear voices, it was just before my second admission to hospital. They were voices of police and the law and judges passing sentence on me. They were therefore very frightening and confusing. I also experience a sort of stasis where my body comes to a stop and I sort of freeze. I attribute this to tension caused by the psychosis of the illness.

I feel very foolish in the over-abuse of cannabis as I know now how fatal it can be for someone with a high intellect. It was most definitely the trigger and the cause of my second episode where you would have thought that I would have learnt. I would strongly advise people of high intellect to steer clear of cannabis as I feel it can often lead to pro-longed periods of psychosis.

After my first admission in 1993 I would often freeze up and be reduced to a sort of shuddering wreck. I used to think that the beats in my heart were flying around all over the hospital. Some of the things that I experienced are really hard to put into words; I spent a lot of time in bed and did not want to surface and hated getting up for medication first thing in the morning.

The most important way in which the nurses helped me was to show sympathy, kindness and patience, despite often being very occupied with other patients. I found occupational therapists most helpful because they helped me to structure my day and find meaningful occupation.

The first medication I took was sulpiride tablets; I found it pretty useless. The miracle happened when I was put on haloperidol orally. It gave me an invisible rope to help pull me out of my psychosis and my general trauma. More recently Clopixol has been better. The side-effects that I experience on haloperidol was a lot of stiffness and more tiredness. With Clopixol, I experience only minimal tired-ness and no stiffness.

The things that keep me well can be described as a four legged stool, namely medication, environment, carers' sup-port and occupation. It is important that the environment where I live is supportive and friendly. My carers are my family and a few friends who have all been terrific and very understanding. Occupation is very important and I try to keep myself busy.

Last week I played golf on Monday, worked Tuesday, Wednesday and Thursday at a local user group. Also on Tuesday and Thursday evenings I went to choir and went to a conference for users and carers about schizophrenia on Friday. On Saturday I spent all day setting up the church and rehearsing for the evening concert at 7.30 which was very enjoyable and a great success. Sunday I slept all day.

The people who are never wrong.

Talk about your anger
share with us your fears
for we are very weary
of your crocodile tears

Very special training
the nurses all have had
on forcing you to face
the fact that you are mad

Lots of funny pills
to take away your ills
make love and life and laughter
practically killed.

'Doctor Doc. my heads a rushing'.
'Quiet there and stop your fussing.
I'm up to my ears in work right now
to our theories you'd do well to bow'.

So don't forget that thorough training
that says to you when you're complaining
take this tablet, and this tablet
cause to my stomach pains your failing.

I keep my mouth tight shut
of feelings such as these
for if I voice them to the Doc.
the staff room ain't at ease.

(A patient)

SUMMARY

Throughout this chapter, various themes have been examined. They include diagnosis, insight, compliance with medication, nonprescription drug use and side-effects. Mental health nurses in both hospital and community settings are in an ideal position to tackle these issues. Effective interventions could significantly improve the health and social functioning of people with schizophrenia. Much emphasis has been placed on the use of educational interventions. Studies have examined the effects of such interventions on:
• Understanding of treatment (Gray *et al.*, 1995).
• Insight into illness (Kemp and David, 1995).

- Attitude towards treatment (Kemp *et al*., 1996).
- Compliance with medication (Pan and Tantum, 1989).

Results from these studies have failed to prove conclusively that educational interventions are effective. However, there is evidence from controlled studies that suggests that significant changes can occur from such interventions. In a study by Kemp *et al*. (1996) significantly improved attitudes to treatment, insight and compliance were demonstrated following a cognitive–educational intervention. Increasingly, these educational interventions are drawing from psychological theories of schizophrenia to design more effective interventions and emphasis has been placed on those that are symptom based.

While the results from clinical trials have yet to emerge, it is interesting to speculate on the effects of educational interventions on, for example, non-prescription drug use.

KEY CONCEPTS

- Schizophrenia is a mental illness characterized by positive, negative and affective symptoms.
- Although schizophrenia has an important genetic component it is clear that environmental factors including obstetric complications and major life events have an important influence on the development of the disorder.
- Assessment is a vital part of designing and delivering effective interventions. Mental health nurses must use assessment tools that are both valid and reliable.
- Pharmacological and psychological play a vital role in both treating the symptoms of schizophrenia and ensuring that people are able to live with the illness.

REFERENCES

Altar CA, Wasley AM, Neale RF, *et al*.: Typical and atypical antipsychotic occupancy of D_2 and S_2 receptors and autoradiographic analysis in rat brain. *Brain Res Bull* 16(4):517–525, 1988.

Amador XF, Flaum M, Andreasen NC, *et al*.: Awareness of illness in schizophrenia and schizoaffective disorder. *Archi Gen Psychiatry* 51(9):826–836, 1994.

American Psychiatric Association: *Diagnostic and statistical manual of mental disorders,* ed 4. Washington, 1994, American Psychiatric Association.

Angermeyer M, Kuhn L: Gender differences in age at onset of schizophrenia. *Eur Arch Psychiatry Neurosci* 237(6):351–364, 1988.

Barraclough C, Tarrier N: *Families of schizophrenic patients; cognitive behavioural interventions*. London, 1992, Chapman & Hall.

Bebbington PE: Life events and schizophrenia. The WHO collaborative study. *Soc Psychiatry* 22:179–180, 1987.

Bebbington PE, Wilkins S, Jones P, *et al*.: Life events and psychosis. Initial results from the Camberwell collaborative psychosis study. *Br J Psychiatry* 162:72–79, 1993.

Bennett J, Done J, Hund B: Assessing the side-effects of antipsychotic drugs: a survey of CPN practice. *J Psychiatr Ment Health Nurs* 2(3):177–182, 1995.

Bentall RP *et al*.: The illusion of reality: A review and integration of psychological research on hallucinations. *Psychol Bull* 107(1):82–95, 1990.

Bentall RP, Baker GA, Havers S: Reality monitoring and psychotic hallucinations. *Br J Clin Psychol* 30(3):213–222, 1991.

Bleuler E: *Dementia praecox or the group of schizophrenias*. New York, 1950, International Universities Press.

Bollini P, Pampallona MJ, Orza ME *et al*.: Antipsychotic drugs: Is more worse? A meta-analysis of the published randomised controlled trials. *Psychol Med* 24(2):307–316, 1994.

Borison R, Rathiraja A, Diamond B *et al*.: Risperidone: clinical safety and efficacy in schizophrenia. *Psychopharmacological Bulletin* 28(2):213–218, 1992.

Boyle M: *Schizophrenia: a scientific delusion*. London, 1990, Routledge.

Brady K, Casto S, Lydiard RB: Substance abuse in an inpatient psychiatric sample. *Am J Drug Alcohol Abuse* 17(4):389–397, 1991.

Brown GW, Harris TO: *Social origins of depression*. London, 1978, Tavistock.

Buchanan A: A two year prospective study of treatment compliance in patients with schizophrenia. *Psychol Med* 22(3):787–797, 1992.

Candido C, Romney DM: Attributional style in paranoid vs. depressed patients. *Br J Med Psychol* 63(4):355–363, 1990.

Canton H, Verriele L, Colpaert FC: Binding of typical and atypical antipsychotics to $5HT_{1c}$ and $5HT_2$ sites: Clozapine potently interacts with $5HT_{1c}$ sites. *Eur J Pharmacol* 191(1):93–96, 1990.

Carlsson A, Lindquist M: Effect of chlorpromazine and haloperidol on formation of 3-methoxytyramine and normetanephrine in mouse brain. *Acta Pharmacol Toxicol* 20:140–144, 1963.

Castle D, Wessley S, Der G, Murray R: The incidence of operationally defined schizophrenia in Camberwell 1965–84. *Br J Psychiatry* 159:790–794, 1994.

Chapman LJ, Chapman JP: The genesis of delusions. In: Oltmanns TF, Maher BA, editors: *Delusional beliefs*. New York, 1988, Wiley.

Claghorn J, Honigfeld G, Abuzzahab FS, *et al*.: The risk and benefits of clozapine versus chlorpromazine. *J Clin Psychopharmacol* 7:377–384, 1987.

Clozapine Study Group: The safety and efficacy of clozapine in severe treatment-resistant schizophrenic patients in the UK. *Br J Psychiatry* 163:150–154, 1993.

Coryell W, Zimmerman M: The heritability of schizophrenia and schizoaffective disorder: A family study. *Archi Gen Psychiatry* 45:323–327, 1988.

Crow, TJ: The two syndrome concept: origins and current status. *Schizophr Bull* 11(3):471–486, 1985.

Cuffel BJ, Heithoff KA, Lawson W: Correlate of patterns of substance abuse among patients with schizophrenia. *Hosp Community Psychiatry* 44(3):247–251, 1993.

Curtis VA, Wright P, Reveley A, *et al*.: Effect of clozapine on *d*-fenfluramine-evoked neuroendocrine responses in schizophrenia and its relationship to clinical improvement. *Br J Psychiatry* 166(5):642–646, 1995.

David A: Insight in psychosis. *Br J Psychiatry* 156:798–808, 1990.

David A, Buchanan A, Reid A, Almeida O: The assessment of insight in psychosis. *Br J Psychiatry* 161:599–602, 1992.

Day JC, Wood G, Dewey M, Bentall RP: A self-rating scale for measuring neuroleptic side-effects. *Br J Psychiatry* 166(5):650–653, 1995.

Day R, Neilson JA, Korten A, *et al*.: Stressful life events preceding the acute onset of schizophrenia: a cross-national study from the World Health Organization.

Cult Med Psychiatry 11(2):123–206, 1987.

DeQuardo JR, Carpenter CF, Tandon R: Patterns of substance abuse in schizophrenia: Nature and significance. *J Psychiatr Res* 28(3):267–275, 1994.

Der G, Gupta S, Murray R: Is schizophrenia disappearing? *Lancet* 335:513–516, 1990.

Diamond RJ: Drugs and the quality of life: the patient's point of view. *J Clin Psychiatry* 46:29–35, 1985.

Dixon L, Haas G, Weiden PJ: Drug abuse in schizophrenic patients: clinical correlates and reasons for use. *Am J Psychiatry* 148(2):224–230, 1991.

Drake RE, Sederer LL: The adverse effects of intensive treatment of chronic schizophrenia. *Compr Psychiatry* 27(4):313–326, 1986.

Duinkerke SJ, Botter BA, Jansen AAI, et al.: Ritanserin selective 5HT$_{2/1c}$ antagonist and negative symptoms in schizophrenia. A placebo controlled double blind trial. *Br J Psychiatry* 163:451–455, 1993.

Eagles JM: The relationship between schizophrenia and immigration. Are there alternatives to psychosocial hypotheses? *Br J Psychiatry* 159:783–789, 1991.

Eagles JM, Whalley LJ: Decline in the diagnosis of schizophrenia among first admissions to Scottish mental hospitals from 1969-1978. *Br J Psychiatry* 146:151–154, 1985.

Fabrega H Jr, Ulrich R, Mezzich JE: Do Caucasian and black adolescents differ at psychiatric intake? *J Am Acad Child Adolesc Psychiatry* 32(2):407–413, 1993.

Falloon IPH: Developing and maintaining adherence to long term drug taking regimes. *Schizophr Bull* 10(3):412–417, 1984.

Falloon IPH, Laporta M, Fadden G, Graham–Hole V: *Managing stress in families.* London, 1993, Routledge.

Farde L, Nordstrom A, Nybrg S, et al.: D$_1$, D$_2$ and 5HT$_2$ receptor occupancy in clozapine treated patients. *J Clin Psychiatry* 55[9 supplement B]:67–69, 1994.

Farde L, Nordstrom AL, Weisel FA, et al.: Positron emission tomographic analysis of central D$_1$ and D$_2$ dopamine receptor occupancy in patients treated with classical neuroleptics and clozapine. *Arch Gen Psychiatry* 49(7):538–544, 1992.

Flannigan CB, Glover GR, Feenet ST: Inner London collaborative audit of admissions in two health districts. *Br J Psychiatry* 165(6):734–742, 1994.

Fleischhacker WW, Meise U, Gunther V, Kurz M: Compliance with antipsychotic drug treatment: influence of side-effects. *Acta Psychiatr Scand* 89[supplement 382]:11–15, 1994.

Galdos PM, van Os JJ, Murray RM: Puberty and the onset of psychosis. *Schizoph Res* 10(1):7–14, 1993.

Garety P, Wessley S: The assessment of positive symptoms. In: Barnes TRE, Nelson HE, editors: *The assessment of psychoses; a practical handbook.* London, 1994, Chapman & Hall Medical.

Garety PA, Hemsley DR, Wessley S: Reasoning in deluded schizophrenic and paranoid patients: Biases in performance on a probabilistic inference task. *J Nerv Ment Dis* 179(4):194–201, 1991.

Gerlach J: Oral versus depot administration of neuroleptics in relapse prevention. *Acta Psychiatr Scand* 89[supplement 382]:28–32, 1994.

Gerlach J, Peacock L: Intolerance to neuroleptic drugs: the art of avoiding extrapyramidal syndromes. *Eur Psychiatry* 10[supplement 1]:27s–31s, 1995.

Gershon ES, DeLisi LE, Harmovit J, et al.: A controlled family study of chronic psychosis. *Arch Gen Psychiatry* 45:328–336, 1988.

Ghaemi SN, Pope HG: Lack of insight in psychotic and affective disorders: a review of empirical studies. *Am J Psychiatry* 139:611–615, 1994.

Gibbon B: Validity and reliability of assessment tools. *Nurse Researcher* 2(4):48–55, 1995.

Goldstein JM, Tsuang MT: The process of subtyping schizophrenia: strategies in the search for homogeneity. In: Tsuang MT, Simpson JC, editors: *Handbook of Schizophrenia, Vol 3: Nosology, Epidemiology and Genetics.* New York, 1988, Elsevier.

Gotesman II, McGuffin P, Farmer AE: Clinical genetics as clues to the 'real' genetics of schizophrenia. A decade of modest gains while playing for time. *Schizophr Bull* 13(1):23–47, 1987.

Gournay K: Schizophrenia: A review of the contemporary literature and implications for mental health nursing theory practice and education. *J Psychiatr Ment Health Nurs* 3(1):7–12.

Gray RJ et al.: The administration of PRN medication by mental health nurses. *Br J Nursi (in press)*, 1996.

Gray RJ, Smedley NS, Miller K, Vearnals S: *The effects of education interventions on people with schizophrenia.* [Unpublished] 1995, The Bethlem and Maudsley

NHS Trust.

Green MF: Cognitive remediation in schizophrenia: Is it time yet? *Am J Psychiatry* 150(2):178–187, 1993.

Hambrecht M, Maurer K, Hafner H, Sartorius N: Transnational stability of gender differences in schizophrenia? An analysis based on the WHO study on determinants of outcome of severe mental disorders. *Eur Arch Psychiatry Clin Neurosci* 242(1):6–12, 1992.

Hammond S: Using psychometric tests. In: Breakwell GM, Hammond S, Fife–Schaw C, editors: *Research methods in psychology.* London, 1995, Sage Publications.

Hare E: Aspects of the epidemiology of schizophrenia. *Br J Psychiatry* 149:554–561, 1988.

Harrow M, Prosen M: Schizophrenic thought disorders: bizarre associations and intermingling. *Am J Psychiatry* 136(3):293–296.

Harvey PD: Reality monitoring in mania and schizophrenia: the association between clinically rated thought disorder and cohesion and reference. *J Nerv Ment Dis* 173(2):67–73, 1985.

Hemsley DR: A simple (or simplistic?) cognitive model of schizophrenia. *Behav Res Ther* 31(7):633–645, 1993.

Hemsley DR, Garety PA: The formation and maintenance of delusions: A Bayesian analysis. *Br J Psychiatry* 149:51–56, 1986.

Honigfeld G, Klett CJ: The nurse's observation scale for inpatient evaluation: A new scale for measuring improvement in chronic schizophrenia. *J Clin Psychol* 21(1):65–71, 1965.

Howe G: *Schizophrenia, a fresh approach.* London, 1986, David and Charles.

Hyttel J, Larsen JJ, Christensen AV, et al.: Receptor binding profiles of neuroleptics. In: Casey DE et al., editors: *Dyskinesia–research and treatment.* Berlin, 1985, Springer Verlag.

Jarman B: Identification of underprivileged areas. *BMJ* 286:1705–1709, 1983.

Johnstone EC, Crow TJ, Frith CD, et al.: Mechanism of the antipsychotic effect in the treatment of acute schizophrenia. *Lancet* I:848–851, 1978.

Jones S, Tallis F: *Coping with schizophrenia.* London, 1994, Sheldon Press.

Kane J, Honigfeld G, Singer J, et al.: Clozapine for the treatment resistant schizophrenic. *Arch Gen Psychiatry* 45:789–796, 1988.

Kaney S, Bentall RP: Persecutory delusions and the self serving bias: Evidence from a contingency judgement task. *J Nerv Ment Dis* 180(12):773–780, 1992.

Kay S, Opler L, Lindenmayer JP: Reliability and validity of the positive and negative syndrome scale for schizophrenics. *Psychiatr Res* 23:99–110, 1988.

Kay S, Opler L, Lindenmayer JP: The positive and negative syndrome scale (PANSS): rationale and standardisation. *Br J Psychiatry* 155(supplement 7):59–65, 1989.

Kelly GR, Mamon JA, Scott JE: Utility of the health belief model in examining medication compliance among psychiatric out-patients. *Soc Sci Med* 25(10):1205–1211, 1987.

Kemp R, David T: Psychosis: Insight and compliance. *Curr Opin Psychiatry* 8(6):357–361, 1995.

Kemp R, Haywards P, Applewhaite G, et al.: Compliance therapy in psychotic patients: randomised controlled trial. *BMJ* 312(7027):345–349, 1996.

Kendell RE, Kemp IW: Winter born v summer born schizophrenics. *Br J Psychiatry* 151:499–505, 1987.

Kendler KS, Glazer WM, Morgenstern H: Dimensions of delusional experience. *Am J Psychiatry* 140(1):59–65, 1983.

Kendley KS: Twin studies of psychiatric illness: current status and future direction. *Arch Gen Psychiatry* 50(11):905–915, 1993.

Kent S, Yellowlees P: Psychiatric and social reasons for frequent rehospitialization. *Hosp Community Psychiatry* 45(4):347–350, 1994.

Kerwin RW, Pilowsky L, Munro J, et al.: Functional neuroimaging and pharmacogenetic studies of clozapine's action at dopamine receptors. *J Clin Psychiatry* 55[9 supplement B]:57–62, 1994.

Kety SS et al.: The significance of genetic factors in the aetiology of schizophrenia: Results from the national study of adoptees in Denmark. *J Psychiatr Res* 21(4):423–429, 1987.

Kety SS, Rosenthal D, Wender P, Schulsinger F: Studies based on a total sample of adopted individuals and their relatives: why they were necessary, what they demonstrated and failed to demonstrate. *Schizophr Bull* 2(3):413–428, 1976.

Knudsen P, Vilmer T: Cannabis and neuroleptic agents in schizophrenia. *Acta Psychiatr Scand* 69:162–174, 1984.

Kuipers L, Leff J, Lam D: *Family work for schizophrenia; a practical guide.* London, 1992, Gaskell.

Lehman AF, Myers CP, Corty CP: Assessment and classification of patients with psychiatric and substance abuse syndromes. *Hosp Community Psychiatry* 40(10): 1019–1025, 1989.

Lewis SW: Congenital risk factors for schizophrenia. *Psychol Med* 19:5–13, 1989.

Liberman JA, Bruce L, Saltz CA, *et al.:* The effects of clozapine on tardive dyskinesia. *Br J Psychiatry* 158:503–510, 1991.

Liberman JA, Safferman AZ, Polack S, *et al.:* Clinical effects of clozapine in chronic schizophrenia: response to treatment and predictors of outcome. *Am J Psychiatry* 151(12):1744–1752, 1994.

Lloyd C: Life events and depressive disorder reviewed: II. Events as precipitating factors. *Arch Gen Psychiatry* 37:541–548, 1980.

Loranger AW: Sex differences in age at onset of schizophrenia. *Arch Gen Psychiatry* 41:157–161, 1984.

Lyon HM, Kaney S, Bentall RP: The defensive function of persecutory delusions: evidence from attribution tasks. *Br J Psychiatry* 164(5):637–646, 1994.

Maier W, Hallmayer J, Minges J, Lichtermann D: Affective and schizoaffective disorders: Similarities and differences. In: Marneos A, Tsuang MT, editors: *Morbid risks in relatives of affective schizoaffective and schizophrenic patients–results of a family study.* New York, 1990, Springer-Verlag.

Mattes JA: Clozapine for refractory schizophrenia: an open study of 14 patients treated up to two years. *J Clin Psychiatry* 50(10):389–391, 1989.

McKay AP, McKenna PJ: The dopamine hypothesis of schizophrenia. *Clinician* 11(4):31–44, 1993.

McNeil TF: Obstetric factors and perinatal injuries. In: Tsuang M.T, Simpson FC, editors: *Handbook of schizophrenia, vol. 3. Nosology, epidemiology and genetics of schizophrenia.* Amsterdam, 1988, Elsevier.

McNeil TF, Cantor–Graae E, Nordstrom LG, *et al.:* Head circumference in 'preschizophrenic' and control neonates. *Br J Psychiatry* 162:517–523, 1993.

Megens AAHP, Niemegeers CJE, Awouters FHL: Antipsychotic profile and side-effect liability of haloperidol, risperidone and ocaperidone as predicted from their differential interactions with amphetamine in rats. *Drug Dev Res* 26(2):129–145, 1992.

Meltzer HY: An overview of the mechanism of action of clozapine. *J Clin Psychiatry* 55[9 supplement B]:47–52, 1994.

Meltzer HY, Bastani B, Kwon KY, *et al.:* A prospective study of clozapine in treatment-resistant schizophrenic patients I: preliminary report. *Psychopharmacol* 99:S68–S72, 1989.

Moore E, Ball RA, Kuipers L: Expressed emotion in staff working with the long term adult mentally ill. *Br J Psychiatry* 161:802–808, 1992.

Morrison AP, Haddock G, Tarrier N: Intrusive thoughts and auditory hallucinations: A cognitive approach. *Behav Cognit Psychother* 23:265–280, 1995.

Mulhall D: *Manual for personal questionnaire rapid scaling technique.* London, 1978, NFER-Nelson.

Negrete JC, Knap W, Douglas D: Cannabis affects the severity of schizophrenic symptoms: results of a clinical survey. *Psychol Med* 16(3):515–520, 1986.

Neuchterlein KH, Dawson ME, Ventura J, *et al.:* The vulnerability/stress model of schizophrenia relapse: A longitudinal study. *Acta Psychiatr Scand* 89(supplement 382):58–64, 1994.

Nicole L, Lesage A, Lalonde P: Lower incidence and increased male:female ratio in schizophrenia. *Br J Psychiatry* 161:556–557, 1992.

Nordstrom AL, Farde L, Nyberg S, *et al.:* D_1 D_2 and $5HT_2$ receptor occupancy in relation to clozapine serum concentration: A PET study of schizophrenic patients. *Am J Psychiatry* 152(10):1444–1449, 1992.

Nyberg S, Farde L, Halldin C, *et al.:* High $5HT_2$ and D_2 dopamine receptor occupancy in the living human brain; a PET study with risperidone. *Psychopharmacol* 110:265–272, 1993.

Nyberg S, Farde L, Halldin C, *et al.:* D_2 dopamine receptor occupancy during low dose treatment with haloperidol decanoate. *Am J Psychiatry* 152(2):173–178, 1995.

O'Callaghan E, Sham PC, Takie N, *et al.:* Schizophrenia after prenatal exposure to 1957 A2 influenza epidemic. *Lancet* 337(8752):1248–1250, 1991.

O'Callaghan E, Sham PC, Takei N, *et al.:* The relationship of schizophrenic births to 16 infectious diseases. *Br J Psychiatry* 165(3):353–356, 1994.

Onstad S, Skre I, Torgersen S, Kringlen E: Twin concordance for DSM-III-R schizophrenia. *Acta Psychiatr Scand* 83(5):395–401, 1991.

Oppenheim AN: *Questionnaire design and attitude measurement.* London, 1984, Heinemann.

Overall JE, Gorham DR: The brief psychiatric rating scale. *Psychol Rep* (10):799–812, 1962.

Owen RR, Beake BJ, Marby D, *et al.:* Response to clozapine in chronic patients. *Psychopharmacol Bull* 25:253–256, 1989.

Pan PC, Tantum D: Clinical characteristics, health beliefs and compliance with maintenance treatment. A comparison of regular and irregular attendees at a depot clinic. *Acta Psychiatr Scand* 79:564–570, 1989.

Pantelis C, Curson DA: The assessment of social behaviour. In: Barnes TRE, Nelson HE, editors: *The assessment of psychoses, A practical handbook.* London, 1994, Chapman & Hall Medical

Parris C, Skagerlind L: Cognitive therapy with schizophrenic patients. *Acta Psychiatr Scand* 89(supplement 382):65–70, 1994.

Peplau HE: Interpersonal relations theory: theoretical constructs principles and general applications. In: Reynolds W, Cormack D, editors: *Psychiatric nursing: Theory and practice.* London, 1990, Chapman & Hall.

Peters *et al*: In: Chadwick P, Birchwood M, Trower, P: *Cognitive therapy for delusions voices and paranoia.* Chichester, 1996, John Wiley & Sons.

Peterson C, Semmel A, von Baeyer C, *et al.:* The attributional style questionnaire. *Cognit Ther Res* 6(3):287–300, 1982.

Piatowska O, Farnill D: Medication—compliance or alliance? A client-centred approach to increasing adherence. In: Kavanagh DJ, editor: *Schizophrenia.* London, 1992, Chapman & Hall.

Pope HG, Jones JM, Cohen BM, *et al.:* Failure to find evidence of schizophrenia in first-degree relatives of schizophrenic probands. *Am J Psychiatry* 139(6):826–828, 1982.

Posey TB: Verbal hallucinations also occur in humans. *Behav Brain Sci* 9(3):530, 1986.

Ram I, Bromet E, Eaton WW, *et al.:* The natural course of schizophrenia: A review of first admission studies. *Schizophr Bull* 18(2):185–207, 1992.

Rifkin L, Lewis S, Jones P, *et al.:* Low birth weight and schizophrenia. *Br J Psychiatry* 165:357–362, 1994.

Rosen A, Hadzi–Pavlovic D, Parker G: The life skills profile: A measure assessing function and disability in schizophrenia. *Schizophr Bul* 15:325–337, 1989.

Rosenthall D: Three adoption studies of heredity in the schizophrenic disorders. *Int J Ment Health* 1(1):63–75, 1972.

Salokangas RKR: First-contact rate for schizophrenia in community psychiatric care. Consideration of the oestrogen hypothesis. *Euro Arch Psychiatry Clin Neuroscience* 242(6):337–346, 1993.

Sandford T: Illicit drug use in psychiatric units and the nursing response. *Mental Health Newsletter.* London, 1995, Royal College of Nursing.

Sellwood W, Tarrier N: Demographic factors associated with extreme non-compliance in schizophrenia. *Soc Psychiatry Psychiatr Epidemiol* 29:172–177, 1994.

Sham PC, O'Callaghan E, Takei N, *et al.:* Schizophrenia following prenatal exposure to influenza epidemics between 1939 and 1960. *Br J Psychiatry* 160:461–467, 1992.

Simpson GM, Angus JWS: A rating scale for extrapyramidal side-effects. *Acta Psychiatr Scand* 212[supplement 44]:11–19, 1970.

Slade PD, Bentall RP: *Sensory deception: A scientific analysis of hallucination.* Baltimore, 1988, The Johns Hopkins University Press.

Smedley NS, Thomas BL: *Reasons for admission to acute psychiatric wards.* [Unpublished] 1995, The Bethlem and Maudsley NHS Trust.

Snowden LR, Cheung FK: Use of inpatient mental health services by members of ethnic minority groups. *Am Psychol* 45(3):347–355, 1990.

Soni SD, Gaskell K, Reed P: Factors affecting rehospitalisation rates of chronic schizophrenic patients living in the community. *Schizophr Res* 12:169–177, 1994.

Takei N, Sham PC, O'Callaghan E, *et al.:* Prenatal exposure to influenza and the development of schizophrenia: is the effect confined to females? *Am J Psychiatry* 152(1):150–151, 1994.

Talbot JA, Bachrach L, Ross L: Non-compliance and mental health systems. *Psychiatr Ann* 16(11):596–599, 1986.

Tarrier N, Harwood S, Yusopoff L *et al.:* Coping strategy enhancement (CSE) a method of treating residual schizophrenic symptoms. *Behav Psychother* 18(4):283–293, 1990.

Thornicroft G: Social deprivation and rates of treated mental disorder. Developing statistical models to predict psychiatric service utilisation. *Br J Psychiatry* 158:475–484, 1991.

Tienari P: Interaction between genetic vulnerability and family environment: The Finnish adoptive family study of schizophrenia. *Acta Psychiatr Scand* 84:460–465, 1991.

Tress KH, Paton G: The assessment of changes in psychpathology. In: Barnes TRE, Nelson HE, editors: *The assessment of psychosis: a practical handbook.* London, 1994, Chapman & Hall.

Tsuang MT, Simpson JC, Kronfol Z: Subtypes of drug abuse with psychosis. *Arch Gen Psychiatry* 39:141–147, 1982.

Tunnicliffe S, Harrison G, Standen PJ: Factors affecting compliance with depot injections treatment in the community. *Soc Psychiatry Psychiatr Epidemiol* 27:230–233, 1992.

Waddington JL: Mechanisms of action of typical and atypical antipsychotic drugs in the treatment of schizophrenia. *Clinician* 11(4):45–54, 1989.

Wender PH, Rosenthal D, Kety SS, *et al.*: Cross fostering: a research strategy for clarifying the role of genetic and experimental factors in the etiology of schizophrenia. *Arch Gen Psychiatry* 30:121–128, 1974.

Winters KC, Neal JM: Delusions and delusional thinking: a review of the literature. *Clin Psychol Rev* 3(2):227–253, 1983.

World Health Organization: *The ICD-10 classification of mental and behavioural disorders.* Geneva, 1992, World Health Organization.

Young JL, Zonana HV, Shepler L: Medication non-compliance in schizophrenia: codification and update. *Bull Am Psychiatr Law* 14:105–122, 1986.

Young HF, Bentall RP: Hypothesis testing in patients with persecutory delusions: Comparison with depressed and normal subjects. *Br J Clin Psychol* 34(3):353–369, 1995.

Zerbin-Rudin E: Endogene psychosen. In: Becker PE, editor: *Human genetik: ein kurzes Handbuck in funf Bande.* Vol. 2. Stuttgart, 1967, Thieme.

FURTHER READING

Barnes TRE, Nelson HE: *The assessment of psychoses: a practical handbook.* London, 1994, Chapman & Hall.

This book describes a range of valid and reliable assessment tools for use in psychotic disorders.

Bentall RP: *Reconstructing schizophrenia.* London, 1990, Routledge.

Boyle M: *Schizophrenia: a scientific delusion.* London, 1990, Routledge.

Both these books present a critique of our understanding of schizophrenia.

Chadwick P, Birchwood M, Trower P: *Cognitive therapy for delusions, voices and paranoia.* Chichester, 1996, John Wiley & Sons.

Fowler D, Garety P, Kuipers E: *Cognitive behaviour therapy for psychosis: theory and practice.* Chichester, 1996, John Wiley & Sons.

Psychological therapies specifically cognitive therapy are becoming increasingly popular for treating psychotic disorders. These two books offer practical advice for clinicians treating delusions, voices and paranoia using cognitive techniques.

Chapter 19

The Management of Violence

Learning Outcomes

After studying this chapter you should be able to:

- Identify the context of the current concerns about violence within the mental health services.

- Outline the main elements of the psychoanalytical, psychological, behavioural, sociocultural, and neurobiological theories on violence.

- Describe the assessment of risk of, cues to and prevention and management of violence.

- Discuss the after-care of those involved in violent incidents.

*T*he subject of violence is vast and, since space is limited, this chapter will concentrate on violence that occurs in the work of the mental health nurse. As the Community Care Act 1990 is implemented more fully, the people being admitted to acute wards and units are those who cannot be managed in the community. In-service user areas are receiving more acutely disturbed people for shorter admission periods. In the author's workplace this has resulted in the most acutely disturbed people being those experiencing 'psychosis'. Research has shown a link between a diagnosis of psychosis and violence (Wessley and Taylor, 1991; Monahan, 1992) and between increased admission rates and violence (James *et al.*, 1990). It is possible, then, tentatively to predict that levels of violence may increase on acute admission wards. This in turn has implications for the nurses on those wards, who are more likely than ever to experience violence and to suffer the psychological trauma associated with it.

Violent behaviour encountered by nurses working in the field of mental health has gained significant attention in the literature since the early 1980s (Shah, 1993). Overall, it appears that violence has increased in mental health care settings.

It is necessary, therefore, for every nurse to become familiar with the current theories about causes of violence, to learn how to assess the risk of violence, to adopt strategies that may actually prevent violence and, despite this, to be able to manage it effectively when it does occur. This chapter will cover these topics together with the care of people following violent incidents. For information about violence to self, see Chapter 17.

DEFINING VIOLENCE AND AGGRESSION

> The sombre fact is that we are the cruellest and most ruthless species that has ever walked the earth; and that, although we may recoil in horror when we read in newspaper or history book of the atrocities committed by man upon man, we know in our hearts that each one of us harbours within himself those same savage impulses which lead to murder, to torture and to war.
>
> *(Storr, 1968)*

Strong words, used to describe violence by the human race. Whether all that Storr has said should be accepted is questionable since, for example, it is known that there are societies that are non-violent (Owens and Ashcroft, 1985). Storr, like other writers at that time, referred to man. It is not clear whether he uses the term to mean the male of the species or mankind. What this statement does provide, though, is an uncomfortable reminder of the possible extremes of behaviour that many of us are capable of.

Defining the concepts of violence and aggression is very difficult because the terms are so often used interchangeably. However, it is important that an attempt is made in each mental health service to agree on a definition. As will be seen later, the monitoring, and subsequent potential for prevention, of violence is dependent on everyone having the same basic understanding of these concepts. It follows, then, that this chapter should identify definitions so that the reader may 'ground' what follows in an understandable way. Siann (1985) suggests that aggression refers to the 'intention to hurt' or '[to] emerge superior to others', but 'does not necessarily involve physical injury'. Violence, according to Siann 'involves the great use of force or physical intensity' usually resulting in physical injury.

Both aggression and violence are at times viewed as legitimate, necessary, acceptable, even admirable. Violence is deemed necessary, during military exercises or in law enforcement and in many sports, not least boxing. What makes this violence palatable is that it is legitimized by its apparent intention to protect, for example, the country, the victim of crime, one's living or one's livelihood. By adding the attribute of protection, the use of physical force that causes harm and pain to other human beings is legitimized, while at the same time the person at whom the force is directed is dehumanized, for example, in war 'the enemy', in law 'the criminal', in sport 'the competition'. These labels detract from the humanness of other persons involved in the confrontational situation and as such makes the use of violence easier (Fromm, 1974).

In the mental health services this is particularly pertinent when health professionals are working with people who may explain their violence in terms of protecting themselves from their perceptions of the evil intentions of others. For example, a person who is experiencing the delusion that their food is being poisoned may behave violently toward the person preparing or serving that food, to prevent what they see as an attempt to kill them. Similarly the person who is detained against their will in hospital, may become violent because they believe that harm is being inflicted upon them.

The relationship between aggression and violence is unclear. It could be said, with Siann's (1985) definitions, that aggression and violence are a continuum and are differentiated by physical force. Therefore, aggression may (but not always) lead to violence.

It is worth noting that, according to the literature, a person's reaction to a stressful situation is influenced by their appraisal of the incident (Mejo, 1990). For this reason distinguishing between violence and aggression may not be that helpful when it comes to the reaction of staff to these events.

VIOLENCE IN CONTEXT

Walker and Caplan (1993), in their comparison between violent crime in the general population and psychiatric in-service user violence, found that the rates were similar, i.e. psychiatric in-service user violence reflected that of the local population in their study.

Of the recorded crime in England and Wales in the year up to June, 1995, 93% was crime against property and 6% was violent crime (violence against the individual, sexual offences and robbery).

This 6% represents 301 400 recorded violent offences. Of these, homicide (murder, manslaughter and infanticide) and serious (life-threatening) offences of violence made up 6% (18 300 offences, 729 of which were in the category of homicide); sexual offences made up 10% (30 000); robbery 21% (62 700) and less serious offences 63% (190 400 recorded offences) (Home Office, 1995).

In comparison to the overall statistics, the figure for people with mental health problems (including mental illness, psychopathic disorder, mental impairment and severe mental impairment) admitted under a restriction order in 1993 for violence against the person totalled 686 (Home Office, 1995). This figure can be broken down by the type of violent act committed:

Murder	89
Homicide	41
Other violence	366
Sexual offences	87
Robbery	103

It can be seen that the number of people with mental health problems convicted of violent assault is very low in comparison to the overall numbers of people commiting violent crimes.

UNDER-REPORTING

For a long time it has been recognized that violence against staff is under-reported (Lion *et al.*, 1981) so the true picture of the rate of assault is never clear. In the author's organization there were 1093 reported violent incidents over a 13-month period (Powell *et al.*, 1994). If nurses are unable to report incidents to colleagues then it follows that they are less likely to inform the police. So most instances, particularly those of a 'less serious nature', go unreported. Hence the Home Office statistics may not be a true reflection of the problem of violence against the person. This means that at best the number of incidents of violence and aggression encountered by mental health nurses can only be guessed at.

A case example would be Nurse A, who goes to help Mrs. B, an 84-year-old person who is experiencing memory loss and extreme confusion, out of bed in the morning. Mrs B.shouts and hits out at Nurse A. Mrs B's finger nails scratch and draw blood on Nurse A's arm. Nurse A tells Mrs.B. who she is and what she is doing and gets on with the job of helping Mrs. B to get up. She is too busy to mention to her colleagues what has happened, 'Anyway', she thinks, 'this happens every day here'.

Would the reader, in Nurse A's position, report this assault to:

- Your colleagues?
- Your line manager?
- The police?
- Other health care staff?

If 'no' has been answered to any of the above groups of people, spend some time considering why. It may be useful to discuss this with colleagues.

CATEGORIES OF VIOLENCE

Fottrell (1980) devised a scale of severity of violent incidents that is widely used as a means to categorize violence in the mental health services. The levels are as follows:

1°— No physical injury.
2°— Minor injury, e.g. bruises, scratches.
3°— Major injury, e.g. large lacerations or broken bones.

While it is useful for reporting purposes to have such a categorization, health service managers may be misled if they receive information that violence in their area is mostly at levels 1° and 2°. They may believe that they do not have a serious problem. However, it has been shown that staff who are exposed to this level of violence often suffer significantly as a result (Whittington and Wykes, 1989).

THEORIES OF AGGRESSION AND VIOLENCE

A number of theories on the development of aggressive behaviour have influenced the treatment of violent people. They can be categorized as psychoanalytical, psychological, behavioural, sociocultural and neurobiological. Current thinking in the field suggests that aggressive behaviour is the result of the interaction of a person's biological, psychological and sociocultural characteristics and that each of these factors must be considered when determining nursing care (Hamolia, 1995).

PSYCHOANALYTICAL BASIS

Psychoanalytical theory suggests that aggressive behaviour is the result of instinctual drives. Freud proposed that two primary drives influence human behaviour, the life force expressed through sexuality and the death force expressed through aggression. He believed that life was a struggle to maintain a balance between the two drives and that behaviour exhibited by humans was simply the result of the more powerful drive (Hamolia, 1995). This theory has limited use today, as Owens and Ashcroft (1985) point out there are humans who live peacefully and who do not display innate aggressive behaviour. This theory also detracts from the notion of the individual being responsible for their own behaviour.

PSYCHOLOGICAL BASIS

According to the frustration–aggression theory (Dollard *et al.*, 1939) aggression occurs as the result of a build-up of frustration. Frustration results when a person's attempt to achieve a desired goal is blocked. These feelings are then reduced through aggressive behaviour. This theory has been criticized for simplifying the complexity of the human spirit and not considering other stressors that might also lead to aggression. In addition, it implies that the absence of aggression is simply caused by the absence of frustration (Hamolia, 1995).

BEHAVIOURAL BASIS

Social learning theory (Bandura, 1977) proposes that aggressive behaviour is learned through the socialization process as a result of internal and external learning. Internal learning occurs through personal reinforcement received when acting aggressively. This may be the result of achieving a desired goal or experiencing feelings of importance, power and control. External learning occurs through the observation of role models such as parents, peers and significant others. Sociocultural patterns that lead to the imitation of aggressive behaviour suggest that violence is an acceptable way of solving problems and achieving status in society. According to this view, activities such as violent crime, aggressive sports and war reinforce aggressive behaviour in individuals (Hamolia, 1995). This may be particularly relevant on in-service user units where violence is frequent. If people have to live in a violent setting and see positive results of violence, they may chose to use this approach themselves.

Morrison (1994) has expanded upon the social learning theory and suggests that a coercive interactional style where the person with mental health problems interacts in a coercive and exploitative manner to maximize self-gain, is a strong predictor of violence and aggression. This theory rests uncomfortably with the current emphasis on empowerment of people with mental health problems, as it suggests that some of these people use violence to get what they want, thus labelling all users of mental health services in a potentially damaging way.

Meloy (1992) suggests that disruptions in early attachment may predispose an individual to violence. Other theories of attachment suggest that aggression arises as a result of early interpersonal relationships that are characterized by insecurity and physical violence. Crittenden and Ainsworth (1989) suggest that the physically abused child becomes hypervigilant to hostile cues. This internal conflict could lead the person to misinterpret the behaviour of others and to respond aggressively.

SOCIOCULTURAL BASIS

Social and cultural factors may also influence the use of violent or aggressive behaviour. Cultural norms help to define acceptable and unacceptable means of expressing aggressive feelings. Sanctions are applied to violators of the norms through the legal system. By this means, society controls violent behaviour and attempts to maintain a safe environment for its members. Unfortunately this prohibition against violent behaviour may also be extended to include any expression of anger, leading to people being prevented from expressing this healthily. A cultural norm that supports verbally assertive expressions of anger will help people deal with anger in a healthy manner. A norm that reinforces violent behaviour will result in physical expression of anger in destructive ways (Hamolia, 1995). Miller (1987) suggests that a person who can integrate their anger as part of themselves will not become aggressive.

Some feminist theorists suggest that violence is the result of the way in which boys and girls are reared. Girls are taught to nurture others while repressing and denying their own needs. Boys are taught unconsciously that to become a 'real man' it is necessary to reject all that is feminine and to repress all feelings, because feelings are feminine, except the one sanctioned emotional outlet open to men, anger. Anger may be expressed aggressively, either verbally or physically (Lloyd, 1995). Aggression may arise then when masculinity is threatened and a willingness to be aggressive is seen as part of what it is to be a man (Lloyd, 1995).

Lloyd goes on to outline the well-documented fact that boys tend to be played with more roughly than girls and that this may be a contributory factor to their greater propensity for aggression.

NEUROBIOLOGICAL BASIS
There has been a flurry of interest recently in the neurobiological basis of violence. Positron emission tomography (PET) scans carried out on the brains of people who have committed violent crimes indicate that there is a link between an abnormality in the brain's chemistry or structure and violent behaviour (Moir and Jessel, 1995).

The chemical abnormality may occur in the neurotransmitters, i.e., the chemicals that are transmitted to and from neurons through synapses. The neurotransmitters most often associated with aggressive behaviour are monoamines, serotonin (5-hydroxytryptamine) and dopamine (3-hydroxytyramine), and the amino acid, gamma-aminobutyric acid (GABA) (Hamolia, 1995).

The structural abnormality may occur in several parts of the brain. The limbic system is associated with the expression of human emotions and behaviours such as eating, aggression and sexual response. It is also involved in the processing of information. Structures commonly included in discussion of the limbic system are the hippocampus, amygdala, cingulate gyrus and hypothalamus. Damage to the limbic system may result in an increase or decrease in the potential for aggressive behaviour (Hamolia, 1995). Moir and Jessel (1995) define violence stemming from damage to the limbic system as 'limbic rage', a type of violence that is explosive in nature where the violent person bitterly regrets their actions afterwards. They suggest that the damage to the limbic system is either innate, caused by head injury, or results from viral infection.

The frontal lobes are the part of the brain where reason and emotion interact. It has been suggested that damage to the frontal lobe of the brain, which mediates purposeful behav-

iour and rational thinking, can result in impaired judgement, personality changes, problems in decision making, inappropriate conduct and aggressive outbursts (Hamolia, 1995).

The temporal lobes play a role in memory and the interpretation of auditory stimuli. The temporal lobe problem most often linked to aggressive behaviour is epilepsy, particularly in those individuals with partial complex seizures (Hamolia, 1995) Aggressive behaviour may occur during a fit when the person is in a state of altered consciousness or after a seizure, because of a transient confusional state. However, Fenwick (1993) suggests that the relationship is far from clear and that aggression in people who have epilepsy is probably due to the associated brain damage caused by repeated seizures.

The links between heavy alcohol drinking and violence are plain for all to see. Alcohol can inhibit fear and thus reduce the person's ability to perceive danger in the same way they would when not intoxicated.

A variety of drugs have also been associated with violent behaviour.

VIOLENCE AND ITS LINKS WITH MENTAL HEALTH PROBLEMS

RATIONALIZING VIOLENCE
Morrison (1993) asserts that violence in psychiatric settings is similar to that in society and should not therefore be viewed as a medical or psychological problem. This idea could be taken further; medicalizing violence may serve to rationalize it, which may increase the feeling that it is 'just part of the job'. Waites (1993), in her work on repeated assaults by family members, suggests that eventually the victim constructs a belief system that constantly rationalizes violence. The medicalization of violence could be seen to parallel this phenomenon, which in effect blames the victim for the assault and in turn may prevent them from seeking help. Organizations have a lot to gain from this, as to rationalize violence may lead to denial of the effects that it has on individuals and abdication of responsibility for caring for those people. Chapman (1990) makes it very clear that violence should not be considered just part of the job.

VIOLENCE AND MENTAL HEALTH PROBLEMS
Much of the literature on violence within psychiatric services focuses on criminal violence committed by people with mental health problems. While being the basic research that helps us to understand violence, this research excludes the day-to-day violence encountered by nurses undertaking their duties. Partly because violence against nurses is very rarely reported to the person's manager, let alone the police, it therefore often remains hidden. (Ryan and Poster, 1993).

The most significant studies carried out to determine the link between mental health problems and violence have been undertaken in America. This needs to be borne in mind when transferring findings across cultures. The author recommends that the reader examine the original study. With this in mind, the study by Swanson *et al.* (1990) demonstrated interesting findings from a survey of 10 000 people who were representative of the population being studied. What this showed was that in a year violent behaviour had developed in 2.1% of people with no diagnosable mental health problem, 12.7% of people with a diagnosis of schizophrenia, 11.7% of people with a diagnosis of major depression, 11% of people with mania or a bi-polar disorder, 24.6% of people who abused alcohol or who were alcohol dependent and 34.7% of people who abused or who were dependent on drugs.

Link *et al.* (1992) found that when people with mental health problems were experiencing hallucinations and delusions, the risk of commiting violent acts was significantly increased, but when they were not experiencing these symptoms their rates of violence reflected that of the general population.

Taylor (1985) notes that approximately 40% of violent offenders experiencing a psychotic episode were acting directly upon delusions, i.e. a false unshakeable belief. Taylor later notes that, despite the common myth, hallucinations are rarely acted upon. She suggests that the strongest link between mental health problems and violence occurs when the person is experiencing 'a delusion of persecution, for example, believing that they are being poisoned, or delusions of passivity or control by other forces' (Taylor, 1985).

Caution is required in interpreting these results and as Sayce (1995) notes 'service users are presumed dangerous even when they have never been violent'. The Swanson *et al.* (1990) and Link (1992) studies cannot be taken as definitive proof that people with mental health problems are more violent than the rest of society. What they do show is a link between altered mental state and an increased risk of becoming violent. Further research in this area is desperately needed, particularly in the UK.

PREVENTION OF VIOLENCE

ORGANIZATIONAL PREVENTIVE STRATEGIES

To acknowledge publicly that violence is a problem is not without its drawbacks, as Lanza (1985) points out, as this may further stigmatize the mental health service and may put off people coming into mental health nursing — a problem that is already apparent (Department of Health, 1994). However, denying that violence is a problem by ignoring it places people in grave danger. The organization has a duty to ensure acceptable and safe working conditions under new Health and Safety legislation (Health and Safety Executive, 1992).

Policy

It is very important that the organization makes it clear that violent behaviour is not acceptable and that it will be dealt with in a swift and effective manner. Not to be explicit about the unacceptability of violence is to condone its continua-tion. To improve the likelihood of preventing violence in the workplace, it is necessary to start with an overall policy that gives explicit details about the following:

- The organization's beliefs about violence toward staff and service users and acknowledgement of its duty to care for staff and service users.
- The support to be provided when a person has been assaulted.
- The action to be taken when a person or their property is damaged through violence.
- The prosecution of the person who is violent.
- The training available in preventing and managing violence and clarity about the type of training that should be undertaken by each member of staff.
- The use of physical restraint techniques and the use of seclusion.

The above points are not exhaustive and each organization may have additional information available. At an organizational level, it is useful to gain information on the sickness rates of nurses, as sickness or absence from work is strongly correlated with stress (Flannery *et al.*, 1991) that violence undoubtedly causes (Dawkins *et al.*, 1985). When there are large numbers of vacancies, agency nursing staff are employed and the use of temporary staff has been strongly correlated with an increase in violent incidents (James *et al.*, 1990).

Monitoring

A central department needs to be responsible for the monitoring of all aggressive and violent incidents within an organization (Box 19.1). Depending on what information is reported, centralized collation of this information can provide details of patterns of violence within units, teams and the organization as a whole. This collated information can then be used as suggested by Murray and Snyder (1991) as the basis of the staff training programme.

PREVENTION OF VIOLENCE IN CLINICAL TEAMS

The team leader or ward manager needs to be aware of the strengths of all those who work in the team, so that their skills may be used effectively at all times. Knowledgeable, assertive leadership of the team can prevent a volatile situation exploding into full blown violence.

The Team Leader or Ward Manager is also responsible for ensuring that the ward milieu is such that it engenders comfort and a respect for people using the facilities. Poorly kept areas may lead people to feel disinclined to keep the area in good repair and also effectively says to the service user 'You are not deserving of a decent environment'. It is also important to keep service users engaged in purposeful, therapeutic activity, rather than leaving them to spend hours in front of the television or wandering around feeling bored.

Managers also need to be particularly aware of the way in which they treat staff. If a manager is caring, thoughtful and supportive then staff are more able to show these qualities to the people with mental health problems that they are

Box 19.1 *Example of monitoring information*

Name of person:
Date:
Clinical area:
Consultant:
Primary Nurse:
Medication:
Reasons for incident: (nurse and service user's perception)
Behaviour prior to incident:
Behaviour during incident:
Behaviour following incident:
Nursing interventions used:
Outcome of nursing interventions:
Medical intervention used:
Outcome of medical intervention:
Was medication given?
Was seclusion used?
Was physical restraint used?
Did anyone sustain physical injury?
Severity of incident (Fotrell's classification):
What follow-up occurred? (e.g. medical treatment, debriefing etc.)

working with. If managers are bullying and punitive, then the staff often behave in this way with the service users.

Consider this case example. Nurse G was asked to attend a study day, which she felt was important for her development. When she approached the team leader to ask permission to attend, the team leader denied her request without listening to her other reasons for wanting to go, saying, 'You don't need that information to work here'. Feeling hurt and angry, the nurse was in the ward area when a service user asked to leave the ward. The nurse told her that she could not leave without a nurse escort. The service user asked if Nurse G could escort them. Nurse G said that she could not because she was too busy. The service user walked toward the door and looked as if she would leave. Nurse G approached the service user and stood in her way. The service user shouted, 'I want to go!' The nurse said that the service user could not leave. With that the service user tried to push past Nurse G, who shouted for help, and the service user was forcibly restrained to prevent her from leaving.

Managers also need to ensure open communication among the team. This can facilitate the clear dissemination of important information to all team members, which is particularly necessary in responding consistently to service users' requests and behaviour. Inconsistency in response leads to confusion in the service user, who is left feeling unsure of their boundaries. In turn, this can lead to an increase in tension and frustration, perhaps even violence, if one staff member says one thing and another says the opposite.

Safe staffing levels are also the manager's responsibility. In situations where managers are finding that all the team can do is to contain the service user group, then they must act upon this and bring the situation to the attention of their line manager.

Managers should also ensure that staff are trained to deal with aggression and violence and that this training is regularly up-dated in the clinical setting.

All nursing staff on in-service user areas need to be aware of current tensions and strains among the service user group. Violence among service users is as frequent as that toward staff and must be given as much attention as prevention of violence to staff. In light of MIND's (1992) Stress on Women Campaign, it will be necessary to ensure women-only spaces where they can be free of the sexual harassment and assault that they often suffer on a regular basis from male service users.

In areas where the facility is a mixed-sex service, then a thorough induction to the clinical area for new service users must stress the respect for the privacy and dignity of all who use the setting and clear guidelines on male and female areas should be communicated both verbally and in writing.

Service users must also be informed of the expectation that they will not harass or intimidate other service users and the consequences of this behaviour made clear. The consequences, of course, must be decided upon by the team. However, some issues are beyond the remit of the team to decide and will be a matter for the police, as in the case of allegations of sexual assault.

SELF-AWARENESS
Stevenson (1991) suggests that nurses should start each day with a personal assessment of their stressors. She notes that additional stressors increase anxiety which, in turn, impairs the ability to respond effectively in emergencies. Stevenson also notes that to maintain therapeutic effectiveness, people must be self-aware. Self-awareness involves being able to note how we affect, and are affected by, others. Self-awareness can also involve the ability to recognize and deal with problems before they get out of hand and start affecting work.

Self-awareness also involves being absolutely aware of one's limitations as a clinician, i.e. being aware and not too proud to admit that one is out of one's depth. This is particularly important when dealing with violence. If the clinical leads colleagues to believe that they can deal with certain situations, when in reality the solution is unknown, then the clinician, the person being cared for and one's colleagues are being placed in danger.

An awareness of an ability to communicate effectively, verbally and non-verbally, to listen to what is being said and to pick up on what is not being said, to understand the non-verbal communication of others and to act upon that information are all vital in prevention of violence.

PERSONAL SAFETY
Prevention of violence also rests upon the nurses' ability to keep themselves safe. What follows is an outline of steps that can be taken to increase personal safety at work (not in any order of priority). The nurse should:
• Always inform colleagues of his or her whereabouts on the ward or in the community.

- Always be familiar with the layout of all rooms and buildings in which work is done (including service user's homes). Be absolutely sure of the location of exits in case of emergency and how locks and catches on doors are released. There is no point being able to find the exit if the door cannot be opened!

- Nurse and service user need to be positioned in a room where both have equal access to the door if things get heated. Blocking a service user in may make them feel trapped or that they have to 'fight' their way out.

- If working in the community, always have a check-in time and make it clear that if there is no check-in by a specified time, then the police should be called immediately.

- Ensure that all the relevant details about a particular person are available before spending time with them, i.e. ensure a good handover of information and ask about any history of aggression or violence.

- Be aware of personal clothing and valuables and its potential to cause harm, e.g. ties, scarves, earrings, nose studs etc.

- Never visit someone in their home alone if it is the person's first contact with the mental health services. (It is often better to ask them to attend the health centre.)

- When out and about in the community, consider carrying a mobile phone or emergency pager that can summon help quickly if needed.

- Be sure to know the precise destination. A person can look vulnerable and could be targeted if they wander around looking lost or fumbling with a street map. Meet up with the local police and become known to them, to establish effective working relationships.

- Think carefully about whether to display nursing status on vehicles. It may attract unwanted attention from people who might think drugs are being carried.

- Think carefully about where to park. If possible, try to park in such a way that when driving away there is no need to reverse or turn around. In an emergency, getting out by reversing can be difficult.

- Park in well-lit areas, and in the dark always walk where there are street lights, if possible.

- Try to avoid wearing or carrying anything that may draw undue attention, e.g. expensive looking jewellery, a smart briefcase or clothes that are completely incongruous to the area being visited.

- Be aware of what in the surrounding environment could be used as a weapon. The author's workplace found that cutlery and crockery were the commonest weapons used. This had major implications for management of the risk of violence at certain times.

- Deploy resources effectively. In the author's workplace it was found that meal times were particularly volatile and also times when there was an increase in the number of people in a particular area, e.g. visiting time. Where this is known, staff can be proactive rather than waiting for a situation to arise.

ASSESSMENT

As part of a comprehensive assessment it is necessary to determine the risk of violence. As is well known, the only real predictor of violence is the previous display of violent behaviour. This information must be elicited at the earliest possible moment. Failure to find out and pass on information about a person's propensity for violence has led to death and to those who have been violent not receiving the most appropriate care, as the Clunis Inquiry makes clear (Ritchie, 1994).

Think about the following case example. Ms C has been referred to the Community Mental Health Nurse Team because she has been wandering about shouting at her neighbours, telling them that the Internet is zapping her energy. Ms C is invited to the team base for an initial interview with a nurse. After a while (when Nurse D feels that Ms C is fairly comfortable with her) the nurse asks, 'Have you ever hurt or physically injured another person, or property?' Ms C replies, 'Of course not'. To make sure that Ms C has understood, the nurse says, 'You have never hurt or injured another person or property'. Ms C replied, 'Only if you count slapping. I didn't really hurt the person'.

Because Ms C has revealed that she has hurt another person, the nurse must ask her to describe what happened. This enables the nurse to identify any pattern or cues to her violence and to judge what situations are most likely to precede violent behaviour.

It is also worth asking if the person has ever wanted to hurt or injure another person or property. (Most of us at some time have violent fantasies; this should not be viewed in isolation from other information gathered.) If a person has wanted to harm another and did not act upon that desire, then they are probably able to identify the negative consequences of behaving violently and thus choose alternative methods of coping in situations where another person might be provoked to aggression or violence.

RISK ASSESSMENT

Monahan (1981) suggests that the questions following (adapted slightly by the author) must be fully answered in an attempt to weigh up the risk of violence.

- What are the person's relevant demographic details?
- What is the person's history of violent behaviour?
- What is the base rate of violence among people within the individual's background?
- What are the sources of stress in the person's current environment?
- What cognitive and emotional factors indicate that the person may be predisposed to cope with stress in a non-violent manner?
- How similar are past situations, where the person has used violence to cope, with those that may arise in the future?
- Who are the likely victims of the person's violent behaviour and how accessible are they?
- What methods and weapons are available to the person to use in violence?

Based on what has been identified so far, the author would add to this list: Is there any evidence of substance misuse?

Even after this careful assessment, Monahan (1988) notes that the best risk assessment would only be accurate for one in three people, i.e. for every person with mental health problems predicted to be violent, two will be violent but their violence will be unpredicted. The demographic predictors of violence are the same for those diagnosed as having mental health problems as for people without such a diagnosis (i.e. age, gender, social class, substance abuse and history). Diagnosis, severity of mental health problem and personality traits are not reasonable predictors.

RISK MARKERS

Steadman *et al.* (1993) suggest the idea of risk markers, which include:

- Characteristics of the social support available to the person.
- Impulsiveness.
- Reactions to provocation.
- Ability to empathize.
- The nature of hallucinations and delusions.

Each risk marker needs to be explored as they may give an indication of the person's propensity for violence.

DEVISING A PROGRAMME OF CARE

When a client has been identified as having a violence problem, then a more thorough assessment will be necessary before a programme of care can be developed to help find alternative strategies for them.

The following will be needed:

1 A detailed description of a recent violent episode, with information on how the person felt physically and emotionally including their thoughts at the time.
2 A list of situations that the person feels are most likely to result in them behaving violently, e.g. not being able to have their needs met immediately, the use of alcohol or drugs etc.
3 Exploration of the person's own understanding of why they think that they become violent.
4 Information on anything that lessens the likelihood of violence, e.g. interaction, medication, environment etc.
5 The individual's personal strengths and signs of other positive coping mechanisms.+

RECORDING VIOLENT INCIDENTS

After every incident the details of what has happened need to be recorded by the mental health nurse in the person's nursing notes. The behaviour of the people involved before, during and after the incident should be carefully documented. As Powell *et al.*(1994) find, most violent incidents are caused by a few people, so it is likely that a person who is violent during their hospitalization will repeat this behaviour. Careful recording can help the nurse to build up a picture of the circumstances that lead to the person becoming violent and to develop strategies for preventing further violence.

Good documentation is essential for any nursing practice (UKCC, 1993). The concept of accountability is implicit in documenting incidents. Nurses can sometimes confuse this with needing to get the record straight for when the 'manager' asks what happened. Lanza (1985) has found that blaming the victim for assault is a common phenomenon in nursing. In a later article Lanza and Carifo (1991) say that 'blaming the victim can maintain the false belief that hospitals are not violent places and that if violence does occur it is the fault of the assaulted person'. The individual who believes that they are going to be blamed will be less likely to ask for help. Thus an organization can deny that help is needed, because it is not being asked for.

MANAGEMENT OF VIOLENCE

When the service user identifies violence as a problem, much can be done to help them find alternative ways to communicate their feelings. By the thorough assessment outlined previously, the nurse and service user will be able to explore the problem in more detail and identify it more exactly (see Case Study).

The nurse and service user need to agree on a goal. The most appropriate would be for Miss J to develop her understanding of why she uses violent behaviour to communicate her feelings. Once she understands, then she can learn alternative ways of coping and avoid causing any further harm to her parents.

ASSERTIVENESS

One important feature of this type of violence is Miss J's inability to communicate her feelings assertively. A strategy

---

Case study: **Management of violence**

Miss J is 22 years old. She lives at home with her parents and has been referred to the Community Mental Health Centre because she says that she can see no future for herself. She becomes aggressive and violent toward her mother and father on a regular basis. She says that they are 'driving her mad' and that she cannot control herself when they start telling her what to do. Nurse K asks Miss J to describe exactly what happened during the most recent violent episode. Miss J described a situation where her father said that she should spend more time reading and less time watching the television. This made Miss J feel very angry and she lashed out at her father, striking him around the head. The nurse then asked Miss J to try to analyze how she was feeling at the time and whether she noticed any physical sensations. Miss J said that she felt angry, annoyed and 'like a child'. She also said that she felt her body become tense and her breathing rapid. Finally, the nurse asked Miss J what her thoughts were at the time of the incident. Miss J said that she could not remember clearly but that she knew she thought her father was nagging her.

On further discussion Miss J said that she felt her parents still treated her like a child. She felt that she could never do anything to please them and that they reinforced this constantly by nagging her.

for improving her ability to communicate assertively would include facilitating her ability to:

- Communicate directly with other people.
- Say no to unreasonable requests.
- State her complaints.
- Express appreciation as appropriate .

(Hamolia, 1995)

If a person feels unable to communicate directly with another they may bottle feelings up, which spill over into subsequent interactions. This can lead to a build-up of tension that can become explosive.

A clinical example would be: Nurse H asks Mr I if he is satisfied with the care and treatment he is receiving. Mr I is very dissatisfied but is afraid that if he tells Nurse H she will see him as a troublemaker and his care will worsen.

When someone does not know how to say no to unreasonable requests, they may end up carrying out activities or shouldering responsibilities that they do not want and cannot cope with. This can lead to an increase in tension and to aggression.

Another example would be: Nurse L asks Mrs M if she would be responsible for showing a new user around the in-patient user unit, and tell the service user what it is like being there. Mrs M feels flattered that she has been asked to do this and agrees. She later feels irritable and snaps angrily at another service user who asks her for a light for a cigarette.

Being able to state complaints is vital, for if we do not protest when we feel that other people are being unreasonable, then we may harbour grudges and hostility that may affect our relationships with others.

A further example would be: Mr N is constantly being asked by another service user for cigarettes. He feels intimidated by this service user and unable to refuse this request. He thinks that the staff should intervene but does not say anything because he is afraid he will look a 'wimp'. He soon becomes the cigarette supplier for most of the Day Centre and becomes increasingly distressed and angry toward staff.

The expression of appropriate appreciation includes being able to say thank you when another person behaves in a way which pleases you, rather than saying thank you constantly.

Communicating assertively can be taught on an individual basis or in a group setting and involves the topics outlined above, together with ideas for alternative ways of behaving. These can be tested out, and how they feel recorded in a journal to be discussed at the next session or group meeting.

Anger management techniques may also be used. The basics of anger management can include being aware of what triggers anger, learning to manage these triggers, noting and controlling physical responses, testing out alternative responses in anger-provoking situations and evaluating these responses for their effectiveness.

LIMIT SETTING AND CONTRACTS

To control the risk of violent outbursts the nurse may find it necessary to use limit setting as a way to contain dangerous behaviour. Limit setting is the non-punitive, non-manipulative act in which someone is told what behaviour is acceptable, what is not acceptable and the consequences of behaving unacceptably. Once a limit has been set it must be consistently reinforced by all staff. If the limit is broken, then the consequences identified must take place (Hamolia, 1995).

Often, when limits are set, the person will test them frequently to see whether staff are prepared to act. This requires that staff are completely consistent in their responses, which will improve the possibility of this intervention working to decrease the undesirable behaviour.

When violence is being used by someone to intimidate or to threaten another to get their own way, then nursing care needs to be aimed at reducing or eliminating the rewards that the service user is getting from behaving in this way. Limit setting in the form of a written contract may also be useful. However, nurses need to be careful about the messages they give. To reward a person for not being violent may actually be as damaging as allowing the violence to continue. For example, if the nurses write in their contract that someone who refrains from violence for 12 hours can then go for a walk with staff and this is witnessed by other service users who have not been allowed out for a walk, they may be left believing that to get out they should become violent!

TIME OUT

When aggression is imminent it may be appropriate to offer the person time out. This may involve taking them to a quiet area of the ward or to their bedroom for a short period where they can calm down in a safe, quiet area. Some clinical areas also have intensive care areas where people who are at risk of displaying violence are nursed over the 24-hour period, their contact with other people being limited to the nurses looking after them. This approach may lessen the need for emergency interventions, and gradual introduction of the service user to the rest of the people in the clinical area can help the user to slowly build up the ability to interact effectively with others without the use of violence.

EMERGENCY INTERVENTIONS

When a violent incident does occur, careful team work is required to de-escalate or defuse the situation with the least damage or injury to those involved.

Several courses of action are available to the nurse confronted by a person who is aggressive or violent. When in immediate danger of being hurt then, if at all possible, the nurse should escape from the situation to get help. There is a set of physical intervention skills that can be used called 'break-away' techniques . These enable the nurse to get out of a variety of holds as quickly as possible and are an essentially non-violent means of escape. They require training and frequent practice to remain effective. Many Trusts now train their staff in these techniques.

In hospital and day care settings the establishment of emergency teams can be invaluable. Such teams can be used to support the work of the regular staff, to provide extra numbers of people if more than one incident occurs and to cover the clinical area while the regular team debrief after an incident. It must be remembered, however, that emergency team members will also need to debrief and should not be sent away before they have had the opportunity to discuss how they feel.

In a situation where a service user is hurting another then, if the nurse is alone, he or she should not physically intervene. The first action must be to summon help. If the nurse goes in alone and gets injured this is not helping the service user who is being attacked. It is also important to scan the environment for anything that could be used as a weapon by the service user.

The author's organization recommends the following actions to be taken in a violent situation (Bethlem and Maudsley NHS Trust, 1994):

1. Calm the situation down by assuming a calm and open posture, standing to the person's side, not face on. Calm down by taking three deep breaths. With each breath out think 'calm'. Help the person to talk about what is troubling them; do not try to interrupt at this stage. Use a soft tone of voice if possible. Take plenty of time. Avoid an audience, i.e. clear the area of spectators or ask a colleague to do this. Allow an increased amount of nurse–client body space. Avoid any sudden movements that may startle the client.

2. Establish understanding communication with the person displaying violence. Convey to the person that an attempt is being made to see their situation as they are experiencing it. Show warmth and continued calmness. Listen carefully to what is being said and let the person know they are being listened to by paraphrasing what they have said, as appropriate. Ensure that names are used. As noted earlier, it is easier to act violently toward a person when they have become dehumanized, so remind them that they are talking to a person.

3. Explore alternative ways to resolve the situation or problem facing the person displaying violence. Begin to help the person address the reasons for their outburst step by step. Offer alternative options to a problem, if necessary. Avoid making the person lose face. If they feel humiliated, then they are unlikely to back down and the situation may escalate to the point where they feel that they must 'win'. This can be extremely dangerous to those involved. Gradually help the person feel that they can reach their goals without the use of violence.

This model of defusing is obviously based around the theory that much violence occurs from frustration or poorly controlled anger.

Where violence stems from the person hallucinating or being caught up in a delusion, then the emphasis is on clear, simple communication that enables the person to feel safe enough to regain contact with the reality of some people. It is particularly important in this case to use the therapeutic relationship, so it is best that someone well-known to the service user carries out the immediate face-to-face defusion.

WEAPONS

If the person is wielding a weapon (which might be anything from a piece of glass to a snooker cue) then nurses must not attempt to physically disarm them. Ask the person to place the weapon down on the floor and to step well away from it; the nurse should never accept an object that is being used as a weapon into his or her hands. If they will not do this, then call the police and secure the area so that the risk to others is minimized. While waiting for the police the nurse may attempt to calm the person enough to be able to encourage them to put the weapon down.

If the nurse is trapped with a person who is wielding a weapon and there is no help available, then, apart from using the defusing skills outlined above, the nurse needs to keep the person in front of them at all times, keeping at a distance and trying to keep them from blocking the doorway. It is probably best not to grab at the weapon as this may cause injury in the process. If the person is about to use the weapon, the nurse might try to prevent this by holding the weapon at its base or by using a coat or jacket or any furniture in the area as a shield.

PHYSICAL RESTRAINT

If all interventions fail to end the violent behaviour then physical restraint may be the only option. The term 'restraint' has many meanings; in this chapter the author means the action of physically holding a person by means of force to immobilize them. The use of restraint as a means to restrict a person's movement and freedom has long been a contentious issue in psychiatry. Its practice is traditional (Drinkwater and Gudjohnnsson, 1989) and has been subject to very little research into its efficacy. Despite this, physical restraint is used frequently throughout the UK.

With the abolition of mechanical restraints such as manacles, straight-jackets and the like, the current method for subduing involves the use of physical, hands-on restraint. This has been sanctioned for use with people who have mental health problems by the Department of Health and Welsh Office (Department of Health and Welsh Office, 1993) in the document *Code of Practice: Mental Health Act 1983*.

Physical restraint of someone is carried out to protect them from themselves or to protect others or property (Department of Health and Welsh Office, 1993). It must be carried out with reasonable force, i.e. 'the minimum necessary to deal with the harm that needs to be prevented' (Department of Health and Welsh Office, 1993). *The Code of Practice* suggests the action outlined in Box 19.3 (adapted by the author):

The author's own research into the experience of physical restraint (Hosking, 1994a) found that service users were terrified by the act of physical restraint, that it made them initially fight more furiously, that it was a humiliating experience and that, in their eyes, it caused irreparable damage to the nurse–service user relationship.

Much has been published on techniques of restraint (e.g. McDonnel *et al.*, 1991; Blumenreich and Lewis, 1993) but little on the use of restraint as an effective nursing intervention.

For many nurses the act of physical restraint is frightening and unpleasant. The incongruity between the caring role and the act of physical restraint may be in part explained by Szasz (1993) who suggests:

> The threat therapeutic zelotry poses to liberty is intrinsic to the dual nature of the state, as a source of both danger and protection.

Dietz and Rada (1983) found that 47% of injuries sustained by staff dealing with violent incidents occurred during physical restraint. These authors also suggest that restraint may in fact escalate violence.

In physically restraining someone, the nurse needs to be aware of the boundaries of his or her professional practice, i.e. the UKCC Code of Conduct (1992) the basis of which is to do good (beneficence) and to do no harm (non-maleficence). The act of physical restraint must only be used in justifiable circumstances, as Ritter (1989) outlines:

Box 19.3

Action to be taken by the team when confronted by violence

- Nominate a team leader to orchestrate the physical intervention.
- Do not intervene physically if you are on your own.
- Remove other people from the scene of the incident.
- Make a visual check for weapons.
- Constantly explain reasons for your actions to the service user and enlist their support for voluntary control as soon as possible. (It is possible that service users by this stage are in a state of high arousal and therefore do not hear nurses explaining what is happening.)
- Nominate staff to assist in control of the person and allocate each staff member a specific task.
- When ready to carry out the restraint the team leader should use a word that signals 'go' to the rest of the team, so that everyone acts at the same time. Do not choose a word such as 'okay'; you may accidentally use it when you do not mean to.
- Aim to restrain the person's arms and legs from behind if possible, immobilize swiftly and safely in a coordinated manner.
- Do not grab the person around the neck.
- Do not place weight on the service user's chest or stomach. This can restrict breathing and induce vomiting, which may cause asphyxiation.
- Never slap, kick or punch.
- Ensure cultural and gender sensitivity when using restraint. A women being restrained solely by men may simulate the act of rape and can be a terrifying experience. There must always be a woman present at the female service user's head so that the patient can see another female who can gently explain what is happening.

The use without legal justification, of direct force...to achieve compliance is a battery.

To prevent the restraint process becoming chaotic it is necessary that nurses become skilled in gentle, safe holding This can only be achieved through effective training. In each organization the form of restraint used is slightly different. There is some uniformity when it comes to the type of holding known as Control and Restraint (C&R) that is generally used in secure units and Special Hospitals. Control and Restraint is, according to Tarbuck (1992):

> A set of physical intervention skills which may be used to control an individual.

What is often unsaid is that Control and Restraint is effective because it works by using a series of 'locks' that cause pain to the individual if they try to resist the hold (McDonnell *et al.*, 1991). Causing pain may be seen to be punitive and may, as Bandura (1973) notes, actually model the aggressive behaviour the person is trying to subdue.

SECLUSION

In the author's workplace, seclusion is defined as 'the forced isolation of a person for an arbitrary period of time' (Thorpe, 1980).

Seclusion has long been a contentious issue (Morrison and le Roux, 1987) and opinion is divided as to its value (Outlaw and Lowery, 1992). Its use has been debated in Britain for many years. Despite this sometimes heated debate, there is still little empirical evidence to suggest that seclusion is an effective intervention (Drinkwater, 1982).

The Context of Use of Seclusion

Seclusion, in the mental health context, has been in existence for hundreds of years. Its use stems from the decline of mechanical restraints and was offered as 'a humane alternative' to these restraints (McCoy and Garritson, 1983). Seclusion is generally used to 'stop impulsive and destructive behaviour' (Grigson, 1984). As identified previously, it involves the forced isolation of the person for an arbitrary period of time (Thorpe, 1980). This forced isolation is presumed to have a calming influence on the person so that they may regain control of themselves and return to the main ward as soon as possible (Kendrick and Wilber, 1986).

Since the mid-1980s there has been rising controversy about the use of seclusion, particularly in Special Hospitals. The death of Michael Martin while in seclusion at Broadmoor (Francis, 1985) re-opened the debate about seclusion. Then the Ashworth Inquiry (Department of Health, 1992) brought the issue of people dying while in seclusion to the forefront. The Ashworth Inquiry recommended that seclusion be abolished and stated:

> [Seclusion] is an inhuman and degrading way to respond to a crisis; it is too often used for minor disturbances or transgression of rules; people are kept in seclusion longer than is necessary to control the initial unmanageability; it is used as a sanction by staff seeking to impose control over service users; there is little or no attention paid to the

psychological and physical effects of isolation on those who are mentally fragile.

(Department of Health, 1992).

Legally, seclusion is not regulated by statute. It is considered to be 'medical treatment' (Department of Health and Welsh Office, 1993). This causes some confusion, as the above document also states 'seclusion is not a treatment technique and should not feature as part of any treatment programme' (Department of Health and Welsh Office, 1993). What this means in practice is that seclusion must only be used in an absolute emergency, when all other means to contain the person have failed.

Ethically, the use of seclusion is fraught and is considered by some to violate the person's basic rights of freedom and dignity (Pilette, 1978) and by others as a tool of social control (Soloff, 1983). Yet in an emergency where extreme harm is being caused, it is the treatment of choice (Brennan, 1991; Wilson, 1993).

The Use of Seclusion

The literature shows that the reasons for seclusion vary greatly. Reasons include to prevent accidental injuries occurring to the confused service user (Kilgalen, 1977), inexperienced ward staff being unable to contain an escalating situation (Morrison, 1989), disruptive behaviour (Myers, 1990), threatened or actual physical violence (Baxter *et al.*, 1989), agitated behaviour without violence (Way and Banks, 1990), screaming, shouting, provocative or disinhibited behaviour (Hafner *et al.*, 1989), verbal abuse toward staff and violence to property (Morrison, 1987), being male and appearing intimidating (Thompson, 1986).

It can be seen that the vast majority of reasons are not legitimate in light of the Mental Health Act Code of Practice (Department of Health and Welsh Office, 1993) which clearly states '[seclusion's] sole aim therefore is to contain severely disturbed behaviour which is likely to cause harm to others'.

This definition is open to wide interpretation of what is 'likely to cause harm to others'. However what is useful is that it excludes harm to self. As the use of seclusion for people who are inflicting injury to themselves can be dangerous (Blumenreich and Lewis, 1993).

Ending Seclusion

The quote from a service user, given below, is taken from Norris and Kennedy's (1992) research into how service users perceive seclusion.

I was scared to death that no-one would come back.

It can be seen from this quote that the ending of seclusion is of importance in reducing feelings of fear brought about by its implementation.

There is some evidence that seclusion is ended only as and when the service user expresses remorse for the behaviour that led to seclusion. It is clear that the ending of seclusion (if it was initially justified) should never in any sense be

linked to the service user expressing remorse or sorrow for any assault or damage that had occurred

(Department of Health, 1992).

There are very few guidelines available to nurses on the cessation of seclusion, probably because of the confusion resulting from not knowing whether seclusion is a punishment, a treatment, or an emergency measure (Tooke and Brown, 1992). The Mental Health Act *Code of Practice* (Department of Health and Welsh Office, 1993) states that observation must take place 'to ascertain the state of the service user and whether seclusion can be terminated'.

The length of time spent in seclusion has been widely reported as varying from 1–2 hours (Russell *et al.*, 1986) to up to 10 hours (Soloff and Turner, 1981). While many research reports focus on the length of time spent in seclusion e.g. Betemps *et al.* (1992), none of them address, in any depth, the issue of when seclusion should end or how that decision is reached.

Critical Exploration

Hosking (1994b) interviewed a group of nurses who used seclusion on a regular basis. From these interviews she found that nurses decided to end seclusion based on the reasons identified in Table 19.1. (It must be noted that this was a small study. However, it may give some insight into issues about the decision to end seclusion.)

Mental state assessment

While an assessment of mental state is important, it has been suggested that seclusion actually maintains the behaviour it is supposed to suppress (Drinkwater and Gudjonsson, 1989), so to assess mental state by looking for the absence of the behaviours identified above may be erroneous and lead to the person spending longer than necessary in seclusion.

Nurses also said that they looked for calmness in the service user. This, they said, would be indicated by the absence of shouting, pacing, banging the door or walls, as recorded on the observation chart. Again, this is an unreliable measure. As has been noted, one of the consequences of seclusion is intense anger. All of the stated behaviours may then be a display of intense anger, rather than a 'disordered' mental state.

Looking for indicators of mental illness can be seen to be similar to what Goffman (1961) describes as 'rituals of degradation' that take place in psychiatric hospital, i.e. focusing on the apparent sickness instead of identifying the person's strengths. This may offer another insight as to why nurses end seclusion based on the absence of 'sick' behaviour, that is, as they are part of the institution, they have been socialized into this type of role.

Severity of the incident

Most of the nurses indicated that their decision to end seclusion was influenced by the severity of the incident that led

TABLE 19.1 Factors instrumental in the decision to cease seclusion

THEME	EXPLANATION OF THEME
MENTAL STATE ASSESSMENT	Nurses looked for an absence of shouting, banging on doors or walls. Assessment of speech and thought content, continuous observation notes read to identify changes in behaviour. Looked for calmness.
KNOWLEDGE OF SERVICE USER	Nurses based the decision on how the service user had reacted to seclusion in the past and on how much resistance the service user put up during physical restraint to be taken to seclusion, i.e. if they were fairly compliant then seclusion would be ended sooner.
RISKS INVOLVED	An assessment of the ward milieu was considered before the person was let out, i.e. would the person in seclusion cause more disruption. One nurse said, 'Well if you have got one person in seclusion and another person who is manic on the ward, it might be best to keep the person in seclusion otherwise there could be chaos'. The risk the service user posed to staff and other service users was considered.
TEAM DISCUSSION	The decision to end seclusion was identified by all nurses as needing to be discussed with the doctor and the duty nurse in charge, i.e. a senior nurse.
GUT REACTION	Several nurses said, 'Well you just know, it's a gut reaction'.
SEVERITY OF INCIDENT	Most of the nurses said that ending seclusion was dependent on the severity of the incident, i.e. how much damage the service user had caused. There was an implication that if the service user had hit a nurse they would be secluded for longer.
SHOW OF REMORSE	Four of the nurses said that if the person had been secluded for doing something 'bad' then they would look for a show of remorse or the service user having 'insight' into his or her behaviour.
ACCEPTING MEDICATION	This was seen to be an indication that the service user had regained some sort of control, i.e. if they were able to accept medication then the risk involved in ending seclusion were less because the service user would be sedated.
SERVICE USER SLEEPING	Several nurses said that if the service user was sleeping in the seclusion room then they would open the seclusion room door and effectively end seclusion while the person was asleep. Sleep was equated with calmness.

up to it. One nurse said, 'Well, if they hit somebody, then they would probably remain in seclusion for longer'. This indicated to the author that there was a misguided, punitive element to this aspect of the decision making. As Storr (1968) notes 'there is little correlation between the severity of the punishment administered and its deterrent effect'.

If the length of time spent in seclusion is related to how severe the incident is, then it may well be perceived as a punishment. That service users do perceive seclusion as a punishment has been repeatedly shown (e.g. Heyman, 1987; Tooke and Brown, 1992; McDonnell *et al.*, 1994). This can only have a detrimental effect on the nurse–service user relationship, as it clearly shows the imbalance of power between the two parties.

Being involved in secluding a person is seen as an unpleasant, anxiety producing act. Menzies (1970) notes that to cope with the intense anxiety caused by the nurse–service user relationship, nurses protect themselves by splitting up their contact with service users. Although Menzies (1970) was referring to splitting up contact by using a task centred approach, secluding a person could be seen as a literal split of contact that may result in reduced anxiety on the part of the nurse.

It is indisputable that dealing with aggression and violence causes stress in nurses (Whittington, 1994). Therefore a decision to prolong a person's stay in seclusion may be related to the nurse's need to reduce their stress to a tolerable level, by keeping the person locked away.

Show of remorse and accepting medication

These themes are linked with the severity of the incident in that they can be seen to be punitive in nature. Several of the nurses claim that the service user should somehow show remorse for the behaviour displayed. One nurse said, 'If they had got insight into their behaviour then I would probably stop seclusion'. This statement implies that a show of remorse is required for the service user to be released. The ending of seclusion should never be based on a show of remorse (Department of Health, 1992).

Demonstration of remorse is closely linked with deciding to end seclusion when the service user accepts medication. Nurses said that this acceptance of medication indicated that the person realized that they were ill and needed treatment. However, both themes display an attitude of paternalism, i.e. 'the protection of individuals from self-inflicted harm, in the way that a mother or father looks after children' (Downie and Calman, 1987). Paternalism is perpetuated by the medical model in psychiatry (Farber, 1993) and as such it is very easy for nurses to slip into this way of interacting with service users.

Offering medication as a precursor to coming out of seclusion appears coercive and may relate to staff anxieties about the risks involved in ending seclusion. As Atkinson (1991) notes:

What is best for the care team should not come before what is best for the service users. People who are in quiet control may look happier than disruptive people, and certainly may be easier to care for, but being quiet and controlled is not necessarily in the person's best interest.

The administration of medication before ending seclusion may also be perceived by nurses as a safety net. It has been shown that health care professionals are not particularly accurate in their prediction of further violence (Wykes, 1994a) and therefore medication may be seen as necessary 'just in case'.

Alternatives for practice
It is clear that the practice of ending seclusion needs further detailed investigation. As the research presented is of limited scope, it is not possible to generalize from the data. However, there are some general recommendations that can be made for practice.
- Information collated on reasons for seclusion in an organization is required. These reasons can then be fed back to nurses at all levels, to ensure that seclusion is being used appropriately
- Nurses need training in the legal and ethical use of seclusion.
- Nurses need to be made aware that they may have engendered anger and fear in the service user and that these emotions need to be distinguished from the dangerous behaviour that led to seclusion in the first place.
- More training may be needed on the prediction of further violence, so that the need to force people to take medication before coming out of seclusion becomes unnecessary.
- Seclusion must never be used as a punishment. In the heat of the moment, when the decision has been made to place a person in seclusion, it may be difficult to think about the ethical and legal implications of this. It is suggested that nurses discuss the use of seclusion among their clinical teams so that they can be clear about the ethical and legal parameters of its use.
- If the ending of seclusion is being delayed because of staff anxieties and stress, then this needs to be investigated and methods found for reducing that stress.
- The use of seclusion clearly shifts the balance of power between the nurse and the service user. Nurses need to be prepared to offer the service user ample time to talk about how they felt about being secluded, to repair some of the potential damage to the relationship caused by this action.

AFTER-CARE

Whittington and Wykes (1989) in their research into the effects of assault on mental health nurses found that most nurses reported symptoms afterwards that were akin to those experienced by disaster survivors, e.g. ruminations about the incident, increased fatigue, increased need to drink alcohol, increased need to smoke, intrusive thoughts, headaches, increased irritability, muscle tension, night awakening, anxiety associated with interaction with people and anxiety associated with the area of attack (Whittington and Wykes, 1989).

CONSEQUENCES OF VIOLENCE
The basis for the nurse–service user relationship according to Reynolds and Cormack (1990) is empathy, i.e. the ability to put oneself in another's shoes and to view their world as they view it (Rogers, 1951). Empathy may be difficult or impossible to achieve when a nurse has been assaulted by a service user. This must ultimately lead to a degeneration in the quality of relationships, which in turn could increase the likelihood of violence and reduce the quality of care.

Like Whittington and Wykes (1989), many other authors have published research on the potential effects of violence for nurses (e.g. Davidson and Jackson, 1985; Engle and Marsh, 1986; Poster and Ryan, 1989abc). These articles make explicit the victim's response to the trauma of violence and how in an organizational and individual sense this trauma may be alleviated.

> My own murderous anger towards another human being was harder to deal with, and traces of it lingered even after I learned my assailant wasn't responsible for his actions
>
> *(Kirschner, 1989).*

This quotation is from an article that gives a first-hand account of a nurse who was assaulted at work by a man who had mental health problems. The intensity of her emotional response to her experience may appear at first to be extreme. However, this response is just one of many strong emotions felt by mental health nurses who are assaulted, or who witness assaults, during the course of their work

Emotions identified most commonly following involvement in a violent or aggressive situation are fear, guilt, powerlessness, anger, denial, dehumanization, outrage, paranoia, confusion and shame. The associated behaviours include avoidance of service users, hypervigilance, blaming oneself, going over the event time and time again in one's mind, sleeplessness or dreaming about the event, not wanting to go to work, tense relationships with colleagues, making formal complaints, not talking about the event to anyone, tearfulness, increased irritability, ignoring service users, dissociation from people and the event and an inability to judge the dangerousness of subsequent potential violent incidents (Whittington and Wykes, 1989; Roberts, 1991; Poster and Ryan, 1993;).

What these authors further suggest is that the effects of violence are similar to those of post-traumatic stress disorder (PTSD), a debilitating anxiety disorder characterized by reaction to a traumatic event that includes 're-experiencing the event mentally, avoidance of the situation or any situation that reminds the person of the event and persistent physiological arousal lasting longer than one month' (Mejo, 1990).

One implication of diagnosing nurses as suffering from PTSD is that the act of diagnosis can lead to evasion of the underlying problem, which appears to be lack of safety for nurses in mental health. Diagnosing the 'sickness' may be a way of avoiding the investigation of underlying problems, which in turn may perpetuate violence.

It is important to remember that witnessing violence may also cause distress (Ryan and Poster, 1991), and support for people who were in the vicinity of the incident must be considered.

DEBRIEFING

Mitchell (1983) devised a process that he called psychological debriefing, which he considers essential to help someone who has experienced trauma to return to normal functioning.

Debriefing is not counselling or therapy. It is a practical way of talking a person through a traumatic event to help them come to terms with it and to prepare them for returning to work. The process of debriefing is outlined in detail in Chapter 25.

This process of debriefing helps the person to ease into recalling the experience in a gentle way, by moving from facts through to feelings, and back to how to cope in the future. It is most appropriate for the debriefers to be people who have similar backgrounds to those who have been involved in the incident. The debriefers must be skilled at using the debriefing technique and have the ability to identify any more serious mental health problems among participants.

One practical difficulty with debriefing is that for each person to speak and go through the process thoroughly it can take anything from 1–2 hours. In the clinical setting this usually is not possible. However, Mitchell and Bray (1990) offer an alternative, which they calls 'defusings'. These generally last for around half an hour and are less structured than debriefing. However, what they do is allow for the ventilation of feelings, which Ragaisis (1994) considers essential for the nurse's ability to 'move forward with life'. They need to occur within 4 hours of the incident whereas debriefing should happen within 72 hours of the incident.

This traumatic event has been labelled as a critical incident (Mitchell, 1985), i.e. 'an extraordinary event that causes extraordinary stress reactions'. More recently Mitchell (1990) redefined this and says that 'any event can be considered a critical incident if it has the ability to distress a person by overwhelming the person's coping ability'. This is not to be confused with 'critical incident analysis' in nursing as devised by Flanagan (1954), which is a learning technique where the student collects 'behavioural data about ingredients of competent behaviour on a profession' (Crouch, 1992).

If nurses do indeed mix up the tasks of critical incident debriefing and critical incident analysis (by talking about management of the service user, staff feelings and what could have been done differently in the situation), they increase the likelihood of people coming away feeling as if it was their fault that the incident occurred. Talking about how you feel at the same time as looking at what could be done differently can easily degenerate into casting blame. If this happens, then it is likely that talking about the incident will be seen as a frightening and unhelpful activity.

Similarly, talking about the future management of the service user while anxieties are running high surely increases the likelihood that clinical decisions are made 'in the heat of the moment' rather than with objectivity.

Discussion of the incident is important. However, discussing the event may increase feelings of anxiety and remind staff of their own vulnerability and so nurses may try to avoid this and say that they 'just want to go home'. This is not the option of choice, as they will go home with all the feelings they have about the incident at the forefront of their thoughts.

It is worth remembering that one of the diagnostic criteria for PTSD is the avoidance of the situation or any situation that is reminiscent of the incident. For the mental health nurse, avoidance of the situation is impossible unless they leave their job. However, avoidance may be observed in the clinical areas as staff staying in the nurses' office and having minimal contact with service users. If they cannot avoid the situation, then they cannot be diagnosed with PTSD and thus may not receive the help that they need (Wykes, 1994b).

On the other hand, by saying that the effects of violence can in some cases induce a mental disorder (PTSD) one may actually increase the likelihood of nurses denying the effects of violence for fear of the stigma of being thought as 'mentally ill'. There has also been a tentative suggestion that the victim of violence may potentially become violent themselves (Collins and Bailey, 1990). This may also increase the anxieties of nurses, particularly in the wake of the Allit inquiry (1994) since now any record of mental illness may be used as a reason for not employing people.

An issue that has not been given much attention is the fact that some nurses may be unable to tell their family and friends about being assaulted because they are ashamed or afraid of causing them anxiety. This has serious implications, for social support is seen as essential for nurses to increase their ability to recover from a stressful event (Hare *et al.*, 1988).

Witnessing a nurse being assaulted may lead to other service users feeling vulnerable because, in their eyes, nurses are supposed to protect them. The nurse may deny their vulnerability, as being assaulted can trigger role confusion, i.e. who needs looking after the most, the people with mental health problems or the nurses? In situations like this, Roberts (1991) has noted that it is almost always the nurse's needs that are disregarded because they are socialized into putting the needs of others first. However, if nurses are experiencing emotional turmoil it is unlikely that they will be of much help to the service users (Turnbull, 1993).

There are several ways in which support to nurses can be offered. Robinson and Mitchell (1993) recommend a critical incident stress debriefing team. the author proposes a model of incident support in Box 19.4.

Ward Managers and Team Leaders need to be properly trained in effective supervision of staff and debriefing of victims of violence. It is important that they take on this role, since debriefers, to be effective, need to have an understanding of the work and environment of the victim (Clark and Friedman, 1992). It is important that nurses receive supervision on a regular basis to reduce the feelings of emotional exhaustion that arise from an accumulation of stress in nursing (Constable and Russell, 1986). Dawson *et al.* (1988) recom-

Box 19.4 *Proposed model of support for staff likely to be involved in violent incidents*

Beforehand:

1 Pre-incident education aimed at managers and team leaders to include all aspects of preventing and managing violence. Also training in 'defusings' (Mitchell, 1990).

When violence occurs:

2 Victim receives medical help.
3 Team 'defuses' while emergency team covers the ward.
4 Victim is seen by immediate manager for support and debriefing.
5 Support group in team on a weekly basis where debriefing of cumulative stresses can take place.
6 Clinical supervision to occur at least fortnightly.
7 Referral to independent counsellor if required.

mends a 'buddy' system whereby when an assault has taken place a nurse who has experienced a similar event, offers support and debriefing. This is said also to decrease staff turnover (Dawson *et al.*, 1988).

Morrison (1987/88) recommends that a Clinical Nurse Specialist is employed specifically to help staff after assault. This person needs to be part of a bigger team and receive good support as, if this is lacking, the work becomes detrimental to the mental health of the debriefer (Talbot, 1990).

If a service user is assaulted the following action must be taken:

• Protect the person from further assault.
• Inform their next of kin, if given permission by the service user.
• Inform the police.
• Provide medical care for any injury.
• Have the incident investigated by the hospital.
• Have the person who carried out the assault removed to a different clinical setting.
• Help obtain legal representation.

In the case of sexual assault the service user must be informed that if they wash or change their clothes, they are destroying evidence that may be used by the police to identify the assailant.

Each organization must have their own policy on dealing with allegations of sexual assault. In the author's organization allegations of sexual assault are always reported to the police, even if the service user does not want this done.

As with nurses who suffer severe psychological consequences following assault, service users are no different. However, in the case of the service user, their symptoms after assault may be labelled by psychiatry as being part of their mental disorder and thus may be ignored or incorrectly treated.

It is very important that the service user is given the same

consideration as the nurse when assaulted, i.e. they need the opportunity to discuss what has happened and they need this opportunity repeated over possibly several months.

Prosecution of Perpetrator of Violence

The prosecution of the service user who is assaultative has always been a controversial subject. There are many reasons for and against the idea. Many nurses say that when they have reported the incident to the police, the police say that they can do nothing because the service user is 'mentally ill' or under a Section of the Mental Health Act 1983. However, it is not for the police to decide whether a case is worth pursuing; this is a matter for the Criminal Prosecution Service. They will judge whether the case should go to court on the basis of whether it is in the public interest.

Even if the service user is not prosecuted, it is important to inform the police that a crime has taken place. They have a duty to record this information and to give you a log number, which you can then use if you choose to claim for damages to the Criminal Injuries Compensation Board.

It is essential that each organization and each team within the organization makes it clear what their policy is on this issue. In the final event, everyone has the right to take civil action against their assailant.

SUMMARY

This chapter has outlined one set of definitions for the terms 'violence' and 'aggression' and has discussed the main theories about these concepts in mental health nursing today. It has been seen that, while violence is a major problem facing mental health nurses, violence committed by people with mental health problems is, relatively speaking, far less than that committed by the general public.

The link between violence and mental health problems has been explored and it can be seen that there is a link between experiencing active symptoms such as hallucinations and delusions and an increased risk of becoming violent, but that this does not always follow. This risk is increased if the person is taking alcohol or unprescribed drugs.

The need for a thorough assessment that attempts to predict the possible risk of violence has been outlined with examples of planning care and interventions for a person who admits to using violence to cope with certain situations.

The prevention and management of violent situations has been covered in some detail with the emphasis being on non-physical intervention wherever possible. The ethical and safe use of physical restraint and seclusion has been explored.

Lastly the consequences of violence for both the service user and the nurse have been detailed, the care that both will need has been identified and a strategy for ensuring appropriate care is available to nurses has been suggested.

KEY CONCEPTS

- There is a misconception that people with mental health problems are highly violent. The reality is that many more people who are not diagnosed as having mental illness are responsible for most violent crime.
- In-patient areas are likely to experience an increase in violent situations following implementation of the Community Care Act 1990 where people are admitted when in acute crisis.
- Organizations must develop policies and strategies to monitor levels of violence to address preventive strategies.
- Self-awareness and steps to ensure personal safety are vital in terms of preventing violence and keeping oneself safe.
- Methods of assessing the risk of violence are useful but the risk of gaining false positives from these assessments is significant. All relevant details including any previous relationship with the service user must be considered.
- When working in an interdisciplinary way with a service user, any history of violence must be communicated to the individual or group of people who will be caring for the service user.
- The psychological consequences of violence for the service user and the nurse cannot be overestimated. Effective, caring support is key to their recovery and well-being.

REFERENCES

Atkinson J: Autonomy and mental health. In: Barker PJ, Baldwin S, editors: *Ethical issues in mental health*. London, 1991, Chapman & Hall.

Bandura A: *Aggression: a social learning analysis*. New Jersey, 1973, Prentice Hall, Englewood Cliffs.

Bandura A: *Social learning theory*. New York, 1977, General Learning Press.

Baxter E, Hale C, Hafner RJ: Use of seclusion in a psychiatric intensive care unit. *Aust Clin Rev* 9:142, 1989.

Betemps EJ, Buncher CR, Oden M: Length of time spent in seclusion and restraint by clients at 82 VA medical centres. *Hosp Community Psychiatry* 43(9): 912–914, 1992.

Bethlem and Maudsley, NHS Trust: *Nursing policies and procedures*. London, 1992, NHS Trust.

Blumenreich PE, Lewis S: *Managing the violent patient: a clinician's guide*. New York, 1993, Bruner Mazel Publishers.

Brennan W: Alone again, naturally. *Nurs Stand* 6(7):46–47, 1991.

Chapman R: Violence is not part of the job. *COHSE Journal* 2(5):10–11, 1990.

Collins JJ, Bailey SL: Traumatic stress disorder and violent behaviour. *J Trauma Stress* 3(2):203–220, 1990.

Constable CJF, Russell DW: The effect of social support and the work environment upon burnout among nurses. *J Hum Stress* 12:20–26, 1986.

Clark M, Friedman D: Pulling Together: Building a community debriefing team. *J Psychosoc Nurs* 30(7):27–32, 1992.

Crittenden PM, Ainsworth MD: Child maltreatment and attachment theory. In: Cicchetti D, Carlson V: *Child maltreatment: Theory and research on the causes and consequences of child abuse and neglect*. New York, 1989, Cambridge Press.

Crouch, S: Critical incident analysis. *Nursing* 37(4), 1991.

Davidson P, Jackson C: The nurse as a survivor. *Int J Nurs Stud* 22(1):1–13, 1985.

Dawkins JE , Depp C, Selzer NE: Stress and the psychiatric nurse. *J Psychosoc Nurs Ment Health Services* 23(11):9–15, 1985.

Dawson J, Johnston M, Kehiayan N, *et al*: Response to patient assault: a peer and support programme for nurses. *J Psychosoc Nurs Ment Health Services* 26(2):8–15, 1988.

Department of Health: *The Community Care Act*. London, 1990, HMSO.

Department of Health: *Report of the Committee of Inquiry into Complaints about Ashworth Hospital*. London, 1992, HMSO.

Department of Health & Welsh Office: *Code of Practice: Mental Health Act 1983*. London, 1993, HMSO.

Department of Health: *Working in Partnership: a collaborative approach to care*. London, 1994, HMSO.

Dietz PE, Rada RT: Interpersonal violence in forensic facilities. In: Lion JR, Reid WH: *Assaults within psychiatric facilities*. New York, 1983, Grune & Stratton.

Dollard J, Doob L, Miller NE, *et al.*: *Frustration and Aggression*. New Haven CT, 1939, Yale University Press.

Downie RS, Calman KC: *Health respect: Ethics in health care*. London, 1987, Faber & Faber.

Drinkwater C, Gudjonsson GH: The nature of violence in psychiatric hospitals. In: Howells K, Hollin CR: *Clinical approaches to violence*. Chichester, 1989, John Wiley & Sons.

Engle F, Marsh S: Helping the employee victim of violence in hospitals. *Hosp Community Psychiatry* 37(2):159–162, 1986.

Farber S: *Madness, heresy and the rumour of angels: the revolt against the mental health system*. Chicago, 1993, Open Court Publishing Company.

Fenwick P: Aggression and epilepsy. In: Thompson P, Cowen P: *Violence basic and clinical science*. Oxford, 1993, Butterworth Heinemann Mental Health Foundation.

Flanagan J: The critical incident technique. *Psychol Bull* 51:327–358, 1954.

Flannery RB, Fulton P, Tausch J, *et al.*: A programme to help staff cope with psychological sequelae of assaults by patients. *Hosp Community Psychiatry* 42(9): 935–938, 1991.

Fottrell E: A study of violent behaviour among patients in psychiatric hospitals. *Br J Psychiatry* 136:216–221, 1980.

Francis E: How did Michael Martin die? *Openmind* 13(3):10–12, 1985.

Fromm E: *The anatomy of human destructiveness*. London, 1974, Penguin Books.

Grigson JW: Beyond patient management: the therapeutic use of seclusion and restraints. *Perspect Psychiatr Care* 22(4):137–142, 1984.

Goffman E: *Asylums*. New York, 1961, Doubleday.

Hafner RJ, Lammersma RF, Cameron M: The use of seclusion: a comparison of two psychiatric intensive care units. *Aust NZealand J Psychiatry* 23:235–239, 1989.

Hamolia, CC: Violence and aggression. In: Stuart GW, Sundeen SJ: *Principles and practice of psychiatric nursing* 5 ed. St Louis, 1995, Mosby.

Hare J, Pratt CC, Andrews D: Predictors of burnout in professional and paraprofessional nurses working in hospitals and nursing homes. *Int J Nurs Studies* 25(2):105–115, 1988.

Health and Safety Executive: *New Health and Safety at Work regulations*. Sheffield, 1992, Health and Safety Executive.

Heyman E: Seclusion. *J Psychosoc Nurs* 25(11):9–12, 1987.

Hosking P: *The experience of physical restraint [dissertation]*. London, 1994a, The Bethlem and Maudsley NHS Trust.

Hosking P: *Ending seclusion. How do you decide?* London, 1994b, The Bethlem and Maudsley NHS Trust.

Home Office: Home Office Statistical Bulletin 95(19): London, 1995, Government Statistical Service.

James DV, Fineberg NA, Shah AJ, *et al.*: An increase in violence on an acute psychiatric ward: a study of associated factors. *Br J Psychiatr* 156:846–852, 1990.

Kendrick DM, Wilber G: Seclusion: organising safe and effective care. *J Psychosoc Nurs* 24(11):26–28, 1986.

Kilgalen RK: The effective use of seclusion. *J Psychiatr Nurs Mental Health Serv* 15(1):22–25, 1977.

Kirschner G: If you scream, I'll kill you. *RN* March:35–36, 1989.

Lanza ML: Factors affect blame placement for patient assault upon nurses. *Iss Ment Health Nurs* 6:143–162, 1985.

Lanza ML, Carifo J: Blaming the victim: Complex (non-linear) patterns of causal attribution by nurses in response to vignettes of a patient assaulting a nurse. *J Emerg Nurs* 7(5):299–309, 1991.

Link B, Andrews H, Cullen F: The violent and illegal behaviour of mental patients reconsidered. *Am Sociol Rev* 57:275–292, 1992.

Lion JR, Snyder W, Merrill G: Underreporting of assaults on staff in a state hospital. *Hosp Community Psychiatry* 32:44–47, 1981.

Lloyd A: *Doubly deviant, doubly damned: society's treatment of violent women*. London, 1995, Penguin Books.

McCoy SM, Garritson S: Seclusion: the process of intervention. *J Psychosoc Nurs Ment Health Serv* 21(8):8–15, 1983.

McDonnell A, Dearden B, Richens A: Staff training in the management of violence and aggression: avoidance and escape principles. *Ment Handicap* 19(3):109–112, 1991.

McDonnell A, McEvoy J, Dearden RL: Coping with violent situations in the caring environment. In: Wykes T: *Violence and health care professionals*. London, 1994, Chapman & Hall.

Mejo SL: Post traumatic stress disorder: An overview of three etiological variables, and psychopharmacologic treatment. *Nurs Practitioner* 15(8):41–45, 1990.

Meloy JR: *Violent attachments*. London, 1992, Janson Aronson Inc.

Menzies E: *The function of social systems as a defence against anxiety*. London, 1970, Tavistock.

Miller A: *For your own good: the roots of violence in child rearing*. London, 1987, Virago.

MIND: *Stress on women*. London, 1992, MIND Publications.

Mitchell JT: When disaster strikes: the critical incident stress debriefing process. *J Emerg Med Serv* 8(1):36–39, 1983.

Mitchell JT: Healing the helper. In: Greene B: *Role stressors and supports for emergency workers*. Washington DC, 1985, Department of Health and Human Services.

Mitchell JT, Bray GP: *Emergency services stress: guidelines for preserving the health and careers of emergency services personnel*. Englewood Cliffs, 1990, Prentice Hall.

Moir A, Jessel D: *A mind to crime: the controversial link between mind and criminal behaviour*. London, 1995, Michael Joseph.

Monahan J: *The clinical prediction of violent behaviour*. Maryland, 1981, US Department of Health and Human Services.

Monahan J: Risk Assessment of violence among the mentally disordered: generating useful knowledge. *Int J Law Psychiatry* 11:249–57, 1988.

Monahan J: Mental disorder and violent behaviour: attitudes and evidence. *Am Psychol* 47:511–521, 1992.

Morrison EF: The assaulted nurse: strategies for healing. *Perspect Psychiatr Care* 24(3/4):120–126, 1987/88.

Morrison EF: Toward a better understanding of violence in psychiatric settings: debunking the myths. *Arch Psychiatr Nurs* 7(6):328–335, 1993.

Morrison EF: Theoretical modeling to predict violence in hospitalised psychiatric patients. *Res Nurs Health* 12(1):31–40, 1989.

Morrison EF: The evolution of a concept: aggression and violence in psychiatric settings. *Arch Psy Nursing* 8(4):245–253, 1994.

Morrison P, le Roux B: The practice of seclusion. *Nurs Times* 83(19):62–66, 1987.

Murray GM, Snyder JC: When staff are assaulted: a nursing consultation service. *J Psychosoc Nurs Ment Health Serv* 29(7):24–29, 1991.

Myers S: Seclusion: a last resort measure. *Perspect Psychiatr Care* 26(3):24–28, 1990.

Norris MK, Kennedy CW: The view from within: how patients perceive the seclusion process. *J Psychosoc Nurs* 30(3):7–13, 1992.

Owens RG, Ashcroft JB: *Violence: a guide for the caring professions*. London, 1985, Croom Helm.

Outlaw FH, Lowery BJ: Seclusion: the nursing challenge. *J Psychosoc Nurs* 30(4):13–17, 1992.

Pilette PC: The tyranny of seclusion. *J Psychosoc Nurs Ment Health Serv* 16:19–21, 1978.

Poster EC, Ryan JA: Nurses' attitudes towards physical assaults by patients. *Arch Psychiatr Nurs* 3(6):314–322, 1989a.

Poster EC, Ryan JA: The assaulted nurse: short-term and long-term responses. *Arch Psychiatr Nurs* 3(6):323–331, 1989b.

Poster EC, Ryan JA: Supporting your staff after a patient assault. *Nurs* 19(12):32, 1989c.

Poster EC, Ryan JA: Workplace violence. *Nurs Times* 89(48):38–41, 1993.

Powell G, Caan W, Crowe M: What events precede violent incidents in psychiatric hospitals? *Br J Psychiatry* 165:107–112, 1994.

Ragaisis KM: Critical incident stress debriefing: A family nursing intervention. *Arch Psychiatr Nurs* 8(1):38–43, 1994.

Reynolds W, Cormack D: *Psychiatric and mental health nursing: theory and practice*. London, 1990, Chapman & Hall.

Ritchie JH: *The report of the Inquiry into the care and treatment of Christopher Clunis*. London, 1994, HMSO.

Ritter S: *Bethlem Royal and Maudsley Hospital manual of clinical psychiatric nursing principles and procedures*. London, 1989, Harper & Row.

Roberts S: Nurse abuse: a taboo topic. *Can Nurse* 87(3):66–69, 1991.

Robinson RC, Mitchell JT: Evaluation of psychological debriefings. *J Trauma Stress* 6(3):367–382, 1993.

Rogers CR: *Patient centered therapy*. London, 1951, Constable.

Russell D, Hodgkinson P, Hillis JA: Time out. *Nurs Times* 82(9):47–49, 1986.

Ryan J, Poster EC: When a patient hits you. *Can Nurse* 87(8):23–25, 1991.

Sayce L: Response to violence: a framework for fair treatment. In: Crichton J: *Psychiatric patient violence; risk and response*. London, 1995, Duckworth.

Shah AK: An increase in violence among psychiatric inpatients: real or apparent? *Med Sci Law* 33:247–57, 1993.

Siann G: *Accounting for aggression: perspectives on aggression and violence*. London, 1985, Allen & Unwin.

Soloff PH: Seclusion and restraints. In: Lion JR, Reid WH: *Assaults within psychiatric facilities*. New York, 1983, Grune & Stratton.

Soloff PH, Turner SM: Patterns of seclusion: a prospective study. *J Nerv Ment Disord* 169:37–44, 1981.

Steadman HJ, Monahan J, Robbins PC, *et al.*: From dangerousness to risk assessment: Implications for appropriate research strategies. In: Hodgins S: *Mental disorder and crime*. London, 1993, Sage Publications Inc.

Storr A: *Human aggression*. Harmondsworth, 1968, Penguin.

Stevenson S: Heading off violence with verbal de-escalation. *J Psychosoc Nurs Mental Services* 29(9), 1991.

Swanson J, Holzer CE, Ganju VK, *et al.*: Violence and psychiatric disorder in the community: Evidence from the epidemiologic catchment. *Area Surv Hosp Community Psychiatry* 41:761–770, 1990.

Szasz T: *Cruel compassion: psychiatric control of society's unwanted*. Chichester, 1993, John Wiley & Sons.

Talbot A: The importance of parallel process in debriefing crisis counsellors. *J Trauma Stress* 3(2):265–276, 1990.

Tarbuck P: Use and abuse of control and restraint. *Nurs Stand* 6(52):30–32, 1992.

Taylor PJ: Motives for offending among violent and psychotic men. *Br J Psychiatry* 147:491–8, 1985.

Thompson P: The use of seclusion in psychiatric hospitals in the Newcastle area. *Br J Psychiatry* 149:471–474, 1986.

Thorpe JG: Time-out or seclusion? *Nurs Times* 76(14):4–6, 1980.

Tooke SK, Brown JS: Perceptions of seclusion: comparing patient and staff reactions. *J Psychosoc Nurs* 30(8):23–26, 1992.

Turnbull J: Victim support. *Nurs Times* 89(23):33–34, 1993.

UKCC: *Records and Note Keeping*. London, 1993, UKCC.

UKCC: *Code of Professional Conduct*. London, 1992, UKCC.

Waites EA: Trauma and survival: post-traumatic and dissociative disorders in women. London, 1993, WW Norton & Company Inc.

Way BB, Banks SM: Use of seclusion and restraint in public psychiatric hospitals: patient characteristics and facility effects. *Hosp Community Psychiatry* 41(1):75–80, 1990.

Walker WD, Caplan RP: Assaultive behaviour in acute psychiatric wards and its relationship to violence in the community: a comparison of two health districts. *Med Sci Law* 33:300–304, 1993.

Wessley S, Taylor P: Madness and crime: criminology versus psychiatry. *Crim Behav Ment Health* 1:193–228, 1991.

Whittington R, Wykes T: Invisible injury. *Nurs Times* 85(42):30–32, 1989.

Whittington R: Reactions to assault. In: Wykes T: *Violence and health care professionals*. London, 1994, Chapman & Hall.

Wilson M: Seclusion practice in psychiatric nursing. *Nurs Stand* 7(31):28–30, 1993.

Wykes T: *Violence and health care professionals*. London, 1994a, Chapman & Hall.

Wykes T: Assaulted nurses 'suffering in silence'. Nurs Stand 8(28):11, 1994b.

FURTHER READING

Cleveland Rape and Sexual Abuse Counselling Service: *Sexual violence against women and children: a practical approach to issue-based training*. Middlesbrough, 1995, Cleveland Rape and Sexual Abuse Counselling Service.
A comprehensive training manual which covers issues to do with rape, child sexual abuse, pornography, personal safety, sexual harassment and gender roles in society. Very useful to those involved in training staff who work with survivors of sexual violence.

Crichton J, editor: *Psychiatric patient violence: risk and response*. London, 1995, Duckworth.
A very readable book containing useful information and practical advice on the subject of violence and the person with mental health problems.

Glendon AI, McKenna EF: *Human safety and risk management*. London, 1995, Chapman & Hall.
This books gives a detailed analysis of risk managment both from an individual and a team perspective. There are suggestions for preparing to train others in risk management.

Walker N, editor: *Dangerous people*. London, 1996, Blackstone Press Limited.
This book offers an overview of the dangerous behaviour displayed by people in society. It has contributions from many experts in the fields of psychiatry, criminal law, academia, the probation service and criminology. The book gives insight into how these fields of study come together to offer services to deal with violent or sexual offenders.

Drug and Alcohol Nursing

Learning Outcomes

After studying this chapter, you should be able to:

- Identify factors that influence the nature and context of drug and alcohol nursing, specifically, personal and professional values, language and criminal justice, and social, cultural and gender issues.

- Describe a framework for categorizing nursing assessment and interventions in addiction.

- List key areas for drug and alcohol assessment in the fields of human development; health and well-being; modifying behaviour; and mental and social health.

- Detail the forms, patterns of use, routes of administration and effects of alcohol and commonly used drugs.

- Distinguish between problem and dependent use.

- Distinguish between effects of substances, of withdrawal and of route of use.

- Describe a model of the process of change.

- Identify the main characteristics of a range of drug and alcohol interventions available to nurses, including prevention and brief intervention, harm minimization, motivational interviewing, relapse prevention, health intervention and solution-focused therapy.

- Identify key areas for development of outcome measurement in drug and alcohol nursing.

*T**his chapter will provide an overview of the nursing role** in assessing and delivering interventions to drug and alcohol users. It will examine the role of specialist and non-specialist intervention within a framework that integrates the core areas of nursing with current good clinical practice in the drug and alcohol field. Information will be provided on the use of all substances regularly encountered in the UK, concentrating on nursing interventions to address problematic and dependent use. There will be an emphasis on the priority areas for nursing, such as health improvement, harm minimization and modifying patterns of addictive behaviour. Commonly used drug and alcohol intervention models will be introduced. Consideration will be given to issues of particular contemporary concern such as hepatitis, HIV, pregnancy and mental health, as well as traditional and newer interventions for alcohol, opiate and stimulant use. The chapter will conclude with an examination of the future for outcome measurement.

Drug and alcohol use stretches across economic, cultural, gender and geographical divides. All societies have their drugs, which in the UK range from the leisurely consumption of tea and coffee to the frantic search for heroin and crack. The use of caffeine and cocaine is seen as totally different, normal and abnormal respectively, but in reality both are stimulants and both are often taken regularly by users to relieve withdrawals and gain a kick. The difference between them is one of degree, of psychological and physical effect, of craving to use, of cost, of availability, of social acceptability and of legal consequences of use. When working with drugs and alcohol it is essential to remember that almost all people are users of some substances at some time. What matters for nurses is the health risk involved, particularly those risks that come from problematic or dependent use. Such risks vary from person to person. They depend not only on the drug itself but also on the way in which it is used and the social and cultural environment in which that use takes place. To address these risks, nurses must have gained insight into their personal and professional values around drug and alcohol use, have developed an awareness of the language used in this area and have some understanding of the social context surrounding drug and alcohol treatment.

PERSONAL AND PROFESSIONAL VALUES

Nurses, in common with the general public, often have strong views about people whose problems with drug and alcohol use bring them into contact with health care services.

Carroll (1993), in an examination of nurses' reactions toward drug users in Scotland, showed that many nurses, such as those working in general hospitals or prisons, have negative attitudes towards users. He found that familiarity with drug users seemed to encourage nurses to be more positive about working with them. This familiarity was primarily gained by direct experience of working with such clients in a helping capacity. Nurses in specialist addiction services had markedly more positive attitudes than their colleagues in general hospitals. Although this may be partially ascribed to such staff self-selecting into a field in which they are interested, it also raises the question of whether other nurses can develop a less negative approach. Much of this is a task for nurse training and development, which needs to explore in depth the past professional experiences that nurses have had of users and enable development of a more informed, positive perspective to care. Personal experiences of drugs and alcohol are equally important here, from past or current use by self, friends, peers or carers. Also worthy of exploration are the effects of the multifarious external influences which may impact on nurses' attitudes and knowledge, such as advertising, media coverage, music, literature, even soap operas. Some nurses will err on the side of over-identification with their clients (They are just like me; I am OK; So what's the problem?). Others will over-differentiate (I am nothing like them; how could anyone be like this?). Such rigid value systems leave little space for the development of an empathic, caring relationship.

LANGUAGE

The addiction field, more than most, suffers from a surplus of linguistic ambiguities and anomalies. These exist within professional and user circles and can be a source of great confusion to the nurse new to the field. A common understanding of behaviour, need, goals and outcome is essential for effective nursing practice. This can best be achieved in nurse–client relationships and professional teams by shared exploration of meaning rather than reliance on definitions from a book. Certain terms, however, are worthy of some definition.

Professional Terminology

The professional language of the drug and alcohol domain is full of vaguely synonymous terms that, in reality, have vastly different meanings depending on who interprets them. Use, abuse, misuse, addiction, dependence, alcoholic, addict, user, substance (use, abuse or misuse) and problem are just some of the common terms employed in an attempt to describe the complexities of this specialism. Different nurses will have their own individual preferences for these terms. This chapter will use some of the above terms interchangeably (with the recognition and indeed hope that readers will question and challenge their potential meaning). In general it is better to avoid the more pejorative terms such as abuse, misuse, alcoholic and addict, unless there is specific reason to use them, and because they are the start of a negative labelling process for clients and their behaviour. The one exception to this is the term 'addiction' (and addictive behaviour), which is presently undergoing a rehabilitation in some circles after years of rejection. It is used frequently in this chapter because of its encapsulation (to a certain extent lay inspired) of the difficulties facing long-term users and their carers, but its use should always arise with the recognition that it could lead to too judgmental an interpretation or too simplistic an explanation of the many physical, psychological and social problems encountered by users. The terms 'substance abuse' and 'substance misuse', on the other hand, are avoided wherever possible as they represent a professional generalization that neither reflects the need for clarity nor the clients' own language.

Jargon, Slang and Drugspeak

Whole books and dictionaries have been written on drug terminology. The media, as so often in this field, casts its stereotyping spell on the language of addiction. For the nurse, it is essential to realize that words and meanings change from user to user, area to area, drug to drug. For many health professionals new to the field there is an enticing lure to 'talk the junkies' talk', but although some sharing of language can increase rapport, too much may cause confusion and contempt and maintains the client in the narrow world of their addiction. For example, one heroin injector may use terms such as 'cooking up' (warming the heroin powder with liquid prior to putting the mixture in a syringe), 'moody gear' (low purity, poor quality heroin), 'cranking', 'jacking up', 'banging up', 'fixing' etc. (injecting), 'clucking' and 'roasting' (experiences of withdrawal); but to another user, particularly from the mouth of a health care worker, such terms could sound foolish or inaccurate. Using purely cold, clinical language is also not always the answer but a balance that ensures that common understanding in everyday words should be aimed for when possible. If in doubt, check meanings with the client.

SOCIAL CONTEXT

Drug and alcohol use, and nursing interventions directed at that use, can only be understood through an appreciation of the wider social issues contextualizing addiction within our society. Interest is steadily increasing in the growth of links between drugs and crime and the delivery of treatment from within the criminal justice system. Equally important are issues of accessibility, equity and diversity in all intervention settings.

THE CRIMINAL JUSTICE DIMENSION

In nursing addictions there is always the awareness of the tension between treatment and social control. Even though it is clear that nursing supplies the former and not the latter, it can be a major challenge to remain an agent of change rather than an instrument of social conformity. The connections between drug use and crime cannot be denied, as is shown by the 70 000 separate crimes committed during the 3 months prior to entering treatment by the 1100 users studied in the National Treatment Outcome Research Study (Task Force to Review Services for Drug Misusers, 1996). This situation raises a number of dilemmas for nursing practice.

Arrest referral schemes, probation liaison initiatives, treatment conditions on sentences and a proliferation of prison detoxification and rehabilitation units are all drawing nurses into the criminal justice arena. This puts nurses alongside other professionals with different agendas.

Multi-agency assessment as recommended by the Advisory Council on the Misuse of Drugs (ACMD) (1991) is the way forward, but can pose grave difficulties over confidentiality. This and other concerns have been clearly described by Goodsir (1993), who warned that 'work involving the disclosure of sensitive information to other professionals who have the capacity to take sanctions against drug users has a potential to be threatening to those being processed by such systems'.

Problems occur particularly for nurses in prisons, in the role of visiting worker or employed health care staff, where there may be a conflict between official (or traditional) reaction to information gained from clients about their drug use and the nurse's wish to encourage openness and honesty in prisoners. One example of this is positive urine testing, which can be used for punishment or therapeutic exploration.

Yet nurses must adapt to these changes in their work and avoid the easy temptation of putting up barriers. Some boundaries are important and there are clear confidentiality guidelines for the profession. But nursing's social responsibilities mean that these boundaries must be balanced with the benefits of joint working and many nurses are finding that such collaboration can, indeed, help rather than hinder the client, if roles and expectations are clearly defined from the start.

ACCESSIBILITY AND DIVERSITY

As well as the treatment–control dilemma, nurses also need to address issues of accessibility, equity and diversity. Many services offered to drug users and drinkers are still restricted in their focus and availability. More recognition is needed of different cultural reactions to drugs and alcohol and of the ambivalence that many pregnant users and mothers have over seeking treatment, because of fear of social or medical service over-reaction. Many drug services remain with their traditional constituency of white, opiate users rather than broadening their role to stimulant users and black users. As the Task Force to Review Services for Drug Misusers (1996) pointed out, such change may not be easy.

> There is a tendency to adopt simplistic views of ethnic minority communities and ways of addressing their needs. Making drug services accessible and appropriate to them is a complex and sensitive task. It requires a comprehensive assessment of needs and work with representatives from local communities to develop carefully tailored service responses. These responses may include ensuring services have people from ethnic minorities on their staff.

These social factors have profound influences on the direction of addictions nursing as a whole, as well as on individual nurse–client relationships. Add the further complications of Government strategies on alcohol taxation and advertising, the different needs of rural and inner-city populations, generational changes in types and patterns of drug and alcohol use, communities' marginalization of many users into social pariahs and society's medicalized 'pill for every ill' response to life stressors, and a vastly complicated picture emerges.

Generalizations about patterns of use are difficult to make. Each area of the country has its own idiosyncrasies, which nurses in local services need to be aware of. The following demographic review from Babor (1994) is as general a view as is possible in this field. 'Substance use tends to be more prevalent in males than in females, in young adults rather than in the elderly and in the lower socio-economic strata rather than the upper or middle classes. With the exception of nicotine, the more addictive the substance (e.g. heroin), the more marginal the user'.

THE NURSE'S ROLE

'The profession of nursing has not formulated systematically organized knowledge about addictions, nor has theory emerged to guide nursing care of individuals, families, and communities experiencing substance abuse problems. Furthermore, limitations in the alcohol and drug abuse scientific community are a result of the narrow research focus on basic science and reliance on research findings more biological than psychosocial in nature. The dominance of the biomedical model has resulted in more research findings that address the physiology of addiction to alcohol and other drugs than in findings that evaluate comprehensive treatment approaches using psychosocial modalities as well as medical treatment. Few studies have examined health or correlates of health – nursing's central focus'. (Sullivan, 1995).

This American perspective on drug and alcohol nursing is not dissimilar to the British situation. Although UK research has started to broaden its focus to wider issues of addictive and health behaviour, there are few instances of a nursing focus on research, either from nurses undertaking research or from research examining nursing interventions. Although this situation is not unique to addictions, it does seem to be a major stumbling block to advancing the cause of nursing in this area. A number of factors have contributed to this state of affairs, some of which are beginning to change. These include:

- The difficulty for the profession to define its role within the complicated sociolegal context outlined above and the strongly medical treatment paradigm that guides most interventions.
- The dearth of national or international nursing theory to guide research and to construct models of intervention.
- The paucity of national nursing initiatives by professional groups or organizations.
- The lack of any national policy agreement as to good practice in drug and alcohol work.

In response to the uncertainties arising from these factors, this chapter introduces a nursing framework for assessment and intervention (Table 20.1). The structure of the framework will then be used in the rest of the chapter to describe the key knowledge and skills required for nursing in this specialism.

The framework combines drug and alcohol nursing as a single area of practice, although some of the interventions described later in the chapter are traditionally used exclusively for specific substances. The debate over joining or separating drugs and alcohol work will undoubtedly continue for many years, with alcohol services often seen as the poor relation from a funding perspective, and many nurses identify much more with one area than the other. However, many health effects and, even more, intervention skills used, are common to drugs and alcohol problems.

TABLE 20.1 Nursing framework for assessment and intervention

Nursing focus area	Key assessment area	Intervention area
Human development	Current drug and alcohol use.	1. Prevention and screening
	Use of different substances. Career of use. Problem use Dependence. Life cycle issues.	2. Brief interventions 3. Support in pregnancy
Health and well-being	Overdose and withdrawal. Route of use. HIV and hepatitis. Risk assessment.	4. First aid 5. Prescribing 6. Minimise harm
Modifying behaviour	Process of change. Relapse behaviour. High risk situations. Addictive beliefs and behaviour	7. Motivational interviewing 8. Relapse prevention 9. Cognitive therapy
Mental and social health	Mental state. Psychiatric complications. Intra and inter personal issues. Social issues.	10. Mental health advice 11. Dual treatment 12. Solution-focused therapy

HUMAN DEVELOPMENT

CURRENT USE

All assessments should explore the client's current use. Central to this are the substances used, quantities and strengths, routes of use, daily frequency, pattern and regularity during past week and month, and the financing of use. Information about use will usually be obtained from the client although carers and other involved parties may also be able to provide some information, particularly if other services are already prescribing drugs for the client. To be able to appreciate the nature of the drug or alcohol use, assessing nurses will need a clear understanding of the range of use and effects of all commonly used substances, as well as of local and cultural variations in patterns of use and drug constituencies. A general guide on most substances is provided below.

Alcohol

Alcohol is widely available, legal to consume from 5 years of age, legal to buy with a meal from age 16 and otherwise from age 18. It is taken orally, for initial relaxation, stress relief, intoxication and disinhibition, prior to its more sedative effects taking over within an hour or two. It can cause major physical damage to most bodily systems, including long-term psychiatric harm.

Amphetamines

Commonly available in many parts of the country; in areas such as South-West and North-East England this is often the most popular drug. Usually in tablet or powder form, about 3–5% pure (the remainder consists of any adulterants dealers can find), taken orally by snorting or by injecting for an initial high, which may continue for several hours; then may be replaced by a lower mood swing if not readministered, although repeated doses increase likelihood of subsequent depression. Can cause cardiovascular problems, sleep and appetite disturbance and eventual exhaustion.

Benzodiazepines

Commonly available around the country, legally and illegally. Mostly temazepam, though diazepam and other variants can be used. Usually in tablet form after recent restrictions on temazepam gel capsule preparations, taken orally or by injecting solubilized crushed tablets or heated gel. Gives powerfully intoxicating effect, which balances out highs of stimulants or placidity of opiates. Overdose can be fatal in combination with alcohol or opiates.

Cannabis

The most commonly used illicit drug, easily obtainable almost anywhere in the country. Usually in broken leaves or black–brown small lumps of resin, taken by smoking with tobacco or herbal cigarettes or smoked in pipes (sometimes through water), or added to cakes and other food. Gives relaxed, often introspective mood, with mild stimulant and hallucinogenic effect from some more powerful types.

Cocaine

Increasingly available in inner cities and some parts of the country. Usually in fine whitish powder, or as small rocks of crack, taken by snorting or injecting powder, occasionally by mixing with cigarettes or inhaling smoke of heated crack. Gives rapid, physical and psychological high, more intense than with most amphetamines, with crack being the most powerful, though short-lived (under 10 minutes). Further repeated doses common, with similar potential to amphetamines for depression, particularly from repeated crack use.

Cyclizine

Used in limited parts of the country. Usually in tablet form taken orally or injected in solution. Gives strong intoxication and high in conjunction with heroin; this combination, pharmaceutically sold as Diconal, was extremely popular with users in the 1970s, until widely restricted, with crushed, solubilized tablets being injected in large quantities.

Ecstasy

Commonly available in most towns and cities; particularly associated with parties and 'raves'. Usually in tablet form, taken orally. Gives a mixture of stimulant and hallucinogenic effects, with increased energy levels; often popular for dancing. Different varieties available, with different constituents increasing particular effects; some are more 'buzzy' (stimulating) and others more 'trippy' (hallucinogenic). Increasing concerns exist about ecstasy related deaths.

Heroin

Commonly available in most parts of the country though sometimes less so in Scotland. Usually in brownish–whitish powder form, about 30–40% pure, and sometimes in ampoule or tablet form. Taken occasionally by snorting, more regularly by inhaling smoke from powder heated on foil ('Chasing the Dragon') or by injecting. Varied chemical constituencies of heroin from different parts of the world dictate whether it has more effect when smoked (heroin base) or injected (heroin hydrochloride). Gives initial high followed by powerful, relaxing, stress- and pain-relieving effect lasting for several hours. Can depress respiratory system. Overdose most likely to occur when tolerance is lowered after a period of abstinence.

Lysergic Acid Diethylamide—LSD

Commonly available in some parts of the country. Usually in tablet, transfer, or microdot form, taken orally. Gives hallucinatory effect, with some variants being extremely powerful once effect comes on after around 20–30 minutes, lasting for several hours.

Methadone

Widely prescribed and often illegally available synthetic heroin substitute. Usually in liquid, tablet or injectable form, taken orally or by injecting. Gives similar effects to heroin but little 'high' and longer but less powerful effect.

Other Drugs

Strong opiates such as morphine, medium ones such as DF118s and weaker ones such as codeine linctus are all used from time-to-time, when available. Also, opiate-like drugs such as Temgesic are widely used in some areas, notably in parts of Scotland. Steroids, for bodybuilding and self-image, are injected or taken orally. Volatile solvent gases and vapours of volatile solvents, such as glue fumes, aerosol sprays and fire extinguisher gases, are inhaled for a short-term powerful intoxication and can cause sudden death syndrome (cardiovascular–respiratory arrest) on first use. Psilocybin is ingested for a hallucinatory effect through the eating of 'magic mushrooms'. Barbiturates, although rarely used now, were popular street drugs of the 1960s and 1970s and have strong sedative and intoxicating effects with a strong possibility of overdose.

Career of Use

Drug and alcohol use is sometimes viewed as a career path developing over time. For health intervention the most important stages on this path are those of problem use and dependence.

Problem Use

The terms 'problem drug use' and 'problem alcohol use' are commonly used to describe the range of physical, psychological and social difficulties that users can experience. It is important to remember that problems can occur in one area of a person's life while other areas can be problem free, that they can arise from first use or long-term dependence and that they can occur with use of one substance while others can be used with no adverse effects. Edwards *et al.* (1994) described alcohol problems as being:

1. Single-episode acute problems or problems arising from chronic long-term drinking.
2. Related to bingeing or more regular intake.
3. Derived from behaviour while intoxicated or from effects post-intoxication.
4. Always self-induced; may affect others.
5. Caused by direct drinking or by responses to the drinker by external social agencies.
6. Caused by the actual ethyl alcohol or contaminants in the drink.

Dependent Use

Dependence is often defined in terms of severity and is described as a syndrome (Edwards and Gross, 1976; WHO, 1993). This can provide a valuable starting point for debate on the whole concept of addiction (Edwards, 1986). It is important that specialist nurses participate in this debate rather than rejecting its medical premise, as sometimes occurs. Yet even non-specialists need to be aware of the central aspects of dependent use. These include compulsion to use, craving, prioritization of use over other behaviour and, above all, the three key factors of neuroadaptation (the ability of nerve cells to become used to the presence of a drug in the brain), tolerance

(a person's ability to become used to the effects of a substance with the result that increasing amounts are required to achieve the same effect) and withdrawal (the body's autonomic response to the removal of the presence of a substance to which it has neuroadapted and gained tolerance). (Johns, 1990)

LIFE CYCLE ISSUES

Adolescence

Most drug and alcohol use starts during adolescence but, because of age boundaries in services, confidentiality issues and the complexities of this period of life, it can be difficult to identify and address problems of use. Ignoring drug and alcohol interventions with this age group can be perilous, as the Health Advisory Service (1994) have pointed out:

> Approximately one in three adolescents who commit suicide is intoxicated at the time of death, and a further number are under the influence of drugs ... the percentage change in alcohol consumption has the single highest correlation with changes in suicide rates. The implications for prevention and intervention are clear: focusing on drug and alcohol use would have a greater impact on adolescent suicide rates than any other primary prevention programme.

Pregnancy

In general, the most harm occurs from use in the early months of pregnancy, although post-natal withdrawal effects can be very unpleasant for the new-born child. Of particular concern are the probable increased potential for neonates to experience low birth weight, perinatal mortality, congenital abnormalities and sudden infant death syndrome. With alcohol there is conflicting evidence as to damage but concern remains as to the possible existence of fetal alcohol syndrome, where excessive drinking is thought to lead to problems such as growth deficiency, facial defects, congenital heart defects and delayed development.

Gender

Drug and alcohol use can raise specific gender problems. Of particular note are issues for some women drug users who may be introduced to injecting by their male partners, who are more likely than men to have a sexual partner that is an injecting user, and whose lack of power in relationships may limit their ability to negotiate less risky behaviours. Of most concern is the sex industry, with some sex workers trading sex-for-drugs and sex-for-money-for-drugs (see Faugier and Cranfield, 1993, for a detailed review of this area).

Families

The effects of use on families can often be more traumatic than on users themselves but many episodes of client contact concentrate on intervention with individuals only. Assessments may raise family issues but they are often not followed up, i.e., the concept of co-dependence is focused on the dependence of partner or child on the user. This may often be useful in exploring family dynamics but a review of this area by Hands and Dear

(1994) concluded that while it may raise awareness of the needs of partners, particularly women, and is supported by a large self-help literature, it can also reinforce negative cultural expectations of women and be seen as 'unnecessarily pathologizing' their lives.

Family members can gain support from organizations such as Alanon (for families of drinkers) and Alateen (for children of drinkers) that back up support to users of Alcoholics Anonymous and Narcotics Anonymous. But it is important that professional interventions also address such areas. The use of genograms, drawn out with the client like a family tree, can be a valuable assessment tool for exploring family issues but such work should be undertaken with caution by nurses untrained in family work as painful conflicts and emotions can easily be aroused. Solution-focused therapy as described later in the chapter is also useful with family work.

INTERVENTIONS

INTERVENTION AREA

Once an understanding of a client's use and related factors has been gained through assessment, nurses have the potential to match a range of interventions to identified need. Indeed such interventions may well begin during assessment. Interventions should be based, whenever possible, on proven effectiveness, and should be reviewed reguarly with the client to ensure that treatment does not just drift on. Recent educational guidelines for good practice for nurses in this field (English National Board, 1996) emphasize that more primary and secondary nursing care teams come into contact with drug users and drinkers than do specialist nurses. Many of the following intervention areas can be developed by nurses in all settings if appropriate training and clinical supervision on reflective practice is provided.

1–PREVENTION AND SCREENING

Prevention of use, particularly among the under-25s, is a high-profile national target (e.g. Tackling Drugs Together, 1995). It can involve many approaches including the increasingly popular peer education. Nurses can become involved in such work but, especially in schools, it is important that drug and alcohol initiatives are not one-off sessions occasionally brought in from outside. Rather they should be integrated into a developmental health education package within the school or Local Education Authority. Such work starting 'early in a child's school career, which is delivered with optimum persistence and intensity and which uses multiple techniques and seeks actively to involve pupils, has good evidence to support its impact' (ACMD, 1993).

Screening in medical or primary health care settings is a more widespread nursing approach. It involves interviewing numbers of patients to question them on specific health areas, in this case most commonly their alcohol use, collecting information on amounts, patterns and frequency of drinking and effects on health. Most of the research published in this area

concentrates on the role of GPs in such work, but nurses in Accident and Emergency, Mental Health and Primary Care Practice also have the opportunity to expand into effective preventive education. In the USA, Sullivan *et al.* (1994) has described the 'unique qualities of nursing practice' which support this role and how nurses 'can reduce the effects of long-term excessive drinking on the individual, the family, and society'.

INTERVENTION AREA 2–BRIEF INTERVENTIONS

The idea of short, structured minimal intervention packages has been developed predominantly in the alcohol field since the 1960s. This work has been comprehensively reviewed by Bien, Miller and Tonigan (1993). They explored a range of approaches including facilitating appropriate referral, encouraging self-referral, screening, single advice sessions, 3-hour assessments, provision of information on the harm caused by drinking and self-monitoring of drinking behaviour. Their review indicated that such time-limited approaches could be successful, if supported by the following six characteristics, which have been given the acronym FRAMES by Miller and Rollnick (1991).

1. Feedback of current health and risks.
2. Responsibility put on the client to change.
3. Advice given explicitly to change.
4. Menu of options offered.
5. Empathic approach taken rather than authoritarian.
6. Self-efficacy (belief in one's ability to achieve a specific task) reinforced.

Utilizing these elements, it is possible for a nurse to increase the likelihood of delaying or reversing the development of harmful behaviour through simple but effective interventions. Examples include clients keeping a drink diary, in which daily drinking behaviour (what, how much, who with, where, when, with what effect and cost) is recorded and reviewed by client and nurse, and using information booklets as a basis for assessment and advice sessions (Heng *et al.*, 1994).

INTERVENTION AREA 3–SUPPORT DURING PREGNANCY

This has been identified as an area in its own right because of the complexities of pregnancy and drug and alcohol use and the importance of all nurses being able to address these when they arise. The creation of specific pregnancy liaison services such as that described by Dawe *et al.* (1992) with links to a Community Drug Team is becoming increasingly popular. But for all nurses it is important to be wary of the high emotions that can exist in client and nurse alike around the pregnancy issue and the fears that clients may hold of social or medical service reactions to their drug and alcohol use. The main intervention areas for nurses are as follows:

1. Providing accurate information to the client and other involved professionals.
2. Encouraging the client to attend ante-natal care.
3. Counselling on contraception and conception.

4. Advising on gradual reduction of sensible, regular use of unadulterated substances.
5. Advising on withdrawal for mother and baby.
6. Encouraging supervised second trimester detoxification.
7. Encouraging healthy diet and lifestyle.
8. Facilitating links with other services.

Withdrawal can sometimes be undertaken without problems. However, there are particular dangers if large amounts of heroin are abruptly discontinued, if withdrawal occurs in the first trimester, if fitting occurs during alcohol or benzodiazepine withdrawal or if withdrawal symptoms are relieved by vast quantities of adulterated street drugs. Further information can be found from the Institute for the Study of Drug Dependence's guide on this area (1995).

HEALTH AND WELL-BEING

OVERDOSE AND WITHDRAWAL

It is important to differentiate overdose and withdrawl from direct effects of substances to match intervention to need effectively. Overdose of combined sedative substances or following lowering of tolerance is a major concern, as can be withdrawal from some substances. Effects may vary according to the nature and purity of the drug used, the individual and the setting they are in, the route of use, underlying physiological conditions and the expectations of users. West and Gossop (1994) compared withdrawal symptoms of all main drugs including alcohol:

> Withdrawal from all drugs of dependence results in mood disturbances...Sleep disturbance also appears to be widely reported... Withdrawal from alcohol, benzodiazepines and opiates is often associated with somatic symptoms. In the former two cases these can involve sweating, tremors and occasionally seizures. Perceptual disturbances have also been reported. In the case of opiates, flu-like symptoms are often reported, including muscle aches and gastric disturbances.

Length of withdrawal can vary depending on the individual and substance. Stimulants tend to have short periods of a 'crash' with subsequent days of fatigue and depression, while sedating substances may have initial symptoms lasting for a week or more with sleep problems and physical unease continuing for days or weeks afterwards. Of particular note here is that opiate withdrawal, though uncomfortable, carries little harm, whereas alcohol and benzodiazepine withdrawal, with the possibility of fitting, needs close monitoring.

ROUTES OF USE

The route of drug use has been shown to have a major effect on harm and dependence. A series of studies in transition of route (e.g. from snorting to injecting) by the National Addiction Centre has highlighted the potential for intervention to reduce harm (e.g. Strang *et al.*, 1992; Griffiths *et al.*, 1994). The possibility of 'freezing' someone's route of use before injecting commences may well therefore reduce or avoid dependence and further harm.

Non-injecting use is by no means safe, rather it is the lesser of two potential harmful routes. Such harm can include damage to nasal membranes from snorting (particularly cocaine), to lungs from inhaling heated cocaine and heroin smoke (and oxidized foil heated up during heroin smoking), skin rashes around the mouth and throat and mouth damage from volatile solvents.

The physical harm caused by injecting not usually elicited by the substance itself but from injuries done to the injection site by equipment or technique, damage to the circulatory system and wider harm to the body caused by infections passed through sharing of used 'works' (injecting equipment). Injuries to the site include common skin infections, abscesses and subsequent ulcers. Injecting into an artery can cause pain and excessive loss of bright- red arterial blood. This usually happens with users who are either inexperienced in site-selection or who have run out of easily accessible veins and are attempting to inject into areas such as the groin. Damage to the circulatory system includes septicaemia, endocarditis and thrombophlebitis. The formation of blood clots may cause deep vein thrombosis; this, along with the loss of fingers or toes, can often happen in users who inject substances that contain chalk (crushed tablets), gel (temazepam or other capsules) or other impurities that do not dissolve in the bloodstream. Damage is more likely when injectors use infected needles, syringes and other paraphernalia used in the preparation of injections, such as spoons and filters. When this involves the receiving of infected blood or drug solution there is a possibility of the two worst banes of intravenous use, HIV and hepatitis.

HIV

Although nursing assessment will be required for the physical manifestations in seropositive users, the most important specific area for drug and alcohol nursing is risk assessment, which focuses information gathering on specific drug and sexual activity and may seek to provide immediate educational responses to clients who identify risk behaviours. Rhodes (1994) describes a number of areas that may need consideration in risk assessment (Table 20.2).

The relationship between drug or alcohol use and sexual risk behaviour is complex but there is little doubt that disinhibiting effects of some substances may lead to a lesser likelihood of safer sex being negotiated or conducted. The Advisory Council on the Misuse of Drugs (1993) recommended that 'at the very least, safer sexual practices should be discussed with a drug user when contact is first made [not least because this may be the only contact made], perhaps in the context of the client's overall risk behaviour'.

Hepatitis B and C

Both strains of hepatitis are of major concern for drug users. Hepatitis B has infected about 50% of UK drug users (Task Force, 1996) while a recent national survey has found that 1243 drug users had been found hepatitis C positive out of 2081 tested, an incidence of 60%, and estimated that up to 400 000 people in the UK may have contracted this virus through injecting drug use (Waller and Holmes, 1995). Clients should be encouraged to take regular tests for hepatitis and nurses should employ risk assessment strategies, although it is not currently thought that hepatitis C can be transmitted sexually. Hepatitis identification brings with it a public health dilemma: that effective treatments for the liver damage it causes have a prohibitive cost. However, the same prevention issues apply regarding injecting behaviour, and general health advice within assessment is also important in areas such as diet and healthy lifestyle. Hepatitis B vaccination should be available for all drug users, and nurses should advocate its provision if it is withheld.

INTERVENTION AREA 4 – FIRST AID

The extra propensity of substance users for overdose, the possibility of deliberate self-harm while intoxicated and the local site damage caused by many injecting users, means that nurses in contact with this client group need more awareness of first aid than in many mental health nursing settings. Nurses working with drug and alcohol users benefit from attending first aid training, with particular importance being attached to wound dressing, dealing with fits and reacting to respiratory arrest. Knowledge of the recovery position is essential and should be taught to clients and carers where any potential for opiate or sedative overdose is identified.

INTERVENTION AREA 5 – PRESCRIBING

Prescribing Practice

The main aims of prescribing are:

1. To stabilize the user through provision of a regular supply of a substitute drug (regular in amount, availability and pharmaceutical purity).

TABLE 20.2 Risk assessment areas

HIV risk associated with injecting drug use	HIV risk associated with sexual behaviour.
Levels of sharing	Drug effects and social risk
Social context of sharing	Levels of sexual activity
Frontloading *	Levels of condom use
Cleaning equipment	Involvement in prostitution
Drug transitions	Sexual behaviour change
	HIV status and sexual behaviour change
	Social context of sexual encounters

*'Frontloading' is a term that describes the transfer of a drug solution from one syringe to another. It can also be termed 'backloading' depending on whether the second syringe is filled from the front by drawing up or from the rear by injecting into the back with the plunger removed. It is an important area not only in its own right but also in its indication of the variety of behaviours that exist which users may not commonly term 'sharing' but which result in passing of potentially infected solutions from one person to another.

2. To take the first steps towards detoxification or, occasionally, maintenance.
3. To draw the client into service contact to commence other health and social interventions.
4. To reduce criminal and other negative drug-related behaviour (by removing the need to obtain drugs or money for drugs).
5. To achieve detoxification.

Good practice in prescribing requires a thorough assessment of current drug or alcohol use and withdrawal symptoms. For substitute prescribing, an initial titrated dose assessment may be undertaken to ensure that the amount given prevents withdrawal symptoms but does not lead to over-intoxication. A strictly monitored supply is essential, through tight regimes in an in-patient setting, through use of carers when possible in home alcohol detoxification and, for opiate prescribing, through specific controlled prescriptions which can be used to restrict chemist dispensation to daily 'pick-ups'.

Urine Testing and Contracts

With opiate prescribing, urine testing is often undertaken to measure compliance. It is commonplace for many users either to sell their prescribed drugs for ones with a better effect or to use extra drugs in addition ('on top') to their prescription. However, it is rarely good practice to stop or reduce prescribing immediately for such behaviour. Rather such conduct should be seen as indicative of the complexities of addiction and, if urines are tested, the result should be used to explore the difficulties a client may be facing in changing old habits, rather than as a punitive tool with which to attempt to force compliance. Having a contract with the client, in writing, from the outset, to cover responses to non-compliance with the prescription is often a more effective way of working and clients should be encouraged to talk openly and without sanction about using extra drugs, rather than being caught out through a test. Having said that, there are drug users who may show no willingness to change. Prescribing services then need to decide whether this is unacceptable and withdraw their help or whether their expectations are too high and that maintenance is a better solution.

Prescribing Options

For opiate use, the most commonly prescribed substitute drug is the opioid, methadone, taken orally in liquid form. Tablets should be avoided as they may be crushed and injected. Lofexidine is gaining popularity for symptomatic relief prescribing, as an alternative to methadone detoxification but lofexidine and clonidine, also used for symptomatic relief, can each cause hypotension. Some services use injectable methadone, which has the benefit of drawing into treatment clients who are not currently able to move away from injecting behaviour. Injectable prescribing has been criticized as perpetuating damaging behaviour and feeding the black market with easily sold drugs but, although it should only be undertaken by experienced services, there are many nurses who feel that with some chaotic, intransigent clients it can be a powerful agent of change. Benzodiazepine prescribing, like its street use, has moved from primary health care to the drugs field. Though beneficial in detoxification, there seems little evidence to support the current medical vogue for widespread longer-term prescribing.

Other prescribing options include daily dispensed oral methadone from large-scale programmes, which is becoming increasingly favoured by the medical mainstream (Ball and Ross, 1991; Farrell *et al.*, 1994), or the more radical use of other substitute drugs, e.g. diamorphine, amphetamine, and cocaine in reefer, oral or injectable form. Many medical services eschew the latter options as being a costly waste with no proven benefit. Proponents of such practices throw the same charge at methadone and assert that giving clients what they want (which often is not methadone) recruits and retains more clients in treatment, with the belief that users will change when they want to and not when services insist. Nurses will hold their own views in this debate, which illustrates the diversity of views and inconsistencies within the so-called British system of prescribing.

For alcohol, the most common substitute is chlordiazepoxide, which is generally considered much safer than the outdated chlormethiazole. Often there is need for concomitant vitamin treatment to address the dietary problems so common with prolonged alcohol use. Disulfiram may be prescribed post-detoxification as a sensitizing drug that discourages relapse through the experiencing of unpleasant symptoms such as nausea and vomiting when alcohol is consumed. History of fitting or severe delirium tremens or poor physical health would usually lead to such work being conducted in hospital, general or psychiatric, depending on local policy. (There are few specialist alcohol units in existence now.) But, as the Medical Council on Alcoholism's Handbook for Nurses, Midwives and Health Visitors shows (Hartz *et al.*, 1990), a well supported home detoxification course can be useful for clients and families, with nurses taking the leading role.

For cocaine and amphetamines there is still little consensus as to best practice but antidepressants such as desipramine may be used to counteract insomnia, depression and craving, and thioridazine is sometimes used to minimize anxiety.

The Prescribing Relationship

Although doctors sign prescriptions, it is nurses who most often work with the client on their regime. For specialist addiction nurses, the prescribing relationship can prove complex as it involves an externally controlled provision of a major factor in the therapeutic relationship. The currency of the relationship often becomes the drug rather than a movement towards change. For the nurse this brings a tension between a discourse based around the level of the prescription, which is often the client's main concern, and the wider therapeutic goals of examining broader health and lifestyle issues, which are often the nurse's agenda.

INTERVENTION AREA 6–HARM MINIMIZATION

Harm minimization interventions concentrate on health factors related to substance use but general health improvement around areas such as diet, sleep disturbance, pain control and

sexual problems should not be forgotten. Areas of intervention may often include:

- Dietary and nutritional advice.
- Exercise.
- Relaxation.
- Anxiety management.
- Sleep advice and therapies.
- Pain control techniques.

The emphasis should be on empowering the user not only to make immediate health improvements but also to learn methods other than (self) medicated treatments. This may include complementary or natural health interventions such as massage and acupuncture, particularly during withdrawal.

Alcohol

With no prescription to retain client contact, and with a far larger number of potential clients available, alcohol workers have created a wide range of harm-reducing interventions. The introduction of standard units to measure the strength of alcoholic drinks has enabled nurses and other workers to conduct much more detailed discussions with clients over alcohol intake. Many clients do not know how much they are drinking and ready-reckoner unit charts available from organizations such as Alcohol Concern can be useful in raising awareness of health damage.

Another major intervention for alcohol is the concept of controlled drinking, which is a strategy to enable the drinker to take control of and cut down, rather than cease, their intake. This can be seen as an option for many drinkers who have a low degree of dependence. Sceptics claim that severely dependent drinkers can never return to a controlled intake (a view similar to that of Alcoholics Anonymous; once an alcoholic, always an alcoholic). However, the very idea of interventions designed to create control and not just create abstinence allows greater scope for nurses, who can work with clients towards agreed drinking goals while simultaneously addressing other problem areas.

 Box 20.1
Hierarchy of goals for drug users

1. Cessation of sharing of injecting equipment.
2. Cleaning used injecting equipment before use.
3. Using sterile equipment only.
4. Injecting one substance only (i.e. not polydrug use).
5. Avoidance of injecting solublized crushed tablets or melted gel.
6. Injecting pharmaceutically pure substances only.
7. No injecting use.
8. Using substances with no (or at least known) adulterants.
9. Avoiding inhaling use (of crack or heroin).
10. Using one substance only.
11. Using in a safe environment.
12. Avoiding tobacco with use.
13. Using in a restricted manner (amount and frequency).
14. Stop using.

Drug-Related Interventions

It is essential to remember that harm minimization interventions for drugs do not just describe HIV-targeted work, which is in fact more specifically termed 'risk reduction'. Harm minimization interventions are aimed at reducing all harm resulting from drug use. Such harm may derive from the direct effects of the drug itself, the route by which the drug is taken or the behaviour associated with the drug use. A useful structure to guide harm minimization work is a hierarchy of goals (Box 20.1).

Harm minimization advice can be given in any arena, from informal contact via outreach work on the street, to formal contact in syringe exchange schemes, GP practices, A&E and even prisons. Examples of practical advice that could lead to clients progressing through the hierarchy of goals are given in Box 20.2.

MODIFYING BEHAVIOUR

THE PROCESS OF CHANGE

Modifying behaviour lies at the heart of addiction work, such as changing from constant alcohol intoxication to sobriety or from heroin injecting to smoking. Yet until recently there has been little analysis done as to the process of change. The leading work in this area recently has been based on a model of this process developed by the US psychologists Prochaska and DiClemente (1983). They described change not as a one-off event but as a gradual process with separate phrases. This idea immediately allows the possibility of intervention at

several stages in any attempt to change. Prochaska and DiClemente have given several different versions of their model of change. Nurses who come across these are advised to use the one that makes most sense to them but here an adapted five-stage model will be used.

FIVE-STAGE MODEL OF CHANGE

Change is not a single event, rather it occurs in stages. Sometimes there is a great desire for change but it is only partially realized. The five-stage model recognizes the different stages that people go through in an attempt to change. (While acquainting themselves with the five stages, nurses new to this model may benefit from considering a behaviour of their own that they wish to change, e.g. smoking, dieting, exercising, changing jobs etc.) In a model, adapted from Prochanska & Di clemento, 1983, as illustrated in Figure 20.1, clients' behavioural change moves from Precontemplation through the other stages to the achieving of a New Behaviour. The accurate assessment of where a client really is within the model regarding any particular behavioural change is essential. At times nurses may move ahead of, or lag behind, the client in working on behavioural change and joint understanding of the true position is essential for change to be followed through.

Description of the Model of Change

Stage 1 Precontemplation
Change has not really been considered and the behaviour is continuing.

Stage 2 Contemplation
Change is being considered but no more than that. This stage may become chronic for some who get stuck in months or years of consideration.

Stage 3 Planning
While change has not yet occurred, active steps are now being taken to prepare for it. This is a more deliberate, focused and dynamic stage than Contemplation.

Box 20.2 *Harm minimization advice*

- Get clean injecting equipment including filters to help keep chalk out of injecting solutions, sterile water, condoms, dental dams for oral sex, and bins for used equipment from syringe and needle exchange schemes.
- Carefully select and rotate injection sites, avoiding arteries and veins. Learn how to inject safely.
- Ensure syringes and needles are clean before use.
- Negotiate safer sex, use of condoms and diversification of sexual repertoire away from risky activities. Beware of the dangers of drug and alcohol related disinhibitions.
- Beware damage caused by other routes of use such as lung cancer through tobacco with cannabis and throat and heart damage from volatile solvents.
- Improve safety by avoiding new or unreliable dealers, not picking poisonous mushrooms, not crushing tablets and not mixing substances.Beware overdose, particularly when tolerance is lowered after abstinence.
- Increase safety by taking LSD with experienced friends and 'chill out' (cool down) and avoid excess clothes like hats to cool down when using ecstasy.
- Keep healthy — there is more to health than safer use.

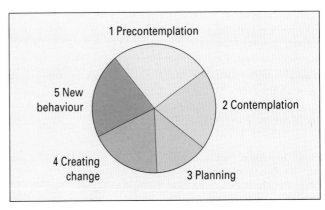

Figure 20.1 Five-stage model of change

Stage 4 Creating change

The person starts to alter what they are doing, thus creating a new behaviour. Change has occurred but needs consolidation to continue.

Stage 5 Achieving new behaviour

Change has occurred and continues. Prochaska and DiClemente term this stage Maintenance (of change) but it is suggested that focusing on a new behaviour rather than the maintenance of change of an old one is an even more positive perspective.

It is essential that this model is seen only as a way of conceptualizing the complications of change rather than as a prescriptive and universal description of the process and that it is seen as:

1. Dynamic, in that people can move backwards and forwards in it.
2. Positive, in that any move towards change, even if not fully realized, is a movement away from previous behaviour.
3. Flexible, in that different people go through different stages for different behaviours at different times.

INTERVENTION AREA 7 – MOTIVATIONAL INTERVIEWING

This is a specific counselling process, with active interventions, usually on a one-to-one basis, designed to develop clients' motivation to bring about change in their lives. It may focus on particular behaviours or the whole process of addiction but is more likely to have effect when targeted in a focused way at particular current issues. It is based on a positive, humanistic view that there is a potential for forward-moving change in all of us and attempts to challenge the thinking and behaviour in clients that blocks their progress to change or contradicts their expressed desire to change. As such it is designed to create a 'cognitive dissonance' in clients in which their claims that change is desired are confronted by behav-

iour that indicates otherwise. As much as possible this confrontation should occur within the client. Although the nurse may use techniques to facilitate this, they should not move into a judgemental and aggressive challenging mode. The dissonance that this creates may produce resistance in the client that Miller and Rollnick (1991) suggest should be rolled with, rather than being either ignored or directly challenged. Therefore, as in some wrestling and martial arts confrontations, the client's own momentum is used to effect change. 'This is not to say that the master is passive. Not at all. He or she adds to the momentum–a little spin, a glance to the side, an extra tug'. Such work is built on eight building blocks as identified by Miller and Rollnick and three main intervention techniques (Box 20.3).

INTERVENTION AREA 8 – RELAPSE PREVENTION

While motivational interviewing focuses on a move to new behaviours, relapse prevention presents the flipside of this process, an attempt to avoid reverting to old ones. It is based on the concept of relapse, an old addiction term usually associated with a return to a previous behaviour pattern, most commonly a reversion to dependent use after a period of abstinence. Within the five-stage model of change relapse can occur at any time. However, because of the connotations of failure that are often associated with the idea of relapse, it is useful with clients to consider any one slip towards the old behaviour (e.g. one drink for an abstinent former drinker) as a lapse which can be easily resolved and which, as was suggested with the model of change, does not mean a return to square one.

The theory of relapse prevention is that, through cognitive–behavioural interventions, the client can learn from such lapses in the past and present and can plan for similar experiences in the future, 'the goal being to teach individuals who are trying to change their behaviour how to anticipate and cope with the problems of relapse' (Marlatt and Gordon, 1985). Success in doing this leads to increased self-efficacy developed through experience of positively coping with adverse or high-risk situations.

High-Risk Situations

These need to be identified in advance and are, most commonly, negative emotional states, interpersonal conflict and social pressure (Marlatt and Barrett, 1994). Other possible danger areas can include negative physical states such as withdrawal, testing out personal control (such as an ex-drinker visiting a pub believing that they can drink only soft-drinks) and responses to urges and cravings. Such situations can occur spontaneously, but as Marlatt and Barrett point out, are often preceded by denial, rationalization, apparently irrelevant decisions to move close to old behaviours (such as going out of the way to drive past a pub) or a lifestyle imbalance in which there are either excessive self-indulgences (wants) or excessive responsibilities (oughts) dominating the client's life, which lead to a desire to escape, i.e. start using again.

Box 20.3 *Motivational interviewing skills*

Building Blocks
1. Giving ADVICE.
2. Removing BARRIERS.
3. Providing CHOICE.
4. Decreasing DESIRABILITY.
5. Practising EMPATHY.
6. Providing FEEDBACK.
7. Clarifying GOALS.
8. Active HELPING.

Intervention techniques.
1. Using open-ended questions.
2. Using active listening, reflecting and summarizing.
3. Using evocative questions.

Wanigaratne *et al.* (1990) provided an excellent description of their relapse prevention programmes for individual and group work in London and included the following interventions:

- Self-monitoring diaries — getting the client to observe and record triggers that result in use and to detail the consequences of use, including physical, emotional, social and financial costs.
- Decision balance sheet — getting the client to record the pros and cons of a behaviour as a basis for deciding whether to continue it. This is useful in assessment and can be recorded in a matrix form with optional additions of pros and cons of changing the behaviour as well as of continuing it.
- Relapse road maps — getting the client to examine past and potential relapses through descriptions of their use as a road map that has danger signs, alternative routes, and blocks and ways of avoiding or diverting from them.
- Cue exposure — getting the client to experience graduated contact with cues to using, for example, substances, equipment and environments and exploring reactions to this and ways of coping with the urges and cravings it brings, thus increasing self-efficacy.
- Substituting behaviours — getting the client to commence new behaviours to take the place of old (e.g. as recreations and more positive addictions such as exercise) and, arguably, support structures such as Alcoholics Anonymous.

INTERVENTION AREA 9–COGNITIVE THERAPY

Although not as established in the field as motivational interviewing and relapse prevention, this area is worth mentioning as it is increasing in popularity because of its focused approach and claims of long-term effect from short-term work. Described in more detail elsewhere in this book, its major theoretical exponent is Aaron Beck (1993). He describes a cognitive model of addiction that has as its main foundation the existence of dysfunctional beliefs. These minimize problems emanating from substance use and maximize difficulties in addressing urges and cravings to use. Cognitive therapy challenges these beliefs.

The approach involves structured sessions, built around mainly open-ended questions that seek to undermine the client's erroneous or limiting belief systems. Once this process has begun, clients are taught to modify their thinking, to cope with painful feelings, to increase the pleasure in their lives and to rehearse cognitive and behavioural responses to high-risk situations. Again this can be linked into the five-stage model of change with which, in the hands of trained nurses, the planning and achieving of behavioural change can be supported by a major internal (cognitive) change.

MENTAL AND SOCIAL HEALTH

CURRENT MENTAL STATE

This area is covered in more detail elsewhere in this book. However, there are some specifically drug and alcohol related psychological issues that may be evident in assessment. These include intoxication, which should be easy to assess with some substances because of smell or 'pinned' pupils (opiates) or restlessness (stimulants, including ecstasy). Often such intoxication results in confusion and lability of mood and, sometimes, aggression, mood changes, and sadness together with aggression. Behavioural manifestations of use include restlessness, agitation, talkativeness, confusion, ataxia, and quiet, introspective detachment; loss of concentration, judgement and memory, and disorientation.

PSYCHIATRIC COMPLICATIONS

As Ghodse (1995) points out, 'The abuse of potent psychoactive drugs does not always produce the desired and sought-after psychic effect but may, on occasion, lead to an abnormal and unwanted mental state'. This can be short-lived as described above or can, at times, continue for long periods with severe mental health problems arising. Often it is the local mental health team, rather than a drug and alcohol agency, that works with clients who have psychiatric problems and continue drugs use. This 'dual diagnosis' (or 'triple' when personality disorder is medically diagnosed) is one in which the original cause (drugs or predisposing mental state) is often obscured and is indeed of little relevance.

INTRA-AND INTERPERSONAL ISSUES

Concentration in the mental health sphere on abnormal states can obscure the fact that many users experience similar personal and relationship problems to the rest of society. Although these can often be dealt with by traditional counselling and mental health interventions described elsewhere in this book, they are worthy of note here as they may be inextricably linked to dependence, and require skilled intervention alongside other addictions work. The potential for some long-term drug and alcohol users to surround themselves with other dependencies, such as destructive relationships, should not be underestimated. At times these may be more positive replacements of substance addiction but they can be equally as destructive.

SOCIAL ISSUES

Although not considered as 'health' issues by the current health–social purchasing divide, the following are areas that need to be addressed by nurses in conducting a full assessment, as they often impact strongly on or are caused by substance use (or alternatively may be an area of strength on which to build), financial difficulties, employment and education, housing or homelessness, legal issues, welfare and benefits, and child care.

Many of these areas are covered in Community Care Assessments from Social Service Care Managers, with whom nurses should ensure good working relationships (often they are based in specialist drug and alcohol services) to effectively advocate for their clients.

INTERVENTION AREA 10–MENTAL HEALTH ADVICE

Although advice on the effects of substance use on mental health may seem straightforward to give (the basic position being that if your health suffers avoid the drug), this is an area much neglected both by specialist addiction services and by mental health nurses. It is therefore worthy of specific emphasis and can be divided into two parts.

Advice During Intoxication

Often intoxication, with the confused, bizarre and sometimes aggressive behaviour which accompanies it, can be easier to avoid than approach. At times this is the best reaction but in some situations such as in A&E departments, with detained patients, or in street agency and outreach locations, intoxicated users need to be dealt with. Usual nursing principles of calm, patient, non-intimidating behaviour apply, with safety the prime factor. Sometimes such users are able to conduct a more therapeutic conversation than when sober, though this should not become a regular interaction. The concept of talking a user down or through their intoxication can be important, particularly when hallucinatory experiences need drawing back to reality. Such work can be time-consuming with little apparent effect but it may occasionally be worthwhile to avoid harm to self or others and may begin a fruitful rapport with a user.

Reducing Harm to Mental Health

As with other harm minimization approaches, the provision of useful advice to users on mental health issues is best conducted through giving accurate information rather than by adopting a tone of moral preaching. Two areas that stand out are, first, the use of excessively intoxicating substances in those users who have a propensity for depression and may act to self-harm while intoxicated (note the connection mentioned earlier between adolescent suicide and substance use) and secondly, the use of stimulant and hallucinatory substances in those users who have the potential for continuing psychosis. The treatment of the latter is addressed below but it may be avoided at times by advice to refrain from or minimize use of substances such as ecstasy, cannabis or LSD, which can be problematic for people who have experienced psychosis in the past.

INTERVENTION AREA 11–DUAL TREATMENT

It is a strange fact of most mental health and addiction treatment services that they are very willing to label a client as having a dual diagnosis but equally unwilling to provide joint care based on that diagnosis. The concept of dual treatment is then a sound one to develop, particularly for mental health nursing, the commonest profession in both types of service. Drake *et al.* (1993) identified a variety of treatment principles for seriously mentally ill patients, with substance use 'the most common co-morbid complication of severe mental illness'.

1. Assertive outreach to engage such clients.
2. Close monitoring to provide structure and social reinforcement.
3. Integration of mental health and addiction interventions.
4. Addressing of wider issues.
5. Safe living environments.
6. Flexible treatment and clinicians.
7. Good timing of interventions.
8. A long-term approach.
9. Optimism.

All these methods should be followed but unless services begin seriously to develop the integration of treatments needed and research into effective outcomes of different treatment settings (drug service, mental health or combined), little progress will be made.

INTERVENTION AREA 12–SOLUTION-FOCUSED THERAPY

This is not an approach exclusive to addiction but it is becoming increasingly popular with drug and alcohol nurses. It avoids any focus on the problems in the client's life, concentrating rather on the search for solutions (Berg, 1991). This is not to deny the existence of problems but the traditional exploration of them is seen as keeping the client and the therapeutic relationship a quagmire where little progress to solution is made. The only reason for problem exploration is to meet clients expectations that they discuss their difficulties. For the nurse practising this approach, every effort should be made to avoid any reference to, or question or reflection on the problem. For most nurses schooled in humanistic counselling this is close to impossible at first.

In the search for a solution there are certain key techniques, as listed below. All of these drive towards an enabling of change within the client. The nurse does not need to know what the problem is. The client knows the problem and needs to find a solution for him- or herself.

1. Identifying what has changed for the better, however small the change.
2. Looking for what is positively different.
3. Searching for positive exceptions to the negative rule.
4. Building on strengths.
5. Exploring 'miracles', 'clients' fantasies of an ideal life.
6. Rating progress, on a scale of 1–10.
7. Setting tasks to work one step up the rating scale.

As with the other major therapy models described in this chapter, considerable training is required for effective practice. However, the concept of moving from a problem focus to an emphasis on solutions is one that all nurses could benefit from.

TOWARDS OUTCOMES IN DRUG AND ALCOHOL NURSING

While the nursing profession has integrated the concept of evaluation into its work for some years now, more progress is needed towards specifically measurable outcomes. This chapter will not attempt to define strict nursing outcomes but will, rather, link the current progress on outcome measurement in the addiction field to some of the nursing interventions described earlier. This is not to say that nurses are unable to create their own outcome measures but to be truly valid these need more research than has been undertaken so far.

The major guide for future outcome measurement for addiction comes from the Department of Health's Task Force Report (1996). This identified three Outcome Domains (drug use, physical and psychological health, social functioning and life context) and a series of measures within each, e.g. reduction in frequency of injecting, arresting deterioration in physical health, reduction in criminal activity. The task for nursing is to develop a similar approach but one that reflects the specific 'nursingness' of interventions, as well as contributing to more generic measures. To achieve such an approach at a clinical level the following guidelines are suggested:

1. Integrate outcome measurement into all stages of the treatment process, before, during and after.
2. Utilize clear, specific and easily measurable behaviours that respond to nursing intervention.
3. Explore different outcome domains, across the four areas of nursing focus discussed in this chapter.
4. Measure outcomes through scales or questions that are unambiguous and scientifically valid.
5. Integrate findings of outcomes into future clinical work.

Building on a detailed outcome review by Marsden (1994) and the recent Task Force recommendations (Table 20.3) provides possible areas for outcome measurement within the nursing framework used in this chapter. These areas are not suggested as being the best nursing outcome domains but, rather, more traditional addiction measures that could reflect nursing intervention as well as input from other disciplines.

TABLE 20.3 Possible nursing outcome areas

Nursing focus area	Key assessment area	Outcome area
Human development	Current drug and alcohol use. Use of different substances. Career of use. Problem use. Dependence. Life cycle issues.	1. Alcohol or drug consumption levels, frequency and mix. 2. Measures of dependence severity. 3. Personal relationships.
Health and well-being	Overdose and withdrawal. Route of use. HIV and hepatitis. Risk assessment.	1. Frequency of sharing and injecting. 2. Detoxification. 3. Physical health.
Modifying behaviour	Process of change. Relapse behaviour. High risk situations. Addictive beliefs and behaviour.	1. Episodes of lapse and relapse. 2. Length of abstinence. 3. Achieving behavioural changes.
Mental and social health	Mental state. Psychiatric complications. Intra- and interpersonal issues. Social and criminal justice issues.	1. Health of Nation Outcome Scores (HoNOS) for mental health. 2. Frequency of crime. 3. Employment or education status.

SUMMARY

Drug and alcohol nursing should be considered as a unified area of practice, as the similarities between the problems raised by alcohol and drugs outweigh the differences. Nurses likely to encounter drug and alcohol users in their clinical practice should explore issues of personal values, language, and the social context of use to be able fully to undertake such work. The increasing links between health and crime make the need to define the role of nursing all the more essential.

The nurse's role in drug and alcohol work is broader than in any other discipline but there is a paucity of nursing theory or research on which to build professional practice. Nursing assessment and intervention with drug and alcohol users should focus on health improvement, harm minimization, modifying behaviour and mental and social health.

Drug and alcohol effects can be directly induced by the substance, can be the result of the route by which the substance is used or can be brought on by withdrawal. Risk assessment for HIV and hepatitis, and broader harm minimization interventions, are key areas for nursing intervention. The most effective way of altering longer-term addictive behaviour relies on cognitive-behavioural models of change in which the commonest intervention areas are motivational interviewing and relapse prevention.

Dual treatment for drug and alcohol users with mental health problems is required to avoid clients falling between addiction and mental health services. Outcome measures need to be developed by nurses over the next few years that clearly demonstrate effectiveness of intervention.

KEY CONCEPTS

- In addictions nursing there is always the awareness of the tension between treatment and social control.
- Nurses likely to encounter drug and alcohol users should explore issues of personal values, language and the social context of use to be able to fully undertake such work.
- Dependence is often defined in terms of severity and described as a syndrome.
- Prevention programmes should be integrated into developmental health education packages in schools or Local Education Authorities.
- The most important specific area for drug and alcohol nursing is risk assessment.
- Harm minimization primarily concentrates on health factors related to the substance use but general health improvement around sleep, diet, sexual problems and pain control should also be included whenever possible.
- Changing behaviour is at the core of addictions work.
- The theory of relapse prevention is that the client can learn from such lapses in the past and can plan for similar experiences in the future.

REFERENCES

Advisory Council on the Misuse of Drugs: *Drug misusers and the criminal justice system. Part 1: community resources and the probation service*. London, 1991, HMSO.

Advisory Council on the Misuse of Drugs: *AIDS and drug misuse update*. London, 1993, HMSO.

Alcohol concern: *Quality in alcohol services: minimum standards for good practice*. London, 1994, Alcohol concern.

Babor T: Overview: demography, epidemiology and psychopharmacology — making sense of the connections. *Addiction* 89(9):1391, 1994.

Ball J, Ross A: *The effectiveness of methadone maintenance treatment. Patients, programs, services and outcomes*. New York, 1991, Springer-Verlag.

Beck A *et al.*: Cognitive therapy of substance abuse. London, 1993, The Guilford Press.

Berg IK: *Family preservation — a brief therapy workbook*. London, 1991, Brief Therapy Press.

Bien TH, Miller WR, Tonigan JS: Brief interventions for alcohol problems: a review. *Addiction* 88(4):315, 1993.

Carroll J: Attitudes of professionals to drug abusers. *BJN* 2(14):705, 1993.

Dawe S *et al.*: Establishment of a liaison service for pregnant opiate-dependent women. *Addiction* 87(6):867, 1992

Drake RE *et al.*: Treatment of substance abuse in severely mentally ill patients. *J Nerv Ment Dis* 181(3):606, 1993.

Edwards G: The alcohol dependent syndrome: a concept as a stimulus to enquiry. *Br J Addiction* 81(3):171–183, 1986.

Edwards G *et al.*: *Alcohol policy and the public good*. Oxford, 1994, Oxford University Press.

Edwards G, Gross M: Alcohol dependence: provisional description of a clinical syndrome. *BMJ* 1:1058, 1976.

English National Board for Nursing, Midwifery and Health Visiting: *Substance use and misuse: Guidelines for good practice in education and training of nurses, midwives and health visitors*. London, 1996, English National Board.

Farrell M *et al.*: Methadone maintenance treatment in opiate dependence: a review, *BMJ* 309:997, 1994

Faugier J, Cranfield S: *Making the connection. Health care needs of drug using prostitutes*. Manchester, 1993, School of Nursing, University of Manchester.

Ghodse H: *Drugs and addictive behaviour – a guide to treatment*. Oxford, 1995, Blackwell Science.

Goodsir J: Civil rights and civil liberties surrounding the use of cocaine and crack. In Bean P: *Cocaine and crack. Supply and use*. London, 1993, Macmillan Press.

Griffiths P *et al.*: Transitions in patterns of heroin administration: a study of heroin chasers and injectors. *Addiction* 89(3):301–309, 1994.

Hands M, Dear G: Co-dependency: a critical review. *Drug Alcohol Rev* 13(4):437, 1994.

Hartz C *et al.*: *Alcohol and health. A handbook for nurses, midwives and health visitors*. London, 1990, Medical Council on Alcoholism.

Health Advisory Service: *Suicide prevention — the challenge confronted*. London, 1994, HMSO.

Heng S *et al.*: Adding value to early client contact. *New dir stud alcohol group* 19:7, 1994.

Institute for the Study of Drug Dependence: *Drugs, pregnancy & childcare — a guide for professionals.* London, 1995, ISDD.

Johns A: What is dependence?. In: Ghodse H, Maxwell D: *Substance abuse and dependence: a guide for the caring professions.* London, 1990, Blackwell.

Marlatt GA, Barrett K: Relapse prevention. In: Galanter M, Kleber H: *The American Psychiatric Press textbook of substance abuse treatment.* Washington, 1994, American Psychiatric Press.

Marlatt GA, Gordon JR: *Relapse prevention, maintenance strategies in the treatment of addictive behaviours.* London, 1985, The Guilford Press.

Marsden J: *Treating alcohol and drug problems: A review of assessment domains, outcome measures and instruments.* London, 1994, Report prepared for the Department of Health.

Miller WR, Rollnick S: *Motivational interviewing — preparing people to change addictive behaviour.* New York, 1991, The Guilford Press.

Prochaska J, DiClemente C: Stages and processes of self change of smoking, and towards a more integrative model of change. *J Consult Clin Psychol,* 51(3):390, 1983.

Rhodes T: *Risk intervention and change — HIV prevention and drug use.* London, 1994, Health Education Authority.

Strang J *et al.*: First use of heroin: changes in route of administration over time. *BMJ* 304:1222, 1992.

Sullivan EJ: *Nursing care of clients with substance abuse.* St. Louis, 1995, Mosby Year Book.

Sullivan EJ *et al.*: The role of nurses in primary care. Managing alcohol-abusing patients. *Alcohol Health Res World* 18(2):158, 1994.

Tackling Drugs Together: *A strategy for England 1995–1998.* London, 1995, HMSO.

Task Force to Review Services for Drug Misusers: *Report of an independent review of drug treatment services in England.* London, 1996, Department of Health.

Waller T, Holmes R: The sleeping giant wakes, hepatitis C: scale and impact in Britain. *Druglink,* 10(5):8, 1995.

Wanigaratne S *et al.*: *Relapse prevention for addictive behaviours: A manual for therapists.* London, 1990, Blackwell.

West R, Gossop M: A comparison of withdrawal symptoms from different drug classes *Addiction* 89(9):1483–1489, 1994.

WHO Expert Committee on Drug Dependence: *Twenty-Eighth Report.* Geneva, 1993, WHO.

FURTHER READING

Berridge V, Edwards G: *Opium and the people: Opiate use in Nineteenth Century England.* New Haven, 1987, Yale University Press.

English National Board for Nursing, Midwifery and Health Visiting: *Project on meeting the education and training needs of nurses, midwives and health visitors in the field of substance misuse.* London, 1995, English National Board.

Gossop M: *Living With Drugs.* London, 1993, Ashgate.

Health Advisory Service: *The substance of young needs. Services for children and adolescents who misuse substances.* London, 1996, HMSO.

Kennedy J, Faugier J: *Drug and alcohol dependency nursing.* London, 1989, Heinemann Professional Publishing Ltd.

• Chapter •

21

Concepts and Treatment
of Eating Disorders

Learning Outcomes

After studying this chapter you should be able to:

- Define an eating disorder.

- Review the incidence and prevalence of eating disorders.

- Describe the completion of a thorough nursing assessment..

- Define the eating patterns and physical, psychological and social behaviours that maintain an eating disorder.

- Define the nature of the therapeutic alliance.

- Compare two approaches to treatment, i.e. in-patient and out-patient..

- Discuss the influence of family therapy and the usefulness of family interventions in treatment..

- Identify possible problem areas for patients and discuss which treatment interventions may be helpful for the patient..

- Develop a strategy for evaluating the care offered.

- Discuss areas that may be useful to research.

CHAPTER OUTLINE

- *Anorexia nervosa*

- *Incidence and prevalence of eating disorders*

- *Nursing assessment, planning and intervention*

- *Bulimia nervosa*

- *Aetiology*

---

*E*ating disorders have been increasing in importance at *the end of the 20th Century. This is because a sister condition to anorexia nervosa, bulimia nervosa, emerged in the 1970s. In the West bulimia nervosa is more common than anorexia nervosa and its influence is spreading globally as Western culture permeates the world. In addition the severity of anorexia nervosa is worsening, the illness runs a more chronic course and the need for impatient beds is rising. Anorexia nervosa is now the third most common chronic illness in adolescence.*

ANOREXIA NERVOSA

Anorexia nervosa, perhaps more than any other psychiatric illness, is the subject of morbid fascination by the press. It has been labelled 'the slimmer's disease'. Unlike any other mental illness it is portrayed in cartoons and in comedy shows. This media attention only serves to trivialize the illness. Both public and professionals discount it as a problem of 'women behaving badly'. There is the assumption that it is under voluntary control and chosen. Those who work closely with sufferers know that this is far from the case. As in any other form of mental illness the sufferers see themselves as having no choice. It is recommended that, to gain some understanding of eating disorders, this chapter is supplemented by reading some of the personal accounts of the illness (Wilkinson, 1981; Wolf, 1994). Sheila Macleod has written an illuminating biography in which she has tried to explain her illness:

I did the only thing I could: I became anorexic. There was nothing conscious or deliberate about my decision, if indeed it can be called a decision at all.

Macleod (1981)

Anorexia nervosa is a severe mental illness. It is the third most prevalent chronic illness in teenage girls (Lucas *et al.*, 1991). The mortality rate is twice that of any other psychiatric illness (Patton, 1988; Sullivan, 1995). The standardized mortality rate lies between 12- and 15-fold that of the general population and the suicide rate is 200 times higher. The illness also has a protracted course. In a classic study, which followed a cohort of Swedish patients over 30–40 years, the median duration of illness was 6 years (Theander, 1985). Unusually for a psychiatric illness there is a greatly increased risk of physical ill health, such as circulatory and gastrointestinal problems and osteoporosis.

HISTORICAL OVERVIEW

Throughout the ages, accounts of girls and women appearing to have no appetite or to be able to exist without eating have appeared. In many ways these resemble contemporary cases of anorexia nervosa. Making a historical diagnosis has its pitfalls (see Russell, 1995, for a detailed summary). The explanations for abnormal behaviour are usually specific to individual cultures (Schmidt and Treasure, 1993). For example, in early Christian societies food restriction and other ascetic practices were understood to show spiritual commitment (Bemporad, 1996). Rudolph Bell in his book *Holy Anorexia* (1985) has researched several historical figures, including Catherine of Sienna, who, he suggests, may have been suffering from anorexia nervosa.

The self-induced starving state became medicalized in the later half of the 19th Century with the separate works of William Gull (1873) and Charles Lasegue (1873). In this context the inability to eat was expressed in terms of vague gastrointestinal symptoms. The emergence of a 'fear of fatness' as an explanation is a modern phenomenon and some cross-cultural psychiatrists, such as Lee *et al.* (1993), suggest that it may be a Western artefact. Lee bases his argument upon their meticulous examination of Chinese cases of anorexia nervosa. Less than half of the cases have ideas about weight and shape as part of their phenomenology. A large proportion resemble the cases of 19th Century anorexia nervosa in Europe, in that there is a focus on somatic, gastrointestinal explanations. Katzman and Lee (1996) suggest that a phobia of 'loss of control' may be an explanation of the behaviour that is less culture bound. Self-starvation has meaning as a method that allows sufferers to be in control.

DIAGNOSES AND DEFINITIONS

Current definitions are given in Table 21.1. Over the last decade the classification of eating disorders has been in a state of flux and is very confusing. The recent trend has been to create subcategories with the result that anorexia nervosa can be divided into two subtypes, restricting and binge–purge. The definition of bulimia includes a specific frequency of bingeing, i.e. twice per week. It is self-evident, and has been found in research studies, that someone who only binges once a week is not very different to someone who binges twice a week. Rather than take a global diagnosis therefore, it is probably preferable to identify problem areas that are causing concern, for example, emaciation, vomiting, rumination etc.

INCIDENCE AND PREVALENCE OF EATING DISORDERS

There is little evidence that the incidence of eating disorders has increased over time (Lucas *et al.*, 1991; Fombonne, 1995). A recent large study in primary care in the UK found the incidence to be 4:100 000 total population (Turnball *et al.*, 1996). Adolescents aged between 10 and 19 were the group at greatest risk with an incidence of 34 per 100 000. The lifetime prevalence rates for all females are 0.5–1.0%. Only 4% are males. There is little evidence of a class bias, although

TABLE 21.1 Current classification and definition (the main points of ICD10 (WHO 1992) and DSM-IV (APA 1996) combined)

Anorexia nervosa	Bulimia nervosa
Body weight at least 15% below that for normal/expected age and height.	Recurrent bouts of overeating at least twice a week over a 3-month period. Large amounts of food eaten in a 2 hour period, more than most would eat during a similar period. Overeating can be defined according to research criteria.
Weight loss is self-induced.	Persistent preoccupation with eating, compulsion to eat. A sense of lack of control over eating.
Self-perception of being too fat.	Use of: self-induced vomiting, laxatives, purging, diuretics, alternating periods of starvation, drugs to stimulate metabolism, appetite suppressants, thyroid preparations, compensatory behaviour to prevent weight gain, exercise.
Absence of three consecutive menstrual cycles when otherwise expected.	Self-perception of being too fat.
Denial of the seriousness of low body weight.	The condition does not occur only during episodes of anorexia; the sufferer can have a normal weight for age and height.

there is a suggestion that those with a greater level of education are at higher risk. (For an example of the clinical features of anorexia see Case study: anorexia nervosa.) The following features are commonly found in people with anorexia nervosa:

- There is usually a severe life event or difficulty as a trigger.
- Predisposing family backgrounds may include a sensitivity to weight and shape and high parental expectations.
- Perfectionistic personality traits are usual.
- Weight loss usually occurs from a mixture of dietary restrictions, in particular, avoiding fats and over-exercise.
- The degree of weight loss may be disguised by wearing layers of clothes.
- There may be no explanation for not eating.
- Sufferers commonly deny that they have a problem and refuse to accept help.

AETIOLOGY

It has been impossible to establish any one factor as necessary and sufficient to explain the onset of anorexia nervosa. The 'catch-all' term is that the aetiology is multifactorial. Furthermore, it is difficult to separate factors that cause the illness from those that enable it to be maintained. It is probable that our culture is one that serves to maintain the illness, which could explain the increasing severity and hence greater prevalence.

SOCIOCULTURAL FACTORS

Many feminist writers have suggested that the changing role of women, leading to major discrepancies in attitudes and expectations between generations, may be of importance (Katzman and Lee, 1996). For a review of this area see Fallon *et al.* (1994). It is uncertain whether this form of difficulty is either necessary or specific for the development of anorexia nervosa.

Dieting

It is unlikely that dieting is a necessary causal factor as anorexia nervosa has been found, and does occur, in cultures in which dieting is rare. Nevertheless, in a culture in which slimness is highly esteemed as a sign of moral virtue, fashionable chic and medical necessity will serve powerfully to maintain the illness.

Psychosocial Stress

Stress has been recognized to be an aetiological factor from the earliest descriptions of the condition (Morton, 1694).

> Mr Duke's daughter in St Mary Axe, in the year 1684, and in the eighteenth year of her age, in the months of July fell into a total suppression of her Monthly Courses from a multitude of Cares and Passions.... From which time her appetite began to abate.

Russell includes this concept in his definition of the illness:

> It may suffice to establish that the patient avoids food and

induces weight loss by virtue of a range of psychosocial conflicts whose resolution she perceives to be within her reach through the achievement of thinness or the avoidance of fatness

(Russell, 1995)

These clinical descriptions are borne out by research (Schmidt *et al.*, 1993b). On the other hand, stress is implicated as important in many functional and organic illnesses and, on its own, it has little explanatory power. It may be the type of stress that is important. Events associated with sexual disgust, so-called pudicity (Schmidt *et al.*, 1993b) or cultural conflict (as described above) may be of specific relevance. On the other hand, it may be that these merely represent typical adolescent issues. An alternative explanation is that it is not the stress *per se* but the way that it is handled that is important. People who go on to develop anorexia nervosa tend to use avoidant coping strategies (Troop *et al.*, 1994).

FAMILY FACTORS

Two schools of family therapy, that of Minuchin (1978) and Selvini-Palazzoli *et al.* (1978) have written with flair and authority about the family factors that may contribute to anorexia nervosa. Minuchin described an interactional pattern that included enmeshment, rigidity, over-involvement and lack of conflict resolution. These models have not proved to be inevitable or specific. Some of the behaviours probably result from concerns about having a child with a chronic severe illness. For example, the degree of enmeshment and over-involvement is not greater than that seen in families with a child with cystic fibrosis. On the other hand, families with a member with anorexia nervosa appeared to be less able to solve problems. This may be as much a maintaining factor as a causal one. The family may have a greater concern about weight and shape issues than the population at large.

INDIVIDUAL FACTORS

The rarity of anorexia nervosa and the fact that it is unusual to have more than one case per family suggests that unique environmental or individual vulnerability factors are causally important.

Genetic Factors

There is a higher risk of anorexia nervosa among family members. Evidence that this is a result of genetic factors rather than a shared environment comes from twin studies which have found that identical twins are both much more likely to have the illness than non-identical twins (Treasure and Holland, 1995).

Psychological Factors

Obsessional personality traits, in particular perfectionism, are common premorbid characteristics. Often this leads to the pursuit of academic or athletic excellence.

PHYSICAL CONSEQUENCES

Anorexia nervosa results in dangerous physical complications. It is important that anyone working with a patient can obtain medical expertise when necessary. It is impossible in this chapter to give more than a brief summary of the complications but the interested reader is recommended to more detailed medical texts (Bhanji and Mattingly, 1988; Treasure and Szmuckler, 1995). Examples of signs you should look out for in anorexia nervosa are shown in Figure 21.1.

INVESTIGATIONS

The most commonly used investigations are blood tests.
• Tests for anaemia and low white cell count are common.

Platelets are low only when weight loss is severe. This indicates that the bone marrow is failing.
• Abnormalities in plasma electrolytes occur if there is vomiting or laxative abuse. (Most commonly, potassium and bicarbonate are decreased; lowered sodium can occasionally occur.) This can lead to circulatory and renal failure.
• Liver function tests can be raised with severe weight loss, indicating liver damage.
• Low urea and plasma proteins indicate severe protein deficiency.

In addition, the electrocardiogram can show a prolonged Q–T interval and U waves. This reflects the effects of salt

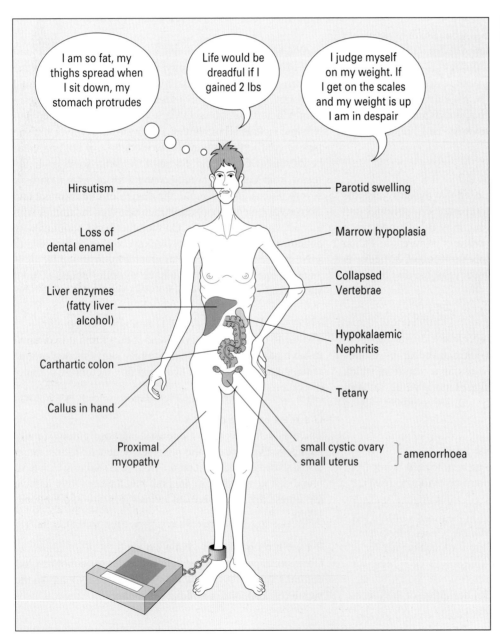

Figure 21.1 The symptoms and signs of anorexia nervosa

imbalance on the heart. Special X-ray scans show severe loss of bone substance, i.e. osteoporosis. This reflects the inability to maintain the balance of bone formation and resorption.

NURSING ASSESSMENT, PLANNING AND INTERVENTION

A complete range of personal details needs to be assessed (Table 21.2).

MODELS OF TREATMENT

Management guidelines have been produced by national groups, e.g. American Psychiatric Association (1993), Royal College of Psychiatrists (1992), Eating Disorders Association (1995). Very little of their content is 'evidence based'; rather, it is based on clinical utility.

Patients with anorexia nervosa are unusual in that they rarely come to seek medical help without any reservations. Their motivation to get help varies. The model of Prochaska and Di Clemente (1986) is helpful in understanding this. In it there are five stages of change:

TABLE 21. 2 Planning for anorexia nervosa

Areas of assessment	Rationale
Safety (usually this is for self; rarely is this an issue for others).	It is unusual for someone with anorexia nervosa to have insight into the dangerousness of the condition. Starvation is the main threat but self-harm is also common, with suicide accounting for half the mortality.
Eating habits, restricting or bingeing. The association of food with the life history.	To determine the pattern and chronology of the eating disorder and to link it with stress to explore the meaning of the symptom.
Weight restriction methods – laxatives, exercise, drugs. Attitudes towards own weight and shape.	To examine for the relevant physical consequences.
What are the patient's physical concerns? How long have they been with no periods? What is their physical stamina? Are there any changes to skin and hair? Physical examination, height and weight, blood pressure, investigations.	To assess the degree of physical damage.
How has the eating disorder affected social life – friends, close relationships, living conditions? How has the eating disorder interfered with education or career prospects?	To establish how the eating disorder has disrupted long-term goals. To explore core values. To examine possible sources of social support.
To examine how the eating disorder has affected mood.	Irritability and temper tantrums, depression and obsessional behaviour are frequently seen and can maintain the problem.
In what way has the eating disorder interfered with financial security?	To discover if the disorder is costing excessive amounts of money. This is usually the case with bulimia nervosa. Is the patient is able to spend money on herself/himself?
In what way has the eating disorder led to an increase in risk taking behaviour, drugs, alcohol, casual sex, stealing. Has it led to getting into trouble with the law?	These sorts of complications are more common in anorexia nervosa of, for example, the binge–purge subtype.
In what way has it interfered with family life? What about the relationship with parents or ability to look after the patient's own children? What is the history of relationships? Are there any relatives with a psychiatric problem or eating disorder? Has the patient experienced losses, personal trauma – abuse, rape. Have there been long running conflicts? Has the patient not been allowed to be the child in the family?	What are the past and current interpersonal difficulties? The precipitating trauma is usually an interpersonal event. Difficulties with earlier relationships may be played out in current relationships, especially in a therapeutic setting.
Summarize the patient's view of the eating disorder. How ambivalent are they? Do they want treatment?	Assess the degree of motivation.

1 Precontemplation — neither interested in nor considering change.
2 Contemplation — considering change.
3 Preparation — being ready to change.
4 Action — embarking on change.
5 Maintenance — sustaining the change.

Over half of the patients with anorexia nervosa who come to the clinic are in the precontemplation and contemplation stages (Ward *et al.*, 1996; Blake *et al.*, 1996). That is, they are not ready to actively change their behaviour. This means that interventions that focus active change will be resisted or ignored. It is usually helpful to involve the family in treatment. This is self-evident in the case of children but may be critical even in adults. This is discussed further below.

THERAPEUTIC ALLIANCE

The resistance to change and rejection of any offers of help and advice can lead to difficulties in the therapeutic relationship unless it is understood. High levels of therapist frustration, treatment resistance and non-compliance are reported by therapists about eating disorder patients (Burket and Schramm 1995). Maladaptive therapeutic relationships are common and include:

- Polarization of therapist's behaviour, resulting in attempts to counteract the anorexic behaviour through indulgence or punishment.
- 'Superparent' – covertly aggressive displays of authoritarian power or superior knowledge, possibly with rescue fantasies.

IN-PATIENT TREATMENT

It has been traditional to use in-patient treatment for anorexia nervosa (for review see Treasure *et al.*, 1995). The basic model is for the nurses to take control of eating away from the patient. How this is done varies. Strict behavioural regimes are no more effective than more lenient approaches. However, there is always a need to balance the reluctance of the patient to change with the nurse's responsibility for the patient's long-term health. Managed care or other forms of health care rationing have led to limitations of the length of in-patient stays in the USA and expectations about treatment, such as a 1 kg per week weight gain in private clinics in the UK.

In-patient treatment for anorexia nervosa is successful in the short term but the relapse rates are high (Mckenzie and Joyce, 1992). Several studies have addressed the issue of therapy to prevent relapse after in-patient treatment. In adolescents, family therapy prevented relapse after in-patient care, whereas individual therapy was more effective in older patients (Russell *et al.*, 1987). This suggests that there may be an interaction between patient characteristics and therapy. Further work in progress at the Maudsley Hospital has not defined which intervention is of most value for the older subgroup. A multicentre study in the USA is examining the use of cognitive behavioural treatment, fluoxetine or combined treatment to prevent relapse in anorexia nervosa. In many parts of the world in-patient admission rates for anorexia are increasing. In part this is the result of readmissions (Williams

and King, 1987; Nielsen 1990; Munk-Jorgensen *et al.*, 1995) whereas those for all other psychiatric disorders are decreasing. Less intensive models of treatment have also been tried. Several centres are using day patient treatment, which is successful for milder cases. However, a proportion of patients with severe illness will require in-patient care.

A few small studies have indicated that out-patient treatment alone can be effective in adult anorexia nervosa (Hall and Crisp, 1987; Channon *et al.*, 1989; Crisp *et al.*, 1991; Treasure *et al.*, 1995). Various forms of out-patient therapy have been tried including dietary advice and cognitive behavioural, cognitive analytical and dynamic therapy. None of the studies have been large enough to detect differences among these types of therapy, although a study in progress at the Bethlem and Maudsley Hospital has found that 'expert' therapy is much more effective than supportive treatment given by trainees.

INVOLVING THE FAMILY

In patients under the age of 18 family therapy was found to prevent relapse after in-patient treatment. However, later research has found that family counselling (which involves the parents being seen on their own for education and support and the child being seen individually) is as effective as family therapy and is preferred by most (Le Grange *et al.*, 1992; Dare and Eisler 1995). Education about anorexia nervosa and emotional support to combat the frustration and irritation from living with this chronic disease can also be provided by carers' support groups. These are frequently used as an adjunct to in-patient therapy. The aims of the group facilitator are to defuse negative emotional reactions such as criticism and hostility and to foster good problem-solving strategies.

DRUG TREATMENT

Various drugs have been tested as adjuncts to in-patient therapy. None has been found to lead to more effective weight gain than standard nursing care. There may be a problem with design in that there may be a ceiling effect. As mentioned above, some of the newer antidepressants that act on 5-HT systems have been found to be effective in open studies. Whether they will prove to be effective in the long term remains to be seen. Palliative treatment, such as potassium replacement or hormone replacement therapy, may be of value in cases with a poor prognosis. Similarly, severe anxiety and distress associated with weight gain can, in some cases, be managed with small doses of phenothiazines.

EVALUATION OF OUTCOME

One of the simplest, yet most difficult, aspects of anorexia nervosa is that the response to treatment, that is, weight gain, is so easy to measure. Although improvement in family functioning or social life can occur without weight gain, these positive benefits may be superficial improvements to please the therapist. It is usual for most aspects to improve as weight increases, unless bulimia develops.

Anorexia nervosa runs a protracted course in the majority of cases. As appears to be the case in all fields of psychiatry, the 'rule' of thirds applies. A third eventually recover, although many of these will have persistent abnormal attitudes to food and body shape. A third will have a poor outcome and remain persistently emaciated, with severe health complications and perhaps requiring hospital care. The other third have a moderate degree of debility. As discussed earlier the mortality is up to 15 times that of the general population. Over the course of 20 years, approximately 20% will have died. Those with a long duration of illness, a severe degree of weight loss and many previous attempts at treatment have a poor prognosis, as do patients with poor social or family functioning before the illness began.

BULIMIA NERVOSA

In 1979 Russell wrote his seminal paper 'Bulimia nervosa: an ominous variant of anorexia nervosa'. This was quickly accepted as a new psychiatric illness and bulimia was incorporated into DSM-111 criteria in 1980 (APA, 1980). Since this time the diagnostic criteria have been more clearly specified and both the US and the WHO systems of classification recognize bulimia nervosa.

Bulimia nervosa appears to be a recent, culture-specific syndrome. It may be a modern expression of distress that, in the past, may have been expressed in conditions such as hysteria, depression or neurasthenia (Russell and Treasure, 1985)(see Case studies on page 318).

EPIDEMIOLOGY
Since its recent description bulimia nervosa has overtaken anorexia nervosa as the most common presentation of eating distress. The number of cases presenting for treatment to primary care has been increasing. Between 1988 and 1993 the number of new cases presenting for treatment increased three-fold. The incidence is 12:100 000 (Turnbull *et al.*, 1996). It is uncertain how much this increase is the result of new cases developing or whether it is because patients and their doctors are recognizing the problem. A large twin study in the USA supports the concept of new cases arising (Kendler *et al.*, 1991). They found that women born before 1960 rarely had bulimia nervosa but the risk of bulimia was much greater in those born after this time. Males account for only 4%. Bulimia nervosa affects women from all social classes. Women between the ages of 20 and 39 are the most common group presenting for care. The following are common features found in people with bulimia nervosa:
- A family history of obesity.
- Events in childhood which damage self-confidence or a secure sense of identity.
- Concern about weight or diet in the family.
- Life events involving relationships triggering the onset of the illness.
- Dieting precedes the illness.
- Impulsive self-harm.

AETIOLOGY

SOCIOCULTURAL FACTORS
The investment of feminine identity in physical appearance is an important factor in bulimia nervosa (Wolf 1992; Kilbourne 1995). Wolf suggests that the campaign for thinness might be part of a male conspiracy to make women feel bad about themselves because men fear the consequences of equality.

Dieting
Dieting is closely linked to bulimia nervosa. In a prospective study of schoolgirls it was found that those who dieted had an 8-fold greater risk of developing bulimia nervosa (Patton, 1988). Other evidence supports this. The emergence of bulimia nervosa as an illness closely parallels the rise of the 'slimming industry'. Dieting is an inevitable precursor in the clinical history. Groups in which dieting is more common, for example models, dancers, dieticians and the obese, have higher rates of the illness.

Stress
Life events and difficulties commonly precede bulimia nervosa (Schmidt *et al.*, 1993b). These usually involve relationship difficulties. The patient is directly involved in the problem, for example there may be a conflict between the subject and one of the parents or friends.

FAMILY FACTORS
Adverse childhood experiences are a common antecedent to bulimia nervosa (Schmidt *et al.*, 1993c). These include physical and sexual abuse and neglect or emotional deprivation. There is, however, no specific link between sexual abuse and bulimia nervosa. The prevalence of abuse in eating disorders is no higher than in other psychiatric illnesses (Palmer and Oppenheimer, 1992).

INDIVIDUAL FACTORS

Genetic
There is much less evidence that genetic factors are as important as in anorexia nervosa (Treasure and Holland, 1995), although evidence from a large twin study suggests that genetic factors do play a role (Kendler *et al.*, 1991). However, the genes may not be specific for bulimia nervosa but load for other risk factors. In families with bulimia nervosa there is a higher risk of depression, substance abuse and obesity.

Psychological
There are several psychological vulnerability factors. Low self-esteem and poor self-identity are common; marked perfectionistic personalities are also found. Frequently there is a tendency towards impulsive behaviour. At its extreme this is manifested as borderline personality disorder.

PHYSICAL CONSEQUENCES

The weight controlling methods are usually responsible for the physical consequences. Vomiting leads to parotid swelling and loss of dental enamel and tooth substance. Traumatic damage to the upper gastrointestinal tract can also occur. The loss of stomach acid leads to potassium loss from the kidney. In turn this can cause tetany and cardiac arrhythmias. The dehydration caused by vomiting can lead to circulatory failure (perhaps shown by fainting), acute renal failure or renal stones. Rebound oedema sets in whenever there is a change in symptoms. Laxative abuse also can lead to a similar picture of salt and water imbalance. Abuse of slimming agents and caffeine can lead to anxiety, sleep disturbance and even a psychotic reaction. The drive to exercise can result in stress fractures or other musculoskeletal injury.

INVESTIGATIONS

Blood tests are needed to monitor the haemoglobin level, which may be raised because of haemoconcentration. Low potassium and high bicarbonate levels are common.

ASSESSING AREAS OF NEED
(See Table 21.3.)

TREATMENT FOR BULIMIA NERVOSA

Patients with bulimia nervosa differ from those with anorexia nervosa in that they are more motivated to seek help. More than 80% are in the action phase. Nevertheless on further assessment they frequently reveal themselves to be ambivalent about giving up their weight control strategies. They would like to stop bingeing but they are reluctant to stop dieting.

THERAPEUTIC RELATIONSHIP

Difficulties with the therapeutic alliance in patients with bulimia nervosa are more openly expressed, in that the patients are frequently late or miss appointments. Many patients appear to be engaged during the session but then fail to keep a diary or any of the other tasks that have been set. Some patients appear very different during, and between, sessions. At times they appear distressed and requesting help and advice and yet the next minute they are rebellious and stubbornly resistant or distant and cut off. This pattern is seen at its most extreme in patients with a borderline personality disorder.

TABLE 21.3 Planning for bulimia nervosa

Areas of Assessment	Rationale
Danger to self.	Patients with BN often have poor impulse control. This leads to self harm by poisoning, cutting, promiscuity, alcoholism.
Weight control methods.	To evaluate physical condition. Apart from laxatives and vomiting, many other drugs and dangerous practices can be used e.g. aspirins, paracetamol, blood letting.
What are the physical concerns: teeth, GI tract?	To discover physical problems and to generate self motivation
How has her social life been affected?	There will be few friends who know about the problem. Difficulties with relationships may exist.
Has her education or career been disrupted?	There may be an inability to work.
How has her mood been affected?	Depression and instability of mood is commonly associated with BN.
What about financial security?	Debts can mount up from large amounts of money spent on laxatives and food. Impulsive shoplifting is common.
What about family life?	Family members may be kept at bay. Children become aware of the eating disorder and may copy the behaviours. Abnormal attitudes to shape and weight may be transmitted to their children.
What about relationships now and in the past?	Has there been a pattern of disturbed relationships. Abnormal experiences with important care-givers will affect your therapeutic relationship. Grief, conflicts, changes of roles may need to be processed.

THE FORM AND CONTENT OF THERAPY FOR BULIMIA NERVOSA

In contrast to the paucity of evidence on which to base management decisions in anorexia nervosa, progress in bulimia nervosa has been impressive. In the USA and UK, most treatment is out-patient based. A study on bulimia nervosa appears in the second volume of *Evidence Based Medicine*. Interestingly, there appears to be a specificity in the response to treatment, in that behavioural therapy and drug treatment show a good initial response with a rapid rate of relapse, whereas cognitive behavioural therapy and interpersonal therapy have more sustained action.

The individual therapies described above are effective but they require trained therapists working with the patient for 18–20 sessions. A recent innovation in the field has been to translate the education and skills training of the most effective form of therapy, cognitive behavioural therapy, into a self-help book (Schmidt and Treasure, 1994). For patients who are motivated and not severely symptomatic (10–20% of cases), following the advice of a self-help book with two psychiatric assessment sessions can lead to recovery (Treasure *et al.*, 1994). In more severely affected patients, if the manual is used as an adjunct to therapy the number of one-to-one sessions can be reduced by over 50% (Treasure *et al.*, 1996). Not only can the therapy sessions be reduced but the need for specially trained therapists has been questioned by the finding that guided self-care with a social worker, with no eating disorder experience, produced reasonable outcomes (Cooper *et al.*, 1996).

These findings suggest that it is appropriate to phase the interventions given to patients with bulimia nervosa. For the first stage, cognitive behavioral self-help can be given with support from a therapist. There are now three self-help books available and it may be helpful to suggest that the patient chooses, or mixes and matches, among these three and any others on the market.

Useful cognitive behavioural self-help books:

- Schmidt U and Treasure JL: *Getting better bit(e) by bit(e)*, Hove, 1993, Lawrence Erlbaum.
- Cooper P: *Bulimia nervosa. A guide to recovery*, London, 1993, Robinson.
- Fairburn CG: *Overcoming binge eating*, New York, 1995, Guilford Press.

A therapist manual, which details how the novice therapist can use a book in the form of motivational enhancement therapy, is now available (Treasure and Schmidt, 1996).

Approximately half of the subjects fail to respond to these non-specialized interventions. They should then be introduced to the next level of therapy, which may be more specialized, such as cognitive behavioural therapy. Those with a severe intensity of symptoms may be helped by an antidepressant that can produce a degree of control, so that psychological work and reflection can take place. Group treatment offers the possibility of a support network, in addition to the ability to reflect on and examine interpersonal difficulties. However, this can pose organizational difficulties. Those with more severe problems, who may also have personality difficulties, may need longer-term therapy which specifically examines the therapeutic relationship, such as cognitive analytical therapy. Therapy with a greater degree of structure such as day-patient care or in-patient treatment may be required for some patients.

EVALUATION

It can be difficult to assess progress in bulimia nervosa as sometimes patients may try to please and appear perfect with diaries and reports of no problems. It is useful to arrange follow-up at 3-monthly intervals to ensure that recovery is complete and sustained.

Even with state-of-the-art treatment, 50% of patients remain symptomatic after 5 years. A long-term follow-up over 10 years has found that many patients gradually lose their symptoms (Johnson–Sabine *et al.*, 1992; Collings and King, 1994).

SUMMARY

Perhaps the best summary for this chapter is a quotation from one of the international experts in this field Walter Vandereycken from Belgium:

> Therapeutic work with eating disorder patients may become a fruitful training experience in developing patience, frustration tolerance, perseverance and flexibility. And it cures you of omnipotent fantasies

(Vandereycken 1993)

The skills needed to deal with this patient group include developing a therapeutic alliance with a patient who is not motivated to change, who has little insight into the severity of their condition, and is reluctant to comply with treatment; these are skills which are needed in all areas of psychiatry.

Case study: **Anorexia nervosa**

L lived with her mother, father and older brother. As far back as she could remember her mother behaved as a 'doormat' for her father, even when he had an affair. Her father was aggressive, demanding and critical, most often with her mother but also with both children at times. Her mother was passive and lacked self-esteem. L also remembered that her mother ate very little at the table. Her maternal grandmother also ate very little and commented on everyone's portion sizes and weight when she visited.

As L reached adolescence she became slightly chubby and immediately went on a diet after a comment from a school friend. She had a boyfriend from the time she was 13. They lived together when she was 17. Her father was somewhat disappointed in this, as he had hoped that she would go on to become a teacher. L became engaged and bought a house, which she struggled to keep spotless. She was somewhat of a perfectionist and could not bear to see anything out of place for long. She accidentally became pregnant and, because she and her partner had not planned to have children for another 5 years, she agreed to a termination. However, following this she felt nauseated and started to cut back on her food. She also began to take up jogging and would be out running most evenings. As the date for the wedding approached L became more and more emaciated. She eventually broke off the relationship.

L had no periods following her termination. She was unable to explain why she could not eat; she stated that she did not feel like it. She was very reluctant to gain any weight. She would not allow anyone to prepare food for her and would spend hours in the supermarket meticulously reading the labels on the packets to check calorie and fat content. Her mother tried for many months to get L to see her general practitioner but she refused, saying there was nothing wrong with her. Eventually she fainted after getting up one morning and so agreed to go to the doctor.

She was admitted to hospital urgently with a body mass index (BMI) of 11.9 kg/m². She was unable to walk up stairs without pulling herself up by the bannister. She had cold, blue fingers and her hair was dry and tended to stick out. She wore many layers of clothes.

She described being frightened of men and had plans to leave hospital and live with her mother. As she engaged with staff, particularly a male member of staff, she was able to describe some of her childhood experiences: fear of abuse from a male friend of her parents, fear that her brother was treating his wife badly, anger with her mother for her passivity. She felt that she had missed out on her childhood by constantly worrying about her mother. She also grieved for the fetus that she had let go.

She gained weight in hospital and after a small relapse she was able to halt her weight loss and work on the issues of her own self-esteem and anger.

Case study: **Bulimia nervosa**

Susan presented for treatment when she was aged 22. Her difficulties with weight and shape were long-standing. She was the youngest child of a family of five. Obesity, high lipid levels and coronary artery disease ran in her family. At the age of 8 she was seen by the school nurse, as she was overweight. Her paternal grandfather had died of a myocardial infarct when her father was 15. Her own father died after having coronary artery bypass surgery when she was aged 11. Susan and two of her brothers were found to have familial hyperlipidaemia. Because Susan resembled her father in appearance, after his death Susan's mother became preoccupied by the need for Susan to diet. The doctors recommended special diets. Susan, however, said all of this would be of no avail until she was ready to change. Her weight continued to increase until, by the age of 18, she weighed 18 stone.

Susan had had difficulties at school because of dyslexia, which was not recognized until she was aged 12. This led to her having poor self-confidence. Her mother became concerned about the discrepancies in teachers' reports—poor performance in examinations but good achievement in class. She therefore organized a private assessment. Nevertheless, even when Susan's disability was recognized, she was given little extra help. In addition, she had marked perfectionistic traits. She would work hard at tasks to ensure that she did them as well as possible. She readily acknowledged that she had extreme black and white thinking. As an example of this she described how when she started her physiotherapy course she would say to herself 'I will kill myself if I fail at this'.

Susan found it difficult to adjust to her father's death. Her mother had protected her as much as possible from the reality of thus event. Susan started to act out in school and at home. She remembers feeling that she must be going mad because she had fantasies about being killed. Her mother considered sending her to boarding school.

At college Susan started to take control over her life and started to diet. Her weight fell from 18 to 10 stone. At the time of leaving college, when she felt uncertain about her future and after a series of life events including the ending of a relationship, she started to binge and vomit. Over the next 2 years this pattern of behaviour escalated and she took several severe overdoses.

KEY CONCEPTS

- Anorexia nervosa is a severe mental illness with a mortality rate of twice that for any psychiatric illness and 15 times that for the normal population; it has a suicide rate 200 times that for the normal population.
- Anorexia lasts on average 6 years and typically affects young women.
- Bulimia nervosa is a new illness and appears to be a form in which distress presents in our culture. The incidence is at least three times that of anorexia nervosa.
- Many factors contribute to the development of anorexia nervosa: genetic factors and a perfectionist personality are predisposing factors, stress and difficulties are triggers and family and cultural factors maintain the illness.
- Dieting is an important risk factor for the development of bulimia nervosa. Early adversity with difficulties in determining self-identity is another risk factor.
- Many of the health difficulties of anorexia disappear after weight gain but osteoporosis may be irreversible.
- The physical consequences of bulimia, such as facial roundness with swollen parotid glands and rebound oedema, may perpetuate the disorder.
- One of the major hurdles in the management of anorexia nervosa is to motivate sufferers to want to recover.
- Early, minimal intervention with cognitive behavioural self-help books is possible in bulimia nervosa.
- A third of cases of anorexia nervosa have a poor prognosis and the majority have some residual symptoms.
- Bulimia nervosa has a relapsing course. Over half the cases remain symptomatic, despite treatment, after 5 years.

REFERENCES

American Psychiatric Association: *Diagnostic and Statistical Manual of Mental Disorders , 3 ed.* Washington DC, 1980, APA.

American Psychiatric Association: *Diagnostic and Statistic Manual of Mental Disorders , 4 ed.* Washington DC, 1994, APA.

American Psychiatric Association: *Guidelines for the treatment of eating disorders.* Washington DC, 1993, APA.

Bell, RM: *Holy anorexia.* Chicago, 1985, University of Chicago Press.

Bemporad JR: Self-starvation through the ages: reflections on the pre-history of anorexia nervosa. *Int J Eat Disord* 19(3):217–237, 1996.

Bhanji S, Mattingly D: *Medical aspects of anorexia nervosa.* London, 1988, Wright.

Blake W, Turnball SJ, Treasure JL: Examining the transtheoretical model of change in eating disorders [In press].

Burket RC, Schramm LL: Therapist attitudes about treating patients with eating disorders. *South Med J* 88:813–818, 1995.

Channon S, De Silva P, Hemsley D, Perkins R: A controlled trial of cognitive behavioural and behavioural treatment of anorexia nervosa. *Behav Res Ther* 27:529–535, 1989.

Collings S, King M: Ten-year follow-up of 50 patients with bulimia nervosa. *Br J Psychiatry* 164:80–87, 1994.

Cooper PJ, Coker S, Fleming C: An evaluation of the efficacy of supervised cognitive behavioral self-help for bulimia nervosa. *J Psychosom Res* 3:281–287, 1996.

Crisp AH, Norton K, Gowers S, et al.: A controlled study of the effect of therapies aimed at adolescent and family psychopathology in anorexia nervosa. *Br J Psychiatry* 159:325–333, 1991.

Dare C, Eisler I: Family therapy. In Szmukler GI, Dare C, Treasure JL, editors: *Handbook of eating disorders:Theory, treatment and research.* Chichester, 1995, John Wiley.

Eating Disorders Association: *Eating disorders: A guide to purchasing and providing services*, 1995, EDA.

Fallon P, Katzman MA, Wooley SC, editors: *Feminist perspectives on eating disorders.* New York, 1994, Guilford Press. New Yord.

Fombonne E: Anorexia nervosa: No evidence of an increase. *Br J Psychiatry* 166:462–471, 1995.

Gull W: Proceedings of the Clinical Society of London. *BMJ* 1:527–9, 1873.

Hall A, Crisp AH: Brief psychotherapy in the treatment of anorexia nervosa. *Br J*

Psychiatry 151:185–191, 1987.

Johnson–Sabine E, Reiss D, Dayson D: Bulimia nervosa: 5 year follow-up study. *Psychol Med* 22:951–959, 1992.

Katzman MA, Lee S: Beyond body image: the integration of feminist and transcultural theories in the understanding of self starvation. *Int J Eat Disord* [In press].

Kendler KS, McLean C, Neale M *et al.*: The genetic epidemiology of bulimia nervosa. *Am J Psychiatry* 148:1627–1637, 1991.

Kilbourne J: In: Fallon P, Katzman MA, Wooley SC, editors: *Feminist perspectives on eating disorders.* New York, 1995, Guilford Press.

Lasegue EC: On hysterical anorexia. *Med Times Gaz* 2:265–269, 1873.

Lee S, Ho TP, Hsu LKG: Fat phobic and non-fat phobic anorexia nervosa:A comparative study of 70 Chinese patients in Hong Kong. *Psychol Med* 23:999–1017, 1993.

Le Grange D, Eisler I, Dare C, Russell GFM: Evaluation of family therapy in anorexia nervosa:a pilot study. *Int J Eat Disord* 12:347–357, 1992.

Lucas AR, Beard CM, O'Fallon WM *et al.*: 50-year trends in the incidence of anorexia nervosa in Rochester, Minnesota: A population based study. *Am J Psychiatry* 148:917–922, 1991.

McKenzie JM, Joyce PR: Hospitalisation for anorexia nervosa. *Int J Eat Disord* 11:235–241, 1992.

Macleod S: *The Art of Starvation.* London, 1981, Virago.

Minuchin S, Rosman BL, Liebman R *et al.*: *Psychosomatic families: Anorexia nervosa in context.* Harvard, 1978, University Press.

Morton R: *Phthisiologia: or, a treatise of consumptions.* London, 1694, Smith and Walford.

Munk–Jorgensen P, Moller–Madsen S, Nielsen S *et al.*: Incidence of eating disorders in psychiatric hospitals and wards in Denmark, 1970–1993. *Acta Psychiatr Scand* 92:91–96, 1995.

Nielsen S: The epidemiology of anorexia nervosa in Denmark from 1973 to 1987: a nationwide register study of psychiatric admission. *Acta Psychiatr Scand* 81:507–514, 1990.

Palmer RL, Oppenheimer R: Childhood sexual experiences with adults: a comparison of women with eating disorders and those with other diagnoses. *Int J Eat Disord* 12:359–364, 1992.

Patton GC: Mortality and eating disorders. *Psychol Med,* 18: 947–951, 1988.

Prochaska JO, Di Clemente CC: Toward a comprehensive model of change. In: Miller WR, Heather N, editors: *Treating addictive behaviours: Processes of change*. New York, 1986, Plenum.

Royal College of Psychiatrists: *Eating disorders*. Council Report CR14, London, 1992. London.

Russell GFM: Bulimia nervosa: an ominous variant of anorexia nervosa. *Psychol Med* 9:429–448, 1979.

Russell GFM: Anorexia nervosa through time. In: Szmukler G, Dare C, Treasure JL, editors: *Handbook of eating disorders: Theory, treatment and research.* Chichester, 1995, Wiley.

Russell GFM, Szmukler GI, Dare C et al.: An evaluation of family therapy in anorexia nervosa and bulimia nervosa. *Archives of General Psychiatry,* 44:1047–1056, 1987.

Russell GFM, Treasure JL: The modern history of anorexia nervosa: an interpretation of why the illness has changed. In: Schneider LA, Cooper SJ, Halmi KA, editors: The psychobiology of human eating disorders: preclinical and clinical perspectives. *Annals of the New York Academy of Sciences,* 575:13–30, 1989.

Schmidt U, Treasure JL: From medieval mortification to Charcot's rose red ribbon and beyond: modern explanatory models of eating disorders. *Int Rev Psychiatry* 5:3–8, 1993.

Schmidt U, Tiller J, Treasure JL: Self-treatment of bulimia nervosa:a pilot study. *Int J Eat Disord* 13:273–277, 1993a.

Schmidt U, Tiller J, Treasure JL: Psychosocial factors in the origins of bulimia nervosa. *Int Rev Psychiatry* 5:51–60, 1993b.

Schmidt U, Tiller J, Treasure JL: Setting the scene for eating disorders:childhood care, classification and course of illness. *Psychol Med,* 23:663–673, 1993c.

Selvini–Palazzoli M, Boscolo L, Cecchin G, Prata G: *Paradox and counterparadox*. New York, 1978, Jason Aronson.

Sullivan, PF: Mortality in anorexia nervosa. *Am J Psychiatry* 152:1073–1074, 1995.

Theander S: Outcome and prognosis in anorexia nervosa and bulimia: some results of previous investigations compared with those of a Swedish longterm study. Conference on anorexia nervosa and related disorders (1984 Swansea, Wales). *J Psychiatr Res,* 19(2–3):493–508, 1985.

Treasure JL, Holland A: Genetic factors in eating disorders. In: Szmukler GI, Dare C, Treasure JL, editors: *Handbook of eating disorders: Theory, treatment and research.* Chichester, 1995, Wiley.

Treasure J, Schmidt U, Troop N et al.: First step in managing bulimia nervosa: a controlled trial of a therapeutic manual. *BMJ* 308:686–689, 1995.

Treasure J, Schmidt U, Tropp N et al: Sequential treatment for bulimia nervosa incorporating a self help care manual. *BrJ Psychiatry* 168:94–98, 1995.

Treasure JL, Szmukler G: Medical complications of chronic anorexia nervosa. In: Szmukler GI, Dare C, Treasure JL, editors: *Handbook of eating disorders: Theory, treatment and research.* Chichester, 1995, Wiley.

Treasure JL, Todd G, Szmukler GI: The inpatient treatment of anorexia nervosa. In: Szmukler GI, Dare C, Treasure JL, editors: *Handbook of eating disorders: Theory, treatment and research.* Chichester, 1995, Wiley.

Treasure JL, Todd G, Brolly M et al.: A pilot study of a randomised trial of cognitive analytical therapy versus educational behavioural therapy for adult anorexia nervosa. *Behav Res Ther* 33:363–367, 1995.

Troop NA, Holbrey A, Trowler R et al.: Ways of coping in women with eating disorders. *J Nerv Ment Dis* 182:535–540, 1994.

Turnbull S, Ward A, Treasure J, Jick H, Derby L: The demand for eating disorder care: an epidemiological study using the general practice research base. *Br J Psychiatry* 196:705–712, 1996.

Vandereycken W: Naughty girls and angry doctors. *Int Rev Psychiat* 5:13–18, 1993.

Ward A, Troop N, Todd G, Treasure JL: To change or not to change. 'How is the question?'. *Br J Med Psychol* 69:139–146, 1996.

Wilkinson H: *Puppet on String*, 1981.

Williams P, King M: The 'epidemic'of anorexia nervosa: another medical myth? *Lancet* i:205–207, 1987.

Wolf N: *The Beauty Myth*. London, 1992, Vintage.

Wolf N: Hunger. In: Fallon P, Katzman MA, Wooley SC, editors: *Feminist perspectives on eating disorders*. New York, 1994, Guilford Press.

FURTHER READING

Brownell KD, Fairburn CG: *Eating disorders and obesity: a comprehensive handbook*. New York, 1995, Guilford Press.
A reference book which is a must for all professionals working with obesity and being eating disorders.

Cooper P: *Bulimia nervosa. A guide to recovery.* London, 1993, Robinson.
Peter Cooper's book gives a clear cognitive behavioural approach to recovery.

Fairburn CG: *Overcoming binge eating.* New York, 1995, Guilford Press.
Chris Fairburn is able to untangle this eating disorder and provide definitive instructions on its treatment.

Garner DM, Garner PE: *Handbook of Treatments for Eating Disorders.* New York, 1997, Guilford Press.
An excellent intensive description of new treatments; if the 1st edition is impressive then the new edition will be well worth waiting for.

Schmidt U, Treasure J: *Getting Better Bit(e) by Bit(e). A survival kit for sufferers of bulimia nervosa and binge eating disorder.* Hove, 1993, Lawrence Erlbaum.
A self-help manual, combining interpersonal and cognitive–behavioural theory to provide a comprehensive step-by-step approach to treating bulimia nervosa.

Schmidt U, Treasure J: *A clinicians guide to getting better bite by bite.* Hove, 1996, Psychology Press.
This is the necessary therapist addition to the self-help manual.

Treasure JL, Troop NA, Ward A: Planning Services for Bulimia Nervosa. *Br J Psychiatry* 169:551–554, 1996.
A clear paper on the necessary processes involved in planning a service.

Szmukler GI, Dare C, Treasure J, editors: *The Eating Disorders: Handbook of Theory, Treatment and Research.* Chichester, 1995. John Wiley & Sons.
This textbook is a must for all those working in the field.

Key Issues in Sexual Health

Learning Outcomes

After studying this chapter you should be able to:

- Identify the barriers that have historically prevented mental health nurses from exploring sexual health concerns with patients.

- Discuss the reasons why sexual health forms an integral part of mental health and well-being.

- Describe the types of knowledge, skills and attitudes that will enable mental health nurses to address sexual health issues with clients.

- Offer a definition of sexuality and identify the key components of sexual health.

- Detail how factors affecting a person's sexual health may impinge on their mental health and how mental health problems can affect sexual health.

- Demonstrate an awareness of the effects of psychotropic medication on sexual functioning.

- Discuss some of the ethical and legal dilemmas relating to sexual health promotion in mental health care.

- Identify the types of sexual risk behaviours that people with mental health problems may practice and the factors that contribute to this.

- Describe the key principles and practice of initiatives to promote sexual health, including educational sessions and introduction of resources such as condoms to mental health settings.

- Show an understanding of how to assess clients' sexual health needs, including assessing for risks and vulnerability in clients engaging in sexual activities.

- Outline research identifying concerns about sexual safety in mental health settings, describe the nurse's role in maintaining a safe environment of care and discuss nurse's role in responding to clients who have experienced sexual harassment, abuse or rape.

CHAPTER OUTLINE

- *The theory–practice gap*

- *Nurses' knowledge and attitudes*

- *Understandings of sexuality and sexual health*

- *Relationship between sexual health and mental health*

- *Relationship between gender and mental health*

- *Sexual activities among people with mental health problems*

- *Sexual health promotion in mental health settings*

- *Developing good practice guidelines*

- *Sexual safety*

- *Mixed-sex wards*

- *Nurse education and training*

- *Sexual Health Link nurses*

*S*exuality and sexual health have never been higher* on the nursing agenda. This is evidenced by the vast increase in the number of publications on the subject. There are increasing numbers of texts on sexual health aimed at nurses and articles in the British nursing press ranging in scope from the history of masturbation (Howe, 1995) to the debate around the appropriateness of mixed-sex wards in mental health settings (Firn, 1995a). In addition, statutory bodies such as the English National Board for Nursing, Midwifery and Health Visiting (ENB) have published sexual health learning packs for practitioners and guidelines for good practice in sexual health education and training (ENB, 1994a; ENB, 1994b).

There are several reasons for this increased attention to and apparent legitimization of sexuality as an important topic in nursing. First, the move towards the provision of holistic care, with a focus upon addressing all a person's needs and not simply the presenting symptoms of their illness, has highlighted the need to address sexual health as an integral part of health. Furthermore, the increased recognition of the nurse's role in health promotion has drawn attention to sexual health issues, while many nursing models have specifically identified sexuality as a key area for assessment and intervention. For instance, the Roper *et al.* (1983) model lists 'expressing sexuality' as one of the twelve activities of daily living.

The emergence of HIV and AIDS has, in many ways, made it impossible to ignore sexual health needs, as the following Case study concerning the sexual relationships between two informal patients demonstrates.

RESPONSES TO PATIENTS' SEXUAL EXPRESSION

In relation to mental health nurses, Thomas (1989) acknowledges that, historically, psychiatric nurses have only addressed sexuality when it has been perceived as a problem, such as a patient masturbating in a public area. This tendency to ignore or turn a blind eye to patients' sexual activities, unless they present as a problem, is not unique to nursing. Research proposals on the subject of sexual health promotion in mental health settings have been submitted to several ethics committees by the author of this chapter. A frequent response from eminent medical personnel has been 'our patients don't have sex'.

When patients have been discovered engaging in sexual activities, the traditional response has been to try to control it. Therefore, most local policies state that sexual relationships between patients are not permitted and staff should intervene to stop any overt expressions of sexuality. These policies tend to give vague or non-practical guidance on how to control sexual expression (Callaghan, 1992). Policies have not been developed that give clear guidelines on how staff should

intervene in such situations. An interesting case, arising in the early 1980s, entailed a student nurse being told that, if she discovered two patients having sex, she should 'prise them apart with a broom'.

Despite this tendency to avoid sexuality, there is a growing body of research based evidence that people with mental health problems:

- Are sexually active (Park Dorsey and Forchuk,1994).
- Experience sexual problems (Bhui and Puffett, 1994).
- Engage in unprotected sex, which carries risks of sexually transmitted disease and unplanned pregnancies (Kelly *et al.*, 1992).
- Have significant gaps in their knowledge regarding safer sex (Goisman *et al.*, 1991).
- Are vulnerable to exploitation and abuse (Cournos *et al.*, 1991).

HEALTH OF THE NATION

The UK Government has also placed the topic of sexuality and related matters at the top of the health care agenda by identifying HIV, AIDS and Sexual Health as one of the five key areas in the Health of the Nation strategy for England and Wales (Department of Health, 1992). In the Key Area Handbook it states:

> Rewarding personal and sexual relationships promote health and well-being. However, sexual activity can also have undesired results such as unwanted pregnancies and the transmission of Human Immunodeficiency Virus (HIV) and other sexually transmitted diseases.

The general objectives of the strategy are detailed in Box 22.1.

THE CHALLENGE FOR MENTAL HEALTH NURSES

These objectives present great challenges for mental health nurses, particularly those working in in-patient settings where there are rarely any clear policy guidelines and where patients have limited access to resources such as condoms, other forms of contraception, and appropriate written information, such as leaflets on sexual health concerns (Royal College of Nursing (RCN), 1996). This chapter will address these issues and will also explore whether it is realistic for mental health patients to experience 'rewarding personal and sexual relationships'

Case study: **Sexual relationships between two informal patients**

A male and a female patient in their late twenties were both in-patients on a unit treating people for obsessive–compulsive disorders. They were observed spending a great deal of time in each other's company, including being alone together in their bedrooms and going away for weekend leave together. The unit was not staffed at night, allowing privacy for the residents. Both patients appeared responsible adults and staff judged them capable of making informed decisions about most aspects of their lives. As such, the issue of their friendship was not discussed as it was not seen to impinge on their presenting symptoms or their care. One day the mother of the male patient told staff he was HIV positive. This caused great concern among the nursing staff, who were worried that the female patient may have contracted the virus, and faced the dilemma of whether to tell her his diagnosis. They were also concerned that they could be held responsible if she had been infected since the staff had not carried out a risk assessment to identify whether the couple were having unprotected sex and whether they both knew the potential risks, and whether either of them felt they were being exploited or coerced. Although HIV was the catalyst for these concerns it was the failure to address sexual health needs that led to the situation developing. In this sense, HIV was presenting a new face to an old problem.

 Box 22.1

General objectives of National health strategy

- To reduce the incidence of HIV infection.
- To reduce the incidence of other sexually transmitted disease.
- To further develop and strengthen monitoring and surveillance.
- To provide effective services for diagnosis and treatment of HIV and other STDs.
- To reduce the number of unwanted pregnancies .
- To ensure the provision of effective family planning services for those people who want them.

within the context of mental health settings, where such behaviour has traditionally been precluded and where there are legitimate concerns about exploitation, vulnerability and consent.

THE THEORY–PRACTICE GAP

Despite the growing number of publications on the subject of sexual health and the elevation of sexuality on the nursing agenda, there is little evidence to indicate that nursing practice has significantly changed. It would seem that in the area of sexual health there is not so much a theory–practice gap as a yawning chasm. For instance, research has shown that even where issues such as sexual abuse and knowledge of contraception are included in the nursing assessment documentation, the majority of nurses leave these sections blank (Park Dorsey and Forchuk, 1994).

Bor and Watts (1993) suggest that talking to patients about sexual matters is as difficult as addressing death and dying. They quote US research that suggests that the following three factors principally account for nurses' reluctance to take a sexual history:

1. Embarrassment.
2. A belief that sexual matters are not relevant to the patient's care.
3. Feeling inadequately trained for the task.

NURSES' KNOWLEDGE AND ATTITUDES

Part of the reason why nurses experience embarrassment and do not recognize the relevance of addressing sexuality may be to do with their level of knowledge of and attitudes towards sexuality. Studies have shown that student nurses have low knowledge levels about sexuality and hold conservative attitudes in comparison with other students. Webb (1985) compared knowledge and attitudes towards sexuality among qualified and non-qualified gynaecological nurses. She found that both groups had considerable knowledge deficiencies and traditional attitudes in relation to sexuality. Webb hypothesized that the gynaecology nurses might be more knowledgeable because their area of work directly related to sexuality issues but she found no evidence that this was the case.

There is also a widespread belief among nurses that patients would not think it appropriate for them to initiate discussions about sexuality. In a study by Wilson and Williams (1988), 25% of oncology nurses had never offered sexual counselling to patients, yet 91% would be happy to do so if the patient initiated the discussion. Wilson–Young (1987) interviewed 100 patients in surgical wards and found that 92% thought discussions on sexuality with health care professionals were appropriate. Therefore, despite the concerns of many nurses, it seems the great majority of patients would welcome the opportunity to discuss sexual concerns. This assertion is supported by a study by Waterhouse and Metcalfe

(1991), who interviewed 73 health employees in a US university. Of these, 92% indicated that nurses should discuss sexual concerns with patients. Those authors acknowledge a number of limitations to the study, not least that the sample was not randomly selected and was not representative of the general population. Nevertheless, they felt sufficiently convinced from their findings to conclude:

> Discussion of sexual concerns initiated by the nurse is valuable for all patients and it is time nurses stopped assuming that clients do not wish to discuss sexuality.

Bor and Watts (1993) also state that negative attitudes towards some sexual lifestyles and practices, such as homosexuality, are a further barrier to communication. Studies carried out in the context of care of people with HIV and AIDS have shown that many nurses have negative attitudes towards gay men and feel them more deserving of their illness than other people with AIDS (Kelly *et al.*, 1988).

Smith (1992) cites a definition of homophobia as 'irrational fear and hatred of anyone or anything connected with homosexuality, or a fear of one's own real or potential homosexuality'. James *et al.* (1994) review the literature and find that many lesbians and gay men fear homophobia from health care providers. They are also concerned about confidentiality, facing hostility and possible physical harm if they reveal their sexual orientation. Researchers also highlight the lack of enquiry into the experiences of lesbian and gay male users of mental health services but reiterate the well-documented fact that many mental health professionals see homosexuality as a problem. Indeed, in the USA homosexuality was listed as a mental illness until the early 1970s (Bancroft, 1979).

The author of this chapter interviewed people with AIDS as part of a research study exploring their emotional and psychological needs. A 28-year-old gay man spoke about how he feared that he would never again be able to be intimate with his partner because of his anxiety about transmitting the virus. This was making him feel very low but he did not feel able to discuss the issue with nursing staff. This was because he could sense that the nurses were not comfortable talking about his homosexuality since, when he had alluded to it on a couple of previous occasions, the nurse had quickly ended the conversation.

UNDERSTANDINGS OF SEXUALITY AND SEXUAL HEALTH

Sexuality is notoriously difficult to define. Most authors favour a broad definition that suggests that it is a multifaceted concept encompassing biological, social, psychological, spiritual and cultural aspects. Thus, Lion (1982) has suggested sexuality includes:

> all those aspects of the human being that relate to being boy or girl, woman or man, and it is an entity subject to lifelong dynamic change. Sexuality reflects our human characteristics, not solely our genital nature.

Like most authors of nursing texts, Lion cautions against accepting definitions of sexuality constructed principally around genital aspects. This definition also highlights the issue of gender, which relates to masculine or feminine characteristics that are socially constructed, and emphasizes how our conception and experience of our sexuality will change throughout life. While many people rightly see their sexuality as an intensely personal construct, it also reflects our relationships to the values, norms and beliefs in our society. As Webb (1985) has stated:

> Sexuality involves the totality of being a person and therefore nurses and patients are only given their full respect as people when nursing care has firm foundations in a truly holistic approach incorporating sexuality as a vital aspect of humanity.

Savage (1988/89) cautions against accepting glib and romantic views of sexuality and points out 'that sexuality can be the vehicle for the expression of power, dependency, hostility or hatred is glossed over'. Therefore, in mental health care we must remember that, while seeking to promote the sexual health needs of our clients, we must also never forget that some clients will have suffered, or will be at risk of suffering, abuse, harassment and exploitation of a sexual nature.

Spend a few minutes writing a sentence begining 'Sexuality is...' that attempts to define what the concept means to you. Are you satisfied with your definition? If not, what is missing? Does it encompass all the aspects that may contribute to sexuality, both positive and negative? Is your definition self-evidently about 'sexuality' or could it be applied to other concepts?

Remember, there is no single 'right' answer, as Webb and Askham (1987) commented:

> "Sexuality" can mean many different things to as many different people, and a single understanding cannot be reached'.

SEXUAL HEALTH

Attempts have been made to try to identify the essential elements of sexual health. The most widely quoted is that produced by the World Health Organization, 1986 (in ENB, 1994b):

1. A capacity to enjoy and control sexual and reproductive behaviour in accordance with a social and personal ethic.
2. Freedom from fear, shame, guilt, false beliefs and other psychological factors inhibiting sexual response and impairing sexual relationships.
3. Freedom from organic disorders, diseases and deficiencies that interfere with sexual and reproductive functions.

Viewed in a critical manner, this is an idealistic definition that would be incredibly difficult for anyone to achieve and maintain, whatever their circumstances. If we consider the circumstances of people with mental health problems, and particularly those in hospital, it would be almost impossible.

In the document *Sexual health: Key issues in mental health*, the Royal College of Nursing (RCN, 1996) adopts the following basic elements of sexual health:
- Absence and avoidance of STDs, including HIV.
- Control of fertility and avoidance of unwanted pregnancy.
- Sexual expression and enjoyment without exploitation, oppression or abuse.

RELATIONSHIP BETWEEN SEXUAL HEALTH AND MENTAL HEALTH

Sexual health and mental health are inextricably woven together. It is clear that many factors affecting a person's sexual health (such as sexual abuse, infection with a sexually transmitted disease, or disfigurement) may precipitate problems requiring help from a mental health professional (Ferguson, 1994). Similarly, a person's mental health problems may impinge on their sexual health either because of the nature of the mental illness or as a result of the treatment. Pinderhughes *et al*. (1972) and Bell (1993) conducted interviews with 122 psychiatric in-patients. They found that:
- Of people with schizophrenia, 47% thought sexual functioning may have contributed to their illness.
- Around one-third felt sexual activity might hinder their recovery.
- Less than half thought their illness had affected their sexual functioning.

Bhui and Puffett (1994) state that there has been insufficient attention paid to the sexual problems experienced by users of mental health services. They undertook a literature search which revealed only five references that arose in the previous 5 years. They found that some psychiatric illnesses that have the potential to become chronic, such as schizophrenia, have their onset during adolescence. This can interfere with an individual's sexual development by disrupting and inhibiting their opportunities to form relationships, to explore their own sexual development and identity and acquire interpersonal social skills necessary for stable relationships. Recurrent episodes of illness are likely to make serious demands on existing relationships and may reduce the attractiveness of the person to current or potential partners because of behavioural disturbances and the social stigma of illness. Finally, failure to develop stable relationships can contribute to low self-esteem and self-worth, further inhibiting the ability of the person with schizophrenia to express him or herself sexually.

It is well recognized that affective disorders can influence sexual desire and arousal. People with manic illnesses may experience sexual disinhibition and increased sexual activity, while people with depressive illnesses and anxiety states commonly report decreased sexual appetite and reduction in ability to become sexually aroused. However, Bhui and Puffett (1994) state that there have been reports of a paradoxical increase in sexual appetite among some individuals with depressive states. Clearly, any recurrent changes in mood are likely to place great demands on maintenance of relationships. Excessive alcohol use and illegal drug use have also been frequently associated with both disturbances in sexual functioning and the maintenance of relationships.

Bhui and Puffett believe that, among people with mental health problems:

> The side-effects of prescribed medication are too often named as the cause of sexual problems, and less attention is directed to other factors which may be amenable to psychological intervention.

This is an important point, since it can be all too easy for health care professionals to pass off sexual problems among patients as being inevitable or secondary to treatment of other symptoms or aspects of the illness. This may be a form of avoidance, given the evidence detailing the difficulties nurses and other professions experience when addressing this issue. However, it is also the case that psychotropic medication can have considerable effects on sexual functioning (Table 22.1).

Clearly, nurses need to be aware of these to inform patients who are concerned about potential effects of drugs on their sexual health and also to help those experiencing problems to understand the possible reasons and to explore solutions.

Bell *et al.* (1993) found that 46 out of 89 (53%) of people with schizophrenia believed that the medication they were taking contributed to sexual problems, with 41 citing antipsychotic medicines as the cause.

TABLE 22.1 Potential side-effects of psychotropic medication on sexual functioning

Drugs	Effects
Neuroleptics	Delayed or absent orgasm Retrograde or absent ejaculation Impaired arousal Sedation Less emotional expression
Antidepressants	Delayed orgasm Priapism Ejaculation delay or failure Depressed sexual response Reduced libido
Benzodiazepines	Reduced arousal Sedation Reduced libido
Lithium	Reduced desire Hyposexuality Less intense or reduced orgasm

(Bhui and Puffett, 1994)

Consider two medications that are commonly administered to patients. It is known they have sexual side-effects: has this possibility discussed with your patients?

RELATIONSHIP BETWEEN GENDER AND MENTAL HEALTH

There are clear differences between the genders in terms of the types and incidence of psychiatric diagnoses. Among the adult population, women are more likely to be diagnosed as mentally ill and more women are admitted to psychiatric hospitals than men. However, these figures are skewed since women live longer than men and therefore a greater number experience dementing illnesses and are over-represented in mental health services for the elderly. Women also use community mental health services more frequently and are more likely to be prescribed psychotropic drugs (Ferguson, 1994).

With regard to diagnoses, rates of schizophrenia are roughly similar between the sexes. However, women are more likely to experience neurotic illness such as anxiety and depression and have much higher GP consultation rates for these problems than men. Some conditions, such as eating disorders, primarily affect women. Ferguson (1994) gives a clear synopsis of the biological and social factors affecting women's mental health.

Men, on the other hand, have a greater tendency to be diagnosed with mania, psychopathy, personality disorders and substance misuse. In addition, they are more likely to be the victims and perpetrators of violent crime and are vastly over-represented in prison. These statistics have led to the claim that, because of the social norms influencing the way men and women can express frustration, anger and distress, women are more likely to be labelled 'mad' while men are more likely to be labelled 'bad'.

Men are also more likely to commit suicide. In 1992 men committed suicide at a rate 4 times that of women. Among men aged between 15 and 24, the rates have increased by 71% in the last 10 years. The UK is the only country in Europe where male rates are rising and female rates falling; some of the explanations for this trend are (Samaritans, 1995):

- Unemployment (affects men more than women.)
- Breakdown in marriages (unmarried men have higher rates than married).
- Choice of means. (Men tend to use violent means or very effective methods such as carbon monoxide from car exhausts.)
- Men's poor use of health services, such as GPs.
- Greater tendency in men to misuse substances, which is itself a high risk factor for suicide (drug users are 20 times more likely to kill themselves, while 15% of alcoholics are believed to commit suicide).
- Changing gender roles challenging traditional roles of men in society, leading to identity crises in vulnerable young men.
- Men's limited ability to express their emotions due to socialization, encapsulated in the common statement that 'big boys don't cry'.

Many of these factors are of a social nature rather than biologically determined. Nurses need to be aware of these issues in order to provide care but also to ensure they are not perpetuating sex role stereotypes, which Webb (1988) defines as 'culturally-dominant conceptions of appropriate sex-role behaviour'. For instance, one mental health service user described how he learnt to control his tears as a boy because otherwise his parents threatened they would 'give you something to cry about'. At school, he refrained from expressing his emotions because boys who cried were bullied. Tragically, when he was admitted to a psychiatric hospital after developing a mental illness aged 19, he observed that male patients who cried were viewed as 'more ill' because this was not seen as an accepted social norm. Therefore, he believed that tearful male patients were more likely to be prescribed treatments such as phenothiazines or ECT (Read , 1992). As a result, he contained his emotions for fear of being judged dysfunctional, even though he was in a therapeutic environment with all the attendant rhetoric about helping clients to express themselves. Ferguson (1994) states that nurses need constantly to examine their assumptions and attitudes to male and female gender roles, to see how this may influence or prejudice the care they provide. In addition, it is part of the nurse's role to help patients recognize when their own gender role expectations may be contributing to their ill-health, such as men who do not feel able to talk candidly and openly about their fears and concerns (Firn, 1995b).

SEXUAL ACTIVITIES AMONG PEOPLE WITH MENTAL HEALTH PROBLEMS

Despite the widespread denial among staff and policy makers (Walker and Frasier, 1994) there is evidence from research conducted in the USA that service users do engage in sexual activities. For instance, Kelly *et al.* (1992) conducted interviews with 60 out-patients in inner city community mental health clinics, 37 (62%) of whom had been sexually active during the previous 12 months. Those men who were sexually active reported an average of 2.3 female partners in the previous month and 13.2 in the previous year. Condoms were used on an average of 18% of occasions. Just 5 female clients (19%) reported having had multiple sexual partners in the previous year.

Although people with mental health problems are sexually active, there have been studies that have shown that people with schizophrenia are less sexually active than members of control groups. Bell (1993) describes a study by Lyketsos *et al.* in 1983 in which 113 clients with schizophrenia were compared to a non-institutionalized control group.

The people with schizophrenia reported significantly less interest in sex, frequency of intercourse and satisfaction with sex. However, this could be, in some part, the result of the lack of opportunity for developing sexual relations and lack of privacy in the institutional setting. This hypothesis is supported by Bell's study in which 40 (46%) of people with schizo-

phrenia living in institutions reported they had stopped sexual relations. Of these, 26 (59%) gave the fact that they were in an institution as the primary reason. When questioned further, 18 of these said it was because admission had caused separation from their partner, 5 cited the lack of privacy and 3 gave other reasons. Bell concluded, 'The common staff attitude that clients with schizophrenia are hyposexual...or that their sexual activity declines as their illness becomes chronic, needs to be confronted'.

In a similar study, Cournos *et al.* (1994) carried out face-to-face interviews with 95 in-patients and out-patients with a diagnosis of schizophrenia and found 44% had been sexually active in the preceding 6 months and 62% of these had had multiple sexual partners. Importantly, they found that sexual activity and having multiple partners was associated with symptoms of more severe illness, including thought disorders and delusions. Among those clients who were sexually active, 50% had exchanged sex for money or goods, while 22% had engaged in same-sex activity during their lifetime and condom use was uncommon. Only 8% of sexually active patients (3 out of 40) reported always using condoms. Among the 21 who exchanged money for sex or goods (such as food or rent) gender differences were identified. Although the number of men and women involved in these activities was similar, men were more likely to buy sex while women were more likely to sell sex, although this was not exclusively the case. Other studies have also reported that condom use is low. Park Dorsey and Forchuk (1994) found that only 5% of clients with chronic mental health problems said they would always use a condom, 5% stated they usually would and 60% said they would never use a condom during sexual activity.

There have also been reports of low knowledge levels among patients regarding sexual risk behaviours. For instance, in the Park Dorsey and Forchuk study 37% said they were 'not at all familiar' with how to use condoms. These figures suggest people with mental health problems are vulnerable to both exploitation and STDs, including HIV.

RISKS OF HIV AND OTHER STDS

Three studies in the USA have sought to determine the rates of HIV seroprevalence among people with mental health problems. Cournos *et al.* (1991) conducted anonymous testing of patients admitted to two psychiatric hospitals in New York. They found that 5.5% (25 out of 451) of patients were HIV positive. Staff were aware of only seven of these infections and had recorded a history of HIV related risk behaviour in just 36% of those with the virus. The majority of the patients were admitted with a psychotic illness. These findings suggest that a proportion of the severely mentally ill are infected with HIV and staff are unlikely to aware of most of those infected. The authors suggest the main implications are that further clarification is needed of the relationship between psychiatric illness and sexual risk taking behaviour, to identify effective prevention strategies.

Two other studies from New York looked at HIV seroprevalence among the homeless with mental health problems. Empfield *et al.* (1993) found an infection rate of 6.4% (13 out of 203) among homeless people in psychiatric hospitals. Once again, anonymous testing of discarded blood samples was used. The strongest predictors of HIV seropositivity were injecting drug use and age under 40. Although the rate was not significantly higher than that reported by Cournos *et al.* (1991) Empfield and colleagues conclude that outreach work is required to reduce risk of acquiring or transmitting HIV among the homeless mentally ill. This conclusion is also reached by Meyer *et al.* (1993), who found infection rates of 5.8% among hospitalized homeless mentally ill, with younger age and being black or Hispanic being most strongly associated with HIV infection.

The rates in the studies reported from samples of in-patients in psychiatric hospitals were roughly similar to those in the surrounding population. This suggests a similar level of risk and a similar pool of infection inside and outside psychiatric hospitals. However, all these studies were conducted in New York and it is not possible to say whether the results are widely applicable.

With regard to other STDs, Kelly and colleagues (1992) found that 20 of 60 people with chronic mental health problems reported that they had been treated for an STD, including syphilis, gonorrhoea, chlamydiosis and herpes. Sexual risk behaviour may, in part, be related to a lack of knowledge among people with mental health problems. Kelly *et al.* (1992) also found substantial deficits in knowledge about sexual risk behaviours among the chronic mentally ill. For instance, 43% believed that heterosexual women cannot get AIDS.

SEXUAL HEALTH PROMOTION IN MENTAL HEALTH SETTINGS

Park Dorsey and Forchuk (1994) examined the notes of 100 patients with severe mental illness and looked specifically at the section on sexually transmitted diseases. In 28 cases this section was blank, while only 4 sets of notes said the patient was aware of the precautions for STDs and that a very disturbing 68 clients were unaware of the necessary precautions (Box 22.2).

These concerns are augmented by lack of national policy guidelines on sexual health in mental health, which could provide a framework for staff in local areas to develop their own policy and practice to meet individual client group needs (Firn, 1994).

There is also a lack of training courses on sexual health promotion in mental health and absence of any distance learning or teaching packs to assist staff to develop their skills and practice in this area. These exist for other client groups, such as people with learning difficulties (McCarthy and Thompson, 1992).

Mental health nurses frequently express concerns about the harmful effects of appearing to encourage or condone sexual expression, in whatever form. As part of the sex education

sessions the author provides for patients, a selection of line drawings is used, detailing different forms of sexual expression and intimacy. Patients are invited to comment on what the picture depicts and whether they would feel comfortable engaging in that activity. The least intimate pictures involve two people holding hands and two people sitting on a couch with their arms around each other, watching television. Virtually all patients agree that these are activities they would find both pleasurable and safe. However, they also state that if they were to do either of things on an in-patient ward, the likelihood is that nurses would ask them to desist.

Among the reasons staff have given for this response are that it is a potential cause of conflict in the ward if patients are seen to be physically attracted to each other, that such activity detracts from their treatment and recovery and that they are concerned about vulnerability and exploitation. While some of these may be genuine concerns, they do not seem to fit with an ethos of individualized care, which recognizes sexual expression as a contributing factor to well-being. Clearly, there needs to be some criteria for staff to assess the individual situation and relationship before deciding on the most therapeutic course of action. This needs to be preceded by a general local debate about sexual expression.

Comfort (1978) noted that:

> the first step in planning any opening up of institutions to sex is full discussion, not between able experts about what would be good for their patients, but between and with patients about what they would like or dislike. The task for staff is to control their own projected anxieties and to avoid impertinent or voyeuristic zeal and the creation of imaginary dangers.

It might be better to include, where appropriate, partners and significant others. For instance, after condoms were introduced to one drug unit, a husband visited and was, first, surprised that his wife was on a mixed-sex ward and, secondly, appalled that condoms were freely available in the toilets. This

Box 22.2

Summary of concerns regarding sexual health promotion in mental health

- Evidence that patients engage in sexual activity that places them at risk of STDs and unplanned pregnancy (Park Dorsey and Forchuk,1994).
- Evidence that significant numbers engage in sex in return for money or scarce goods, raising concerns about exploitation (Cournos *et al.*, 1994).
- Evidence that homeless people with mental health problems may engage in more sexual risk behaviours (Empfield *et al.*, 1993).
- Studies showing that people with mental health problems have significant gaps in their knowledge regarding risk of sexual activities and use of condoms (Kelly *et al.*, 1992).
- Limited access to resources such as condoms and genito-urinary and sexual health clinics or family planning services.
- Limited access to appropriate written information such as leaflets.

led to him demanding to know from staff whether his wife had been admitted to a 'knocking shop'.

It is a well-recognized principle that health promotion initiatives need to be targeted at groups at risk and presented in ways that are accessible and meaningful to the lifestyles and experiences of those groups. Thus, sexual health promotion guidance, videos and training packs exist for people with learning difficulties (e.g. McCarthy and Thompson, 1992). In the experience of the author of this chapter, while the type of information provided in these resources is appropriate to the needs of people with mental health problems, these do not identify with the characters and images depicted in these resources. This can affect their ability to engage with the subject and may give them the impression that it is not a concern relevant to their lifestyle. It is therefore very important that resources are developed and sensitive and effective training and education implemented that address knowledge deficits and empower clients to negotiate safe and comfortable forms of sexual expression.

SEX EDUCATION PROGRAMMES FOR PEOPLE WITH MENTAL HEALTH PROBLEMS

Goisman *et al.* (1991) conducted a pilot workshop for 50 clients with schizophrenia, schizoaffective disorder and major mood disorder; the workshop consisted of three, 1-hour sessions on sex education, AIDS information and condom use. They reported that among those who completed pre- and post-course questionnaires there were considerably increased knowledge levels and an increase, in the following 6 months, of clients requesting information on sexual health issues and asking for condoms. This small study suggests that some changes in knowledge and intention to reduce sexual risk behaviours is possible among this client type, even following relatively short educational sessions. Further work needs to be done to substantiate these findings and also, most importantly, to see whether it leads to any reduction in actual risk-taking behaviours.

As Herman *et al.* (1994) report, there is little evidence on the efficacy of risk reduction interventions for clients with serious mental illness. They attempted to address this by devising an intervention consisting of 10 group sessions covering HIV and AIDS information, demonstrations of condom use, techniques for managing high risk situations, communication and assertiveness lessons, skills building and development of personal awareness of own high risk situations. The intervention included role-play, modelling, group discussion and use of videotapes.

Some 45 patients attended the sessions and a post-group evaluation questionnaire indicated that 89% were more likely to use a condom during sex, and 75% were less likely to have sex with someone they did not know; 77% of parents reported they would speak to their children about HIV.

These findings suggest that such interventions can lead to increased intention to modify risk behaviour, but they do not demonstrate whether any actual changes in behaviour resulted.

Goisman *et al.* (1991) refer to a study where staff predicted that patients would find it difficult to tolerate 'sexually charged material' and would experience a worsening of symptoms. However, the evaluation found that patients with chronic mental illness were able to complete the programme without worsening of psychopathology and most welcomed the opportunity to learn about sexual health issues.

This mirrors the author's own experience of carrying out sex education sessions with this client group. Topics have included:

- Forming relationships.
- Contraception and family planning.
- Negotiating safer sex, including how to say no.
- STDs.
- HIV and AIDS.
- Legal concerns.
- Being sexual in mental health settings.

Brief questionnaires completed by participants after the sessions indicate that the overwhelming majority find them very useful. The following guidelines and safety measures have been adopted:

1. Ask staff in the care area sensitively to ensure that anyone with a history of perpetrating or experiencing sexual abuse or anyone with false beliefs about sexuality is excluded. Topics may be more safely and effectively addressed on a one-to-one basis.

2. It is important to set out ground rules, preferably negotiated with participants beforehand.

3. Make groups open, in the sense that anyone can leave at any time without giving an explanation. This allows space if a person becomes distressed. Concerns must be followed up.

4. If a client leaves the group they cannot rejoin and no one can join after the group has started. This prevents disruption and enables people to feel more comfortable about disclosing information about themselves.

5. Make clear who the client can approach for help or further information after a session.

6. Ensure sessions take place in a private, quiet room where other clients cannot wander in.

7. Use methods such as line drawings (see McCarthy and Thompson, 1992) to avoid jargon and to get around the fact that language about sexuality can be confusing and that some words and terms may cause offence.

8. Be aware of cultural differences in attitudes and values towards sexuality and be sensitive to these; e.g. some people may have religious objections to condom use.

9. Invite an experienced member of staff from the care setting into the group so that they can advise the facilitator if a patient is distressed or appears to be expressing delusional ideas.

10. Teaching methods should also be sensitive to the fact that people may have limited concentration as well as anxiety and social withdrawal. Utilize methods that will be interactive and engage people rather than use 'chalk and talk' type lectures.

11. Keep sessions relatively short and focused – 30 to 45 minutes may be sufficient. It is better to have few short sessions than

one or two longer ones. This helps to reinforce the message and assists participants to maintain concentration.

12. Consider whether to divide groups according to different functional levels as suggested by Goisman *et al.* (1991). The author's experience is that a range of abilities can be tolerated and may be helpful, as long as it is not too wide.

13. Try to keep a roughly equal balance between sexes in a group because over-representation by members of one sex can inhibit those of the other sex from expressing themselves.

14. Consider having two facilitators, one male and one female, to be able to respond to questions from both sexes and to encourage questions about men's or women's specific concerns.

PROVISION OF CONDOMS AND OTHER RESOURCES

The evidence presented so far clearly shows that a significant number of both in-patients and out-patients engage in sexual activities that place them at risk of unplanned pregnancies and STDs. Most authors agree that it seems unrealistic to think that patients can be educated, coerced or restrained from engaging in sexual activities, even if this were thought a desirable option. Another way of attempting to eliminate these risks is by enabling patients to use condoms correctly whenever they engage in penetrative sex.

However, the actual practice of making condoms available in mental health settings presents many challenges. Often staff say they do not know how actually to go about making condoms available and are concerned about legal issues. Some of these practical, ethical and legal concerns include:

• Concerns about accessibility. Should the condoms be freely available in dispensers or should staff have some control about how many are given out and to whom?

• Should condoms be provided as free goods or should patients have to pay for them, for example via a vending machine? Does the adoption of vending machines as part of a normalization approach, work against need for open access?

• Should condoms be kept in the care area or is it sufficient and less controversial to have information about how and where to obtain them, for example from local GUM clinic, GP or commercial outlet?

• If condoms are not available in each care area, are machines in visitors' toilet, out-patient departments or hospital social club appropriate?

• Should condoms be sold in the hospital shop? (One professor of psychiatry remarked that he considered it absurd that the hospital shop sold cigarettes to patients but did not sell condoms with their potential to prevent ill health. However, his views were not universally shared by his colleagues!)

• Will the provision of condoms, or even discussion of sexual issues, lead to an increase in sexual activity?

• How will concerns and possible offence to patients and, to some extent, to staff be taken into account?

These questions need to be addressed by each local area with regard to their specific client group and the type of mental health setting.

Winship (1995) describes the introduction of condoms into a drug dependency unit located within a psychiatric hospital. Even though it had been demonstrated that the client group in the unit were at risk transmissible agents such as HIV from and hepatitis through unsafe sexual practices, the introduction of condoms was not without problems and challenges. The proposal met with resistance from staff for two main reasons. First, they feared that having condoms available would generate sexual arousal among clients and lead to increased sexual activity. Secondly, the policy of the unit was that sexual relations between clients were not permitted and therefore the availability of condoms sent out a mixed message.

Condoms were initially kept in the office and only brought out for education sessions or if clients asked for them. Because of concerns that clients were embarrassed by having to negotiate this restricted access, they were eventually placed in the male and female toilets, allowing free access by clients. Winship emphasizes the need to frame the introduction in a wider programme of health education. The unit held education sessions on sexual health and also used posters, leaflets, videos and teaching materials to complete a comprehensive package of sexual health promotion measures.

Despite the initial fears of staff, the recorded incidence of sexual intercourse involving patients was lower in the year following the initiative than in the previous year when condoms were not available. This correlates with research findings evaluating sex education in school, which demonstrate that this does not increase sexual activity and may promote safer sex practices (Health Education Authority, 1994). Less positively, Winship reports that on the last three occasions of clients having sex before his article was published, none reported using condoms.

Clearly, open access to condoms is not a complete solution to sexual risk behaviour. There is evidence that people with mental health problems hold similar negative views towards condoms as those of the general population, including perceiving them as messy, likely to reduce pleasure and an unwelcome interruption during foreplay, which reduces usage (Health First, 1996). These issues need to be addressed by further research and during education sessions with clients.

Think of a sexual health promotion initiative that could be introduced to your care area. This could be the introduction of resources such as condoms, producing a leaflet targeted at your client group or a sexual health session aimed at clients or colleagues. When you have chosen, use the following mnemonic (SMART) as a framework for planning your initiative:

• Specific — what exactly do you hope to achieve? List your aims and objectives.

• Measurable — how will you know if you have achieved your intended outcomes?

• Achievable — is the initiative realistic? If not, do not be afraid to narrow the focus.

- Resources — what will you need in terms of funding, support from peers and superiors, time away from regular work etc.? Specify how you will aquire them.
- Timetable — plan out target dates for each critical stage.

DEVELOPING GOOD PRACTICE GUIDELINES

The recognition and acceptance that clients engage in sexual activities makes it imperative that staff have clear guidelines that provide a framework within which they can respond sensitively and sympathetically, in a manner that does not deny the patient's right to be sexual but also ensures that there is no harm to any patients in the unit.

Although a few authors continue to insist that patients should be prevented from engaging in sexual activities, the broader recognition that sexual relationships can contribute to mental health and emotional well-being means that many mental health services will wish to consider how to manage and respond to clients expressing their sexuality. It is not appropriate, nor possible, to provide prescriptive guidance that applies to every form of mental health service. For example, there will be different issues to consider in an acute in-patient intensive care unit compared with a community drop-in mental health centre. Similarly, the issues arising in a an adolescent unit will not be the same as those in a residential unit for the elderly mentally ill. This is not to say that any of these client types do not have sexual needs but that they will express these needs differently and the responses will require tailoring to meet them.

Whenever clients are known, or thought, to be engaging in sexual relationships, management and care decisions need to be based upon individual assessment of specific circumstances. The principal role of the nurse is to assess whether consent is given by both parties to the sexual relationship. An important consideration will be whether either client is detained under a Section of the Mental Health Act, as this may indicate they are unable to make informed judgements. In addition, the following factors may assist in the assessment:

- Is there any suggestion or evidence of coercive, exploitative or threatening behaviour in relation to the sexual activities?
- Are both parties in complete control of their sexual behaviour or could their current mental health problem be influencing their behaviour in a manner that may cause regret or harm?
- Are patients able to understand any risks to physical health such as STDs or unplanned pregnancies?
- Where are the sexual activities taking place, and in what context, and does this interfere with the care or well-being of other clients?
- Are there any relevant legal issue pertaining to the sexual activities, for example age of consent, that require consideration?

Some people have raised the concern that any hospital setting must be viewed as a public place. Therefore, it could be argued, men having sex with men would be illegal and sex between men and women would fall foul of the public decency laws. However, it is by no means clear that, for instance, a hospital bedroom in a psychiatric hospital is viewed as a public place within the particular laws governing sexual activities. Nurses may be wise to consult the Trust solicitors for their views. However, a draft report by the Special Hospital Services Authority (SHSA, 1993) took legal advice that found that, under European law, it is probably illegal to prevent two consenting adults detained in a Special Hospital from engaging in sexual intercourse.

Many nurses will have come across patients masturbating in view of staff, residents and visitors. However, many nurses would agree that even if a client cannot lock him or herself in a room, their bedroom may be considered an acceptable place for them to masturbate in as long as they are not able to be viewed by passers-by.

The RCN state in two separate publications (RCN, 1994; RCN, 1996) the importance of nurses recognizing the legitimacy of sexual partners of the same sex. The author was also involved in writing a policy on sexual relationships for a mental health Trust that acknowledged its commitment to no discrimination against clients on the basis of sexual orientation. As such, it was explicitly stated that the same criteria for assessing how to respond to sexual activities between patients should be applied, regardless of the sex of either party. However, it should be remembered that the age of consent for men having sex with men is 18 years, compared with 16 years for sex between men and women.

As the assessment of sexual relationships is such a complex issue, it is preferable that care and management decisions are not taken by individual nurses, but follow consultation within the multidisciplinary care team and consider the client's expressed views and wishes.

Whenever possible, it is preferable that sexual health needs are explored as part of the overall assessment procedure and are frequently reviewed. The aims of this assessment will be:

1. To enable the client to express any concerns or ask any questions about sexual health issues.
2. To enable the nurse to identify any concerns about a client's sexual health, that may either be relevant to their mental health problems or may make the client vulnerable to exploitation and harm.
3. To advise the client regarding any policies and expectations regarding expression of sexuality.
4. To enable the client to take as much responsibility as possible for the expression of their sexuality in an informed manner.

Information arising from this assessment that is relevant to the client's care should be recorded in the appropriate place in the notes. If it is decided that it is not appropriate to carry out a detailed assessment of sexual health needs, because a client has delusional beliefs of a sexual nature for instance, this should also be recorded and the reasons stated. The aim of this is to reduce the reported incidence of sexual health sections of assessment forms being left blank (Park Dorsey and Forchuk, 1994).

Consideration also needs to be given to the issue of sexual activities between a patient in a psychiatric hospital and a partner who is not a client. Some organizations have called for the provision of 'safe private spaces for service users to engage in consensual, intimate activities' (RCN, 1996). Such facilities may be thought appropriate for clients to meet with partners, particularly if the client is likely to have a prolonged stay in hospital and has limited opportunities for leave. In such a scenario, the nurse would still need to be sure the client was able freely to consent to sexual relations, even with an established partner.

To be able to respond to sexual health needs of clients in the ways outlined, consideration needs to be given to the appropriate mix of male and female staff in each care area. This is in recognition of the right of clients to discuss issues around sexuality with a nurse of either sex.

In the UK it is a criminal offence for a male nurse to have a sexual relationship with a female patient (Ritter, 1989). Any sexual activity between a member of staff and a patient will almost certainly be viewed by an employer as a serious disciplinary offence that could result in dismissal and the individual being reported to their professional organization for misconduct.

Occasionally a patient may make sexual advances to a nurse and Ritter (1989) notes that the approach is most commonly by a male patient towards a female nurse. This may be for a number of reasons including a desire to form a relationship, an expression of hostility and a threat, or because the patient misconstrues the interest and compassion demonstrated by the nurse as an indication of sexual attraction. For such situations, there is a need to set clearly defined boundaries and objectives to emphasize and maintain the relationship on a professional, therapeutic level. Nurses working in the community are particularly open to approaches of a sexual nature and need to respond decisively to any suggestion, and to maintain boundaries, since they may be vulnerable to assault or allegations of sexual impropriety. Ritter (1989) emphasizes the value of self-awareness skills, regular clinical supervision and support and use of role-play as ways to help nurses avoid or manage such situations. The importance of policies that support sensitive care relating to clients' sexual health needs has been emphasized by a number of authors (e.g. Park Dorsey and Forchuk,1994).

Consider the case study Sexual safety.

SEXUAL SAFETY

It is extremely important that nurses feel sufficiently confident and skilled to carry out a sexual health assessment, including a history of any previous abuse. Park *et al.* (1994) report a study in which 70% of women who were out-patients at a psychiatric hospital reported previous abuse when asked directly, but only 6% had volunteered this information without being asked. In their own study of patients' notes, they found that 66% of assessment charts were left blank with respect to history of abuse. They postulate that this reflects nurses' discomfort with the topic.

There is a growing body of evidence indicating that a disturbing and unacceptable number of female clients are subject to sexual harassment, assault and rape while in-patients in psychiatric hospitals (MIND, 1992). While it is not possible to put an accurate figure on the extent of the problem, a US study found that over 70% of clients had been threatened with violence and 38% sexually assaulted. Of the latter, 27% had been assaulted by members of staff (Batcup and Thomas, 1994). In the UK, Thomas *et al.* (1992) report a study that found that 27% of clients were concerned for their safety in a London psychiatric teaching hospital. There has been a report of a person with a history of being sexually abused being constantly harassed in hospital (Hughes, 1992) while one appalling report detailed the case of a woman who had been admitted to a psychiatric hospital after experiencing a sexual assault in the street. The next morning she suffered another serious sexual assault, this time by a male patient (Altounyan, 1993). It is most worrying to note that male nurses have also been reported following allegations of sexual harassment of female clients and that these reports are increasing (UKCC, 1993).

Mental health settings should provide a therapeutic and safe enviroment for the care and treatment of the mentally distressed. Sometimes an intervention that alleviates this distress cannot be found but, at the very least, it should be possible to prevent the client from sustaining further harm caused by other clients or staff. These reports suggest that patients are vulnerable to sexual harassment, assault and rape and MIND (1992) report that on some occasions when this has occurred, staff have not fully investigated or reported the matter.

The RCN (1996) have stated that nurses manage the environment of care and must therefore take the lead in ensuring services are as a safe as possible and in protecting vulnerable, confused and disinhibited clients. Whenever sexual harassment or assault is threatened or occurs, nursing staff should follow these basic principles while taking into account any local policies or guidance:

1. Intervene to stop an incident developing and take steps to prevent a recurrence. (This will involve moving one client;

Case study: **Sexual safety**

A 35-year-old man with enduring mental health problems had lived for the last 5 years in a hostel. He was managing well with the support of a CPN and taking a monthly depot injection. He informed the CPN that he had started visiting the local public toilets where he engaged in unsafe sex, including anal intercourse with other men without a condom. He said he visited the toilets because he had not been able to form any other sexual relationships. What are the principal legal and ethical issues the CPN needs to consider? How may the CPN assist the client to meet his sexual needs in the most safe and fulfilling manner?

where possible it is preferable this should be the perpetrator.)

2. Ensure that the incident is reported to appropriate organizations and individuals, such as the senior manager responsible for the unit, and to the police. Some organizations have policies stating police must always be informed, while others list criteria upon which a decision can be made.
3. Provide appropriate and sensitive support and counselling for complainant or victim, which may include use of outside agencies such as Rape Crisis and genito-urinary services.
4. Provide support and counselling for the alleged perpetrator.
5. Follow local guidance with regard to the collection of evidence without prejudice.
6. Wherever possible, give clients involved opportunity to choose the sex of the staff member providing support and counselling.
7. Ascertain who the clients would like informed about the incident and do not disclose to family and friends of the complainant (or victim) or perpetrator without their consent.

If a client reports an incident that occurred in their home or elsewhere in the community that is not part of the Trust's property, the role of the nurse is slightly different. The key responsibility is to explore what assistance the client wants in coming to terms with their experience. In particular, establish whether the client wants it explored as part of the therapeutic relationship or if they also want to report the matter. If the client does decide to inform the police, the nurse can advise regarding police procedures and act as advocate and support. Regardless of whether the incident is reported, the nurse should explore with the client how to minimize the possibility of a recurrence of the harassment or assault.

MIXED-SEX WARDS

With the exception of Special Hospitals, mixed-sex wards are now commonplace in psychiatric hospitals. Most authors state that the principal theory behind their introduction was the move towards 'normalization' in mental health service provision. Supporters of this argument state that since men and women mix freely in society, this should also be the case in mental health settings. However, it is not the social norm to sleep, wash, eat and dress in close proximity to strangers of the opposite sex. In addition, the concerns about women's safety have led to criticism of blanket provision of mixed-sex accommodation on the grounds that this is not the most therapeutic and safe for all patients (Firn, 1995a). Thomas *et al.* (1992) interviewed 150 male and female in-patients and found that while 57% were happy with mixed-sex accommodation, almost 1 in 5 (19%) would have preferred single-sex accommodation. Among the women interviewed, 27% expressed a clear preference for single-sex wards. The main reasons for this were a perception that there would be less violence and more privacy in women-only wards.

Firn (1995a) has argued that the normalization rationale for mixed-sex wards is not relevant to acute mental health care in the 1990s, when length of patient stay is being constantly reduced and rehabilitation issues are addressed in the community. Those who have been critical of calls for single-sex wards have suggested that it would mark a return to the days when patients in psychiatric hospitals only met at Christmas. However, proponents have asserted that single-sex wards do not represent segregation, but choice for those who would prefer such accommodation. Viewed in this manner, single-sex wards represent a response to the need to ensure the safety and dignity of clients and prevent harm and distress in modern mental health care.

It is the role of nurses to facilitate the provision of private areas for men and women, even in mixed-sex wards. This is necessary to maintain social convention and prevent distress (Ritter, 1989). This may be difficult depending on the environment and culture of the wards. Some wards have therefore designated specific areas as 'women-only spaces' (Thomas *et al.*, 1992)

Think of a mixed-sex psychiatric care setting in which you have worked. In what ways could the environment have been modified in order to improve the dignity and safety of different sexes and minimize the potential for distress, harassment or assault?

NURSE EDUCATION AND TRAINING

The need for education and training for nurses in all aspects of sexuality to be provided at pre- and post-registration has been widely documented (RCN, 1996), while it is also widely accepted that, during nurse training programmes, there is a tendency for sexuality to be limited to issues such as human reproduction (Park Dorsey and Forchuk, 1994). Herman *et al.* (1994) attempted to train 40 mental health staff who had volunteered to run sessions on HIV prevention with their client group. They found a major obstacle was that most of the mental health professionals had received very little education or training around sexuality and most expressed discomfort about the topic. It is clear that if this was the response among a group who had volunteered to do work in this area that this problem is likely to be widespread.

Webb (1988) says her study demonstrated a need for curriculum development in relation to sexuality, to raise awareness and knowledge levels. She points out that some experimental studies have shown that workshops or sessions on sexuality in nursing and medical students' curricula can increase knowledge, and there is some evidence that this leads to more liberal attitudes.

Therefore, curriculum development requires opportunities for nurses to explore their own attitudes and values relating to sexuality and reach a level of 'self-acceptance and comfort'. Savage (1998/89) warns that she has yet to meet anyone who is 'entirely at ease with their own sexuality' and questions whether this is a realistic statement. We should therefore be careful not to over-simplify what is a complex subject. However, it is clear that nurses need to develop self-awareness about their own values and beliefs around sexuality and how these may impinge upon the care they provide.

Webb highlights that nurse lecturers themselves are unlikely to be entirely comfortable with the subject and that they should teach and facilitate it openly, recognizing that they, too, are likely to require support and possibly further training to be effective. Finally, consideration of issues around sexuality needs to be incorporated throughout the curriculum to reflect that it is intrinsic to all aspects of care and cannot be compartmentalized into one or two study blocks. However, comprehensive guidelines for good practice in teaching nurses have been prepared and are available from the English National Board for Nursing, Midwifery and Health Visiting (ENB, 1994b).

Ritter has stated that if the necessary skills to address sexual health do not exist within the nursing care team, at least one of the first-level nurses should attend appropriate post-registration training to address this skills deficit. This person should also be able to transfer the knowledge and skills to colleagues and act as a resource (Ritter, 1989).

SEXUAL HEALTH LINK NURSES

The author has experience of establishing a Sexual Health Link Nurse scheme in a mental health Trust, which was an attempt to ensure that each care setting had a person with the necessary knowledge and skills to respond to sexual health issues raised by staff or clients. The ward manager was contacted in each unit in the Trust, both in-patient and community, and asked to nominate a member of staff. This resulted in 42 nurses and one occupational therapist being proposed for the link nurse role. Two days, training on sexual health issues in mental health was provided and at the end of the second day the participants identified their key responsibilities. These were as follows:

1. Receive new policies and guidelines relating to sexual health and ensure all staff and, where appropriate, clients are aware of the contents and implications.
2. Ensure appropriate written information such as leaflets and posters are available in the care setting and are accessible to clients and staff.
3. Ensure the educational needs of clients and staff are met through the facilitation or arrangement of appropriate training and health education sessions.
4. Keep updated regarding new treatments, approaches to care and prevention issues and disseminate this information to clients and staff as appropriate.
5. Ensure that all new staff and clients are aware that the Link Nurse is available to respond to any concerns related to sexual health and can provide information about other resources and services.

By being a resource for both staff and clients in the care setting, Link Nurses have a valuable role in ensuring sexual health issues are adequately addressed. They can draw upon the support and assistance of a lecturer–practitioner to enable them to fulfil their roles. A recurring programme of training days is planned, in conjunction with the Link Nurses, to enable them to keep updated on latest knowledge and practice, develop new skills and to meet to exchange information and provide mutual support.

SUMMARY

Interest in issues around sexuality and sexual health are higher on the nursing agenda than ever before. This is the result of a combination of factors including the shift in philosophy towards holistic nursing care and the emphasis on the nurse's role in health promotion. In addition, the emergence of HIV, coupled with increasing evidence that people with mental health problems engage in sexual activities that place them at risk of STDs, has forced mental health professionals to address sexual health needs, which were previously ignored. Finally, *The Health of the Nation* (Department of Health, 1992) identifies sexual health as a key target area and lists a number of objectives aimed at reducing the incidence of STDs, HIV and unplanned pregnancies. Furthermore, this document states that rewarding personal and sexual relationships is conducive to health and well-being.

Sexual health is extremely difficult to define but its most basic elements include the control of fertility and avoidance of unplanned pregnancy, absence and avoidance of STDs, including HIV, and sexual expression and enjoyment without exploitation, oppression or abuse (RCN, 1996).

Despite the increased awareness of the importance of the nurse's role in promoting sexual health, there is little evidence to indicate that nursing practice has significantly changed. Research shows that many nurses do not address this area of care even when it is directly related to their field of practice, such as nurses working in gynaecology (Webb, 1985). Studies have suggested this is the result of a number of factors including embarrassment, feeling inadequately skilled and a belief that patients will not consider the promotion of sexual health relevant to their care (Bor and Watts, 1993). However, evidence suggests most patients would welcome the opportunity to discuss concerns around sexual health with nurses, although this should still be approached in a manner sensitive to different cultural and religious beliefs and attitudes.

Research suggests that many nurses' attitudes are traditional and their knowledge base is poor. There is an identified need for nurse education to incorporate sexuality and sexual health throughout pre- and post-registration curricula and to ensure sexual health promotion is not left to one or two individuals and compartmentalized into certain sessions such as human biology or reproduction. For this to happen, nurse lecturers will also need to feel comfortable and confident about addressing the subject.

A person's mental health problems may impinge on their ability to develop and maintain sexual relationships, and psychotropic medication can affect sexual functioning (Bhui and Puffett 1994). In addition, factors affecting a person's sexual health, including abuse or infection with an STD, can also impinge on their mental well-being (Ferguson, 1994). There is insufficient attention paid to these issues, which should be addressed during nursing assessments.

A growing body of evidence has found that people with long-term mental health problems engage in sexual activities that may place them at risk of an STD or unplanned pregnancy. Studies in the USA suggest that rates of HIV infection in psychiatric hospitals are at similar levels to those in the general population (Cournos *et al.*, 1991). A disturbingly high number of patients may also engage in sex in return for money or goods such as cigarettes (Kelly *et al.*, 1992). These findings raise serious concerns about exploitation and vulnerability, particularly when considered alongside evidence that many clients have significant gaps in their knowledge about sexual health issues and have limited access to resources such as condoms (Park Dorsey and Forchuk,1994). These issues pose considerable challenges for mental health nurses, who need to take the lead in assessing levels of knowledge and risk, facilitating educational sessions where required, promoting a safe environment and devising clear policies and guidelines for responding to issues such as sexual abuse and harassment (Goisman, 1991; Firn, 1994). In addition, consideration needs to be given to introducing resources such as condoms to mental health settings, alongside training for staff to enable them to respond to complex ethical and legal dilemmas arising from practice in this area and a positive recognition that clients have sexual needs and are sexually active (Winship; 1995).

While the promotion of sexual health is an integral part of a holistic approach to mental well-being, the need to maintain safety is paramount. The incidence of sexual abuse and assault experienced by clients in mental health settings, particularly women, is completely unacceptable (RCN, 1996; MIND, 1992).

Such concerns demand a strategy for maintaining sexual safety and promoting sexual health in mental health services. Nurses are in a prime position to initiate and influence change in conjunction with other professionals and service users and their representatives. This issue cannot be addressed in a piecemeal, *ad hoc* fashion but requires a coordinated strategy, which will include the development of clear policy and practice guidelines, integration of sexuality and sexual health within professional education and training, service development to maintain safer environments including a critical review of mixed-sex accommodation, and provision of regular staff support and supervision. In addition, further research and audit is required to evaluate the effectiveness of nursing interventions in the field of sexual health along with the dissemination of findings and examples of good practice.

KEY CONCEPTS

- The attainment of sexual health is an integral part of mental and physical health and well-being.
- Defining sexuality is extremely difficult and mental health nurses need to assist individuals to recognize what sexual health means for them.
- Recent evidence indicates that people with mental health problems are sexually active, have high rates of sexual risk behaviours and that nurses have a crucial role to play in maintaining sexual safety and preventing harm.
- Mental health problems can impinge on sexual expression and well-being while concerns about sexual health can initiate or contribute to mental health problems.
- When clients have been observed expressing their sexuality, mental health nurses' traditional response has been characterized by attempts to ignore or control the behaviours.
- Current programmes of education and training for nurses have not prepared them to promote sexual health, with low knowledge levels identified and traditional attitudes expressed.
- Mental health nurses have a crucial role to play in assessing clients' sexual health needs and enabling clients to experience rewarding sexual relationships without fear of exploitation, abuse or ridicule.
- Good practice guidelines are urgently needed and nurses need to take a central role in their development.

REFERENCES

Altounyan B: Sex on the ward. *Nurs Standard* 7(24):20–21, 1993.

Bancroft J: *Human sexuality and its problems.* Edinburgh, 1979, Churchill Livingstone

Batcup D, Thomas B: Mixing the genders, and ethical dilemma: How nursing theory has dealt with sexuality and gender. *Nurs Ethics* 1(1): 41–50, 1994.

Bell CE, Wringer PH, Davidhizar R, Samuels ML: Self-reported sexual behaviors of schizophrenic clients and non-institutionalised adults. *Perspect Psychiatr Care* 29(2): 30–36, 1993.

Bhui K, Puffett A: Sexual problems in the psychiatric and mentally handicapped populations. *Bri J Hosp Med,* 51(9): 459–464, 1994.

Bor R, Watts M: Talking to patients about sexual matters. *British Journal of Nursing,* 2(13): 657—660, 1993.

Callaghan P: Sex and the psychiatric nurse. *Bethlem and Maudsley Gazette,* Spring, 15–17, 1992.

Comfort A, editor: *Sexual consequences of a disability.* Philadelphia, 1978, George F. Stickley.

Cournos F, Empfield M, Horwath E, *et al.* HIV seroprevalence among patients admitted to two psychiatric hospitals. *Am J Psychiatry* 148(9):1225–1230, 1991.

Cournos F, Guido JR, Coomaraswamy S, Meyer–Bahlburg H, Sugden R, Horwath E: Sexual activity and risk of HIV infection among patients with schizophrenia. *Am J Psychiatry,* 151(2): 228–232, 1994.

Department of Health. *The health of the nation.* London, 1992, HMSO.

Empfield M, Cournos F, Meyer I, *et al.* HIV seroprevalence among homeless patients admitted to a psychiatric inpatient unit. *Am J Psychiatry* 150(1):47–52, 1993.

ENB: *Caring for people with sexually transmitted diseases, including HIV disease.* London, 1994a, English National Board for Nursing, Midwifery and Health Visiting.

ENB: *Sexual health education and training: guidelines for good practice in the teaching of nurses, midwives and health visitors.* London, 1994b, English National Board for Nursing, Midwifery and Health Visiting.

Ferguson K: Mental health and sexuality. In: Webb C, editor: *Living sexuality: issues for nursing and health.* Harrow, 1994, Scutari Press.

Firn S: No sex please.... *Nurs Times* 90(14):57, 1994.

Firn S: Hobson's choice. *Nurs Times* 91(10):56, 1995a.

Firn S: Peril of the stiff upper lip. *Nurs Times* 91(25):60, 1995b.

Goisman RM, Kent AB, Montgomery EC, Cheevers MM, Goldfinger SM: AIDS education for patients with chronic mental illness. *Community Ment Health J* 27(3):189–197, 1991.

Health Education Authority: *Health update 4: Sexual health.* London, 1994, Health Education Authority.

Health First: *Sexual health promotion in mental health,* 1996. Report of a research study available from Health First, 15 St. Thomas' Street, London SE1.

Herman R, Kaplan M, Satriano J, Cournos F, McKinnon K: HIV prevention with people with serious mental illness: staff training and institutional attitudes. *Psychosoc Rehabil J* 17(4):97–103, 1994.

Howe J: A natural remedy. *Nurs Standard* 8(29):46–47, 1995.

Hughes P: Therapeutic for whom? *The Guardian,* 2 July, 1992.

James T, Harding I, Corbett K: Biased care? *Nurs Times* 90(51): 28–31, 1994.

Kelly JA, Murphy DA, Bahr GR, *et al.:* AIDS/HIV risk behavior among the chronic mentally ill. *Am J Psychiatry* 149(7):886–889, 1992.

Kelly JA, St. Lawrence JS, Hood HV, Smith S, Cook DJ: Nurses' attitudes towards AIDS. *J Contin Educ Nurs* 19(2):78–83, 1988.

Lion E: *Human sexuality in the nursing process.* New York, 1982, John Wiley.

Lyketsos G, Sakka P, Mailis A: The sexual adjustment of chronic schizophrenics: a preliminary study. *Br J Psychi* 143, 376–382, 1983.

McCarthy M, Thompson D: *Sex and the 3Rs: Rights, responsibilities and risks. A sex education package for working with people with learning difficulties.* London, 1992, Pavilion Books.

Meyer I, McKinnon K, Cournos F, *et al.*:HIV seroprevalence among long-stay patients in a state psychiatric hospital. *Hosp Community Psychiatry* 44(3):282–284, 1993.

MIND: *Stress on women: policy paper on women and mental health.* London, 1992, MIND Publications.

Park Dorsey J, Forchuk C: Assessment of the sexuality needs of individuals with psychiatric disability. *J Psychiatri Ment Health Nurs* 1:93–97, 1994.

Pinderhughes C, Grace B, Reyn L: Psychiatric disorders and sexual functioning. *Am J Psychiatry* 128(10):96–102, 1972.

RCN: *The nursing care of lesbians and gay men: an RCN statement. Issues in nursing and health, number 26.* London, 1994, Royal College of Nursing.

RCN: *Sexual health: key issues in mental health.* London, 1996, Royal College of Nursing.

Read J: Real men do cry. *Openmind* 55:14, 1992.

Ritter S: *Manual of clinical psychiatric nursing principles and procedures.* London, 1989, Harper & Row.

Roper N, Logan W, Tierney A: *Using a model for nursing.* Edinburgh, 1983, Churchill Livingstone.

Samaritans: *Behind the mask: men, feelings and suicide.* London, 1995, Samaritans.

Savage J: Sexuality: Expectations of nurses. *Radic Community Med* Winter, 19–22, 1988/89.

Smith GB: Homosexual psychiatric patients. *Psychosoci Nursi ment Health Serv* 30(12):15–21, 1992.

SHSA: *Advisory committee on patient relationships in special hospitals: Interim report.* 1993, Special Hospitals Services Authority.

Thomas B: Asexual patients. *Nurs Times* 85(33):49–51, 1989.

Thomas B, Liness S, Vearnals S, Griffin H: Involuntary cohabitees. *Nurs Times* 88(49):58–60, 1992.

Walker S, Frasier D: HIV and the long-term mentally ill. *Nurs Standard* 8(16):51–53, 1994.

Waterhouse J, Metcalfe M: Attitudes toward nurses discussing sexual concerns with patients. *J Adv Nurs* 16:1048–1054, 1991.

Webb C: *Sexuality, nursing and health.* Chichester, 1985, John Wiley.

Webb C: A study of nurses' knowledge and attitudes about sexuality in health care. *Int J Nurs Studi* 25(3):235–244, 1988.

Webb C, Askham J: Nurses' knowledge and attitudes about sexuality in health care – a review of the literature. *Nurs Educ Today* 7:75–87, 1987.

Wilson ME, Williams HA: Oncology nurses' attitudes and behaviors related to sexuality of patients with cancer. *Oncol Nursi Forum* 13:39–43, 1988.

Wilson–Young E: Sexual needs of psychiatric clients. *J Psychosoci Nursi ment Health Serv* 25: 30–32, 1987.

Winship G: Condoms on the ward: Sexual health education in psychiatric treatment settings. *Ther Communities* 16(3):163–169, 1995.

FURTHER READING

Armstrong E, Gordon P:. *Sexualities.* London, 1992, Family Planning Association.
A training resource that gives advice about how to plan and implement teaching programmes on sexuality and details tried and tested exercises.

Carlson GA, Greeman M, McClellan TA: Management of HIV positive patients who fail to reduce high-risk behaviors. *Hospi Community Psychiatry* 40(5):511–514, 1989.
Discusses the ethical dilemmas for staff posed by patiens with mental health problems and HIV who do not adopt safer sexual practices.

Fegan L, Rauch A, McCarthy W: *Sexuality and people with intellectual disability.* Sydney, 1993, Maclennan and Petty.
An Australian publication written by a psychologist and coordinator in a Family Planning Association that explores many aspects of sexual health, with advice on developing policies and providing sex education to address the needs of people with intellectual disabilities.

Foucault M: *The history of sexuality: An introduction.* Harmondsworth, 1984, Penguin.
This is an intellectually challenging book, which explores changing attitudes towards sexuality from the 17th Century and challenges the assumption that because sexuality is now much more visible and openly discussed we are less sexually repressed than our predecessors.

Kalichman SC, Kelly JA, Cournos F et al.: HIV seroprevalence among long-stay patients in a state psychiatric hospital. *Hosp Community Psych* 44(3):282–284, 1993.

Knox H: *SEXplained...The Uncensored Guide to Sexual Health.* London, 1995, Knox.
Written by a clinical nurse specialist, this source book provides factual information and advice, in a question and answer format, on sexually transmitted diseases, contraception and safer sex.

Lawler J: *Behind the screens: Nursing, somology and the problem of the body.* London, 1991, Churchill Livingstone.
Based largely on a PhD by an Australian Associate Professor of Nursing, this book draws on interviews with nurses to combine an academic discourse on 'the body' with an exploration of the way nurses manage the bodies of others while delivering nursing care.

McKinnon K, Cournos F, Meyer-Bahlburg H, *et al.*: Reliability of sexual risk behavior interviews with psychiatric patients. *American Journal of Psychiatry* 150(6):972–974, 1993.
Examines the reliability of tools used to assess sexual risk behaviours in people with mental health problems.

Payne A, editor: Sexual activity among psychiatric inpatients: International perspective. *J Forensic Psychiatry* 4(1):109–129, 1993.
A collection of short articles from different countries discussing policy and clinical practice issues relating to sexual health concerns in secure environments.

Webb C, editor: *Living sexuality: Issues for nursing and health.* London, 1994, Scutari Press.
Eleven chapters by specialists in the field of sexuality (almost all of whom are nurses), which link research and nursing care in specific areas ranging from young men's experiences of testicular cancer to women's health in old age.

World Health Organization Regional Office for Europe. *Concepts for sexual health.* Copenhagen, 1986, World Health Organization.

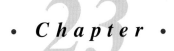

· *Chapter* ·

Child, Adolescent and Family Mental Health Nursing

Learning Outcomes

After studying this chapter you should be able to:

- Define childhood mental health.

- Discuss the role of child mental health nurses.

- Compare and contrast the various theoretical views on child development.

- Describe common childhood mental health problems and disorders.

- Show an understanding of current social and political influences in the field.

- State the basic principles of child protection.

- Demonstrate an appreciation of the differences between child and adult mental health.

- Outline main interventions used in child, adolescent and family mental health nursing.

CHAPTER OUTLINE

- *History of child and adolescent mental health nursing*

- *Development of children, adolescents and families*

- *Mental health problems in children and adolescents*

- *Contemporary sociopolitical influences*

- *Child protection*

- *Applying nursing principles in the assessment of mental health of children and adolescents*

- *Therapeutic intervention*

hild and adolescent mental health nursing is a specialty that has increased in importance with the political understanding that the mental health of children foreshadows the mental health of adults. In 1989 the UK adopted The United Nations Convention on the Rights of the Child. This defines a child as a human being below the age of 18 years unless, under the law that applies to the child, majority is attained earlier (Newell, 1991).

The Department of Health (DoH) states that 'there is nothing more important than maintaining the mental health of children and young people. Happy, stable young people are more likely to become happy, stable parents who in turn are able to provide a safe and secure upbringing for their children' (Health Advisory Service (HAS), 1995).

According to the HAS (1995) the mental health of children and young people is indicated specifically by:
- A capacity to enter into and sustain mutually satisfying personal relationships.
- Continuing progression of psychological development.
- An ability to play and to learn, so that attainments are appropriate for the age and intellectual level.
- A developing moral sense of right and wrong.
- The degree of psychological distress and maladaptive behaviour being within normal limits for the child's age and context.

HISTORY OF CHILD AND ADOLESCENT MENTAL HEALTH NURSING

Child and adolescent mental health nursing has a relatively short history, despite awareness since the earliest times of the psychological well-being of children. The 16th and 17th Centuries saw many doctors and others trying to understand the

page

disorders suffered by disturbed children. Explanations consistent with the times did not get much beyond being possessed by spirits.

The 18th Century saw the rapid expansion of institutional care and many more children were admitted to asylums. For instance, at the Bethlem Hospital almost 5% of its patients were young people under 20 years of age. The 19th Century witnessed a growing interest in childhood insanity and increasing amounts of unusual cases were published; by the middle of the century childhood madness was a regular feature of the literature.

Admission criteria were based on the inability of the parents or carers to contain the child at home, rather than the ability of professionals to effect improvement in hospital. At first nurses became custodians, then surrogate parents. Children were dependent on nurses to meet their basic needs; nurses ensured that children were adequately fed, clothed, had sufficient rest, received some form of education and were constructively occupied. This led nurses to develop knowledge, skill and attitudes that helped contain and control children. Wards were often highly ordered and routine centred and were emotionally blunt environments. Doctors and others were regarded as therapists and were responsible for treatment, while nurses were there to provide care. However, it soon emerged that containment and the development of a philosophy that ensured a therapeutic environment was not only essential but frequently proved to be the therapy that brought about change.

Nurses were achieving some success in working with mentally disordered children. In 1799 a 3-year-old child was admitted to the Bethlem Hospital because she had developed convulsions and become anxious, cried, kicked, bit and had lost control of her bowels and bladder. She was admitted for 4 months and placed under the care of a nurse; she learned to control her bladder and bowels 'by great attention and perseverance on the part of the nurse' (Parry–Jones, 1994).

The psychological development of children has been studied extensively since the start of the 20th Century. This has informed clinical practice and underpinned the creation of the child guidance movement. The first clinic was opened in 1927 and represented a shift in thinking to that of a more psychosocial perspective and attempts were increasingly made to prevent mental disorder. Most clinics were operated by teams of psychologists, social workers and psychiatrists with indistinct and overlapping roles. The child guidance movement 'conceived its task to be primarily that of adjusting the growing individual to his own environment ... rather than ... curing a mental illness or treating a psychiatric patient' (Keir, 1952). By 1994 there were approximately 139 community facilities for children with mental health problems (Kurtz *et al.*, 1994).

Nurses continued to be limited to hospital care and were bound, on the whole, to the medical model. Mental hospitals developed out-patient services for children, the Tavistock Clinic in 1926 and the Maudsley Hospital in 1930. Then, in 1947, 20 years after the commencement of the child guidance movement, children's in-patient units were opened. By 1994 there were approximately 62 such units for children in Britain (Kurtz *et al.*,

1994). Nurses were employed to care for disturbed children. Children admitted fell into two broad groups, those who were aggressive and probably suffered what we now call conduct disorder and those who appeared to be psychotic, including those with autism.

Nurses, like others, found that the skills learnt in hospital could be adapted and used in community settings and consequently mental health nursing has become more accessible, with over 62% of community services employing child and adolescent mental health nurses (Kurtz *et al.*, 1994). There is a specialist child and adolescent mental health nursing qualification (ENB603) available in a small number of centres, which has ensured 34% of clinics and all but four of the in-patient units have a specialist nurse.

Nurses are prepared by specific training to perform tasks other members of the child and family consultation team have traditionally done. These include (HAS, 1995):

- Special interview techniques suitable for eliciting information from children of all ages and their families.
- A working knowledge of child development.
- A knowledge of dynamics of families, groups and systems and how these affect individuals in them.
- Understanding of the particular impact of major events on children's lives, e.g. abuse, bereavement.
- An awareness of how a professional's own life experiences informs their approach to others.
- Familiarity with manifestations of serious or potentially serious psychiatric disorder.
- Sufficient knowledge and ability to apply appropriate psychologically based therapies and psychiatric treatments.

Historically, child and adolescent mental health nurses have been concerned about their lack of recognition in child psychiatry (Pothier *et al.*, 1985). Nursing in child and adolescent mental health has developed rapidly, being one of the specialties to have its own qualification. It now provides nursing to children and their families in a variety of residential, community and other settings.

DEVELOPMENT OF CHILDREN, ADOLESCENTS AND FAMILIES

To work effectively, child and adolescent mental health nurses must clearly understand normal child development. This is important not only at the point of assessment but also in planning interventions that are realistic and achievable.

THEORETICAL CONSIDERATIONS
To work effectively, child and adolescent mental health nurses must clearly understand normal child development. This is important not only at the point of assessment but also in planning interventions that are realistic and achievable. The practice of child and adolescent mental health nursing is based on biological, psychological and social sciences and systems theories (Clunn, 1991).

Since the 1960s, the proportional influence of nature and nurture on individuals' development has been much debated. Although classic theories of child development have supported the argument that biology played a cental role in development, Nagel pointed out in the late 1950s that 'development was both a process and the product of a process' (Clunn, 1991).

Life span theory, which first became established in the 1970s, concludes that rather than being discontinuous, individual development continues throughout life. Proponents of this theory held the premise that change and stress were the main causes of mental ill health. The implications were enormous as people began to believe in their potential for change, irrespective of the effects of childhood traumas, which had previously been viewed as permanent. Life span theory has also contributed to the understanding that the family is one of the most important influences on a young person's development.

The major differences between child development and life span theories are that in the former, infancy and childhood are regarded as the formative years for an individual's development, which is regarded as linear, whereas in the latter, development is seen as a life-long process which is influenced by stressful events such as illness, death, divorce, accidents and migration.

Theories of Development

The following classical theories contribute to our understanding of young people (Figure 23.1).

Personality development

Bee (1985) sets out the three alternative explanations for the development of the personality by outlining the biological, social learning and psychoanalytical theories. Biological approaches to child development take into account the concepts of temperament and personality traits; it is assumed

Figure 23.1 Developmental life cycles

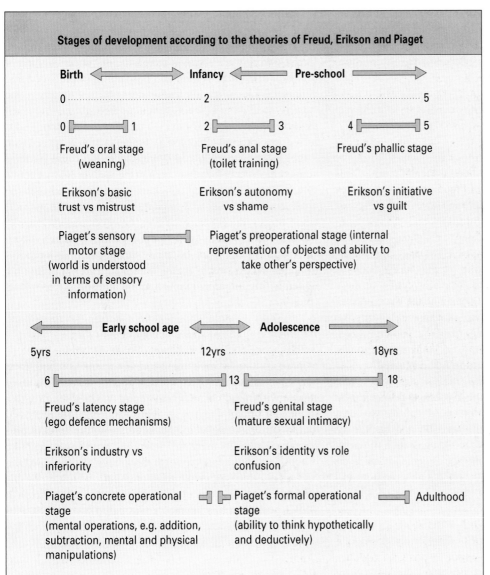

Stages of development according to the theories of Freud, Erikson and Piaget

Birth ⟷ Infancy ⟷ Pre-school

0 .... 2 5

0 ⊢———⊣ 1   2 ⊢———⊣ 3   4 ⊢———⊣ 5

Freud's oral stage (weaning)   Freud's anal stage (toilet training)   Freud's phallic stage

Erikson's basic trust vs mistrust   Erikson's autonomy vs shame   Erikson's initiative vs guilt

Piaget's sensory motor stage (world is understood in terms of sensory information) ⟶ Piaget's preoperational stage (internal representation of objects and ability to take other's perspective)

⟵ Early school age ⟷ Adolescence ⟶

5yrs .... 12yrs 18yrs

6 ⊢———⊣ 13   13 ⊢———⊣ 18

Freud's latency stage (ego defence mechanisms)   Freud's genital stage (mature sexual intimacy)

Erikson's industry vs inferiority   Erikson's identity vs role confusion

Piaget's concrete operational stage (mental operations, e.g. addition, subtraction, mental and physical manipulations) ⟷ Piaget's formal operational stage (ability to think hypothetically and deductively) ⟶ Adulthood

that every individual is born with a specific temperament or innate characteristic pattern of responding to the physical and social environment. These patterns shape the developing child's interactions with the world around him or her. In turn, these affect other people's behavioural responses to the child, which may lead to the development of psychopathology (Clunn, 1991). Evidence for this theory has been investigated since the mid-1970s; recent research findings confirm the basis for the theory and have further challenged traditionally held beliefs that personality is shaped in the first 5 years of life. It is now generally accepted that, despite early trauma or deprivation, the development of a healthy personality is possible as long as experiences later on in life are good and nurturing.

Social learning theories

The basis of all social learning theories is the importance attached to learning through the environment, other people and experience. Learning is a process that shapes the development of individuals. Bandura, perhaps the earliest and most well known social learning theorist wrote 'Except for elementary reflexes, people are not equipped with inborn repertoires of behaviour. They must learn them. New response patterns can be acquired either by direct experience or by observation' (Bee, 1985).

Such theories place importance on parents as the main mediators by which children's behaviour and style of interaction is reinforced (Rutter and Cox, 1985).

Psychoanalytical theories

Although there are many psychoanalytical theories, this section will concentrate on those of Freud and Erikson, as they regard development as sequential. Freud believed that the first 5 years of life were the most important and the character formed during that time was consistent throughout life (Clunn, 1991). Freud's theory involves five psychosexual stages during which a particular erogenous zone (or part of the body) is predominant. Freud believed that during the course of these stages, three aspects develop that constitute the basic personality, the first being the id or the store of instinctual energy, the second being the ego, the thinking, planning, and organizing part of the personality, and the third being the super ego, the conscience, which channels the id into acceptable forms of behaviour, according to parental and societal rules (Bee, 1985).

Erikson's theory emphasizes the psychosocial stages as he was more interested in the development of identity. He takes into account development throughout life and his theory comprises eight stages (from birth to old age), each of which is shaped partly by the cultural and social demands made on the developing child but also by the child's own physical and intellectual abilities (Bee, 1985).

Theories of attachment and bonding

Research into the development of security or insecurity in a child's early attachment draws upon aspects of psycho-analytical theory such as the proposition that children's early

relationships with their main care-giver greatly influences the quality of their relationships throughout life (Bee, 1985). According to Bowlby, attachment refers to 'the quality of the affectional ties between infant and parent that develops over time' (Clunn, 1991).

Rutter (1980) suggests that infants are born with a predisposition to behave in ways which will promote closeness and contact with their main care-givers. Rutter (1980) has identified three central concepts on which all attachment theorists agree. These are:
1 Bonding is seen to involve a reciprocal, behavioural interaction, with both parent and child playing an active role.
2 For bonding to occur both environment and emotional development in the child are important.
3 The development of attachment relies on social learning principles.

Research findings on the development of attachment have been well documented. In developing his theories of attachment, Bowlby emphasized the central role of families in relation to children's mental health. (Clunn, 1991).

Cognitive development theory

Piaget's work was central in increasing our understanding of this area of child development. His findings confirmed that children think differently from adults and that they have the capacity to learn spontaneously, mainly through activities such as play, which is to be regarded as crucial for children's cognitive development (Bee, 1985). Piaget (1975) proposed four stages from birth up to young adulthood. Research findings support the assumption that children themselves play an active role in the development of their cognitions and that the changes occur sequentially as a result of interaction with the environment. Recent research does, however, contest Piagets' use of stages, as an information-processing approach is considered to better explain cognitive development as a process of acquiring and generalizing basic strategies that involve remembering, organizing information and solving problems (Bee, 1985).

Theories of moral development

Both Piaget (1975) and Kohlberg (1964) viewed the development of children's moral reasoning in conjunction with their cognitive maturation. Kohlberg's theory comprises three stages, within each of which there are two or three progressive levels of moral reasoning (Hogarth, 1991). He theorized that moral reasoning in infants begins with the level of pre-conceived morality in the first stage, i.e. 'what I want and like is good' and progresses to stage three, level three, called the 'universal ethical principle of orientation', which is considered to be the most abstract and difficult to attain. Hogarth (1991) points out that his theory was based on research with boys and cites research carried out on girls' responses to the same questions, which yielded different findings.

The development of a concept of self

It is known that in the first few months of life, an infant cannot distinguish between him- or herself and other people. However, between about 18 and 24 months children develop a sense of themselves as being separate from others with their own intentions and feelings. This has been validated by research on infants' self-recognition (Clunn, 1991). In early childhood children begin to place themselves in comparative categories of age, size and gender based on their physical attributes and capabilities. By school age, the self concept includes the individual's views and beliefs, which become incorporated and modified through the process of adolescence. An important aspect of the development of the concept of self is the development of self-esteem. Although the development of an individual's self-esteem is a continuing process, starting in infancy through to adulthood, acquiring a sense of self-worth is considered a major developmental task in childhood (Barker, 1995) particularly as young people with mental health problems often have difficulties in the development of self-esteem. Development of self-esteem has important implications for protective factors against mental health problems.

Developmental life cycles

Life can be seen as a process to be negotiated, including the expansion, contraction and realignment of relationships in order to support the entry, exit and development of the family members in a functional way. As Figure 23.2 shows, this corresponds with the stages commonly used as a model for representing the development of the family life cycle in Western societies (Carter and McGoldrick, 1989).

PARENTING TASKS AND SKILLS

The tasks facing parents are many and the skills required to achieve them are complex, particularly given the ability

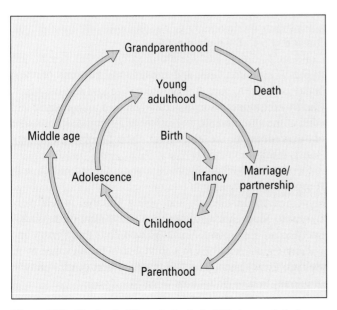

Figure 23.2 The family life cycle (typical of Western societies)

needed to adapt to the infant as she or he progresses to adulthood. There are several aspects of parental behaviour towards the developing child and adolescent that seem particularly important to enable healthy progression to adulthood, such as warmth, emotional closeness, consistent and authoritative means of control, and congruent clear and good communication as well as an adequate level of cognitive stimulation (Bee, 1985). Parents are themselves influenced by a number of important factors, which include the growing infant's temperament and developmental abilities. Hogarth (1991) has identified a number of needs that a growing child and adolescent has in becoming a well adjusted adult. These include love and commitment; close supervision and structure; attainable expectations and standards about behaviour; opportunities to develop psychosocial and cognitive skills; and to learn to make decisions and to cope with increasing autonomy and responsibility. In addition there are physical needs such as opportunities to maintain adequate physical health and provision of a safe environment.

ON BEING GOOD ENOUGH

Recent years have seen increasing emphasis on parents and other adults in care-taking roles for young people. Issues about the nature of parenting, which are necessary to enable the development of well adjusted youngsters and adults, and the type of social or professional input needed to enable this, have been high on the political agenda. Parenting and its associated aspects have been closely studied particularly by child and adolescent mental health professionals for almost three decades. Winnicott (1965) coined the phrase 'the good enough parent' to indicate that perfect parents do not exist but that good enough parents are able to provide and facilitate an environment in which the child's development is promoted and which is sensitive to the child's growing needs. It seems that there is agreement among professionals that the basic needs of a growing child and adolescent, which must be met by good enough parents, include basic physical care, affection, continuous security, stimulation of innate potential, guidance and control, and opportunities for taking responsibility according to age and maturity. Research findings have confirmed that just as child and adolescent development is largely affected by parenting (Cooper, 1985), the reverse is also true and parenting is now seen to be much influenced by the reciprocal interaction between child and parent (Rutter and Cox, 1985). The reciprocal nature of parenting is now seen as a means of doing things with children rather than to them, including communicating, problem solving and relationship continuity (Quinton and Rutter, 1988). It is now widely accepted that parenting cannot be viewed just in terms of the dyadic parent–child relationship in isolation but in context of wider social relationships and networks. In other words, parenting is seen in an ecological perspective (Belsky, 1984) which requires that attention is given to the emotional, psychological, social and physical resources available to parents within their wider context.

THE EFFECTS OF CLASS AND CULTURE

While there is considerable difference in child rearing practices across class and culture, which themselves are continuing to change according to wider societal expectations, there is an overall assumption that children's development must not be hindered or obstructed (Cooper, 1985) and it is believed that most 'good enough' parents would agree on what constitutes good enough parenting. Rutter and Cox (1985), on reviewing research findings into parenting styles that proved more effective in enabling development of well adjusted adults, concluded that an authoritative–reciprocal parenting style in which a combination of firm limit-setting, recognition of children's rights, encouragement of their independence by shared decision making and an ability to put their needs first, on the whole seemed to be associated with the development of adults who have an awareness of social responsibility and a low level of aggression, high self-esteem and a degree of self-efficacy.

The primary task of the family is to facilitate the transitions that a developing infant has to make to become an adult, while also coping with its own transitions through the developmental stages of life and the stresses that often occur such as bereavement, loss, illness, divorce, new relationships, change of jobs, unemployment and migration. Many mental health professionals tend to view child and adolescent mental health in the context of family mental health and take into account the developmental tasks achieved by the family when making assessments and planning interventions (Barker, 1995) as it is assumed that a good adjustment to family life in childhood precedes a good adjustment of young people and adults as members of society.

MENTAL HEALTH PROBLEMS IN CHILDREN AND ADOLESCENTS

Mental health problems are best seen as difficulties in the child's mind, which may arise from any number of congenital, constitutional, environmental, family or illness factors. Nurses will meet children who show a range of conditions, from emotional and behavioural problems to severe and persistent mental disorder. The prevalence of diagnosable mental disorder (now ICD10 or DSM1V) in the child population is estimated to be as high as 25% with 10% of children having moderate or severe problems (HAS, 1995).

On the basis of the HAS (1995) figures it is generally accepted that in a population of 250 000, of which 20–25% is aged under 18 years, there would be between 5000 and 12 000 children with mental health or psychiatric disorders at any one time.

PROBLEMS OF CHILDREN

Mental health problems fall broadly into the following groups.

Mild Childhood Problems

Mild childhood problems such as sleep and feeding difficulties, unhappiness, anxiety and social problems, bed wetting and faecal soiling, over-activity, temper tantrums, behaviour problems, and abdominal pain without physical cause present frequently to health visitors, GPs and school nurses. Children with such ailments are often referred to child and family consultation services to be seen by the team, which may include a child mental health nurse. The children may show extremes of 'normal' behaviours or give clues to the child's or family's underlying problem. Whatever the cause, the effect is usually distressing and unpleasant for all involved.

Emotional and Conduct Problems

Emotional and conduct problems are found in around 10% of children and up to 20% of adolescents. Persistent fears, anxiety states, phobias and psychosomatic disorders, low mood and antisocial behaviour are all relatively common (HAS, 1995).

Childhood Depression

Childhood depression has recently been the subject of much professional and media attention. Graham and Hughes (1995) in their report *So Young, So Sad, So Listen* say that up to 5% of children under 12 suffer distress and about 2% of these are 'depressed'. They say that in a school of 1000 pupils about 50 would be seriously depressed each year. Major depressive disorders are now regarded as commoner than previously thought with 1% in middle childhood and 2–5% in mid adolescence.

Unipolar or Bipolar Disorders

Unipolar or bipolar disorders are rare before puberty but increase in frequency during adolescence. Hypomania when it presents in teenagers is often dramatic, difficult to treat and very challenging to work with.

Conduct Disorders

Conduct disorders include children who steal, truant, are aggressive, cause fires and those who, because of their behaviour, fail to socialize or internalize and resolve anger. Childhood conduct disorder is clearly linked with juvenile and adult crime, drug and alcohol misuse and, untreated, has major consequences for the individual, their family and society (HAS, 1995).

Hyperactivity

Hyperactivity in toddlers and young children is relatively common. Most children from time to time are restless, distractible and inattentive. However, when it is the primary and dominating characteristic in a child who is handicapped by it, then it becomes attention deficit disorder. Between 1% and 2% of primary school children are affected.

Developmental Disorders

Developmental disorders such as language delay and autism can cause major problems. Autism is experienced by 3–8 children per 10 000 and of these only 10–15% are likely to be able to lead independent lives.

Obsessive–compulsive Disorder

Obsessive–compulsive disorder occurs in up to 2% of adolescents.

Suicide and Deliberate Self-harm

Suicide and deliberate self-harm in childhood is relatively rare but the rate has been increasing since the mid-1980s. Suicide accounted for 0.5% of deaths in the 5–14 year age group in 1989. Suicidal ideation is common in adolescents and the incidence of suicide attempts, while much lower, is still a significant problem; 3% engage in acts of deliberate self-harm at some time during their adolescence (HAS, 1995).

Eating Disorders

Eating disorders such as anorexia nervosa occur in about 1% of 15–19-year-old girls, with a peak onset at 16. It also occurs in children as young as 6 years and is thought to be increasing. Bulimia nervosa is more common but occurs in later adolescence (HAS, 1995).

Psychotic Disorders

Psychotic disorders are rare. Schizophrenia, for instance, is difficult to diagnose in children. Early-onset schizophrenia occurs before 18 and very early onset before age 13. Psychotic disorders in children and adolescents are usually severe, highly unpredictable and more difficult to work with than those which occur in adulthood (HAS, 1995).

Post-traumatic Stress Disorder

Children and adolescents experience an adult-like PTSD. However, there is uncertainty as to the extent children share the symptoms described in adults (HAS, 1995).

Drug and Alcohol Use and Misuse

Recent surveys have highlighted concern about children who use or misuse drugs and alcohol (HAS, 1995). The Health Education Authority conducted a survey of young people aged 9–15 years and found that by 15 years of age 16% of males and 14% of females had tried cannabis, 5% and 2% had used LSD; 4% and 2% amphetamines and solvents, 3% and 1% tranquilisers and Ecstasy. Heroin and cocaine had been used by 1% of both males and females (Health Education Authority, 1992).

Atypical Psychosexual Development

Children develop their gender and sexual identity in highly individual ways. How and why this process becomes distressing for the child is the subject of much controversy. Most young people experience no difficulty, while others experience a turbulent and painful transition to adult maturity.

FACTORS INFLUENCING MENTAL HEALTH

It is important for nurses to be aware of the research based findings about risk and protective factors in child and adolescent mental health, as these may well affect the nature and style of interventions that are made. Risk factors are 'circumstances that make the development of a disorder more likely' (Barker, 1995).

Risk factors interact with each other in a complex way and it is generally believed that a child and adolescent mental health problem is more likely to occur when there is more than just a single risk factor involved. The following list of the main risk factors is by no means comprehensive:

- Accidents in or outside the home that cause neurological and physical injuries. These are thought to predispose young people to developing mental health problems or learning difficulties (Barker, 1995).
- Specific developmental delays including speech and communication difficulties (Pearce, 1993).
- Physical illness especially affecting the nervous central system; there is a greater risk for children with epilepsy (Pearce, 1993) and the risks are increased for children who are repeatedly ill and have several admissions to hospital (Barker, 1995).
- Each of the above may predispose a child to early academic failure in school, which is a risk factor in itself.
- Abuse and neglect, ill treatment, failure to meet children's physical, emotional and psychosocial needs and violation of their rights have been strongly associated with mental health and academic problems (Barker, 1995).
- Family discord and breakdown. The rates of childhood mental health problems can be as high as 80% in the first year after divorce (Pearce, 1993). Marital discord and disharmony as well as overt parental conflict and inconstant parenting and hostile relationships are known to lead to increased rates of emotional and behavioural problems in children and adolescents (Pearce, 1993; Barker, 1995).
- Mental health problems, particularly depressive illnesses, in the mother (Pearce, 1993).
- Parents who are socially isolated or have few social supports (Rutter and Cox, 1985).
- When one parent is a criminal or when there are delinquent siblings in the family, rates of delinquency increase (Rutter and Cox, 1985).
- Cumulative effects of stress, such as when young children and adolescents experience more than two adverse life events close together — this results in them being at increased risk of developing emotional and behavioural problems (Pearce, 1993).
- The experience of being fostered with a number of different placements over a long period and other forms of institutional care (all of which tend to happen when children come into the care of local authorities) — these have been found to predispose children to higher rates of emotional and behavioural problems and school failure (Wolkind and Rutter, 1985).

- Deprived environmental surroundings such as poor housing (Rutter and Cox, 1985), and living in inner city areas with high levels of environmental threat, such as assaults or burglaries — these have also been found to be associated with higher rates of mental health problems in both children and adolescents (Cox, 1993; Hogarth, 1991).
- Schools with poor organization, unclear discipline, high teacher turnover, low staff morale, lack of or unclear policies on dealing with bullying and a general lack of recognition of children as individuals — these have also been found to have powerful influences on the rates of mental health problems in young people (Cox, 1993; Wolkind and Rutter, 1985).

These risk factors are commonly associated with many children and adolescents, yet interestingly some manage to develop as well-adjusted individuals without suffering a recognizable mental health problem. This seems to be because of protective factors at play for these young people. Protective factors are defined as the opposite of risk factors as they 'reduce the likelihood of a disorder appearing' (Barker, 1995).

The most powerful protective factor is positive self-esteem; the development of positive self-worth and self-image is a central developmental task of children, which continues into adulthood (Quinton and Rutter, 1988). Increased self-confidence and belief in one's own ability to affect what is happening and to deal with stressful situations in a problem-solving manner, are all part of high self-esteem.

Other protective factors are:

- A secure, affectionate and stable relationship with at least one parent or constant adult figure who functions in the role of care-giver (Barker, 1995, Pearce, 1993).
- Good and successful experiences including achievement in activities requiring special skills or academic achievement (Quinton and Rutter, 1988).
- An adaptable temperament, constituting the ability to accept changes, rules and frustration without upset (Barker, 1995).
- An improvement in family and environmental circumstances, even if it occurs later in the development of a child or adolescent, will serve to lessen the effect of earlier adverse circumstances (Barker, 1995).
- Girls generally have lower rates of behavioural and emotional disorders than boys and are more likely to elicit protective behaviour from parents and care-givers (Barker, 1995; Quinton and Rutter, 1988).

CONTEMPORARY SOCIO-POLITICAL INFLUENCES

Every child and adolescent mental health nurse must be fully aware of the Children Act 1989 or the Children Act (Scotland) 1995 legislation, as it embodies society's views of how needs of children and adolescents must be met and how they can best be protected. There are numbers of publications outlining the responsibilities of all professionals who work with children and families (Department of Health, 1991a; Department of Health, 1995). In addition to providing guidance on protecting children and young people, the Children Act 1989 covers, for example, disputes between parents about the future of their children, the needs of children with disabilities and the onus on professionals to develop and promote services to prevent family breakdown. It aims to strike a balance between encouraging family autonomy while protecting the rights of children. Important principles that it states are as follows:

> ... the welfare of the child is of paramount consideration in court proceedings;
>
> Wherever possible children should be brought up and cared for in their own families;
>
> Children should be safe and protected by effective intervention if they are in danger;
>
> When dealing with children, courts should ensure that delay is avoided and may only make an order if to do so is better than to make no order at all;
>
> Children should be kept informed about what happens to them and should participate when discussions are made about their future;
>
> Parents continue to have parental responsibility for their children even when their children are no longer living with them. They should be kept informed about their children and participate when decisions are made about their children's future;
>
> Parents of children in need should be helped to bring up their children themselves;
>
> This help should be provided as service to the child and family and should: be provided in partnership with the parents; meet each child's needs; be appropriate to the child's race, culture, religion and language; be open to effective independent representation and complaints procedures; and draw upon an effective relationship between the local authorities and other agencies, including voluntary agencies.
>
> *(Department of Health, 1991b)*

The implications for child and adolescent mental health nurses include not only having a full working knowledge of local child protection procedures, which involves regular updating, training and clinical supervision, but also the following:

- Appreciation of the importance of cooperating and working in conjunction with the Social Services and Education departments.
- The ability to offer services both to parents and children that listens to and empowers them, gives them appropriate information, takes into account children's wishes and feelings and enhances parents' abilities to meet their children's needs.
- The importance of identifying children in need and of referring them to the local Social Services department. A child is defined as being in need if he or she is:

unlikely to achieve or maintain or to have the opportunity to achieve or maintain, a reasonable standard of health without provision of ... services by local authority; ... health or development is likely to be significantly impaired, or further impaired without the provision of such services, and if the child is disabled. [Section 17 (10)].

(Department of Health, 1991b)

The Act requires that any assessments or treatments given to children and adolescents are with the consent of those with parental responsibility and that a more mature child or adolescent has the right to make an informed choice before medical or psychiatric treatments are carried out. A definition of the only circumstances allowed by law for restricting the liberty of a person under 18 in a hospital is given:

1. The child has a history of absconding, is likely to abscond if not detained and is likely to suffer 'significant harm' if s/he were allowed to leave, and/or
2. If s/he is not detained s/he is likely to injure him- or herself or other persons.

The law allows for a person under 18 to be detained for no more than 72 hours, whether consecutively or in aggregate in any period of 28 days. To detain a child beyond this time he or she must be detained under Mental Health legislation or a Secure Accommodation Order (Sampson, 1993).

The rights of children and their families who use mental health services and the standard of service they can expect are outlined in *The Patient's Charter – Services for Children and Young People* (Department of Health, 1996).

CHILD PROTECTION

Every child and young person has a right to a life free from abuse but each week at least four children in Britain will die as a result of abuse or neglect (Meadow, 1993). Experience suggests that this is 4 or 5 times more common than 10 years ago, probably because of increased public and professional awareness and better recognition (Meadow, 1993). There are 45 000 children on local authority Child Protection Registers at any given time and many of these children and young people will present to child mental health nurses at some stage.

Child abuse, defined simply, is 'any treatment of a child in a way that is unacceptable in a given culture at a given time' (Meadow, 1993).

Sexual abuse of children is one of the most high profile areas of abuse. Sexual abuse occurs:

when dependent developmentally immature children and adolescents participate in sexual activities that they do not fully comprehend, to which they are unable to give informed consent.

(Meadow, 1993)

Emotional abuse of children is generally more difficult to determine, because it is based on judgements of the quality of parenting. Some regard a child as abused if he or she has a behavioural problem to which the parents fail to respond appropriately or if they refuse to seek and accept professional help. Emotional abuse also exists when parents are persistently neglectful, hostile or rejecting of their children.

Nurses have a duty to inform the social services of the local authority if they receive an allegation of abuse from anyone about any child or they have any suspicion whatsoever. Each health authority or Trust will have a child protection policy, a designated and named nurse and detailed procedures to follow. It is important to discuss immediately any concerns with a senior colleague and ensure contemporaneous record keeping.

Children and young people will sometimes disclose abuse to a nurse, typically a nurse with whom they have established or are establishing a trusting relationship. They may ask the nurse to treat the information in confidence. Of course children have the same general right as adults to expect confidentiality but this does not automatically apply in all circumstances. The UKCC Code of Conduct says that the disclosure of confidential information is permissible if such disclosure is in the wider public interest. They go on to say explicitly that disclosure of child abuse is in the public interest.

To disentangle the complexity of child protection and child mental health work, it is sometimes helpful to see these issues separately, i.e. that protection of the child from harm is predominately the responsibility of the social services and responsibility for the mental health care of the child rests with the health service.

Each setting that provides a service for children with mental health problems, whether it be community or hospital based, will have local policies and procedures to guide staff in many complex and challenging situations; it is important that all staff have access to them.

APPLYING NURSING PRINCIPLES IN THE ASSESSMENT OF MENTAL HEALTH OF CHILDREN AND ADOLESCENTS

PROCESS OF REFERRAL

The source of a referral of a child or adolescent with mental health needs is especially important because the referrral is usually made by someone other than the young person concerned. When considering the process of referral, in addition to ascertaining who has made the referral, it is important to clarify what questions need to be answered, who else is involved, how much more information is needed in addition to that which has been provided and what has been done regarding the referred problem so far. Most importantly it is essential to clarify that the family or carer of the young person concerned knows about the referral and has consented to it. Even if nurses are not directly involved at the point of referral it is important that they are aware of the process and of the details of the referral of each case that they become involved in, as the referral process can itself make a significant difference to the way in which a case is handled and the outcome of intervention (Selvini Palazzoli *et al.*, 1980).

PURPOSE OF ASSESSMENT

Assessment formats vary according to the type and nature of child, adolescent and family mental health service. The method of assessment will also depend on the overall philosophy of the team, clinic and the resources available, as well as any specific therapeutic, training or research interests held. Assessment aims to clarify the family's view of the problem, including specific concerns on the child and family's level of functioning. Methods of assessment in child and adolescent mental health service include history taking from parents or carers, interviews with the whole family, individual interviews with the child or adolescent, interviews with siblings and others such as foster carers, observation of the play or activity centred interaction between parent and children or family members and physical and mental health examinations of the young person. Nurses need to develop a clear framework for the initial assessment, as this serves to structure the process. The assessment process needs to be discrete from treatment or therapeutic intervention, although many of the skills used in the assessment are just as valid in later work.

The assessment procedure (see Case studies) should also allow an opportunity for the young person and their family to clarify what changes are hoped for, what type of help is sought, the level of motivation and commitment for the expected changes, as well as the appropriateness of any intervention that may be offered. For this to occur, the assessment process needs to be viewed as an exercise not only in information gathering but also in giving information. Clunn (1991)

points out that, without a clearly planned assessment procedure that includes a formulation or working model of the problems that are presented as well as agreed goals, the therapeutic process can easily become unnecessarily complex and confusing. Furthermore, a thorough and clear framework for the assessment process enables families to become clearer about their goals. It is sensible to base the decision about which intervention to implement on the young person and the family's goals, as making an agenda to work to their goals rather than the professionals' is likely to positively affect the outcome of the intervention (Reimes and Treacher, 1995; Nelson–Jones, 1982).

Nurses aim to observe, assess, formulate hypotheses and set well defined goals, while responding to the complex social and developmental needs of the child. They need to be able to design flexible and creative solutions to difficult problems, while bearing in mind that behaviour has to be seen in the context of the family, society and culture. In reaching a 'way of thinking' about children it is important to appreciate how children are different from adults. Maddison and Kellehear (1982) describe these differences.

Children present mental ill health in very different ways from adults. All children grow and develop in physical, psychological and social dimensions. Children experience the world around them in ways difficult for adults to understand.

Children and young people may not have reached the level of sophisticated thought and speech required by the adult world. They may be telling the adults around them about their internal experiences by acting out distress in their day-to-day behaviour. Therefore, when children or adolescents act in odd or bizarre ways, it is important to avoid focusing exclusively on the behaviour.

The vast majority of children live within a group, usually their family. Children are not only 'shaped' by the adults

---

Case study: **Assessment — leading to more appropriate intervention**

Kylie, a 3-year-old girl, and her mother were referred by the GP because of the mother's concerns about Kylie's behaviour. The GP reported that the mother had found it even harder to cope with the child since the arrival of her younger sister, now 13 months old. The whole family (including the father) were seen for an assessment by the nurse, during which they were interviewed together to observe the interaction between the family members, and then the mother was seen alone to take a history. This assessment highlighted that the child actually had no mental health problems herself and was a bright, contented and well adjusted little girl but that the mother was extremely anxious and felt very hopeless because of marital problems. The nurse gave the family feedback and a plan for further help.

Case study: **Assessment — allowing aims to be clarified**

Fiona, 5 years old, was referred by her GP, who gave the presenting problems as behavioural difficulties, a degree of learning disability and reported that the parents found it increasingly hard to cope with her. The excessive demands Fiona made on her parents were making it difficult for them to give attention to her two older sisters. The nurse carried out an initial assessment with the parents only and was able to determine that they actually preferred not to receive treatment immediately for Fiona's behavioural problems. They believed that she needed a fuller assessment of her developmental needs and felt that previous diagnoses of learning disability and secondary behavioural problems were not accurate. The parents had read a great deal about child mental health problems and had wondered whether or not their child was autistic. A specialist assessment led to a diagnosis and formulation that not only satisfied the parents but clarified the child's future educational and developmental needs.

around them but have a strong influence on how those adults behave. Therefore it is crucial to place the child in context and see them as part of the whole. A health professional will not be able to understand the child without meeting, listening to, observing and making an attempt to understand the family.

The literature, research and clinical experience support the view that all family members, including children, contribute to adaptive as well as maladaptive interactions (Wright and Leahey, 1987). In contrast to adult psychiatry, where an appreciation of the cause and the treatment is essential, with children it is crucial to think of what the problem means to the individual and family, how it is maintained and what relationship it has to all the family members. The nurse needs to be aware that all childhood problems have complex causes and effects and it is often more illuminating to look to the visible effects to aid understanding.

It is important not to believe you can 'rescue' the family from the distress they suffer. It is empowering for parents and for their children to help them solve their own problems to their own satisfaction.

Families may present to child mental health nurses because they have exhausted their ideas of how to solve a problem. It can be productive to alter their understanding of the problem. Doing this enables the family to try new solutions, which, in turn, helps them to progress.

The context in which children live has been discussed, together with the fact that their presenting problems (whatever they be, behaviours, moods, thoughts or perceptions) may be caused by and have effects on those around them. Therefore it seems clear that, in some circumstances, it may be possible to bring about change in the child by bringing about change in the family or home.

Child mental health nurses routinely use nursing hypotheses as tools to help understand the complex nature of childhood mental health problems. Before seeing a child, after assessment and at regular stages throughout contact, a nursing hypothesis is a useful way to formulate explanations about how an individual child has established and is maintaining a particular problem or need.

INITIAL ASSESSMENT ENGAGING FAMILIES

Non-attendance for appointments in child and adolescent family mental health services is a common problem and for this reason a number of factors have been identified that have been shown to reduce it:

- Telephoning families, in addition to writing to them with the appointment, just before the assessment date.
- Ensuring that the waiting time between referral and first assessment appointment is neither too long, i.e. over 8 weeks, or too short, i.e. below 3 weeks (Subotsky, 1993).
- Providing clear information about the agency the family has been invited to attend and the process of assessment (Reimers and Treacher, 1995).
- Carrying out pre-assessment home visits as these can be reassuring for families who are often concerned about the stigma attached to bringing their child or adolescent to a mental health service.

Pre-assessment home visits can provide an opportunity for the child and adolescent mental health nurse to engage the family to clarify their concerns, reassure them regarding any fears or anxiety about the process of attending the hospital or clinic and thereby enable better preparation for attendance for the formal assessment and subsequent intervention appointments. Pre-admission home visits are a common feature of in-patient units for young people and enable child and adolescent mental health nurses to both gather and give crucial information about

---

Case study: **Engaging the family — escort to initial assessment**

Billy, 5 years old, Kate his 8-year-old sister and their mother were referred by their GP for the children's continual fighting, non-compliance with mother's requests and physical aggression towards her. The mother had received treatment from the local mental health team for periods of depression and agoraphobia. On reading through the referral and getting extra information from the GP it became apparent that the mother did not go anywhere unescorted, particularly with the children as they were both so difficult to manage. The nurse contacted social services to which the family were known and which had, for a number of years, provided a family support worker. The nurse spoke to the family support worker's supervisor and followed this up with a letter, explaining the importance of the mother and the two children being escorted by the support worker. This would enable the family to attend the appointment, which involved a long journey for them. The family were subsequently enabled to attend further treatment appointments.

Case study: **Engaging the family — support for the home situation**

Mohamed was referred by his social worker for an assessment of his aggressive and self-harming behaviour, both at school and at home. Mohamed was a 6-year-old boy in a family of seven children, aged between 11 months and 12 years, which lived on income support in a high-rise block of flats on a council estate. On the day of the initial assessment, the social worker telephoned just after the appointment time to inform the team that the child had absconded, yet again, earlier in the day but that the mother still wished to come and therefore had requested another assessment appointment. The nurse suggested to the team that, before another assessment appointment was sent, it should be clarified with the social worker that the family would be provided with transport, child care assistance and any support needed. This would help to ensure that the mother could give more attention to the referred child on the day of the appointment so that she and Mohamed could actually get to the interview. This action was followed by successful attendance.

and to the young person concerned and to clarify whether proceeding with assessment with a view to in-patient admission would be the next appropriate step. For some families, their ability to get to appointments can be a practical issue, particularly when the families are large, they have a long distance to travel, include children who are very young or, indeed, where they have been referred not at their own request but by social services because of concerns about ability to care for their children. The practical issues involved include child care arrangements, transport and sheer physical effort of getting to the appointment. These things can only be overcome by a child and adolescent mental health nurse planning carefully before the assessment appointment about practical ways in which the family's attendance can be facilitated. (See the Case studies for examples of typical situations.)

Once a family has arrived for an initial assessment appointment, a number of important skills are used to build rapport (Nelson–Jones, 1982). Needless to say communication skills that are used when engaging families in assessment and subsequent intervention sessions are very important. Taylor (1991) highlights the importance of patients' perceptions of health professionals and how they are likely to be more responsive to a health professional who seems warm, who answers their questions and gives them information. Some of the important elements of non-verbal communication skills include making eye contact at appropriate moments, turning towards the family members and leaning slightly forward, adopting the tone of voice of those being interviewed and active listening to their concerns. Taylor (1991) recommends adopting a friendly stance, rather than a professional business-like one, to communicate supportiveness and spending some time talking about neutral topics to engage family members. It is also important to find out how the family members recieve information and to clarify other concerns or worries that have not been mentioned.

COMMUNICATION WITH CHILDREN AND ADOLESCENTS

The skills used in engaging families are just as important when engaging children and adolescents during individual assessment interviews. However, a number of other issues need to be considered, as it can be daunting for a young person to come to a mental health setting with their family, let alone to sit in a room on their own being interviewed by a stranger. The physical aspects such as room size, seating and distance between the nurse and the young person are important, and provision of toys or drawing paper and pens for younger children is helpful. The type of language that the nurse uses should also be consonant with the young person's cognitive and communication abilities. Using humour and conveying empathy through verbal and non-verbal behaviour can be extremely effective as long as they are used appropriately. Even though the young person may have been introduced to the interviewer alongwith their family, it is worthwhile making a reintroduction, stating name and job as clearly as possible as it is likely that the young person may not have taken this in

at first, or may not have understood it. Clunn (1991) recommends that nurses adopt a relaxed conversational tone of enquiry when interviewing young people and avoid any rigid questionnaire-style format. However, it is also important to have some clear aims and objectives when interviewing. Below is a framework that provides guidance on carrying out initial interviews with children and adolescents. This clearly needs to be used flexibly bearing in mind the interviewee's age and ability and the context in which they are seen.

- Find out the young person's perceptions of why they are here and if they say they do not know or are unclear, make sure it is explained who made the referral and what the concerns were. This should be done in a way that does not make the child feel blamed or guilty.

- It is extremely useful to find out what the young person enjoys doing and what their hobbies and recreational activities are as this can serve not only to make them become less anxious but will provide valuable information about other aspects of their life.

- Ask about school, the subjects that they like and dislike and how they find the teachers and the timetable; friends are important, including whether the young person has best friends, who they are closest to at school or in the neighbourhood and the activities that they engage in with their friends. It is useful to ask them to name their friends and give a brief description of the type of person that they are.

- Family relations are important, so ask about relationships with siblings and parents, who they are closest to and family activities or outings that have occurred in the past or recently.

- The young person's perception of the family's view of the problems is also important and whether they agree or disagree with parental and family concerns about their behaviour. It is important to find out whether the young person perceives family members as being punitive and unreasonable or supportive and caring.

- The range of emotions the young person is able to express or articulate is an important aspect of their development, so it is extremely useful to find out what sorts of things make them happy, sad, angry, what they do about it and what the consequences are. For example, how do they deal with worries, who do they seek comfort from, if at all.

- Asking the young person to name three wishes is a common technique but must be used carefully, as many young people who have been to helping agencies have been asked the same question several times over.

- Finding out what the best and worst things the interviewee thinks could happen to them is useful in clarifying their fears and hopes. Determine whether the young person has any questions, not just at the end but at relevant points in the interview. At the end, find out if there is anything that they wish to add or talk about that have not been discussed.

- With young children it is useful to engage them in the interview by telling them that there will be play and talk for some time and allow them within reason to choose which they want to do first. With older children and adolescents make sure they know why the interview is taking place (i.e. to get their views on things) and how long it is envisaged the interview lasting. If a specific intervention has already been requested as part of the referral or by the family, it is extremely important to find out the young person's view on that and on attending the department or clinic in the future.

HISTORY TAKING FROM PARENT

Most methods for taking histories from parents tend to follow a traditional medical format, which has proved to be effective. It is important for nurses to remember that, just because a particular question has been asked, it does not mean that a clear response will be forthcoming. The principles of engaging and basic communication skills are just as important when interviewing parents. Clunn (1991) has provided a useful table of the developmental data that need to be obtained from parents; the following format contains aspects of this and other questions the authors have found helpful in assessment.

- Obtain a summary of the parents' current concerns and get specific example of the problems. For example, with aggressive behaviours, what the antecedents are, the actual behaviour and how long it actually lasts, what the consequences are and how family members respond.
- Information on pregnancy and delivery is important, particularly if there were complications in either.
- Physical developmental milestones, such as the age at which the child began to sit, crawl, walk, talk, was toilet trained and was weaned, what the sleeping and eating pattern is like, the child's current vocabulary (particularly important for pre-school children) and the child's self care-skills.
- The family history, such as the parents' own upbringing, occupation, relationships, extended family contact and social supports and their current daily routine — these are all important in mapping out broader influences on the young person's life.
- Psychosocial milestones, such as the young person's relationship with other family members, adults and peers. Ability to separate and attend school, academic progress, life events and coping strategies and hospitalizations are all relevant.
- Parental perceptions are very important. For example, how the parent describes and perceives the child and what sort of attributions they make, what they feel works and does not work in response to the concerns about the young person's behaviour.
- Clarify what coping strategies the parents have used and how they believe they and other family members have been affected by the presenting problems.

THERAPEUTIC INTERVENTION

The role of child and adolescent mental health nurses in therapeutic interventions can vary depending on the setting and their specialist interests. On residential units, child and adolescent mental health nurses will have defined roles as primary and associate nurses and have full responsibility for the nursing care provided to a number of young people during their admission. Child and adolescent mental health nurses working in child guidance clinics or out-patient departments will have full responsibility for the caseload they carry (which tends to be more than providing nursing care to the referred young person, as the care and treatment offered will often involve the parents and whole family and wider networks, such as schools). In each of these situations the child and adolescent mental health nurse works both as an individual and as part of a wider team. This can be a source of challenge as well as tension. Child and adolescent mental health nurses have developed their skills and interests in a variety of therapeutic interventions, while also continuing with their day-to-day tasks of managing the environment and providing individual nursing care.

Therapeutic interventions are made by nurses when they carry out clear and effective communication with their colleagues and comprehensive liaison with the young person's network including the parents, schools, and social services and education departments. In addition, the very process of building a relationship with a young person as a primary or associate nurse and facilitating the therapeutic milieu (on day or residential units) are in themselves an important intervention. A number of core skills and principles are involved in building therapeutic relationships with young people, which involve managing issues relating to the dynamics among staff and young people, among colleagues within the same setting and among agencies. These principles and issues are dealt with next and apply to nurses working in a variety of settings, although the feelings and dynamics that come into play are often not as intense as in the community or out-patient setting, where the young person and family are only seen for a maximum of 2 hours at a time, compared with the duration of face-to-face contact that nurses have with young people and their families in day and residential units.

PRINCIPLES OF THERAPEUTIC RELATIONSHIPS WITH YOUNG PEOPLE AND MANAGING DYNAMICS

There is no doubt that working with children and adolescents with mental health problems has the potential to arouse extremely powerful feelings in the nurse and other professionals. A number of principles and skills are important when building therapeutic relations with young people, which include the following (Ney and Mulvihill, 1985):

- Self-restraint is required to ensure that the nurse does not give in to the strong urge to nurture the young person and provide all that is perceived to have not been provided by their parents. This is unrealistic and alienates the young person from the parents and the parents from the staff.
- Optimism and realistic expectation is a prerequisite. With many common problems there is little evidence at first sight of the severity of the impairment caused, which makes it very easy to develop unrealistically high expectations.

Helping a young person to change and make the most of their potential takes time and occurs slowly. It is therefore important for the nurse to have steadfast hope and engender this in their colleagues, the young person's family and the professional network. This sense of hope will be conveyed and experienced by the young person as supportive encouragement and a belief in their ability to change.

- The ability to tolerate the young person's ambivalence to the health professional's willingness to be available for them and to be helpful, is crucial to facilitate a healthy and therapeutic relationship. Many young people with mental health problems, while desperately wanting empathy, warmth and understanding, will simultaneously reject these things before they themselves have to bear the pain of being rejected. Nurses need to have the strength to retain confidence and belief in themselves while also continuing to respond consistently and to communicate willingness to contain the powerful projections of feelings that the young person finds impossible to tolerate. It can often take a long time before the young person develops sufficient trust to allow the nurse to help set realistic and achievable goals to work towards change (Hoxter, 1983).

- The ability to reflect on the feelings that the young person arouses in the nurse and the nature of the relationship is also important, as the feelings that are aroused provide information about how the young person is feeling and how he or she has experienced, and relates with, other people. Together with this, the nurse needs to be able to work not only with the transference (the whole range of emotions that the young person has experienced in other important relationships and brings to the current one) but also with the counter-transference (the nurse's own hopes, expectations, fears and emotions from other relationships, as well as the reactions of the nurse as a consequence of experiencing the young person's transference) (Salzberger–Wittenberg, 1988). This will enable the nurse to use the therapeutic relationship with the young person effectively, to help them change and reintegrate into their own family and community in as adaptive a way as possible.

Case study: Re-integrating with peer group

Elizabeth, aged 10, quickly and easily formed relationships with the staff members on admission to the in-patient unit. She would spend all of her recreational time either in her bedroom listening to music or talking to other nurses and inviting them to join in games, while distancing herself and rejecting all her peers from her games. The primary nurse spoke to Elizabeth about this after 2 weeks and helped her to identify playmates and days and times when she felt able to join in, as a starting point, together with the nature of support that the nurse should provide for these predetermined activities. In this way Elizabeth continued to be able to enjoy a solitary activity listening to music, while reducing the amount of time spent inappropriately with adults and increasing that with her peer group.

Child and adolescent mental health nurses have the challenging task of ensuring that they do not foster the young person's inappropriate dependency on themselves, while also remaining constantly available and able to contain the many emotions that the young person will experience and project. The importance of development of self-esteem and a sense of self-worth has been demonstrated earlier as a protective factor against mental health problems. Nurses are in a prime position to enable this to occur for the young people that they work with by providing unconditional, positive regard for the young person as a whole (while helping them to change the behaviours impairing their development) and by assisting them to achieve and maintain friendly peer relationships and facilitating reintegration into school and community life (see Case study). These involve the nurse having to remain supportive while also encouraging age-appropriate independent behaviour, in a firm and reassuring manner. This can only occur after obtaining the young person's trust and having classified their motivation to work towards these goals, at a pace that he or she can tolerate (Wilkinson, 1983).

The range of extreme feelings that can be aroused in nurses and other professionals working with young people can lead to complex dynamics within staff groups and between agencies. Hoxter (1983) has highlighted the phenomena, endemic in this specialty: the urge to feel angry and frustrated with colleagues and the wish to find somebody to blame for the young person's predicament.

WORKING WITH DISTURBED AND DISTURBING CHILDREN

The demands placed on nurses who work with disturbed and disturbing children are high. Some people find it difficult to accept that childhood is not automatically a happy and carefree time for all.

Children and young people admitted to in-patient units represent a group of extremely disturbed and dependent individuals, especially following the development of improved community services. The stress levels are high in light of the child's unpredictability and propensity to act-out, often in dramatic and challenging ways. There are methods to reduce stress by taking active steps to 'look after' yourself. On most in-patient units there are several recurring themes that warrant attention.

Each staff team must ensure it has a sufficient number of people with specific training in child and adolescent mental health nursing. These people should have developed creative solutions to problems in a variety of settings, which reduce anxiety by speedily resolving challenging behaviours. This promotes a clear sense of direction, resourcefulness and an atmosphere of containment. Containment in this context reduces anxiety.

Supervision for all staff is a fundamental building block of support in child mental health. As well as ensuring adequate appraisal and personal development, it is a forum where relationships with the children and young people can be explored and understood. This will hopefully bring about improved work performance.

Wilkinson (1983) describes some of the emotional reactions that are experienced by nurses in the field. Anger is commonly felt, that the lives of children can be destroyed by problems or that parents can sometimes appear uncaring. Some nurses can feel despair and sadness, while others have feelings of love for particular children and this in turn makes them feel guilty. Acknowledgement of these powerful feelings is a positive first step. Some nurses are able to verbalize them to a manager, supervisor or colleague. Others may act out their feelings in team meetings or with peers or the children. These aspects need to be closely monitored, sensitively challenged and explored, otherwise the dynamics can become emotionally burdened and occasionally unhealthy.

INDIVIDUAL WORK

Various talking and creative therapies are used with children, despite the recent emphasis on family approaches. Individual psychotherapeutic techniques have a very important part to play, although, of course, it would be too simplistic to use one strategy to help all children. Some difficulties are more amenable to particular help, while some children and young people just prefer individual therapy.

Nurses will use both play and individual sessions in therapeutic ways with children. It is important to assess the developmental level of a child's verbal and communication skills before embarking on any goal-directed work.

A useful guide is given by Graham (1993):

- *Voluntary attendance.* Often children are brought to treatment because a parent wants it. It is usually best to seek commitment from the child to come for the sessions, except in some specialist units — where it is thought to be crucial to insist on attendance.
- *Establish the pattern of attendance.* It is important to give the child a plan, how many sessions? Where will they be held?
- *Clarify the reason for the sessions.* It is important to explain the purpose of the session, in age appropriate detail to the child. Don't assume that the child will know what it is that is supposed to happen. Most adults will know that the session is for them 'to talk about their problems', but a child may not.
- *Defence mechanisms.* In trying to make sense of the child's world, the nurse will probably make particular use of the concept of unconscious defence mechanisms — means by which the child protects itself from emotionally unbearable thoughts. It may be unwise to confront these head on, but to convey a sense of acceptance of the feelings, may mean the child needs to use them less.
- *Making connections.* Make connections rather than make dynamic interpretations, which the child may not have the degree of abstract thought to use. It can be more helpful to make connections linking situations, time frames, feelings and behaviours, etc.
- *Making clarifying suggestions.* Make tentative suggestions to 'help make sense' of the situation. If the child rejects a particularly relevant suggestion, explore how upset the child would be if it were true.
- *Observe the child in the session.* Look carefully at how the child behaves and reflect on aspects of the child's manner which help explain or clarify the process. This also gives the child feedback about how others perceive him or her.
- *Respect for the child.* Demonstrate that you are taking the child seriously and attend to what they say and do. Take a lively interest in their world, experiences, thoughts and feelings. Appear genuinely glad to see them, smile and praise all aspects of positive change or coping.
- *The silent or unresponsive child.* Many children find it very difficult to talk about their feelings at all. Sometimes with older adolescents, reflecting on the silence is helpful. Otherwise the use of some technique to encourage expression, such as drawing and play can also be effective.
- *Explore feelings.* Whatever is going on, spend time exploring how the child makes you feel. This may even be shared with the child to enable them to see the emotion at a distance, before being able to own it.
- *Ending the sessions.* Expect a variety of protests toward the end of a series of sessions. Denial may be followed by anger and sadness. These are not new 'problems' but reactions to loss which are protective and self-limiting.

(Reproduced by permission of Oxford University Press)

PLAY

We all play; it helps us learn and develop and enhances life. Children have been described as passing through stages of play development. The first 5 years of life see a child's rapidly changing ability to play. In the first year a child will explore themselves in a solitary manner, in the second year will play in parallel among other children and in the third year they may play the same game but be involved in their own part of it. At 3 years they are able to play cooperatively, with just another child to begin with, then with larger groups and more complicated activities and games, involving complex rules and ritual.

Play therapy is largely founded on the work of Axeline, who developed it in the 1940s. It has become more widely used only since the 1980s. Carroll (1996) presents a concise overview of its development and position today.

The British Association of Play Therapists define it as 'the dynamic process between child and therapist, in which the child explores, at his or her own pace and with his/her own agenda, those issues past and current, conscious and unconscious, that are affecting the child's life at present'. The child's inner resources are enabled by the therapeutic alliance to bring about growth and change. Play therapy is child centred, in which play is the primary medium and speech is the secondary medium.

There are two main types. Directive play therapy is used to control and direct the child's play to a particular objective. The play materials are carefully chosen and play is kept on course to meet a desired outcome. In non-directive play therapy, the sole responsibility rests with the child. The child takes their play wherever it goes; it is unique and gives the child a sense of control.

Nurses are well placed to use play therapeutically. Play can be planned and implemented that, for instance, exercises judgement, improves concentration, tests memory and aids socialization. Play can also help children to structure their thoughts more logically or to learn to relax and have fun.

GROUP THERAPY

Group therapy with children and adolescents falls into two main categories, experiential or educative groups. The experience of children and young people in groups shows several important differences from that of adults. Adolescents, in particular, often react with swings from rebellion to submission. Young people may demonstrate a variety of testing, acting out and resistance behaviours. These include shouting, hostility and open displays of anger, all of which may represent an inability to articulate an emotion or a need to avoid bringing a painful conflict into awareness. Well run and theoretically sound group experience provides children with clear boundaries and a safe place to express their turmoil. This provides them with a sense of containment, which is the foundation of the security that is a prerequisite of growth and change.

Age is clearly a factor in setting out group therapy practice. Participants should be broadly similar in terms of development. This allows the focus of the group to be meaningful to all. For example, leaving home and becoming an autonomous individual may be the present struggle for a 17-year-old but would not be shared by a 13-year-old. Sex is also a relevant factor; children at particular ages, e.g. 12–14-year-olds, do better in single sex groups.

Ghuman and Willmoth (1994) studied an adolescent in-patient group for 12 years and made the following observations, which help in understanding the adolescent group process. Common themes run through teenage groups. Issues of trust and confidentiality continually arise; the group members repeatedly go through periods of silence and over-activity, speech and acting-out behaviour centred around the conflict over reality, and their feelings, needs, wishes and fears. Teenagers display a variety of resistance, ego defences and varying degrees of ambivalence.

Groups with children and adolescents need to have clear limits and boundaries. Rules about conduct need to be explicit and transgressions in speech or behaviour need to be confronted. The group needs to be semi-structured; sitting in silence expecting young people to take the lead will often just ensure silence continues. Introducing and guiding topics may provide the support they need to begin exploring pertinent issues realistically. The use of reflection and link making are important but traditional dynamic techniques, such as interpretation and symbolism, should be used cautiously by experienced staff. For instance, suggesting to an angry 16-year-old that the reason he smashed a window was because he was disappointed that his mum failed to visit might make a useful link (between his emotions and his behaviour). However, to suggest that the smashed window was symbolic of his smashed relationship with his mum (however true) would probably result in anger, rejection and further hostility.

Role modelling, pro-social behaviour and direct communication are essential. Helping young people articulate clearly and directly is giving them an important tool with which to test reality and solve problems.

BEHAVIOURAL PSYCHOTHERAPY

Wilkinson (1983) and Herbert (1994) provide a comprehensive outline of behavioural psychotherapy theory and its many applications in treatment of child and adolescent mental health problems. Behavioural work involves the application of learning theory to design individually tailored techniques to help the young person change the behaviour that is obstructing their development. Behavioural work with children and adolescents includes applications of classical and operant conditioning theories, as well as of social learning principles and modelling. For child and adolescent mental health nursing, the application of social learning is common, as much of the young person's behaviour is acquired by observation. Child and adolescent mental health nurses have to be aware of their behaviour and interactions with young people and staff to ensure that they provide healthy role models. Age-appropriate social behaviours can be learned through observation and modelling and therefore the social skills that nurses take for granted in their day-to-day interactions provide a rich source of observational understanding. Also, appropriate expression of emotions, such as the ability to express anger without violence, sadness or disappointment without blame, and happiness without overexcitement, are all things that young people not only observe but can participate in and learn from.

Operant condition techniques have proved extremely useful in the day-to-day management of nursing care and intervention to help young people modify inappropriate social behaviour. The commonest form involves the use of star charts, with the young person earning stars for each period they have managed not to exhibit the targeted unacceptable behaviour. The stars accrue value over time and a certain number earn a particular reward, which may be social or material, chosen by the young person. Such interventions rely heavily on the use of positive reinforcers and nurses need to be aware that even negative attention in the form of scolding or getting angry can provide reinforcement for a young person's inappropriate behaviour. It is therefore essential that 'ABC' analysis of the behaviour is made over a period of time. This involves recording the:

1 Antecedents, i.e. what was going on before the behaviour occurred.
2 Behaviour, i.e. the actual behaviour itself, what the young person does and for how long.
3 Consequence, i.e. what happened as a result of the young person's behaviour and the responses from others.

This will allow a programme to be developed with more appropriate reinforcers and the withdrawal of reinforcers, such as attention, when inappropriate behaviours occur (Herbert, 1987).

Classical conditioning techniques also have their use when young people have developed phobic reactions to particular objects or situations that cause them debilitating anxiety. This technique involves the nurse listing a hierarchy of fear-provoking situations, drawn up together with the young person, who is also taught relaxation techniques. As this is incompatible with anxiety it is therefore self-reinforcing (Wilkinson, 1983). With children and adolescents, the process of desensitization is then used, in which the young person is encouraged to expose themselves to successively more fear-provoking situations, according to the list drawn up earlier, while also practising relaxation. With classic conditioning techniques, the level of motivation and commitment to change that the young person has is more important than with operant techniques, as the initial anxiety that is felt can, when confronting things such as a fearful situation and object, itself be off-putting. With operant techniques, young people thrive on reinforcers such as positive attention, approval, and much notice being taken of their day-to-day, ordinary achievements.

PARENT TRAINING TECHNIQUES

Parent training refers to educative interventions with parents that aim to help them cope with and more effectively manage the problems they experience in relation to their children's behaviour (Callias, 1994). Since the mid-1970s a number of parent training methods have been developed (Forehand and McMahon, 1981; Patterson, 1982; Ney and Mulvihill, 1985; Herbert, 1988; McAuley, 1988; Webster–Stratton, 1991). Although the methods of parent training vary a great deal, e.g. group training using videotaped scenarios of parent–child interaction as devised by Webster–Stratton (1991), individualized parent training with one-to-one attention from the therapist and *in vivo* training (Forehand and McMahon, 1981) they all draw on social learning theory. While the majority of parent training packages have been developed to help parents deal with antisocial behaviour in their children, this approach has also been effective in families where children have been abused and neglected (Gent, 1992). The principal objectives of parent training packages are to help parents to identify the behaviours they find difficult to manage while also encouraging them to notice and reward their child's positive prosocial and ordinary, appropriate behaviour. By teaching parents to set clear consistent limits and provide firm but warm supervision, parents are made aware of the potency of attention and are taught to use this contingent upon the child's behaviour.

Many nurses provide parent training, often without realizing it, through the course of their day-to-day interactions with parents, such as handing over when parents collect or leave their child at the day or residential unit. This provides opportunities for helping the parents to manage specific situations (such as mealtimes or play activities) or tasks (such as getting the young person to school) by providing practical advice on the management of the child's behaviour based on the nurse's experience of which interventions the young person has responded to. By way of their interactions and responses to young people, in front of the parents, the nurse can model patterns of behaviour informally so that parents have the opportunity to learn from observation.

Wilkinson (1983) highlights the important role that nurses play by involving parents in the planned treatment of their child and the support that they can provide to parents by using their skills of empathizing, while being firm and communicating clearly. Gent (1992) describes how nurses, as therapists, can use a particular parent training technique that was developed in the USA by Forehand and McMahon (1981). This involves the use of a one-way screen and feedback loop between connecting rooms. The parent can be given encouragement and instructions (by the therapist on the other side of the screen, through an earphone) during direct interaction with their child. This method, while aiming to improve parents' ability to manage children more effectively, has the secondary objective of improving the quality of interaction between parents and children, so that children start to experience their parents in a warm, consistent, and approving way. Although the sessions are carried out in the clinic, regular homework tasks are set and monitored. By discussion and through problem-solving techniques, generalization to natural home and social situations is encouraged. This way of working with parents has been criticized. The main criticism is that it involves middle-class value judgements and can make parents feel patronized. However, the experience of nurses using this technique is that, when they employ their skills to build therapeutic relationships with the parents and work in collaboration with them, this results in the children, the parents and the therapist deriving satisfaction from the progress made in enhancing parent–child relationships. Clinical experience of the technique has been shown to be much more effective with children than with adolescents. All of the parent training packages mentioned have been developed for children up to about 10 years of age.

FAMILY THERAPY

Most schools of family therapy were developed in child and adolescent mental health settings, e.g. Minuchin's structural family therapy and Haley's strategic family therapy. The fundamental concept underpinning all the schools of family therapy is that the family is seen as a system. Each member's behaviours, interactions and relationships have an effect upon, and are themselves affected by, the others. To help part of the system (i.e one family member) to change, the whole system (the family) has to be helped to change. Traditionally, family therapy was thought to involve seeing the whole family together, the therapist supervising through a one-way screen, and with a break midway through the session for feedback. The thinking has evolved to accept the usefulness of approaches that involve working with whichever parts of the family are most motivated and willing to change through therapy and without necessarily using the supervision structures provided by the one-way screen. Treacher (1988) argues the increasing need for therapists to apply an integrative approach when working with families rather than using one model.

Family therapy approaches have been applied to a broad range of child and adolescent mental health problems including behavioural problems, eating disorders and self-harm and in situations where stressful events have occurred, such as child abuse and neglect, fostering and adoption, and loss through illness or death or divorce. Wilkinson (1983) has described the role of nurses and the implications for them when conducting family therapy on day or residential units. She contrasts this with family case work, which involves working in a less formal way, by focusing specifically on the young person's problems and conducting sessions in the home, such as facilitating clear communication and management skills. Wilkinson also cautions nurses about becoming involved in work with families without having developed the necessary skills to establish and maintain therapeutic contact with them. This can result in families feeling alienated and withdrawing the young person completely from treatment. Often child and adolescent mental health nurses are best placed to help families come to terms with the degree of change that the young person has made in treatment and the continuing needs that will have to be met.

MEDICATION MANAGEMENT

Medication has a small but significant contribution to make in the treatment of some childhood mental disorders. The indications for drug use in children are often very different from those in adults. Children differ in their response to drugs.

Hyperkinetic disorders have been demonstrated by extensive research to respond, in the short term, to drugs classed as stimulants (although it is not known if, or what, they stimulate) such as dexamphetamine.

Aggressive behaviour and *conduct disorder* have shown short-term improvement in controlled trials with chlorpromazine and haloperidol. Lithium, propranolol and carbamazepine may be useful in controlling extremes of aggression but there have been few studies undertaken and the long-term effects are unknown. Except in the management of a psychiatric emergency, benzodiazepines should not be used because in children paradoxically they lead to aggression.

Affective disorders — childhood depression has not on the whole been shown to respond to antidepressants, however in some serious cases it might still be tried. *Obsessive–compulsive disorder* has been found to improve significantly in young people treated with clomipramine. Recent trials of fluoxetine have also shown positive results. *Anxiety* is a problem for some children, which has not been improved in clinical trials with drugs. *Bipolar affective disorders* respond to antipsychotic medication and mood can be stabilized with lithium or carbamazepine.

Autism does not usually respond to medication. Drugs can sometimes be used to control distressing problems. Haloperidol, fenfluramine and naltrexone have shown some impact on *stereotypic, ritualistic behaviours* and other problems.

Enuresis is improved in 40% of children on tricyclics such as imipramine but the child nearly always relapses when drugs are discontinued.

Eating disorders in children and young people show little improvement when treated with medication. *Anorexia nervosa* is not improved by antidepressants but *bulimia nervosa* may be helped slightly by these drugs.

Tourette's syndrome and *tics* are reduced with haloperidol, pimozide and, possibly, clonidine.

Sleep disorders such as night-waking and night terrors can be rapidly treated with trimeprazine but only in the short-term. Hypnotics can be hazardous in children and are best avoided.

Schizophrenia in children and young people and how it can be treated with medication has been the subject of little research. Doubts about the efficacy of antipsychotic drug use in children exist. Clinical experience suggest the traditional neuroleptics such as chlorpromazine, haloperidol and sulpiride are useful in symptom control. Recent studies with clozapine seem to suggest that for treatment-resistant adolescents (as young as 12) their response is possibly better than, or at least similar to, that in adults. Side-effects may occur with the same frequency. However, the most serious side-effect, agranulocytosis, may be slightly more of a risk.

When working with young people under 18 who receive medication for a mental health need the nurse should consult specialist literature on the subject.

SUMMARY

Research indicates that up to 20% of children suffer significant degrees of mental disorder but much of it is amenable to the independent intervention of child mental health nurses. All young people below the age of 18 have a right to expect mental health service providers that are able to deliver care appropriate to their age, level of development and family circumstances. It seems clear that to focus on the mental health of children is not only neccesary to alleviate their distress, promote healthy development and minimise dysfunction but it is cost-effective in terms of diverting people away from the adult psychiatric services, reducing delinquency and social problems.

Child mental health nursing is relatively new. Nurses need a good working knowledge of child development and systems theory and an appreciation of how they inform most aspects of working with children.

The factors that are known to increase the risk of disorders are explored, alongside those that are known to be protective. Children are by definition vulnerable, and working in this field imposes special responsibilities on nurses, such as that of surrogate parent, advocate, child protector and childrens law expert.

Each of the common childhood disorders are outlined briefly and the methods in which child mental health nurses need to conceptualize and work with the problems and needs presented are discussed. Nurses work in teams, with children across a spectrum of need, from those who cause their parents concern, when they exhibit healthy, adaptive emotional and behavioral responses which are appropriate for their age and context, to those adolescents who develop severe and enduring mental illness.

KEY CONCEPTS

- Investment in the mental health of children is an investment in them, their children and future generations.
- Childhood mental health can only be understood in the context of a child's development.
- The prevalence of mental disorder in the child population is estimated as being as high as 25%.
- Factors that influence the mental health of children are not the same as those that influence the mental health of adults.
- The experience of childhood is culturally and socially determined. However, the welfare of the child is always paramount.
- Mental health nurses require a different set of skills and abilities to work effectively with children and their families.
- Mental ill health in children and families is best viewed systemically and not from a linear or medical perspective.

REFERENCES

Barker P: *Basic child psychiatry.* Oxford, 1995, Blackwell Science.

Bee H: *The developing child.* New York, 1985, Harper & Row.

Belsky J: The determinants of parenting: a process model. *Child Development* 55:83–96, 1984.

Bowlby J: Attachment and loss (Vol 1), *Attachment.* New York, 1969, Basic Books.

Bowlby J: Attachment and loss (Vol 1), *Separation, anxiety and anger.* New York, 1973, Basic Books.

Bowlby J: Attachment and loss (Vol 1), *Loss, sadness and depression.* New York, 1980, Basic Books.

Callias M: Parent training. In: Rutter M, Taylor E, Hervos L, editors: *Child and adolescent psychiatry: modern approaches.* Oxford, 1994, Blackwell.

Carroll J: Play therapy. *Young Minds Magazine* 24, 1996.

Carter B, McGoldrick M, editors: *The changing family life cycle: a framework for family therapy.* Boston, 1989, Allyn & Bacon.

Clunn P: *Child psychiatric nursing.* St Louis, Missouri, 1991, Mosby Year Book.

Cooper C: Good-enough, border-line and bad enough parenting. In: Adock M, White R, editors: *Good-enough parenting – a framework for assessment.* London, 1985, BAAF.

Cox A: Preventative aspects of child psychiatry. In: Garralda M: *Managing children with psychiatric problems.* London, 1993, BMJ publishing group.

Department of Health: *Working together under the Children Act 1989: a guide to arrangements for inter-agency co-operation for the protection of children from abuse.* London, 1991a, HMSO.

Department of Health: *The Children Act 1989: an introductory guide for the NHS.* London, 1991b, HMSO.

Department of Health: *Child protection: clarification of arrangements between the NHS and other agencies,* London, 1995, HMSO.

Department of Health: *The Patient's Charter — Services for children and young people.* London, 1996, HMSO.

Forehand R, McMahon R: *Helping the noncompliant child: a clinician's guide to parent training.* New York, 1981, The Guilford Press.

Gent M: Parenting assessment: the parent/child game. *Nurs Stand* 8(29):31, 1992.

Ghuman H, Wilmoth E: Group psychotherapy setting, structure and process. In: Ghuman H, Sarles R: *Handbook of adolescent inpatient psychiatric treatment.* New York, 1994, Brunner/Mazel.

Graham P: *Child psychiatry: a developmental approach.* Oxford, 1993, Oxford University Press.

Graham P, Hughes C: *So Young, So Sad, So Listen.* London, 1995, Royal College of Psychiatrists.

Health Advisory Service: *Child and adolescent mental health services: together we stand. The commisioning, role and management of child and adolescent mental health services.* London, 1995, HMSO.

Health Advisory Service: *Children and young people: substance misuse services. The substance of young needs. Commissioning and providing services for chil-dren and young people who use and misuse substances.* London, 1996, HMSO.

Health Education Authority: Tomorrow's young adults: 9–15 year olds look at alcohol, drugs, exercise and smoking. London, 1992, MORI.

Herbert M: *Behavioural treatment of children with problems: a practice manual.* London, 1987, Academic Press.

Herbert M: *Working with children and their families.* London, 1988, British Psychological Society.

Herbert M: Behavioural methods. In: Rutter M, Taylor E, Hervos L, editors: *Child and adolescent psychiatry: modern approaches.* Oxford, 1994, Blackwell.

Hogarth C: *Adolescent psychiatric nursing.* St Louis, Missouri, 1991, Mosby Year Book.

Hoxter S: Some feelings aroused in working with severely deprived children. In: Baston E, Szug L, editors: *Psychotherapy with severely deprived children.* London, 1983, Routledge & Kegan Paul.

Keir G: Symposium on psychologists and psychiatrists in the child guidance service, 3: A history of child guidance. *Br J Ed Psychol* 22:5–29. 1952.

Kohlberg I: Development of moral character and moral ideology. In: Hoffman M, Hoffman I, editors: *Review of child development research (Vol 1).* New York, 1964, Russell Sage Foundation.

Kurtz Z, Thornes R, Wolkind S: *Services for the mental health of children and young people in England: a national review.* London, 1994, Maudsley Hospital and South Thames Regional Health Authority.

Maddison D, Kellehear K: *Psychiatric nursing.* Edinburgh, 1982, Longman Group.

McAudey R: Parent training: clinical applications. In: Falloon IRH, editor: *Handbook of behavioural therapy.* New York, 1988, Guilford Press.

Meadow R, editor: *ABC of child abuse.* London, 1993, BMJ Publishing Group.

Nelson–Jones R: *The theory and practice of counselling psychology.* London, 1982, Cassell Educational Ltd.

Newell P: *The UN Convention and children's rights in the UK.* London, 1991, National Children's Bureau.

Ney PG, Mulvihill DIL: *Child psychiatric treatment.* Kent, 1985, Croom Helm.

Parry-Jones W: History of child and psychiatry. In: Rutter M, Taylor E, Hersov L: *Child and adolescent psychiatry: modern approaches.* Oxford, 1994, Blackwell Scientific.

Patterson GR: *Coercive family process.* Oregon, 1982, Castalia Publications.

Pearce J: Identifying psychiatric disorders in children. In: Garralda M: *Managing children with psychiatric problems.* London, 1993, BMJ Publishing Group.

Piaget J: *The development of thought: equilibration of cognitive structures.* New York, 1975, Viking Press.

Pothier P, Norbeck J, Laliberte M: Child psychiatric nursing: the gap between need and utilisation. *J Psychosoc Nurs* 23(7):18, 1985.

Quinton D, Rutter M: *Parenting breakdown: the making and breaking of intergen-erational bonds.* Hants, 1988, Group Publishing Co.

Reimers S, Treacher A: *Introducing user-friendly family therapy.* London, 1995, Routledge.

Rutter M: Attachment and the development of social relationships. In: Rutter M, editor: *Scientific foundations of developmental psychiatry.* London, 1980, William Heinemann Medical Books Ltd.

Rutter M, Cox A: Other family influences. In: Rutter M, Hervos L, editors: *Child and adolescent psychiatry: modern approaches.* Oxford, 1985, Blackwell.

Salzberger–Wittenberg I: *Psycho-analytic insight and relationships – a Kleinian approach.* London, 1988, Routledge & Kegan Paul.

Sampson, K: Acting with restraint. *Nurs Times* 89(38):40–43, 1993.

Selvini Palazzoli M *et al:* Hypothesing, circularity and neutrality: three guidelines for the conductor of the session. *Family Process* 19:3–12, 1980

Subotsky S: Psychiatric treatment for children – the organisation of services. In: Elena Garralda M, editor: *Managing children with psychiatric problems.* London, 1993, BMJ Publishing Group.

Taylor SE: *Health psychology.* New York, 1991, McGraw-Hill.

Treacher A: Family therapy: an integrated approach. In: Street EW, Dryden W,

editors: *Family therapy in Britain.* Milton Keynes, 1988, Open University Press.

Webster–Stratton C: Annotation: strategies for helping families with conduct disordered children. *J Child Psychol Psych* 32:1047–1062, 1991.

Wilkinson T: *Child and adolescent psychiatric nursing.* Oxford, 1983, Blackwell Scientific.

Winnicott DW: *The maturational processes and the facilative environment.* New York, 1965, International Universities Press.

Wolkind S, Rutter M: Socio-cultural factors. In: Rutter M, Herslov L, editors: *Child and adolescent psychiatry: modern approaches.* Oxford, 1995, Blackwell.

Wright L, Leahey M: *Families and psychosocial problems.* Springhouse, 1987, Keith Lassner/Springhouse Corp.

FURTHER READING

Schoen Johnson B: *Child, adolescent and family psychiatric nursing.* Philadelphia, 1995, Lippincott Co.

    This text provides good coverage of the subject. It looks at mental health need and how nurses can apply the nursing process with children. It details the main theories that inform our work. It explores what factors place children at risk of mental ill health and presents in sections each of the common disorders and treatment modalities.

Clunn P: *Child psychiatric nursing.* St Louis, Missouri, 1991, Mosby Year Book.

    A useful introduction to the theoretical and philosophical foundations of child mental health nursing. It goes through relevant child development and applies it to common childhood disorders.

Hogarth C: *Adolescent psychiatric nursing.* St Louis, Missouri, 1991, Mosby Year Book.

    This book provides an overview of adolescent development, mental disorder and mental illness in teenagers. It is particularly helpful for nurses working in in-patient units.

Garralda M, editor: *Managing children with psychiatric problems.* London, 1993, BMJ Publishing Group.

    This is an excellent first text which provides a concise and easy to read guide to child mental health issues. It covers treatments and has an outline of service provision.

West P, Sieloff Evans C: *Psychiatric and mental health nursing with children and adolescents.* Gaithersburg, Maryland, 1992, Aspen publications.

    This book follows a needs based approach and provides chapters on nursing intervention for children with particular problems as opposed to disorders. It uses the nursing process and gives good guidance about using nursing diagnoses.

Rutter M, Hervos L, editors: *Child and adolescent psychiatry: modern approaches.* London, 1985, Blackwell.

    By far the most comprehensive research based review of child psychiatry. It is written by eminent authorities from around the world and provides an outline of current research and up to date clinical details and is nearly always a good place to start an exploration of the literature about most child mental health disorders

Care of the Elderly

page

Learning Outcomes

After studying this chapter you should be able to:

- Describe the nature and extent of mental health problems experienced by older people.

- Explode some of the myths and stereotypes surrounding the older person and mental health.

- Identify and describe the elements of a comprehensive nursing assessment for the older person with mental health needs.

- Discuss the major biopsychosocial theories of ageing.

- Utilize knowledge gained to enhance therapeutic nursing interventions with elderly mentally ill patients and their carers.

- Understand the interplay between different agencies, interprofessional working methods and the requirements of good interprofessional relationships for the benefit of the patient and their families.

- Discuss the relevant research that has taken place that has been used to improve the quality of care for the elderly mentally ill patient.

CHAPTER OUTLINE

- *Context of care*
- *Myths and stereotypes*
- *Theories of ageing*
- *Physical aspects of care*
- *Assessment methods and tools*
- *Functional illness*
- *The dementias*
- *Cultural and ethnic needs*
- *Carers' needs*
- *Elderly abuse*
- *Women and ageing*
- *Men and ageing*
- *Interpersonal interventions*
- *The environment of care*
- *Counselling*
- *Standards and quality outcomes*

*A*s the population of older people in the world increases, concerns about the health of and delivery of health care to these elderly people become increasingly important. Stereotypes and myths often depict the elderly as a homogeneous group. On the contrary, the older adult is an individual combination of multiple interpersonal developmental and situational experiences. The population of England and Wales has 19% women and 13% men over the age of 65; 13% of elderly women are over 85 compared with only 6% of elderly men (Office of Population Censuses and Surveys, 1993).

The proportion of older people in our society is constantly growing; in the UK the proportion over 65 has trebled since the beginning of the 20th Century. By the year 2001 there will be an increase of 4% in those over 65, of 20% among those aged 75–79 and of 31% in those aged 80–84, with a 46% increase in those older still (Department of Health, 1990). The chance of admission to a psychiatric unit is greatly increased in later life with approximately 1 in 4 adults admitted being over 65. Research indicates that this is only the tip of the iceberg, as the vast majority of mental health problems among elderly people are managed by carers in the home.

The complexity and interaction of the needs and problems of old age are often underestimated and understated. Mental health in later life depends on a number of factors. These include physiological and psychological status, personality, social support systems, economic resources and life style.

A familiar comment made by nurses working in elderly care settings is 'I only give basic nursing care, such as feeding patients'. From a psychiatric nursing perspective, this involves an understanding of communication skills, psychomotor skills, hallucinatory and delusional experiences, orientation, dependence, anxiety, trust, hostility, mood (particularly depressed affects), feeding techniques both physical and psychological, nutritional and hydration needs, digestion, preventive and curative aspects of elimination problems and ethical aspects of care delivery (Cormack, 1986) to name but a few of the skills and considerations nurses need in their repertoire.

The application of a 'holistic' model of care in a strong multidisciplinary framework has been shown to be beneficial in elderly care settings. Holistic nursing is a phrase that has found its way from the USA but it is not necessarily the same as a problem-solving approach to individualized patient care. Although there is some common ground, there are some basic philosophical differences. Holism implies doing things 'with' the patient, rather than doing things 'for' the patient. The extent of mental disorders in the elderly appears considerable; therefore nurses and other health care professionals will be increasingly responsible for caring for older adults.

CONTEXT OF CARE

Community care has had a major impact on the care provided for the elderly mentally ill population in the UK. While there are differences throughout the country similarities can be found in every area. Health care has a price and elderly people everywhere are suffering from this new culture. Social services and health care services have always worked together in a supportive climate, which has encouraged interprofessional working and peer group support.

The climate has changed to one in which health and social care have had to become separate entities. This is not conducive to community care for anyone needing these services; for the elderly it is positively life threatening. New models and frameworks for practice are occurring despite the new legislation and clinicians, social workers and other agencies are still maintaining services throughout the country despite policies and agendas which are actually detrimental to health and to good quality of life.

The changes laid out in the White Paper *Caring for People* (Department of Health, 1990) emphasize the role of needs assessment which, with good case management, is intended to form 'the cornerstone of high quality care'. This legislation means that a series of assessments by health care workers and social services will now have to be made to provide a comprehensive package of care to meet the needs of elderly people. This process holds a number of variables that are creating real difficulties for the individuals requiring services. Older people are now being subjected to a form of means testing to identify whether or not they can afford to pay for their own services, from a daily home help to a residential nursing home. Some individuals are being asked to consider selling their properties and to use other capital, which they may have worked for over the years, to pay for their nursing and social care.

On a positive note, new methods of working have brought in case management and the Key Worker, which can help to provide individualized care and comprehensive follow-up after discharge from hospital. Most older people are cared for in their own homes by informal carers. Formal carers from the health and social services are often employed to support the existing structures and to offer support to the main carers. This practice ultimately allows the older person to stay at home for as long as possible.

MYTHS AND STEREOTYPES

Some myths and stereotypes will be discussed in this section with the intention of exploding them through discussion and analysis of their origins. Older people suffer a number of negative stereotypes – images that do not accurately represent their everyday realities and aspirations. Such stereotypes are constructed from a complex blend of sensory images. There is a tendency for human beings to oversimplify and to construct an image where a part is represented as a whole – hence we have the ageist stereotype of 'the dirty old man'. Such notions must be understood in terms of a historically formed 'disgust function', through the development of a heightened sensitivity to bodily demeanour and functions as part of civilizing processes and through the dynamics of power struggles between the established and outsiders, i.e. those with norm defining power and those without (Elias, 1994).

Many of the statements listed in Box 24.1 have a common link, 'infantilization'. They share an assumption that old people are like children. Older people patently are not children; none the less in contemporary Western society old age is often popularly associated with childhood through both verbal and visual images. This association is variously constructed; for example, there is the remarking of parallels between old age and childhood seen in the writings of Dylan Thomas:

First voice: All over the town, babies and old men are cleaned and put into their broken prams and wheeled onto the sunlit cockled cobbles or out into the backyards under the dancing underclothes and left.

(a baby cries)

Old man: I want my pipe and he wants his bottle.

(Dylan Thomas, Under Milk Wood, 1954)

In this image the two social categories, positioned at either end of life, share the experience of dependency. This myth creates a structure which excludes elderly people from their status as adults and in turn their personhood, through effectively obliterating their life history and social identity and reducing them to the level of their physical and mental disabilities.

A number of movements have sought to combat age discrimination in labour markets, to abolish mandatory retirement age and oppose ageist language and negative stereotypes of the elderly. The best known are The Gray Panthers, Age Concern and Help The Aged. The images of positive ageing they seek to advance amount to a deconstruction of the image of old age as necessarily a phase of bodily decline. The dominant ideology of Western culture depicts what old age should be for individuals, thus creating a self-fulfilling prophecy for many people.

Ageism is endemic in society and resides within us all; indeed it exists in the minds of those who have themselves become old. They will have learned that to be old is to conform to these stereotypes and to accept the ascribed elderly role in the social order. This is the nature of ageism; it pervades the attitudes, thinking and expectations of young and old alike. In the nursing context, it is important to not only be aware of the effects of ageism on the individual but also how to combat these and speak out against ageist practices and policies.

The good news about old age is that most elderly people enjoy a healthy life, untroubled by incontinence, dementia and other disorders. Suffering with Alzheimer's becomes more of a risk the older we become. However, research into new treatment methods are showing signs of breakthroughs in treatment approaches and methods. It is nearly always possible to treat the diseases and disabilities that older people experience and there is no reason why it should be assumed that disease in old age is untreatable ... although such assumptions are often made.

THEORIES OF AGEING

A comprehensive review of theories is beyond the scope of this chapter. However, theories relevant to the psychiatry of old age will be discussed. Ways of defining ageing and explaining the causes and consequences of the ageing process are based on three major approaches:
1. The biological theories of ageing.
2. The psychological theories of ageing.
3. The sociological theories of ageing.

No one theory can include all of the variables that influence ageing and people's response to it. It is difficult to separate the effects of stress, disease processes and specific age-related changes. Theories of ageing may help, however, to clarify

Box 24.1 *Some common myths and stereotypes*

- We will never be old ourselves.
- Modernization is good for old people.
- Sickness and disability come with old age.
- Old people are sweet and kind and at peace with the world.
- Old people are weak and helpless.
- Old people don't have sex.
- Old people are boring and forgetful.
- Old people are unproductive.
- Old women are a burden on everyone.
- Old age begins at 60.
- Old people don't have any feelings.
- Old people are past being consulted about anything, including their own lives.

some of the physical and mental changes experienced by the older person.

BIOLOGICAL THEORIES

Biological theories of ageing can be broken down into two broad categories:
1. Developmental—genetic theories (primary ageing).
2. Stochastic theories (secondary ageing). (Busse *et al.*, 1989).

Primary ageing refers to the declines in function that are genetically controlled, while secondary ageing refers to the changes occurring as a result of acquired disease and trauma. If the events related to secondary ageing could be prevented, life would be extended but because of primary ageing, decline and death are inevitable.

The wear and tear theory suggests that structural and functional changes may be speeded up by abuse and slowed down by care. From a physiological standpoint, ageing is viewed developmentally, beginning with conception and leading to decline and death. Problems associated with ageing are the result of accumulated stress, trauma, injuries, infections, inadequate nutrition, metabolic and immunological disturbances and prolonged abuse. This concept of ageing is seen in widely accepted myths and stereotypes regarding the older person, as noted in such phrases as 'He's doing well for his age', or 'What can you expect at that age?' Recent research on the value of exercise and cognitive stimulation in later years refutes the basic premise of this theory, since both body and mind seem to benefit from use and stimulation.

Stress Adaptation Theory

The stress adaptation theory (Seyle, 1956) emphasizes the positive and negative effects of stress on biopsychosocial development. As a positive influence, stress may stimulate a person to try new, more effective ways of adapting. A negative effect of stress would be inability to function because of feeling overwhelmed. The balance of positive and negative stress must be examined. Although it is often assumed that stress accelerates the ageing process, there is little evidence to support that conclusion. Stress may drain a person's reserve capacity, physiologically, psychologically, socially and economically, which in turn can lead to an increased vulnerability to illness and injury.

PSYCHOLOGICAL THEORIES

Psychology has accumulated an enormous body of knowledge relating to mental stability and change in later life. This information has not been integrated into a viable comprehensive theory. The main areas that have been studied by psychologists can be placed in three broad categories—cognition, personality and coping mechanisms.

Erikson's Stage of Ego Integrity

Erikson's theory of human development (Erikson, 1950) identifies tasks that must be accomplished at each of the eight stages of life. The final task related to the stage of life identifies reflection about one's life and accomplishments and is identified with ego integrity. If there is a sense of failure, despair results. The end result of resolving the conflict between ego integrity and despair is acquired wisdom. Erikson's stages are intended as an approximation of the main struggles encountered at each period of life.

Those whose life journeys have been relatively successful will be able to place their lives in context and view the last stages of their lives more philosophically. They will feel that their losses are unfortunate but will tend to be more successful in finding ways around them that enable them to remain essentially optimistic. Those who are unsuccessful will tend to view the ageing process as catastrophic, unfair and debilitating and their pessimism will restrict their ability to cope adequately with the realities of old age.

Life Review Theory

Lewis and Butler (1974), have discussed a variety of methods of reinforcing life-review activity, including keeping scrapbooks and family albums, writing autobiographies, constructing genealogies and summating life work. Lewis and Butler have proposed that life-review activities, aside from benefiting elderly patients, may also have positive benefits for listeners as well. Life review occurs in all age groups to varying degrees. However, within the age group of older person, life review can become more focused and concentrated. Older people can have a vivid memory for past events and can recall early life experiences with great clarity. They appear to review and sort earlier life events and experiences to better understand their present circumstances.

An approach used to enhance life review, at either an informal or formal level, may involve the development of reminiscence groups to provide a forum for initiating the process and to provide feedback during the review. The life review may have positive or negative consequences. Anxiety, guilt, fear and depression may surface if the person is unable to resolve or accept old, unresolved problems. Studies by Gorney (1968) showed that people in their 60s and 70s engaged in a 'life review' reminiscence and that people in their 80s and 90s engaged in a 'life review' resolution . It has also been suggested that people dissatisfied with their past life engage in life review to a greater extent than those who are satisfied (Coleman, 1974).

SOCIAL THEORIES OF AGEING

Broadly speaking, the sociological theories of ageing examine the relationship of the older person to society and the role and status of the older person.

Disengagement Theory

This theory evolved from studies conducted by the University of Chicago on human development. It postulated that older adults naturally withdraw from active exchange with each other as part of the normal ageing process (Cumming and Henry, 1961) This was assumed to be a sign of psychological well-being and adjustment on the part of the elderly.

This theory did not consider the multitude of differences among the elderly population or the numerous factors external to the elderly person that could make withdrawal the only solution, e.g. loss of role, status, financial security, and friends and relatives.

The theory has major implications. Stereotypes could be reinforced, including the idea that older people only enjoy the company of people their own age and that retirement facilities should prohibit intergenerational living arrangements. This, of course, excludes older people from the mainstream of society.

Social Role Valorization

This theory goes quite a long way to addressing some of the concerns raised by the previous theory. The major themes of this theory address the problems associated with loss of role for the individual and the negative repercussions that occur following these losses, on individual, systems and societal levels. The process of devaluation begins and the individual begins to suffer the consequences of this process, which are at best highly unpleasant and at worst life curtailing. These consequences can be very subtle and health care workers can often be blind to them. The major themes are:

- The role of the unconscious.
- The relevance of role expectancy and role circularity to deviancy making and unmaking.
- The concept of positive compensation for devalued people.
- The developmental model and the importance of personal competency enhancement.
- The power of imitation.
- The dynamics and relevance of social imagery.
- The importance of personal social integration and valued social participation especially for people at risk of devaluation.

From a nursing perspective there are a number of points that can be directly addressed within the framework of good practice. The dynamic of role expectancy and role circularity is often referred to as a 'self-fulfilling prophecy' and here refers to the language used about people, their personal appearance, signs and symbols displayed around the people and the activities that are offered and provided for people.

The important assumptions underlying the developmental model are that all people have the potential for positiveness at all stages of their lives, no matter how old or impaired they are.

Imitation is one of the most powerful learning mechanisms known. This dynamic should be capitalized upon, in a positive way, especially for the benefit of devalued persons, so that they can use the models provided to help them function in a more appropriate and, hopefully, valued way. Further reference will be made to this theory in the section on nursing interventions with this client group (Wolfensberger, 1991).

Modernization Theory

The status of older people is high in static societies and tends to decline with rapid social change. Cogwill and Holmes, (1972) modernization theory suggests that the status of older people in any society is inversely related to the level of industrialization in that society. With the growth of industrial society, the powers and the prestige of the elderly are reduced.

These sociological theories described above have various degrees of validity, and, since in sociology, as well as in biology and psychology, there are no overarching theories that incorporate them all, they must all be taken into account to construct a meaningful understanding of the processes taking place.

PHYSICAL ASPECTS OF CARE

Many psychiatric symptoms in the elderly patient can be missed or become less obvious through physical complications. This can make diagnosis more difficult and therefore reduce the likelihood of appropriate care and treatment being offered (Burr and Andrews, 1981).

MANAGEMENT OF CONTINENCE

Incontinence can be a problem for elderly patients and has profound psychological, medical and social ramifications. There are many causes and presentations; treatments available depend on individual needs and circumstances.

Great sensitivity and understanding are required by the carers and professionals who are helping the older person. This is the most important part of an effective management programme; maintaining dignity and self-respect throughout any procedure is essential and time and patience should be exercised at all times.

To simplify the descriptions of behavioural treatment strategies, consideration will be given to two general categories.
1. People who are functionally intact, living independently and able to manage their own treatment.
2. People with significant cognitive or physical impairments that contribute to and, in some cases, cause the incontinence. These people need a considerable amount of direct care to meet their needs.

The commonest types of incontinence found among patients are:
• Stress incontinence.
• Urge incontinence.
• Mixed incontinence.

A fourth type of incontinence, called overflow incontinence, can occur. In most elderly people there will not be a single cause with a single treatment; several interacting factors will be responsible. Hence continence will most likely be achieved when physical, mental, environmental and social causes are all considered and corrected where possible.

Why Incontinence Happens

Mechanical obstruction may cause incontinence; prostate disease is a common cause of obstruction in men, fibroids in women; acute urinary tract infections and other acute illnesses may render an older person incontinent, as can reduced mobility for any reason. Diabetes may cause incontinence as a result of the increased flow of urine. Constipation may act as an obstruction to the flow of urine. Drugs that lower the level of consciousness impair the ability to plan for continence by making regular visits to the lavatory and allowing enough time to visit it; diuretics may overwhelm a failing control system; some drugs cause constipation and alcohol has a diuretic effect. Depression can compromise self-care and anxiety can make the person feel as though they want to pass urine all the time. (A few deep breaths before passing urine can help a person suffering anxiety to relieve their bladder more effectively).

The regulation of fluid intake can have a significant effect on the control that an older person has. Older people need 1.5—3.0 litres of fluid a day. Many drink too little because of:
• Decline in the sense of thirst with increasing age.
• Physical handicap making preparation of drinks difficult.
• Mental decline making preparation of drinks difficult.
• Fear of incontinence fluid restriction tends to make incontinence worse because concentrated urine is more irritating, prone to infection and any leakage smells worse).

Provided that an adequate total amount is taken in 24 hours, timing may be arranged to avoid 'accidents', e.g. by restricting fluids after about 6 p.m.

Patients who are aware of their need to pass urine, and have severe frequency or urgency, may be helped by nearby commodes and small hand held urinals. Patients who are not aware of their need to pass urine, either because of mental impairment or loss of bladder sensation, will need protective clothing. Many different types are available to suit the needs of the patient.

Frequent toileting and prompts to use the toilet will help to maintain any bladder control that the person may have and also encourage them to maintain their independence. A baseline chart can be used to establish the usual patterns for individual patients. In some cases it can form the basis of a toileting programme. Regular checks can be made with patients, perhaps on a 2-hourly basis, when toilet facilities can be offered. During the night disturbance should be kept to a minimum, perhaps with checks being made at 2 a.m., with a view to keeping the patient dry along with a single night visit to the lavatory.

Many people can be helped to maintain their self-respect and dignity through effective management of continence. There are various ways in which this can be achieved, some of which have been discussed. Incontinence is something that can affect people of any age but it is more prevalent in the older age group; further advice, help and support can be gained from contacting local groups such as the Disabled Living Centres and the Association of Continence Advisors.

EATING AND DRINKING

The enjoyment and appreciation of food can occupy a large amount of an older person's time. Making mealtimes as enjoyable and leisurely as possible will help to encourage a relaxing environment. Many older people with mental health problems will refuse to eat or drink, because of either a depressive illness or due to some paranoid or delusional ideas about the food being poisoned. As dietary changes can affect older people quite dramatically, it is essential that a certain level of nutrition is maintained at all times. Sometimes it may well be necessary to stay continuously with a patient, offering small sips of fluids or something light to eat, to ensure that a toxic condition does not arise. Tempting patients with their favourite foods may help to stimulate their appetite.

ASSESSMENT METHODS AND TOOLS

Assessment methods can vary greatly depending on individual preference. However, certain fundamental principles should be followed to ensure that the patient receives appropriate care and treatment (Box 24.2).

Ethical considerations also must be considered in the context of assessment. It has been suggested that the best way to take a comprehensive assessment of a patient is by taking a blank piece of paper and recording as much information as possible from the patient. This form of assessment could probably be attempted by those with a vast amount of experience in working with the elderly. However, for the purpose of identifying specific aspects of health and ill health, an assessment tool will provide a clear framework for the assessor that will also protect the patient from any undue violation of their privacy.

At the level of individual assessment, definitions can clarify need and need assessment. Shared understanding of these concepts is essential to the multidisciplinary ethos required in this specialty. Needs assessment is a staged process conducted by a care professional, which begins with the identification of specific difficulties, accounts for the presence and efficacy of current help (therefore assessing unmet need normatively), recognizes perceived need and, finally, specifies the type of help required to meet those needs.

Standardized assessment tools are widely employed by those working with the elderly mentally ill. Such tools include behaviour and dependency ratings, for example the Clifton Assessment Procedure for the Elderly (CAPE) (Pattie and Gilleard, 1979; Pattie, 1981), mental status questionnaires, e.g.

the CAPE and the Mini Mental State Examination (Folstein *et al.*, 1975) and general tests of intellectual or cognitive functioning.

ASSESSMENT METHODS

A multidisciplinary framework should always be utilized for assessment of the elderly mentally ill, as a number of services are usually required to provide a comprehensive package of care. Interprofessional working methods should be used with the focus on the similarities between professions, rather than the differences, i.e. working towards making life better for the patients and their families.

Where needs exist, assessment and referral would be desirable to further the general objectives of care for the elderly person, described by Wright (1985) as follows:
- The maintenance of health and independence.
- Social integration.
- A satisfactory domiciliary and caring environment.
- The relief of the burden carried by families and friends in providing long-term care for an older person.

Assessment methods need to adopt an approach that addresses needs, rather than a framework focusing solely on problems or a cure model. The work of Bond and Reed (1991) suggests that the models and frameworks currently used are based on cure models and, when cure is not possible, it is patients who have failed the system; it is they who are considered 'hopeless' cases.

To ensure that 'care' is taking place, nurses must be able to work within a value system that encourages the identification of needs, identifies the strengths of the patient and recognizes the futility of a total cure model in elderly care settings.

Gaining a full and comprehensive assessment requires the use of excellent nursing skills, such as active listening, prompting and probing when necessary and confronting and challenging interventions–of course, within a framework that is supportive and genuine.

Concentrated discussion and conversation may be very uncomfortable for the older person and the nurse needs to use discretion when collecting data for the initial assessment, as the patient may not find it possible to sit for any length of time in an 'interview' setting.

The nurse's ability to collect useful data will depend greatly on how comfortable he or she feels during the interaction. As in any situation with two people, genuine interest and concern will be noted by the other party and the tone and level of the conversation will be set accordingly.

Although older people differ in their willingness to reveal life histories and personal experiences, most desire relationships with others and are anxious to share information with interested parties. Allowing the patient to 'tell their story' can give the nurse the opportunity to assess subtle changes in long-term and short-term memory, decision making ability, judgement making patterns and orientation to time, place and person. Often, this approach will encourage building a rapport with the older person, which may be more difficult when using a more formal approach with specific questions.

Box 24.2	***Principles of assessment***

- Patient centred.
- Takes time; the longer the assessment, the fuller and more comprehensive an assessment will be achieved.
- Multidisciplinary approach.
- A wide variety of sources should be used for the assessment — patient, carers, friends, multidisciplinary team.
- An assessment framework needs to be identified. (Models, developed from your ward team; frameworks, which identify the elements that fit with your team's philosophy.)

ASSESSMENT TOOLS

The development of assessment tools has greatly increased the scope of determining the severity of mental illness in older people and also of identifying their care and treatment needs. The more commonly used rating scales have been designed for assessment of mood, cognition, behaviour and self-care. More recently assessment tools have been used that also look at the needs of carers.

Behaviour Assessment Scale of Later Life

The behaviour assessment scale of later life (BASOLL) was developed to improve the efficiency and quality of the service provided by a busy urban service for the elderly mentally ill (Brooker *et al.*, 1993). The aims of the BASOLL were twofold:

1. To identify significant behavioural problems to begin the process of care planning.
2. To provide a checklist of behavioural symptomatology for the major psychiatric disorders of old age, which can be used either to alert staff to the need for specialist assessment or to provide information to aid diagnosis.

The tool includes sections on self-care, mobility, sensory impairment, behavioural indices of dementia, depression and paranoid disorders, evidence of challenging behaviour and continence. Mood disturbance includes items on sleep disturbance, complaints of feeling depressed, suicidal ideas, obsessionality, appetite disturbance, suspiciousness, hallucinations, delusions and paranoia.

The BASOLL is a broad-based instrument that has been found to be helpful in care planning with a diverse group of elderly patients. There are two formats that can be used: the interview version, which takes about 40 minutes to complete, and the checklist version.

Clifton Assessment Procedures for the Elderly

The Clifton Assessment Procedure for the Elderly (CAPE) incorporates both cognitive and behavioural measurements of disability. It was devised as a brief measure of psychological functioning for chronic psychiatric patient groups and has been validated against the outcome of day hospital and day centre care. The assessment scales consist of a cognitive assessment scale (CAS) and a behaviour rating scale (BRS). A grading system is offered linking disability and dependency to need for care.

CAS has three parts:

1. Information and orientation. This contains 12 subcategories and has been shown to be valid on its own.
2. Mental ability subscale.
3. Psychomotor test.

Scores of 7 and below are usually associated with an organic diagnosis and scores above this with a functional illness.

BRS is an 18-item scale with 4 subscales:

1. Physical disability.
2. Apathy and inactivity.
3. Communication difficulties.
4. Social disturbance.

The CAPE scale takes only a few minutes to administer and can be used easily by all health care professionals.

Needs-Led Assessment

The concept of need and the practice of needs-led assessment are each subject to a wide range of interpretations, to the likely detriment of individual assessments and multidisciplinary working. The assessment of a person's difficulties can be unpopular with practitioners and may be seen as incomplete in itself, as suggested by anecdotal and other evidence (Barrowclough and Fleming, 1986; Harding *et al.*, 1987). As a result, there is a move towards focusing assessment on the things that a person can do and likes to do (Centre for Policy on Ageing, 1990). Some of the concerns with assessing difficulties alone (i.e. assessing dependency) are that such assessments are necessarily problem focused (for example, focusing on impairment, what a person cannot do or what abilities they have lost), entailing a number of negative connotations This is particularly true for people with dementia.

Strengths–Needs Analysis

An assessment that utilizes a strengths–needs analysis provides a comprehensive, patient-centred assessment that highlights the personal strengths of the individual.

Providing a profile of strengths and needs (an example is shown in Box 24.3) can help to provide a framework of assessment that considers abilities as well as impairments and

Box 24.3 *Strengths–needs analysis*	
STRENGTHS	NEEDS
• Healthy.	• To eat at regular times.
• Mobile.	• To lock door and carry a key when going out.
• Interested in keeping busy.	
• Likes to look attractive.	• To use watch, clock, calendar and daily paper to orientate self.
• Talented painter.	
• Financially secure.	
• Very caring family.	• To change underwear every day.
• Socializes every day.	

defines impairments as needs to be met, rather than problems to be eliminated. Other measures examine service provision as well as need and also look at the environment, thereby going beyond examining function to assess the adequacy of current service provision and potential for future services (Brewin, 1992).

FUNCTIONAL ILLNESS

Levels of functional illness in the elderly are high. The prevalence of severe clinical depression among this age group is a major concern to health care workers. Careful assessment is required because of the possibility of a wrong diagnosis of a dementing illness being made, as some of the signs and symptoms are similar, e.g. poor memory and changes in eating habits and general behaviour.

Depression in the elderly differs from that in younger people. It may begin with decreased interest in normal activities and a lack of energy. There may be an increased dependence on others; conversation may focus entirely on the past. There may be multiple physical complaints with no diagnosable cause. The person may have pain, especially in the head, neck, back or abdomen with no history or evidence of a physical cause. Other symptoms in the elderly include weight loss, paranoia, fatigue, gastrointestinal distress and often a refusal to eat or drink, with life-threatening consequences. Older people with depression are more likely to respond to questioning with annoyance or silence or short unresponsive answers. Irritability and hostility are characteristic responses.

Many older people are loath to complain of 'nervous problems', since they may look upon these as lack of moral fibre. Not only may they not mention their feelings of misery and anxiety but they may actually deny having any symptom that could be looked upon as nervous in origin. However, they may complain of physical symptoms that can be seen as respectable, such as constipation, abdominal pain, headaches and a whole variety of sensations that are the results of anxiety (see Case study: Functional illness).

In the elderly as with others, it is important to bear in mind the possibility of depression swinging towards mania, either because of the natural history of the condition or the therapy used for depression. The combination of an antidepressant and electroplexy often quickly relieves depression but unless used with great care, it can result in mania replacing the depression.

MANIA AND HYPOMANIA

These are not common conditions in the elderly but do occur, particularly in atypical forms. Distractibility is important when caring for these patients. Having a knowledge of the patient's likes and interests may help to manage situations that could become difficult, e.g. a patient may decide to dance naked in the snow and if told not to do this, it is quite likely that he or she will try to do it all the more. If, instead of trying to insist that the patient should not, an interesting alternative is offered, it is very likely that the patient will forget about any previous plans and follow the initial lead. The term 'hypomania' (see Case study: Hypomania) describes a relatively minor type of mania and is probably commoner than the extreme, flamboyant manifestations of this condition.

This is not an uncommon expression of mania in the elderly; there is a mixture of manic, depressive and paranoid symptoms, all interwoven.

An increase in the incidence of depression has been found among the very aged (75 years and over) (Newman, 1989). This is of special concern, as it is a major factor leading to institutionalized care and suicide. Diminished physical vigour, functional incapacity, aberrant or atypical behaviour, persistent refusal of food and fluids, perceived loss of control, lack

---

Case study: Functional illness

Miss Lucy May was admitted to hospital after taking an overdose of paracetamol. Following recovery, she said that she had taken the overdose because of intolerable pain in her neck. This pain had prevented her from sleeping for years and was now more than she could stand.

She had had the pain in her neck on and off for a period of 11 years but this had not worried her until a few months prior to her suicide attempt. She had consulted the family doctor, who prescribed analgesics. These had no effect and she was referred to a physician, who ordered a whole range of investigations. No cause for her pain was discovered and she was referred to a psychiatrist, who considered her to be suffering from mild anxiety symptoms and prescribed a minor tranquilliser.

When she recovered from her suicide attempt a detailed history was taken, which revealed considerable evidence of a depressive illness. She was treated with electroconvulsive therapy and antidepressants, rapidly improved and became symptom-free. She said she had never felt so well for years.

Case study: Hypomania

Mrs Cantini was Italian, 68 and had never suffered with any psychiatric illness until her husband became ill. He was admitted to hospital following an attack of delirium tremens. His wife remained at home with her widowed daughter. The day following her husband's admission to hospital she suddenly became very excited and started speaking at a very fast rate. She said that she felt unbelievably well but was worried about the Germans who were coming to get her. She said that her husband would get better but while saying this looked very sad and she wept.

It was very difficult to assess her symptoms at home and she was admitted to hospital. Further examination revealed symptoms of both hypomania and depression with ideas of persecution. She was elated and depressed at the same time and continued to express fears that the Germans were coming to get her.

A course of electroplexy was decided upon and after four treatments she reverted to her normal self. She remained well for 6 months and then had a recurrence of symptoms, which responded quickly to electroplexy. She has remained well since then.

of a strong family support network, loneliness, social isolation and withdrawal, are a few of the essential warning clues to life-threatening behaviour in the elderly, particularly the very aged (Coleman and McCulloch, 1985).

ANXIETY DISORDERS

The treatment and care of older people with anxiety disorders can be particularly difficult because of the overlap with depression or medical illness.

Generalized Anxiety Disorder

The central feature of this disorder is excessive and persistent anxiety, typically over a period of months or years. The symptoms cluster into the following three categories:

1. Motor tension — trembling, muscle tension, restlessness.
2. Autonomic hyperactivity — shortness of breath, rapid heart rate, sweaty or cold clammy hands, dry mouth, dizziness, digestive disturbances, frequent urination and trouble swallowing or 'lump in throat'.
3. Vigilance and scanning — feeling on edge, exaggerated startle response, difficulty concentrating, insomnia and irritability.

Many older people with this disorder may also present with features of depression. A mixed picture of the symptoms and course of treatment can make proper assessment and specific treatment difficult (Box 24.4). A major problem that can occur with the older person is that the disorder is treated symptomatically, which can lead to patients being prescribed many different types of medication (Sheikh and Swales, 1994)

Panic Disorder

This disorder is characterized by recurrent episodes of severe anxiety and fear (panic attacks) manifested by a multitude of somatic and cognitive symptoms, examples of which are described in generalized anxiety disorder, above. Although there have been relatively few studies completed with the elderly population, it is recognized as a major life-threatening disorder, as some long-term studies have shown older men who have experienced panic disorder for a long period of time

suffering from major cardiovascular problems.

The most frequent mental health complications of anxiety disorders include depression, alcoholism and prescription drug abuse and, particularly in panic disorder, a high risk of suicide (Sheikh and Swales, 1994).

THE DEMENTIAS

Dementia is a chronic disease with substantial morbidity, complicated presentations and very serious effects on families and care-givers. The care of a patient with dementia is therefore complex, requiring multidisciplinary evaluation, a plan of care and continual reassessment. For practical purposes, dementia in elderly patients can be attributed to:

- Alzheimer's disease (AD).
- Multiple cerebral infarction.
- Mixed AD and multi-infarct dementia (MID).
- Senile dementia of Lewy body type.
- Dementia in Parkinson's disease.
- Dementia in alcoholism.
- Causes secondary to other brain lesions–tumour, trauma etc.
- Causes pathologically unexplained–toxic or metabolic; vitamin lack; pseudo-dementias etc.

ALZHEIMER'S DISEASE

Some of the causes that have been postulated as giving rise to Alzheimer's disease are: environmental factors (including aluminium, ionizing radiation, food neurotoxins) and acute organic brain syndrome caused by viruses or head injuries. There is a substantial genetic contribution to the risk of developing Alzheimer's disease. In some instances of Alzheimer's disease the gene probably responsible is on chromosome 21. There is a wealth of evidence to suggest that the disease shows familial clustering. People with a blood relative affected have an increased risk of developing the disease (Van Dujin, 1995).

Alzheimer's disease and senile dementia of the Alzheimer type (SDAT) both have an insidious onset and a prolonged course, sometimes running for 20 years. For the majority of people suffering from dementia the need for acute management should seldom arise. Many older people become ever more forgetful and adapt gradually and graciously to their limitations, while their families and friends perceive them simply as starting to show their age rather than as demented. A little more help is offered and more support every few months.

Health care professionals are often initially involved with a person suffering from dementia as a result of a crisis in their situation. The clinical picture of dementia obviously differs from individual to individual. However, there are some common characteristics that can be observed over time, in differing degrees. These include memory failure, lack of concentration, some visuospatial disturbance, mild dysphasia, emotional disturbance and personality changes. This is how one husband described the onset of his wife's dementia:

Box 24.4 *Differences between anxiety and depression*

DEPRESSION	ANXIETY
Depressed mood worse a.m.	Anxious mood worse p.m.
Lack of energy.	Agitation.
Terminal insomnia.	Initial insomnia.
Feelings of guilt.	Panic attacks and phobias.
Patients might appear more dependent and clingy.	Patients tend to have poorly adjusted personalities.
Usually have a history of regular cycles of depression.	Irregularly recurrent with incomplete periods of remission.

I didn't really notice, until much later, but looking back, now, I can find things that happened... she used to be a good card player, you see, especially at solo whist; she belonged to a club, went every week, twice a week, and several times she was forgetting the number of the cards, and, she had a pretty good memory for that, for knowing which cards are out, and eventually she could only remember the face cards. Looking back it was the beginning; in fact, that was so many years ago, ten years anyway, but eventually she had to leave; then she gravitated to bingo, but even that was getting too much for her, but we didn't think no more of that, either, for some reason, but eventually it just gradually came; she would just stand in the kitchen, and wonder why she was there; she was going to do something and just didn't remember what she was there for; this was the time I began to get anxious about her; she could still do things but she forgot very often where she was and what she was going to do, and since then it's just been a gradual process. Now she can't do a thing, now I've got to get her out of bed, and wash her, and dress her, every morning, and take all her wet things off every morning; it's a wet bed, but as I say the whole thing has come on so gradually over the years, and well at the moment, you see it's all right, during the day, mostly, except it's a one sided affair, really...

This gradual loss of competence represents one dimension in the development of dementia. However, it is not necessarily the one that family members may initially pick up, nor is it by any means the only dimension. This is how one woman described the early changes she noticed in her husband:

Well he started on the motorists, what business had they parking in front of the door, and telling them to take their cars away or he would get the police. He would also use very bad language... it would be about beginning at that time, you see, and with the children too, that came. We have a little garden and of course if the children came near the garden, he would tell them to clear out and things like that, and threaten them; once a ball came into the garden and instead of handing it back, he pitched it right across the road... and not so long ago, he threw a hoe at one of the children in the street; and then I had a neighbour at the other end of the street and she came along and said he had threatened their son, and when she spoke to him he threatened her... but however, since then she's recognized that he's not just normal... anyway, in fact, I said to him, "I'll have no friends left in the street if you carry on like this..." well for a long time he'd always had a bad memory for names, for people; he would come in and he would say to me, "I saw,..." and then he would stop and he wouldn't remember who it was. I had to guess who it was, and because I couldn't, he would get himself into a rage... and other things, he never did much shopping at all, except for his papers, and he'd get me two pints of milk; well sometimes he would come back with four, you know with two cartons instead of one, and just recently he said, well, he would get the milk, but where's the flagon?

For this woman the change in character, the bad temper and the impulsive reactions were odd and upsetting; it was the appearance of 'new' behaviour that indicated all was not well,

rather than the disappearance of existing skills (Gilleard, 1984). There has been a minimal amount of work completed in relation to the psychological needs of people with dementia and how, carers and professionals, can best meet these needs. However, the work of Tom Kitwood and his colleagues from the dementia care group in Bradford have started to address these needs through the person-centred approach to care called Dementia Care Mapping.

DEMENTIA CARE MAPPING

The new culture of caring for people with dementia recognizes first and foremost the person, not the illness. It is important to have a clear and complete understanding of the person's abilities, tastes, interests, values and spirituality. This is an observational method, which provides a detailed evaluation of care given by members of staff to dementia sufferers. This assessment aims to adopt the perspective of the client, examining the quality as well as the quantity of the interactions and activities, judging their impact on the individual's sense of well-being. Within this new culture it is also imperative to recognize the feelings, concerns and vulnerabilities of the people doing the caring and to help individuals transform these into positive resources for the work to be done. The sense of well-being and personhood is what matters most when caring for someone with dementia. Kitwood and Bredin (1992) emphasizes four factors which contribute to well-being:

1. A sense of personal worth — we are valuable to others.
2. A sense of agency — we can make things happen.
3. Social confidence — we can reach out to others and there will be a response.
4. A sense of hope — despite setbacks, life goes on.

The Dementia Research Group in Bradford has developed training and education packages that are dynamic, developmental, humanistic and creative, thus moving away from the technical frame of reference to a person-centred framework (Kitwood, 1988.).

The equation used in this framework is:

$$D = P + B + H + NI + SP$$

Dementia (D) in an individual may be considered to be the result of a complex interaction between five main components:

P = Personality
B = Biography
H = Physical health
NI = Neurological impairment
SP = Social psychology

Personality here means the temperament of each individual, the resources that the person has had available all of their life and their emotional problems. Biography refers to what has happened to the person throughout their life, the risks, losses, adventures, opportunities and relationships. Often the sum total of these in an older person would certainly overwhelm many people in the prime of life.

Physical health is very important, as often people with dementia cannot let us know when they are in pain or discomfort but will instead display strange or antisocial behaviours. Also there are several conditions causing confusion (such as urinary tract infections or constipation) that can be treated through medical intervention.

Neurological impairment is the part of the equation that is most discussed. However, in terms of how people with dementia are cared for, it is the least relevant part of the equation.

Finally, there is the social psychology component of the equation. This is considered to be the domain in which personhood lies, i.e. the day-to-day picture of what is happening to the individual, how the person is responded to, whether or not there are helpful and enabling responses from others.

Dementia Care Mapping actually 'maps' the behaviours and responses of the person with dementia over a period of time and highlights deficits in good care practice, which can then be rectified. It is also an invaluable tool in effective care planning based on meeting the individual needs of the person with dementia. The qualities described in Box 24.5 need to be valued and developed within services to ensure that good practice is taking place.

The old culture of dementia care (Box 24.6) encompassed the view that, on a functional level, the person was undergoing a decline. In the new culture of dementia care the decline in abilities still exists but there is an emphasis on the increase in personhood development, which involves highly skilful interventions from the care staff working with the patients. Carers and professionals who are adequately resourced, personally as well as practically, will be the most successful in having a direct and significant effect on the well-being of those they are caring for.

MULTI-INFARCT DEMENTIA

Dementia caused by multiple brain infarcts is called multi-infarct dementia (MID), or atherosclerotic dementia, and is relatively rare (Hachinski, *et al.*, 1974). This disease is considered to appear when a certain volume of infarcted brain tissue, at least 50—100 ml, is present. As a consequence of the many cerebral events, the course of the disease is usually stepwise. As with all vascular disease the risk factors, such as hypertension and obesity, need to be modified, and other possible causes, which may be treatable, need to be investigated.

CREUTZFELDT–JAKOB DISEASE

Creutzfeldt–Jakob disease (CJD) was first described in 1921, when an unusual spongy appearance of the brain was discovered on post mortem, in six cases. It is a rare, rapidly progressive, dementing illness, affecting both sexes, with an onset usually after the age of 55. It is usually fatal, with a clinical course rarely exceeding 6 months in duration. There have been many connections made with animals over the year—sheep have a form of spongiform encephalopathy, which has been recognized for the last 250 years and in recent times, cattle have also been found to have developed a form of spongiform encephalopathy. The theory proposed is that the cattle had been exposed to the sheep encephalopathy, scrapie, through the consumption of rendered sheep remains as part of their diet. A number of theories of aetiology have been postulated including:

- Spongiform encephalopathy may be a primary hereditary disorder.
- A mutation may be an effect of a virus or other agent, which then causes the production of an abnormal protein and causes the illness (Esmonde, 1994).

The possibility of transmission of the disease through the consumption of animal products cannot be ruled out, but this route this is somewhat unlikely, in view of the occurrence of CJD in life-long vegetarians.

PICK'S DISEASE.

This was first described in 1892 as a dementing disorder with prominent personality and character alteration. The typical features are disintegration of the personality and the development of uncharacteristic traits coupled with a loss of cognitive function. The distinctive feature, which gives this disease its name, is the atrophy of, predominantly, the frontal and

Box 24.6 *Old and new cultures of dementia care*

Old culture of dementia care	New culture of dementia care
Dementia care is a backwater; it makes high demands and little challenge.	Dementia care is a rich area requiring staff with very high ability and resourcefulness.
It is suited to those with low abilities and few qualifications.	It challenges human ability to its limits.
Caring involves providing a safe environment, meeting basic personhood needs (food, warmth, etc.) and giving physical care.	Caring for someone with dementia involves maintaining a range needs besides physical.

Box 24.5 *Positive dementia carer qualities*

- Inner quietness.
- Lowered psychological defences.
- Empathy.
- Ease in making contact.
- Stability and resourcefulness.

temporal lobes, and the presence of ballooned neurones, known as 'Picks' bodies. Insight is impaired quite early and often there is a development of a fatuous euphoria or apathy alternating with periods of restlessness.

DIFFUSE LEWY BODY DISEASE

This has only recently been recognized as a cause of dementia (Crystal *et al.*, 1990). The illness bears many resemblances to Alzheimer's disease but probably may be differentiated clinically on the basis of more marked agitation, visual hallucinations and delusions. Parkinsonian symptoms also occur early. As Lewy bodies are also found in Parkinson's disease, it is postulated that the two diseases may have a common causation.

HUNTINGTON'S DISEASE

This dementia is an inherited condition with an onset usually after the age of 30 and rarely after the age of 70 (mean age 41 years). Characteristics of the disease include progressive chorea, psychological changes and dementia, although not necessarily in that order. There is no diagnostic test available as yet. However, it is possible to see typical changes in the brain on a CT scan. With the recent advances in molecular genetic techniques, it is now possible to offer presymptomatic testing to individuals at risk, in some cases with an accuracy of prediction of likelihood of involvement as low as 2% and in others, as high as 98%.

DEMENTIA AND PARKINSON'S DISEASE

About 20% of people who suffer from Parkinson's disease develop dementia (Brown and Marsden, 1984).

This type of dementia has specific clinical and psychological characteristics and is now believed to be associated with specific neuropathological changes. Depression is common in Parkinson's disease and may give the appearance of a pseudodementia, relieved by antidepressant treatment. It has been observed that this type of dementia occurs at a much later age and patients are more likely to suffer from toxic confusional states following any pharmacological intervention. Apathy and depression seem to characterize the dementia of Parkinson's disease. Visual hallucinations, often with little or no affective component, are common.

PSEUDODEMENTIA

In this condition, symptoms of disorientation and memory loss occur and mimic dementia. In contrast to dementia, the clinical course of the condition is relatively short and it has a defined date of onset. The concept of pseudodementia has become increasingly controversial in recent years. Today the term generally is used to describe reversible cognitive changes of depression, which are sometimes confused with progressive dementia in older patients. A relatively short course of antidepressants can significantly improve this condition.

BEHAVIOUR PATTERNS IN DEMENTIA

There are a number of behaviour patterns associated with dementia. Two common ones are wandering and dysphasia.

Wandering

Patients who have a dementing illness often present with wandering behaviour, which can be distressing for those relatives who are concerned for their safety. People will wander for many different reasons. The behaviour does not just 'occur'; there are known precipitating factors (see Box 24.7).

Reduced social interaction, and increased cognitive impairment and agitation are probable sources of wandering behaviour. It has been suggested that wandering can replace social interaction for some cognitively impaired people. If so, unchecked wandering adversely may affect the preservation of social skills. Conversely, it may be possible to reduce wandering by heightening social opportunity. Wandering is sometimes a sign of agitated depression. Restlessness towards nightfall ('sundowning') and nocturnal roaming by patients who are unaware of the time and are bored as well as restless are a particular strain on carer (Lowenstein, 1982).

Expressive and Receptive Dysphasia

People with a dementing illness will often experience a degree of dysphasia, either by not being able to express themselves coherently through the normal channel of communication, i.e. speech, or by not understanding what is being said to them in a receptive way. Therefore it is important to use very simple, short sentences during conversation and not to ask too many questions or complicate the issues being discussed. The person otherwise will become agitated and anxious, wanting to respond to you but unable to find the right words or expressions.

CULTURAL AND ETHNIC NEEDS

The needs of elderly people from different cultural and ethnic backgrounds is a sadly neglected area. A major factor influencing the lack of information available is the lower uptake of services by this age group. A number of probable reasons for this exist, including more expansive family

Box 24.7

Why patients wander

- Trying to find home.
- Trying to find the toilet.
- Feeling hungry.
- Experiencing pain.
- Acute medical or environmental trigger–stress or loss.
- Experiencing boredom.
- Side-effects of drugs or withdrawal.

networks, preference for alternative medicine and the stigma attached to mental illness.

The elderly black population is growing, as first generation immigrants reach their 60s and 70s. The stronger family networks that are apparent in the Asian, African and Afro-Caribbean populations will also significantly change as the values of the younger generations conform more to Western culture, e.g. social mobility will result in members of extended families living further apart.

A convenient stereotype, which is often used to justify the lack of services for this group, is that 'they want to look after their own' (Walker and Waqar, 1994). Older people from different cultural backgrounds will have different ways of expressing sorrow, pain and grief and will often talk about their spiritual life in relation to their suffering. They may not have a withdrawn personality or be suffering from somatic complaints they may talk about their guilt or unworthiness. It is important to involve as many members of the family as possible to determine general patterns of conduct, so that abnormal behaviour can be identified.

Many other cultures give older people a higher status within the family network; the elderly provide a role as arbitrators in many major family disagreements or for decisions concerning marriage and domestic functions. There is a social stigma against leaving one's elderly relatives in institutional care. There are very few elderly mentally ill patients as permanent residents in psychiatric hospitals in Libya and India.

Vulnerability to psychiatric difficulties becomes more prevalent as people age; older people from different ethnic backgrounds are at particular risk. These older people have often suffered deep-seated multifaceted loss, through leaving their homeland, of social role and status, of a familiar and safe environment, and of easy verbal communication, sometimes even with younger members of their own family. Past persecution and maltreatment and forgetting learned languages in old age also enhance the risk of paranoid feelings and may generate a vicious circle of fear and hostility. A term used to describe the situation that these elderly persons often find themselves in is 'triple jeopardy' (Norman, 1985). They are not merely in double jeopardy by reason of age and discrimination, but in triple jeopardy, at risk because they are old, because of the physical conditions and hostility under which they have to live and because services are not easily accessible to them.

With these facts in mind, it is crucial to encourage members of the family, friends and others to be involved in the care process for the older person. Support and encouragement should be offered to the family about how well they have been managing and how their experience and knowledge about caring will be really useful in giving the correct care and treatment to their relative.

CARERS' NEEDS

The needs of carers can vary enormously, as the family unit itself no longer conforms to the traditional format. Family carers are recognized as providing most of the care required by the elderly person, with professionals offering only a small amount of support and active treatment, often when the situation has become intolerable, or overwhelming for the carers. Early intervention by professionals in the family situation can prove to be helpful and can often prevent a crisis situation occurring.

The identification of carers' needs can actually help the carer continue in their role and use the services that are available. A useful model that has been adopted for this purpose comes from the Admiral Nursing Service, which was set up with the sole purpose of looking after carers. The nurses focus on the coping strategies of carers and on health promotion and education needs, and work within a stress management model (Zarit *et al.*, 1985). Having the support of an identified person can often encourage carers to continue in their role with the family member at home and avoid the need for hospitalization. Encouraging carers to make use of services such as respite and day care facilities can often help them to continue to meet their own needs and to retain some of their independence.

Meeting other carers can also reduce the feelings of isolation, which might be pronounced, and sharing experiences with each other can be an educational resource and support second to none.

The Carers (Recognition and Services) Act 1995, describes local authorities' duties in relation to carers. Under the Act a carer is entitled, on request, to an assessment when the local authority carries out an assessment of the person cared for, in respect of community care services.

ELDERLY ABUSE

There has been an increasing recognition in the UK, particularly since the mid-1980s, that elderly people are at risk of all forms of abuse. The prevalence of abuse in the population over 65 has been estimated to be approximately 5% (Ogg and Bennett, 1992; Kurrle *et al.*, 1992). It has been consistently found that dementia sufferers are more likely to experience abuse, although their increased risk may be explained only partly by their cognitive impairment (Homer and Gilleard, 1990). It is estimated that a person with Alzheimer's disease is at least twice as likely as a non dementing older person living in the community to be subjected to physical abuse. There is a whole spectrum of abuse, from verbal and psychological to physical, financial and sexual abuse. Recourse to the law may be required to protect the person. The Mental Health Act 1983 (Sections 2 and 3) may be used to admit patients who are considered at risk of abuse. However, in most cases of suspected or actual abuse of people with dementia their need is usually for protection from abuse rather than compulsory treatment in a psychiatric facility as governed by the Act. The admission requirements under the Act are sometimes fulfilled, for example, where the patient is exhibiting seriously aggressive behaviour towards their carer, a factor that has been repeatedly shown to have an association with reciprocal physical abuse of the dementia sufferer (Coyne *et al.*, 1993)

WOMEN AND AGEING

Women predominate among elderly people, especially in the very old age group. Older women are more likely to be widowed and, in the UK and other developed countries, to live alone. Generally, women are more likely to be disadvantaged in terms of poorer health and higher levels of functional disability. They have fewer financial and other material resources and, because of their living arrangements, have less access to kin as informal carers and are more reliant on state health and welfare services. However, older women have the advantage of their friendship networks and the social support, that they can rely on from friends.

Throughout the EC, with the exception of Denmark, elderly women have lower incomes and living standards than men. Older women are almost twice as likely as elderly men to have an income at or below the poverty threshold. Official figures underestimate the income disadvantage of elderly women when the household, family or taxation unit is the unit of analysis.

The main sources of income for older people in the UK are the state, earnings, interest on savings and non state pensions. Average total income for women in this country in 1993 was given as a median of £61 with an upper quartile of £91 per week (Arber and Ginn, 1994). Women's disadvantage could be alleviated by redistributive state pensions supported from taxation, as in Denmark. However, in the UK the opposite trend is taking place with a huge shift towards private pension schemes. Many more statistics exist that confirm the levels of poverty in which elderly women live in the UK, however, it is only necessary to highlight these concerns to understand their significance in relation to the mental health of older women and the effects of such constraints.

Good health is essential to independence, especially the capability for self-care such as eating, bathing and personal mobility (e.g. negotiating the stairs and walking outside of the home). People with a higher level of functional disability or cognitive impairment will require more practical support and personal care from either informal carers or the state.

Women generally have acquired the skills that will influence their ability to form intimate relationships from an early age. Women not only have more friends on average than men in later life but the quality of their friendships tends to differ too. Women's friends are often their close confidants, with whom troubles and joys, and anxieties and hopes can be shared, whereas elderly men tend to rely on their wives to fulfil this role (Fischer and Oliker, 1983).

From a nursing perspective it is crucial to allow women to form meaningful, intimate relationships while they are being cared for and for the nurse to nurture any opportunity for friendships to grow. This form of intervention can have a significant positive effect on the emotional and mental health of the individual and therefore can be seen as proactive measure in maintaining a sense of well-being.

MEN AND AGEING

Men have some obvious advantages in terms of their financial and social status as they get older but a very significant disadvantage is the lack of a social network following retirement. On an emotional level, men are more likely to discuss practical events and shared interests with other men and often there is a huge area left concerning their feelings, doubts and sorrows, with no possibility for them to come to terms with their situation and who they are. Men suffer the same amount of grief, disillusionment, unfulfilled expectations and losses as women but are often unable to find a way to unburden themselves from their feelings.

For many men the social roles they have occupied throughout their lives have been created through their occupations and status. The family roles that men have occupied are also important but the evidence, which is growing, suggests that friendships are as important–if not more important–to older people than family ties (Wenger, 1990).

INTERPERSONAL INTERVENTIONS

Communicating with older people can involve a wide range of skills from simple, obvious ones such as showing an interest in the person through active listening, touch and body language, to more complex techniques such as validating people's feelings and challenging and confronting interventions. The latter are not often discussed within the context of the elderly mentally ill as it is often assumed that 'old people are kind and sweet and at peace with the world' or 'old people are past being consulted about anything, including their own lives'. The power of stereotyping can have a tremendous effect on the treatment and care options available for individuals and, in turn, on the level of communication that occurs between two individuals.

Coping strategies and defence mechanisms have been in place for a long time but that does not mean that an attempt should not be made to explore them. However, this requires sensitivity on the part of the nurse and effective skills relating to the older person. The story-telling technique discussed earlier has tremendous potential for opening up previously closed doors. There are some fundamental requirements for this process to take place effectively:

• Time.
• Genuine interest on behalf of the nurse.

• A good understanding of communication techniques.
• A supportive relationship.

Older people, like anyone else, will acquire strategies to defend themselves from painful or intolerable feelings. These strategies can often be so developed and crystallized within the person that he or she is known for them and descriptions arise such as 'cantankerous' or 'manipulative' or, on the other hand, 'sweet' and 'cute'. It would be at the least foolish and at worst damaging to try to communicate effectively with older people without using their terms of reference. This means speaking plain English and not confusing issues with jargon or interpretations that will mean nothing to the patient and encourage the breakdown of the interaction.

Touch can have a very powerful effect on individuals who are often feeling isolated, misunderstood and frightened. A wider discussion around the different types of touch that nurses can use therapeutically with patients is discussed in Chapter 28, Complementary Therapies and Mental Health Nursing.

VALIDATION THERAPY

The underlying assumptions behind validation therapy are that all behaviour has meaning, that early, learned emotional memories replace intellectual thinking in the disoriented very aged and that the disorientated very aged return to the past to try to resolve unreconciled conflicts.

Naomi Feil completed a series of studies using validation therapy techniques with remarkable results (Feil, 1982). Behaviours that were considered 'difficult to manage', such as wandering and shouting, were explored using the interpersonal techniques of validation and the responses showed the distressed older person being calmed and comforted with 'someone finally listening'.

Validation therapy (Box 24.8) is a process used to communicate with disoriented elderly people by validating and respecting their feelings in whatever time and place is real to them at that given moment, even though this may not correspond with our reality, here and now (Bleathman and Morton, 1988). Sceptics have claimed that validation 'colludes with delusion'. This is an erroneous understanding of validation. At no time does the nurse agree with false or questionable facts stated by the older person. What the nurse does is:

1. Acknowledge memories as being memories.
2. Acknowledge the reality of feelings, in conjunction with how these feelings affect a person, regardless of the correctness of the facts.

Offering an approach that helps to open doors to the inner life of the older person is therapeutic, helpful, meaningful and useful. Validation accepts a person's memories and fantasies as important, because they are essential components of a person's life and are necessary to understand motivation and behaviour. Naomi Feil is so convinced of the importance of validating feelings to facilitate the resolution of one's life that she has added a ninth developmental stage to Erikson's Developmental Framework, specifically for the very old, namely that of 'resolution versus vegetation' (Jones, 1985).

REMINISCENCE THERAPY

Reminiscence is a normal activity of old age. It is normal for an older person to look back over his or her life and to review its ups and downs, perhaps dwelling especially on the good things and trying to put it all in perspective. For many people the sharing of memories can be stimulating and enjoyable. Reminiscence work can be considered as using two different concepts, recreational and therapeutic. Basically, the aims of reminiscence are to provide an opportunity for old people to relate meaningful aspects of their life to others and in so doing to help them re-establish a sense of personal identity. This also enables the older person to form links between the past and the present and hence make a more realistic appraisal of the current situation and improve orientation.

Both forms of reminiscence work require sensitivity, as one person's joy can be another's disappointment. Some individuals choose to keep their memories intact and do not use reminiscence positively, i.e. they have bad memories but they have no wish to come to terms with or forget them. Others

Box 24.8

Examples of common behaviours that can be dealt with using validation techniques

Patient-centre behaviour	recommended response
1. 'Nurse, someone's stolen my cardigan'.	Ask 'who', 'what', 'where', and when' type questions, not 'why'. Affirm the feelings of loss, as though everything has been stolen or taken from the patient. This behaviour is often a symbol for expressing such feelings of loss.
2. 'Take me home nurse. I want to go home'.	Ask such questions as: 'What do you miss about home?', 'What do you want to do at home?' and 'Does this place remind you at all of home?'.
3. 'The little ones are turning, learning' (typical of severe disorientaion).	Some good questions might be, 'You're thinking about your children and all the work and fun had as they grew up?' and 'Did you like being a father/ mother?'

may avoid looking back at any bad past memories and choose to wear rose-tinted glasses when reflecting on their past.

Recreational reminiscence can involve talking with one person or a small group of people about their past but with quite a lot of control staying with the older people themselves. It might involve listening to some old time music or looking at some old photographs or a film. Some external reminiscence aids can be useful for this kind of work and it is thought to be more beneficial to have some sensory stimulation attached to the verbal cues, to aid memory recall (Jacques, 1992).

Therapeutic reminiscence involves a different format, which is focused and structured more by the therapist. This form of therapy can be very powerful for the patients and it should be considered carefully before patients are encouraged. There are several indications where therapeutic reminiscence could be considered, particularly in relation to any abnormal grieving response that an individual may have. As many older people find it easier to recall long-term memories than recent events, this kind of work can be used with people who have some cognitive decline and can help to restore a sense of equilibrium for the individual. It has been used to reduce loneliness, bolster self-esteem, improve mood, increase cognitive functioning and enhance life satisfaction (Baker, 1985).

THE ENVIRONMENT OF CARE

The environment has a profound effect on the nature of the interactions and relationships within its boundaries. Assessment units that contain broken furniture and broken windows, with little in the way of homely comforts, have been shown to harbour increased violence and antisocial behaviour. Within elderly-care settings it is important to make the environment as homely as possible, with good lighting, and practical seats (not too low), arranged in small circles with private areas available for people who want to spend time on their own. Patients should be encouraged to bring in their own belongings, such as photographs and personal effects.

Music and television should be optional for the patients but not automatically switched on for no apparent reason. Daily newspapers available are useful to help orientate people and to discuss current affairs and items of interest, along with other pieces of reading material, perhaps from the hospital library. Large-print books and talking books are useful for people with visual impairments.

Organizing groups for patients can be stimulating, socializing and therapeutic. Community groups run within the ward can encourage patients to be involved in the decisions that are being made. Activity groups need a separate area to be run effectively and therapeutic groups should regulary utilize the same room, at the same time of day, to provide consistency.

The format of these groups depends on the needs of the patients and should be flexible enough for the focus to change accordingly. For example, an anxiety management group may be held over a month to meet the needs of the patient group arising at that particular time. Another group could be started

following this, looking at health promotion.

Noise in a hospital environment can be a constant irritant to patients. It is good practice to have an area considered 'quiet' and night nurses, particularly, should be aware of noises that could disturb patients. Night time can often be very difficult for patients who may not be able to sleep. However, it could be a useful opportunity for nurses to offer time for patients to talk about their troubles.

Mealtimes are an important part of the patient's day and can provide important insights into the mental health of a patient. It is important to make the dining area a pleasant place to eat and to try to make the food look as appetizing as possible. Having the menu written for the patients can help them in their choice of food.

COUNSELLING

Counselling is based on the idea that to talk about a problem is helpful, which is why counselling is sometimes referred to as a 'talking cure'. However, it is more than this. Counselling is based on the belief that all behaviour, however odd or irrational, has meaning. The meaning might be difficult to decipher but will usually be found to have something to do with the inner emotional life of the individual. Counselling seeks to discover this meaning.

There may be an assumption that counselling older people is essentially similar to counselling any other age group but even a cursory examination should suggest otherwise. Simple communication with the elderly is often not straightforward. Poor hearing, poor eyesight, general ill health and low morale through loneliness and grief all affect the older person's ability to respond to counselling interventions (Scrutton, 1989). The absence of a full and coherent developmental psychology of old age has not helped to dispel the ageist message. Sigmund Freud, himself wrote that:

> psychotherapy is not possible near or above the age of 50, the elasticity of the mental processes on which the treatment depends is as a rule lacking; old people are not educable

(Freud, 1905)

This may account for the obvious neglect of counselling facilities available for the older person. Still other factors have influenced the slow development of counselling techniques for the older person, such as the medicalization of old age, social policy and powerful myths and stereotypes that prevail, such as old people 'just want to sleep and be peaceful'.

Counselling agendas of the elderly broadly encompass these themes: the loss of significant people, the loss of the parental role, retirement, loss of financial status, declining physical abilities and poor health, loss of independence and the effect of attitudes on the experience of old age. This is not an exhaustive list and each individual will have a different agenda, depending on their personal experiences. However, these themes are of sufficient importance to contribute to emotional and social distress at some level in most older people. At the very least they can cause the individual to worry and if this worry is not adequately dealt with this in turn can lead to stress and then to physical and mental illness, to social disengagement and ultimately perhaps to stress-induced confusional states.

Counselling can be offered to older people in many different forms, through therapeutic and social reminiscence and during meaningful activities. It is not always an appropriate option to hold an isolated counselling session, which the older person may find strange and threatening. However, this does not mean that older people cannot benefit from skilful counselling. It is often the context in which it is provided that can determine the outcome.

Counselling the ill is more difficult than counselling the well, not least because of their reduced ability to think clearly, to make judgements, to arrive at sound decisions, to determine a course of action and generally to fight their own battles. In situations where the mental state of older counsellees is of major concern, for example in depression, extreme social loss or grieving and in excessive emotional stress, counselling can be a means of determining the origins of this mental state and helping individuals to face and come to terms with their feelings.

STANDARDS AND QUALITY OUTCOMES

Research over the last 30 years has consistently criticized elderly care environments as being of poor quality, lacking resources, having low staff levels and giving minimal activity or structure in the daily lives of those being cared for. Recent studies suggest that care may have become more rather than less rigid (Smith, 1986; Green, 1992). The emphasis has been on humane containment for a group of people waiting to die and therefore were not worth bothering with. Providing the quality of care was acceptable, the quality of life was seen as of little consequence (Age Concern, 1990; Green, 1992). A review of nursing research in the elderly and mental health suggests certain strategies that have a positive influence on mental health and well-being and are also conducive to a 'caring organization' (Roberts, 1990). The strategies cited include:
- Individual therapy.
- Control over choice.
- Reinforcement.
- Socialization.
- Movement and choice.

Subsequently, research to identify the indicators of good quality care has taken place (Gilloran *et al.*, 1993). The major concepts are:
- Autonomy.
- Maintaining individuality.
- Respecting dignity.
- Recognizing the need for privacy.
- Maintaining choice.
- Encouraging independence.

It has been noted that these are abstract concepts and that, to measure quality of care, indicators are needed. These might include, for example, whether patients are allowed to eat or go to the toilet at their own pace, to choose where they sit for a meal and to decide at what time to go to bed and get up in the morning, rather than have these aspects of their lives dictated by the needs of the ward regime.

Meaning and purpose in activities are two other indicators of quality that must be considered when caring for the elderly mentally ill patient group. Given the right circumstances older adults can improve aspects of their intellectual functioning, or, at least, maintain existing functions, through stimulating and challenging activities (Baltes and Willis, 1982; Lauder, 1993).

Several research studies have identified those factors found to have a positive influence on the mental health of the older person. These include movement, touch, reminiscence, cognitive therapy, group and individual therapy, empathetic communication, control over choice, reinforcement and socialization. Nursing research on mental health in the older person is still in the early stages; it is important to continue to validate nursing practice through research. The use of certain methods in therapeutic practice must be justified and alternatives must be explored where appropriate.

SUMMARY

Caring for older people with mental health problems is a complex, dynamic process. We are moving away from the image of nursing older people being a task oriented role.

Research and developments in care and treatment are paving the way towards a new image, requiring knowledgeable reflective practitioners. We will be old ourselves one day, and who knows who will be caring for us. Our care practice should be based on evidence that it is helpful and therapeutic; the more evidence based practice is in place, the less task orientated practice will be seen.

We are living longer and the issues of good quality health care in later life are here to stay. Nursing provides the perfect arena for identifying factors which can contribute to the well being of older people. We should pursue the quest for good quality care and always question our practice: remember, we will be old ourselves one day.

KEY CONCEPTS

- Older people need to be supported as valued members of society.This can be encouraged through the use of positive language and the promotion of meaningful activities.
- Every individual needs a comprehensive assessment to ensure that necessary care and treatment options are offered.
- Carers must be supported in their role and their views and opinions need to be valued and used for the benefit of their relatives.
- We must examine and reflect on the nursing care that we provide to this group of patients and change our practice accordingly.
- Personhood can increase with people who have a dementing illness, this should be capitalized upon.
- Meaningful activities are beneficial for older people with mental health problems.
- Counselling interventions in various forms should be offered as common practice in mental health settings.
- Physical health must be maintained and physical needs must be met to provide good psychiatric nursing care.
- Many mental health difficulties in older people can be fully resolved through skilful care and treatment.
- Caring for the elderly mentally ill population requires excellent psychiatric nursing technique with the ability to adapt and develop new practices to meet the needs of the patient group.

REFERENCES

Age Concern: *Left behind? Continuing care for elderly patients in NHS hospitals — a review of Health Advisory Service reports.* London, 1990, Age Concern.

Arber S, Ginn J: Women and ageing. *Rev Clin Gerontol* 4(5):349, 1994.

Baker NJ: Reminiscing in group therapy for self worth. *J Gerontol Nurs* 11(7):21, 1985.

Baltes PB, Willis S: *Enhancement of intellectual functioning in old age. Ageing and cognitive process.* New York, 1982, Plenum.

Barrowclough C, Fleming I: *Goal planning with elderly people.* Manchester, 1986, Manchester University Press.

Bleathman C, Morton I: Validation therapy with the demented elderly. *J Adv Nurs* 13(4):5–11, 1988.

Bond S, Reed J: Nurses assessment of elderly patients in hospital. *Int J Nurs Stud* 28(1): 55–64, 1991.

Brewin C: Measuring individual needs for care and services. In: Thornicroft G, Brewin CR, Wing JK, editors: *Measuring mental health needs.* London, 1992, Gaskel.

Brooker DJR *et al.*: The behavioural assessment scale of later life (BASOLL). A description, factor analysis, scale development, validity and reliability data for a new scale for older adults. *Int J Geriatr Psychiatry* 8: 747–754, 1993.

Brown RG, Marsden CD: How common is dementia in Parkinson's disease. *Lancet* (2):1262–1265, 1984.

Burr J, Andrews J: *Nursing the psychiatric patient.* London, 1981, Baillière Tindall.

Busse EW, Blazer DG, editors: *Handbook of geriatric psychiatry.* New York, 1989, Van Nostrand Reinhold.

Centre for Policy on Ageing: *Community life: A code of practice for community care.* London, 1990, Centre for Policy on Ageing.

Cogwill DO, Holmes LD: *Aging and modernization.* New York, 1972, Appleton Century Crofts.

Coleman PG: Measuring reminiscence characteristics from conversation as adaptive features of old age. *Int J Aging Hum Devel* 5(7):281, 1974.

Coleman PG, McCulloch AW: The study of psychosocial change in late life: some conceptual and methodological issues. In: Munnichs JMA, Mussen P, Olbrich E, Coleman PG, editors: *Lifespan and change in a gerontological perspective.* New York, 1985, Academic Press.

Cormack D: Psychogeriatric nursing in 2005. *Nurs Times* 82 (37):39–41, 1986.

Coyne AC, Reichman WE, Berbig LJ: The relationship between dementia and elder abuse. *Am J Psychiatry* 150(11): 643, 1993.

Crystal HA, Dickson DW, Lizardi JE, Davies P, Wolfson LI:Antemortem diagnosis of diffuse Lewy body disease. *Neurology* 40(6):1523–1528, 1990.

Cumming EH, Henry WE: *Growing old: The process of disengagement..* New York, 1961, Basic Books.

Department of Health: *Caring for people. Community care in the next decade and beyond.* London, 1990, HMSO.

Elias N: *The established and the outsiders.* London, 1994, Sage.

Erikson E: *Childhood and society.* New York, 1950, WW Norton.

Esmonde TFG: Creutzfeldt–Jakob disease and other degenerative causes of dementia. In: *Principles and practice of geriatric psychiatry.* Chichester, 1994, Wiley & Sons.

Feil N: *Validation: The Feil method.* Cleveland, 1982, Edward Feil Productions.

Fischer C, Oliker S: A research note on friendship, gender and the life cycle. *Soc Forces* 62(8):124, 1983.

Folstein MF, Folstein SE, McHugh PR: Mini mental state: a practical method for grading the cognitive state of patients for the clinician. *J Psychiatr Res* 12(9):189, 1975.

Freud S: *On psychotherapy.* London, 1905, Hogarth Press.

Gilleard CJ: *Living with dementia.* London, 1984, Croom Helm.

Gilloran A *et al.*: Measuring the quality of care in psychogeriatric wards. *J Adv Nurs* 18(5): 269, 1993.

Gorney JE: Experiencing and age: patterns of reminiscence among the elderly. University of Chicago, 1968, Dissertation.

Green S: Outcome measures for the elderly. *Int J Health Care Qual Assur* 5(4):17–22, 1992.

Hachinski VC, Lassen NA, Marshall J: Multi-infarct dementia. A cause of mental retardation in the elderly. *Lancet* 2(8):207–210, 1974.

Harding K, Baldwin S, Baser C: Towards multi-level needs assessment. *Behav Psychother* 15(6):134, 1987.

Homer A, Gilleard C: Abuse of elderly people by their carers. *BMJ* 301(14):1359, 1990.

Jacques A: *Understanding dementia.* London, 1992, Churchill Livingstone.

Jones G: Validation therapy: a companion to reality orientation. *Can Nurse* 81(3):20–23, 1985.

Kitwood T: The technical, the personal and the framing of dementia. *Soc Behav* 3(1):161, 1988.

Kitwood T, Bredin K: Towards a theory of dementia care: personhood and well being. *Ageing & Society* 12(4):269, 1992.

Kurrle SE, Sadler PM, Cameron ID: Patterns of elder abuse. *Med J Aust* 57(10):673, 1992.

Lauder W: Health promotion in the elderly. *BJN* 2(8):401–404, 1993.

Lewis MI, Butler RN: Life review therapy: Putting memories to work in individual and group psychotherapy. *Geriatrics*. 29(11):165–173, 1974.

Lowenstein R: Disturbances of sleep and cognitive functioning in patients with dementia. *J Neuro Ageing* 3:371–377, 1982.

Newman JP: Aging and depression. *Psychol Aging* 4(2):150, 1989.

Norman A: Triple jeopardy: growing old in a second homeland. Centre for Policy on Ageing. London, 1985, Dorset Press.

Office of Population Censuses and Surveys: *Population trends 74.* London, 1993, HMSO.

Ogg J, Bennett G: Elder abuse in Britain. *BMJ* 305:998, 1992.

Pattie AH: A survey of the Clifton assessment procedure for the elderly. *Br J Clin Psychol* 20(2):173, 1981.

Pattie AH, Gilleard CJ: *Manual of the Clifton assessment procedures for the elderly (CAPE).* Sevenoaks, 1979, Hodder & Stoughton Educational.

Roberts B: Nursing research in geriatric mental health. *J Adv Nurs* 15(9):1030–1035, 1990.

Scrutton S: *Counselling older people.* London, 1989, Edward Arnold.

Seyle, H: The stress of life. New York, 1956, McGraw–Hill.

Sheikh JI, Swales P: Prognosis of anxiety disorders. In: Copeland JRM, Abou–Saleh MT, Blazer DG editors: *Principles and practice of geriatric psychiatry.* Chichester, 1994, John Wiley and Sons Ltd.

Smith G: Resistance to change in geriatric care. *Int J Nurs Stud* 23(1):61–70, 1986.

Thomas D: *Under Milk Wood.* London, 1954, Dent.

Van Dujin CM, Hofman A, Kay DWK: Risk factors for Alzheimer's disease: A collaborative analysis of case control studies. *Int J Epidemiol* 1995 (in press).

Walker R, Waqar IU: Asian and Black elders and community care: a survey of care providers. *New Community* 20(4):635, 1994.

Wenger GC: The special role of friends and neighbours. *J Aging Stud* 4(2):149, 1990.

Wolfensberger W: Social role valorisation. A proposed new term for the principle of normalisation. *Ment Retard* 12(6):234, 1991.

Wright S: Tearing down walls — a nurse specialist in the care of the elderly. *Nurs Mirror* 161(2):48–49, 1985.

Zarit S, Orr NK, Zarit JM: *The hidden victims of Alzheimer's disease —families under stress.* New York, 1985, University Press.

FURTHER READING

Blakemore K, Boeham M: *Age, race and ethnicity.* Philadelphia,1994, Open University Press.
> *An interesting book, useful for reference purposes.*

Copeland J, Mohammed T, Abou–Saleh Blazer DG: *Principles and practice of geriatric psychiatry.* Chichester, 1994, John Wiley & Sons.
> *A useful reference book, covering a wide range of issues relating to the mental health of older people. Particularly useful in relation to cultural and ethnic variations, and also interprofessional working.*

Levy R, Howard R: *Developments in dementia and functional disorders in the elderly.* Petersfield, 1995, Wrightson Biomedical Publishing Ltd.
> *A neat volume presenting a comprehensive account of the recent advances and current controversies in the study and treatment of the dementias, memory impairment, depression and other functional disorders in the elderly.*

Scrutton S: Counselling older people. London, 1989, Edward Arnold.
> *An excellent book–comprehensive, with many case vignettes. Offers many approaches to a very complex problem. Also useful relating to other professionals and carers.*

Chapter 25

Care of the Survivor

<table>
<tr><td>

Learning Outcomes

After studying this chapter, you should be able to:

- Recognize and identify the clinical features of post-traumatic stress disorder.

- Compare and contrast two psychological models of traumatic sequelae.

- Understand the process of assessment of post-trauma reactions.

- Review critical incident stress debriefing.

- Describe the theoretical basis of behavioural and cognitive interventions and how they can be applied to the survivor of trauma.

- Critically analyse current research on effectiveness of behavioural and cognitive behavioural interventions.

</td></tr>
</table>

CHAPTER OUTLINE

- *Psychological reactions following traumatic incidents*

- *Prevalence of psychological disturbance following a traumatic incident*

- *Psychological models of post-traumatic stress*

- *Assessment of survivors of trauma*

- *The management of acute trauma: critical incident stress debriefing (CISD)*

- *Treatment of long-term reactions*

*T*he aim of this chapter is to introduce nurses to the psychological reactions that arise following traumatic incidents. The initial part describes the psychological sequelae of trauma, then identifies competing psychological models and looks in detail at the assessment process for individuals who have chronic reactions. Following this, interventions are described for the acutely traumatized and also cognitive–behavioural therapy for those with chronic or long-term difficulties. Case studies of clients who have received such therapy from the authors will be used to illustrate clinical points. Finally, the efficacy of these approaches is briefly discussed, with a note on supervision.

The authors recognize that many of the symptoms of post-traumatic stress described in this chapter are also experienced by adult survivors of child sexual abuse (CSA). However, there are so many additional complexities that it is believed child sexual abuse should be considered separately. While many of the therapy techniques described in this chapter are applicable to CSA, treating survivors of child sexual abuse requires a much more multimodal approach (Herman, 1995). Therefore, discussions have been confined to traumas in adulthood.

PSYCHOLOGICAL REACTIONS FOLLOWING TRAUMATIC INCIDENTS

Psychological difficulties following trauma have been noted in the literature for many years. Samuel Pepys, writing in his diaries in 1666, describes the emotional turmoil he felt following the Great Fire of London (Daly, 1983). Since this time a whole body of literature has emerged describing the features of post-trauma reactions following a wide range of traumatic events such as rape (Rothbaum *et al.*, 1992), physical assault (Richards and Rose, 1991), road traffic accidents (Muse, 1986), war (Kulka *et al.*, 1990), child sex abuse (Mcleer *et al.*, 1988) and major disasters (Green *et al.*, 1990). It is not only those actually involved in traumatic events but also those witnessing such events, for example police, fire and ambulance personnel and nurses, who may suffer from psychological distress (Hodgkinson and Stewart, 1991).

Post-traumatic reactions and mental health difficulties that can occur following a trauma can be seen as acute and chronic. One of the most prevalent chronic reactions is post-traumatic stress disorder (PTSD), which became a psychiatric diagnosis (DSM III) in 1980, mainly as a result of research into the effects of the Vietnam War on US veterans.

While involvement in or witnessing a traumatic event usually leads to psychological disturbance only for a few days, this may persist for months or years. There are many related feelings that may occur, for example, guilt, depression, shame, helplessness and hopelessness. It is not clearly established why some people develop long-term psychological difficulties following trauma and others do not. However, the more traumatic the event, the more likely an individual is to experience long-term psychological disturbance, the so-called dose response (Foy *et al.*, 1984). Further, in a number of studies social support and the personal meaning an individual gives to an event have been found to buffer the effects of the traumatic incident (Joseph *et al.*, 1992). PTSD is defined according to DSM IV (American Psychiatric Association, 1994) as in Box 25.1.

There is some evidence that PTSD does not always occur in isolation and many researchers have found coexisting mental health disorders, such as major depression, drug and alcohol misuse, obsessive–compulsive disorder, personality disorder, phobias and generalized anxiety disorder (Keane and Wolfe, 1990; Green, 1994).

PREVALENCE OF PSYCHOLOGICAL DISTURBANCE FOLLOWING A TRAUMATIC EVENT

The prevalence of PTSD has been investigated both in the general population and in specific 'at risk' groups. Studies that have investigated PTSD in the general population have found between a prevalence of 1% and 9% (Helzer *et al.*, 1987; Davidson *et al.*, 1991; Breslau *et al.*, 1990). Studies that have focused on particular at risk groups, however, have found much

higher rates of PTSD. For example Rothbaum *et al.* (1992) studied 95 rape survivors and found that 94% had most symptoms of PTSD 1 week after the assault, 64% 1 month later and 47% at 3 months post-assault. Orner (1993) studied soldiers who had served in the Falklands War and found that 60% of his sample were experiencing symptoms of PTSD. Kilpatrick and Resnick (1993) found that 35% of women had PTSD following an aggravated assault. These studies and other reviews of prevalence of PTSD (e.g. Davidson and Fairbank, 1993; Green, 1994) suggest that psychological disturbance following a traumatic incident is a major, current mental health problem.

PSYCHOLOGICAL MODELS OF POST-TRAUMATIC STRESS

A number of psychological models have been proposed in the literature to explain the development and maintenance of psychological sequelae of a traumatic incident.

BEHAVIOURAL MODEL

The behavioural conceptualizations of PTSD that have been proposed in the literature (Keane *et al.*, 1985) have relied heavily on Mowrer's (1947, 1960) two-factor learning theory. In essence, Mowrer's theory consists in classical and instrumental learning. Classical conditioning involves stimulus–stimulus learning, where a previously neutral stimulus occurs at the same time as an aversive one (called the unconditioned stimulus, UCS). The UCS always elicits an unconditioned response (UCR) and, following repeated pairings, the neutral stimulus then provokes the same response, becoming a conditioned stimulus (CS). The response is now termed a conditioned response (CR) and occurs in the absence of the original stimulus.

The second element in Mowrer's theory, instrumental conditioning, is where a being behaves in whatever way is necessary to avoid and escape from the aversive stimulus (UCS or CS). Thus, avoidance and escape are learnt behaviours, which are reinforced and maintained by arousal reduction.

Keane *et al.* (1985) argue that the above model can account for the acquisition and maintenance of psychological disturbance following a traumatic event. Thus, the individual exposed to a traumatic event (UCS) elicits increased physiological arousal and psychological distress (UCR). Previously neutral external environmental cues or reminders (sights, sounds, smells etc.) and internal stimuli (thoughts and feelings) that were present at the time of the trauma become conditioned stimuli (CS), which produce high levels of physiological arousal and psychological distress (CR). The individual tries to avoid and escape these cues, as a way of reducing arousal, but they in fact maintain the psychological disturbance in the long term.

Further, Keane *et al.*, (1985) posit that higher order conditioning and stimulus generalization can account for the wide range of stimuli that evoke arousal and distress in PTSD. Stimulus generalization proposes that similar responses can be elicited by neutral stimuli that resemble the original stimulus.

Box 25.1

Definition of involvement in a traumatic event

The person has been exposed to a traumatic event in which both of the following were present:

First, that the event or events involved actual or threatened death or serious injury, or a threat to the physical integrity of others;

Secondly, the person's response involved intense fear, helplessness, or horror.

(American Psychiatric Association, 1994)

Although the authors propose an adequate theoretical account, it is not without its critics (Foa *et al.*, 1989). The main difficulties with this model are that it fails to account for the wide range of symptoms, such as guilt or depression, that are so often present in individuals exposed to a traumatic event. Further, this model only accounts for abnormal, rather than normal, responses.

COGNITIVE AND INFORMATION PROCESSING MODELS

Cognitive and information processing models have been proposed to account for post-trauma reactions (Chemtob *et al.*, 1988; Krietler and Krietler, 1988; McCann *et al.*, 1988; Foa *et al.*, 1989; Creamer *et al.*, 1992; Janoff–Bulman, 1992). Essentially, these models argue that cognitive variables (e.g. expectations, assumptions, attributions, attitudes, beliefs etc.) play an important role in understanding survivors' post-trauma responses.

One of the most comprehensive models of psychological disturbance following a traumatic incident has been developed by Foa *et al.* (1989). Fundamentally, they argue that psychological disturbance occurs as a result of the individual's failure to process the traumatic event. They rely heavily on the work of Lang (1979) and suggest that fear is a cognitive structure, which has three principal elements:

1 Information about the feared situation.
2 Information about the person's verbal, physiological and behavioural responses.
3 Interpretive information about the meaning the stimuli has for the person and their responses.

Foa *et al.* (1989) argue that fear structures are differentiated from other cognitive structures by the element of threat. Further, they argue that PTSD is differentiated from other disorders because the trauma is of monumental significance and violates previously held views of safety. Thus situations and stimuli that were previously thought of as safe are considered dangerous. Importantly, Foa *et al.* incorporate uncontrollability and unpredictability into their model and suggest that the more unpredictable and uncontrollable a traumatic event, the more likely it is that PTSD will develop.

Foa and Kosak (1986) argue that two conditions are necessary to change this fear structure and hence produce fear reduction:

First, fear-relevant information must be made available in a manner that will activate the fear memory.... Next, information made available must include elements that are incompatible with some of those that exist in the fear structure, so that a new memory can be formed. This new information, which is at once cognitive and affective, has to be integrated into the evoked information structure for an emotional change to occur.

Therefore the authors propose that cognitive–behavioural interventions are the treatment of choice for PTSD, in that behavioural interventions are aimed at activating the fear structure and cognitive interventions at modifying the meaning elements (Rothbaum and Foa, 1992).

A more cognitive model has been proposed by Janoff–Bulman (1985, 1992), who argues that psychological disturbance following a trauma is accounted for by the 'shattering' of an individual's core assumptions or cognitive schema. Cognitive schema is defined as 'a mental construct that represents organized knowledge about a given concept or type of stimulus' (1992). She highlights three core or fundamental assumptions, which are shared by most people, that are particularly affected following a traumatic incident. These are:

1 The world as benevolent.
2 The world as meaningful.
3 The self as worthy.

In terms of the world as benevolent, Janoff–Bulman argues that most people perceive the world as a good and safe place. Further, she argues that people believe the world to be meaningful and comprehensible. Drawing on Lerner's (1970, 1980) 'just world hypothesis' i.e. people get what they deserve, she contends that people perceive that they have control over negative events and states. 'A meaningful world is one in which a self-outcome contingency is perceived; there is a relationship between a person and what happens to him or her' (1992).

The third assumption, that the self is worthy, is related to the view that people evaluate themselves in positive light, i.e. we think of ourselves as good, worthy, benevolent and moral beings. From these core assumptions comes a sense of invulnerability. While people are aware that negative events can and do happen, they underestimate the likelihood of these events occurring to themselves. Janoff–Bulman (1992) cites considerable evidence that these positively biased assumptions are generally shared by most individuals and, while they are illusory, they are adaptive and beneficial for good mental health.

The argument that these core assumptions are 'shattered' by a traumatic experience and account for the psychological disequilibrium that follows, is put succinctly by Janoff–Bulman (1992) as:

The essence of trauma is the abrupt disintegration of one's inner world. Overwhelming life experiences split open the interior world of victims and shatter their most fundamental assumptions. Survivors experience 'cornered horror' for internal and external worlds are suddenly unfamiliar and threatening. Their basic trust in their world is ruptured. Rather than feel safe, they feel intensely vulnerable.

Cognitive and information processing models suggest that interventions aimed at modifying or re-evaluating assumptions about the self, the world and the traumatic event are likely to ameliorate many of the more distressing PTSD symptoms.

PSYCHODYNAMIC MODEL

The most influential psychodynamic model is proposed by Horowitz (1986). The basis of this model is that the individual has a number of schemata or cognitive maps of the self and world, established by experience. These schemata allow the individual to process information in an automatic and unconscious manner. In the event of traumatic experience, the information is at odds with the existing schema (e.g. the loss of a loved one is clearly at odds with schemata of self and world in which the loved one plays an important role). Horowitz's model establishes that the individual's cognitive processes are thereafter engaged in trying to assimilate this 'aberrant' or contrary information into previously stable schemata. Horowitz contends that, to assimilate this information, trauma creates two opposing sets of internal processes, 'intrusion' and 'denial'. Thus the individual oscillates between these two states, i.e. thinking about the trauma and avoiding thinking about it, determined by the individual's distress or failure to incorporate the trauma into the psyche. Here denial is seen as a defence against intrusion.

Further, Horowitz argues that denial manifests itself in terms of emotional numbness and avoidance of thoughts, activities and stimuli that resemble the trauma. Intrusion manifests itself through re-experiencing phenomena (intrusive thoughts, nightmares etc.). This process of intrusion and denial is seen as 'working through' the trauma and eventually results in the individual incorporating this new information into their cognitive schemata. Horowitz argues that when old and new information are matched and revised this is known as the 'completion tendency' and states that at this point 'Inner models or schemata are congruent with the new information about the self and world, and with the actual external situation to the extent that it is represented accurately in that new information' (Horowitz, 1986).

Horowitz's model contends that the above process is a normal and predictable stress response syndrome that occurs after a serious life event and that psychopathology only occurs if this process is 'prolonged', 'blocked' or exceeds tolerable intensity (Horowitz and Kaltreider, 1980). Psychodynamic interventions, therefore, concentrate on enabling the individual to integrate the new information in terms of their pre-existing beliefs.

ASSESSMENT OF SURVIVORS OF TRAUMA

When interviewing a survivor of a traumatic experience, many challenges are faced. These include obtaining an accurate picture of the presenting difficulties, forging an initial therapeutic alliance with the client and developing an agreed, effective treatment strategy.

THE PROCESS OF ASSESSMENT

The interpersonal qualities necessary for effective assessment include good interviewing skills, which do not necessarily come naturally. Anybody can ask questions. However, interviewing is not just about questions. It is a process that allows a client to express their needs fully while giving an accurate picture of the problems they face. A good interviewer will not only finish an interview having achieved both these aims but will also have a client who is confident about the therapeutic partnership.

INFLUENCE

In any interview there is a power differential between the therapist and the client. The therapist is the expert and the provider. The client is the 'sick' person seeking help. However distasteful this analysis might seem, it is inevitable that clients will be influenced by their own expectations of the therapists, the interview and the roles they perceive for the therapists and themselves. Factors such as gender and race have a similar 'inevitable influence' on the interview. Therapists can try to understand these but they are difficult to control.

Other influences are more easily dealt with. Principal among these are the therapist's expectations of the client. Three beliefs are most important:

1. The client is trying to cope, even if their behaviours appear highly dysfunctional or bizarre.
2. The client is responsive and will work with the therapist in a therapeutic alliance.
3. The client is honest and their account is an accurate picture of how things are for them.

A client will usually try to live up to what they think the therapist expects of them, so if these suppositions are expressed by the therapist both explicitly and implicitly this will start to encourage the trust and confidence necessary for mutual cooperation.

INTERVIEWING – GENERAL SKILLS

An interview has a beginning, a middle and an end. In the beginning the therapist should say what is going to be done. This is then done and recapitulated at the end of the session.

Planning

Before starting, consider what is known about the client, the interview goals and where the interview is going to take place to make the process comfortable and effective.

Introduction and Orientation

Introductions should be clear and practised. A good introduction includes the name of both therapist and client, the role of the therapist and the purpose of the interview. An excellent introduction also includes the intended duration of the interview.

Interpersonal Skills

Much has been written about the correct interpersonal behaviours (e.g. eye contact, non-verbal language) in interviews and it is not the intention here to provide an exhaustive text on the subject. However, there are a number of important points to note. Handling high levels of emotion (almost always present in interviews with trauma survivors) requires considerable empathy and understanding. This is a key skill. Without retreating from a client's expressions of emotion and while learning to empathize and not restrict the client's emotional release, make sure the interview moves on towards its goal. Displaying attention verbally and non-verbally is also important but do not neglect note-taking. Eye contact must be broken in order to write, since all the information given cannot possibly be retained without taking notes. Non-intrusive note-taking is a skill that should be practised often. Also, demonstrate that close attention is being paid to the client by frequently recapitulating information gathered. Feeding this back to the client gathers more information and shows them that there is a definite commitment to getting an accurate picture of their problems.

Information Gathering

To gather assessment information we must ask questions. The golden rules when asking questions are:
• Clarity.
• Single, not multiple questions.
• No leading questions.

In other words, ask clear questions, one at a time, without giving the answer away with the question.

Endeavour to enable clients to talk about their own problems from their own point of view. To do this, use a questioning funnel (Figure 25.1), containing both open and closed questions.

Start off with a general open question, for example, 'Could you tell me what your main problems are?' Once a client has described one or more areas of difficulty, for example 'flashbacks and nightmares', respond with a specific open question, such as, 'Can you tell me a bit more about the flashbacks?' Then move into more specific or closed questions, such as, 'How often do they occur?' or, 'How long do they last?'.

At each stage, funnel information on relevant topics provided by the client towards answers that enable the formulation of accurate problem descriptions. Seek frequent clarifications by reflecting back and checking information with the client.

In this way an interview is conducted, not an interrogation. The aim is for a free flow of information to be provided by the client on topics they consider to be important. However, they will have to be directed to areas that may also need to be assessed but this comes later and should always be by the use of open questions, moving down to closed questions only when there is a need to confirm detail.

The Ending

The ending is as essential a part of the interview as any other. People remember best what is said first and last, so endings can leave a lasting impression. Three things must be done:
1 Summarize the key points of the interview.
2 Organize the next steps and ensure that they are agreed and clearly understood.
3 Close the interview on time.

Endings provide the opportunity to reinforce the therapeutic relationship that is hoped will result in a successful therapy outcome for the client. Both client and therapist must leave the interview with a shared agreement of what went on in it and, most importantly, what is going to happen in the future.

THE CONTENT OF THE ASSESSMENT

The Event

Many people coming for an assessment interview will expect that the therapist will want them to talk about the initiating trauma. Indeed, many people have a great urgency to do so. However, as many, if not more, people are reluctant to discuss events in depth, for fear of the emotional reaction they will feel. Sometimes they fear their story will be too disturbing for the therapist to tolerate.

A dilemma the therapist has, therefore is whether to concentrate on the person's reactions to the trauma (which will usually be the main reason for their seeking help) or to focus on the event itself. The authors' view is that post-trauma reactions are the most important facts to gather. Focusing too much on the event too soon is potentially destructive for therapy. Therapy will usually involve a gradual confrontation with the traumatic memories. To start this process too early could sensitize the client and destroy any subsequent attempts at effective therapy.

However, one clearly cannot ignore the event. Clients would have very little confidence in the therapist if he or she paid no attention whatsoever to the trauma itself. A careful balance must be struck, therefore, between the 'here and now' and the past memory. One way to do this is to acknowledge at the beginning of the interview that talking about the trauma will be painful for the client and to make it clear that it is not necessary at this stage to get a very detailed account of the

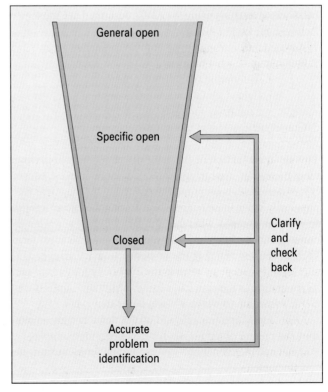

Figure 25.1 The question funnel

traumatic event. Although the therapist must communicate the fact that the event is of central importance and will be addressed as a fundamental part of treatment, for assessment purposes the emphasis is firmly on the impact of the trauma on the client's life.

The Impact

Using the process of question funnelling described earlier, determine the major impact of the trauma on a person's well-being. Start with the four Ws:

1 What is the problem?
2 Where does it happen?
3 When does it happen?
4 With whom is it better or worse?

The client is given the opportunity to specify his or her main difficulties. Therefore the four Ws are used to move down the question funnel to get more detail. For example, the main problem may be identified as 'phobic avoidance'. It is necessary to know where and when this occurs and if the presence of other people makes it better or worse.

Next, elicit more detail by asking about:

1 The frequency of the problem (how often).
2 The intensity of the problem (how bad, for example use a simple 0–8 scale).
3 The duration of the problem (how long-lasting).

Here, information is being gathered on how often the client avoids situations or objects, how fearful they are and how long their fear lasts.

Once this much detail has been gleaned, conduct a detailed behavioural analysis using the ABCs described in Chapter 29, Behavioural Psychotherapy.

1 Antecedents — triggers, precursors, situations etc.
2 Behaviour — what happens:
   • Autonomic (the physical reaction).
   • Behaviour (what a person does).
   • Cognitive (thoughts and images).
3 Consequences — the results of the above.

This detailed section of the assessment consists in giving a clear picture of what triggers the avoidance (places, people, behaviours, television programmes etc.), what the client feels physically when these triggers occur, what they do as a result, (e.g. avoid, escape), what they think or imagine and what the consequences of this are. Consequences can be short term, such as feeling relief if the response to a TV trigger is to successfully escape by turning the TV off, or long term, such as frustration at the restrictions such a strategy imposes on a client's freedom to watch TV whenever they want.

Other useful questions expand on this detail and give a more rounded picture of the impact for the client; for example:

• Onset and maintenance — when did the problem start; has it fluctuated?
• Modifying factors — what makes it better?
• Handicap to life — what impact does the problem have on the client's activities of daily living?
• Why is help being sought now — what has prompted the client to seek help now?
• What does the client want — how would the client be able to know that the problem was improving; what do they really want to change?
• Past treatment — what has or has not helped in the past?
• Drugs, alcohol and caffeine — what is the current intake of these substances and how are they affecting the client's health?

Mental State

It is always essential to be able to assess a client's mental state. The most common psychological problem likely to be seen alongside PTSD is depression. Moderate levels of depression seem to respond well to therapy aimed at PTSD but severe depression may require adjunctive treatment such as anti-depressants. Checks to assess suicidal ideas and intent, which must always be asked about and responded to if present, are particularly important.

Specific Symptoms of PTSD

PTSD has three major groups of symptoms, intrusions, avoidance and hyperarousal (see Box 25.2). The therapist needs to be aware of these in the assessment so that if the client is not forthcoming in any of these areas, he or she can be monitored. An open question is still used to begin with and questioning should be tied in to aspects of the client's previous account (the three areas of PTSD are usually closely associated). However, if flashbacks, for example, have not been mentioned, they must be asked about; if poor concentration and irritability have not been referred to, these should be checked again before closing the interview, to see if these areas constitute a problem.

> ### Box 25.2 Clinical features of post-traumatic stress disorder
>
> **Re-experiencing symptoms**
>
> e.g.   intrusive thoughts and images
>   nightmares
>   flashbacks
>
> **Avoidant and dissociative symptoms**
>
> e.g.   avoidance of thinking about the trauma
>   phobic avoidance
>   detachment from others
>
> **Hyperarousal symptoms**
>
> e.g.   sleep disturbance
>   hypervigilance
>   irritability

Summarizing Assessment

This problem-focused approach to assessment will enable the gathering of accurate information on how the client views their own problems. The client's account must always be viewed as primary. However, within the assessment it must be remembered that PTSD symptoms are complex, so all potential problem areas should be examined.

MEASUREMENT

The process of empirically validating therapy, which is central to the philosophy of cognitive–behavioural therapy, requires practitioners to use clinical measurement as part of their routine clinical practice. Health before and after therapy should be assessed to show how effective the therapist is being, to give clients feedback on their progress and to develop a body of knowledge that will help the therapist and others deliver the most effective help to those that need it.

There are many scales available. It is suggested that three parameters require measurement:

1 Specific client-centred problems, for example:
   'Flashbacks, occurring three times a day causing me to feel physically anxious and leading me to lose concentration and to distract myself by thinking of other things'. These can be measured by asking the client to rate the severity of the identified problem on a simple 0–8 scale as used in the Exposure Therapy case study .

2 Measures of handicap.
   These measure the impact of a client's problem within key domains of their life. Commonly these domains are work, home life, social leisure, private leisure and personal relationships (Marks, 1986).

3 Measures of specific symptoms and general health.
   A number of 'off the shelf' questionnaires are available, which allow the comparison of clients with others. Some measures have cut-off points, above which clients are regarded as having clinically significant problems. The most common measures are the Impact of Events Scale (IES) (Horowitz *et al.*, 1979) where a score greater than 26 is considered clinically significant and the General Health Questionnaire 28, GHQ-28 (Goldberg and Williams, 1988) where a score of 4 or more is significant. Other measures include the Post-traumatic Symptom Scale, PSS (Foa *et al.*, 1993) and the PTSD subscale of the SCL-90 (Saunders *et al.*, 1990).

It is appropriate to ask a client to fill in a range of symptom-specific and general health questionnaires after the assessment interview and then regularly throughout the therapy programme. Usually, one intermediate measurement point mid-therapy is sufficient, followed by measures at the termination of active therapy and at regular follow-up points. Measures should be discussed with the client and compared and contrasted with previous scores.

THE MANAGEMENT OF ACUTE TRAUMA: CRITICAL INCIDENT STRESS DEBRIEFING

Critical incident stress debriefing (CISD) is essentially the provision of an opportunity for acutely traumatized individuals to vent their feelings and thoughts about the incident, while receiving advice and guidance on the symptoms they are experiencing and how to get help for them. Developed by, among others, Mitchell (1983) and Dyregrov (1989) it has become the standard initial response to trauma and most disaster plans provide for CISD after a major incident. Most debriefings are group events but it is possible to use the same techniques with individuals, in cases where the traumatic event has only involved one person. Mitchell's original debriefing model has seven stages (Box 25.3).

As the above shows, there is a considerable overlap between phases. When involved in a debriefing it is well nigh impossible to separate the individual phases as neatly as outlined by Mitchell. Clients move from facts to feelings and reactions and then back again continually through the debrief. The authors have found a simpler model, developed by Letts and Tait (1995) of London's Metropolitan Police, to be nearer to the reality of a debrief. After the introduction, this has merely three further stages: facts, feelings and future.

Box 25.3 ***Mitchell's debriefing model***

1. Introduction
The purpose of the debriefing, the roles of debriefers, the rules of the group.

2. Facts
Clients participating on a group basis are encouraged to outline to each other what actually happened during the traumatic incident.

3. Thoughts
The clients' thoughts during an incident, the meaning these thoughts gave to their experience.

4. Reactions
The feelings experienced by clients are explored in this section, for example, fear, helplessness, loneliness etc. and the decisions they took in the incident.

5. Symptoms
Physical and emotional symptoms at the time of the incident and afterwards.

6. Teaching
'Normalizing' clients' reactions, preparations on what to expect in the future.

7. Re-entry
Summarizing the debriefing and arrangements made for further contact with the debriefer or other helpers.

THE INTRODUCTION

Participating clients will probably have had no previous experience of a critical incident stress debriefing so it is essential to make an early impression in the introduction. The debriefers must establish their own backgrounds, their relevant expertise and the ground rules for the debriefing. A debrief is not a counselling session. Explicit aims and rules should be stated.

Aims

1 Obtain or put together a clear factual understanding of the events.
2 Discuss impressions, reactions and feelings.
3 Decrease individual and group tensions.
4 Receive information on current and future reactions.
5 Know how to access further help.

Rules

1 No one is forced to speak.
2 The debrief is confidential.
3 No one is on trial.
4 People may feel temporarily worse — 'the cost of recovery'.
5 No breaks during the meeting (all toilet breaks pre-meeting).
6 The meeting belongs to the clients, not the debriefers. Participating clients will get out of it only what they put in.

FACTS

CISD is not an operational debrief. However, without the facts of an incident clients cannot properly understand their reactions. The best way to open up a debrief is to step back after the introduction and hand the meeting over to the group to say what actually happened. In a group of people, despite them having experienced the same event, no two people will have the same memory of what happened. The facts stage is the time during which to get the whole picture. Everyone should be involved in putting this together, wherever and however they were involved.

Facts include the clients' own sensations (sights, sounds, smells etc.) and most importantly what they did in response to these sensory inputs. Their thoughts about the incident as it is unravelled are of greatest importance. Most people who have experienced an accident or other traumatic event describe time as 'standing still'. This is because, when we think we might be under threat, the brain focuses all its attention on the potential threat. A vast amount of cognitive activity goes on in a small amount of time, leaving survivors with an impression of an event lasting many times longer than it really did. In a debrief, getting survivors to talk about what they were thinking at the time of the incident is extremely important because of this large amount of mental activity. Another reason thoughts are important is because the meaning an event had will be very significant in helping process the experience emotionally.

FEELINGS

Very often facts can seem safe but feelings appear more challenging. However, it is the feelings (guilt, fear, helplessness etc.) that need to be explored if the debriefing is to achieve its aims. This is the stage where clients can really get a sense of shared experience. The isolation of people who are afraid to admit their feelings can be broken down by a skilled debriefer facilitating mutual sharing and comparing of emotional experiences. During this stage in a debrief, an individual client discovers that there are many similarities between how he or she and others are feeling.

Mobilizing group support is important to give succour to those clients who may be distressed. It is always better to try to assist the group to comfort a fellow member, than for the debriefer to do it themselves.

This process of getting members to support each other is an especially important one for groups of people who work together. If people see how their colleagues are feeling, they will have a better understanding of a workmate's needs in the days and weeks after a debrief. The debrief works on team building.

FUTURE

In many debriefs, once the scene has been set and the natural initial reluctance to speak overcome, the debriefer can settle back to a watchful attitude, only intervening to clarify, reflect or gently push the discussion in a particular direction. However, the third stage, Future, is much more active. It is the debriefer's role here to summarize what the clients have said and use this information to describe what they might expect in the future. A debriefer must demystify the emotional, physical and behavioural reactions to a traumatic event, normalizing them. Without making cast-iron predictions about the future, the debriefer should inform participants what reactions, recovery and readjustment to expect.

Clients' attention is directed towards good practice in recovery. Identifying appropriate sources of social support is a crucial exercise as is cautioning against dysfunctional avoidance. The debriefer can outline simple principles, such as encouraging people to organize a gradual return to normal duties so that they may gradually overcome fears of returning to a workplace where there has been a traumatic incident.

Finally, the debriefer should ensure that the clients are aware of what professional support services are available to them after the debrief. Some people may request individual counselling for further ventilating of their anxieties and this should always be available.

KEY DEBRIEFING SKILLS AND COMPETENCIES

A summary of the key skills the authors believe are necessary for effective debriefing is given in Box 25.4. Most of them are about managing a group of people to facilitate the best exchange of information so that, for example, no one person dominates, the debriefer achieves the best balance between direction and free flow and the aims of the debrief are met.

FOLLOW-UP

In the authors' view CISD interventions are incomplete without structured follow-up. Research has indicated that by 1 month after an incident the greater part of natural recovery has taken place. In Rothbaum *et al.* (1992), the follow-up of rape survivors showed that if they had not recovered by 1 month, survivors were likely to have persistent symptoms of PTSD for many months, possibly years.

Follow-up is best done by individual assessments of need, based on a discussion with the survivor about the pattern of their current symptoms compared to those arising immediately after the incident. If there is any indication of PTSD, a structured assessment can be carried out as outlined earlier.

Clearly, if the acute symptoms persist 1 month after a traumatic incident and a picture of traumatic intrusions, avoidance and hyperarousal has established itself, survivors should be offered therapy for PTSD, as outlined below.

TREATMENT OF LONG-TERM REACTIONS

While the above is a useful intervention, up to 25% of individuals may go on to develop more chronic or long-term problems. As stated above, if symptoms continue for more than 1 month post-trauma, it is likely that therapy will be required.

The theoretical models described earlier have been used as a basis for treatment interventions. The psychodynamic approaches have been used in the treatment of PTSD (Bustos, 1992), However, there is a paucity of controlled research demonstrating its efficacy (Fairbank and Nicholson, 1987). Although our discussion of treatment is limited to behavioural and cognitive interventions, many psychodynamic approaches emphasize the use of imagery. In reviewing behavioural, psychodynamic and biological treatment approaches, Fairbank and Nicholson state 'direct therapeutic exposure to the memories of trauma emerged as the treatment technique common to all three theoretical models'. The approaches with the most empirical evidence of efficacy are behavioural and

cognitive (Solomon *et al.*, 1992). The fundamentals of behaviour therapy are detailed in Chapter 29; this chapter will focus on how these and other techniques can be applied to the individual who has psychological difficulties following a traumatic incident.

The development of behavioural and cognitive–behavioural interventions for PTSD has been based on the following key principles (Hackman, 1993):
1 The empirical validation of treatment.
2 A treatment focused on the 'here and now'.
3 The use of explicit, agreed and operationally defined treatment strategies.
4 The specification of treatment goals (usually chosen by the patient) to bring about desired life change.
5 The use of collaborative therapeutic strategies between patient and therapist.

The following section provides the practising clinician with current, available evidence of behavioural and cognitive–behavioural interventions in the treatment of post-traumatic stress disorder. After the assessment and before any therapy is considered, a clear treatment rationale is essential. The following rationale is the one the authors use.

CLIENT AND NURSE IN PARTNERSHIP – THE RATIONALE

It is extremely important that an active and collaborative treatment programme based on cognitive or behavioural principles is preceded by a clear and understandable rationale. Clients will only engage in therapeutic exercises if they understand fully the principles of the approach. As well as being a fundamental ethical principle, therefore, informed consent is a crucial criterion for clinical success.

The best rationales are progressive, in that they build up a complex model gradually by presenting elements of the rationale, one at a time. The rationale for cognitive behavioural therapy of PTSD is based on a visual representation of the emotional processing model (Figure 25.2). Here, the mind is depicted as a factory.

Stage 1
Initially, draw a basic outline of a factory, as a model for the mind. The client is prompted to suggest what a factory does (processes raw material) and then to identify the mind's raw material i.e. the sensory inputs from eyes, ears etc.

Stage 2
Together, agree that machinery in factories usually takes this raw material from one side to another, processing it along the way. This machinery is depicted as a conveyor belt on the diagram. The processed inputs are stored in memory, represented as a cupboard at the end of the conveyor belt. The process of getting from one end of the belt to the other is referred to in the rationale with the client as thinking.

Box 25.4 *Debriefing: key skills and competencies*

Clear giving of introductions.
Mixing facilitation and direction.
Information-seeking by reflection.
Drawing in reluctant participants using others in the group.
Ability to tolerate and allow free flow of expressed emotion.
Comparison of commonalities and discussion of differences.
Using the group to direct support to others.
Meeting the needs of all, not just the voluble.
Summarizing effectively.
Explaining anxiety and emotional processing clearly.

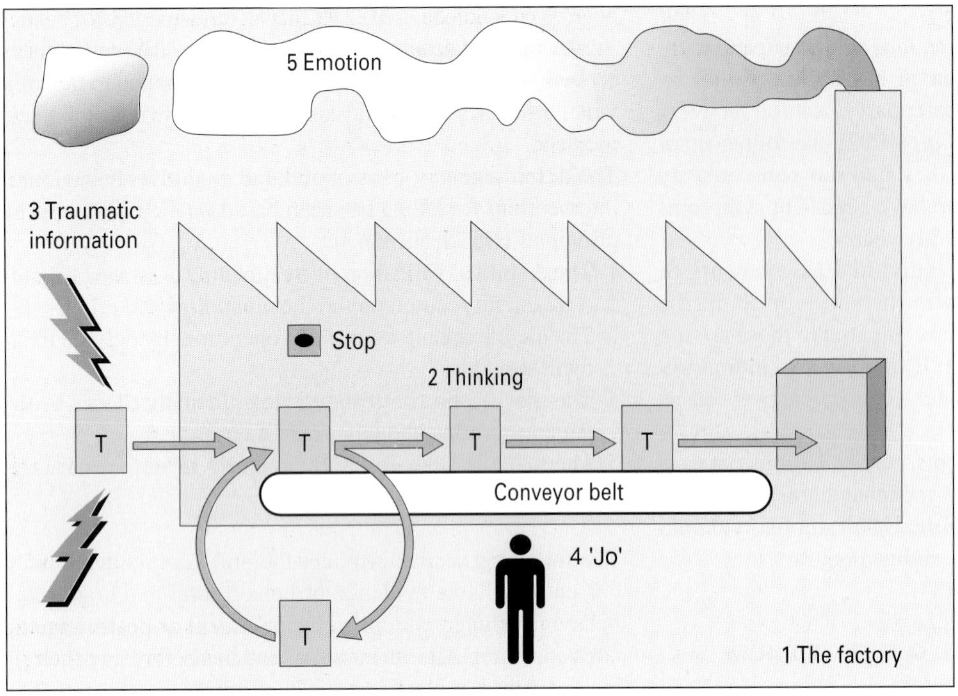

Figure 25.2 The rationale

Stage 3

Now, take the client through what happens when a traumatic incident occurs and when the mind receives a huge input of disturbing sensory 'raw material'. This can be represented as a large box at the beginning of the conveyor belt. The client is asked what they would do with this information. Most clients with PTSD immediately identify with a desire to stop the conveyor belt and halt the processing. This can be depicted as the emergency stop button, present in every factory. At this stage the traumatic information topples off the conveyor belt and is outside the processing environment.

Stage 4

Using examples from the client's own history, it can be shown how triggers and reminders re-activate the process, causing flashbacks and intrusions. These latter are represented on the diagram by Jo, a factory operative, placing the traumatic material back on the conveyor belt. Now the client is prompted for their usual response when experiencing intrusions (escape, avoidance, distraction etc.), pressing the stop button once again resulting in the vicious circle of intrusion and avoidance characteristic of PTSD. When the client is able to identify this pattern as their current coping response to traumatic memories, move on to Stage 5. It is, however, extremely important at this key stage that an empathic and understanding approach with the client is demonstrated and that this current strategy is not derided. Avoidance is an appropriate attempt to cope with short-term distress; unfortunately, it gives no long-term relief.

Stage 5

Now, ask the client what the alternative would be. The aim is to help the client understand the costs and benefits of thinking about the traumatic incident. The costs are the emotions

and distress, which are pollutant by-products of thinking about the incident, illustrated as smoke issuing from the factory chimney. The benefits are in breaking the vicious circle, reducing flashbacks and getting the processed memory into storage.

Stage 6

At this stage in the rationale, explain the therapy or therapies felt to be appropriate. Where exposure is being suggested the rationale would be that avoidance is useful in the short term but not the long term; that the best way to break the vicious circle is by confrontation with the thing that frightens us, and this is called 'exposure'. Exposure should be graded, prolonged, repeated and done as homework so that anxiety decreases, called 'habituation'.

A graph of approach–avoidance anxiety peaks (expressed as subjective units of distress, SUDS) with the habituation curve superimposed is used to explain the decline in anxiety over time produced by prolonged exposure (Figure 25.3).

EXPOSURE THERAPY

Behavioural–cognitive interventions nearly always include an element of exposure therapy. Fundamentally, exposure therapy is a therapeutic intervention that is used where anxiety is maintained by avoidance behaviour. As was outlined in the rationale, one of the hallmark symptoms following a trauma is fear and avoidance. The individual feels anxious when thinking about or confronted by reminders of the trauma, hence, to relieve this anxiety or distress, the individual avoids these cues, or avoids thoughts or feelings of the trauma. Avoidance brings about short-term relief but long-term maintenance of the problem. (For more detailed discussion see Chapter 29, Behavioural Psychotherapy). To break this cycle the client is asked to confront rather than avoid these thoughts, feelings, and stimuli until anxiety subsides, a process called habituation. Exposure, therefore, is the therapeutic confrontation of feared stimuli until anxiety subsides.

The two principal methods of exposure are:

1 Imaginal exposure.
2 Live exposure.

For an effective outcome, most clients require both forms of exposure.

Imaginal Exposure

Imaginal exposure involves repeatedly confronting the memories of the traumatic incident until the client's level of distress or fear is reduced. The client is asked to 'relive' their trauma in the presence of a therapist. The client recounts the entirety of the trauma in the first person, in the present tense and in as much detail as possible. To obtain this detail, the client is asked to describe in full the stimulus elements (what they saw, what they smelt, what they heard, what they tasted, etc.), the response elements (i.e. thoughts, feelings and behaviours) and the meaning element (what the trauma meant to them, e.g. 'I thought I was about to die'). The session is recorded and the client is instructed to listen to the tape daily for 1 hour between sessions.

Clearly it is distressing to the individual, but, so that the event is 'emotionally processed', the client is gently encouraged by the therapist to continue. When distress has decreased to a level of at least 50% (this usually takes between one and three sessions) subsequent sessions are focused on a technique called 'rewind and hold' (Richards and Rose, 1991). This involves identifying, between the client and the therapist, critical parts of the trauma that continue to evoke high levels of distress. Crucial parts of the trauma may include elements such as an image (e.g. the face of a rapist), a thought (the belief that they were about to die) and a series of scenes including images, thoughts and feelings. Thus the client is instructed to go through the scene and then rewind to the critical point and expand on this aspect, again describing it in detail. The client is then asked to hold the image until anxiety or distress decreases. Again, the session is recorded and the client is asked to listen to the tape daily, between sessions.

Although the duration is variable, imaginal exposure takes approximately five weekly sessions. A treatment session takes about 90 minutes to complete, 60 of which should be devoted to imaginal exposure and the remainder to reviewing, feedback and setting homework. Imaginal exposure is a relatively simple technique but requires a high level of expertise from the therapist to build a trusting rapport and to manage the session effectively. Clients are often highly distressed and a clear rationale is essential, as is an empathic approach. In summary the principles of imaginal exposure are as follows:

1 First person, present tense.
2 Detailed.
3 Stimuli (i.e. what they saw, heard, smelt etc.).
4 Response (how they felt, thought and acted).
5 Meaning elements (what the incident meant to that individual).
6 Sessions recorded for repeated homework.
7 Prolonged (sessions of at least 45–60 minutes duration).

Following imaginal exposure, avoidances of situations and objects may remain unchanged, and hence live exposure is used to reduce problems in this area.

Live Exposure

Live exposure involves the confrontation of feared or avoided situations, or objects, that are impairing the individual's life. For example, a survivor who has been physically assaulted in the street may avoid going out alone; the survivor of a transport disaster may avoid entering places where escape is difficult; a survivor of a road traffic accident may avoid driving. In live exposure, one of the first tasks is for the therapist and the client to determine a hierarchy of feared and avoided situations, starting with the least anxiety-provoking, confronting it until anxiety-reduction occurs and then moving on to the next one, until the client reaches the top of the hierarchy. In a similar vein to imaginal exposure, live exposure needs to be prolonged, in that the client needs to stay in the situation for an hour. Furthermore, it needs to be repeated, i.e. clients need to practise their tasks for at least 1 hour daily. In summary, the main principles of live exposure are as follows:

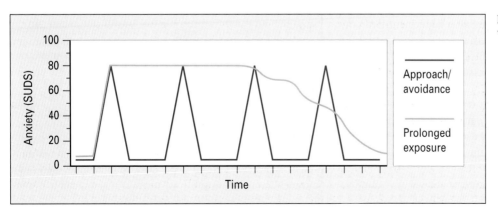

Figure 25.3 Approach/avoidance versus prolonged exposure

- Graded.
- Repeated.
- Prolonged.
- Practised regularly (daily) as homework.

COGNITIVE INTERVENTIONS

Cognitive models of trauma reactions (detailed earlier) emphasize the importance of the role the cognitive process may have in an individual's response to a traumatic event. Further, these models focus on how the development and maintenance of post-trauma reactions may be mediated by cognitive processes, and suggest that therapy should be aimed at modifying cognitive schemata. In brief, cognitive therapy aims to educate the survivor to identify and monitor thoughts, beliefs and assumptions about themselves, the world and the traumatic event. Clients are taught to identify the logical errors in their thinking and to find more realistic and helpful alternatives to their current way of thinking.

Cognitive therapy is a structured, collaborative, problem-oriented and time-limited approach. It draws upon Socratic questioning methods and guided self-discovery, enabling the survivor to view their negative thoughts, beliefs and assumptions as hypotheses to be validated in a scientific and systematic manner. Thus the survivor is encouraged to re-evaluate and modify their thoughts through a variety of cognitive interventions and to find more realistic and helpful alternatives to their current way of thinking.

Cognitive and cognitive–behavioural interventions for PTSD have recently been incorporated in the literature. This has come about because it has been argued that, although exposure may reduce fear and anxiety, it may not reduce other emotional reactions such as depression, guilt, shame, low self-esteem etc., which are commonly found in clients with PTSD (Pitman *et al.*, 1991; Solomon *et al.*, 1992; Resick and Schnicke, 1992). Thus more recent literature has recognized the importance that thinking or cognitions have in the maintenance of these negative emotions and has argued that cognitive behavioural interventions, such as stress inoculation training and cognitive therapy, may help in modifying or re-attributing such thinking and thereby reduce these negative reactions.

There are increasing numbers of articles detailing the application of cognitive therapy for survivors of trauma (Thrasher *et al.*, in press; Parrott and Howes, 1991; Kubany, 1994; Resick and Schnicke, 1992). The latter have identified cognitive interventions or particular issues with specific types of trauma and highlight a plethora of techniques to challenge dysfunctional thoughts, beliefs and assumptions.

Case Studies

The following case studies give a detailed view of how therapy is conducted. The first case study uses an exposure technique alone, the second demonstrates the value of cognitive interventions.

Effectiveness of Behavioural and Cognitive–Behavioural Interventions in Treating PTSD

There is increasing empirical evidence that the treatments described above are promising in both the short and long term for survivors of trauma. A number of single case studies using behavioural or cognitive–behavioural techniques for survivors of rape (Lovell, 1992) and physical assault (Thrasher *et al.*, in press; Richards, 1989), burns (Lovell, 1991) and for war veterans (Keane and Kaloupeek, 1982) have shown them to be effective.

Case study: **Exposure therapy**

Jean was a 35-year-old married woman, employed by a security firm to collect money from public houses and deposit it at the bank. On the day of the incident, Jean had parked her car outside the bank. She was about to wind her window up when a man approached the window who said he had a gun and would not harm her if she carried out his instructions. He ordered her to drive. About 15 minutes later he asked her to park beside a garage surrounded by blocks of flats.

He asked Jean for the key to the safe, which was in the boot of the car. Jean, believing she was at risk, was anxious and fumbled for the keys. The assailant became increasingly agitated and angry and began to verbally abuse her. At this point she became convinced that she was about to be killed. She found her keys, handed them over and the assailant opened and emptied the safe of its contents. He then came back to the car, handcuffed Jean to the steering wheel, and told her that someone was watching her and if she attempted to shout for help she would be harmed. The episode lasted no more than 3–4 minutes. For about 20 minutes following the robbery Jean sat in the car, terrified and distressed and, although a number of people walked past, she was too frightened to ask for help.

She saw an elderly couple leave a flat opposite and believed that they were unlikely to be part of the abduction. She called to them and asked them to call the police. Although they were aware that she was handcuffed, they initially refused to help, saying that they did not want to get involved because they were going to their daughter's for tea; to call the police would make them late. Jean became extremely distressed as she was convinced that either the assailant or an accomplice were now watching and as soon as the couple moved, she would be killed. She repeatedly begged the couple who eventually reluctantly agreed to help. The police came, she was taken to the local hospital where she was treated for shock and was allowed home a few hours later. It was only on reaching hospital that she felt safe.

For a week after the incident Jean was not able to leave the house. She returned to work but had to be accompanied there and back by her partner, though this need petered out over a 4–5 month period. A year following the incident she was referred by her GP for psychological treatment of her chronic post-traumatic stress disorder. At the assessment she complained of being constantly irritable and argumentative, which was affecting her relationship with her partner and children. Her irritability was also causing difficulties at work. She had frequent, intrusive, distressing and unwanted thoughts and images of the trauma up to 20 times daily and

(continued)

In terms of controlled studies, the efficacy of these treatments is more demonstrable. Keane *et al.* (1989) compared imaginal exposure with a waiting list control for Vietnam veterans suffering from PTSD and found imaginal exposure to be superior. Resick and Schnicke (1992) treated survivors of sexual assault using cognitive processing therapy (CPT) and compared this treatment to a waiting list control. In brief, CPT consists in asking the client to write an account of the trauma and then, in later sessions, focusing on particular issues using cognitive interventions. The authors found that CPT reduced many of the symptoms of PTSD in a relatively short time.

Foa *et al.* (1991) have completed the most sophisticated studies in PTSD to date. They compared survivors of rape and randomized them to prolonged exposure, stress inoculation training, supportive counselling or to a waiting list control. The results found prolonged exposure and stress inoculation training to be superior to supportive counselling and waiting list in reducing PTSD symptoms. Further, they found that at post-treatment, prolonged exposure was superior to stress inoculation training but at 3-month follow-up prolonged exposure was better than stress inoculation training.

Case study **Exposure therapy** *(continued)*

occasional nightmares. Reminders, such as TV programmes, media reports, or someone talking of being assaulted would cause her to feel anxious. She described sleeping much more (up to 12–14 hours daily) to escape from thoughts and feelings of the incident. Jean avoided talking or thinking about the incident. Further she felt low with tearfulness, impaired concentration and a loss of interest in previously enjoyed hobbies and activities.

Jean was able to drive to work alone but avoided walking, shopping, crowded places or visiting anywhere alone. Whilst at work travelling from business to business, she had become increasingly hypervigilant. For example if a car was behind her for more than 2–3 minutes she would become anxious, write down the car number and then take sharp turns to ensure she was not being followed. Although she was able to deposit money at banks, she avoided the bank where she had been abducted.

Thus the impact of trauma impaired every area of her life. As part of the assessment, one clinical measure used was a problem and goal rating (Marks, 1986). Jean was asked to define her problem in her own words and rate how this interfered in her life and to define four goals she would like to achieve at the end of treatment (see Figure. 25.4). Jean was treated with exposure therapy after accepting the treatment rationale. Although she was apprehensive about recollecting the trauma, she understood the rationale and agreed to therapy.

During the first session of imaginal exposure Jean, while obviously distressed, gave a clear and detailed account of the incident. She rated her level of distress during the session as 8 (using a 0–8 point rating scale, where 0 denotes no distress or anxiety and 8 extreme distress or anxiety). The session was audio-taped and Jean was instructed to repeat the imaginal exposure as homework, using the tape as a guide, for an hour a day and to keep a recording of her distress and anxiety on a homework sheet. Time was devoted at the end of the session to discussing the treatment, to receiving and giving feedback on the treatment session, and to plan for and pre-empt any difficulties with homework.

At session two, Jean reported that she had been able to complete her homework daily and, though she had found it difficult, felt a sense of achievement. Her anxiety and distress rating decreased over the week from 6 to 2. During this session Jean was asked to identify the most critical parts of the trauma: these were as follows:

1. The point when the assailant became agitated and verbally abusive, i.e. where she believed she would be killed.
2. The point where she believed the assailant or accomplice were watching her and where the elderly couple initially refused to help.

The first scene was expanded on in great detail via imaginal exposure. Using the 'rewind and hold' technique described earlier Jean was instructed to 'hold' the image, describing in detail her thoughts, feelings, etc. She was then asked to 'rewind' this image and hold it again. She was asked to repeat this procedure until the session was finished. Again the session was audio-taped and Jean was asked to carry out homework as before.

At session five Jean was asked to complete the self-rated clinical measures that had been done at the assessment. These measures and her verbal report of her general health showed considerable gains as a result of the therapy. Her mood had improved, she no longer experienced intrusive thoughts and images or nightmares and her sleep pattern had returned to its previous 7–8 hours nightly. Jean was pleased with her progress, though she felt that her avoidances and her hypervigilance had not changed. It was agreed that the next stage of treatment would target these areas using live exposure.

A repeat of the treatment rationale was given and therapist and patient together devised a graded hierarchy of feared and avoided situations. It was decided in that session to commence live exposure, with Jean tackling small crowds in a local area accompanied by the therapist. Jean was to stay in situ for an hour. At the beginning of the session Jean rated 7 and by the end of an hour she was rating 2. She was pleased with her progress and as homework, Jean felt that she could try to repeat the session daily with her partner and then alone. By the 7th appointment Jean had achieved her homework targets with only minimal anxiety. The next two sessions consisted in going to the bank, sitting outside and progressing to depositing money there.

The final session involved going shopping in central London. Jean completed all these tasks alone as homework on a daily basis.

At the end of therapy Jean had improved by about 85% and felt that her difficulties had been resolved. She was no longer avoiding any situation, regularly went shopping alone, deposited money in the bank where the incident took place and, while she was vigilant at work, this was felt to be a reasonable safety precaution. She was no longer depressed, and did not feel anxious or fearful when reminded of the event or have intrusive thoughts or images. She was no longer irritable, with consequent improvement in her relationships with her partner and children. She re-started her previously enjoyed interests and hobbies.

Jean completed therapy and was encouraged to continue doing the things she had practised during sessions and as homework. As with any therapeutic intervention follow-up is crucial, therefore Jean was seen at 1, 3, 6 and 12 months after completion to ensure all the gains she had made during therapy were maintained. When Jean was last seen at 12 months she was symptom free.

Case Study: **Cognitive–behavioural therapy**

John was 28 years old, married and a policeman. While on duty, he had been asked to attend a domestic argument between a man and a woman. When he and a colleague arrived, they could hear shouting. They were unable to gain entry and broke the door down. Inside they found the man holding a knife at his partner's throat. The partner already had multiple stab wounds and clearly required urgent medical attention. The assailant informed the police that if they did not leave immediately he would cut her throat. John attempted to talk to him and believed the man to be relaxing his grip, but suddenly he stabbed his girlfriend in the throat. They managed to disarm the man, and administered immediate first aid to the woman, but she was dead by the time the ambulance arrived.

John immediately began to suffer symptoms and 6 months later was referred by his welfare department for treatment of his PTSD. At assessment, John was visibly distressed when talking about the incident. He reported that he had frequent nightmares and intrusive thoughts and images for much of the day. He had difficulty in handling any sharp knives. Even looking at them provoked considerable anxiety. He felt fearful at work, particularly about disarming someone. Although it had not arisen since the incident, he knew that there was a possibility of a similar incident occurring.

Following an assessment and rationale, John was treated using imaginal and live exposure in a similar way as described in the previous case study. At the end of 10 weeks of treatment he had made a significant improvement, in that nightmares, intrusive images and thoughts had decreased in intensity and frequency. He was able to handle sharp knives and attend confrontational situations at work with minimal anxiety. However, he continued to feel extremely guilty and depressed and his feelings that he had caused the incident did not diminish. He continued to be plagued by feelings of guilt with self-statements such as 'If only I had acted quicker she would still be alive' or 'If I had taken a different course of action, the woman would still be alive today'. These feelings led to a sense that he had failed in his duty and was thus an incompetent policeman. He felt that he was responsible for the woman's death.

It was felt that the most effective way of dealing with these feelings was to use cognitive therapy. A rationale of treatment was given and the first thing done was to identify and elicit the negative thoughts and beliefs that were producing this level of guilt and subsequent depression. The main thoughts identified were that 'it was my responsibility that the girl died'. John was asked to rate how much he believed this thought to be true on a 0–100 scale (0 = this thought is not at all true, to 100 = this thought is completely true). John believed this thought to be 80% true.

There are many cognitive techniques to challenge negative or unhelpful thoughts and the following method is only one way of modifying negative thinking (Beck *et al.*, 1979; Hawton *et al.*, 1989) In brief, a series of questions were used to allow John to re-evaluate his thoughts in a more rational or objective way. These questions centred on issues such as 'Are you taking responsibility for something that was not your fault? If a similar event happened to a colleague of yours and they took the same actions as you, what would your response be?' In answer to the latter question John said, 'In fact a similar situation did happen to a colleague of mine a few years ago and I said to him that he had acted correctly. Like my own situation there was every indication that the man was going to surrender the weapon'.

(continued)

A study by Richards *et al.* (1994) compared individuals exposed to a range of traumas and gave half the group imaginal exposure followed by live exposure, and the other half live exposure first, followed by imaginal session. Their results showed a 60–80% improvement in overall symptomatology, which was maintained up to 1 year afterwards.

Although there are few controlled studies and many have focused on a specific type of trauma, the results are promising and suggest that, currently, behavioural and cognitive interventions are the treatment of choice for survivors of traumatic events. However, it is unclear whether exposure based treatments are superior to cognitive treatments or whether a combination of behavioural and cognitive treatments is the optimal therapy. Research is currently investigating this issue in the USA and the UK.

SUPERVISION

Helping the survivors of trauma can be intensely emotionally challenging for any clinician. During therapy, practitioners witness the effects of trauma and hear highly detailed accounts of extremely distressing events. They run the risk of suffering from vicarious traumatization.

It is essential to set up supervision networks and personal strategies to help therapists manage their own feelings. In the same way that such reactions are normalized in acutely traumatized clients, therapists should not pretend that they can remain immune from their own emotions. Distressing events produce distress, whether directly or indirectly experienced.

Supervision should be regular and allow therapists to debrief themselves similarly to the CISD procedure described earlier. There should be a safe environment for therapists to facilitate their own factual, cognitive and emotional debriefing.

Case Study **Cognitive–behavioural therapy (continued)**

As the session proceeded it became evident to John that he was not totally responsible for the death of the young girl and consequently was not an incompetent policeman. John was asked what statement he could use to challenge this thought, in the light of a more objective evaluation of the thought. He said, 'Given the circumstances I acted correctly. Although I wish the girl had not died, there was nothing I could have done to prevent her death'. John was able to recognize that while he wished the woman had not died, the reality was that he had responded to the situation in the correct manner and in fact had used the correct first aid procedures. Importantly, at the end of the session he reported that the colleague who was with him, together with his immediate boss, had praised him for his handling of the situation and his competence in the first aid he had administered. He was asked to re-rate his belief in the original negative thought (he rated 15%) and how much he believed his alternative thought (he rated 85%). Following this session his sense of guilt decreased and he no longer believed he was an incompetent policeman. John was followed up at 6 months with no resurgence of symptoms.

Figure 25.4 Problems and goals (see Case study: Exposure therapy)

Main problem

1 Unwanted thoughts and images about the trauma. Avoiding walking or going out alone. Irritability with family, and sleeping too much. Hypervigilant, car numbers.

Pre	Mid	Post	1M	3M	6M	12M
7	3	1	1	0	0	0

This problem upset me and/or interferes with my normal activities.

0	1	2	3	4	5	6	7	8
does not		slightly/ sometimes		definitely/ often		markedly/ very often		very severely/ continuously

Goals

1 To walk, drive and shop alone every day with minimal anxiety

Pre	Mid	Post	1M	3M	6M	12M
8	7	1	2	1	0	0

2 To be able to let a car pass without checking or writing numbers down

Pre	Mid	Post	1M	3M	6M	12M
7	5	0	0	0	0	0

3 To take money to the bank alone

Pre	Mid	Post	1M	3M	6M	12M
8	5	0	0	0	0	0

4 To sleep for 7–8 hours nightly, undisturbed

Pre	Mid	Post	1M	3M	6M	12M
6	0	0	0	0	0	0

My progress towards acheiving each target regularly without difficulty:

0	1	2	3	4	5	6	7	8
complete success		75% success		50% success		25% success		no success

SUMMARY

Psychological distress following a traumatic event can lead to short- and long-term mental health problems. A number of theoretical models have been proposed to account for the maintenance and acquisition of psychological disturbance. In some individuals post-traumatic stress disorder may occur. In the short term, much distress is normal and healthy. Not all individuals require therapy *per se* and a debriefing model has been given for use with individuals immediately after a trauma. However, for those that develop long-term difficulties behavioural–cognitive therapy is an extremely effective intervention.

KEY CONCEPTS

- Post-traumatic stress disorder (PTSD) is a chronic disabling problem characterized by:
  - Intrusive memories of the initiating traumatic event.
  - Avoidance of these memories, together with objects and situations that are reminders of the event.
  - Physiological hyperarousal such as sleep disturbance, irritability and poor concentration.
- PTSD is thought to be a problem for between 1% and 9% of the population in general and up to 50% of those experiencing traumatic events such as disasters, sexual assault, crime and combat.
- Information-processing models of PTSD suggest that the key PTSD symptoms arise from a conflict between the traumatic experience and the individual's core beliefs about themselves and the world, leading to incomplete processing of the new traumatic information.
- Acute anxiety symptoms are common after traumatic events but, for most people, are short-lived and can be effectively managed using critical incident stress debriefing (CISD) techniques.
- If significant distress persists beyond 1 month post-trauma it is likely that therapy will be required.
- Assessment of PTSD should be client-centred and use a process of question-funnelling from general, open questions to specific, closed questions to elicit details of all symptoms and areas of client distress.
- Therapy should be empirically validated by regular administration of client specific, handicap and symptom measures, repeated before and after therapy.
- A combination of imaginal and real life exposure to trauma-related images and avoidances is a highly effective treatment for PTSD.
- Cognitive techniques that assist people to integrate their traumatic experiences with their core beliefs also appear to be very effective.
- Nurses engaged in therapy with traumatized clients risk being vicariously traumatized and must ensure that they have regular, structured and effective supervision.

REFERENCES

American Psychiatric Association: *Diagnostic and statistical manual of mental disorders.* Washington, 1994, American Psychiatric Association.

Beck A, Rush AJ, Shaw BF, Emery G: *Cognitive therapy of depression.* New York, 1979, The Guildford Press.

Breslau N, Davis GC, Andreski P, Peterson E: Traumatic events and post-traumatic stress disorder in an urban population of young adults. *Arch Gen Psychiatry* 48(3):216, 1990.

Bustos E: Psychodynamic approaches in the treatment of torture survivors. In: Basoglu M, editor: *Torture and its consequences.* New York, 1992, Cambridge University Press.

Chemtob L *et al.*: A cognitive action theory of post-traumatic stress disorder. *J Anxiety Disord* 2(3):253, 1988.

Creamer M, Burgess P, Pattison P: Reaction to trauma: a cognitive processing model. *J Abnorm Psychol* 101(3):452, 1992.

Daly RJ: Samuel Pepys and post-traumatic stress disorder. *Br J Psychiatry* 148(July):64, 1983.

Davidson JRT *et al.*: Post-traumatic stress disorder in the community: an epidemiological study. *Psychol Med* 21(3):713, 1991.

Davidson JRT, Fairbank JA: The epidemiology of post-traumatic stress disorder. In: Davidson JRT, Foa E, editors: *Posttraumatic stress disorder: DSM IV and beyond.* Washington, 1993, American Psychiatric Press.

Dyregrov A: Caring for helpers in disaster situations: psychological debriefing. *Disaster Manage* 2(2):25, 1989.

Fairbank JA, Nicholson RA: Theoretical and empirical issues in the treatment of PTSD in Vietnam veterans. *J Clin Psychol* 43(1):44, 1987.

Foa E *et al.*: Treatment of posttraumatic stress disorder in rape victims: A comparison between cognitive–behavioural procedures and counselling. *J Consult Clin Psychol* 59(5):715, 1991.

Foa E, Kosak MJ: Emotional processing of fear: Exposure to corrective information. *Psychol Bull* 99(1):20, 1986.

Foa E, Steketee G, Rothbaum BO: Behavioural/cognitive conceptualisations of post-traumatic stress disorder. *Behavi Ther* 20(2):155, 1989.

Foa E, Riggs DS, Dancu CV, Rothbaum BO: Reliability and validity of a brief instrument for assessing post-traumatic stress disorder. *J Traum Stress* 6(4):459, 1993.

Foy DW *et al.*: Etiology of posttraumatic stress disorder in Vietnam veterans: analysis of premilitary, and combat exposure influences. *J Consult Clin Psychol* 52(1):79, 1984.

Goldberg DP, Williams P: *A user's guide to the General Health Questionnaire.* Windsor, 1988, NFER-Nelson.

Green BL: Psychosocial research in traumatic stress: an update. *J Trauma Stress* 7(3):341, 1994.

Green BL *et al.*: Buffalo Creek survivors in the second decade: stability of stress symptoms. *Am J Orniopsychiatry* 60(1):43, 1990.

Hackman A: Behavioural and cognitive psychotherapies: past history, current applications and future registration issues. *Behav Cognit Psychother* 21(suppl.1), 1993.

Hawton K *et al.*: *Cognitive behaviour therapy for psychiatric problems: a practical guide.* New York, 1989, Oxford University Press.

Helzer JE, Robbins LN, McEvoy L: Post traumatic stress disorder in the general population. *New England J Med* 317(26):1630, 1987.

Herman JL: Complex PTSD: A syndrome in survivors of prolonged and repeated trauma. In: Everely GS, Lating, JM, editors : *Psychotraumatology—Key papers and core concepts in post-traumatic stress.* Plenum Press, 1995, New York.

Hodgkinson PE, Stewart M: *Coping with catastrophe: handbook of disaster management.* London, 1991, Routledge.

Horowitz MJ: *Stress response syndromes,* ed 2. New York, 1986, Jason Aronson.

Horowitz MJ, Wilner N, Alverez W: Impact of event scale: a measure of subjective stress. *Psychosom Med* 41(3):209, 1979.

Horowitz MJ, Kaltreider NB: Brief psychotherapy of stress response. In: Karsasu T, Bellack L, editors: *Specialised techniques in individual psychotherapy.* New York, 1980, Brunner/Mazel.

Janoff–Bulman R: The aftermath of victimisation: rebuilding shattered assumptions. In: Figely CR, editor: *Trauma and its wake.* New York, 1985, Brunner/Mazel.

Janoff–Bulman R: *Shattered assumptions*. New York, 1992, Free Press.

Joseph S *et al.*: Crisis support and psychiatric symptomatology in adult survivors of the Jupiter cruise ship disaster. *Br J Clin Psychol* 31(1):63, 1992.

Keane TM *et al.*: A behavioural approach to assessing and treating posttraumatic stress disorder in Vietnam veterans. In: Figeley CR, editor: *Trauma and its wake: the study and treatment of posttraumatic stress disorder*. New York, 1985, Brunner/Mazel.

Keane TM *et al.*: Implosive (flooding) therapy reduces symptoms of PTSD in Vietnam combat veterans. *Behav Ther* 20(2):149, 1989.

Keane TM, Kaloupek D: Imaginal flooding in the treatment of posttraumatic stress disorder. *J Consult Clin Psychol* 50(1):138, 1982.

Keane TM, Wolfe J: Comorbidity in post-traumatic stress disorder: an analysis of community and clinical studies. *J Appl Soc Psychol* 20 (21):1776, 1990.

Kilpatrick DG, Resnick HS: PTSD associated with exposure to criminal victimisation in clinical and community populations. In: Davidson JRT, Foa E, editors: *Posttraumatic stress disorder: DSM IV and beyond*. Washington, 1993, American Psychiatric Press.

Krietler S, Krietler H: Trauma and anxiety: the cognitive approach. *J Trauma Stress* 1(1):35, 1988.

Kubany ES: A cognitive model of guilt typology in combat-related PTSD. *J Trauma Stress* 7(1) 3, 1994.

Kulka RC *et al.*: *Trauma and the Vietnam generation: report of findings from the National Vietnam Veterans Readjustment Study*. New York, 1990, Brunner/Mazel.

Lang PJ: A bioinformational theory of emotional imagery. *Psychophysiol* 16(6):495, 1979.

Lerner MJ: The desire for justice and reactions to victims: social psychological studies of some antecedents and consequences. In: Macaulay J, Berkowitz L, editors: *Altruism and helping behaviour*. New York, 1970, Academic Press.

Lerner MJ: *The belief in a just world*. New York, 1980, Plenum.

Letts C, Tait A: Post raid debriefing. *Occupational Health* 47 (12):418–421, 1995.

Lovell K: Post-traumatic stress management. *Nurs Stand* 11(6):30, 1991.

Lovell K: The reality of rape. *Nurs Times* 88(25):52, 1992.

Marks IM: *Behavioural psychotherapy: Maudsley pocket book of clinical management*. Bristol, 1986, Wright.

McCann L, Sakheim DK, Abrahamson DJ: Trauma and victimization: a model of psychological adaptation. *Counsel Psychol* 16(4):531, 1988.

Mcleer SV *et al.*: Post-traumatic stress disorder in sexually abused children. *J Am Acad Child Adolesc Psychiatry* 27(5):286, 1988.

Mitchell J: When disaster strikes: the critical incident stress debriefing process. *J Emerg Med Serv* 8(1):36, 1983.

Mowrer OH: On the dual nature of learning: a reinterpretation of 'conditioning' and 'problem solving'. *Harv Educat Rev* 17(4):102, 1947.

Mowrer OH: *Learning theory and behaviour*. New York, 1960, Wiley.

Muse M: Stress-related, posttraumatic chronic pain syndrome: behavioural treatment approach. *Pain* 25:389, 1986.

Orner R: Post-traumatic stress syndromes among British veterans of the Falklands war. In: Wilson JP, Rapheal B, editors: *International handbook of traumatic stress syndromes*. New York, 1993, Plenum Press.

Parrott CA, Howes JL: The application of cognitive therapy to posttraumatic stress disorder. In: Vallis TM, Howes JL, Miller PC, editors: *The challenge of cognitive therapy: applications to nontraditional populations*. New York, 1991, Plenum Press.

Pitman RK *et al.*: Psychiatric complications during flooding therapy for post-traumatic stress disorder. *J Clin Psychiatry* 52(1):17–20, 1991.

Resick PA, Schnicke MK: Cognitive processing therapy for sexual assault victims, *J Consult Clin Psychol* 60(5):748, 1992.

Resick PA, Schnicke MK: *Cognitive processing therapy for rape victims: a treatment manual*. Newbury Park, 1993, Sage Publications.

Richards DA: Hidden scars. *Nurs Times* 85(22):66, 1989.

Richards DA, McDonald R: *Behavioural psychotherapy: a handbook for nurses*. Oxford, 1990, Heinemann.

Richards DA, Rose JS: Exposure therapy for post-traumatic stress disorder: four case-studies. *Br J Psychiatry* 158(June):836, 1991.

Richards DA, Lovell K, Marks I: Post-traumatic stress disorder: evaluation of a behavioural treatment program. *J Trauma Stress* 7(4):669, 1994.

Rothbaum BO *et al.*: A prospective examination of post-traumatic stress disorder in rape victims. *J Trauma Stress* 5(3):455, 1992.

Rothbaum BO, Foa E: Cognitive–behavioural treatment of posttraumatic stress disorder. In: Saigh P, editor: *Post traumatic stress disorder: a behavioural approach to assessment and treatment*. New York, 1992, Macmillan.

Saunders BE, Arata CM, Kilpatrick DG: Development of a crime-related post-traumatic stress disorder scale for women within the symptom checklist-90-revised. *J Trauma Stress* 3(3):439, 1990.

Solomon SD, Gerrity ET, Muff AM: Efficacy of treatments for posttraumatic stress disorder: an empirical review. *JAMA* 286(5):633, 1992.

Thrasher SM *et al.*: Cognitive restructuring in the treatment of post-traumatic stress disorder: two single cases. *Clin Psychol Psychiatry* (in press).

FURTHER READING

Foy DW: *Treating PTSD: cognitive–behavioural strategies*. New York, 1992, Guildford Press.

  A comprehensive book which explains CBT treatments in PTSD in detail. Chapters are written across trauma types by experts in the field.

Green B: Psychosocial research in traumatic stress: an update. *J Trauma Stress* 7:341–362, 1994.

  A well-written paper that highlights up-to-date research on various aspects of PTSD.

Richards DA: Hidden scars. *Nurs Times* 85(22):66–69, 1989.

  A single case-study which describes PTSD and gives a clear account of exposure therapy.

Saigh P: *Posttraumatic stress disorder: a behavioural approach to assessment and treatment*. New York, 1992, Macmillan.

  An excellent source book that details the history, prevalence, assessment and behavioural treatment of PTSD.

Solomon SD, Gerrity ET, Muff AM: Efficacy of treatments for posttraumatic stress disorder: an empirical review. *JAMA* 268:633–638, 1992.

  A comprehensive and critical review of controlled studies of treatments used in PTSD (e.g. medication, behavioural and cognitive–behavioural therapy and psychdynamic therapy).

Forensic Psychiatric Nursing

Learning Outcomes

After reading this chapter you should be able to:

- Gain an insight of the environments in which the forensic psychiatric nurse works.

- Understand which competencies and skills are shared by the psychiatric nurse and the forensic psychiatric nurse and which are not.

- Better understand a number of specific clinical presentations for which the forensic psychiatric nurse has to provide treatment and management.

- Gain a brief insight into mentally disordered offenders as a client group distinct from 'generic' psychiatric clients.

- Appreciate and discuss the need constantly to balance the therapeutic and security regimes and how each conflicts with the other.

- Understand the need for a wide variety of assessment and management skills.

- Gain an insight into the process and areas for care planning assessment, implementation and evaluation.

- Discuss and show by example the nursing interventions required in treatment and management of the mentally disordered offender.

*T*his chapter endeavours to give the reader an* insight into the role of the forensic psychiatric nurse (FPN) and the interventions used by an FPN in the care and management of mentally disordered offenders in various secure settings. The generic base for forensic psychiatric nursing, the core elements of its brother 'general' psychiatry, is covered in the rest of this book. While the other chapters can and do devote themselves to major topics, the aim of this one is to look at the profession as a whole and to highlight certain areas within it. Here the authors aim to explain something of the development of current forensic psychiatry, the environments and how they interlink with and complement each other, problems and behaviours of this client group, specific nursing interventions and innovative practices and developments within the specialty.

The overriding theme is that there is no single model of forensic psychiatric nursing that encompasses the range of approaches utilized by this growing specialty. As a result there is a need to take a holistic approach to nursing interventions. This is exemplified by the importance placed on the concept that 'the patient is not the problem — *the problem* is the problem' (Barker, 1995). Thus the patient with schizophrenia or the person who behaves dangerously is not the problem. Rather it is the dangerous behaviour itself or the schizophrenic presentation and effects that create problems and which need to be addressed to assist the patient to achieve mental well-being. This is neither new nor particularly controversial but it is worth emphasizing that it should form the basis for any and all nursing activities.

The description of the range of skills, competencies and approaches given in this chapter by no means exhausts the variety of approaches currently practised in the field. This chapter does, however, describe areas of nursing practice found in a broad range of secure establishments.

The vast majority of forensic psychiatric nurses consider forensic psychiatric nursing to be a specialty in its own right. The only stumbling block to prevent autonomous professional status is that there is no professional qualification, equivalent to the Registered Mental Nurse (RMN), for the forensic psychiatric nurse. There are, as might be expected in a specialist field, numbers of post basic educational courses available at diploma and degree level. Many argue that an independent FPN qualification is not necessary as the current RMN and Registered Mental Handicap Nurse (RMHN) are adequate. Undoubtedly, this will continue to be debated among managers, nurses and educationalists. However, some graduate and postgraduate Forensic Psychiatric Nursing courses have been established, e.g. the BA in Forensic Nursing, based at the Robert Gordon University, Aberdeen and run in conjunction with the State Hospital, Carstairs.

It is the authors' intention that this chapter will help you to form your own ideas and points of view about this growing and increasingly important specialty within nursing.

While the function of forensic psychiatric nursing seems obvious and bound to public opinion and scrutiny, the role is something of a complex one. The overall function could be described as providing health care for people with a recognized mental disorder under conditions of special security (high, medium and low) required to protect the public from their dangerous, violent or criminal propensities. While this view is somewhat simplistic, it captures the essence of the FPN's function.

The role or roles of the FPN, however, are more complex. When questioning the role of the FPN it would help to understand what a generic psychiatric nurse is and does. In his inaugural speech, Professor Barker (1995) said that the practice of psychiatric nursing is a complex of interpersonal relations given the form of care, human meeting human, and that the content of these meetings, interactions, exchanges and mutual influence are the processes by which it is carried out. Interpersonal relations represent the proper focus of nursing.

It could, therefore, be considered that the basic skills of both are the same, the differences being that the forensic nurse performs these in a locked environment, behind closed doors. It is the application of the nurse's skills within that environment and the nursing interventions delivered within the context of a client's offending behaviour and dangerousness, that separates FPNs from their generic colleagues

FORENSIC ENVIRONMENTS

There are four main types of environment where forensic nursing is performed. These will be described in general terms, as the differences between specific locations are as numerous as the locations themselves.

PRISONS—PENAL SYSTEM

Prisons in England and Wales can be divided into two categories: local or training, with the latter including the dispersal prisons. All local prisons (Box 26.1) are closed, while training prisons can be either open or closed and invariably house a lower category of prisoner. There are currently eight maximum secure or 'dispersal' prisons. These are organized and equipped to accommodate the most dangerous and high risk prisoners, who invariably have long sentences. Female prisons are organized similarly; HMP Durham has a unit for women who require special security and who present specific problems and are serving long sentences.

Considering that a large proportion of the overall prison population is drawn from the socially disadvantaged, unemployed, unemployable, inadequate and rootless members of society, it is no surprise to find that large numbers of this population have a psychiatric disorder classifiable in terms of ICD-10 (World Health Organisation, 1992).

No prison, or part of a prison, is recognized as a hospital for the purposes of the Mental Health Act 1983. (For further information on the Mental Health Act 1983 see Chapter 8).Therefore, except in cases of life threatening emergencies, prisoners cannot be treated without their consent. This, obviously, poses serious problems if there is a delay in transferring a prisoner to a hospital under Sections 47 or 48 of the Mental Health Act (Department of Health and Social Security, 1983). In an attempt to alleviate these problems, some prisons have contracted-in a psychiatric service, as opposed to simply buying sessional work from a consultant psychiatrist.

Box 26.1 *Local prison health care provision*

This example comes from the Forensic Service based at the Hutton Centre in Middlesbrough.

The Hutton Centre Forensic Services, in collaboration with the Forensic Service at St. Nicholas's Hospital in Newcastle, provide a wide-ranging, fully staffed, multidisciplinary team to attend to the needs of the mentally disordered offender in prison. The contract drawn up between the various parties ensures that a prisoner with a mental illness receives the care appropriate to his or her needs, in the shortest possible time, from the staff most suited to respond. The contract team, which would be found in any hospital setting, comprises consultant psychiatrists, psychologists, social workers and community psychiatric nurses from both forensic services, all working on a coordinated sessional basis. They work closely with the prison health care staff in providing advice and support in carrying out day-to-day care.

This multidisciplinary team provides care to a wide range of needs in three prisons in the north east of England; one is a Category A maximum secure prison, the second is a local prison with a high security female wing and the third is a Remand Centre that has a large adolescent population.

HIGH SECURE PROVISION

The high security psychiatric hospitals stand at one extreme of the range of provision for the violent and offender patients.

(Royal College of Psychiatrists, 1980)

The three special hospitals for England and Wales, Ashworth, Broadmoor and Rampton, provide 'conditions of special security' for people who are subject to detention under the Mental Health Act 1983 and who are also dangerous (Department of Health and Social Security, 1977). Carstairs State Hospital provides a similar service for Scotland and Northern Ireland, while Dundrum Hospital caters for the Republic of Ireland.

Security is obviously the main distinguishing feature of the special hospitals with its main objective being to prevent patients absconding. It involves maintaining a perimeter wall or fence with a sophisticated system of entry to the campus, including detection devices, airlocks, electronic doors and other precautions to prevent unauthorized access or egress and items being brought in that would compromise the security regime. The internal security is just as stringent, with well established routines of locking and of monitoring patient movement and activity. Inside the walls exists what could be described as a small, self-contained, institutional version of village life with all the needs of the 'villagers' being met on one site.

The level of security applied to a patient should always be the *minimum* level that is compatible with safety and good management (Department of Health and Home Office, 1992). The practicalities mean that special hospitals take three types of patient:

1. Those patients who would present a significant and immediate danger to the general public, were they to escape.
2. Those who prove unmanageable and dangerous to staff in hospitals lower in the security hierarchy.
3. Those who need some significant degree of security on a long-term basis.

The above measures ensure that the security of the perimeter is of a very high standard, while that of different parts of the interior can be varied according to requirements. These are appropriate to the patients' mental well-being, progress in treatment and rehabilitation, and present and potential dangerousness.

Decisions on levels of security should be taken with the maximum of information about factors such as:

- Seriousness of previous aggressive behaviour.
- Severity of mental disorder.
- Type of mental disorder and its prognosis.
- Length of time the patient is expected to be at risk of behaving aggressively.
- The range of therapeutic and educational services available.
- Knowledge of the original offending behaviour.

There are many managerial issues surrounding the care of the individual in the secure setting. Those which have immediate implications for the therapeutic as well as the secure regime are considered below. The management of patients in secure provision is achieved by three easily identifiable, interrelated factors:

1. Physical security.
2. Quality of nursing care.
3. Patient motivation.

Physical Security

The physical security of special hospitals has always been affected by the penal system. It is difficult to determine just how much of the security provided by the special hospitals matches that of the high security, dispersal (Category A) prisons, as there are several degrees of security in both types of institution. In the early 1980s the (Deparment of Health and Social Security) claimed that all special hospital patients were subject to the same degree of security provided for Category A prisoners. In 1961, the Ministry of Health Working Party (Ministry of Health, 1961) put forward a definition of the objectives of security:

the public must be provided with strong protection against the more serious risks and with adequate protection against the lesser risks.

Despite all special hospital patients being subject to security regimes commensurate with that of Category A prisoners, one difference arises that applies to all levels of secure facilities. All high and medium secure forensic establishments, in trying to balance security and treatment, have a gradient system of security inside, and sometimes outside, the secure campus. This internal level of security is dependent upon a variety of subjective and clinical issues: degree of dangerousness chronicity, mental stability, appropriateness for discharge and preparation for discharge, among others. It is widely accepted that the physical confinement of patients is for the protection of the public. Secure institutions, however, also have a duty to protect patients and staff within the establishment. Elements of such internal security may include frequent counting and searching of patients, monitoring patient movement by CCTV and centralized radio control, and the use of medication to minimize violent and disruptive behaviour. The latter is particularly contentious, although the association between security and medication was explicitly expanded in a policy statement issued by the Royal College of Psychiatrists (1980):

the prompt but appropriate judicious use of medication where it is properly indicated is another measure related to security.

Quality of Nursing Care

From the beginning of the 19th Century it has been recognized that the quality of nursing care is linked directly with security. In the high secure forensic hospital, responsibility for both security and nursing is vested in the nursing staff. Difficulties experienced by staff in combining these two functions were reported to the Estimates Committee (House of Commons, 1968).

As forensic psychiatric nursing has generic psychiatric nursing at its core, the issue of quality of nursing is a common feature (see Chapter 9).

Patient Motivation

The effects of the institution itself in modifying patient motivation were noted by the Hospital Advisory Service (Royal College of Psychiatrists & DHSS, 1977) in its report on Broadmoor. The number of long stay patients, vulnerable to institutionalization, who wished to return to unsupported life outside decreased after a decade. Positive patient motivation deriving from a cooperative approach may assist in reducing the level of security that would otherwise be necessary. It is a stated nursing expectation that achievement of patient acceptance of and participation in the planning, implementation and evaluation of the treatment programme is paramount. Lack of patient insight into their condition or treatment programme prejudices the patient's active and willing acceptance.

In the forensic environment this problem can be further compounded. For example, forensic patients, who are in hospital with an indefinite date of discharge and consequent perceived lack of direction or goal, exclude themselves from voluntary therapy sessions, primary nursing interventions and any of the 'contractual' relationships.

Forensic staff need to tread with caution at all stages of the treatment programme, as patient management requires not only conventional treatment but principles of basic security and interpersonal safety. It is crucial that security and safety should not be compromised in the name of achieving (possibly unrealistic) patient needs.

MEDIUM SECURE PROVISION

In the late 1950s the then Minister of Health, Enoch Powell, appointed a working party (the Emery Committee) to consider security in psychiatric hospitals and the future tasks of special hospitals (Ministry of Health, 1961). Its members clearly recognized the consequences of the 'therapeutic community, open door' policy and observed that:

1. Security precautions cannot be disposed of for all psychiatric patients.
2. Security precautions are a necessary part of treatment for the sake of the patient as well as the public.
3. The maximum security provided by special hospitals should not be used if suitable facilities can be made available locally.
4. Patients should be treated near their homes, insofar as this is possible, to maintain links with the local community.

Emery and his colleagues had pointed out the need to introduce local secure facilities, not necessarily high secure ones but certainly something between that and the open ward or the locked ward of old. Despite medium secure provision being conceived in the early 1960s, the reality did not occur until

after the publication of the Glancy (Department of Health and Social Security, 1974) and the Butler (Home Office and Department of Health and Social Security, 1975) reports. Both reports saw a network of regional security as essential to solving problems of management and in placement of the mentally disordered offender and those presenting significant management problems in conventional psychiatric hospitals.

The two committees had different remits. The Butler Committee dealt with mentally disordered offenders as a whole while the Glancy Committee also looked at disturbed patients already within the NHS who required more secure provision.

The Butler and Glancy Reports and the DHSS Guidelines (Department of Health and Social Security, 1975) provided general principles, but each regional team found it necessary to create its own concept of medium secure provision before moving to the planning stage. Those Regional Health Authorities that already had a resident forensic psychiatrist took account of existing facilities, population density and the size of the region before deciding on a service model and site for a permanent unit.

Medium Secure Unit (MSU) is now used instead of Regional Secure Unit (RSU) because, since the demise of Health Authority Regions in April 1996, the 'Regional' nomenclature is no longer pertinent. The first purpose-built Medium Secure Unit to open was the Hutton Unit (now Centre), St Luke's Hospital, Middlesbrough, in November, 1980.

Each of the previously designated regions now has at least one MSU within its boundaries. These units vary in size from 20 to 100 beds. The type of patient admitted, however, invariably will be the same across the country.

Obviously, at any time, should the patient's mental state or behaviour warrant it they can be referred to staff in other services, i.e. from MSU to special hospital or from MSU to MSU, to enable them to be nearer their families.

Just as in special hospitals, the patients in MSUs will also be detained under the Mental Health Act 1983 and, although not unheard of, it is very rarely that a patient comes in on an informal or remand basis.

The MSU forms the focal point of a comprehensive forensic psychiatric service, which comprises multidisciplinary services to both in-patients and out-patients across a wide range of environments, ranging from the patient's home to generic psychiatric hospitals, prisons and special hospitals.

Attention has been drawn to a profound need for longer-term, medium secure beds. Burrow (1993b) points out that addressing this need would focus more effectively on strategies for the group of patients who lie between needing maximum secure and short-term medium secure accommodation.

The Hutton Centre in Middlesbrough has recently opened a 13-bed ward to provide longer-term care for exactly this client group. Whereas most MSUs have a proposed maximum length of stay, usually around 2 years, this ward caters for patients who require treatment under conditions of medium security for longer periods. This is, as far as the authors know, the first and only such ward of its kind in the country, in the NHS. The delivery of this service without the recreational resources of the larger special hospitals has provided particular challenges to the FPN in maintaining an adequate quality of life for clients. The need to maintain these standards in a smaller and less well resourced environment presents even greater challenges.

COURT DIVERSION SCHEMES

It has long been contended that too many mentally ill have been given custodial sentences for what would seem to be errors of judgement resulting from an aspect of their mental illness. This has obviously created problems not only for the person who, while suffering from a manifestation of mental illness, now has to endure the stressors of prison but also for an already overcrowded penal system. Such a person enters a potentially hostile environment where very few others care about or understand the mentally ill. The issue of placement before being sent to prison therefore becomes of paramount importance. The alternatives are clearly special hospitals or MSUs, though in many cases such people do not require that level of security or any security at all (Box 26.2). What is needed is a treatment environment of lower security for the perpetrators of the 'non serious' offences. Of this group only a small proportion require admission to a forensic unit, the rest being adequately managed in general psychiatric units, or, at the most, a short-term, low security ward.

INTERLINKING OF SERVICES

There is obviously a degree of cross-service and cross-cultural mixing, from patients and innovative working practices to staff exchanges. One immediate area is the transfer of patients from high secure facilities to medium secure ones to assist them with their rehabilitation and eventual discharge. The working relationships between both sites has to be open, honest and in the patient's best interest at all times. One innovation in this area is the Clinical Service Agreements, which have been drawn up between certain special hospitals and some of the MSUs. The transition from high to medium secure must be a mutually facilitated affair, including the patient at all stages of the process.

The role of the nurse during this transitionary period, in both high and medium secure sites, is to offer and supply:

- Continuity of care and therapeutic direction.
- A seamless service to all concerned parties – patient, family and carers, and care teams from both sites.
- Effective communication networks between care delivery teams.
- Support to the patient and his or her family.
- Professional advice on clinical issues.
- Examples of previous care to assist in the promotion of evidence based treatment programmes.

OFFENDING BEHAVIOUR AND CRIME

To try to give a broad view of the sorts of offences that the forensic psychiatric nurse may encounter from any one patient group, a listing was made on a specific day of the immediate in-patient population of an MSU. Clearly, the balance of offending behaviours would change as the patient group changes but the list is representative of the range encountered. Table 26.1 shows the range of offences of 42 in-patients. (There are obviously a number of multiple offences here). It is worth pointing out that 20% of these patients have committed a form of homicide and that there are 67% cases of violence against another person (adult and child). (The 'nil' section are non-offender patients).

TABLE 26.1 Index offence snapshot — MSU

Murder – manslaughter (including diminished responsibility)	10
Attempted murder	1
Aggravated bodily harm Grievous bodily harm Assault	11
Arson	7
Rape, sexual assault	7
Firearms offences	2
Child sexual assault	3
Theft, burglary	3
Armed robbery	1
Poisoning	1
Nil	3
TOTAL	49

> **Box 26.2**
> ### *A specimen personality profile*
>
> A personality profile of a typical patient diverted from the Magistrates' Court to the psychiatric in-patient services *could* read like this:
>
> Single; homeless male with a chronic, serious and enduring mental illness. He would have a history of in-patient treatment; usually detained.
>
> There will also be a history of recidivistic behaviour, usually for minor offences, e.g. theft, public order etc.

THE FORENSIC PSYCHIATRIC NURSE

The image of the Forensic Psychiatric Nurse has changed over the years but more rapidly since the 1970s. With the change in image has come a change in role and a change of status among colleagues, both within psychiatry and nursing in general.

This is demonstrated in a document published by the Royal College of Nursing (Tarbuck, 1994), which states which core competencies are inherent in psychiatric nursing. It then goes on to state the advanced nursing interventions that forensic psychiatric nurses have to offer; these are shown in Table 26.2 – a number of key skills are explicitly identified with the FPN (Box 26.3).

Box 26.3 *Key competencies of the forensic psychiatric nurse*

1. Assessment of offending behaviour.
2. Assessment of dangerousness.
3. Management of dangerousness.
4. Management of personality disorders with associated offending behaviour.
5. Risk assessment.
6. Understanding associated ethical issues in the management of the mentally disordered offender.

Table 26.2 Forensic nurse advanced interventions

1. Assessment of dangerousness.
2. Management of dangerousness.
3. Anger management.
4. Behavioural therapies.
5. Cognitive therapies.
6. Counselling (and its variants).
7. Family therapy.
8. Group therapy.
9. Loss and bereavement counselling.
10. Psychodynamic and psycho therapies.
11. Rehabilitation therapies.
12. Risk assessment and management.
13. Social skills training.
14. Setting of quality standards and auditing the care delivered in low, medium and high security mental health care settings.
15. Teaching health and social service colleagues about forensic mental health care.
16. Undertaking research, and cooperating with the research of others.
17. Publishing good practices in forensic care and management.
18. Providing clinical, resource and site management in low, medium and high security settings.
19. Commissioning new secure units commensurate with the best advice available.

The remainder of this chapter will explore these competencies, illustrated (where possible) by case studies. (For simplicity of explanation and to aid enhancement and illustration, a number of competencies have been amalgamated).

EXAMPLES OF NURSING INTERVENTIONS

COMPETENCY 1

For many years there has been a search to determine whether there is a link between crime and mental illness. Obviously this tended to focus both on mental disorders in the prison population and on the criminal activities of psychiatric patients.

Assessment of Offending Behaviour

Studies of patients at the pre-admission stage conclude that those with a mental illness are more likely to commit violent offences prior to admission to a psychiatric environment (Tardiff and Sweillam, 1980). Lindqvist and Allbeck (1990) and Sosowsky (1978, 1980) in their studies of discharged psychiatric patients showed that such patients have a greater likelihood of offending compared to the general population. Staff should concentrate upon relationships between specific mental illnesses and offending behaviours. This will enable staff to identify symptoms, appropriate treatment and those occasions when the offending behaviours are likely to reappear.

THE NURSE'S ROLE IN MULTIDISCIPLINARY TEAM ASSESSMENT

It is essential for the multidisciplinary team to establish a clear understanding of any potential for future re-offending. Through skilled observation and accurate, unbiased documentation, a detailed and meaningful compilation of relevant life events and indicators of offending behaviour can be produced. This allows the team to assess the possibility of the patient offending or re-offending in the future. To justify a leading role in the assessment process, the nurse must be able to state clearly what is being predicted and how those conclusions have been reached (Monahan, 1981). To prevent incidents recurring there must be stringent monitoring and supervision. Risk assessment should be clearly defined, with particular concerns for the individual being acted upon promptly and efficiently.

Pre-Admission Assessment – the Nurse's Role

Requests for assessments (Box 26.4) to a forensic service can originate from many sources, e.g. prisons, police, Crown and Magistrates' Courts and other psychiatric units. The method of referral for assessment is generally by written request, or by telephone in urgent cases. Once the initial request is received an assessment is carried out both by the consultant psychiatrist and by nursing staff (see the Case study: Pre-admission assessment). This can be done jointly or, more usually, as two separate assessment interviews. When considering unusual or extremely

Pre-admission nursing assessment

Box 26.4

The assessment is compiled from the nursing, medical and other professional agencies' notes, discussions with professionals currently involved in the person's care and with the individual him- or herself. The assessment follows a specific format. As well as basic details, which include age, last known and current address etc. a full developmental history is sought. This is very wide ranging and looks at many features of the individual's background.

It includes:
- education and any associated problems;
- IQ;
- relationships with family, friends and peers;
- employment details;
- management of finances;
- any past hobbies and interests;
- sexual development;
- past hospitalization; major operations, physical illnesses;
- psychiatric problems; treatments; attempts to harm self; any substance abuse;
- current and past offences, plus any periods of imprisonment.

The reason for the referral should also be included in this section. The assessing nurse should attempt to ascertain any problems and stressors either from the notes or the individual during the assessment.

During the initial interview with the patient, the nurse will obtain verbal data but also use observational skills to elicit information. The aspects addressed during this part of the assessment should include:
- appearance;
- personal hygiene;
- any present physical difficulties.

Details of current mental state include:
- mood level;
- ability to communicate;
- concentration;
- eye contact;
- facial expressions and other non-verbal messages;
- diet and sleep pattern plus any related problems;
- level of orientation and any strange beliefs and feelings.

Although the nurse may have written information about the patient's relationships with relatives, friends and peers, he or she should try to determine how the patient views their relationship with others.

Any current hobbies or interests can be identified. It is Important to know home and possible discharge address, as well as the expected support from others on discharge.

The assessing nurse should look at present treatment with the view to:
- the level of cooperation;
- estimated level of insight;
- progress or deterioration;
- medication and current behaviour.

Case Study: **Pre-admission assessment**

Background

David Smith was assessed by an MSU following a request to the Forensic Service from a local prison, where he was on remand awaiting sentencing. David was arrested by the police after wandering around the town, randomly assaulting people and causing damage to property.

He is in his late 30s with a history of mental health problems from his early 20s. These began, he recalls, when he started to believe that neighbours were spreading rumours and were harassing him. He also believed that a local radio station was broadcasting personal information about him and that his neighbours were trying to break into his flat with an axe. He claims that he was dismissed by both the police and Social Services.

David has had many previous admissions to psychiatric hospitals in the past. He had made a number of serious attempts at self-harm and had abused many substances over a number of years. He has a history of both visual and auditory hallucinations, experiencing paranoid ideation occasionally. He also has a criminal history, some of which involves violence towards people.

At the time of the assessment by the Forensic Team, David had no insight into his current situation. He was experiencing auditory and visual hallucinations and suffering paranoid ideas. Beliefs regarding his neighbours and the local radio station persisted and he felt that the only way he could gain recognition for his plight was to explain it to some 'higher authority', a judge for example. Therefore he perceived his arrest as somewhat fortunate. However, in the assessment he said that if the judge did not act on his 'appeals' then he would have to 'take the matter further'. He would not give any indication as to what this entailed or what, if anything, he had planned.

While in prison David began to refuse to take any food or fluids and began to lose weight. He was assessed while in prison and it was evident that his mental state was deteriorating further, so he was transferred to a Medium Secure Unit on Section 48/49 of the Mental Health Act 1983.

The nursing perspective

The assessment interview with David proved a little difficult but not impossible. He appeared confused on occasion, obviously responding to auditory hallucinations with extremely poor concentration.

The nursing staff used the following styles in this assessment:
- A firm (but not threatening) manner with short questions. David had obvious difficulties in staying in one place and kept wandering away.
- Nursing staff allowed him a degree of freedom to walk around the room as he wished, thus reducing his anxieties about the interview without him becoming aggressive or threatening.
- An open approach was used with David — he was given full information as to where the staff came from and the point of the assessment.

After some considerable time, however, it was decided that because of David's mental state a more thorough assessment was needed. When the report was produced one recommendation for David was that he should be admitted to the MSU for a period to:
- Have his medication reviewed.
- Allow the completion of a thorough assessment and his dangerous presentation over a longer period of time.
- Ensure the assessment of his offending behaviour in relation to his mental state and the possibility of his re-offending in the future.

difficult individuals, a psychological assessment may also be required.

Once all information is gathered it should be correlated and a thorough report prepared, including conclusions and recommendations. This is then discussed at a full multi-disciplinary meeting. Suitability for admission will only be considered after other possible avenues for treatment have been considered and discussed fully. It is crucial that as much information as possible regarding offences and offending behaviour is gathered at the time of the assessment as this will act as a baseline for any future plans regarding offending behaviour.

COMPETENCIES 2 AND 3

In the clinical setting, the business-orientated health service, risk management has come to mean a systematic method of recognizing risks in advance and reducing them to a minimum, by examining data and trends from the clinical setting. This should result in, and ensure, safe clinical practice, or at least a reprieve from blame in the event of a disaster, clinical or otherwise.

The Assessment and Management of Dangerousness (a Brief Insight)

A major element of risk management, risk assessment, is associated with assessment of dangerousness, though not exclusively. The term 'risk assessment' implies a systematic process that can be monitored, reviewed and developed to suit changing needs.

In the secure setting, risk assessment is a very important element of patient management (especially if somebody gets it wrong). The major assessment is for dangerousness towards self or others. There needs to be some degree of certainty about a patient's level of dangerousness, as this is particularly relevant to their ongoing treatment programme as well as determining whether they are ready for discharge. Furthermore, knowledge of a patient's degree of dangerousness is imperative in deciding their day-to-day management, level and type of security, and observations required, to determine reactions to stress and other possibly problematic situations and to monitor progress.

Unfortunately, thanks to the popular press, schizophrenia has become the mental illness most associated with the 'crazed killer'. Headlines such as 'frenzied attack', 'maniacal', 'dangerous psycho' all serve to fuel the public imagination. The evidence to support or dispute this is, in itself, conflicting. On the one hand, there is the view that people with schizophrenia are more likely to commit violent crimes than either people with other mental disorders or the population in general (Taylor and Gunn, 1984) while Lindqvist and Allbeck (1990) show that people with schizophrenia commit many more non-violent crimes than violent ones and those that are deemed to be violent are of a minor nature.

The Ritchie Report on Christopher Clunis (Ritchie *et al.*, 1993) stated that it was highly likely that people suffering from schizophrenia who are likely to offend may have become distanced from those with the task of monitoring their condition. The nurse must be aware constantly of the patient's mental health and also have an awareness of episodes of the illness when re-offending, particularly of a violent nature, is likely. If the antecedents are clearly identified and the nurse caring for this type of patient is aware of particular, individual circumstances that are relevant to the patient's history, then with a regular, consistent and quality approach to interventions re-offending will be minimized, effectively managed and hopefully avoided.

What is Dangerousness?

There are numerous definitions of dangerousness (Home Office, Department of Health and Social Security, 1975; Scott, 1977; Walker, 1978). All revolve around the threat, whether real or the propensity to cause serious harm to another. What is evident and more important to the forensic nurse in the clinical setting, is that dangerousness can be coloured by an observer's subjectivity. What an observer thinks about a person, based on what he has said or done (in the past as well as currently) rather than something measurable, may result in judgement about what might happen, rather than what the person is.

Possibly, different leading questions are required in current clinical practice. Health Professionals should stop asking, 'Is the patient dangerous?' and start determining whether the patient 'might behave in a dangerous manner in certain circumstances'.

This latter stance then leads into other avenues of clinical investigation, which can include the following:
- What is the situation?
- What stimuli are necessary?
- What stressors is the patient experiencing?
- How does the dangerous reaction reveal itself?
- How can the dangerous reaction be prevented?
- What techniques and skills need to be utilized?

All these questions need to be asked in the context of the patient responding dangerously to a particular set of stimuli.

The Assessment

Risk assessment has, over the years, become an intrinsic part of most nursing models of care and is tailored to suit the model, which in turn is chosen for its suitability for a particular patient group. Many incorporate histories, responses to certain stimuli, interactions in given situations, levels of functioning and the patient's own perceptions. The assessment of dangerousness is, however, largely the remit of separate testing aimed at exploring recurrence, treatment needs and treatment potential (Pollock and Webster, 1990) in relation to a patient's behaviour and dangerousness.

The nurse's role in the assessment is crucial to gaining an overall picture, as it is only the nurses who monitor the patient's behaviour day and night. The nurse is continually examining the effects of interactions, environment, stimuli, and stressors on the patient's behaviour thus providing important data for assessment of current and future risk (Box 26.5).

Assessment of dangerousness can be broken down into three distinct stages (based on McClelland, 1995).

General history

This should be detailed; criminal, psychiatric and developmental history is required. The history can be taken either formally by psychiatrists, psychologists or nurses, or informally via the day-to-day interactions of the nursing staff. Information can be sought from the patient, their family and friends and even (if relevant and appropriate) victims. Looking at childhood factors as part of the developmental history would highlight any adolescent predispositions towards violent attitudes and behaviour. Detailed information about the index offences or specific behaviours (if a non-offender) should be a prerequisite and a basis for any assessment. Details often overlooked in an assessment are the time, date and location of the offending or dangerous behaviour. This information raises awareness of the patient 'celebrating' anniversaries and also has relevance to possible future discharge arrangements. Details about the victim (age, sex, race and relationship to the offender) should also be included in the assessment. The patient's mental state, both at the time of offending and at interview, will look at stress levels, level of arousal and indications of any psychosis. Establishing a trusting relationship early is essential for a clear, unbiased history. The initial, formal, history taking sessions serve to pave the way for more structured or informal one-to-one sessions.

Information required should also include the patient's aptitude with weapons, their reported and actual access to them, possible weapon collecting behaviour and methods of disposing of them, and any impulsiveness in relation to violent or criminal behaviour.

Box 26.5

Items to be considered in the assessment of dangerous behaviour

1. How does the patient's mental illness correlate with their violent behaviour?
2. How does the patient explain the causes of their violent and dangerous behaviour? (e.g. is it delusion or hallucination based)
3. Can the patient accept the clinical team's explanation of the causes and understand them?
4. How does the violent or dangerous behaviour change with intervention from the clinical team?
5. Are there any other possible causes that may be linked to this behaviour other than the primary diagnosis? (e.g. substance abuse)
6. Has the patient a degree of insight into their behaviour and the need for care and treatment?
7. Do your colleagues share your opinions of the patient's presentation and the severity of the dangerous or violent behaviour and its causes and antecedents?
8. Were there any environmental factors that contributed to the violent or dangerous behaviour?
9. Would a change of care regime bring about any changes to this presenting behaviour? (positively or negatively)
10. Are there any indications why the patient chose a particular victim?
11. Are there any 'trends' evident in the type of victim, which can act to identify potential victim types or groups?

(Chiswick, 1995)

Nature of offending behaviour

The second stage of this crucial assessment is an evaluation of cognitive, affective and situational factors that would motivate the person to commits acts of violence or aggression. As with other parts of the assessment, a holistic approach is necessary as this will aid the most effective assessment of the patient's dangerousness. This stage will look at the patient's perception of any incidents and their version of the events as well as the official account gleaned from deposition papers. The patient's perception both of themselves and their victims, how they expresses remorse (if at all) and any indication of repetitive behaviour in either the near or distant future are important to the predictive nature of the assessment. This element of the assessment will also be pursued by other members of the clinical team looking for evidence of psychopathy, psychosis and other types of personality or behavioural dysfunctions. This continues after any recognized formal stage has been completed.

Predictors

The final stage looks at the prediction of future violence in various environments and what strategies can be employed in any treatment mode. The security level, accommodation and degree of supervision is considered as a result of the information gained from the assessment. How the patient responds to a treatment regime, their immediate environment and how they cope with any stressors they have encountered since admission, will all enable the nurse to make an objective prediction of the patient's compliance levels in the future as well as in the present (see Case study: Prediction of dangerousness). The holistic approach continues during this stage (as during every other) by discussing with the patient all information to determine their reactions and feelings that have bearing on the prediction of future care, treatment and levels of dangerousness.

COMPETENCY 4

The area of offending behaviour and psychopathic disorder is well documented; there is further indication that criminal behaviour is both persistent and serious (Hare *et al.*, 1988). Hart *et al.* (1988) showed that after incarceration, re-offending is likely to occur within 12 months because of the difficulties encountered in supervision.

Management of Psychopathic Behaviours

Follow-up studies of male psychopaths discharged from forensic psychiatric establishments shows that there is an estimated 75% re-offending rate of a violent nature (Harris *et al.*, 1991).

It is evident from studies that to make any impact on the psychopath's offending behaviour will present the care team with major problems (Table 26.3). However, holistic care and group therapies addressing such issues as anger control, victim empathy, assertion and social skill, are important especially when linked with individual work. This should focus on issues such as looking at remorse, victimology, stress management and coping strategies, which all endeavour to make a

Case study: **Prediction of dangerousness**

Background

Terry is in his early 40s, and currently in a high secure special hospital. His first contact with the law and psychiatric services came when he was in his 20s and he began to have fantasies and vivid dreams about killing people. He was admitted to a local psychiatric unit under Section 2 of the Mental Health Act, 1983 for assessment. While he was there his mental state and behaviour deteriorated dramatically and he seriously assaulted a fellow patient with a pool cue.

He was transferred to high secure services following an emergency referral and assessment. During the early years in the special hospital, he presented as volatile and unpredictable, with his assaults being impulsive and indiscriminate. The severity of these assaults increased culminating in the attempted rape and murder of a female member of staff.

Terry spent the next couple of years on a very intensive regime in the special hospital. This was intended to reduce the amount of stimulus to below the level that triggered his assaultive behaviour. There were long periods when he had to be nursed in seclusion. Throughout this period of intensive high secure care, to accompany the nursing interventions that were addressing Terry's psychosis and unpredictable behaviour, the medical staff were endeavouring to determine which combination of medication was suitable to meet his immediate needs.

As Terry become less psychotic and more in touch with reality, the staff were able to ascertain the causes of his assaultive behaviour. It became apparent that years of drug abuse had caused his psychotic breakdown. His assaultive behaviour was as a result of his delusional belief that people wanted to kill him because of some perceived indiscretion against society and that the letting of blood (the murder fantasies) increased his power over women. He accounted for an auditory hallucination by asking, 'Why do they have to come to me to die?' The intensity of the hallucinatons fluctuated, reaching an unbearable point at the peak of his assaultive behaviour.

As the years progressed, Terry's mental state became more stable and his psychosis diminished, so his assaultive behaviour decreased and his immediate security requirements diminished to such a degree that he was transferred to ward where he was allowed more personal freedom and autonomy. Currently, Terry has been on the same medication for a number of years as this has been successful in reducing his psychosis. His assaultive behaviour has decreased to the occasional verbal outburst, which nowadays only rarely results in his becoming physically aggressive. The occasional deterioration in his mental state is quickly remedied by a temporary increase in his medication.

Despite the dramatic changes in Terry's presentation and mental state the general opinion of the multidisciplinary clinical team is that Terry should remain in a high secure environment for some years yet before his referral and possible transfer to a medium secure setting is considered.

When Terry was admitted to the high secure hospital he was considered to be chronically dangerous (Chandley and Mason, 1995) and unlikely to be well or safe enough to be nursed other than in a high secure facility. Over the years Terry has improved sufficiently to now be considered suitable for (eventual) possible transfer to an MSU. However, whether he will ever be ready for discharge into the community is another issue, for the distant future, and a lot of work is required before that stage.

The nursing perspective

In treating Terry over the years the nurses have had continually to assess his mental state, in some cases on a day-to-day basis. This gave some indication of how Terry was going to respond to them at any particular time or situation. By compiling a dossier of dangerous and assaultive behaviours, the staff can have a record of not only how often Terry has assaulted people, but also a comprehensive picture of the antecedents of this behaviour. It also serves as a valuable reference of indicators of mental state deterioration. This evidence-based practice aids the clinical team in the constant struggle to maintain a safe environment for Terry, the staff and his peers while delivering the treatment necessary and appropriate to his immediate needs. At times an element of risk taking is necessary; this is where the dossier is invaluable. Any degree of risk taking needs to be evidence based.

---

psychological change (Brett, 1992) by initiating actions that target the patient's propensities to offend (Burrow, 1993).

There are many personality disorder presentations. What follows acts as an example of one manifestation of this difficult diagnostic group, deliberate self-mutilation.

The Nurse Management of Self-Mutilation

Self-mutilation is a recognized feature of patients diagnosed with psychopathic or borderline personality disorder. The predominant form of mutilation is multiple cuts typically to the forearms but any other part of the body may be used. This is associated with self-burning with cigarettes, repeated overdoses or rapid, large intakes of alcohol or drugs.

Wounds are usually inflicted by broken glass, knives, razor blades or needles. The use of such implements obviously creates a problem for secure environments. The presence of such implements compromises the security regime yet, despite concentrated efforts by nursing staff, patients still manage to

TABLE 26.3 Characteristics of psychopathy

1. Displaying charm and good intelligence — superficially.
2. No evidence of any delusion or irrational thinking.
3. Displays of unreliability.
4. Regularly untruthful and insincere.
5. An inability to learn by mistakes.
6. Poor judgement.
7. Suicide gestures — but rarely carried out.
8. Specific loss of insight regarding behaviour.

(Cleckley, 1976)

---

acquire such 'tools'. This is done by stealth, theft, by acts of property damage and sometimes with the assistance of their peers.

Purpose of self-mutilation

There is a view, corroborated by reports in the literature, that patients who mutilate themselves do so as a result of dysfunctional emotional and coping strategies. A number of the more classic reasons have already been stated. It has been reported (Kafka, 1969; Lester, 1972; Gardner and Butler, 1975; Gardner and Gardner, 1994) that a series of experiences is common to self-mutilators.

Damage to a person's personality results in a cluster of characteristics, which include:
- Feelings of numbness.
- Depersonalization or detachment from surroundings.
- Chronic anxiety.
- Impaired self-esteem.
- Difficulty forming meaningful relationships.
- Hopelessness or helplessness.
- Physical aggression preferred as opposed to verbal expression (usually aimed at self).
- Rage.
- Intrusive, overwhelming thoughts and urges.
- Nightmares.
- Impulsiveness.

Any one, or a combination of any, of these feelings persist until the patient has performed the act of mutilation. This brings feelings of relief from whatever psychological pressure had built up and peace with him- or herself.

One common feature of self-mutilators is that the patient is able (consciously or in a pseudofugue state) to disassociate from the area of mutilation and therefore feels no pain regardless of the depth of the wound The action of cutting and the ensuing blood-letting acts as a catharsis for the patient, enabling them to cope with life and its turmoils again, albeit temporarily in most cases.

Re-opening wounds before and after they have healed, biting out sutures and staples and physically ripping wounds open (sutures and all) are all too common occurrences. Even when the drastic resort of placing a plaster cast over the arm has been used it has been known for the patient to destroy this systematically to gain access to the wound underneath. Similarly it has been known for a patient to secrete a cutting implement (a piece of broken razor, a sliver of glass) into an open wound prior to suturing. It is therefore readily at hand to produce in moments of isolation to carry out this 'necessary' act even after being searched for such implements.

Role of the nurse

It is worth considering at this point the range of experiences the self mutilator is reported to be going through, to try to pave the way for the nurse's understanding of the individual's possible reasons for performing such an internalized aggressive act. It is widely accepted that childhood abuse (physical and sexual) results in an emotionally damaged adolescent and adult. Obviously, the amount of damage is proportional to the amount of abuse, which also affects the amount of treatment required.

The ultimate aim of all treatment programmes should be to alleviate and address the underlying cause of the self-mutilative behaviour rather than focusing on the behaviour in isolation. There is no single correct way to deal with self-mutilative behaviour. The general principles in the management of personality disorders referred to earlier need to be observed. Approaches will depend upon the patient, the patient's skill base, and the therapeutic relationship between patient and staff and the environment and its regime. Approaches to care could include:
- The 'We won't tolerate that sort of behaviour here' approach, though this is not highly recommended as it could engender a response of defiant (self) destructive behaviour.
- Giving the patient extra attention — 'Lets talk it through' — with a view to expressing feelings verbally rather than physically. It could fail, however, if the patient refuses to cooperate.
- Medication. This may be helpful to alleviate any underlying tension but does little or nothing to resolve the psychological need to mutilate and may just result in more determined mutilation next time.
- A structured, behavioural-based management approach. 'Inappropriate behaviours e.g. mutilation) will be discouraged while encouraging more appropriate responses to applied reinforcers that are scientific and research based'.
- Ross and McKay (1979) suggest *not* stopping the mutilation behaviour when it occurs (unless it becomes life threatening) thus reducing the severity of the damage. This is supported by a proactive psychotherapeutic approach to the underlying causes.

Consistency is the key in any form of nursing intervention. These interventions must target needs that have been identified by both patient and nurse. It would be sensible to assume that interventions that enable the patient to express emotion in a less damaging way may include anger, anxiety, assertion training; raising self-esteem and strengthening ego structures. Similarly, counselling could be employed to assist the patient to come to terms with past damaging events, i.e. sexual or physical abuse, and help them to come to terms with the causes for their self-mutilation. Staff must be aware, however, that during the intensive stage of any therapeutic intervention the incidence of self-mutilation may well increase for a period. No matter what strategy is employed, an element of clinical risk-taking is always necessary, especially if one adopts Ross and McKay's approach.

Many people (Crabbe, 1983; Burrow, 1991ab) have looked at this area in an attempt to define the dilemma raised. It has already been accepted that, irrespective of the offence committed, the patient is in need of treatment (rather than punishment) in a therapeutic environment (rather than a penal one) and that the level of security should be the minimum to safeguard the patient, the staff and the public.

Risk Assessment (Therapeutic Risk Taking in a Secure Environment)

It is evident that a large part of the forensic nurse's role centres on control and the maintenance of the local security regime. Counting, searching and monitoring all work to enforce and reinforce this role. Despite security underpinning every aspect of the establishment's existence, many nurses have been involved in development of innovative care and treatment.

An example of therapeutic risk-taking in this context is the use of patient freedom within the secure environment and the operation and practice of a leave system (Box 26.6). Most special hospitals now operate a system whereby certain patients are allowed escorted leave outside the perimeter wall, while others are allowed unescorted leave within the secure campus. This system of extended leaves is inherent to the rehabilitation process in an MSU regime. Internal (or ground) leave is now an accepted risk-taking feature of life in a secure setting. Obviously, the criteria for leave vary from hospital to hospital and between high and medium secure units but the common denominators are mental stability, increased self-responsibility, trust and progress towards discharge. Within an MSU where there is no secure campus, only a perimeter fence surrounding the actual building or part of it, the risk is obviously greater that patients may abscond from either escorted or unescorted leave. What follows is an example of a leave programme for a patient in an MSU and the nurse's role.

The benefits to the patients on a leave programme include:
- Motivation (or re-motivation) — the patient feels that at long last progress he can measure is being made.
- Feelings of trust and responsibility are reinforced.
- Some semblance of control regained over one aspect of life.
- Raised self-esteem.
- The chance to interact with people other than immediate peers and staff.

In most MSUs a leave system has been developed to assist the patient's rehabilitation and continuing treatment. It is based on a four-tier system (five, if no leave is counted). (The system and terminology will not be the same in all settings; this is the system in operation in the author's own MSU.)

Obviously, granting (or suspension) of any leave programme is a multidisciplinary decision with the nurse playing a key role in balancing risk with therapeutic value. The nurse should always discuss the appropriateness and conditions of the leave programme with the patient and, after consultation with colleagues, mutually formulate an agreed programme of graduated leaves. It is inadvisable to try to encourage or let the patient attempt to complete the programme too soon. Observation, continuing assessment and discussion with the patient is essential to ascertain whether they are coping with added stressors placed upon them during this programme (see Case study: Risk taking—a leave programme). There is no set time period for a leave programme. It should proceed according to the progress the patient makes within both it and the overall treatment regime.

For some nurses a patient's index offence may evoke feelings within them that will hinder the development of a truly therapeutic relationship with their patients, if not dealt with in a constructive way. It is, therefore, very important for forensic nurses to strive to show faith, trust and respect for patients despite their past and present behaviour.

Ethical Issues in the Management of the Mentally Disordered Offender

Forensic nurses have a responsibility to take an active role in promoting this patient group in the rest of society, by consciously raising the status of patients to that of people deserving of appropriate health facilities and treatments. The outdated notion that labels mentally disordered offenders as 'criminal lunatics' or 'deviants' hinders the progress of forensic psychiatry.

It can be seen that a conflict of interests arises immediately, in that the demands of the public regarding a mentally disordered offender run counter to meeting his or her needs effectively. At any secure facility the first thing that is evident is perimeter security followed by internal security measures. It has become a part of the forensic nurse's role to supervise, regulate and ensure the continued functioning of the secure environment that enables effective treatment to take place. The

Patient leave profile

Box 26.6

Escorted ground leave
The patient is allowed to go into the immediate grounds of the hospital, outwith the security of the Unit, with staff escort. This is usually for a set time each day.

Unescorted ground leave
This is follows when the patient has completed the escorted phase without causing the escorting staff any concern.

Escorted full leave
The patient has now progressed to an important part of the treatment and re-integration programme. This is where he or she is allowed to leave the grounds of the hospital with staff. This stage usually, though not always, runs side-by-side with the previous one, thereby raising self-esteem and a sense of responsibility. Obviously, if a patient is subject to a restriction order (Sections 41 or 49) then prior permission must be sought from the Home Secretary, accompanied with a detailed proposed plan of outings.

Unescorted full leave
Here the patient is allowed to leave and return to the MSU campus, i.e. outwith the parent hospital grounds. Upon leaving the Unit a detailed description of the patient's clothing and travel itinerary are all recorded. By this stage the patient will have consistently displayed mental stability, no evidence of any dangerous or offensive behaviour and a willingness and responsibility to work towards discharge.

Case Study: **Risk taking — a leave programme**

Background

Frank was on leave from a general psychiatric hospital when he committed an offence that resulted in him being charged with attempted murder. After a period in prison he was transferred to an MSU where he was eventually detained under Sections 37/41 of the Mental Health Act 1983 for treatment and rehabilitation.

An initial assessment concluded that Frank was suffering from paranoid psychosis, displaying symptoms of paranoia, namely suspicious behaviour, irritability and isolation. He also expressed persecutory beliefs that his thoughts were being broadcast to others by the television and radio.

Following an extensive treatment programme Frank's mental state improved and he was being maintained at a suitable level. After assessing the potential risk of absconding and danger to the public, the Multidisciplinary Team decided that the next stage of his rehabilitation would be to allow Frank escorted leave within the hospital grounds. A care plan was formulated, specifying the criteria and length of time for which the leave would be permitted. This was gradually increased, which is consistent with all leave programmes.

The second stage of leave required HO approval due to legislation. This leave was fully escorted leave into the community; the third stage was unescorted ground leave and the fourth and final stage was full unescorted leave.

Nursing perspective

Frank progressed through the first three stages of leave without incident. He behaved appropriately at all times and made no attempt to evade the escorting nurses. His next goal is full unescorted leave. As with all periods of leave, they are planned and discussed before they take place. On return from leave Frank was given the opportunity to discuss any problem areas identified or encountered. Positive feedback was given, along with advice on how to resolve any problems that arose.

The nursing skills used in the implementation of Frank's care plan included:
- Encouraging Frank to take responsibility for initiating the leave.
- Assessing Frank's mental state by observation and discussion prior to each leave.
- Assessment of verbal and non-verbal communications that may suggest a threat of either dangerous behaviour (i.e. a repetition of his offending behaviour) or of him absconding while in the grounds unescorted.
- Offering support and education to resolve actual or perceived problems around using his leave.
- Positive reinforcement in discussion with Frank regarding correct utilization of his leave and displays of appropriate attitude towards his responsibilities within the scope of the care plan and its implementation (i.e. reporting his destination and proposed time of return to staff; no attempts to abscond or to breach the security regime; returning by the time agreed; reporting to staff any problems he may have encountered either with the leave in general or in situations arising during it).
- An open and honest relationship being maintained between Frank and a named nurse so that areas such as 'therapeutic risk taking' and Frank's responsibilities within this process can be discussed freely.

conflict is that this custodial role interferes with and is undertaken irrespective of any therapeutic activity the staff are involved in.

This interest in the patient's well-being can be put under tension at times when a remand or convicted prisoner with a history of asocial behaviour is transferred in. Considerations should be given by nursing staff to the following key issues.

1. Is there the potential for conflict between patient and patient, patient and staff or staff and patient following the admission of certain offender groups, which brings with it the potential for importation of prison culture?
2. Are there possible areas for manipulative behaviour?
3. Is there violence among the patients for reasons other than illness?

In the prison culture where nurses are identified as 'screws' the relationship is determined by security requirements rather than caring, which is a source of conflict in itself in the early days after admission. The nurse must be aware of this potential conflict and the ethical issues that may arise from it. This culture brings with it an inherent distrust for therapeutic activities and the rationale and nursing philosophy behind them. Nursing staff should be vigilant at all times to prevent an over-prevalence of this damaging and threatening culture.

One cannot assume that forensic nurses have never attempted to come to terms with this role conflict. They are certainly qualified, as nurses, to focus upon a specific group of mental disorders. However, there is no formal training in restrictive custody for professional registration and similarly there is no basic training in the management of offending behaviours.

It is in the patient's interest that nursing staff regularly and rigorously monitor behaviour for any signs of deterioration and that the patient is protected from the influences and exploitation of their more manipulative, dangerous or unscrupulous peers.

Some nurses' instinct may be to dislike their client group; others may, from time to time, be affected by the stressors encountered in managing such a demanding patient group. Many may believe, from the infamy surrounding their deeds, that certain offenders will not benefit from treatment or release.

For forensic nurses there is no acceptable argument that allows them to 'conscientiously object' to working therapeutically with mentally disordered offenders. Similarly, it is unacceptable to perceive therapeutic custody as any form of punishment.

Clinical supervision, as discussed in Chapter 10, must be regarded as a necessity for the FPN. This will help lessen the effects of these dilemmas and conflicts and ensure that they do not lead to the development of an unhealthy perspective or inappropriate relationships that will compromise the FPN's role.

SUMMARY

This chapter opened by asking whether there is a need for a professional qualification, equivalent to the RMN, effectively resulting in five basic nurse qualifications being available:

1. Psychiatric Nurse.
2. General Nurse.
3. Children's Nurse.
4. Learning Disability Nurse.
5. Forensic Psychiatric Nurse.

As experienced forensic psychiatric nurses, the authors have their opinions and feelings on this issue, but it is best left for the reader to draw his or her own conclusions from what has been read about skills and competencies, and about the client group and the problems associated with its management, both organizational and clinical. It is worth pointing out, however that if the reader wishes to gain an insight into the developments in this field, then look no further than the nursing journals, especially mental health ones. These regularly include contributions from the people who are considered, by their peers, to be 'product leaders', and also from the very staff that this chapter has highlighted, those who work in the clinical setting.

Hopefully, after completing this chapter the reader will be able to understand and appreciate:

• The development of current day forensic psychiatry and its interface with general psychiatry and other disciplines and agencies.
• The environments and how they interlink with and complement each other.
• The problems and behaviours of this the group dealt with.
• Specific nursing interventions within the specialty.

KEY CONCEPTS

The overall function of forensic psychiatric nursing could be described as:
• Providing health care for people with a recognized mental disorder within conditions of high, medium or low security.
• Protecting the public from such patients' dangerous, violent or criminal propensities.
• Providing conditions of intensive nursing care for those who require this for their self- destructive or other management problems of a non-offending nature.
• Acting in a rehabilitative and assessment role, by providing a 'stepping stone' for patients who are progressing down the security hierarchy on their way to eventual discharge.
• Providing a holistic approach to the treatment and management of the mentally disordered offender, an approach which is best described as 'a complex of interpersonal relations'.
• Needing continually to balance security and risk with therapy and patient needs.
• Providing skills and competencies necessary to maintain high standards of care delivery within the secure setting
• Assessing dangerousness and dangerous behaviour in both current and potential clients.
• Taking a proactive and evidence based approach to the management of dangerousness.
• Assessing offending behaviour for current and future treatment regimes.
• Assessment of the client, especially where there is an element of 'therapeutic risk taking'
• Managing behaviours of patients with personality disorders.
• Having a sound understanding of ethical issues in regard to the management and treatment of the mentally disordered offender.

REFERENCES

Barker P: *Healing lives; mending minds*. Professorship inaugural lecture, Department of Psychiatry, University of Newcastle, 1995 (Unpublished).

Brett TR: The Woodstock approach: One ward in Broadmoor Hospital for the treatment of personality disorder. *Criminal Behav Ment Health* 2:152, 1992.

Burrow S: Inside the walls. *Nurs Times* 89(37):38, 1993.

Burrow S: The treatment and security needs of special hospital patients: a nursing perspective. *J Adv Nurs* 18:1267, 1993.

Chandley M, Mason T: Nursing chronically dangerous patients: ethical issues of behaviour management and patient health. *Psych Care* 2(1):20, 1995.

Chiswick D: Dangerousness. In: Chiswick D, Cope R, editors: *Seminars in practical forensic psychiatry*. London, 1995, Royal College of Psychiatrists.

Cleckley H: *The mask of sanity*. St. Louis, 1976, Mosby.

Crabbe G: Care or control. *Nurs Times* 84(28):19, 1983.

Department of Health and Home Office: *Review of social services for mentally disordered offenders and others requiring similar services*. Reed Committee Report, London, 1992, HMSO.

Department of Health and Social Security: *Report of the working party on security in NHS psychiatric hospitals*. Glancy report, London, 1974, HMSO.

Department of Health and Social Security: *The National Health Service Act*. London, 1977, HMSO.

Department of Health and Social Security: *The Mental Health Act 1983*. London, 1983, HMSO.

Garner R, Butler G: Learning from acts of deliberate self harm: a study of self inflicted injury in a secure unit. *Psych Care* 1(5):197, 1994.

Gardner AR, Gardner AJ: Self mutilation, obsessionality and narcissism. *Br J Psych* 127:127, 1975.

Hare RE, McPherson LM, Forth AE: Male psychopaths and their criminal careers. *J Cons Clin Psychol* 56:710, 1988.

Harris GT, Rice ME, Cormier CA: Psychopathy and violent recidivism. *Law Hum Behav* 15:625, 1991.

Hart SD, Kropp PR, Hare RD: Performance of male psychopaths following conditional release from prison. *J Cons Clin Psychol* 56: 227, 1988.

Home Office and Department of Health and Social Security: *Report of the committee on mentally abnormal offenders*. Butler committee Report, London, 1975, HMSO, Cmnd 6244.

House of Commons: *Second report from the estimates committee: the special hospitals and the state hospital*. London, 1968, HMSO.

Kafka J: The body as a transitional object: a psychoanalytical study of a self mutilating patient. *Br J Med Psychol* 42:207, 1969.

Lester D: Self mutilating behaviour, *Psychol Bull* 78(2):119, 1972.

Lindqvist P, Allbeck P: Schizophrenia and crime: a longitudinal follow up of 644 schizophrenics in Stockholm. *Br J Psych* 157:345, 1990.

McClelland N: The assessment of dangerousness: a procedure for predicting potentially dangerous behaviour. *Psychiatr Care* 2(1):17, 1995.

Ministry of Health: *Special hospitals: Report of working party*. Emery report, London, 1961, HMSO.

Monahan J: *Predicting violence: an assessment of clinical techniques..* Beverly Hills, 1981, Sage.

Pollock N, Webster C: The clinical assessment of dangerousness. In: Bluglass R, Bowden P, editors: *Principles and practices of forensic psychiatry*. Edinburgh, 1990, Churchill Livingstone.

Royal College of Psychiatrists: *Secure facilities for psychiatric patients: a comprehensive policy*. London, 1980, Royal College of Psychiatrists.

Royal College of Psychiatrists & DHSS: Guidelines on the care and treatment of mentally disordered offenders, news and notes (suppl) *Br J Psychiatry* April, 1977.

Ritchie, JH, Dick D, Lingham R: *The report of the inquiry into the care and treatment of Christopher Clunis; presented to the Chairman of North East Thames and South East Thames Regional Health Authorities*. London, 1993, HMSO.

Ross R, McKay H: *Self mutilation*. Toronto, 1979, Lexington Books.

Scott PD: Assessing dangerousness in criminals. *Br J Psychiatry* 131:127, 1977.

Sosowsky L: Crime and violence amongst mental patients reconsidered in view of the new legal relationship between the state and the mentally ill. *Am J Psychiatry* 135:33, 1978.

Sosowsky L: Explaining the increased arrest rate among mental patients: a cautionary note. *Am J Psychiatry* 137:1602, 1980.

Tarbuck P: *Buying forensic mental health nursing: a guide for purchasers*. London, 1994, Royal College of Nursing.

Tardiff K, Sweillam A,: Assault, suicide and mental illness. *Arch Gen Psych* 37:164, 1980.

Taylor PJ Gunn J: Violence and psychosis: effects of psychiatric diagnosis on conviction and sentencing of offenders. *BMJ* 289:9, 1984.

Walker N: Dangerous people. *Int J Law Psychiatry* 11:37, 1978.

World Health Organization: *The ICD-10: Classification of mental and behavioural disorders*. Geneva, 1992, WHO.

FURTHER READING

Chiswick D, Cope R, editors:*Seminars in practical forensic psychiatry*. 1995. Gaskell.

This is a concise account of practical aspects of forensic psychiatry. Key points are summarized and case studies are used as illustrations.

Faulk M: *Basic forensic psychiatry*. Oxford, 1988, Blackwell Scientific.

Dr Faulk has set out in a clear, concise manner issues that are pertinent to the management and treatment of the mentally disordered offender. This is invaluable reading for staff who are either new to this field, or as a reference for those already working in it.

Herbst K, Gunn J, editors: *The mentally disordered offender*. Oxford, 1991, Butterworth Heinemann/Mental Health Foundation.

This book follows the progress of the mentally disordered offender through the system of prison, hospital and community offering areas for debate and investigation. The editors do not arrive at any clear conclusions and this

allows the reader to question further what been has read.

Morrison P, Burnard P, editors: *Aspects of forensic psychiatric nursing*. Aylesbury, 1992, Avebury.

By using a collection of small studies the editors aim to raise and succeed in raising issues that they feel needed clarification. This collection highlights the dichotomous conflict encountered by staff working within the field of forensic psychiatry, and the need for 'therapeutic orientation' while acting as 'social policemen'. Invaluable reading for all forensic nursing staff.

Vaughan PJ, Badger D: *Working with the mentally disordered offender in the community*. London, 1995, Chapman & Hall.

This book offers an in-depth examination of a variety of areas involved in working with this client group including risk assessment, social supervision, primary and secondary interventions.

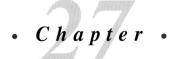

• *Chapter* •

Psychopharmacology

Learning Outcomes

After studying this chapter you should be able to:

• Identify the role of the nurse in psychopharmacological treatments.

• Describe pharmacokinetics and problems of polypharmacy and drug interactions.

• Discuss the mechanism of action, clinical use, and adverse reactions related to antianxiety and sedative–hypnotic drugs.

• Discuss the mechanism of action, clinical use, and adverse reactions related to antidepressant drugs.

• Discuss the mechanism of action, clinical use, and adverse reactions related to mood stabilizing drugs.

• Discuss the mechanism of action, clinical use, and adverse reactions related to antipsychotic drugs.

• Describe mental health nursing practice issues including patient education, promotion of patient adherence and the use of drugs in the control of behaviour.

*U*ndoubtedly the use of pharmaceutical interventions* has enabled many people with mental illness to be both integrated into the community and to maintain independent living. Traditional historical accounts suggest that the pharmaceutical developments of the 1950s encouraged the massive therapeutic and political changes that took place over the following decades. Unfortunately the expectations of pharmaceutical developments to cure, or even treat, mental illness effectively far exceeded the therapeutic gains and limited success that were actually achieved. Inevitably such disappointment, together with the harmful and unwanted side-effects of most of the prescribed medications, produced disillusionment and a backlash against psychiatry and orthodox treatments from service users, some health professionals and the public.

Instead of unnecessary, repressive pharmacological interventions, critics call for empowerment of service users, a continuum of care, and a range of treatments and therapies, including talking therapy, tailored to individuals. All of these are to be framed in personal and social rather than medical terms. Some service users feel so strongly about using medication to treat mental illness that they have called for the setting up of self-help groups for people who wish to withdraw from major tranquillizers (Rogers *et al.*,1993). Mental health nurses are often placed in a difficult position regarding the controversies around pharmacological interventions; acting as the patient's advocate, allowing patients freedom of choice and adhering to their preferences or wishes, often conflicts with giving medication, particularly if it has to be given by force.

The introduction of Project 2000 training with an emphasis on health as opposed to illness has also encouraged many nurses to move away from a biomedical model and to embrace a more health-orientated perspective. While such an approach has many advantages, critics suggest that it does not equip nurses for the realities of caring for people with mental illness and has often encouraged them to hold hostile views about the role of medicines. Concerns have been raised over the level of knowledge and understanding of the drugs commonly used to treat mental illness. Gournay (1996) suggests that at a basic level there is a real concern for nursing educators to think about how medication management can be taught more effectively and comprehensively. However, it is not only Project 2000 graduates who lack the required knowledge. Research continually shows that qualified mental health nurses are often not able to detect even serious side-effects or adverse reactions to neuroleptic medications (Bennett *et al.*, 1995).

ROLE OF THE MENTAL HEALTH NURSE

Psychopharmacology presents many challenges and contradictions for mental health nurses. This chapter describes some of the general principles of drug treatment in psychiatry and discusses some of the main issues facing mental health nurses in contemporary practice. The chapter tries to present a balanced view of drug treatment and how it is complementary to the wide range of psychosocial and interpersonal interventions now used by mental health nurses. Significant advances have been made with drug treatments and these often improve the patient's functioning, allowing other psychological therapies and nursing interventions to take place. However, the knowledge and skills of mental health nurses are also used to encourage patients to take medication in the first instance or to continue with their treatment, for example, by helping to address the problem of a negative attitude to mental illness and to accepting drug treatment. In their day-to-day work most mental health nurses would argue that they adopt an eclectic approach when responding to people's needs and problems. Giving medication is an important aspect of the nurse's work with clients but it is rarely a single isolated event. It is only one of a range of interventions currently used.

Without denying the problems associated with pharmacological treatments, it is important neither to belittle the benefits that have been achieved nor to ignore the opportunities that exist. The government's policy on the provision of community care for people with mental illness and the decision to close many psychiatric hospitals present mental health nurses with many new challenges. The effective use of prescribed medicines is of considerable importance in facilitating the discharge of patients with mental illness back into the community. Medicines are often thought to be essential to maintain independent living and improve quality of life, though the evidence is far from conclusive. For example, research has shown that overall community functioning does not improve in 40–60% of medicated patients (Wallace *et al.*,1988). Relapse resulting from non-compliance with medication is often cited as one of the main reasons people are readmitted to hospital (Thomas, 1996). In a retrospective study of admissions to psychiatric hospital, 43.2% were associated with non-compliance

to treatment (Kent and Yellowlees, 1994). The cost of non-compliance with treatment among people with schizophrenia is estimated at around £100 million per year in Great Britain (Davies and Drummond, 1993).

The shift to provide mental health services in more accessible community-based settings and the reduction of in-patient beds means that, for the most part, only the most severely ill people are now admitted to acute wards. When admission to hospital is required, it is seen as part of the patient's overall treatment plan. Since contemporary mental health services no longer have the in-patient ward as the main focus, the aim of the admission is to stabilize the patient and to discharge them into the community as quickly as possible. As already stated, common reasons for admission include relapse resulting from non-adherence to medication. This requires assessment and close supervision of the patient's drug regime. Another reason for acute admission, particularly in inner city areas, is patients with first episodes of major psychiatric disorder. Patients with acute mental health problems are often very vulnerable and will require careful assessment and the administration of medication to control acute symptoms and alleviate distress. Recent research suggests that people with severe mental illness often have high rates of alcohol and drug abuse (Gray and Thomas, 1996). The management of patients with a dual diagnosis presents many problems for mental health nurses, not least the ability to assess them accurately.

ASSESSMENT
Psychotropic drugs treat symptoms of mental illnesses. They can alter the thought, mood and behaviour of patients, thereby having the power to improve an individual's functioning and well-being. However, not all inappropriate behaviours are treated by drugs and not every personality trait identified in a client is a symptom of illness to be targeted for drug treatment. Similarly, for a significant proportion of patients, other therapies have been found to be just as effective as drug treatment. This means that it is essential to obtain baseline data about each patient before commencing drug treatment. Assessment is a systematic method of collecting information about an individual. Assessment is carried out by all the professionals involved in care. Whereas it will be the responsibility of the psychiatrist to carry out a full mental state examination of the patient, culminating in a diagnosis and the prescription of medication, the nursing assessment focuses on the person's response to illness and identifies those problem areas or needs that will require psychosocial interventions.

Patients with severe and enduring mental illness are often prescribed complex treatment regimens, including polypharmacy of antipsychotics. Officially recommended doses and frequencies of dosing are sometimes ignored, which often results in lack of coordination, missed doses and lack of therapeutic effect. These problems have become so commonplace that the Bethlem and Maudsley Trust has set up a National Medication Review Clinic. The clinic is run by a psychiatrist, mental health nurse and pharmacist, who review all aspects of an individual's medication including drug safety, cost, efficacy, adherence and understanding, and drug suitability. A side-effect profile is compiled using LUNSERS, the Liverpool University Neuroleptic Side-Effect Rating Scale (Day *et al.*, 1995). This is a self-rating scale, which patients find easy to complete in 5–20 minutes. It can be used easily and is but one such rating scale that may be of assistance to nurses. The main points are that nurses should undertake systematic assessments of the side-effects of medication and that they should seek to gather their data as accurately as possible. Other rating scales, such as the abnormal involuntary movement scale

(AIMS) that assesses such movements (National Institute of Mental Health, 1975), may assist them in this (see Box 27.1). Another medication assessment tool for nurses to use in taking a drug history is described in Box 27.2.

COORDINATION OF TREATMENT PROGRAMMES

The broad aim of mental health services is to improve the functioning of people suffering from mental health problems. Improvement in functioning is brought about by devising a

---

Box 27.1

Abnormal involuntary movement scale (AIMS)

A simple method to determine tardive dyskinesia symptoms
Total score equals the sum of the items

Patient identification: _____ Date: _____
Rated by: _____ Treatment period: _____

- Either before or after completing the examination procedure, observe the patient unobtrusively at rest (e.g. in waiting room).
- The chair to be used in this examination should be a hard, firm one without arms.
- After the patient is observed, he or she may be rated on a scale of 0 (none), 1 (minimal), 2 (mild), 3 (moderate), and 4 (severe) according to the severity of symptoms at time of interview.
- Ask the patient whether there is anything in his mouth (e.g. gum, sweet)and if there is, ask him or her to remove it.
- Ask the patient about current dental condition. Ask if dentures are worn. Do teeth or dentures cause any bother now?
- Ask the patient whether he or she notices any movement in mouth, face, hands, or feet. If yes, ask for a description of such movement and to what extent it currently causes bother or interferes with activities.
- 0–1–2–3–4 Have the patient sit in a chair with hands on knees, legs slightly apart, and feet flat on floor. (Look at entire body for movements while in this position.)
- 0–1–2–3–4 Ask the patient to sit with hands hanging unsupported. If male, between legs; if female and wearing a dress, hanging over knees. (Observe hands and other body areas.)
- 0–1–2–3–4 Ask the patient to open mouth. (Observe tongue at rest within mouth.) Have him or her do this twice.
- 0–1–2–3–4 Ask the patient to protrude tongue. (Observe abnormalities of tongue movement.) Have the patient do this twice.
- 0–1–2–3–>4 Ask the patient to tap thumb with each finger as rapidly as possible for 10 to 15 seconds separately with right hand then with left hand. (Observe facial and leg movements.)
- 0–1–2–3–4 Flex and extend patient's left and right arms (one at a time).
- 0–1–2–3–4 Ask the patient to stand up. (Observe in profile. Observe all body areas again, hips included.)
- 0–1–2–3–4 *Ask the patient to extend both arms, outstretched in front with palms down. (Observe trunk, legs, and mouth.)
- 0–1–2–3–4 *Have the patient walk a few paces, turn, and walk back to chair. (Observe hands and gait.) Do this twice.

*Activated movements

Box 27.2

Medication assessment tool

1. Psychiatric medications–for each medication ever taken by the patient obtain the following information:
a. Name of drug
b. Why prescribed
c. Date started
d. Length of time taken
e. Highest daily dose
f. Who prescribed it
g. Whether it was effective
h. Side-effects or adverse reactions
i. If it was taken as prescribed; if not, explain
j. If anyone else in family has been prescribed this drug; if so, for what reason and was it effective.

2. Prescription (non-psychiatric) medications for each medication taken by the patient in the past 6 months and for major medical illnesses if more than 6 months ago, obtain the following information:
a. Name of drug
b. Why prescribed
c. Date started
d. Highest daily dose
e. Who prescribed it
f. Whether it was effective
g. Side-effects or adverse reactions
h. If drug was taken as prescribed; if not, explain.

3. Over-the-counter (non-prescribed) medications–for each medication taken by the patient in the past 6 months, obtain the following information:
a. Name of drug
b. Reason taken
c. Date started
d. Frequency of use
e. Whether it was effective
f. Side-effects or adverse reactions.

4. Alcohol, caffeine, nicotine and street drugs
a. Name of substance
b. Date of first use
c. Frequency of use
d. Summarize effects
e. Adverse reactions
f. Withdrawal symptoms

treatment plan, which can include dimensions such as psychopharmacology, social skills training, cognitive therapy, assistance with housing and finance and other necessary interventions. These various treatments require coordination and tailoring of the programme to the individual. Mental health nurses, through the nurse–patient relationship, are ideally placed to fill this coordinating role.

ADMINISTRATION OF MEDICATION

The administration of medication is recognized as an important part of the mental health nurse's role. It requires not only making sure that the correct prescription is administered safely but, according to the United Kingdom Central Council for Nursing, Midwifery and Health Visiting (UKCC, 1992), thought and professional judgement directed to the following:

1. Confirming the correctness of the prescription.
2. Judging the suitability of administration at the scheduled time of administration.
3. Reinforcing the positive effect of the treatment.
4. Enhancing the understanding of patients in respect of their prescribed medication and the avoidance of misuse of these and other medicines.
5. Assisting in assessing the efficacy of medicines and the identification of side-effects and interactions.

Most NHS Trusts will have local policies for the administration of medication. Nurses are expected to familiarize themselves with these policies and conform to their direction. Some Trusts allow first level nurses to administer certain listed medications that have not been prescribed by a medical practitioner. In such circumstances the nurses must be able to justify the administration and be accountable for the action taken.

MONITORING DRUG EFFECTS

Mental health nurses must be knowledgeable about pharmacology to evaluate the effects of psychopharmacological drugs. These include their influence on patients' symptoms of illness, side-effects and adverse reactions. Certain observations are often required before a patient commences drug treatment, to ensure that a baseline reading is available and deviations are identified as soon as possible. In addition to taking observations on temperature, blood pressure and weight, in some circumstances nurses are now expected to use electrocardiography both prior to patients starting drug treatment and after the treatment has become established, particularly where doses are above the recommended level and while they remain high. The Royal College of Psychiatrists (1996) have recently issued guidelines for the use of electrocardiography in relation to neuroleptics, antidepressants and lithium.

PATIENT EDUCATION AND COUNSELLING

It is good nursing practice to inform patients about the medicines they are to receive and to warn them about the potential side-effects. It is also important to provide similar information for relatives and carers. Mental health nurses should contribute fully to information-giving. Whenever possible verbal information should be backed up with written material. Nurses should make time available to enhance information giving with discussion, allowing patients, relatives and carers plenty of opportunity to ask questions.

INTERDISCIPLINARY CLINICAL RESEARCH DRUG TRIALS

Medicines are subject to human testing prior to licensing and established products may be investigated for new indications. Registered medical practitioners may prescribe unlicensed products for individual patients on a 'named patient' basis. As a member of the multidisciplinary team, the nurse may be involved on several levels, including administering the drug and monitoring its side-effects through to being the principal investigator in the drug trial. All NHS Trusts have their own ethical procedure for carrying out drug trials. It is essential that clinical investigators obtain the prior approval of the local ethical committee before commencing a trial. The ethical committee ensure the product under investigation has received a clinical trial certificate or clinical exemption certificate. For a fuller account of the ethics of drug trials see *Psychiatric Drugs Explained* (Healy, 1993).

PRESCRIBING MEDICATION

Following the report of the Government's Advisory Group on Nurse Prescribing (Department of Health, 1989) nurse prescribing legislation was passed in 1992. This allowed community nurses, with appropriate training, powers to prescribe a limited number of drugs, medicines and appliances. Two years after the bill was published, the Department of Health implemented pilot testing at eight sites. An evaluation of the sites has been carried out and the results are awaiting publication. In the meantime the Department of Health has decided that further testing is required before the case for nurse prescribing is proved. This decision has been strongly criticized by nursing organizations, which argue that across the UK many nurses are already effectively prescribing under local protocols. In some psychiatric hospitals nurses are currently issuing and administering specified drugs to patients under local protocols.

PHARMACOKINETICS

Pharmacokinetics is the study of the action of a drug in the body over a period of time and the movement of that drug both within, and out of, the body. There are four major aspects of pharmacokinetics: absorption, distribution, metabolism and excretion.

Drugs taken orally must first be dissolved in the gut fluid before being absorbed and passed into the bloodstream (absorbtion). Tablets also need to disintegrate before dissolving, which delays the onset of the drug's effects. Intravenous drugs enter the body directly and are thus not absorbed in any way. Drugs given intravenously act much more quickly.

Once in the blood, the drug becomes distributed around the body (distribution). Some of the drug stays in the blood but it usually moves, by diffusion, to different 'compartments' such as the brain or the heart. A measure of this distribution process is volume of distribution; a large volume of distribution (>50 litres) indicates that most of a given dose of a drug is outside the blood and being held in tissue compartments.

As soon as a drug enters the body, the process of removing it from the body begins. This usually involves chemical modification of the drug by the liver (metabolism) to render it less active and to allow it to be excreted by the kidneys (excretion). A few drugs (lithium, for example) do not need to be metabolized before being excreted. Rates of metabolism and excretion are often combined in the term 'clearance'. The clearance of a drug is simply the rate at which the drug is inactivated or removed from the body. The main measure of clearance is the half-life; this is the time taken for the concentration of drug in the blood to fall by a half.

It is important to know a drug's half-life both because this gives an indication of the rate of clearance and because the half-life determines how long it takes to achieve a steady state of concentration. Steady state is said to occur when the amount of drug excreted equals the amount ingested, and it is reached after approximately four to five half-lives. Until steady state is attained, the drug level continuses to rise, and changes after each dose — this means that, until the achievement of steady state, the optimal dose cannot be determined and neither is a blood level reading accurate in determinig a proper dose range. (This is why, after starting administration of lithium, a blood level reading is not taken for 3–4 days.) It may take longer to reach steady state in the elderly because slower liver metabolism and excretion tend to prolong a given drug's half-life.

Another significant aspect of half-life is frequency of dosing. Usually a drug with a half-life of 24 hours or more can be administered once a day after steady state has been reached; a drug with a shorter half-life may need to be administered more often to achieve constant clinical effects. Termination of drug treatment is also affected by half-life. In general, the effects of drugs with a long half-life can last a long time (sometimes weeks) after the last dose. The cessation of drugs with a short half-life usually must be tapered (discontinued gradually over several days or weeks). In general, all psychoactive drugs should be discontinued by slow tapering (over 2 weeks or more).

Over this chapter focuses on the adult patient, however, children and the elderly are also frequently given psychoactive drugs. Generally, adults and children metabolize drugs similarly, although children exhibit a variable response to these drugs. Children must receive lower drug doses because of the smaller volume of distribution corresponding to their lower body weight.

The elderly and newborn are particularly sensitive to psychotropic drugs. For the elderly, drug distribution, hepatic metabolism and renal clearance are all affected by age. If a pregnant woman takes psychoactive drugs before delivery, the infant may experience withdrawal symptoms unless the baby is detoxified from the drug. The infant whose mother takes psychoactive drugs generally should not be breast-fed, although some drugs are thought to be safe to use (Duncan and Taylor, 1995). Patients with liver disease are extremely sensitive to most psychoactive drugs and patients with renal impairment are particularly sensitive to lithium. In both cases, clearance is slowed, making the effect of given doses much greater than would normally be expected.

DRUG INTERACTIONS

Drugs can interact with each other on two levels:
1. Pharmacokinetic — one drug interferes with the absorption, metabolism, distribution, and excretion of another drug, thus raising or lowering the levels of the drug in the blood and tissue.
2. Pharmacodynamic — one drug combines with another to increase or decrease the drugs' effects on an organ system.

Concurrent use of drugs (polypharmacy) can enhance a specific therapeutic action, may be necessary to treat concurrent illnesses and can counteract unwanted effects of one of the drugs being used. Unfortunately, problems have been associated with concurrent drug use; confusion between therapeutic efficacy and side-effects and development of drug interactions, are just two. In general, polypharmacy in psychiatry should be used only when necessary and with caution. Box 27.3 lists guidelines for polypharmacy and Box 27.4 alerts the nurse to patients at a higher risk for drug interactions. The British National Formulary should always be consulted to see if a drug interaction occurs. This reference gives an up-to-date view of the rapidly accumulating data on drug interactions and indicates which interactions are clinically important.

Box 27.3 *Guidelines for polypharmacy*

1. Identify specific target symptoms for each drug.
2. If possible, start with one drug and evaluate effectiveness and side-effects before adding a second drug.
3. Be alert for adverse drug interactions.
4. Consider the effects of a second drug on the absorption and metabolism of the first drug.
5. Consider the possibility of additive side-effects.
6. Change the dose of only one drug at a time and evaluate results.
7. Be aware of increased risk of medication errors.
8. Be aware of increased cost of treatment.
9. Be aware of decreased patient compliance in the after-care setting when the medication regimen is complex.
10. In follow-up treatment, eliminate as many drugs as possible and establish the minimum effective dose of the drugs utilized.
11. Patient education programmes regarding concomitant drug regimens must be particularly clear, organized, and effective.
12. Patient follow-up contacts should be more frequent.

Box
27.4

Increased risk factors for development of drug interactions

- Polypharmacy
- High doses
- Geriatric patients
- Debilitated or dehydrated patients
- Concurrent illness
- Compromised organ system function
- Inadequate patient education
- History of non-compliance
- Failure to include patient in treatment planning

Patients often fail to report over-the-counter medications when asked about current medications. Nurses must be sure to obtain this information.

BIOLOGICAL BASIS FOR PSYCHOPHARMACOLOGY

All communication in the brain involves neurones 'talking' to each other at synapses. These nerve cells are the basic func-

tional unit of the nervous system and the study of this communication process forms the basis of much of the neurosciences. The following description is simplified to present a very basic frame of reference from which to view the rather overwhelming complexity of neuropharmacological mechanisms.

The synapse is a narrow gap separating two neurones (the presynaptic cell and the postsynaptic cell) at a transmission site (Figure 27.1). During neurotransmission a chemical neurotransmitter is released from a storage vesicle (reservoir) in the presynaptic cell, crosses the synapse and is recognized by the receptor on the postsynaptic cell membrane (this recognition is called binding). Receptors are the cellular recognition sites for specific molecular structures such as neurotransmitters, hormones and many drugs. Thus their action is selective for specific chemicals. The neurotransmitter can therefore be considered a key that fits exactly into a lock (the receptor). Neurotransmitters, the chemical messengers that travel from one brain cell to another, are synthesized by enzymes from certain dietary amino acids or precursors. At the synapse, neurotransmitters act as receptor activators (agonists) or, very rarely, inhibitors (antagonists) and trigger complex biological responses within the cell. The chemical remaining in the synapse is either reabsorbed ('reuptake') and stored by the presynaptic cell or is metabolized (inactivated) by enzymes, one of which is monoamine oxidase (MAO).

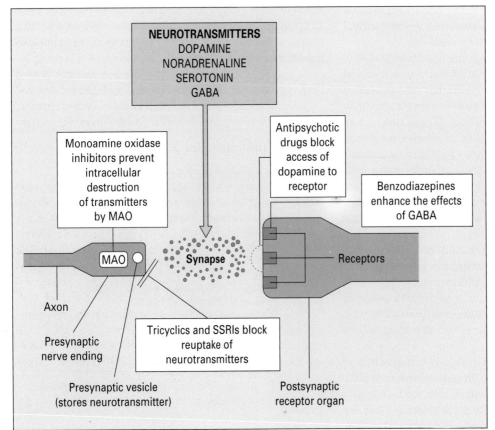

Figure 27.1 Neurotransmission of the synapse

Examples of neurotransmitters include dopamine, 5-hydroxytryptamine (5-HT, or serotonin), noradrenaline, gamma-aminobutyric acid (GABA) and acetylcholine.

Many psychiatric disorders are thought to be caused by an over-response or an under-response somewhere in the complex process of neurotransmission. For instance, psychosis is thought to involve excessive dopamine neurotransmission. Depression and mania are thought to result from disruption of normal patterns of neurotransmission of noradrenaline, serotonin and other neurotransmitters. Anxiety is thought to consists in a dysregulation of GABA and endogenous antianxiety chemicals.

If a particular psychiatric illness is known to result from too much or too little neurotransmission in a particular neurotransmitter system and if the mechanism of action of the psychiatric drugs is understood, then some order in the various pharmacological strategies used in psychiatry can be recognized. This process of cell-to-cell communication at the synapse can be affected by drugs in several important ways:

- Release: More neurotransmitter is released into the synapse from the storage vesicles in the presynaptic cell.
- Blockade: The neurotransmitter is prevented from binding to the postsynaptic receptor.
- Receptor sensitivity changes: The receptor becomes more or less responsive to the neurotransmitter.
- Blocked reuptake: The presynaptic cell does not reabsorb the neurotransmitter well, leaving more neurotransmitter in the synapse and therefore enhancing or prolonging its action.
- Interference with storage vesicles: The neurotransmitter is either released again into the synapse (more neurotransmitter) or is released to metabolizing enzymes (less neurotransmitter).
- Precursor chain interference: The process that 'makes' the neurotransmitter is either facilitated (more neurotransmitter is synthesized) or disrupted (less neurotransmitter is synthesized).
- Synaptic enzyme interference: Less neurotransmitter is metabolized, so more remains available in the synapse.

Not all of the above strategies have yielded clinically relevant treatments. Several have, however, and these are emphasized in this chapter (see Figure 27.1) Antipsychotic drugs block dopamine from the receptor site; tricyclic antidepressants and selective serotonin reuptake inhibitors (SSRIs) block the reuptake of noradrenaline and serotonin and regulate the areas of the brain that manufacture these chemicals; monoamine oxidase inhibitors (MAO inhibitors or MAOIs) prevent enzymatic metabolism of noradrenaline and serotonin, and benzodiazepines potentiate GABA.

Understanding this process has led to the variety of treatment approaches in pharmacotherapy that attempt to change or modify one or more of the steps in neurotransmission. Unfortunately, to date the actions of psychopharmacological drugs are not confined to the specific brain areas that are thought to be associated with psychiatric symptoms. Often, the drugs interact with many receptors other than the ones they are specifically aimed at. These drugs spread throughout the body, causing unwanted drug reactions or side-effects and undesirable drug interactions during concomitant drug therapy. Current psychopharmacological research attempts to understand better the cause of psychiatric illness at the neurotransmission level and the increased specificity of psychopharmacological drugs. The major stumbling block in this approach is that effective drugs have been discovered largely by chance. This means that most of our ideas on the causes of psychiatric illness are based on discovering what exactly an effective drug does and them assuming the disease process must be the reverse of the drug's activity. This 'backwards' process is far from satisfactory.

ANTIANXIETY AND SEDATIVE–HYPNOTIC DRUGS

This section divides antianxiety and sedative–hypnotic drugs into two categories, the benzodiazepines and non-benzodiazepines. The latter group includes several classes of drugs. The benzodiazepines are the most widely prescribed drugs in the world and since the 1960s they have almost entirely replaced the barbiturates in the treatment of anxiety and sleep disorders. Their popularity is related to their effectiveness and wide margins of safety. In recent years their popularity has declined because of their potential to cause tolerance and dependence.

BENZODIAZEPINES
The major indications for the use of benzodiazapines are generalized anxiety disorder, anxiety associated with other psychiatric diagnoses, sleep disorders, anxiety associated with phobic disorders, post-traumatic stress disorder, alcohol and drug withdrawal, anxiety associated with medical disease, skeletal muscle relaxation, seizure disorders and the anxiety and apprehension experienced before surgery.

Mechanism of Action
The benzodiazepines are thought to reduce anxiety because they are powerful potentiators of the inhibitory neurotransmitter, GABA, although the role of GABA in anxiety is not yet clear. A postsynaptic receptor site specific for the exogenous benzodiazepine molecule has been discovered. The search for a naturally occurring antianxiety chemical has recently resulted in the discovery of an endogenous benzodiazepine-binding inhibitor (DBI). The benzodiazepine molecule and GABA do not compete for the same receptor site. However, the benzodiazepines do compete with DBI for a role in neurotransmission, indicating that DBI may be the antianxiety neurotransmitter. Research in this field promises to provide a great deal of information in the future.

Clinical Use

The benzodiazepines are the drug treatment of choice in the management of anxiety, insomnia and stress-related conditions. The target symptoms for use of these drugs are listed in Box 27.5. Major studies are beginning to show that higher-dose benzodiazepines, particularly alprazolam, a triazoloben-zodiazepine, appear to have specific antipanic effects in the treatment of panic disorder.

The specific types of benzodiazepines have no significant clinical advantages over each other. Some of the differences suggested for the use of these drugs can be attributed more to marketing strategies than clinical efficacy. Prescribing decisions can be made, however, on the basis of whether or not the drug breaks down into active metabolites that effectively extend drug half-life (Table 27.1). Duration of action after a single dose can be relatively brief, depending on how rapidly the drug is metabolized and how extensively it is distributed to body tissues (in turn, this is based on lipid solubility). Duration of action at steady state can be much longer. Differences in half-life can be clinically useful. For example, patients with persistent high levels of anxiety should take a drug with a long half-life. Patients with fluctuating anxiety might be better off with short-acting drugs.

When used as hypnotics the benzodiazepines ideally should induce sleep rapidly and their effect should be gone by morning. The rate of absorption of the different benzodiazepines from the gastrointestinal tract varies considerably, thus affecting the rapidity and intensity of onset of their acute effects. Temazepam, diazepam and clorazepate are absorbed fastest, whereas prazepam and oxazepam are absorbed slowest. Antacids or food in the stomach slows down this process. The formulation of all drugs alters their absorption rate; liquids are absorbed more quickly than tablets or capsules. Any of the benzodiazepines can be an effective sedative–hypnotic when administered at bedtime.

Benzodiazepines can be used to suppress the alcohol withdrawal syndrome. The concomitant use of alcohol and benzodiazepines can be dangerous because it produces extreme sedation and respiratory depression.

Box 27.5

Target symptoms for antianxiety and sedative–hypnotic benzodiazepines

Psychological
Vague sense of irritability and uneasiness
Sense of impending doom or panic
Insomnia

Physical
Flushed skin
Hot or cold flushes
Sweating
Dilated pupils
Dry mouth
Nausea or vomiting
Diarrhoea
Tachycardia, palpitations
Dizziness, light-headedness
Shortness of breath
Hyperventilation, with paraesthesias
Tremor
Restlessness
Headache
Urinary frequency

TABLE 27.1 Benzodiazepines

DRUG	Approximate equivalent dose	Dose range (mg/day)	Duration of action	Licensed as hypnotic?	Licensed as anxiolytic?	Forms available
Alprazolam	0.5	0.75–3.0	M	N	Y	tabs
Bromazepam	3	3–60	M	N	Y	tabs
Chlordiazepoxide	10	30–100	L	N	Y	tabs, caps
Clorazepate	7.5	7.5–22.5	L	N	Y	caps
Diazepam	5	5–30	L	Y	Y	tabs, liq, inj
Flunitrazepam	0.5	0.5–2.0	L	Y	N	tabs
Flurazepam	15	15–30	L	Y	N	caps
Loprazolam	1	1–2	S	Y	N	tabs
Lorazepam	1	1–4	M	Y	Y	tabs, inj
Lormetazepam	1	0.5–1.5	S	Y	N	tabs
Nitrazepam	5	5–10	L	Y	N	tabs, liq
Oxazepam	15	45–120	M	Y	Y	tabs
Temazepam	10 (mg)	10–40	S	Y	N	caps/tabs, liq

S = <12 hours (short)   M = 12–24 hours (medium)   L = <24 hours (long)

Some patients may need to take antianxiety drugs for extended periods, however the drugs have their drawbacks, of which dependence is the most importance, and should always be used with non-pharmacological treatments for the patient with chronic anxiety. Psychotherapy, behavioural techniques, environmental changes, stress management and an ongoing therapeutic doctor–patient relationship continue to be important in the treatment of anxiety disorders.

Most experts believe that treatment with benzodiazepines should be brief, used during a time of specific stress. The British National Formulary recommends 2–4 weeks. Those drugs with a long half-life (longer than 18–24 hours) can be given once a day. Drugs with a short half-life (8–15 hours) need to be given more frequently; they can be taken as required for increased symptoms of anxiety, at the time such symptoms occur. The patient should be observed frequently during the early days of treatment to assess target symptom response and to monitor side-effects so that the dose can be adjusted.

Some patients do require long-term antianxiety medication treatment but this should be avoided where possible. In long-term use, tolerance develops (higher doses are needed to give the same effect) and dependence or addiction are very often seen. Both of these problems are more common with potent, short-acting drugs such as lorazepam. In general, benzodiazepines should be used intermittently and for short periods.

Concentrations of benzodiazepine drugs in the blood have not yet been firmly correlated to clinical effects. All benzodiazepines are rapidly absorbed by mouth. The injectable benzodiazepines such as lorazepam and midazolam have been proved reliable when administered in the deltoid muscle and lead to rapid and predictable rises in the blood level when used intravenously. (NB diazepam should not be given intramuscularly since it damages tissue and has erratic absorption.) When given intravenously, administration should be slow (over 1 minute) and direct, not mixed in an IV infusion, because plastic tubing absorbs the drug and the drug can precipitate when mixed with saline or dextrose.

Another clinical indication for the use of benzodiazepines is as a sedative–hypnotic to improve sleep. Insomnia (poor sleep) includes difficulty falling asleep, difficulty staying asleep and awakening too early. It is a symptom with many causes and often responds to non-pharmacological strategies such as talking about problems, increased daytime exercise and physical comfort measures at night. Drugs to induce sleep have their place but should be used with discretion and are never a substitute for good nursing care.

Adverse Reactions

Because the benzodiazepines have a very high therapeutic index, overdoses of benzodiazepines alone almost never cause fatalities. The effect of benzodiazepines can be reversed by the specific antagonist, flumazenil. Side-effects of benzodiazepines are uncommon, dose related and almost always harmless. Table 27.2 summarizes these reactions and nursing considerations. The benzodiazepines generally do not live up to their reputation of being strongly addictive if they are discontinued very gradually, if they have been used for appro-

TABLE 27.2 Benzodiazepine side-effects and nursing considerations

Side-effects	Nursing considerations
Acute/common	
Drowsiness, sedation	Encourage activity, avoid driving.
Ataxia, dizziness	Caution with activity, beware falls.
Feelings of detachment	Encourage socialization.
Increased hostility	Observe carefully and be alert for signs of disinhibition.
Anterograde amnesia	Patient cannot recall events that occur when drug is active.
Long-term/common	
Tolerance to effects	Use only short-term whenever possible.
Dependency	Do not use in those with alcohol misuse.
Rebound insomnia/anxiety	Discontinue very slowly.
Rare/idiosyncratic	
Weight gain	Encourage weight control.
Headache	Give paracetamol.
Confusion	Reduce dose.
Gross psychomotor impairment	Reduce dose.
Depression	Withdraw therapy where possible; may give an antidepressant.
Paradoxical rage reaction	Withdraw therapy.

Box 27.6 *Benzodiazepine withdrawal syndrome*

Usually worsens several days after taper begins, increases over several weeks, then subsides. Minimize by slowing taper.

Mild Symptoms	Severe symptoms
Tremulousness	Psychosis
Insomnia	Seizures
Dizziness	
Headaches	
Tinnitus	
Anorexia	
Vertigo	
Blurred vision	
Agitation	
Anxiety diarrhoea	
Hypotension	
Hyperthermia	
Neuromuscular irritability	

priate purposes and if their use has not been complicated by other factors such as chronic use of barbiturates or alcohol.

Tolerance does develop to the sedative effects of benzodiazepines but it is unclear whether induced sleep or antianxiety effects promote tolerance. These drugs should be discontinued relatively slowly to minimize withdrawal symptoms and rebound symptoms of insomnia or anxiety. The general rule is a decrease by 5% of the dose each 1 to 3 days, although this varies. All benzodiazepines, regardless of half-life, should be discontinued by tapering. When these drugs are discontinued too rapidly or are stopped precipitously, especially after prolonged use of high doses, a benzodiazepine withdrawal syndrome can occur as described in Box 27.6. If this occurs, the dose must be raised until symptoms are gone and then tapering can be resumed at a slower rate.

An elderly patient is more vulnerable to side-effects because the ageing brain is more sensitive to sedatives and because hepatic metabolism of benzodiazepines is slowed in the elderly. Dosing ranges from quarter to half of the actual daily dose (see current BNF). The benzodiazepines with no active metabolites (see Table 27.1) are less affected by liver disease, the age of the patient, or drug interactions. Use of benzodiazepines during pregnancy, especially during the first trimester has been associated with infant cleft lip and cleft palate, multiple congenital deformities and intrauterine growth retardation. When used late in pregnancy or during breast-feeding, these drugs have been associated with floppy infant syndrome, neonatal withdrawal symptoms, poor suckling and hypotonia.

NON-BENZODIAZEPINES

The advantages of the benzodiazepines compared with most other antianxiety and sedative–hypnotic agents have led to greatly decreased use of some of the older, more dangerous non-benzodiazepines such as barbiturates.

Non-benzodiazepine anxiolytics and sedative–hypnotics, listed in Table 27.3, are used when alternatives to benzodiazepines are sought or when preferred by clinicians or patients. Two exceptions to this are zopiclone and zolpidem, which are licensed for short-term (up to 28 days) treatment of insomnia. Structurally unrelated to benzodiazepines, zolpidem and zopiclone appear to bind more selectively to neuronal receptors involved in inducing sleep. They are usually well-tolerated and appear to have little antianxiety, anticonvulsant, or muscle-relaxant properties. Side-effects include daytime drowsiness, dizziness, a metallic taste (zopiclone) and diarrhoea (zolpidem).

The barbiturates have been largely replaced by the benzodiazepines, the former are still sometimes used. However, barbiturates have numerous disadvantages to their antianxiety effects: tolerance develops, they are more addictive, they cause serious, even lethal withdrawal reactions, they are dangerous in overdose and cause central nervous system (CNS) depression and they can cause a variety of dangerous drug interactions.

The propanediol drug, meprobamate, has also dropped in popularity. Its adverse effects, drug interactions, potential for abuse and withdrawal syndromes are similar to those observed with barbiturates. Also, many studies show meprobamate to be no more effective than a placebo.

Chloral hydrate can cause gastrointestinal irritation and causes a variety of drug interactions. Tolerance, physical dependence, addiction, and a withdrawal syndrome are all problems. It is available in an number of guises (Table 27.3)

Antihistamines, especially hydroxyzine and promethazine, are usually not as effective as the benzodiazepines; they cause sedation but do not cause physical dependence or abuse. A disadvantage of the antihistamines is that they lower the seizure threshold.

Propranolol blocks beta-noradrenergic receptors both centrally and in the peripheral cardiac and pulmonary systems. This drug probably decreases certain physiological symptoms of anxiety, especially tachycardia, rather than centrally acting on anxiety. More research is needed to define a proper role for propranolol in the treatment of anxiety.

Buspirone, a non-benzodiazepine anxiolytic drug, has been the subject of much discussion. It appears to be a potent antianxiety agent with no addictive potential but its anxiolytic effects take a week or more to develop. Buspirone is effective in the treatment of anxiety and does not exhibit muscle-relaxant or anticonvulsant activity, interaction with CNS depressants or sedative–hypnotic properties. It is not effective in the management of drug or alcohol abuse.

ANTIDEPRESSANT DRUGS

Research on the biology of depression has led to many discoveries and even more questions. It has been proposed that either serotonin or noradrenaline or both are reduced in depression and that an excess of noradrenaline is produced in mania. The biological understanding of antidepressant drugs supports this theory: MAO inhibitors 'inhibit' the metabolism of these neurotransmitters and tricyclic antidepressants and even more specifically, the SSRIs block their reuptake at the presynaptic neurone. Both these mechanisms allow more neurotransmitter to remain in the synapse, thereby solving the perceived functional 'deficit' in depression. Several factors challenge the simplicity of this theory: 25% to 30% of people who are depressed do not respond to antidepressant drugs and several new drugs that seem to be effective antidepressants do not appear to affect noradrenaline or serotonin levels. There is also evidence that antidepressants regulate the locus ceruleus, the part of the brain that makes most of the noradrenaline.

The primary clinical indication for use of antidepressant drugs is major depressive illness. These drugs are also useful in the treatment of panic disorder and nocturnal enuresis in children. A variety of preliminary research studies suggest that they are useful in attention deficit disorders in children and in narcolepsy. The SSRIs are receiving attention for their effectiveness in treating bulimia and for their apparently low side-effect profile and toxicity. The tricyclic antidepressant (TCA) clomipramine (Anafranil) and the SSRIs, fluoxetine (Prozac), fluvoxamine (Faverin) and paroxetine (Seroxat), have been

shown to be effective in obsessive–compulsive disorder. Table 27.4 shows the side-effect profiles of these medications.

Patients who respond to the initial course of treatment with antidepressants should continue taking the drugs at the same dosage for at least 6 months afterwards. This is known as continuation treatment. If they are symptom-free during this time, they can then be tapered off the medication. Patients who have relapses after the continuation-treatment is ended may require long-term or even life-long maintenance medication to prevent recurring depression (Depression Guideline Panel, 1993). Patients who have had three or more episodes of major depression have a 90% chance of having another and are therefore potential candidates for long-term maintenance antidepressant medication. The maintenance medication given is generally of the same type and dosage found to be effective in the acute phase of treatment.

TRICYCLIC ANTIDEPRESSANTS
The tricyclic drugs have been the mainstay of the treatment of depression for several decades They have undoubted efficacy and their adverse effects are well known but they are poorly tolerated and toxic in overdose, Potentially better alternatives have led to a decline in the use of tricyclics over the past 5–10 years.

TABLE 27.3 Antianxiety, sedative hypnotic drugs — non-benzodiazepines

Drug	Brand name	Duration of action
	Barbiturates	
Amylobarbitone	(sodium) Amytal	L
Quinalbarbitone	Seconal	L
	Propanediols	
Meprobamate	Equanil	M
	Chloral derivatives	
Chloral hydrate	Noctec	S
Chloral betaine	Welldorm	S
Triclofos sodium	-	S
	Antihistamines	
Promethazine	Phenergan	M
Diphenhydramine	Medinex	M
	Beta-blockers	
Propranolol	Inderal	S
	Anxiolytic (5-HT₁ agonist)	
Buspirone	Buspar	S
	Imidazopyridine	
Zolpidem	Stilnoct	S
	Cyclopyrrolone	
Zopiclone	Zimovane	S
	Thiamine derivative	
Chlormethiazole	Heminevrin	S

S = <12 hours (short)   M = 12–24 hours (medium)   L = <24 hours (long)

Mechanism of Action

TCAs include some drugs that are structurally dissimilar, however, the drugs in this class are quite similar in their clinical effects and adverse reactions. They are divided into several categories, tertiary amine tricyclics (or parent drugs), secondary amine tricyclics (or metabolites) and a newer non-tricyclic (or heterocyclic) group of drugs.

Clinical Use

Antidepressant drugs are listed in Table 27.4. Elderly patients and patients with a concomitant physical illness may require lower doses of these drugs than physically sound adults and careful assessments for side-effects while they are taking the drugs. For patients with an acceptable cardiac history and an ECG within normal limits, TCAs are safe and effective in the treatment of acute and long-term depressive illness.

Unfortunately, all antidepressants must be taken for 3–4 weeks or longer before a full therapeutic response is evident. Table 27.5 describes the target symptoms for these drugs in the approximate order of the time it takes for each symptom to begin to improve. When caring for suicidally depressed patients, it is important to remember that they become more motivated and begin to look better long before their subjective depressive feelings and suicidal thoughts are relieved. The nursing care plan must include suicide assessments and suicide precautionary measures for weeks after these patients begin to look less depressed.

Two of the tricyclic antidepressants, imipramine and nortriptyline, have been rigorously studied in relation to blood plasma levels, which have been correlated with clinical response.

TABLE 27.4 Antidepressant relative adverse effects

Drug	Brand name	Sedation	Cardio-toxicity	Anticholinergic effects	Forms available
Tricyclics (in order of introduction)					
IMIPRAMINE	Tofranil	++	+++	+++	tabs, liq
AMITRIPTYLINE	Tryptizol	+++	+++	+++	tabs/caps, liq, inj
DESIPRAMINE	Pertofran	+	++	++	tabs
NORTRIPTYLINE	Aventyl	+	++	++	tabs
PROTRIPTYLINE	Concordin	−	+++	++	tabs
TRIMIPRAMINE	Surmontil	++++	+++	++	tabs, caps
DOXEPIN	Sinequan	+++	++	++	caps
DOTHIEPIN	Prothiaden	+++	+++	++	tabs, caps
CLOMIPRAMINE	Anafranil	++	+++	++	tabs/caps, liq, inj
LOFEPRAMINE	Gamanil	+	+	+	tabs
AMOXAPINE	Asendis	++	+	++	tabs
Atypical antidepressants					
VILOXAZINE	Vivalan	+	+	+	tabs
MIANSERIN	Bolvidon/Norval	+++	−	+	tabs
TRAZODONE	Molipaxin	+++	+	−	caps, liq
MAPROTILINE	Ludiomil	++	++	++	tabs
NEFAZODONE	Dutonin	+	−	+	tabs
VENLAFAXINE	Efexor	+	−	+	tabs
Selective Serotonin Reuptake Inhibitors (SSRIs)					
CITALOPRAM	Cipramil	−	−	−	tabs
FLUVOXAMINE	Faverin	+	−	−	tabs
FLUOXETINE	Prozac	−	−	−	caps, liq
SERTRALINE	Lustral	−	−	−	tabs
PAROXETINE	Seroxat	+	−	−	tabs
Monoamine Oxidase Inhibitors (MAOIs)					
ISOCARBOXAZID	Marplan	+	++	++	tabs
PHENELZINE	Nardil	+	+	+	tabs
TRANYLCYPROMINE	Parnate	-	+	+	tabs
Reversible Inhibitor of Monoamine Oxidase A (RIMA)					
MOCLOBEMIDE	Manerix	-	-	-	tabs

The monintoring of plasma levels for most other antidepressants, although less a extensively researched area, also sometimes used (Orsulak, 1989). Plasma level guidelines are helpful, since individual patients metabolize drugs at different rates. The monitoring of a plasma level can help keep the dose within the therapeutic range, and also ensures that enough drug is in the patient's system to be effective. Some drugs, particularly nortriptyline, have a 'therapeutic window' (the range within which the drug is considered to be therapeutic) and a plasma level below or above the range limits results in a decrease in antidepressant effectiveness. Blood for a plasma level check should be drawn 8–12 hours after a single (usually bedtime) dose. Measuring the level soon after drug ingestion results in an artificially high level, representing the peak of drug metabolism rather than the average steady-state plasma level. There is still a considerable amount of debate over the usefulness of TCA level monitoring (Taylor and Duncan, 1995a) and this technique is used much less often in the UK than in the USA.

It is estimated that about 25% of patients with depressive illness have chronic or recurrent symptoms. These patients may benefit from a maintenance regimen of antidepressant drugs. A TCA that has been successful in the past for a particular patient may be continued indefinitely. Full treatment doses are usually required.

Adverse Reactions

The nurse should know the common side-effects of the tricyclic antidepressants and their nursing treatments, as described in Table 27.6. Most of these side-effects cause minor discomfort but some can produce serious illness. These drugs have no known long-term adverse effects; tolerance to therapeutic effects does not develop and persistent side-effects often can be minimized by a small decrease in dose. Because TCAs do not cause physical addiction, psychological dependence or euphoria, they have no abuse potential. Their long half-life (24 hours or longer) allows them to be conveniently administered once a day, at night for most people. If the bedtime dose interferes with sleeping or causes nightmares (both very rare) the dose should be given in the morning or divided into several doses throughout the day. This, however, may lead to daytime sedation.

Patients with bipolar illness may be switched into mania by TCAs. They should be watched closely for increased activity, greater difficulty concentrating and eating and decreased sleeping patterns. All antidepressants can precipitate mania.

Because TCas are among the most toxic substances available when taken in excessive amounts, overdoses and suicide attempts using them are extremely serious and require emergency medical attention. Ingestion of 1000 to 3000 mg can be lethal. This may represent barely a 1-week supply of medication. For in-patients, mouth checks may be necessary. Even for out-patients who are not suicidal, antidepressants should be prescribed in small amounts and frequent assessments should be made. Accidental overdoses in children whose parents are taking an antidepressant are unfortunately common and often lethal. The health teaching and care of these patients should include an assessment of household members, and patients should be cautioned to keep these drugs in the childproof bottles received from the pharmacy, to keep the drugs out of the reach of children, and to discard leftover drugs when pharmacotherapy is completed.

Most patients develop tolerance to the side-effects of antidepressants and most side-effects are dose related; thus they can be minimized by increasing the dose gradually when the drug is first prescribed. This gives the patient time to adjust physiologically to the drug. This is especially true when antidepressants are used to treat panic disorder. Patients with panic disorder are particularly sensitized to any drug side-effects that remind them of symptoms of anxiety or panic attacks (e.g. rapid heartbeat, dizziness, nausea, blurred vision). In the case of severely depressed patients or those who are suicidal, doses are generally increased more rapidly to minimize the time it takes to reach steady state and therapeutic effectiveness.

TCAs, like all psychotropic drugs, should be avoided if possible during pregnancy, especially in the first trimester. However, these drugs have been given throughout pregnancy without harmful effect on the fetus and their use should be considered if a pregnant woman is severely depressed, especially if suicide is a risk.

SELECTIVE SEROTONIN REUPTAKE INHIBITORS

SSRIs not only represent a new approach to the treatment of depression and perhaps other disorders but also may provide a safer treatment option. The SSRIs inhibit the reuptake of serotonin at the presynaptic membrane. This results in an increase of available serotonin in the synapse and therefore at the postsynaptic membrane. Thus these drugs promote the neurotransmission of serotonin in the brain. Their selectivity for serotonin means they do not have significant effects at the transmission sites of other neurotransmitters and therefoe have fewer side-effects (Charney *et al.*, 1990).

TABLE 27.5 Antidepressant target symptoms

Onset of drug effect	Symptom
Week 1	Insomnia, anxiety — *especially if drug is very sedative* Appetite disturbance
Week 2	Fatigue Somatic complaints Agitation Retardation
Week 3	Low mood Suicidal thoughts Subjective feelings of depression — *anhedonia, poor self-esteem, pessimism, helplessness, guilt, sadness*

TABLE 27.6 Tricyclic antidepressant side-effects and nursing considerations

Side-effects	Nursing considerations
Central nervous system	
Drowsiness	Build up dose slowly. Give drug at night. Drowsiness tends to wear off. Change to a different drug if it persists. Avoid driving.
Confusion	Quite common in the elderly. Change to a different drug.
Lowered seizure threshold	Avoid amoxapine, maprotiline. Increase dose slowly with others.
Tremor, ataxia	Quite rare; tolerance develops.
Extrapyramidal side-effects	Rare, except with amoxapine.
Mania	Occurs with all antidepressants, especially in patients with bipolar disorder. May have to stop drug.
Psychosis	More common in elderly, may be related to anticholinergic effects.
Gastrointestinal	
Heartburn, nausea, vomiting	Administer with or after meals or at bedtime.
Constipation	Encourage fibre intake. May give stimulant laxative.
Dry mouth	Very common, tends to wear off. May change drug if severe.
Haematological	
Leucopenia, thrombocytopenia	Very rare but should be monitored as routine practice.
Agranulocytosis (very low neutrophil count with fever and malaise; may be fatal)	Very rare. Discontinue drug and admit to hospital and ? isolate. Intravenous antibiotics usually needed. Never give drug again. Use a different chemical class in future.
Hepatic	
Hepatic toxicity — jaundice, abnormal LFTs, fever	Abnormal LFTs quite common but usually benign. If jaundice develops, discontinue drug. Give a drug from a different class.
Endocrine	
Amenorrhoea	Rare — only with amoxapine.
Menstrual irregularities	Rare — change to different class.
Ophthalmic	
Blurred vision	Quite common but tends to wear off. May change drug.
Cardiovascular	
Postural hypotension — dizziness	Increase dose slowly. Monitor BP sitting and standing. May change drug. Tends to wear off.
	Not dangerous and tends to wear off. Reassure patient.
Tachycardia	Baseline ECG needed for comparison. Withdraw drug if any ECG changes noted during treatment.
ECG changes	Rare but avoid using tricyclics in patients with recent MI or in heart block. May also avoid if any cardiac problems present.
Sudden death	
Cutaneous	
Rash, photosensitivity	Rare. Give antihistamine, change antidepressant.
Genitourinary	
Changed sexual desire, delayed orgasm	Effect is unpredictable. Change drug, moclobemide has few sexual adverse effects.
Urinary retention	Withdraw drug immediately. Switch to trazodone or an SSRI.
Withdrawal syndrome	
Malaise, dizziness, anxiety	Common if treatment >6 weeks. Withdraw over 2–4 weeks.
Intoxication syndromes	
Overdose	Treat aggressively. Transfer to general hospital.
Anticholinergic intoxication — confusion, anxiety, seizures	Withdraw all anticholinergic drugs. May give physostigmine to reverse effect.
Miscellaneous	
Weight gain, tinnitus, allergic reaction	Rare. Change drug or give smaller dose. Give chlorpheniramine if allergic reaction is severe.
Sweating	Common, especially at night. Try a drug from a different class.

TABLE 27.7 SSRI adverse effects and nursing considerations

Side-effects	Nursing considerations
Nausea	Give after meals or at bedtime. Tends to wear off. May use cisapride.
Diarrhoea	Ensure adequate hydration. Use antidiarrhoeals.
Insomnia	Give in the morning.
Dry mouth	Quite rare; wears off.
Nervousness, anxiety	Use relaxation techniques. Reduce dose. Tends to wear off.
Headache	Use paracetamol. Change drug if problem persists.
Male sexual dysfunction	May use cyproheptadine or drug holiday. May be dysfunction-beneficial in premature ejaculation.
Female sexual dysfunction	May use cyproheptadine or drug holiday.
Drowsiness	Quite rare, wears off.
Sweating	Quite rare, wears off. Use loose-fitting cotton clothing.
Rash (fluoxetine)	Withdraw drug.
Hypertension (venlafaxine)	Withdraw drug.

A recently introduced antidepressant, venlafaxine (Efexor) raises the levels of serotonin and noradrenaline. Hence it has a broader spectrum of pharmacological activity and is therefore called a non-selective uptake inhibitor or SNRI (serotonin–noradrenaline reuptake inhibitor). This dual action is claimed to be unique and to offer improved efficacy. However, there is little to support either claim. Besides, most TCAs can be termed SNRIs because they usually affect serotonin reuptake (e.g. clomipramine) and are metabolized to compounds that affect noradrenaline reuptake (e.g. desmethylclomipramine).

The SSRIs have antidepressant effects comparable to those of the other classes of antidepressant drugs, yet without significant anticholinergic (constipation, dry mouth), cardiovascular (hypotension, arrhythmias) and sedative side-effects. They also do not cause weight gain, thus making them more acceptable to patients with bulimia and to other individuals who are concerned about gaining weight. In addition, they are relatively safe in overdose. These properties have made them very popular in the short period of time that they have been available, even though they are much more expensive than many of the older tricyclic compounds. The SSRIs frequently cause nausea and agitation and so are poorly tolerated by some patients. Debate continues on the question of whether the SSRIs are, in general, better tolerated than TCAs. Table 27.7 lists the side-effects of and nursing interventions for the SSRIs currently available. The next few years will undoubtedly see several new SSRIs approved and marketed.

MONOAMINE OXIDASE INHIBITORS

MAOIs are very effective antidepressant and antipanic drugs that have been perhaps under-used and overly feared. The MAOIs currently used in psychiatry are listed in Table 27.4. Because of the potential for a hypertensive crisis when tyramine-containing foods and certain medicines are taken along with these drugs, careful health teaching combined with relia-

bility of patients is quite important. The patient must avoid certain foods, drinks, and medicines, must know the warning signs, symptoms and even treatment of a hypertensive crisis (Box 27.7) and must be taught the commoner side-effects of MAOIs (Table 27.8). For various indications these drugs are effective and are safe when used as prescribed. They generally cause fewer anticholinergic, sedative, and cardiovascular effects than TCAs. They are non-addictive (with the possible exception of

Box 27.7 *Signs and treatment of hypertensive crisis during MAOI medication*

Warning signs
Increased blood pressure, palpitations, frequent headaches

Symptoms of hypertensive crisis
Sudden elevation of blood pressure
Explosive headache–occipital; may radiate frontally
Head and face are flushed and feel 'full'
Palpitations, chest pain
Sweating, fever
Nausea, vomiting
Dilated pupils
Photophobia
Intracranial bleeding

Treatment
Withhold next MAOI dose
Do not lie patient down (elevates blood pressure in head)
IM chlorpromazine 100 mg, repeat if necessary. (Mechanism of action: blocks norepinephrine)
IV phentolamine, administered slowly in doses of 5 mg. (Mechanism of action: binds with norepinephrine receptor sites, blocking norepinephrine)
Fever: Manage by external cooling techniques

TABLE 27.7 MAOI adverse effects and nursing considerations

Adverse effect	Nursing considerations
Postural light-headedness, dizziness	Advise patient to take time when standing up. Use support tights. Reduce dose.
Constipation	Encourage high fibre diet. May use bulk-forming laxatives.
Delayed orgasm	Reduce dose. Separate dose and sexual activity by as much time as possible.
Muscle twitching	Quite rare. Reduce dose; oral thiamine may help.
Drowsiness	Increase dose slowly. Tends to wear off. Reassure patient.
Dry mouth	Not usually common or severe. Tends to wear off.
Fluid retention	Rare. May use low dose thiazides.
Insomnia, agitation	Seen mostly with moclobemide and tranylcypromine. Reduce dose.
Urinary hesitancy, retention	Stop drug.
Hypertension	Stop drug.

tranylcypromine) and tolerance does not develop to therapeutic effects; however, safety in pregnancy has not been established.

The patient should be on a restricted diet several days before beginning the medication, while on the medication and for 2 weeks after stopping the medication. No more than one MAOI should be given at a time. Neither should MAOIs be used along with other antidepressants except in limited cases and under expert supervision.

Tyramine is an amino acid released from proteins in food when they undergo hydrolysis by fermenting, ageing, pickling, smoking and spoiling. It is deactivated by MAO in the gut wall and liver. When MAO is inhibited, tyramine may reach adrenergic nerve endings, causing the release of large amounts of noradrenaline and producing a hypertensive reaction. Also, sympathomimetic drugs act on the neurotransmission process by releasing noradrenaline from the storage vesicles in the presynaptic nerve ends. Because monoamine oxidase has been inhibited when MAOIs are used, large amounts of noradrenaline are released and a severe hypertensive reaction can occur. Chlorpromazine–an antipsychotic drug–and the alpha-adrenergic blocking agent phentolamine bind to the noradrenaline receptor sites, preventing noradrenaline stimulation and resolving the hypertensive crisis.

A new MAOI, moclobemide, has recently been marketed. It is novel because it is a reversible MAOI or RIMA (reversible inhibitor of monoamine oxidase A). Moclobemide, unlike older MAOIs, only temporarily inhibits MAO and is easily dislodged from its MAO binding site by tyramine. The tyramine reaction is much reduced and so there are no dietary restrictions. Hypertensive episodes usually only occur when very large amounts of tyramine are ingested. Moclobemide also seems to have a lower side-effect profile than the current MAOIs (Fitton *et al.*, 1992). It remains to be seen if the current MAO inhibitors will continue to be used for certain patient populations or if they will be used less frequently for depression and other disorders now that reversible MAOIs are available.

MOOD STABILIZING DRUGS

Mood stabilizing drugs are widely used in bipolar affective disorder and other related conditions. Lithium is still the most used agent but carbamazepine and sodium valproate are becoming more popular. Other drugs (e.g. clozapine) may also have a role in the treatment of bipolar disorder.

LITHIUM

Lithium, a naturally occurring element, was noted to have medicinal properties during the 19th Century when it was found to be present in the waters of some European mineral springs. It was described as having antimanic properties in 1949 and has been used as a mood stabilizer since that time. Today it is readily and safely administered under careful clinical guidelines and has an important clinical role as a mood stabilizer in the treatment of cyclical affective disorders.

Mechanism of Action

The exact mechanism of action of lithium is not fully understood but many neurotransmitter functions are altered by the drug. It has been suggested that lithium corrects an ion exchange abnormality, alters sodium transport in nerves and muscle cells, normalizes synaptic neurotransmission of noradrenaline, serotonin and dopamine, increases the reuptake and metabolism of noradrenaline and changes receptor sensitivity for serotonin. Its clinical effectiveness is likely to be the combined result of several of these complex actions.

Clinical Use

Acute episodes of mania and hypomania and recurrent bipolar illness are the most frequent indications for lithium treatment. Other disorders with an affective element, such as recurrent unipolar depressions, schizoaffective disorder, catatonia and alcoholism are sometimes effectively treated with lithium, especially when they are periodic or cyclical. In addition, lithium has been reported to be effective in treating non-affective disorders such as aggressive conduct disorder, borderline personality disorder and eating disorders. In general, lithium is not effective in the initial treatment of an acute depressive episode but can be given with antidepressant drug treatment in refractory cases to good effect. Box 27.8 lists the target symptoms of mania and depression for lithium therapy.

Before treatment with lithium, a complete history and physical examination are required, with special attention to the kidneys (lithium is excreted by the kidneys) and the thyroid. Regular medical check-ups (Box 27.9) are essential while the patient is on maintenance lithium treatment. In high doses, lithium may cause renal damage and reduce renal function. It also frequently causes hypothyroidism, even at therapeutic doses.

In acute episodes, lithium is effective in 1–2 weeks but it may take up to 4 weeks or even a few months to treat the symptoms

fully. Sometimes an antipsychotic agent is used during the first few days or weeks of an acute episode to manage severe behavioural excitement and acute psychotic symptoms. In a maintenance regimen, lithium decreases the number, severity and frequency of occurrence of affective episodes. However, mild mood swings or the recurrence of affective symptoms are not uncommon while on lithium maintenance. These problems usually respond to a temporary increase in lithium dose, antipsychotic or antidepressant medication or short-term psychotherapeutic support. The maintenance dose for each patient must be individualized and may vary from time to time. The therapeutic range of lithium is usually held to be 0.5–1.0 mmol/litre of plasma. Box 27.10 lists factors predictive of a lithium response.

Lithium therapy usually is started with 400 mg daily until steady state is reached, usually in 3–4 days. In the UK, modified release tablets (Priadel, Camcolit) are used because the peak level is then lowered (causing fewer adverse effects) and the effect prolonged (allowing once daily dosing). After 3–4 days, a blood level reading is taken in the morning, 12 hours after the last dose. Because of the low therapeutic index of lithium, toxic blood levels can be reached quickly in certain circumstances. Also, because lithium is a salt, the sodium and fluid balance of the body affects lithium regulation. It is essential clinical practice to monitor serum blood levels regularly (every week for the first month, then every 3 to 6 months) so that the dose can be regulated and to teach the patient about lithium toxicity symptoms and issues regarding salt and fluid intake. Dehydration must also be studiously avoided as this too may result in lithium toxicity.

The dose is increased until bipolar symptoms are reduced, until side-effects are too great or until the upper limit of the therapeutic blood level is reached. The therapeutic range used to be considered to lie between 0.6 and 1.4 mmol/litre for adults but lower levels are now thought appropriate (see above). After

Target symptoms for lithium therapy

Mania/Depression
Irritable
Expansive
Euphoric
Manipulative
Labile with depression
Sleep disturbance (decreased sleep)
Pressured speech
Flight of ideas
Motor hyperactivity
Assaultive or threatening
Distractibility
Hypergraphia
Hypersexual
Persecutory and religious delusions
Grandiose
Hallucinations
Ideas of reference
Catatonia
Sadness
Pessimistic
Anhedonia
Self-reproach
Guilt
Hopelessness
Somatic complaints
Suicidal ideation
Motor retardation
Slowed thinking
Poor concentration and memory
Fatigue
Constipation
Decreased libido
Anorexia or increased appetite
Weight change
Helplessness
Sleep disturbance (insomnia or hypersomnia)

Examinations before and during treatment with lithium

Before treatment
Renal: urinalysis, urea, electrolytes, 24-hour creatinine clearance, history of renal disease in self or family, diabetes mellitus, hypertension, diuretic use, analgesic abuse.
Thyroid: TSH (thyroid stimulating hormone), T4 (thyroxine), T3 RU (resin uptake), T4 I (free thyroxine index), history of thyroid disease in self or family.
Other: Complete physical examination and history, ECG, fasting blood sugar, complete blood count.

Maintenance lithium considerations
Every 3 months: assess lithium level (for the first 6 months).
Every 6 months: reassess renal status, lithium level, TSH.
Every 12 months: reassess thyroid function, ECG.
Assess more often if patient is symptomatic.

Box 27.10 *Factors predicting lithium responsiveness*

Positive response
Family history of mania or bipolar illness
Positive response of family member to lithium
Prior manic episode
Onset of illness with mania
Alcohol abuse
Cyclothymic personality features (numerous periods of mood disturbances but lacking symptom severity and duration to meet DMS-IV bipolar diagnostic criteria)
Euphoria and grandiosity
Diagnosis of primary affective disorder
History of treatment compliance with pharmacotherapy

Negative response
Rapid cycling (more than two episodes a year)
Thought disorder with depression and paranoia
Anxiety
Obsessive features
Onset after age 40

Box 27.11 *Lithium side-effects*

Acute, common and usually harmless
CNS: Fine hand tremor (50% of patients), fatigue, headache, mental dullness, lethargy
Renal: Polyuria (60% of patients), polydipsia, oedema
Gastrointestinal: Gastric irritation, anorexia, abdominal cramps, mild nausea, vomiting, diarrhoea (dose with food or milk; further divide dose)
Dermatological: Acne, pruritic maculopapular rash
Cardiac: ECG changes, usually not clinically significant, may be persistent
Body image: Weight gain (60% of patients); can be persistent

Long-term, adverse and usually not dose related (patient usually can continue to take lithium)
Endocrine: (1) Thyroid dysfunction—hypothyroidism (5% of patients); replacement hormone may be necessary (2) Mild diabetes mellitus—may need diet control or insulin therapy
Renal: (1) Nephrogenic diabetes insipidus—decreasing dose can help; patient must drink plenty of fluids; thiazide diuretics paradoxically reduce polyuria and may be helpful (2) Microscopic structural kidney changes: (10% to 20% of patients on lithium for 1 year); usually does not cause significant clinical morbidity

Lithium toxicity, usually dose related
Prodrome of intoxication (lithium level e.g. 2.0 mEq/litre): Anorexia, nausea, vomiting, diarrhoea, coarse hand tremor, muscle fasciculations, twitching, lethargy, dysarthria, hyperactive deep tendon reflexes, ataxia, tinnitus, vertigo, weakness, drowsiness
Lithium intoxication (lithium level e.g. 2.5 mEq/litre): Fever, decreased urine output, decreased blood pressure, irregular pulse, ECG changes, impaired consciousness, seizures, coma, death

the patient has had a good response to lithium, the maintenance lithium dose usually may be set lower to maintain a therapeutic blood level. Adjusting the dose is a simple procedure because there is a precise correlation with 12-hour plasma level; if 400 mg/day gives 0.3 mmol/litre, 800 mg/day should give 0.6 mmol/litre.

In geriatric patients or those with medical illness, a serum lithium level of 0.6–0.8 mmol/litre is recommended. Use of lithium in pregnancy is not recommended. Various congenital abnormalities have been reported in babies exposed to lithium *in utero*, particularly during the first trimester. In the later stages of pregnancy, the lithium plasma level is very difficult to control and thyroid problems may occur in the new-born.

Adverse Reactions
Although lithium is used often, it is a challenge to patient education for nurses and other clinicians. Usually patients are treated with lithium for several years and various physiological and environmental factors can rapidly raise their blood levels of lithium above the therapeutic limit. Patients must be taught the difference between acute and long-term side-effects and the signs of lithium toxicity (Box 27.11). Patients must also be taught the common causes for an increase in lithium level and ways to maintain a stable therapeutic level as described in Box 27.12. Lithium toxicity is an emergency situation. Management of serious toxic states is outlined in Box 27.13.

Lithium treatment failure can occur, even at therapeutic blood levels of lithium. Several alternatives to the use of lithium alone include the addition of some anticonvulsants for manic breakthrough and the addition of antidepressant drugs for depression breakthrough. Electroconvulsive therapy (ECT) for either mania or depression is also effective and should be

Box 27.12 *Stabilizing lithium levels*

Common causes for an increase in lithium levels
1. Decreased sodium intake
2. Diuretic therapy
3. Decreased renal functioning
4. Fluid and electrolyte loss: sweating, diarrhoea, dehydration, fever, vomiting
5. Medical illness
6. Overdose
7. Non-steroidal anti-inflammatory drug therapy

Ways to maintain a stable lithium level
1. Stable dosing schedule by dividing doses or use of sustained-release tablets
2. Adequate dietary sodium and fluid intake (2 to 3 litres/day)
3. Replace fluid and electrolytes during exercise or gastrointestinal illness
4. Monitor signs and symptoms of lithium side-effects and toxicity
5. If patient forgets a dose, a dose may be taken if less than 2 hours have elapsed; if longer than 2 hours, the dose should be skipped and the next dose taken; never double up on doses

considered, particularly when the suicide risk seems high. Most importantly, there is no psychopharmacological substitute for a strong therapeutic relationship, patient education, psychodynamic intervention and regular maintenance evaluations.

ANTICONVULSANTS

Carbamazepine (Tegretol), marketed since the 1950s as an anticonvulsant, was also seen to have mood stabilizing effects on patients with temporal lobe epilepsy. Research has demonstrated that carbamazepine is helpful in the treatment of acute mania and in the long-term prevention of manic episodes when lithium is ineffective or contraindicated (Glod and Mathieu, 1993). The effect of carbamazepine builds up slowly over 10 days or so of administration. Other psychiatric applications of carbamazepine, although still experimental, include the treatment of borderline personality disorder, schizophrenia and schizoaffective disorder. Side-effects include skin rash, sore

Box 27.13 *Management of serious lithium toxicity*

1. Rapid assessment of clinical signs and symptoms of lithium toxicity; if possible, obtain rapid history of incident, especially dosing, from patient; explain procedures to patient and offer support throughout.
2. Withhold all lithium doses.
3. Check blood pressure, pulse, rectal temperature, respiration, level of consciousness. Be prepared to initiate stabilization procedures, protect airways, provide supplemental oxygen.
4. Assess lithium blood level immediately; assess electrolytes, BUN, creatinine, urinalysis, complete blood count when possible.
5. Run electrocardiogram; monitor cardiac status.
6. Limit lithium absorption; if acute overdose, provide an emetic; nasogastric suctioning may help because lithium levels in gastric fluid may remain high for days
7. Vigorously hydrate: 5 to 6 litres/day; keep electrolytes balanced; use IV line and indwelling urinary catheter.
8. Patient will be bedridden: monitor range of motion, frequent turning, pulmonary toilet.
9. In moderately severe cases:
   a. Implement osmotic diuresis with urea, 20 g IV two to five times per day, or mannitol, 50 to 100 g IV per day.
   b. Increase lithium clearance with aminophylline, 0.5 g up to every 6 hr and alkalinize the urine with IV sodium lactate.
   c. Ensure adequate intake of sodium chloride to promote excretion of lithium.
   d. Implement peritoneal or haemodialysis in the most severe cases. These are characterized by serum levels between 2.0 and 4.0 mEq/litre with severe clinical signs and symptoms (particularly decreasing urinary output and deepening CNS depression).
10. When appropriate: interview patient; ascertain reasons for lithium toxicity; increase health teaching efforts; mobilize postdischarge support system; arrange for more frequent clinical visits and blood level checks; assess for depression and suicidal intent; consider concomitant antidepressant drug treatment and supportive non-pharmacological therapy.

throat, mucosal ulceration, low-grade fever, drowsiness, vertigo, ataxia, diplopia, blurred vision, nausea, vomiting, hepatotoxicity and a temporary and benign 25% decrease in the white blood cell count. A rare but serious problem is carbamazepine-induced agranulocytosis, a significant decrease in the white blood cell count that does not return to normal. Therefore full blood counts are monitored regularly.

Carbamazepine is administered initially at 200 mg/day and can be gradually increased to as much as 1600 mg/day or higher. Modified release tablets (Tegretol Retard) can be given twice daily and may be better tolerated. Maintenance doses range from 200 to 1600 mg/day. Therapeutic serum levels seem to lie within the range 6–12 mg/litre with neurotoxic side-effects more common above 10 mg/litre. Caution is advised when carbamazepine is used along with haloperidol for the control of excited psychosis (since plasma levels of haloperidol may be reduced) and with lithium (since neurotoxicity may be potentiated).

Another anticonvulsant medicine used in psychiatry is sodium valproate (Epilim). This drug has been shown to be effective in the manic phase of bipolar disorder and schizoaffective disorder, even in patients who had failed to respond to or who had been unable to tolerate conventional drug therapy (McElroy *et al.*, 1989). This drug is well tolerated in general, particularly if once-daily modified release tablets (Epilim Chrono) are used. The most common side-effects include gastrointestinal complaints such as anorexia, nausea, vomiting, and diarrhoea; neurological symptoms of tremor, sedation, and ataxia; increased appetite and weight gain. Very rare but serious side-effects include pancreatitis and severe hepatic dysfunction. Liver function and haematology levels are checked monthly during the first 6 months of therapy, and then every 3–6 months.

Valproate is begun at 500(MR) mg/day in single daily doses until a serum level of 50–100 mg/litre is achieved. Response usually occurs in 1–2 weeks. Valproate is not safe for use during pregnancy. It can be used in long-term maintenance alone or with other drugs such as lithium, antipsychotics or antidepressants.

Others

A few other drugs have occasionally been shown to be effective mood stabilizers. The calcium antagonists verapamil and nimodipine can sometimes bring about dramatic improvement but their use is limited by the occurrence of hypotension. The atypical antipsychotic clozapine also appears to be an effective mood stabilizer. In rapid cycling bipolar affective disorder, high dose thyroxine is sometimes used.

ANTIPSYCHOTIC DRUGS

Antipsychotic drugs are some of the most widely used medicines, being used in schizophrenia, bipolar disorder, severe anxiety and the manic phase of manic-depressive illness. After years of stagnation new drugs have been developed and are to be brought onto the market. These have the potential to be more effective and better tolerated. It is likely that the 1990s will be seen as a turning point in the treatment of psychosis.

MECHANISM OF ACTION

The antipsychotic drugs are dopamine antagonists and block dopamine (D2) receptors in various pathways in the brain.

Their effectiveness is thought to be the result of their ability to block dopamine D2 receptors in the limbic system, which is the emotion-generating part of the brain. Unfortunately, they also block other dopamine receptors, including D2 receptors in other parts of the brain. This explains some of their side-effects and the differences in tolerance to desired and undesired drug effects. Most recently two atypical antipsychotic drugs, clozapine and risperidone, have offered an alternative to the traditional antipsychotic drugs for the treatment of

TABLE 27.9 Antipsychotics: equivalent doses and relative adverse effects

Drug	Approx eqiv dose (mg)	Sedation	Extra pyramidal	Anticholinergic	Cardio vascular
Phenothiazines					
Chlorpromazine (Largactil)	100	+++	++	++	+++
Promazine (Sparine)	200	+++	+	++	++
Methotrimeprazine (Nozinan)	25	+++	++	++	++
Thioridazine (Melleril)	100	+++	+	+++	+++
Pipothiazine (Piportil)	?	++	++	++	++
Depot only					
Pericyazine (Neulactil)	10	+++	+	+++	+++
Fluphenazine (Moditen)	2	+	+++	++	+
Perphenazine (Fentazin)	10	+	+++	+	+
Prochlorperazine (Stemetil)	15	+	+++	+	+
Trifluoperazine (Stelazine)	5	+	+++	+/–	+
Thioxanthenes					
Flupenthixol (Depixol)	3	+	++	++	+
Zuclopenthixol (Clopixol)	15	++	++	++	+
Butyrophenones					
Haloperidol (Serenace)	3	+	+++	+	+
Droperidol (Droleptan)	1	++	+++	+	+
Benperidol (Anquil)	0.25	+	+++	+	+
Trifluoperidol (Triperidol)	1	+	+++	+	+
Oxypertine					
Oxypertine (Integrin)	5	+	++	+	–
Substituted benzamide					
Sulpiride (Dolmatil)	200	–	+	–	–
Diphenylbutylpiperidines					
Fluspirilene (Redeptin)	?	+	++	+	+
Depot only					
Pimozide (Orap)	2	+	+	+	++
Dibenzazepines					
Loxapine (Loxapac)	10	++	+++	+	++
Clozapine (Clozaril)	50	+++	–	+++	+++
Benzisoxazole					
Risperidone (Risperdal)	2	+	+/-	+	++

refractory schizophrenia. The success of clozapine in particular has cast doubt over the long-held theory that blockade of D2 receptors is necessary for an antipsychotic effect.

CLINICAL USE

The most frequently prescribed antipsychotic drugs are listed in Table 27.9. With the exception of clozapine (Meltzer, 1993) these drugs do not differ from each other in terms of overall clinical response at equivalent doses; they all have an equal chance of effectively treating the target symptoms of psychosis. In treating negative symptoms of schizophrenia (lack of volition, poor self-care, social withdrawal), clozapine and risperidone may have some advantages over older drugs. What distinguishes the chemical classes of the antipsychotic drugs is the extent, type and severity of side-effects produced. Therefore an understanding of the side-effects of each class of drug becomes a major nursing focus when caring for patients receiving antipsychotic medications.

Past success with a psychiatric drug in a patient or in a patient's first-degree relative may be the first reason to select a particular antipsychotic drug. The most common cause of treatment failure in acute psychosis is an inadequate dose. The most common cause of relapse seems to be patient non-compliance with maintenance drug therapy.

The major uses for antipsychotic drugs are in the management of schizophrenia, organic brain syndrome with psychosis and the manic phase of manic–depressive illness. The occasional use of autipsychotics may be indicated in severe depression with psychotic features or in severe anxiety, particularly when the patient may have a tendency towards drug or alcohol dependency. Non-psychiatric uses for antipsychotic drugs include treatment of vomiting and vertigo and as an adjunct to analgesics for pain relief.

The clinical symptoms of psychosis that are considered the major target symptoms for pharmacotherapy with the antipsychotic drugs are listed in Box 27.14. The initial nursing care plan should address drug dose, target symptom response and observed side-effects and their treatment, along with patient safety, education and reassurance. The relationship the nurse establishes with the patient who is very psychotic forms the basis for an ongoing therapeutic alliance, and such active non-pharmacological treatment of the residual or negative symptoms of psychosis is more successful when the patient's behaviour, mood, and thought processes begin to show improvement with pharmacotherapy.

Clozapine (Clozaril) differs markedly from standard antipsychotic drugs in that it more selectively blocks specific types of dopamine neurotransmitter receptors. Clozapine is a relatively poor D2 receptor antagonist. Despite this, the clinical effects of clozapine in treating positive and negative symptoms are superior to those of other classes of antipsychotic drugs (Barrett *et al.*, 1990). Clozapine also causes few, if any, acute extrapyramidal side-effects and only very rarely gives rise to tardive dyskinesia. It has been shown to be more effective for many patients who are non-responders to adequate trials of standard antipsychotic drugs. It is also indicated for patients who are responders

to standard antipsychotics but who have developed intolerable extrapyramidal side-effects. Clozapine does not worsen pre-existing tardive dyskinesia and in some cases, symptoms of tardive dyskinesia improved after the standard antipsychotic had been discontinued and clozapine therapy had been initiated (Littrell and Magill, 1993). Unfortunately, clozapine does cause orthostatic hypotension (which is treatable (Taylor *et al.*, 1995), tachycardia, sedation) anticholinergic reactions, weight gain and a paradoxical hypersalivation, especially during sleep). There is a seizure risk that increases with dosage and often a rapid return of psychotic symptoms when the drug is discontinued.

The most serious adverse effect of clozapine is agranulocytosis, which occurs in approximately 1–2% of patients (this is 10 to 20 times greater than with standard antipsychotic drugs). This risk continues to increase during the first 4 months of treatment, then declines gradually but never entirely disappears. After a year the risk is similar to that seen with other antipsychotics. Weekly full blood counts to monitor any decline in white cell count and clozapine prescriptions 1 week at a time are needed for the first 18 weeks of therapy. After this, only fortnightly testing and dispensing are required. After a year some patients may be eligible for monthly monitoring.

A lowered white cell count recovers if the drug is stopped in time. Once a patient has this problem with clozapine,

Box 27.14 *Antipsychotic drug target symptoms*

Appearance
Bizarre or dishevelled
Poor hygiene, poor nutrition

Behaviour
Hyperactivity
Bizarre actions
Hostility, assaultiveness
Insomnia
*Motivation — poor
*Social functioning — poor

Mood and affect
Flat affect
Agitation
Anxiety and tension
Intellectual functioning — poor
*Unrealistic planning
*Lack of insight
*Poor judgment

Thought processes
Loose associations
Delusional ideas
Hallucinations
Suspiciousness
Negativism

*Residual symptoms: not highly responsive to traditional antipsychotics.

reinstatement of the drug is contraindicated. Clearly, the requirement for blood testing adds a significant cost to the treatment of patients taking clozapine. For the schizophrenic patient who needs this drug and can be monitored for agranulocytosis and does not need concomitant drugs that also lower white blood cell count (such as carbamazepine), clozapine may make a significant difference in treatment outcome. A great many chronically ill patients have now derived substantial benefit from the use of clozapine. The increased drug cost is usually fully offset by the reduction in the need for care that results from the use of clozapine.

Finally, while clozapine does reduce the negative symptoms of schizophrenia, patients taking this medication still need help with other aspects of their psychosocial functioning. Psychoeducation, social skills training, group support and other rehabilitative interventions are beneficial in improving the overall level of functioning and the resulting quality of life.

Risperidone (Risperdal), another new atypical antipsychotic, is similar to clozapine in some respects but does not require frequent blood monitoring. As an atypical drug, it has a low incidence of extrapyramidal symptoms. Unlike with clozapine, this atypical feature disappears at high (16 mg/day) doses. It is likely that risperidone is not as effective as clozapine in refractory schizophrenia. Its main advantage is that it is free from extrapyramidal side-effects at therapeutic doses (4–8 mg/day). This may make it better tolerated.

Sertinole and olanzapine are two new atypical drugs. They do not cause extrapyramidal symptoms or problems related to high prolactin levels. Both are at least as effective as older drugs and may, like clozapine and risperidone, have improved efficacy against negative sy,ptoms. Only clozapine has proven efficacy in refractory schizophrenia.

GENERAL PHARMACOLOGICAL PRINCIPLES

Dosage requirements for individual patients vary considerably and must be adjusted as the target symptom changes and side-effects are monitored. Initially the patient is dosed several times a day and the daily dose can be raised every 1–4 days until symptoms improve. Some patients respond in 2–3 days, some take as long as 2 weeks. Full benefits may take 6 weeks or more. Parenteral high doses can be used initially to control a highly excited or dangerous patient. Response to clozapine may take several months.

When the patient has been stabilized for several weeks, the daily dose can be lowered to the lowest effective dose. The half-life of most antipsychotic drugs is greater than 24 hours, so the patient can be dosed once a day after steady-state is reached (approximately 4 days). Bedtime dosing allows the patient to sleep through side-effects, when they are at their peak. After 6–12 months of stable maintenance drug therapy, the patient can be slowly tapered from medication to assess the need for continued drug treatment. Some schizophrenic patients require a lifetime of continual medication management. A patient who is unresponsive to an adequate trial (6 weeks at a proper dose) frequently responds to another chemical class of antipsychotic drug, so a second drug trial usually is given.

Most antipsychotic drugs can be administered by oral and intramuscular routes. Some drugs can be given as intramuscular depot injections; in these cases the drug (e.g. fluphenazine) is esterified (to fluphenazine decanoate) and dissolved in a viscous oil, which acts as a reservoir of drug. After the injection, the drug slowly dissolves into the blood over a period of weeks. Depot injections improve patient compliance and can greatly reduce rates of readmission to hospital.

Details of the currently available depot injections are given in Table 27.10.

A very wide range of doses of antipsychotics is used; the reasons for this are unclear. Certainly, individual response varies considerably. However, there is little firm evidence to support the use of megadose therapy (>1000 mg/day chlorpromazine equivalents) and this kind of therapy greatly increases the risk of adverse effects and even sudden death. The Royal College of Psychiatrists has issued guidance on the monitoring of patients on high doses of antipsychotics and this can be found in the current British National Formulary (BNF).

Antipsychotic drugs do not cause chemical dependency, nor is there tolerance to their antipsychotic effects over time.

TABLE 27.10 Depot antipsychotics

DRUG	BRAND NAME	TEST DOSE (mg)	DOSE RANGE week?(mg)	DOSING INTERVAL (weeks)	COMMENTS
Flupenthixol decanoate	Depixol	20	12.5–400	2–4	Mood elevating; may worsen agitation
Fluphenazine decanoate	Modecate	12.5	6.25–50	2–5	Avoid in depression. High EPSE
Haloperidol decanoate	Haldol	25*	12.5–75	4	High EPSE, low incidence of sedation
Pipothiazine palmitate	Piportil	25	12.5–50	4	? Lower EPSE
Zuclopenthixol decanoate	Clopixol	100	100–600	1–4	Useful in agitation and aggression

(adapted from Taylor and Duncan, 1995b)

* Test dose not specified by manufacturer

Because of their wide therapeutic index, overdoses of these drugs ordinarily do not result in death, and therefore they have a very low suicide potential. Because they do not produce euphoria, they also have a very low abuse potential. Antipsychotic drugs are not respiratory depressants but produce an added depressant effect when combined with drugs that produce respiratory depression. Therefore patients who also may be taking drugs such as benzodiazepines must be carefully observed. The interpretation of the effects of antipsychotics on the fetus is inconclusive. It is always best to avoid any drug during the first trimester, although what is best for a psychotic pregnant mother must be carefully considered.

ADVERSE REACTIONS

The side-effects of antipsychotic drugs are many and varied and demand a great deal of attention from the nurse. Table 27.11 gives a comprehensive list of side-effects that includes risk factors and treatment considerations. Some side-effects are merely uncomfortable for the patient; most are easily treated but some are life-threatening. The nurse should refer to this list frequently but should pay particular attention to the extrapyramidal symptoms (EPS) both in the short term and long term. It is important to minimize the patient's fears, increased sense of stigmatization and possible non-compliance with drug treatment through effective patient education and support (see Critical Thinking about Contemporary Issues).

Acute EPS side-effects are common, effectively treated and rarely dangerous consequences of drug treatment. These effects are a direct result of an antipsychotic's effect on dopamine receptors. Drug strategies to treat EPS include lowering the dose of the drug, changing to an antipsychotic drug with a lower profile for that side-effect (Table 27.11) or administering one of the anticholinergic drugs listed in the BNF. These drugs are administered with antipsychotic drugs if acute extrapyramidal symptoms occur. Since tolerance to these symptoms usually occurs in the first 3 months of antipsychotic drug treatment, drugs to treat EPS are used only during the first 3 months and then discontinued. Long-term use usually is not necessary and may increase the risk of tardive dyskinesia (an irreversible condition consisting in abnormal movements of the lips, tongue and neck or trunk).

Unfortunately this common, long-term extrapyramidal symptom currently has no effective treatment, although research continues in this area. Therefore primary preventive measures are important (Dillon, 1992; Lohr and Caligiuri, 1992). (Figure 27.2). The abnormal involuntary movement scale (AIMS) or LUNSERS should be a part of every patient's treatment. A serious and potentially fatal (14–30% mortality) EPS of dopamine-blocking agents is neuroleptic malignant syndrome, and is described in Table 27.11.

Because of their importance in managing patients treated with psychotropic medications and the problems they present the clinician in making the appropriate diagnosis, medication-induced movement disorders are now to be coded on Axis I of the DSM-IV (American Psychiatric Association, 1994). Although they are labelled 'medication-induced', it is often difficult to establish the causal link between medication exposure and the develop-

ment of movement disorders because some of these disorders occur in the absence of medication exposure. Nonetheless, the following disorders are to be listed on Axis I:
1. Neuroleptic-induced parkinsonism.
2. Neuroleptic malignant syndrome.
3. Neuroleptic-induced acute dystonia.
4. Neuroleptic-induced acute akathisia.
5. Neuroleptic-induced tardive dyskinesia.
6. Medication-induced postural tremor.
7. Medication-induced movement disorder not otherwise specified.
8. Adverse effects of medication not otherwise specified.

Currently, the correlation between plasma levels of antipsychotic drugs or serum dopamine receptor binding and clinical response has yet to be determined but these tests hold promise for refining drug selection and dosing regimens. Psychopharmacological research has just begun to discover chemical classes of antipsychotic drugs that have mechanisms of action highly specific for the target symptoms of psychosis and yet do not produce a variety of unwanted side-effects. Research is no longer based on finding new dopamine antagonists but on finding drugs that resemble clozapine in pharmacology and efficacy but which have fewer, less severe adverse effects.

MENTAL HEALTH NURSING PRACTICE

The place of drugs in the treatment of psychiatric disorder is well established. According to current knowledge, drug treatment is the most effective intervention for many psychiatric disorders. It is therefore essential for mental health nurses to possess the necessary knowledge and skills to carry out the interventions associated with psychopharmacology safely and effectively. Nurses have accumulated a great deal of information about the use of drugs in modern psychiatric practice. Recent developments not only include pharmacological advances but also those interventions that address the needs of the person on the receiving end. These include educational programmes, seeking attitude change and sometimes the need to control behaviour.

PATIENT EDUCATION

In 1972, Raphael's survey of the views of people with mental health problems highlighted medication was a source of concern and that patients wanted information about drugs and their side-effects (Raphael, 1972). Twenty years later a survey carried out by Rogers *et al.* (1993) on 516 people who were users of mental health services shows that the situation has changed very little. People are often ill-informed about the psychotropic medications they are taking. Rogers *et al.* suggest that one of the reasons patients feel ill-informed about their treatment is that psychiatrists continue to be paternalistic and are fearful of telling patients about the potency of the drugs they prescribe and their side-effects. Although some

TABLE 27.11 Antipsychotic side-effects and nursing considerations

Side-effects	Nursing considerations
Central nervous system	
Drowsiness and sedation	Build up dose slowly. Give drug at night. Drowsiness tends to wear off. Change to a different drug if it persists. Avoid driving. May use sedative drug if sleep disturbance is troublesome.
Confusion	Quite common in the elderly. Change to a different drug.
Lowered seizure threshold	Avoid the more sedative drugs and clozapine. Increase dose slowly with others.
Extrapyramidal side-effects (EPSE)	Tolerance develops slowly. Use anticholinergics PRN or change to a drug with lower risk of EPSE. Educate patient about risks of EPSE and available treatments.
a) Dystonia — sudden muscle spasms anywhere but especially in neck, back and eyes	Acute dystonia occurs in first few days of treatment. Give parenteral anticholinergic +/– respiratory support.
b) Akathisia — feeling of inner restlessness, pacing, dancing feet	Common and unpleasant. Responds poorly to anticholinergics. Give propranolol or clonazepam. Change antipsychotic. Try to distinguish true akathisia from anxiety states.
c) Parkinsonism — tremor, rigidity, muscle stiffness, monotone voice, shuffling gait	Usually wears off and responds well to anticholinergic medication. Change antipsychotic if effect persists.
d) Tardive dyskinesia (TD) — unusual movements around mouth and neck and shoulders. Tardive dystonia and akathisia may also occur	Ranges in severity from socially embarrassing to severely disabling. Related to length of use of antipsychotic drug, made worse by anticholinergics. May be irreversible and is often difficult to treat. Increasing dose gives temporary relief, withdrawing drug may reveal hidden TD. Clozapine does not cause TD and may improve symptoms in those who already have it.
e) Neuroleptic malignant syndrome(NMS) — muscular rigidity, fever, tremor, tachycardia, sweating, stupor. Raised CPK and white cells. May be fatal.	Usually very rapid development and so considered a medical emergency. Discontinue all drugs and transfer to (intensive) medical care. Dantrolene and bromocriptine may be used but main treatment is symptomatic. All antipsychotic drugs may cause NMS. If NMS occurs with one drug, use one from a different class, preferably low potency, once symptoms of NMS have fully resolved. Clozapine may be best choice. Do not use depots.
Gastrointestinal	
Constipation	Encourage fibre intake, may give stimulant laxative PRN if severe.
Dry mouth	Very common with some drugs, tends to wear off. May change drug if severe.
Heartburn, nausea, vomiting	Rare side-effects. Administer with or after meals or at bedtime.
Haematological	
Leucopenia, thrombocytopenia	Rare but blood should be monitored as routine practice. Mandatory monitoring with clozapine (weekly, then fortnightly then monthly).
Agranulocytosis (very low neutrophil count with fever and malaise; may be fatal)	Very rare. Discontinue drug and admit to hospital and? isolate. Intravenous antibiotics usually needed. Never give drug again. Use a different chemical class in future.
Hepatic	
Hepatic toxicity — jaundice, abnormal LFTs, fever	Abnormal LFTs quite common but usually benign. If jaundice develops, discontinue drug. Give a drug from a different class.
Endocrine	
Hyperprolactinaemia; amenorrhoea; menstrual irregularities; sexual difficulties: low libido, impotence, anorgasmia	Occurs with all drugs apart from clozapine. High prolactin levels do not always result in adverse effects. If side-effects are troublesome, use lower dose, change drug or use amantadine or bromocriptine (but beware of drug-induced psychosis).
Ophthalmic	
Blurred vision	Quite common anticholinergic effect, which tends to wear off. May change drug to one with lower anticholinergic potential.

TABLE 27.11 Antipsychotic side-effects and nursing considerations (cont)

Side-effects	Nursing considerations
Cardiovascular	
Postural hypotension, dizziness	Occur frequently with chlorpromazine, thioridazine and clozapine. Tend to wear off. Increase dose slowly. Monitor BP sitting and standing. May change drug.
Tachycardia	Not dangerous and tends to wear off. Reassure patient, may give propranolol.
ECG changes	Baseline ECG needed for comparison. Withdraw drug if any ECG changes noted during treatment. ECG essential in patients on high dose neuroleptics.
Sudden death	Rare but avoid using antipsychotics in patients with recent MI or in heart block. May also avoid if any cardiac problems present.
Cutaneous	
Rash, photosensitivity	Rare with most drugs but common with chlorpromazine. Sun screen needed in summer. Give antihistamine, change drug.
Genitourinary	
Changed sexual desire, delayed orgasm	Effect is unpredictable, probably most frequent with thioridazine and chlorpromazine. Lower dose, change drug, or give amantadine or bromocriptine if related to hyperprolactinaemia.
Urinary retention	Withdraw drug immediately. Switch to drug with lower anticholinergic potential.
Miscellaneous	
Weight gain,	Common with all drugs but especially clozapine. Give dietary counselling.
Tinnitus, allergic reaction	Rare. Change drug or give smaller dose. Give chlorpheniramine if allergic reaction is severe.
Sweating	Uncommon. Try a drug from a different class
Withdrawal syndrome	
Malaise, dizziness, anxiety	Common if treatment > 6 weeks. Withdraw over 2–4 weeks.
Intoxication syndromes	
Overdose	Treat aggressively. Transfer to general hospital.
Anticholinergic intoxication — confusion, anxiety, seizures	Withdraw all anticholinergic drugs. May give physostigmine to reverse effect.

research has been carried out examining information-giving among medical staff (Ballard and McDowell, 1990), very little work has been carried out among mental health nurses. Most of the available literature comes from the recent research interest in patient satisfaction surveys. For example, Shields *et al.* (1988) report that lack of information is a constant criticism made by patients on psychiatric wards.

One of the commonest concerns of relatives is not knowing how to cope with someone who has a mental illness or how to solve problems–for example, what to do when a patient refuses to take his or her prescribed medication. Brooker *et al.* (1994) report the success of training a group of CPNs in the application of psychosocial interventions set up to address these problems. The content of the training programme included interaction with the client and family, communication skills enhancement, family problem-solving, family education and dealing with drug compliance. People with mental health problems and their families benefit from educational programmes about mental illness and how to cope with it, including use of medication and its side-effects. The effectiveness and replicability of techniques of patient and family education have been demonstrated (Gamble, 1994).

However, many mental health nurses receive little teaching about psychotropic drugs during the curricula of their basic training. The Mental Health Nursing Review (Department of Health, 1994) suggests that it is essential that nurses are fully conversant with the aims, possible side-effects and contraindications of each prescription they administer. There is a compelling need for training courses to be reviewed and for the training needs of mental health nurses, in relation to patient education about medication, to be identified. Courses teaching techniques, which have been shown to be effective, should be widely available to enhance the skills of mental health nurses.

PROMOTING PATIENT ADHERENCE
Non-adherence to prescribed medication is one of the major determinants of outcome for patients with schizophrenia (Bebbington, 1995). Patients who do not take their medications as prescribed are more likely to relapse (Linn *et al.*,1982), be readmitted to hospital (Green,1988) and spend a longer of period of time in hospital (Caton *et al.*, 1985). The cost of non-adherence among people with mental illness in Britain is estimated at £100 million per year (Davies and

Drummond, 1993). Bebbington (1995) suggests that non-adherence may occur in up to 50% of people with schizophrenia who are prescribed neuroleptics. Much research has been carried out to examine the demographic variables associated with non-adherence. It has been shown that non-adherence is commoner in young people, particularly if male and from certain ethnic groups. Patients' and relatives' beliefs about mental illness and about the usefulness of medication

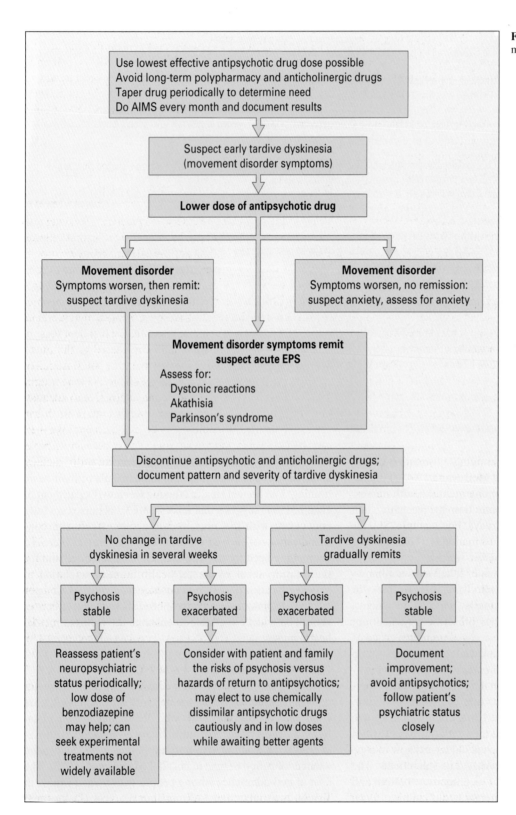

Figure 27.2 Preventitive measures for tardive dyskinesia

are of considerable importance. However, some of the problems with non-adherence may well stem from the failings of professionals. A collaborative approach is needed if nurses and patients are to reduce misunderstandings and improve adherence to prescribed medication. Nurses and workers in other disciplines must examine the treatment plan in the light of the user's perspective, choice and needs. They must listen to and take notice of users who frequently complain of being prescribed complex drug regimens and too many drugs, and of lack of information and poor accessibility to staff with positive attitudes. For example, Woof and Goldberg (1988) observed that CPNs asked questions about symptoms in a language and tone associated with an ordinary social enquiry rather than discussing strategies for dealing with problems. Turner (1993), examining the standard and content of nurse and client contacts during the administration of depot drugs, suggest an overall variation in the standards of care observed. Although some clients received nursing care of an acceptable and, at times, excellent standard, others found that nurses minimized contact with them at injection time, and therefore did not make effective use of this opportunity for interaction with patients; i.e. nursing assessment did not take place, neither was the opportunity taken to explore other important issues with the patient.

Before addressing the problem of non-compliance Piatkowska and Farnhill (1992) suggest that therapists should examine their own attitudes, assumptions and practices. They argue that contemporary views are replacing compliance with concepts such as 'therapeutic alliance' or, at least 'adherence' to medication. Such concepts emphasize respect for patients' rights, the need for informed decision making and a sense of control in the treatment situation. Adopting this approach, mental health nurses are ideally placed to improve patient adherence.

Understanding non-adherence from the patient's perspective will allow the nurse to anticipate any problems and intervene appropriately. For example, many patients decrease or completely stop taking their medications as soon as they start feeling better. If they have a bad day, they may take medication again for a day or two. Explaining to these patients how the medication works in the body and the need for maintaining therapeutic levels of the medicine in the bloodstream may help patients better understand their illness and adhere to the treatment plan. Still other patients may fear that the medications are addicting and that they will become dependent on them, or are embarrassed about the stigma of being on a psychiatric medication. Clarifying the use of the medication and the positive impact it can have on all aspects of the patient's life may help to reframe the issue of taking medication, in a way that promotes adherence. Kemp *et al.* (1996) carried out a randomized control study using a cognitive–behavioural intervention, which they entitled 'compliance therapy', to determine whether they could improve adherence to treatment in acutely psychotic patients. Twenty-five patients received compliance therapy and showed significantly greater improvements in their attitude to drug treatment and in their

insight into illness and compliance with treatment, compared with the control group. Furthermore, these gains persisted for 6 months. In the study, compliance therapy was provided by a psychiatrist assisted by a clinical psychologist. However, the authors believe that compliance therapy is eminently suited for adaptation to typical busy clinics and intend to examine the ease with which the technique may be taught to a range of health professionals. Nurses would be ideally placed to provide such therapy. The nurse–patient relationship and the strength of the therapeutic alliance could play an extremely important role in exploring users' ambivalence to treatment, in encouraging users to discuss their fears, problems and concerns about medication and in assisting them to focus on adaptive behaviours.

THE USE OF DRUGS IN THE CONTROL OF BEHAVIOUR

The Mental Health Act 1983 Code of Practice (1994) suggests that the control of patient behaviour by medication requires careful consideration. The appropriate use of medication to reduce disturbance and excitatory symptoms in order to carry out other interventions can be an important adjunct to a patient's treatment programme. However, medication which begins as purely therapeutic may, by prolonged routine administration, become a method of restraint. Each patient must be reviewed regularly. It should be considered at the outset whether, where medication would have to be administered by force, it would be lawful and therapeutic in the longer term. Medication should not be used as an alternative to adequate staffing levels or skills mix levels. Medication or its threatened administration should never be used as a punitive measure or to enforce good behaviour. The nurse should never withhold a drug that the patient needs and the use of medication.

RAPID TRANQUILLIZATION

Rapid tranquillization consists in the administration of sedating medication to control disturbed behaviour. Figure 27.3 is an algorithm for rapid tranquillization, the aim of which is to alleviate distress and produce a calming effect on the patient in the shortest possible time (Pilowsky *et al.*, 1992). Local policy will determine indications for use. Nurses must observe, and monitor carefully, vital signs including temperature, pulse and blood pressure. The decision to inject a patient against his or her will may be completely justified by the clinical situation (Thompson, 1994). However, the procedure will inevitably be carried out during high emotional arousal and careful consideration needs to be given to preparation, postprocedural action and debriefing.

GOOD PRACTICE IN THE ADMINISTRATION OF DEPOT NEUROLEPTICS

Psychotropic medications are commonly used in the treatment

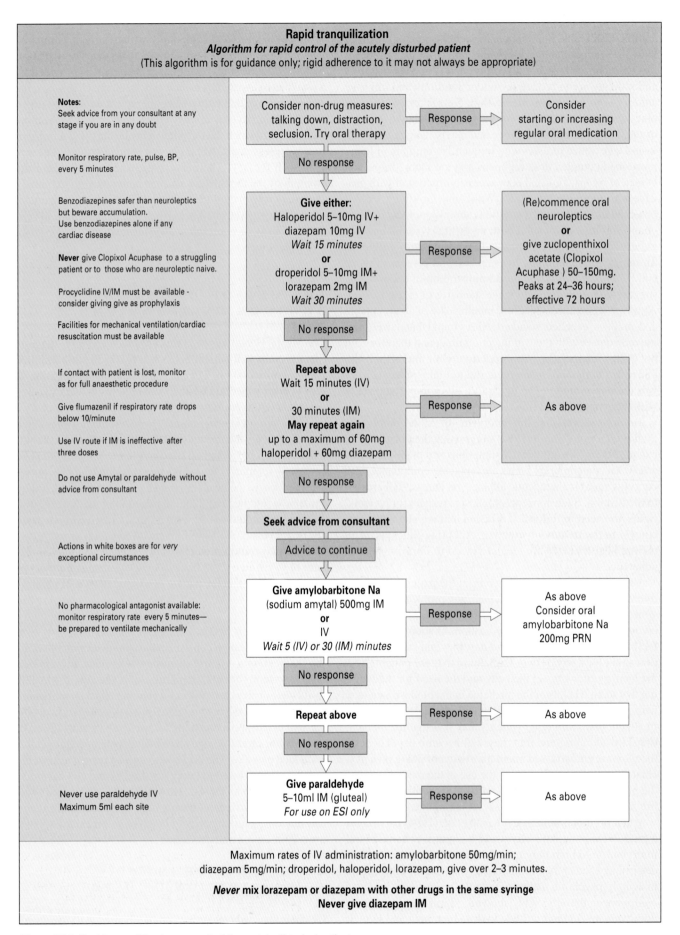

Rapid tranquilization
Algorithm for rapid control of the acutely disturbed patient
(This algorithm is for guidance only; rigid adherence to it may not always be appropriate)

Notes:
Seek advice from your consultant at any stage if you are in any doubt

Monitor respiratory rate, pulse, BP, every 5 minutes

Benzodiazepines safer than neuroleptics but beware accumulation.
Use benzodiazepines alone if any cardiac disease

Never give Clopixol Acuphase to a struggling patient or to those who are neuroleptic naive.

Procyclidine IV/IM must be available - consider giving give as prophylaxis

Facilities for mechanical ventilation/cardiac resuscitation must be available

If contact with patient is lost, monitor as for full anaesthetic procedure

Give flumazenil if respiratory rate drops below 10/minute

Use IV route if IM is ineffective after three doses

Do not use Amytal or paraldehyde without advice from consultant

Actions in white boxes are for *very* exceptional circumstances

No pharmacological antagonist available: monitor respiratory rate every 5 minutes—be prepared to ventilate mechanically

Never use paraldehyde IV
Maximum 5ml each site

Consider non-drug measures: talking down, distraction, seclusion. Try oral therapy → Response → Consider starting or increasing regular oral medication

No response

Give either:
Haloperidol 5–10mg IV+ diazepam 10mg IV
Wait 15 minutes
or
droperidol 5–10mg IM+ lorazepam 2mg IM
Wait 30 minutes → Response → (Re)commence oral neuroleptics **or** give zuclopenthixol acetate (Clopixol Acuphase) 50–150mg. Peaks at 24–36 hours; effective 72 hours

No response

Repeat above
Wait 15 minutes (IV)
or
30 minutes (IM)
May repeat again
up to a maximum of 60mg haloperidol + 60mg diazepam → Response → As above

No response

Seek advice from consultant

Advice to continue

Give amylobarbitone Na
(sodium amytal) 500mg IM
or
IV
Wait 5 (IV) or 30 (IM) minutes → Response → As above Consider oral amylobarbitone Na 200mg PRN

No response

Repeat above → Response → As above

No response

Give paraldehyde
5–10ml IM (gluteal)
For use on ESI only → Response → As above

Maximum rates of IV administration: amylobarbitone 50mg/min; diazepam 5mg/min; droperidol, haloperidol, lorazepam, give over 2–3 minutes.

Never mix lorazepam or diazepam with other drugs in the same syringe
Never give diazepam IM

Figure 27.3 Rapid tranquillization–control of the acutely disturbed patient

of psychiatric disorders. Since the greater part of care is now delivered in the community, it is essential that mental health nurses and practice nurses possess knowledge and skills related to psychopharmacology. In response to recent developments in the field, the Department of Health in collaboration with the Royal College of Nursing has produced good practice guidelines for the administration of depot neuroleptics ((Department of Health, 1994). The document describes the skills and knowledge mental health nurses and practice nurses need to provide services that meet the user's requirements. The document makes nine recommendations that nurses can follow to deliver competent nursing care and to place the user at the forefront of services. The document can be obtained from BAPS Health Publications Unit, DSS Distribution Centre, Heywood Stores, Manchester Road, Heywood, Lancs, OL10 2PZ.

SUMMARY

This chapter has examined developments in psychopharmacology and their relevance to mental health nurses. Although there has been an increase in the range of therapeutic interventions now on offer, psychopharmacology remains the mainstay of British psychiatry. For many psychiatric disorders, drug therapy is the most effective means of treatment in our present knowledge. If mental health nurses are to administer drugs effectively, these drugs must be given safely and with knowledge of their pharmacological actions and proposed therapeutic effects. The necessity of adequate knowledge including dosage, the route and frequency of administration, likely side-effects and length of treatment will be even more important as and when mental health nurses take on the responsibility of prescribing drugs.

KEY CONCEPTS

- Psychopharmacology is the fastest growing treatment in the current practice of psychiatry.
- The mental health nurse makes a unique contribution to the implementation of psychopharmacology.
- Benzodiazepines, the most widely prescribed class of drugs, have almost completely replaced other classes of antianxiety and sedative–hypnotic agents.
- Antidepressant drugs are effective, non-addictive but can be lethal in overdose.
- The various classes of antipsychotic drugs have similar therapeutic effects but are dissimilar in side-effect profiles. Side-effects are varied and can be disabling and life-threatening.
- The mood stabilizer, lithium, is effective in the treatment of bipolar illness in short- and long-term treatment regimes.
- Clozapine and risperidone are new antipsychotic agents with positive clinical effects. Patients taking clozapine need to be closely monitored for agranulocytosis, which is the drug's most serious side-effect.
- Important issues related to psychopharmacology and mental health nursing practice include patient education and promoting patients' adherence to their pharmacological treatment plan.

REFERENCES

American Psychiatric Association: *Diagnostic and statistical manual*, ed 4. Washington EC, 1994, American Psychiatric Association.

Ballard CG, McDowell AWT: Psychiatric in-patient audit — a patient's perspective. *Psychiatr Bull* 14(11):674–675, 1990.

Barrett N, Ormiston S, Molyneux V: Clozapine: a new drug for schizophrenia. *J Psychosoc Nurs Ment Health Serv* 28(2):24, 1990.

Bebbington PE: The content and context of compliance. *Int Clin Psychopharmacol* 9 supplement 5:41–50, 1995.

Bennett J, Done J, Hunt B: Assessing the side effects of antipsychotic drugs: a survey of CPN practice. *J Psychiatr Ment Health Nurs* 2:177–182, 1995

Brooker C, Falloon I, Butterworth A, Goldberg D, Graham-Hole V, Hillier V: The outcome of training community psychiatric nurses to deliver psychosocial interventions. *Br J Psychiatry* 164:222–230, 1994.

Caton CL Koh SP, Fleiss JL, Barrow S, Golstein JM: Rehospitalization in chronic schizophrenia. *Hosp Community Psychiatry* 43(3):140–144, 1985.

Charney DS, Krystal JH, Delgado PL, Heninger GR: Serotonin-specific drugs for anxiety and depressive disorders. *Annu Rev Med* 44:437, 1990.

Davies LM, Drummond MF: Assessment of costs and benefits of drug therapy for treatment-resistant schizophrenia in the United Kingdom. *Br J Psychiatry* 162:38–42, 1993.

Day JC, Wood G, Dewey M, Bentall RP: A self-rating scale for measuring neuroleptic side-effects: Validation in a group of schizophrenic patients. *Br J Psychiatry* 166:650–653, 1995.

Department of Health: *Report of the advisory group on nurse prescribing*. London, 1989.

Department of Health: *Working in partnership: A collaborative approach to care. Report of the mental health nursing review team*. London, 1994, Department of Health.

Depression Guideline Panel: *Depression in primary care*, vol 2. *Treatment of major depression. Clinical practice guidelines*, no. 5. (AHCPR publication no. 93-0551). Rockville, MD, 1993, US Department of Health and Human Services/ Public Health Service/ Agency for Health Care Policy and Research.

Dillon NB: Screening system for tardive dyskinesia: development and implementation. *J Psychosoc Nurs Ment Health Serv* 30(12):3, 1992.

Duncan D, Taylor D: Which antidepressants are safe in breastfeeding mothers? *Psychiatr Bull* 19(9):551–552, 1995.

Fitton A, Faulds D, Goa KL: Moclobemide: a review of its pharmacological properties and therapeutic use in depressive illness. *Drugs* 43(3):561, 1992.

Gamble C: The Thorn nurse training initiative. *Nurs Stand* 15(4):31–35, 1994.

Glod CA, Mathieu J: Expanding uses of anticonvulsants in the treatment of bipolar disorder. *J Psychosoc Nurs Ment Health Ser* 31(10):37, 1993.

Gournay K: Setting clinical standards for care in schizophrenia. *Nurs Times* 92(7):36–37, 1996.

Gray R, Thomas B: Effects of cannabis abuse on people with serious mental health problems. *Br J Ment Health Nurs* 2(1):230–233, 1996.

Green JH: Frequent rehospitalisation and non-compliance with treatment. *Hosp Community Psychiatry* 39(9):963–966, 1988.

Healy D: *Psychiatric drugs explained*. London, 1993, Mosby.

HMSO: *Mental Health Act Code of Practice*. London, 1993, Department of Health and Welsh Office.

Kent S, Yellowlees P: Psychiatric and social reasons for frequent hospitalisation. *Hosp Community Psychiatry* 45(4):347–350, 1994.

Kemp R, Hayward P, Applewhaite G, Everitt B, David A: Compliance therapy in psychotic patients: randomised control trial. *BMJ* 139:778–783, 1996.

Linn MW, Klett CJ, Cafey EM Jr: 1996. Relapse of psychiatric patients in foster care. *Am J Psychiatry* 139(8):778–783, 1982.

Littrell K, Magill AM: The effect of clozapine on preexisting tardive dyskinesia. *J Psychosoc Nurs Ment Health Serv* 31(9):14, 1993.

Lohr JB, Caligiuri MP: Quantitative instrumental measurement of tardive dyskinesia: a review. *Neuropsychopharmacol* 6(4):231, 1992.

McElroy SL, Keck PE, Pope HG, Hudson JI: Valproate in psychiatric disorders: literature review and clinical guidelines. *J Clin Psychiatry* 50(1):23, 1989.

Meltzer HY: New drugs for the treatment of schizophrenia, *Psychiatr Clin Am* 16(2):365, 1993.

Orsulak PJ: Therapeutic monitoring of antidepressant drugs: diagnostic update. *Ment Illn Neurol Disord* 3:1, 1989.

Piatkowska O, Farnill D: Medication–compliance or alliance? A client-centred approach to increasing adherence. In: Kavanagh DJ, editor: *Schizophrenia: an overview and practical handbook*. London, 1992, Chapman & Hall,

Pilowsky LS, Ring H, Shine PJ, *et al.*: Rapid tranquilisation–a survey of emergency prescribing in a general psychiatric hospital. *Br J Psychiatry* 160:831–835, 1992.

Raphael W: *Psychiatric hospitals viewed by their patients*. London, 1972, King Edward's Hospital Fund for London.

Rogers A, Pilgrim D, Lacey R: *Experiencing psychiatry: Users' views of services*. London, 1993, Macmillan, in association with Mind Publications.

Royal College of Psychiatrists: *Psychiatr Bull* 326–330, 1996.

Shields PJ, Morrison P, Hart D: Consumer satisfaction on a psychiatric ward. *J Adv Nurs* 13(3):396–400, 1988.

Taylor D, Duncan D: Plasma levels of tricyclics and related antidepressants: are they necessary or useful? *Psychiatr Bull* 19(6):549–550, 1995a.

Taylor D, Duncan D: Antipsychotic depot injections — suggested doses and frequencies. *Psychiatr Bull* 19(6):355–356, 1995b.

Taylor D, Reveley A, Faivre F: Clozapine induced hypotension treated with moclobemide and Bovril. *Br J Psychiatry* 167:409–410,1995;

Thomas B: Rethinking acute in-patient care. *Aust NZ J Ment Health Nurs* 5:10–17, 1996.

Thompson C: Consensus statement on higher-dose antipsychotic medication. *Br J Psychiatry* 164:448–485, 1994.

Turner G: Client/CPN contact during the administration of depot medications: implications for practice. In: E White, C Brooker, editors: *Community psychiatric nursing: A research perspective*, vol 2. London, 1993, Chapman & Hall.

UKCC: *Standards for the administration of medication*. London, 1992, UKCC.

Wallace CJ, Donahoe CP, Boone SE: Schizophrenia. In: Hersen M, editor: *pharmacological and behavioural treatment: An integrative approach*. New York, 1988, Wiley.

Wooff K, Goldberg D: Further observations on the practice of community care in Salford: differences between community psychiatric nurses and mental health social workers. Br J Psychiatry 153:30–37, 1988.

FURTHER READING

Bazire S: *Psychotropic drug directory 1996*. Salisbury, 1996, Quay Books.
An invaluable reference for all psychopharmacological issues and problems.

Kerwin R, Taylor D: New antipsychotics: a review of their current status and clinical potential. *CNS Drugs* 6:71–82, 1996.
A review of the pharmacology, efficacy and toxicity of the new atypical antipsychotics.

Taylor D: Clozapine – 5 years on. *Pharm J* 254:266–263, 1995.
A comprehensive, readily understood review of the use of the atypical antipsychotic clozapine.

Taylor D, Lader M: Cytochromes and psychotropic drug interactions. *Br J Psychiatry* 168:529–532, 1996.
An explanation of the pharmacokinetic interactions commonly seen in psychiatry.

· *Chapter* ·

28

Complementary Therapies and Mental Health Nursing

---

*T**he Medical Faculty at the University of Rome* convened the world's first congress on Alternative Medicine in 1973 with a programme covering 135 different therapies. In 1994, in the UK alone over 300 different forms of alternative therapies were being practised.

Complementary therapy is a fairly recent term for what otherwise has been called alternative or traditional therapy. The term 'complementary' is used to suggest a closer working partnership between orthodox medicine and other forms of treatment, each recognizing the need for the other.

The chapter aims to cover many complementary therapies, particularly those where research has proved their worth in nursing. Mental health and well-being has not received as much interest as physical health but is, the authors believe, an area where the re-introduction of complementary therapies will develop.

The World Health Organization (WHO) has declared its intention to actively encourage practitioners of traditional medicines to provide health for all by the year 2000. For too long the systems of traditional and modern medicine have gone their separate ways in mutual antipathy, yet their goals are identical, i.e. to improve the health of mankind and thereby the quality of life. Only a closed mind would continue to assume that each has nothing to learn from the other.

Traditional medicine exists in cultures around the world and dates back hundreds of thousands of years. The WHO's definition of traditional medicine includes all forms of health care that fall outside the official health sector. These include formalized traditional systems of medicine such as Chinese medicine, the practice of traditional healer, biofeedback, chiropractic, neuropathy, homoeopathy and even Christian Science. In the UK this definition would mean the inclusion of over 60 therapies. These can be broadly classified (West, 1980):
• Physical therapies, such as herbal medicine, homoeopathy, manipulation (e.g. osteopathy), reflexology, aromatherapy.
• Oriental therapies (e.g. yoga, t'ai chi).
• Systemic therapies (e.g. acupuncture).
• Sensory therapies (e.g. art, music, dance).
• Psychological therapies, for example psychotherapy, hypnotherapy, dream therapy and humanistic psychology (gestalt, primal work) to identify only a few.
• Paranormal therapies (faith healing, exorcism, radionics etc.).
• Diagnostics such as palmistry and astrology.

The ability to communicate with someone else, whether by verbal or non-verbal means, is central to any form of care and is at the core of all the therapies described here. What is considered is not only what a nurse may be doing with or to somebody but how it is carried out.

REVIVING INTEREST

Modern society is renewing interest in natural remedies and ways of protecting the mind to promote health. Scientific reductionism is being challenged with a broader concept of health. Every person is seen as unique and a highly complex physical and spiritual being. People are becoming more aware of their physical environment, particularly in the context of the devastating and contaminating effect Western society is having on the food we eat and the air we breathe. Methods of soil cultivation, and of food production and preservation have all increased the shelf life of food but at the cost of reduced quality and freshness. Practically everything we eat has been tampered with chemically in some way, which may prove to be harmful to our bodies (Mellor, 1978).

Which magazine in 1981 surveyed people who had received alternative therapies during the previous 5 years. Two out of every three people said that they had been receiving conventional treatment that had not helped or had caused side-effects. Side-effects are a concern to many people taking modern medicines and a growing hazard of the powerful chemicals used in modern drugs. It has been estimated that prescribed medications will cause two out of every five patients to suffer side-effects, with an even greater number showing levels of dependency. In addition, the cost of modern medicine is such that it has to be rationed because of its effects upon the country's resources (Stanway, 1979).

The move to community medicine brings an opportunity to return to a level of care that meets the needs of a community, beginning with the family, with primary health care teams providing that care. While the medical world is in transition, complementary therapies are filling the gaps it has left. People are becoming interested in regaining control over their treatment and the medicines they take.

THE PHILOSOPHY OF NATURAL HEALING

Millions of people across the world have gathered remedies for common ailments from their own environments. As recently as the 1850s, plant extracts and organic compounds were in common use as antiseptics, before the introduction of chemicals.

Our bodies are made up of numerous cells that have now been studied at molecular level, though even this depth of knowledge cannot explain the atomic energy fields that may exert influence from one cell to another. What we consider solid tissue is being broken down and replaced continuously. The scientific reductionistic approach has yet to explain what

controls these energy fields. There appears to be some superior, almost mystical controlling force that enables body functions to work in harmony most of the time. From this perspective, life events and bodily functions are considered to be subject to the ordinary laws of cause and effect and the influence of a superior world. Likewise, ailments can be seen to derive from external and internal disruptions, whether dietary, genetic, psychological or otherwise. Once these wider concepts of health and illness are appreciated, it becomes clearer why people the world over have been practising different forms of medicine, some alien to us, for thousands of years.

A HISTORICAL PERSPECTIVE

The treatment of emotional instability dates back to primitive man. Both Hippocrates (460–370 BC) and Galen (AD 130–200) wrote of psychiatric problems and advised anyone troubled by 'the passions' to find a wise adviser.

Yoga has been practised for thousands of years and is known to affect certain parts of the body. The Ancient Greeks knew the importance of colour in healing and yet not until the Romans was it proved that human skin could detect and respond to colour and was much more sensitive than previously thought possible.

From the dawn of mankind, women have been regarded as a potent source of life and power and in many cultures have become the embodiment of life and health. Prescriptions for stopping pain, pots for plant distillation and surgical tools have been found in archaeological excavations dating as far back as 5500 BC.

WOMEN AS HEALERS
From the earliest times, women have been seen as the progenitors of new life and therefore viewed as the life source. It was women who could produce new life and were therefore seen as the life source. The male role in procreation was not immediately obvious; nurturing and caring for a new life appeared to be related solely to the female body. Women were therefore associated with life and death and with caring for and healing the sick.

Achterberg (1990) describes women's position in society as a good measure of the development of civilization. Until 2000 BC, women were involved in all aspects of civilization. If unmarried they were priestesses, while the remaining majority owned and worked their own property and were often employed as physicians. Women began to lose esteem when more became known about the biology of procreation. Creation myths began to involve both sexes, rather than the birth of the world coming solely and magically from a female divinity. Sumer, possibly the most ancient of civilizations, ended with disorder, injustice and inequality and an unbalanced ecology. The male attributes of hunting and war overtook the more female attributes of birth and life represented by farming.

Around 500 BC, geological events caused temperatures to

fall and, with the Iron Age drew to a close, male gods of war began to increase in significance as civilization clambered for more fertile and safer ground. The seasons were changing and entire villages were being threatened with disaster through famine and sickness. Healing was considered a secondary occupation to a more masculine dominated occupation of hunting, war and invasion.

Greek tradition has often formed the epitome of healing practice, with the Greek physicians considered forefathers of modern medicine. Greek mythology presented women as lesser gods but there were healing goddesses in abundance. Greek women (e.g. Helen of Troy) were known to have mood and mind altering medicines in their repertoire, such as verbena, adiantum and wine, burned sulphur, poppy juice and evening primrose. Some scholars believe women were largely responsible for the initial development of surgical techniques and medicinal therapeutics, which made Greek medicine the most advanced in the ancient world (Achterberg, 1990).

Medieval times saw a gradual decline in domestic treatments. The awareness that came from observing the seasons, living close to the earth and observing the relationship between them began to disappear from general knowledge. As Christianity became the dominant system of religion, beliefs in the spirits of the earth gradually disappeared. Amulets and idols, banned by the Church, were replaced by shrines and relics, saints, with their own healing properties.

BOTANIC REMEDIES THROUGH HISTORY

It is impossible to be certain when plants were first used medicinally. Tens of thousands of years ago, people would use their sense of smell, as well as sight, to determine whether a plant would induce vomiting, diarrhoea or sleep, or could invigorate. Burning plants with food introduced herbs as taste enhancers and brought recognition of their aromatic qualities. Smoking is considered to have been one of the first forms of treatment with herbs and was often used to drive out evil spirits (Tisserand, 1989).

Maretheus, a renowned Greek physician, recognized that aromatic plants, especially flowers, had either stimulating or sedative properties. He identified roses and hyacinths as being refreshing and invigorating for a tired mind. Most flowers with fruity or spicy scent are considered to have similar properties. Plants with blue flowers, such as valerian and lavender, are sedative and red plants like cinnamon and cloves are found to be warming and stimulating. However, this generalization cannot be taken as a firm rule; it is more likely that the colour of the plant's essence (essential oil) better indicates its use.

In the 16th Century, herbalism was still the dominant form of healing. Paracelsus (1493–1541) laid the foundation for the more extensive use of minerals such as iron, mercury and antimony in medical practice, which overtook the botanical remedies. Paracelsus coined the word 'laudanum' for his preparations of powdered gold and pearls used in his study of alchemy. He was the first to direct that if a man was deficient in blood, he should be given iron. Paracelsus was the first physician–alchemist to work with minerals as medicinal preparations and laid the foundations for future homoeopathic practice.

As herbalism was declining in Europe, the settlers in America amalgamated their knowledge of herb lore with the Native Americans, who had been using plants for centuries. Samuel Thompson (1769–1843) is famous for popularizing ancient Indian remedies and for establishing herbal schools and botanical societies all over the USA. In 1864, Dr Coffin was instrumental in establishing the National Association of Medical Herbalists in Europe, having brought back the bulk of his knowledge from America.

HERBALISM

During the Plague, fires were ordered every evening and pungent smells (e.g. from sulphur, hops, pepper and frankincense) used to help with fumigation . Perfumed candles were used in hospitals and pomanders hung from silver chains around people's necks, aromatics being the best form of antiseptic available at the time.

The 17th Century was such a golden age for English herbalists that popular herbal medicine was soon cultivated by charlatans and quacks. Herbal medicine began to lose respect and reputation, particularly with the rise of apothecaries and chemical medicines. Research into the properties of herbs and essential oils moved to Europe and in particular to France. The area around Grasse in southern France became and still remains a centre of cultivation and production of essential oils. Cosmetics were used as antiseptics and Renee Gattefosse (a chemist) researched and reported the antiseptic properties of herbs, and is the person to whom has been attributed the introduction of the word aromatherapy. Gattefosse's book *Aromatherapie* published in 1937 reported substantial research on the use of essential oils but momentum was lost during the Second World War. Herbal remedies fell from favour although were still used by the poor for self-treatment.

PSYCHOLOGICAL ASTROLOGY

The influence of the planets has also been proposed for hundreds of years. Nicholas Culpeper (1616–1654) was perhaps the greatest of the astrologer–physicians. His astrological abilities earned him little respect but he is well known for his knowledge of herbs.

Medicine and astrology are said to be inextricably linked. Until the 18th Century, astrology was a part of a doctor's training and an essential element in the treatment of disease. Box 28.1 shows some of the historical links between astrology and medicine.

The melancholistic humour in the 15th and 16th Century, when ideas about hermetic philosophy and alchemical gold were at their peak, was associated with Saturn in the birth chart. There was a belief that to be truly creative and inspired, the artist or philosopher had to be melancholic. The term means something a little less pathological than today's term

Box
28.1

Astrological links with medicine

Hermetic medicine
Astrological medicine was first formalized in the writings of Hermes Trismegistos. Hermes Trismegistos is also the name applied by the greek Neoplatonists to the Egyptian god Thoth. The writings put forward the view that man reproduces himself in miniature through the structure of the universe.

The four humours
Hippocrates proposed that man's character was a result of balance of the four humours, blood, phlegm, black bile and yellow bile. These four were loosely linked to astrology and the four signs of water, earth, fire and air.

Herbal remedies
The Arabs were the first to associate herbs with specific signs or planets.

are confronted with. Psychiatric hospitals are full of people who are carrying everyone else's burdens (Greene, 1988).

The splitting process is also characteristic of Gemini, Sagittarius, Scorpio and Capricorn. These signs are wildly opposite in nature and tend to split in reverse ways. Usually Scorpio and Capricorn take on the bad side of the split, while Gemini and Sagittarius will project this darkness outside, although it is not always as straightforward. Greene (1988) goes on to discuss Kleinian theory as having a close affinity to the esoteric model of alchemy.

CG Jung's interest in alchemy was chiefly responsible for the drawing together of psychology and astronomy. Jung's work insofar as it relates to astrology, concentrates on those people who are missing out on a dimension of life (Parker and Parker, 1990).

Like astrologists, modern psychologists and psychiatrists are concentrating more on improving techniques and consolidating research considered generally beneficial to patients rather than debating various schools of thought.

'depression' (Greene, 1988). There have been periods in history when melancholia has been considered romantic and fashionable. The melancholic poets such as Keats, Byron and Shelley experienced long periods of black moods, leaving them brooding and unable to work, interspersed with inspirational bouts and furious periods of activity.

Melanie Klein's (1975a) theory on the depressive position suggests that the emergence of the child's ego can be disrupted, producing an arrest in development that appears in the adult psychology. The paranoid–schizoid condition has its origins in the child who is unable to contain opposite emotions such as love and hate at the same time. The ego is not yet strong enough to cope with the tensions and offers no faculty of reason. Klein (1975b) suggests that tension builds between feelings of love and hate about another person and that then these two feelings are split. Klein's description of the paranoid-schizoid person suggests that theirs is a psychological state that cannot integrate good and bad feelings. It is a way of perceiving life as distorted and split, with no one (including oneself) being allowed to be whole. It is a natural state at a certain stage of childhood but in adulthood can be life-destroying.

These powerful primitive (childhood) feelings, encompassing rage and the desire to devour and destroy, are considered to belong to the domain of human experience associated with Pluto (Greene, 1988). Pluto is a symbol of primitive instinctual need. One hates the person one loves, as they are seen to possess the ability to hurt and humiliate through withdrawal. Saturn on the other hand, is more to do with the realistic acceptance of human limitations, enabling the person to deal with the world and recognize its opposites. This is a frequent phenomenon of psychotherapeutic work. People identify with all the blackness and ugliness in the family, unwittingly carrying this in themselves and projecting it onto other people, and then try to fight or convert the evil they

INDIVIDUAL THERAPIES

In this section the authors cover only some of the many therapies available but in so doing are not professing or promoting any one above another. The overall aim is to give nurses an increased awareness of what is available and what might be considered beneficial in formulating treatment strategies for patients.

THE INTERPRETATION OF DREAMS
Today, dreams are usually discussed in connection with the work of Freud and Jung, while dream lore of antiquity has almost been forgotten. Greek physicians saw in dreams an indication of bodily and psychosomatic disturbance. Dreams served to offer an orientation in life and warn of fateful future events. In spite of its elusive quality, truth is sought in dreams (Strunz, 1994). Popular dream interpretation was subject to as sophisticated an approach as is found with in-depth modern psychoanalysis.

Falk and Hill (1995) describe the effects of dream interpretation for a group for a women going through divorce. They compared 22 women, aged between 22 and 57 years of age and undergoing separation or divorce, in a short-term dream interpretation group. These women were compared to a group of 12 women on a waiting list, used as the control group. All the women were asked to complete several questionnaires looking at anxiety, depression, coping, insight and self-esteem ratings. The results indicate that the sample group differed in terms of better self-esteem and insight from the control group.

IMAGERY
Since the 1970s there has been an increased interest in man's ability to form images or related mental representations of external experiences, or internal memories and emotions.

Joseph Shorr is considered a pioneer in using imagination as a basis for psychotherapeutic intervention. Child psychologists have long been aware of imagery as a vehicle through which thought and behaviour manifest themselves. Television leaves little to the imagination but not so the radio, which allows the mind to take action and relate images to the unfolding words of a story. Imagery may well be a powerful ingredient that unites perception, motivation, emotion, subjective meaning and realistic and abstract thought (Shorr, 1983).

Waking imagery consists in asking patients to imagine a situation. In doing so, all people reveal how they view the world. Essentially each person willing to reveal an image, reveals an element of themselves, how they see the world and how they see others.

HYPNOSIS

Hypnosis has always been a controversial topic. Healing through the use of trance states again goes back to antiquity. The Ebers papyi, (ancient documents over 3000 years old) describe the hypnotic procedures used by Egyptian soothsayers, Hindu fakirs, Persian magi, Indian yogis and the Greek oracles, all having similar methodology.

Until 1530, no explanation was sought beyond divine intervention for trance states. Anton Mesmer (1734–1815), an Austrian physician whose work on the subject gave hypnosis its alternative name of mesmerism, offered a view on animal magnetism but was subsequently found to have plagiarized the work of an Englishman, Richard Mead (1673–1754). Mead was directly influenced by the work of his patient, Isaac Newton. His idea was of a fluid through which the planets influenced human health, thought of as a transparent odourless gas that envelops the body. He started to treat patients with magnets applied to painful areas. The Marquis de Puysegur (1751–1815) continued Mesmer's work in France. Puysegur discovered that bringing on a crisis in patients did not necessarily cure them but, by allowing them to remain responsive to the hypnotist's wishes, patients were more able to control their symptoms.

In 1880 Dr Joseph Bruer discovered by accident that patients in trances were more easily persuaded to speak freely. Freud later joined Bruer in investigating hypnosis in clinical cases. The use of hypnotism in the early 19th Century stimulated debate and provided the basis for Freud's theory. His interpretation of dreams (1900) and subsequent works, are the widest theories on the human mind and its development. In Britain, it was largely the 1914–18 War that revived the use of hypnosis, through its positive effect on repressed traumatic experiences.

Milton Erikson (1901–1980) was probably the most influential hypnotherapist. Erikson attempted to enter into the patient's personal view of the world and carried out his treatment from the patient's perspective. From his work has developed neurolinguistic programming (NLP), described as a communication skill and a new psychology (O'Connor and Seymour, 1990). Erikson was founding president of the American Society for Clinical Hypnosis and travelled extensively giving lectures and seminars, leading to a world-wide reputation of being a successful and sensitive therapist. A simple secret was his astute observation of patients' non-verbal communication and behaviour patterns. Erikson also used language in deliberately vague ways so that patients could apply their own meanings and interpretation to what he said. The Milton model is a method of using language to induce a trance state where the patient is in close contact with hidden resources. O'Connor and Seymour (1990) define a trance state as where a person is at their most natural and highly motivated to learn from the unconscious in an inner directed way. It is considered neither a passive state nor one under another person's influence but works through the cooperation of patient and therapist. A person in a trance state is usually still; eyes are closed, the pulse is slower and the face is relaxed. Blinking and reflexes are also slower or absent and the breathing rate is slower. The therapist will use a prearranged signal to bring the patient out of a trance or will lead them out by what is being said. The patient may also spontaneously return to normal consciousness.

A therapist's view of working with clinical hypnotherapy
Judith Clark is a Senior Drug Worker holding Diplomas in Iridology and Nutrition and in Clinical Hypnotherapy and an Advanced Certificate in Alcohol and Other Drug Studies:

I was working in Australia in Rehabilitation and Addictions and then went through half my Occupational Therapy training before becoming quite unwell myself. I underwent my own therapy and eventually decided to work independently with clinical hypnotherapy in Australia. My philosophy is that with addictions, denial is an aspect that needs to be addressed. A person who is addicted uses denial so that they can justify the harm they are doing to themselves and to those around them. In order to keep doing this they need to deny and repress their emotions, to such an extent that this denial goes beyond their conscious awareness and becomes unconscious. In counselling, you try to address reality with people on an intellectual, rational level, whilst battling against all these defence mechanisms. Hypnotherapy takes a person beyond the conscious level and goes underneath the wall of defences that have been built up over time; it goes straight to an emotional feeling level. This allows people to realize that they can feel again without being knocked out by that. I've seen such amazing changes in people through the use of hypnotherapy, it allows a person to be honest with themselves at last; this then allows for reaching a level of acceptance and forgiveness. It gives them a freedom to recover.

This all happens on a voluntary basis. Where I worked people elected to have either acupuncture, relaxation and massage, hypnotherapy or whatever. We would sit down with people in a group and discuss the options and explain exactly what would happen and what would be expected to happen in a session and the possible effects. For a few days after a session people often feel worse; it's a painful process as they are looking at things they've kept hidden for so long. But it's the realization that this pain is going to end and there is another way of looking at things. Things really can change and this is where the healing takes place. It's about accessing these emotions, enabling people to feel and accept them, work through the difficulties and then to reach a level of acceptance and forgiveness. By working through I mean this might take a series of six sessions, once a week.

Perhaps if I tell you of this 50-year-old man I saw – he was a real biker, with a bald head, tattoos and only half a leg, all those stereotypical macho images. He was a Vietnam veteran and a heroin addict. In treatment he described carrying round a heaviness that was with him all the time. Through using hypnotherapy I was able to take him back to his experiences in Vietnam and guide him to a path were he could explore his emotions about what happened there and find some answers for himself. There was one particular incident, where he and his troop were marching through the jungle and came across some children that were burning from a bomb explosion. The children were burning alive, so he had to shoot them to get them out of their misery. All his life he had real difficulty associated with all the guilt around that horrific incident. He had children of his own but couldn't understand how they wanted to love him; he said "How can they love me when I'm responsible for that?" It took three or four sessions to get back to that experience and for him to allow the children in and get their forgiveness in his mind, and for him to say what he needed to say to them. It finally allowed him to move on, to give them a symbol of peace, which he choose as a bright light; he gave them peace and they gave him forgiveness. He described feeling able to walk around without their ghosts – he could now move on.

It's wonderful to see those changes; people are killing themselves every day carrying around so much distress, that hypnotherapy is not about re-exposing them to distress, it's about changing their perspective of things and dealing with the hidden emotions that shape their perceptions. People's faces and skin become freer and looser, not really a physical change; its quite hard to describe it in words. It's about enabling a person to let go of their suffering, I've been through it myself – I don't think I could have worked like that if I hadn't.

I suppose there is a danger in nursing to want to rescue people and give them answers rather than allowing people to find the answers for themselves. Nurses want to make people feel better whilst in our care. Basically it's about trust and honesty, that the person is allowed to feel and say things they've not allowed themselves to think and feel for years, and not to feel rejected by their thoughts, that's important. If you can work with someone at an emotional level, their whole perception and outlook on life widens and they can see the fuller picture, in technicolour as it were rather than black and white.

Harmful Effects of Hypnosis

It may be that psychological and physical illness can be precipitated through the use of hypnosis. Someone undergoing hypnosis might describe feeling different and the hypnotist has an important role to play in interpreting this feeling or sensation as part of the debriefing process. Some unpleasant physical sensations can result from maintaining a person in one position over a period of time. Hypnotic suggestion has been shown to alter metabolic rate, so physical fitness needs to be enssured before entering a trance state. A person who suffers any form of distress after minimal exercise is not recommended to try hypnosis as heart rate and oxygen consumption can be affected. There is only one person recorded in the UK as suspected of dying following a hypnotic state – this occured after being subjected to the imagery of being hit by a bolt of lightening. Although it is not clear that the hypnosis was the cause, it is surely sensible never to induce harm or subject patients to any unnecessary risk.

HUMOUR

Humour has been identified as an important strategy for both nurses and patients in dealing with the stress of coping with illness. Described anecdotally as the 'best medicine' (alongside a good night's sleep), humour and laughter have become specifically identified as beneficial, both physiologically as well as psychologically.

James (1995) describes the use of humour as a holistic nursing intervention and a skill nurses could utilize more frequently. Richman (1995) writes of the five principles of using humour as a therapeutic tool. These are presented as:
- Humour enhances the helper–patient relationship.
- Humour is life affirming.
- Humour increases social cohesion.
- Humour is an interactive process.
- Humour reduces stress.

Humour, like any other intervention, needs to be used with sensitivity. An awareness of when it is inappropriate is essential, as someone's sense of humour is personally honed and influenced by social and cultural factors. It cannot be assumed that everyone will find the same situation hysterically funny. Christie (1995) associates the ability to use humour with the creative process and suggests that humour helps put people in touch with painful and often subconscious emotions, allowing improved insight and communication.

MUSIC THERAPY

Gautheir and Dallaire (1993) define music therapy as the controlled use of music and its elements to help the psychological, physiological and emotional integration of the individual or group in the course of treatment. They describe two methods of music therapy:
1. The active mode, where the patient actively takes part by playing an instrument or singing.
2. The passive mode, where the patient is required to listen to music.

When introducing music therapy, an initial assessment of the patient is required to discover and monitor the degree of acceptance, as significance can vary according to the moment, memories and situation (Gauthier and Dallaire, 1993).

Galmany (1993) theorizes that music therapy enhances and promotes a pleasurable experience, as it reactivates the fetal experience of auditory contact with the outside world but most importantly with the mother. This infralinguistic level of communication (through rhythm, sonic and visual traces) is where music infiltrates and activates unconscious and conscious memories of pleasure and comfort.

From published reports, music therapy appears to be of use to all age groups. Goddaer and Abraham (1994) describe how relaxing music played at meal times in nursing homes helped to reduce the prevalence of agitated behaviour by 63% and verbal aggression by 70%.

HOMOEOPATHY

The practice of homoeopathy dates back to the earliest times of health care provision and has undergone many changes in the value placed upon it by different societies, cultures and health care systems. The word homoeopathy is derived from two Greek words, *homois* meaning similar and *pathos* meaning suffering. The combination of these two words represents a very concise description of the homoeopathic method of remedy selection. The principle of like treating like was first acknowledged in the time of Hippocrates. Paracelsus in the 15th Century wrote 'You bring together the same anatomy of herbs and the same anatomy of the illness into one order. This simile gives you an understanding of the way in which you shall heal'.

A considerable body of research data exists to demonstrate the efficacy of the use of homoeopathy with plants, animals and humans. Although the characteristic homoeopathic approach to disease has been recognized throughout history, it was not until the German physician Samuel Hahnemann (1755–1843) first experimented with the principles in a methodical and scientific way that a strong homoeopathic movement developed. Hahnemann was appalled by the crude treatments of the 18th Century and began to look at different, more holistic, forms of treatment. During this time mentally ill patients were treated like wild animals and placed in madhouses, which resembled torture chambers. Hahnemann wrote:

> I never allow an insane person to be punished either by blows or any other kind of corporal chastisement because there is no punishment where there is no responsibility and because the sufferers deserve only pity and are always rendered worse through such rough treatment and never improve
>
> *(Hahnemann, 1994)*.

Homoeopathy soon spread rapidly throughout Europe, India, Russia, Canada and America and most countries had established journals and hospitals before the turn of the 20th Century.

Homoeopathy and Mental Illness

Most homoeopathic doctors advise that homoeopathic medicine does not help in the complex disorders of schizophrenia and manic depressive illnesses. However, the less dramatic but often just as distressing disorders, which arise from depression and anxiety, might well gain considerable help from homoeopathic treatments. An appropriate remedy can often help patients overcome mild or moderate degrees of such reactions and reduce or avert their need for stronger antidepressants or anxiety-relieving medications. Severe depressive illness with associated delusions or strong negative thoughts and suicidal ideation often require more intensive input than homoeopathic treatments can offer.

A combination of therapies has been reported as particular useful, for example homoeopathy and psychotherapy. It is now widely acknowledged that increased understanding of how symptoms have developed, of the conflicts contributing to them and of ways in which habitual anxieties can be changed, are all very helpful to the therapeutic process. In general, having diagnosed the cause of mental disturbance with a positive approach to family and partner's contribution, there is often a very positive response to homoeopathic remedies (Vitkhoulas, 1986).

Some of the most valuable remedies for relieving the tensions and stresses of the disturbed mind have been found to be Gelsemium, Ignatia, Lycopodium, Natrum Mur, Nux vomica and Pulsatilla. Three case studies show the use of different homoeopathic remedies.

Potency Levels in Homoeopathy

Remedies are used at various potencies, determined by the degree of dilution. The first potency (1c) is made by adding one part of the pure mineral to 99 parts of an alcohol solution.

Case Study: **Homoeopathy — Aurum for depression**

A 34-year-old woman presented with a history of depression from the birth of a second child two and a half years previously. The depression came on soon after the birth and made her feel suicidal and indifferent to everything and everybody. She had lost interest in sex, felt desperate and hopeless and cried incessantly. Eventually this subsided and she was able to return to work, but she had still not fully recovered. She shouted at her children most of the time and everything was an enormous effort for her. Her physical health was quite good but she suffered from joint pains in both her hips, all her fingers and toes and in her jaw. She was prescribed Aurum 10m in view of the severity of her depression and this resulted in observable improvement. Two weeks later she felt less depressed, was able to laugh again and found sleep more refreshing. A month later she was feeling much better and reported that she was again enjoying sex and that her joint pains had improved. No further remedy was required and 2 years later there had been no recurrence of depression.

This mixture is then succussed (shaken vigorously). To achieve the second potency (2c) one part of this mixture is then added to 99 parts of the alcohol solution, and again succussed. This process is continued indefinitely to achieve the desired potency. The most common potencies employed in clinical practice are shown in Table 28.1.

The Arndt–Shultz Law

Hahnemann's belief in the minimum dose is supported by the Arndt-Shultz law, which states, in reference to general biological activity, that large stimuli tend to harm or destroy, lesser stimuli tend to inhibit, while small stimuli tend to encourage.

Case study: **Homoeopathy — Pulsatilla for depression and tension**

An 18-year-old female was seen because she had been feeling low, worn out and depressed since completing her A level examinations. She felt dizzy and had a generalized pressure in her head, did not want to go out and was feeling black, despairing and tense. She worried that there was something very wrong with her and that she was dying. She described crying all the time and could not sleep, was off her food, not particularly thirsty, could not tolerate heat and suffering from chest pain when she breathed in. Pulsatilla 10m was prescribed and when seen two weeks later there was a marked improvement. Over the subsequent year she showed no further symptoms.

Case study: **Homoeopathy — a series of remedies for depression and anxiety**

A woman aged 40 attended the homoeopath with her husband, having lost all her confidence and interest in anything over the past 6 months. She was severely depressed and would wake early in the morning crying and worrying. She had lost her appetite and consequently lost 19 kg in weight. Her hair was beginning to fall out, which was an added stress and worry to her. She appeared to be very insecure and was physically clinging on to her husband. All of her problems had begun soon after her daughter had left home, since when she had never felt well.

She was prescribed Lycopodium, which was given in a 10m potency. Two weeks later she was feeling much better with only two bad days that week. However, 2 weeks later she was again nervous and tearful. Kali Carb was prescribed in a high potency particularly because she was afraid of being alone. A further 2 weeks later she was less irritable and not so exhausted but still had little confidence on her bad days. Pulsatilla was prescribed and 2 weeks after this she was much more relaxed and smiling for the first time. She was seen twice more and her confidence and well-being grew. At 6 months follow-up, she said that she would never look back.

AROMATHERAPY

The therapy of aromas consists in the use of organic essences of plants for healing and the maintenance of health and vitality (Table 28.2). The aromas come from appropriate parts of plants, such as the wood from the sandalwood tree, the petals of roses, the peel from lemons, the leaves from rosemary and berries from the juniper bush, to name but a few. These are put through a process of distillation where the volatile odiferous substance is captured. It is the extracted liquid which is known as the essential oil, and this can have many uses. The powerful links between our sense of smell and our emotions play the largest part in the success of aromatherapy and it is through these that the oils have the power to calm troubled emotions.

During the 1980s public interest in Britain began to focus on the attainment of good health. More and more people started looking for natural methods of dealing with stress and all its symptoms, together with ways of ensuring healthy living through diet, lifestyle and relaxation. Once again people are turning their attention to removing the actual causes of disease and illness and away from simply concentrating on remedies to make existing symptoms go disappear. Now, if anything, emphasis is on health promotion and illness prevention, which is where aromatherapy has a large part to play.

The stresses and strains of living in the 20th Century take their toll on everyone. Job uncertainty, financial pressures and other demanding situations are a part of everyone's life. To relieve stress people sometimes turn to alcohol, drugs or food, all of which have their side-effects, which only serve to depress even more. Aromatherapy is a useful way of helping to halt this downward spiral by re-establishing balance and harmony within the body's system. In addition, it is completely natural and has only positive effects. Many of

---

TABLE 28.1 Potencies used in homoeopathy

Dilution ratio	Centesimal series	Decimal series
1/10 or 10-1	1x	–
1/100 or 10-2	2x	1c
1/1000 or 10-3	3x	–
1/10,000 or 10-4	4x	2c
10 - 12	12x	6c
10 - 24	24x	12c
10 -60	60	30c
10 - 2,000	not made	m (= 1,000c).

TABLE 28.2 Some common oils and their effects

Essential oil	Physiological effect
Basil:	Helps relieve and clear a weary mind after excess concentration
Benzoin:	Gives a warm lazy sensation, as if basking in the sun
Bergamot:	Good for revitalizing when feeling worn out and generally a bit down
Camomile:	A calming oil, best used for agitation or restlessness
Cedarwood:	Gives a sense of grounding and reassurance
Clary-sage:	Relaxing to the point of euphoria
Geranium:	A great balancer, restores harmony and equilibrium.
Jasmine:	A calming serene oil which uplifts, soothes
Lavender:	Relaxing to the point of drowsiness
Mandarin:	A soothing oil particularly good for dealing with a knotted, stressed and upset stomach
Melissa:	Works with deep anxiety; helps with black, negative thoughts
Patchouli:	Gives a sense of warmth and friendliness
Rosemary:	Can revive a weary body
Rose:	A renowned healer, it gives a sense of being centred and made whole again
Rosewood:	Gives a cheering and rosy feeling
Sandalwood:	Can help protect and preserve energy and give courage to carry on
Tangerine:	A nerve tonic
Vetiver:	The oil of tranquillity
Ylang- ylang:	Gives a mellow feeling, it can relax and uplift at the same time.

the essential oils described here have a relaxing effect and each oil acts in its own unique way. Some can relax the body to the point of inducing sleep, while others relax and yet revitalize at the same time.

TOUCH

Using the hands to touch and heal is an ancient art and seen as an essential nursing skill. It is a logical extension to the nurse's role of giving intimate physical contact and care. However, the Eastern and Western worlds have very different views on the effect and importance of physical contact.

The use of touch in nursing according to Sims (1986) can be divided into four categories:

1. Instrumental touch — seen as a deliberate physical contact made as part of a procedure, such as supporting a patient in walking.
2. Expressive touch — seen as spontaneous and affective in nature, such as a hug or gentle squeeze for the purpose of comforting someone feeling unhappy. Verbal response has been shown to increase with the use of expressive touch with the elderly (McCorkle, 1974; Hollinger, 1986).
3. Therapeutic touch — involves the transference of energy from one person to another with the intention of healing (Macrae, 1987).
4. Systematic touch — seen as synonymous with massage, with the intention of enhancing the receiver's well-being.

Therapeutic touch is described by Krieger (1975) as an energy field interaction in which the therapist assumes the deitative state of awareness called centring and places their hands 2–4 inches from the body of the patient. To provide a theoretical rationale for therapeutic touch, Kreiger has drawn on two concepts originally cited in an Eastern philosophical system common to Buddhist and Taoist thought. Kreiger believes individuals are able to deliberately and consciously transfer energy to another individual whose energy flow is depleted. The transfer of energy surrounding the individual can be perceived and directed through the hands (Jurgens, 1993).

The Rogerian conceptual model also draws upon the assumption that energy fields are fundamental units of the individual and their environment. Rogers (1970) believes that when a nurse treats a patient, each has an energy field pattern that affects the other's environment and that the intent of nursing practice is to strengthen the coherence and integrity of the human energy field and to divert and redirect patterning of the human and environmental energy fields for maximum health potentials.

Some studies have shown that the use of therapeutic touch has a significant effect on reducing anxiety states and promoting relaxation (Kreiger *et al.*, 1984; Heldt, 1981; Quinn, 1975). Touch is often advocated by nurses as an important means of communication, showing support and empathy and establishing rapport. Communication theorists have stressed that communication consists not only of the verbal content of the message but also the relational factors that are conveyed with it, mainly by non-verbal cues.

In some settings, patients can often be deprived of the benefits of touch and physical contact, which in turn can further increase a sense of perceptual deprivation and isolation. In some elderly care settings and acute psychiatric settings the use of touch falls into the category of systematic touch. In the care of the elderly, use of pets and pet therapy have been used successfully and found not only to reduce hypertension but also anxiety states and agitation.

PROFESSIONAL CONDUCT AND FUTURE PRACTICE DEVELOPMENTS

There is increasing evidence to suggst a significant increase in the number of people receiving complementary therapies. However, complementary therapies are still regarded in the UK with suspicion. Society has tended to depend solely on the prevailing mode of orthodox scientific medicine although it has been shown, from a historical perspective, to lead to stagnation and prejudice. With its increased use, public awareness of complementary therapies as an additional element of choice in health care treatments has reached significant proportions in the population, with a major change in attitude.

A word of warning is needed when discussing the potential use and abuse of complementary therapies. So many self-help books and non-academic texts have been published that Pope's aphorism 'a little learning is a dang'rous thing' needs to be heeded. At present there is nothing to prevent anyone setting up a clinic as an astrologer, healer or psychotherapist regardless of their professional training standards and qualifications. Personal recommendations and a careful check on a person's credentials are always of value to avoid worthless consultations and spending money on tricksters.

A major concern remains the standard of training in the UK. What is required is systematic instruction to give individuals both general and specialist skills. At present there are organizations and bodies in existence that ensure those people who practice have the necessary level of training to be considered competent.

A consumer checklist has been compiled (Royal College of Nursing, 1993) because of a massive increase level of interest in complementary therapies, as shown by the number of enquiries recieved. Nurses are often asked by patients which therapies would be most beneficial and it is therefore important that they know how to find out about therapies and offer the best advice. Table 28.3 outlines some of the pertinent questions to consider.

As training programmes for individual therapies are being drawn up to ensure that European Community directives are met, it is unlikely that therapies will be banned. However, there are directives that will affect the use of herbal, homoeopathic and nutritional remedies.

The need for improved educational standards, together with a code of practice for therapists, is now being acknowledged. This trend is likely to continue, with more therapies following the route of osteopathy, which was regulated in 1995. This regulation of therapies should help to ensure that the practice of complementary therapies within the National Health Service, either by health service staff or other professional therapists, will be safe and of a high quality. Provided nurses ensure that they use complementary therapies that are researched based, this trend of increasing use will continue.

SUMMARY

Complimentary therapy has been of interest to many nurses for a long time now, and it seems at last is being recognized alongside more traditional and medical interventions in the treatment of the mentally ill. Within the chapter we have not been able to look closely at many of the therapies on offer and there remains limited literature on the uses of complimentary therapies on mental health but most specifically severe mental illness.

There appears to be a surge of interest not only among nurses but also amongst the general public and therefore the patients we meet in the clinical practice. Nurses are in a position to brace the changes and meet the future embracing the use and application of such therapies, and to research and evaluate their effectiveness.

TABLE 28.3 Questions to ask about complementary therapies

Is the therapy available on the NHS?
Can the GP delegate care to the therapist?
What insurance cover does the therapist have?
Is the therapist a member of a recognized body with a code of practice?
What are the therapist's qualifications and length of training?
How long has the therapist been practising?
What is the cost of the treatment?
How many sessions should you expect?

KEY CONCEPTS

- Complementary therapies can be used by nurses alongside more orthodox forms of treatment for people with mental health problems.
- Complementary therapies have a historical foundation that has influenced the development of contemporary health care provision.
- The contemporary world is increasingly interested in natural healing and remedies that do not have severe side-effects.
- Nurses are approached for information and advice about complementary therapies and therefore need to have access to information.
- Research into complementary practices has produced some encouraging results in the improvement of physiological, psychological and emotional responses.
- The holistic philosophy of an individual's health and well-being fits well with the use of complementary therapies and regards each patient as unique.

REFERENCES

Achterberg J: *Woman as healer*. London, 1990, Random Century Group Ltd.

Christie GL: Some psychoanalytical aspects of humour. *Int J Psychoanal* 75(4):479–489, 1995.

Falk DR, Hill CE: The effectiveness of dream interpretation groups for women undergoing a divorce transition. *J Assoc Stud Dreams* 5(1):29–42, 1995.

Galmany NN: Musical pleasure, pt 2. *Int J Psychoanal* 74:383–391, 1993.

Gattefosse RM: *Aromatherapie: Le huiless essential hormones vegetales*. Paris, 1937, Giradot.

Gauthier PA, Dallaire C: Music therapy. *Can Nurse* 89(2):46–48, 1993.

Goddaer J, Abraham IL: Effects of relaxing music on agitation during meals among nursing home residents with severe cognitive impairment. *Arch Psychiatr Nurs* 8(3):150–158, 1994.

Greene L: *Dynamics of the unconscious — seminars in psychological astrology*. Harmondsworth, 1988, Penguin.

Hahnemann S: *Organon of medicine*. London, 1994, Victor Gollancz.

Heldt P: Effect of therapeutic touch on anxiety level of hospitalised patients, *Nurs Res* 30(**3**):32–37, 1981.

Hollinger LM: Perception of touch in the elderly. *J Gerontol Nurs* 6(12):9–13, 1986.

James DH: Humour: a holistic nursing intervention. *J Holist Nurs* 13(3):239–247, 1995.

Jurgens A, Meehan TC, Wilson HL: Therapeutic touch as a nursing intervention. *Holist Nurs Pract* Nov 2(1):1–13, November, 1993.

Klein M: *Envy and gratitude*. London, 1975a, Hogarth Press.

Klein M: *Love, guilt and reparation*. London, 1975b, Hogarth Press.

Kreiger D: Therapeutic touch the imprimatur of nursing. *AJN* 75(5), 1975.

Macrae J: *Therapeutic touch – a practical guide*. London, 1987, Arkana.

McCorkle R: Effects of touch on seriously ill patients. *Nurs Res* 23:125–132, 1974.

Mellor C: *Guide to natural health*. Hertfordshire,1978, Mayflower Books.

O'Connor J, Seymour J: *Introducing neuro-linguistic programming. The new psychology of personal experience*. Kent, 1990, Mandala.

Parker D, Parker J: *The new complete astrologer,* 4 ed. Hampshire, 1990, Mitchell Beazley.

Quinn JF: Therapeutic touch as an energy exchange — testing the theory. *Adv Nurs Sci* 6(2):42–49, 1984.

Richman J: The lifesaving function of humour with the depressed and suicidal elderly. *Gerontologist* 35(2):271–273, 1995.

Rogers ME: *The theoretical basis of nursing*. Philadelphia, 1970, FA Davies.

Royal College of Nursing: *Complementary therapies — a consumer checklist*. London, 1993, Scutari.

Shorr J: *Psychotherapy through imagery*. New York, 1983, Thieme-Stratton.

Sims S: Slow stroke back massage for cancer patients. *Nurs Times* 82(13):47–50, 1986.

Stanway A: *Alternative medicine*. Aylesbury, 1979, Penguin.

Strunz F: The dream as a tool in diagnosis healing and life orientation in antiquity. *Fortschr Neurol Psychiatr* 62(10) 389–98, 1994.

Tisserand R: *The art of aromatherapy,* 9 ed. Frome, 1989, Daniel Company.

Vithoulkas G: *The science of homoeopathy*. London, 1986, Thorsons.

West R: Alternative medicine: prospects and speculations. In: Black N, Boswell D, Gray A *et al.*: *Health and disease*. Scotland, 1980, Open University Press.

FURTHER READING

Baseley G: *A country compendium.* Bucks. 1979, WH Allen.
> *A small book which, although now considered outdated, gives valuable information on all aspects of health through nutrition.*

Greene L, Sasporatas H: *Dynamics of the unconscious. Seminars on psychological astrology.* London, 1988, Arkana/Penguin.
> *Liz Greene is always a fascinating read. Some excellent essays are presented in this book which covers astrology from a psychological perspective.*

Gauquelin M: *Neo-astrology. A Copernican revolution.* London, 1991, Arkana/Penguin.
> *More hardcore than Liz Greene but still fascinating.*

Gordon L: *A country herbal.* London, 1980, Webb & Bower.
> *A quick and easy reference guide to herbs and their uses.*

Hyde M: *Jung and astrology.* Kent, 1992, Aquarian/Thorsons.
> *This book offers information on Jung and his thoughts on the importance of astrology in helping understand the mind.*

Launet E: *Edible and medicinal plants of Britain and Northern Europe.* London, 1981, Hamlyn.
> *Rather specialized but still interesting, especially if you fancy a bite when you are out!*

Leyel CF: *Culpeper's English physician and complete herbal remedies.* California, 1971, Wiltshire Book Company.
> *Culpeper's original works are presented in this book, which is interesting for its historical information.*

Petulengro L: *The roots of health. Romany lore health and beauty.* London, 1968, Pan Books.
> *This specialist book is old but remains an excellent overview of the history of health.*

Page M: *The Observer's book of herbs.* London, 1980, Fredrick Warne.
> *Another good reference book on herbs and their properties.*

Rankin–Box DF: *Complementary health therapies: a guide for nurses and the caring professions.* London, 1988, Croom Helm.
> *The first book on complimentary therapies aimed specifically at nurses.*

Behavioural Psychotherapy

<table>
<tr><td>

Learning Outcomes

....

After studying this chapter you should be able to:

• Understand of the basic theory behind behavioural psychotherapy.

• Understand the aetiology and epidemiology of the major disorders.

• Define problems and goals in behavioural terms.

• Understand how to monitor anxiety levels recorded by clients.

• Apply the theory to practice using case examples.

</td></tr>
</table>

*T*his chapter will provide knowledge of the history of behavioural psychotherapy, its uses and some of the basic techniques needed to help clients run their own treatment programmes, as well as more specific information on the more common types of disorder that can be treated using this approach. Students should seek out a trained therapist if they wish to gain knowledge of more advanced techniques that may be used or if they wish to practise these techniques. Supervision of clinical practice is essential for any student, even for those with training in the techniques, and should be arranged before entering into clinical work.

A BRIEF HISTORY

There are a number of historical instances in which techniques closely resembling current or recent behavioural practices have been used, which predate behavioural psychotherapy. Real-life exposure for fear reduction only became common practice in behavioural psychotherapy in the late 1960s. Behavioural psychotherapy was developed from early work by researchers, such as Pavlov, who were trying to analyse behaviour patterns in animals and humans (Pavlov, 1927). Pavlov conditioned dogs to exhibit behaviours when presented with certain stimuli; in one case the ringing of a bell caused dogs to begin salivating as he had conditioned them to associate the sound of the bell with the presentation of food (classical conditioning). He then rang the bell without presenting food and found that after a number of times the conditioned response, i.e. salivation, waned. This process was called extinction. His theories could not explain all behaviours, however, and it was left to other researchers to try to fill in the gaps. Thus new theories developed, e.g. two-stage learning theory (Mowrer, 1950; Miller, 1951) and social learning theory (Bandura, 1977). Joseph Wolpe was the first to effectively use behavioural psychotherapy in treatment when working in the 1950s. He developed a treatment called systematic desensitization. This involved the client practising relaxation while imagining anxiety-provoking stimuli.

Up until the 1970s behavioural psychotherapy had been the domain of the psychiatrist and psychologist. However, in 1972 Isaac Marks began a training programme at the Maudsley Hospital to teach nurses the techniques. Marks recognized that therapists were relatively few for the future workload. Since nurses made up the largest proportion of health service personnel, he proposed that they could be used as the main therapist using little or no supervision. His studies demonstrated that nurses were able to attain the same results as psychiatrists and psychologists and the fact that they were cheaper to employ gave more weight to his arguments for a full-time training course for nurses. Nurses have since been trained at a number of centres around the country.

Behavioural psychotherapy is made up of numerous interventions which aim to change client's attitudes and behaviours. Therapeutic techniques work in three main ways. First, reducing anxiety, e.g. exposure therapy (in real life or in imagination), ritual (response) prevention, cognitive restructuring, coping tactics, and mental cultivation of reassuring thoughts. Second, through impulse reduction, e.g. self-monitoring and self-regulation, covert sensitization, satiation and aversion. Third, by developing new behaviours, e.g. social skills training, sexual skills training, modelling, shaping, contracting, role rehearsal and education.

These techniques, used in combination, can treat a wide range of problems such as phobic disorders (Marks, 1971; Öst, 1989b), obsessive–compulsive disorder (Marks *et al.*, 1975), sexual dysfunction and alternative sexual practices (Hawton, 1985), habit disorders (Azrin and Nunn, 1973), social skills deficit, chronic fatigue syndrome (Butler *et al.*, 1991), post-traumatic stress disorder (Lovell and Richards, 1995), conversion disorders and physiological problems related to behavioural or psychological medicine (irritable bowel syndrome, pain management). Further advances are being made in the area of serious mental illness using these techniques with clients who have psychotic disorders (Tarrier, 1994).

This chapter will focus on the most commonly used technique, i.e. exposure therapy. Exposure therapy is frequently used to treat anxiety disorders. Through education and training, behavioural psychotherapy aims to enable clients to design and run their own exposure programmes.

TREATMENT RATIONALE

To explain the basic principles of exposure therapy and the way in which it works, it is first useful to consider how anxiety problems are maintained in clients. In some cases the origin of the anxiety can be identified, e.g. developing a phobia of dogs following being bitten by one as a child or the onset of obsessive cleaning and hand washing following the birth of a baby. However, many clients are not able to identify the origins of their fear and so it is important that clients understand the systems that maintain and reinforce their problems at the time of presentation, thus enabling them to understand the way in which their treatment will reduce these problems. This will be the focus of this section.

There are many models that can be used to explain the maintenance of anxiety disorders. One of the simplest ways is through the three systems model that postulates that anxiety is made up of three elements namely:

1. Autonomic component — the physical arousal symptoms of anxiety.
2. Behavioural component — the actions performed by the person when anxious.
3. Cognitive component — the catastrophic thoughts and fears present when anxious.

By using these three systems in a flexible way, it is possible to demonstrate clearly to clients the process of fear maintenance. To increase client understanding the model should be adapted to suit the client's presenting problem. For the purposes of this explanation a simple, specific phobia will be used as an example of the model (Figure 29.1).

In most anxiety disorders there is a trigger (or cue) for the anxiety. In the above example this would be the sight of, say, a spider. However, it may not always be the spider *per se* that is the trigger. It may be places where spiders live, such as sheds and garages, or a piece of fluff on the carpet that is mistakenly interpreted as being a spider. In other disorders the triggers will vary also. In agoraphobia the fear of panic in public places is triggered by things such as shops, restaurants, trains and buses. In obsessive–compulsive disorder (OCD) the triggers are even more diverse and range from obvious cues such as dirt, germs and other contaminants, to more rarely seen examples such as sharp objects, children and electrical appliances. The model, as mentioned above, should be adapted to suit the client's description of the problem. For instance, most clients with obsessive ruminations describe the intrusive obsessive thought as the trigger. This then cues their fear and anxiety that, in turn, leads to the obsessive behaviours. This adaptation of the model would have only three components, as the trigger and thought are one and the same. The process outlined in Figure 29.1 occurs almost instantaneously and no part of the cycle is any less important than the others. Different clients will describe the events in different orders. Once the client has applied their own particular physical symptoms, thoughts and behaviours to the

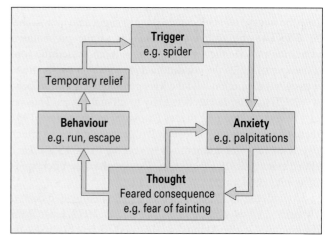

Figure 29.1 The three systems model of fear maintenance

model it is important to relate this process to their anxiety or distress. This can be done by plotting the anxiety levels over time and relating back to the model (Figure 29.2).

Figure 29.2 shows how anxiety is triggered and rises as the client is exposed to the feared situation or object and as the fearful thoughts become more exaggerated. Common anxiety symptoms experienced may be palpitations, tension, headaches, dizziness, sweating, feelings of being unreal or being in unreal surroundings (depersonalization and de-realization) and shaking. As the anxiety or distress rises there comes a point where the physical symptoms can no longer be tolerated or the client believes that the feared consequence is about to happen. It is at this point that the client will perform a behaviour designed to reduce this distress. This behaviour usually take three forms:

1. Avoidance or escape — if the situation is causing high anxiety the person may escape from it. This will cause a reduction of anxiety as the feared stimulus is removedand will probably then lead to avoidance of that, or similar, situations in the future as the reduction of the anxiety, i.e. the reward of feeling better, reinforces the behaviour.

2. Reassurance — the person may try to rationalize their fears and thoughts, to convince him- or herself that everything is going to be all right, or they may ask others to reassure them.

3. Rituals — the person may feel that they can prevent the feared consequence happening by performing certain behaviours; e.g. if someone feels that they have become contaminated and fears that they may pass something on to others, they may wash in a ritualistic fashion; or if they fear they have neglected to do something that may endanger others, they may check and re-check things.

Once these behaviours are performed, the distress and anxiety will decrease until the next time that a trigger is encountered. For clients to understand the treatment rationale, it is important to relate it to their anxiety levels and behaviour and

to point out that these behaviours merely offer temporary relief from symptoms.

It should be explained that to overcome their fears they must expose themselves deliberately to the object or situation that provokes the fear. They should remain with the fear (and the cause) as their anxiety mounts. At the point where they would normally reduce the fear by escaping from the situation or using anxiolytic (anxiety reducing) rituals, they should remain in the situation and stay with the anxiety until it declines of its own accord (habituation). This is demonstrated in Figure 29.3. In severe cases this may take as long as 1–2 hours but the time generally diminishes with more repeated practice. By using a hierarchy of feared situations clients can grade the self-exposures and work through them gradually.

The element of repeated practice is also very important when using exposure therapy. In essence, exposure therapy is about the client learning to cope with anxiety until it no longer bothers them. As when learning any new thing, it becomes easier the more times it is practised, e.g. driving a car, attending job interviews. Clients' behaviours have been learned as a way of coping with their anxiety. Exposure therapy offers them the chance to learn new, less handicapping methods.

THE STAGES OF TREATMENT

In this section of the chapter the stages of treatment will be outlined and some of the issues arising from them will be discussed.

ASSESSMENT

The first stage when considering behavioural psychotherapy as a treatment option is thorough assessment of the client and their problems. Obviously different people will work in slightly different ways within the specialty of behavioural psychotherapy but the following section hopes to outline the type of information the nurse should seek, before determining

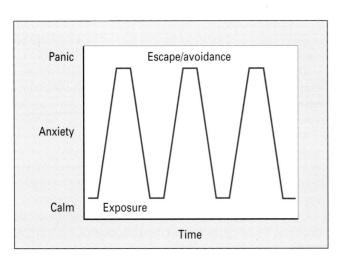

Figure 29.2 Anxiety fluctuations with behaviour

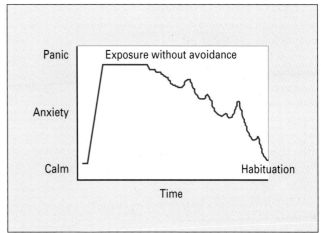

Figure 29.3 Anxiety pattern with exposure and habituation

whether the treatment is suitable for a client and their problem.

The assessment stage can be broken down into several areas, which are described under the following general headings:

- Problem assessment — focuses on gathering information about the presenting problem, including a behavioural analysis. This will allow the therapist to decide whether the problem suits the criteria for treatment.
- Mental state assessment — will determine the client's ability to participate in a treatment programme based on their current mental state.
- Client assessment — will focus on issues such as motivation to do the therapy and issues that may interfere with therapy.

Problem assessment can use information from a number of sources such as old case notes, referral letters and reports from agencies involved in client care. However, the main way of gathering data for assessment of a problem is usually through interview. Interview allows the therapist to focus on areas pertinent to the therapy and to the client, to gain information not previously recorded, as well as to make observations while with the client. For the purposes of the initial assessment therapists should assume that clients are being honest about their problem, that they wish to work in a collaborative way and that they are trying to cope with their problems. By the end of the assessment the therapist should aim to have:

- Gathered information about the client's problem, its impact on their lives and the lives of those around them.
- Given the treatment rationale, along with an informed account of possible difficulties and prognosis.
- Determined whether behavioural psychotherapy is the appropriate treatment for the client's problem.

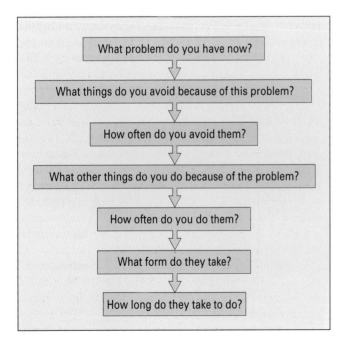

Figure 29.4 Funnelling pattern at assessment interview

- Allowed the client to make an informed decision about whether they wish to proceed with treatment.
- Educated the client about the treatment environment and resources available.
- Discussed future options if the treatment is not suitable for the existing problem.

The initial stages of the assessment interview should focus specifically on the present state of the client's presenting problem, since the causes of the problems are seldom clear and there still will be arguments within the field as to what the exact nature of anxiety disorders is. Many clients will want the therapist to know how the problem started but to determine suitability it is essential to gather data about the form of the problem now. Later in the interview information about the problem onset can be collected. The interviewer should start by asking open-ended questions that allow the client to start talking about their problems, e.g. 'Please tell me about the problem that is affecting you at present?' As the client provides information, this will also provide cues for the therapist to ask closed questions to gain specific problem data. Overall the interview should follow a funnelling format to gain information (Figure 29.4).

This funnelling system is often referred to as the 5 Ws approach:

1. What is the problem?
2. Where does it occur?
3. When does it occur?
4. Who makes the problem better or worse?
5. Why does the problem occur?

It is also useful to look at the frequency of the problem, and at the intensity of the symptoms and their duration.

Following the initial information-gathering about the problem, the client can be asked to recall a specific event at the time when they first became anxious (providing it relates to their problem). From this a behavioural analysis can be performed. The information needed for this analysis is a breakdown of the behavioural, cognitive and autonomic elements of the incident. The incident can be further broken down into the antecedents, the incident itself and the consequences, i.e. before, during and after. At each stage the client should be questioned about the three systems of anxiety (Table 29.1).

This behavioural analysis will give the therapist information about likely reactions to future self-exposure exercises and help when applying the treatment rationale, as the model presented can be personalized using data from this analysis.

Although behavioural psychotherapy tends to focus on the presenting problem, it is useful for the therapist to question the client about the onset of the problem, any precipitating factors, and how it has fluctuated over time, i.e. has it worsened steadily and have there been any symptom-free periods? Coupled with this is the investigation of the use of modifiers. These can include medication, alcohol, illicit drugs, smoking and caffeine, as well as the use of a good luck charm or talisman. These may have significant effects on the way the problem presents and may also influence the efficacy or form of treatment.

Questioning on past treatment may reveal further information about the client and their motivation to participate in treatment. Clients who have sought referral to a unit or service are usually motivated to change and have recognized that they have a problem. Other clients who have been persuaded to seek treatment by family or other health care professionals may not be so motivated. This is not always the case and careful questioning will give the therapist insight into motivational issues. By eliciting the past treatments that a client has had, the therapist will be able to make predictions about issues that may arise in the future; e.g. a client who has had therapy before, but did not attend many of the sessions is likely to be a poor attender in the future. Clients who have done well in previous treatment episodes are likely to do well again but greater attention may need to be paid to preventing relapse rather than educating them about techniques.

A mental state examination should be done to check how the problem affects mood, suicidality, irritability, energy levels, libido, memory, concentration, sleep, weight and appetite. This is outlined in more detail in Chapter 5.

From the data collected the therapist will be able to make a judgement about the suitability of behavioural psychotherapy for the client's problem. Clients who appear unmotivated may need to fulfil contingencies before beginning treatment; i.e. they may be asked to complete some minor exposure tasks or re-read information about the treatment and then contact the therapist to discuss it. Contingencies are tasks or clear boundary definitions designed to test the client's motivation and ensure that they are clear about what is required for the treatment. Other clients will refuse treatment.

There are some general criteria which can act as guidelines for the therapist. These include:

- The presence of severe depression and suicidal thoughts and impulses will cause lack of motivation and create risks for treatment, and clients who are suffering from these problems should seek treatment for them before beginning self-exposure therapy.
- High levels of benzodiazepines (5 mg diazepam daily or equivalent), consumption of high levels of alcohol and use of illicit drugs will mask anxiety symptoms, thus delaying or preventing habituation from occurring.
- Organic conditions such as dementia, poor physical health and acute psychotic symptoms will reduce compliance and understanding of the self-help principles, and clients will need to be carefully assessed if they present with these symptoms. Clients well maintained on medication or who are presently not actively psychotic may still be treated.

Further considerations with regard to local policies and geographical access to services will need to be made, e.g. the client's ability to get to appointments. Treatment will usually be offered if:

- The problem can be defined in terms of observable behaviour.
- The problem is current and predictable.
- The therapist and client can agree on clearly defined behavioural goals.
- There are no contra-indications (see above).
- The client understands and accepts the rationale and treatment. Treatment should not be started without client consent.

The form of treatment can vary depending on what a particular service offers. Most services tend to offer out-patient clinics and community care or domiciliary visits. There are some units that offer in-patient or residential treatment. Out-patient treatment services tend to consist of individual therapists working in existing departments, such as psychology or community mental health care settings. Other departments have been specifically set up to run only a behavioural psychotherapy service but these are fewer in number. Even rarer are residential or in-patient units that offer these specialist services. It is estimated that there are 100–150 full-time equivalent nurse therapists with specialized training in the United Kingdom at present, and that to meet national needs there needs to be 1800 such nurses (Gournay, 1995). However, many nurses have learned basic behavioural psychotherapy skills without completing specialized courses and at present many specific phobics and agoraphobics are treated in community settings by nurses. In the future, nurse training may look specifically towards behavioural psychotherapy techniques as an answer to some anxiety problems, rather than the more generic approaches taught currently. In the meantime, courses such as the ENB 650 in Adult Behavioural Psychotherapy continue to serve in the training of specialized therapists.

TABLE 29.1 Behavioural analysis

Antecedents

Behaviour	What were you doing before the incident?
Cognitions	What were your thoughts at the time?
Autonomic	How did you physically feel?
Others	Where were you? Who was with you? What was happening?

Behaviour

Behaviour	What did you do during the incident?
Cognitions	What were you thinking as things were happening?
Autonomic	How did you feel during the incident? What symptoms did you experience?

Consequences

Behaviour	What did you do?
Cognitions	What were you thinking?
Autonomic	Once it was over, how did you feel?

EDUCATION

It is important that the client is advised on what the treatment entails before consenting to it. This not only means providing information and education about their present problem and the treatment rationale for dealing with it but also other information that may affect their ability receive the treatment or influence their decision to start. Many clients wish to know why they are affected with their problem. This is a difficult question to answer as therapists are unsure themselves why these fears develop. In some cases a specific event is linked with onset and helps the therapist by providing a likely cause to the problem but in others the onset is slow and insidious with no obvious causal factors. Different schools of psychiatry will give differing reasons as to why a person presents with a problem. Increasingly, combinations of these theories are being used to explain the development of anxiety disorders. The most commonly used models at present are the cognitive and behavioural models, which are used either individually or in combination. Because of the diverse possible reasons for clients' problems, it is probably more useful for the nurse to remind clients of maintaining factors rather than those that caused onset.

Another common question is 'What are my chances of getting better?' Here the nurse should provide realistic information to the client regarding what improvement the latter can expect. Many units use audit measures and will be able to give average outcome results. However, these should be linked to diagnosis, as there may be subtle differences between diagnostic groups; e.g. obsessive–compulsive disorder generally takes longer to treat than specific phobias to maintain the same level of improvement. Also, the level of compliance and motivation may well influence treatment outcomes and the nurse should try to provide factual information and not make promises that may not be able to be kept. Many textbooks contain information about treatment and outcome results, as well as about problems in treating these types of disorders (Marks, 1987). It is important that information should be:

- Factual and, if possible, based on research findings.
- Presented clearly and concisely in a form that the client can understand.
- Realistic about possible problems that may arise and the amount of time and effort that will be needed to overcome them.

PLANNING

Treatment should be planned in a structured fashion. This can be done by getting the client to indicate a hierarchy. A hierarchy should consist of an ordered list of objects or situations that the client feels unable to face, has difficulty facing or that cause high levels of anxiety. Ideally this list should consist of 15 to 20 items. This may be possible in the case of a specific phobia such as a fear of spiders but such a short list is less likely with a complex case of obsessive-compulsive disorder, where a client may have hundreds of rituals associated with one behaviour. For instance, when getting up, washing and dressing in the morning, a client may go through a myriad of washing, checking and reassuring rituals and may take anything up to 6 hours to carry out a task that would take the average person up to 1 hour to complete. Therefore, in these more complex cases, it is essential that the list covers larger groups of behaviours, rather than giving specific examples. This is demonstrated in Box 29.1 with a simplified item hierarchy.

When actually treating the problem, these items in the hierarchy can be further broken down into specific individual homework goals. In this way the client will not be flooded by their fears but will be able to work through them in a graded fashion.

To further structure treatment and monitor its efficacy it is important to use some kinds of measurement. Measuring allows us to obtain a baseline and convert subjective statements made by clients, for example 'I feel awful and tense', into objective scores on a numbered scale, thus allowing changes to be noted accurately. This can be done by defining Problems and Goals and rating them. This section details one method of doing this – it is not the only method and can be adapted to suit different clinical areas. Before beginning assessment of the problem and the client's progress, it is useful to give the client a rationale for proceeding. Measurement serves a number of purposes benefitting the client, the nurse and the organization that they work for. Benefits include the following:

- The ability of client and nurse to track progress across a number of measured clinical areas, e.g. mood, anxiety, problem impact and goal attainment, and thereby adjust therapy to suit the client's particular needs.
- The client can track their degree of improvement and see where more effort needs to be made, or areas where the problem has been overcome. This may help to improve motivation and confidence and gives the client feedback.
- The use of measures as an audit tool will enable a service to give referrers and clients accurate information about prognosis and chances of success. It also helps the service to justify what it is presently doing and to develop new innovations in treatment for the future based on this knowledge.

Box 29.1

An example of a problem hierarchy in a case of obsessive–compulsive disorder

Highest anxiety

1. Touching items contaminated with urine, blood, faeces or other bodily fluids causes anxiety and ritualistic behaviour.
2. Wearing items of clothing for more than one day causes anxiety and ritualistic behaviour.
3. Touching other people or other people's items causes anxiety and ritualistic behaviour.
4. Touching, washing own body causes anxiety and ritualistic behaviour.

Lowest anxiety

5. Touching daily objects that are not known to be contaminated causes anxiety and ritualistic behaviour.

Problems and Goals are a basic but effective way of measuring a client's problem and their progress in achieving their goals for treatment. They constitute a case-specific measure, as the problem statement and the goals relate purely to the client and have been designed by the client with the aid of the nurse. Other validated questionnaires are not case specific as they can be applied to any client.

Problem statements should be defined in collaboration with the client and use his or her own words. They should consist of:

1. Feared consequence, e.g. panic or heart attack.
2. Antecedent, e.g. going more than 1 mile from the house.
3. Behaviour, e.g. avoidances.
4. Consequence, e.g. restriction of daily life.

An example of a problem statement in a case of agoraphobia might be 'fear of a heart attack on going more than 1 mile from home alone, leading to avoidance of going out and crowded situations, resulting in restricted social, work and home life'. The problem can then be measured by both client and therapist by choosing a number from the scale that corresponds most closely to the severity of problem in their view (see Figure 29.5).

Two problem definitions are usually sufficient, though clients with multiple problems may need more. If a client has several problem behaviours that are all related to one theme, the nurse should try, through discussion, to get them grouped together as one problem rather than as several different ones.

Like problems, goals are defined in collaboration with the client using his or her own words. They should be things that clients would like to do, but cannot or find difficult because of the problem. It is useful to have a variety of goals but when explaining how to define them to the client it should be emphasized that the goals should be seen as things they wish to achieve by the end of treatment, i.e. in 6 months to 1 year's time depending on the length of treatment and whether follow-up is offered. Goals should be identified from the problem definition, stated positively, and above all be realistically achievable. The goal definition should contain the following:

1. Behaviour, e.g. shopping.
2. Conditions, e.g. alone or at busy times.
3. Frequency, e.g. twice per week.
4. Duration, e.g. for 1 hour.

Examples of goal statements in a case of agoraphobia might be:

• Go shopping in a large supermarket store alone at 9 a.m. twice a week for 1 hour.
• Walk 3 miles to parents with baby and stay for 1 hour twice a week.
• Go to the pub and socialize with three friends for the evening once a week.

The goal can then be rated by both client and therapist on a scale such as that in the example shown in Figure 29.6.

Goals can be an important tool in starting the therapeutic process because they encourage realistic expectations from therapy, focus the client on the possibility of change, stress the client's active role in therapy and provide structure to therapy.

Other measures that can be used as standard include the Fear Questionnaire, Work and Social Adjustment Scale and Beck Depression Inventory. Others may be used when appropriate for the client's problem, e.g. Social Situations Questionnaire, Compulsion Checklist, Obsessive–Compulsive Time Discomfort And Handicap or Conventional Sexual Activity (Marks *et al.*, 1986). Other validated measures are given in Chapter 5.

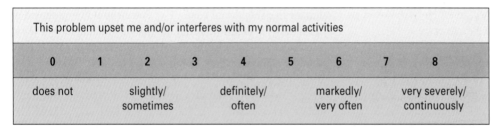

This problem upset me and/or interferes with my normal activities								
0	1	2	3	4	5	6	7	8
does not		slightly/ sometimes		definitely/ often		markedly/ very often		very severely/ continuously

Figure 29.5 An example of a problem rating scale

My progress towards achieving the goal regularly without difficulty:									
	0	1	2	3	4	5	6	7	8
Discomfort	none		slight		definite		marked		very severe
Behaviour	complete success		75% success		50% success		25% success		no success

Figure 29.6 An example of a long-term goals rating scale

All measures should be made at regular intervals to monitor progress and maintenance of gains. Usually these intervals are assessment or pre-treatment, mid-treatment and discharge, and 1 month, 3 months, 6 months and 1 year follow-up. To administer measures correctly the nurse should always explain the measure clearly to the client in advance and check their understanding. When repeating measures the nurse should do so without the previous ratings being seen to reduce subjectivity, i.e. the previous rating influencing the client's or nurse's current rating of the problem. If the measure is rated by both client and therapist and the ratings are markedly different, then the nurse should check for misunderstandings by either party, e.g. misunderstanding of the problem or of the rating scale. When rating, the nurse should note down measurements first without the client seeing them. The client should then complete their ratings. This prevents data contamination, i.e. the client being influenced by what the nurse has recorded or the opposite. If ratings differ by more than 2 points on a 0–8 scale, or a similar amount on a comparable scale, then the issue should be discussed as to why each person rated the way they did.

Homework goals are also an important way in which the treatment can be structured. If we consider treatment as a ladder leading to the attainment of long-term goals, then homework goals are the rungs of the ladder that will enable the client to climb to the top and see success. The hierarchy should list the areas that the client experiences difficulty with. To begin the programme, the client should select one that would be useful for them to overcome and that causes them at least some discomfort. They should try to start as high up the hierarchy as is realistically possible. The ritual or avoidance can be defined as a problem, e.g. 'Repeated checking of electrical appliances for fear of harming others'. From this, the client and nurse can create the self-exposure task using the same method as for the treatment goals, for example:

1. Behaviour — use electrical items.
2. Conditions — without checking afterwards.
3. Frequency — five times a day.
4. Duration — for at least 1 hour.

Examples of self-exposure homework goals for obsessive–compulsive disorder are:

- Use the toaster for 10 minutes daily without returning to check.
- Switch light switches on and off repeatedly five times a day for 5 minutes without counting or returning to check.
- Turn the fire on and off 10 times a day and not return to check for at least 1 hour.

Homework tasks that have been devised should then be recorded on a daily goal sheet. The goals can be rated on a scale similar to that shown by Figure 29.7, to indicate how much distress the client feels.

Clients rate their anxiety or distress before they start the exposure exercise, during it, and just before they finish it. They should also note any comments. Examples of homework diary sheets can be found in many texts or can be designed to suit the service in which the nurse works.

IMPLEMENTATION

The best way to tackle fears is through self-exposure exercises. The client and nurse agree weekly targets, which the client then records in a daily diary. There may be more than one exercise that the client can do to face one item on the hierarchy, and so the programme may have many exercises to be completed for the week. It is best to start with 3–4 exposures for the first few days and then gradually to add to them.

Avoidance of the anxiety prevents exposure to the feared thoughts. Rituals or reassurance stop exposure by reducing the anxiety. Avoidance, rituals and reassurance prevent clients from confronting their feared thoughts and situations and from learning that their fears may not actually be realized. Treatment involves confronting the feared thought, object or situation (self-exposure) long enough for the anxiety to fall away to a significant extent (see below). However, this alone is unlikely to be successful if the client continues to cancel out or neutralize their anxiety with compulsive behaviours. So, as well as self-exposure the client should stop cancelling out the anxiety (response prevention) and, rather, should prolong the exposure. A course of exposure entails clients exposing themselves, via graded exposure excercises, to what they fear without resorting to avoidance and rituals or seeking reassurance. These exercises should be prolonged to allow enough time for anxiety to decline; a fall in anxiety levels of at least 50% should be aimed at before terminating the exposure procedure. This usually takes 1–2 hours but may take longer in exceptional cases. Exposure should be repeated at least daily, if not more often. In this way the client will learn more quickly. Finally, the exposures should be carried out by the client alone. Some homework goals may be done with other people initially, so that they can help and support the client. However, at some stage the client needs to find out if they can cope alone.

When designing exposure tasks the client should try to actively seek out feared situations and thoughts rather than wait for things to happen and then try to deal with them. Response prevention needs to be consistent and continuous

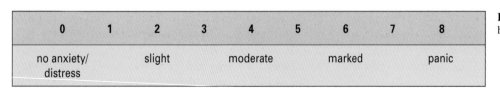

Figure 29.7 An example of a homework goals rating scale

for maximum benefit to the client.

If, during exposure, the client gives in to the urge to avoid, ritualize or seek reassurance, they should repeat the exercise of self-exposure (re-exposure). For example, if a client fears contamination and, to reduce that fear, washes their hands repeatedly, exposure would consist in intentional self-contamination and avoidance of washing. If the urge to wash becomes too great to resist, the client can re-contaminate by touching a 'contaminated' object, so ensuring the continuation of the exposure.

Clients neutralize their anxiety or discomfort by asking relatives and friends for reassurance should desist from so doing; indeed, they should ask those from whom they are seeking support to answer each such request by saying 'Hospital says no answer' in an emotionless, bored voice. Reassurance gained by clients in this manner does not help in the long run, and the temptation to give such support should be firmly resisted, even if the client is irritated or forceful. If, after having said 'Hospital says no answer' to five of the client's requests for reassurance, only to find that the client still persists, the recipient of the appeals should walk away. Non-hospital units can develop their own phrases for with-holding reassurance.

It is worth mentioning the technique of imaginal exposure at this point. Imaginal exposure should follow the same rules of being graded, prolonged, repeated and frequent. However, rather than entering the actual situation, the client should be asked to create vivid visual and sensory images of the feared items on their hierarchy. They can do this by talking through the imagined situation in the first person and present tense for example 'I am walking'. This then sets up a running commentary of the exposure that can be recorded and used for repeated homework exposures. When doing the commentary the client should try to include not only descriptions of what is happening using all of their senses but also the feelings they are experiencing. This technique has been found to be useful in the treatment of clients with post-traumatic stress disorder (PTSD) and is also beneficial in cases where the feared stimulus is not readily accessible, e.g. fears of flying or thunder.

The most preferable way of organizing a course of treatment is where sessions are regular and frequent, e.g. 1 hour each week. This means that the total treatment period is relatively short (8–12 weeks). At first, appointments should be made often e.g. weekly for out-patients and daily or on alternate days for in-patients. The nurse can offer guidance and support to the client in the first stages of their self-help treatment. This ensures that any difficulties are dealt with and that the client is engaging correctly in treatment; it also shows the nurse's commitment. As treatment progresses and the client becomes more adept at the techniques and at problem solving, the intervals between sessions can be lengthened. This also allows the client to become more independent and reduces any nurse dependency that may have developed. It will also prepare the client for the lead-up to discharge and follow-up.

The ideal environment for therapy is a quiet, undisturbed room with plenty of natural light and comfortable seating. This is not always available but should be sought where possible. All possible resources should be used and any equipment needed should be prepared and brought to the session to avoid interruptions.

Treatment can take several forms. Out-patient treatment is the commonest form of therapy. Even clients with extreme rituals or avoidances can usually attend out-patient sessions if accompanied and this is a good test of their commitment to therapy. This approach is thought by many to be the best option. The nurse–client relationship is undiluted and the nurse is able to focus solely on the individual and his or her particular problems and idiosyncrasies. Domiciliary visits tend to take place only in exceptional circumstances. Generally, clients will only have residential or in-patient treatment if the handicap is extremely severe, they have no support network or if they live so far away that it is impractical to have out-patient treatment; however this can often be overcome by using phone contact. In these cases clients may be admitted to begin treatment. When they have made gains and are less handicapped, they can return home to continue therapy.

There has been a move over the years to conduct therapy with minimal intervention from the nurse, mainly to improve cost-effectiveness. Some have suggested that clients can be treated purely with a self-help manual. Ghosh *et al.* (1988) found similar results for computer-assisted, therapist-assisted and self-help manual treatments. The great majority of sessions should, therefore, involve problem-solving and home-work planning, with therapist-accompanied exposure being used only rarely. The nurse may, rarely, accompany a client during exposure where it is not possible to persuade the client to start self-exposure. The nurse should start fading out his or her presence during the first exposure session. There is little justification for accompanying the client during exposure beyond the second session. It is important for clients to learn, by then, that they can be exposed to their fears alone and do not need a nurse physically present for support.

EVALUATION

Review of progress at regular intervals is essential when dealing with anxiety disorders. Nurses, in most cases, act as guides, supports and educators in helping clients to help themselves by self-exposure. They teach clients about the rationale for the treatment, help them to plan and implement it and help them to evaluate their performance and redesign the programme as necessary. At each session the nurse and client should review the self-exposure homework goals that have been recorded between sessions. From the diaries it is possible to tell if habituation is taking place or whether further exposures are needed. Client and nurse can negotiate future programme goals as well as reviewing and solving any difficulties that may have arisen between the sessions. In the light of new information, the nurse and client may wish to reassess their appraisal of the problem before continuing to develop further exposure goals. Other complications, such as lowered mood or suicidality, will also need to be addressed by reassessing the client's ability to carry through a treatment programme. Regular mental state checks are advised in most cases, as severe anxiety caused by exposures can have a significant effect on mood.

SPECIFIC PROBLEMS

In this section some of the major conditions that are treated with behavioural psychotherapy are discussed.

OBSESSIVE–COMPULSIVE DISORDER (OCD)

An obsession is a persistent thought, image or impulse that is intrusive, repetitive and unwanted. It causes distress, feels senseless, is usually resisted and is beyond the client's control. Obsessions are generally recognized as being the product of one's own mind and not imposed from without. The content of the obsession is usually repugnant, worrying, blasphemous, obscene or nonsensical. Common themes are dirt, contamination, sex, religion, aggression or violence, orderliness and socially unacceptable actions.

In two studies involving non-clinical populations, thoughts and impulses, with all the characteristic intrusive qualities of obsessions, occurred in 88% of a 'normal' population. This suggests that it is not the thought that is the problem but the person's response to it. Most of us can dismiss such intrusive thoughts and impulses but clients with an obsessional problem are unable to do this and the thought causes extreme anxiety and distress. They then try to deal with the anxiety by ignoring or suppressing the thought or neutralizing it with some other thought or action (compulsive ritual).

A compulsion is a repetitive, purposeful and intentional act that is performed according to certain rules or in a stereotyped way. The act is designed to neutralize discomfort or prevent some dreaded event or situation occurring. Most often such an act is partly acceptable but the client recognizes that it is excessive, unreasonable or exaggerated. The act is performed with a sense of subjective compulsion that is coupled with a desire to resist the compulsion. Resisting leads to a sense of mounting tension, which can be relieved immediately by yielding.

Stern and Cobb (1978) looked at types of rituals in 45 subjects and found the following percentages for rituals:

Cleaning	51
Repeating	40
Checking	38
Orderliness	9
Hoarding	2

Obsessions can occur without rituals but most rituals are preceded by obsessions. Welner *et al.* (1976) found that of 150 patients, 69% had obsessions and compulsions, that 25% had obsessions only and that 6% had compulsions only.

It is estimated that 10.8% of the general population have obsessive–compulsive symptoms but only 0.05% have OCD. OCD accounts for approximately 2% of adult psychiatric clients. The mean age of onset is 22 years and 92% of clients develop their symptoms between the ages of 10 and 40 years. The mean age of presentation is 34. There are no differences in the occurrence of the disorder between sexes.

It is thought that OCD tends to occur more in people who have always had meticulous and perfectionist personalities. However, most people with such traits never develop OCDs and 30% of patients never had them. Many obsessional problems start from a period of depression but continue after the depression has lifted. Depression is a complication in 33% of people with obsessive–compulsive problems.

The problem is thought to be maintained by the act or thought that cancels out the intrusive thought or image (Figure 29.8.).

The client has an intrusive thought that causes anxiety or distress. They then try to cancel or neutralize this thought with

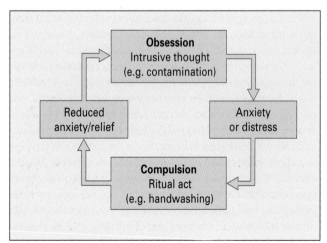

Figure 29.8 A behavioural model of OCD

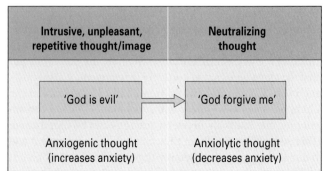

Figure 29.9 An example of neutralizing thoughts in OCD

some other thought or action, in this case hand washing. This reduces the anxiety caused by the thought but the relief from the compulsive act is only short term and the more the person does this, the more frequent and intense the thought, resulting in more frequent rituals. One can see how the anxiety raised by particular fears will lead to particular avoidances or rituals, e.g. fear of dirt leading to washing, doubting leading to checking, fears of harming others leading to reassurance seeking and fears of injury leading to touching. Although these are compulsive acts, the same is true for thoughts (Figure 29.9).

See the following case study of a woman with OCD.

Exercise 1 Using the case study, construct an exposure hierarchy that it is the client would elicit. Following this, define the problem and set some long-term goals. Finally, using these, design at least one homework goal that the client could use.

Exercise 2 With a colleague, repeat Exercise 1 using a role-play to develop skills. For this exercise, client's problem can be assessed in the form of a role-played interview before progressing to defining goals.

PHOBIAS

Phobias occur when a person has a persistent and irrational fear of a specific object, activity or situation. This results in an urge to avoid the phobic stimulus. The fear generally has a specific focus and is the most common presentation of the anxiety response, with biological, cognitive and behavioural elements. Most clients with phobias recognize that their fear is excessive or unreasonable but this does not prevent phobias causing severe handicap. There are three general categories of phobias – specific (or simple) phobias, agoraphobia and social phobia.

Specific Phobias

A specific phobia is an irrational fear of a single object or situation (excluding those avoided as a consequence of agoraphobia) that occurs whenever that stimulus is presented. There is avoidance that is associated with the feared situation. The most common fears are those of small animals, e.g. dogs, snakes, spiders. Others include claustrophobia, height phobia, vomit phobia, flying phobia, thunder phobias and blood–injury phobias. It is estimated that 76 people per 1000 have a phobia but only 2 phobias per 1000 are disabling (0.2% of the population). Onset for most phobias is in childhood. Animal phobias are present in most children prior to puberty but generally disappear as the child gets older. Those left with animal phobias tend to be female. The male to female ratio in specific phobics is 1:1.7.

Grouped with specific phobias are those fears known as illness phobias. These are usually characterized by an intense fear of dying or having illnesses such as cancer, heart disease and AIDS. Clients will constantly ruminate that they may have one of these illnesses and may avoid anything that will trigger off these ruminations, e.g. reading medical articles or broadcasts. They may also develop ritualistic behaviours such as

---

Case study: A woman with obsessive–compulsive disorder

Kate is a 37-year-old unemployed woman who lives with her husband and two children. She has had a 10-year fear of contamination from faeces and urine. She avoids using public toilets and touching taps directly (she uses kitchen towels to turn taps on and off). She avoids touching objects in her own house, such as bathroom utensils, cupboards, door handles, TV controls and the washing machine. Stains or marks, particularly brown ones, on items or seats cause her anxiety and she constantly has to check such items. She washes her hands up to 50 times a day depending on what she is doing and the level of contamination. If she feels badly contaminated she will shower. This can take up to 2 hours and happen more than once a day. When washing, she washes different parts of her body one at a time, but not always in the same order. She seeks reassurance from others that what she is doing is right and acceptable, and reassures herself by convincing herself that things are not contaminated. If she touches a contaminated objects she feels disgusting and dirty. She fears that she will pass this on to others. Her anxiety symptoms include tachycardia and palpitations, sweating, hyperventilation and shaking and she fears that the anxiety will harm her. She has given up work and no longer socializes or has other people in the house because of her fears. The family life has been affected dramatically and when her children and husband come into the house they have to change immediately and wash or shower.

Onset was at age 27, following the birth of her second child. She takes antidepressant medication as her mood is low, and she is fed up with the problem. She has no thoughts of suicide.

---

checking their body, asking others for reassurance, or asking for repeated examinations and second opinions. These phobias mark the bridge between specific phobias and OCD but differ from hypochondriasis in that the fears have a specific focus and are not diffuse. It has been noted by some authors that these types of fears tend to follow what is fashionable. For instance, some years ago one of the commonest illness fears was of venereal disease but this is now rare and has been superseded by the fear of AIDS.

One type of phobia that results in differing autonomic responses is the fear of blood, injury or injection needles. In these cases there is a diphasic response. At first sufferers get the typical anxiety symptoms of anxiety, such as tachycardia, sweating, tightness in the chest and shaking. This rapidly changes as blood pressure drops to levels low enough to cause fainting. A slightly modified treatment approach is required. Applied tension combined with graded exposure has proven to be an effective treatment for blood–injury phobia. It aims to alter the patient's physiological responses that maintain the phobia. The second phase of the diphasic response consists in a rapid drop in blood pressure and, consequently, the cerebral blood flow. The client feels dizzy and eventually faints. To reverse this, the client needs to learn a coping skill that can be applied quickly and easily in most situations. Applied tension produces an increase in blood pressure and cerebral blood flow by tensing the gross body muscles. By learning to identify the early signs of the fall in blood pressure, clients can use the tension technique before fainting occurs. Exposure to a large array of blood–phobic situations helps to reduce fear of the – and this is further strengthened when applied tension is used at this time (Marks, 1988). In cases where the fainting response is absent, self-exposure or imagination, will usually suffice. See the case study of a man with a specific phobia.

Exercise 1   Using the case study, construct an exposure hierarchy that might be elicited by the client. Following this, define the problem and set some long-term goals. Finally, using these design at least one homework goal that the client could use.

Exercise 2   With a colleague, repeat Exercise 1 using a role-play to develop skills. For this exercise an assessment of the client's problem can be prepared in the form of a role-played interview before progressing to defining goals.

Agoraphobia

Despite the common assumption that agoraphobia is a fear of open spaces, this is, in fact, not the case. Agoraphobia is a fear of being in public places (from the Greek *agora* meaning market place or public place) especially when alone or where escape might be difficult or help not available should some-thing happen. Sufferers avoid crowded shops and precincts, trains, buses, lifts and other public situations. Typically they describe a 'fear of fear' and avoid feared situations in case they bring on panic. Two-thirds of agoraphobics are women and generally onset is between 18 and 35 (average age 28 years). Agoraphobia occurs in 6 people per 1000 (0.6% of the general population).

Commonly associated with agoraphobia is the presence of panic disorder and generalized (free-floating) anxiety. This may be fairly constant or may vary greatly from day to day. This lasting, generalized anxiety may merge into panics. These panics may strike at any time of the day or night and are thought to be exacerbated by stressful events and situations. Panics can vary greatly in both intensity and duration. Common symptoms include severe palpitations, constricted chest, shooting pains in the arms and chest and blurred vision. These symptoms usually last between 5 and 10 minutes but in some cases may continue for an hour or more.

Agoraphobia has been well researched over the years because of the large number of cases. Research has included telephone assessment and treatment for severe housebound agoraphobics using a comparison between exposure therapy and relaxation. Exposure was found to have a significant effect but not to the same level as face-to-face contact (McNamee *et al.*, 1989). In 1984 Rachman introduced the idea of the 'safety signal perspective' for agoraphobia, when he argued that much of agoraphobic behaviour was geared towards achieving and maintaining safety or a sense of safety.

Case study: **A man with a specific phobia**

Gary is a 23-year-old engineer with a 4-year fear of being or feeling sick. He lives with his girlfriend in their rented flat. Because of his fear, he checks food (he has stopped eating meat because it may not be cooked properly) and always looks to see that food is within the sell-by date and is well cooked. He checks that foods are not off and tries not to eat foods that he feels may clash. He keeps notes on the foods he has eaten already. He avoids places where people might be sick, e.g. ferries, pubs and accident sites, as well as people who are drunk. On holiday flights, if there is turbulence, he sits in an aisle seat. When shopping, he checks expiry dates on food 4–5 times and will leave packets out on his return home in case he wants to check them again. He questions his girlfriend and shop assistants about the food and may even rummage in the bins to find out the sell-by date of something he has eaten. The problem is worse in the morning on waking as he feels he is going to be sick. He has not vomited for 4 years. Other triggers for his fear include physical illness, being stuck in traffic jams and the sounds of ambulances. Anxiety symptoms include shaking, sweats, nausea, increased heart rate, deep breathing and rigid posture.

The problem started 4 years ago after a bout of gastro-enteritis. He takes no medication and does not drink alcohol. Impact on his social life is severe. He is unable to eat out at restaurants and cannot go to the pub or parties with his friends. At home he has wasted hundreds of pounds worth of food through overcooking or throwing it away. He feels generally happy and has no suicidal intent or ideation. His concentration has diminished because of his pre-occupation with food. He does eat regularly and has not lost weight, though his diet is affected by the problem.

Case study: **A man with agoraphobia**

David is a 34-year-old unemployed man who lives in a rented bedsit with three other people. He has had a 10 year fear of going out of the house alone in case he panics. He avoids public places such as shops and pubs. He is unable to use public transport and when out has to be accompanied by a friend or family member. Even when accompanied he will not go into a shop more than a few feet and will stay near exits. He cannot use lifts, escalators or go onto the first floor of any building. When in public places he feels hot, has palpitations and hyperventilation and fears that he will have a heart attack. He carries beta-blockers prescribed by his GP, but very rarely uses them as his anxiety decreases once he is no longer confronted by an anxiety- generating situation. He also carries a bottle of water and some sweets to suck if he becomes anxious. At home he has panics up to 3 times a day with no identifiable triggers. He has had to give up his job as a gardener and cannot look after his own back garden. He is unable to shop alone and tends only to go to local shops. He no longer socializes and his relationship with his girl-friend has ended because of the problem.

David has low mood because of the social isolation and has a poor sleep pattern because of panics. He takes antidepressant medication for his mood and to help him sleep. He has poor concentration and is more irritable than he used to be. He has not had thoughts of committing suicide but at times thinks he would be better off if he did not wake up in the morning.

He used this model to explain the onset of agoraphobia and make suggestions about how these perspectives could be assessed.

See the case study of a man with agoraphobia.

Exercise 1   Using the case study, construct an exposure hierarchy that might be elicited the client. Following this, define the problem and set some long-term goals. Finally, using these design at least one homework goal that the client could use.

Exercise 2   With a colleague, repeat Exercise 1 using a role-play to develop skills. For this exercise, an assessment of the client's problem cna be prepared in the form of a role-played interview before progressing to defining goals.

Social Phobia

Most of us have in our teenage years experienced anxiety and the fear of feeling awkward or embarrassed in a variety of social situations. However, these feelings generally decrease with time. Only when this normal anxiety become so severe, with an increase in avoidances and a resulting handicap in a person's life, can it be talked about in terms of a social phobia. In the general population, 0.5% of people are badly handicapped by social fears. Onset is usually in late adolescence and there are no differences between the sexes.

Social phobics fear situations in which others may look at them or may form an opinion (usually negative) of them. It is not the crowd *per se* that they fear but more the fact that the members of that crowd may evaluate them negatively. This may be for a number of reasons. Many clients report a fear of saying the wrong thing or looking stupid when they are in public, a fear partly shared by agoraphobics. However, there are a number of features peculiar to social phobia that distinguish it from agoraphobia. First, social phobics tend to report different autonomic symptoms rather than the palpitations, hyperventilation and dizziness or faintness of agoraphobia. They more commonly report blushing, hot flushes, shaking and sweating, to the point where they are unable to write in public or wear make-up to hide their blushing. Secondly, there is commonly an inability or difficulty in maintaining eye contact with others and when in social situations there are avoidant behaviours. Clients with agoraphobia will tend to avoid a situation if they predict that they may panic. Social phobics will also avoid situations that may evoke panic but more commonly do enter the situations providing they are able to perform certain behaviours, e.g. sitting with their backs to people, sitting in poorly lit areas or having alcohol to help them relax. It is important, when assessing clients, that the nurse ensures correct analysis of the problem i.e., social phobia or social dysfunction (Stravynski and Greenberg, 1989). Social dysfunction consists in difficulty in initiating and maintaining social contact resulting from skills deficit. Clients presenting with social dysfunction will require social skills training in addition to self-exposure therapy.

Social phobics present a number of challenges to the nurse, which are not experienced when treating other anxiety disorders (Butler, 1985). It is not always easy to define specific tasks in advance that can be repeated or graded, because of the variable and unpredictable nature of social situations. Where possible, the nurse and client should try to pick exposures that are going to vary the least. Prolonging exposures in social situations can also be difficult. Although a client may be in social situations on a daily basis, it is unlikely that many of these will last the hour required for exposure. Even those that do, are unlikely to involve speaking to others for the duration of the exposure. Therefore, where exposures cannot be prolonged, they should be repeated much more frequently. It is important to ensure that the client is engaging in exposures, i.e. they maintain eye contact and are conversing with others and are not avoiding. Lastly, many clients with social phobia will not be able to get proof that their fears are irrational. For example, if agoraphobic clients, who fear fainting or dying of a heart attack, expose themselves to their feared situations and afterwards realize that they have not died or fainted, they are more likely to challenge their irrational fears and learn from the experience. However, the same is not always true for clients with social phobia. If they fear negative evaluation from others, how are they to get proof that this has not occurred or, if they feel hot, how can they prove that they were not blushing? If they ask people if they were blushing this could be deemed as seeking reassurance. It may be useful in these situations to use role-play to rehearse situations

---

> *Case study:* **A woman with social phobia**
>
> Jane is a 27-year-old student studying mathematics at university. She has had a 7-year fear of losing control or collapsing when in social situations. In these situations she gets feelings of depersonalization and derealization and tenses her muscles as a reassurance that she will not lose control. She panics whenever she has to go out into such situations. She avoids classrooms, parties, waiting rooms, interviews, public transport, cinemas, using telephones, busy high streets, dentists, doctors and hairdressers. She is unable to write, eat and speak in public. The problem is worse in larger crowds and especially if people do not know of her difficulties. She tends to try to hide herself in these situations and does not like bright lighting as she can then be seen easily. She does not like to be a focus and so seats herself away from the centre of attention and will not sit opposite others. When out, she checks for easy exits, but there is little seeking of reassurance from others. She does, however, reassure herself on occasions. The problem is worst prior to her periods or when she is with assertive people. The effects on her life are profound. She is in danger of losing her place at university through non-attendance for lectures and feels unable to work if she were to have to get a job. Her social life has gone and relationships with friends have stopped due to her not having contact with them.
>
> Onset of the problem was at 10 when she felt under pressure socially at home and was teased and bullied at school. She takes diazepam 2 mg tablets prior to socializing or will have at least 6 pints of lager a day to avoid social anxiety. Her mood feels 'OK' at present, but concentration is very poor.

and give feedback to the client or use videotape to analyse their performance. The use of cognitive challenging techniques may also be beneficial.

See the case study of a woman with social phobia.

Exercise 1   Using the above case study, construct an exposure hierarchy that might be elicited by the client. Following this, define the problem and set some long-term goals. Finally, using these design at least one homework goal that the client could use.

Exercise 2   With a colleague, repeat Exercise 1 using a role-play to develop skills. For this exercise an assessment of the client's problem cna be prepared in the form of a role-played interview before progressing to defining goals.

OTHER PROBLEMS

This section briefly covers some of the other disorders mentioned earlier in this chapter. Post-traumatic stress disorder has recently come to prominence. Following the traumatic events of the capsizing of the Zeebrugge ferry, the Bradford City and Hillsborough football disasters and the Kings Cross fire, it was found that some survivors were suffering from collections of symptoms. These consisted of heightened arousal, avoidance and dissociation, and symptoms of re-experiencing the traumatic event. Recent research has showed that exposure therapy and cognitive–behaviour therapy have significant effects on these symptoms and nurses are learning techniques to help clients with these problems. Developments have been rapid and public sector industries, such as building societies, have also recognized the need for therapists who can help the victims of traumatic events. Disorders and the treatment techniques associated with them are explained in more detail in Chapter 25.

Chronic fatigue syndrome has been recognized as a problem in its own right for some years now. The syndrome is characterized by long-term fatigue that may last months or even years. Fatigue is more acute in the short term following exertion, and pain in joints and muscles is often experienced. The origins of these symptoms are unclear but many clients report onset following viral infections. Treatment takes a dual approach of gradually building up a programme of graded exercise to re-establish a daily routine that may have been previously avoided due to the fatigue felt. The second part of the treatment process looks at the client's cognition about their problem and through restructuring helps them to readjust their view of this. Treatment research has showed the effectiveness of these techniques and a number of papers and books are now available.

Although not a new area of treatment, behavioural psychotherapy for sexual dysfunctions has proved very successful. Disorders such as erectile failure, premature ejaculation, vaginismus and loss of sexual interest respond well. Common techniques include sensate focus (non-genital and genital) and orgasmic re-conditioning. Hawton's book on sex therapy gives a thorough account of these techniques (Hawton, 1985).

Other areas where behavioural techniques have been found to be useful are, behavioural medicine, i.e. behavioural treatments for organically based problems. These have included bowel re-training for irritable bowel syndrome and problem-solving and imaginal exposure in the use of pain management.

TREATMENT ISSUES

This section will introduce some of the issues that the nurse must bear in mind when conducting therapy.

GENDER ISSUES

The present drive for single-sex wards and the aims of increasing the rights of women within mental health services raise issues for nurses working one-to-one with clients. Occasionally female clients, and more rarely male clients, will express a preference for a nurse of the same sex. This is commoner with sexual dysfunctions or clients suffering from PTSD following rape or physical or sexual abuse as an adult or child. Although the client's wishes should be adhered to in these cases, it may be of benefit that the nurse discusses with the client the reasons for the choice. First, it may give the nurse more insight into the problems the client is suffering and, secondly, it may help to challenge some of the taboos about nurses working with clients of the opposite sex. The possibility that male nurses may not be able to understand a female point of view about sexual matters is likely to be true, more often than not, if they do not get chance to work with female clients and have the opportunity to the issues they face. Generally, however, it is accepted that the more comfortable the client feels, the more successful assessment and treatment is likely to be.

CULTURE AND RELIGION

Culture and religion can have effects on the way in which treatment evolves, when dealing with certain exposure tasks or in sex therapy. In cases where a form of treatment runs counter to religious or cultural beliefs, the nurse should consult with cultural or religious advisers before proceeding. In many cases, religious advisers can be people known to the client and they will often be able to give the go-ahead for treatment or suggest compromises. Cultural obstacles to treatment can be sometimes more difficult to circumnavigate and in these cases the nurse should comply with the client and advisors and not go ahead with the therapy.

ETHICS

There are a number of ethical issues that can occur during treatment. These issues may be with the nurse–client relationship or may be treatment-related. It is important for nurses to recognize factors that will influence treatment. Nurses are regarded by clients as being professionals, which puts them in a position of power. Client have to tell them a great deal about themselves, while the nurses is likely to disclose very little of this information. The client has to trust the nurse and this trust can be abused if the nurse is not aware of ethical constraints. The UKCC Code of Professional Conduct acts as a guideline for nurses in these cases, and the concomitant use of supervision is essential. A second problem arises when the treatment rationale requires a client to do something that it may be unethical for the nurse to agree to; e.g. someone with PTSD following a sexual assault in a dark alley at night may avoid any possibility of such a situation arising but ethically the nurse cannot expose the client to the danger of a repeated attack through doing self-exposure tasks in dark alleys at night. In these cases imaginal exposures may be used. Similar ethical dilemmas have been mentioned under culture and religion.

FOLLOW-UP

The first year following treatment is the time when clients are at the greatest risk of relapse and, therefore, follow-up should be offered where possible to guide and support clients through this difficult time. Follow-up appointments at intervals that can be varied to suit clients are most useful and further measurement can be carried out at fixed points (as mentioned under planning treatment). Follow-up obviously will vary depending on the resources that a service has to offer but most services are able to offer advice on relapse prevention. Relapse prevention should be introduced towards the end of treatment and can consist of techniques that the client may find useful in the future, as well as offering clear, concise advice on what to do in the case of a treatment setback. Many packages of this type can be found that have been shown to be effective (Öst, 1989a). Follow-up also helps to collect further data for research into the efficacy and longevity of treatment.

CO-THERAPISTS (OR KEY WORKERS)

Co-therapists can assist and support the client through difficult phases of treatment. If a co-therapist is a family member, this may also help the family to adjust to the client's change. Where possible they should be used to help with continuity of therapy between sessions and after discharge. With the introduction of the Care Programme Approach and its legal implications for the care of clients after discharge from hospital, there will be an increase in use of Key Workers (co-therapists) in the community. However, most clients with anxiety problems do not come under sections of the Mental Health Act and, therefore, the implications for nurses working with these clients may not be legally defined. Where possible, co-therapists should also receive training and education about behavioural psychotherapy, if they are not familiar with the techniques involved, to assist clients with the maintenance of their programmes. Supervision will also be essential for co-therapists if they are to learn and develop their skills.

SUPERVISION

Supervision is very important to the nurse. The nursing profession has developed the role of the nurse by accepting responsibility and accountability for clinical practice. This has meant a move towards monitoring nursing practice through audit, but for nurses to reflect upon their own practice it is essential for methods of supervision to be in place. Nurses who have trained in behavioural psychotherapy often work autonomously. To maintain objectivity in their work, they recieve supervision for the purposes of reflection and feedback on their clinical practice, and of developing new knowledge and personal and professiona skills to apply to their work. Discussion and analysis of issues within the work area can also take place. There are many models of supervision that cover clinical practice, as well as other issues such as personal and professional development, education, and management (Faugier, 1994). The need for supervision should be met and nurses who wish to receive it should seek it out. Difficult clinical cases and conflicts in therapeutic relationships can cause a great deal of stress to nurses and their clients. These issues can be discussed and analysed in supervision and support can be given. This is particularly true for nurses treating clients with PTSD, who can be very distressed by the issues they have to deal with, particularly if they can relate them to their own experiences.

HEALTH PROMOTION

Part of the nurse's role is that of health promotion. It could be argued that using self-exposure programmes is contrary to health promotion. It is well known that stress and anxiety in excess are not good for humans but this is in the long-term and behavioural treatments are of relatively short duration. However, it is important for the nurse to act as a health educator when treating clients. Education about treatment has already been mentioned and, as well as this, nurses should be prepared to use their role as educators in other areas such as medication, diet, exercise, sexual behaviours, substance abuse or whatever is applicable to the area of practice where nurses work. Nurses should use research findings to provide clients with the most up-to-date information.

Recently, there have been advances in the use of computers to help clients treat themselves. As well as this, the setting up of self-help groups for the treatment of anxiety disorders has increased the availability of help to clients with no access to mental health services. This can only be a good development for those who have anxiety problems. Many of these new developments base their treatment principles on behavioural psychotherapy techniques. These current developments may lead to many people treating themselves in the future, without ever having to see a health professional.

SUMMARY

The characteristics of behavioural psychotherapy are that it is problem oriented and works by identifying problem areas that are then worked on through a treatment strategy. It is structured and active, in that the client is involved in the design of their own treatment programme. Daily homework tasks need to be carried out between treatment sessions.

Treatment is directed, with homework goals being aimed at the problems identified. The treatment techniques are based on extensive research into psychological methods (empirically based) and treatment generally lasts for between 8 and 10 weekly treatment sessions for out-patients and 8 to 12 weeks for in-patients, making it short term. The approach is collaborative. Problems and targets are agreed and rated by therapist and client and homework goals are mutually designed and agreed. Therapists, through the use of education and guidance, help clients to become their own therapist so that they may tackle their problem and any future ones that may arise.

The process of therapy follows closely that of the nursing process (assessment, planning, implementation and evaluation).

Behavioural psychotherapy is the treatment of choice for phobic disorders, obsessive–compulsive disorder, sexual dysfunction, alternative sexual practices, habit disorders and social skills deficit.

There is need for more trained specialist nurses in this field and for basic nurse education courses to include more teaching and practice of skills for these techniques, to meet future demands.

KEY CONCEPTS

The characteristics of behavioural psychotherapy are that:
- It is a collection of techniques that aim to modify the behaviour that the client finds unacceptable or that is unwanted.
- It is derived from the work of empirical psychological research.
- It educates the client, their family and their co-therapist to design and run their own treatment programmes.
- It is generally short-term therapy, lasting 8—12 weeks or sessions.
- It uses a collaborative approach.
- It uses measurement of agreed problems and targets and daily homework goals and other rating scales to monitor and evaluate care.
- Its main treatment method is exposure therapy and the prevention of anxiolytic rituals and avoidances.
- It is becoming increasingly widespread and is being used to treat a growing range of problems.

REFERENCES

Azrin NH, Nunn RG: A method of eliminating nervous habits and tics. *Behav Res Ther*, 11:619–628, 1973.

Bandura A: *Social learning theory.* Englewood Cliffs, 1977, Prentice Hall.

Butler G: Exposure as a treatment for social phobia: some instructive difficulties. *Behav Res Ther*, 23(6):651–657, 1985.

Butler S, Chalder T, Ron M, Wessely S: Cognitive behaviour therapy in chronic fatigue syndrome. *J Neurol, Neurosurg Psychiatry* 54:153–158, 1991.

Faugier J: Thin on the ground. *Nurs Times* 90(20):64–65, 1994.

Ghosh A, Marks IM, Carr AC: Therapist contact and outcome of self-exposure treatment for phobias: A controlled study. *Bri J Psychiatry* 152:234–238, 1988.

Gournay K: Management of anxiety states. *Nurs Times* 91(45):29–31, 1995.

Hawton K: *Sex therapy: A practical guide.* Oxford, 1985, Oxford University Press.

Lovell K, Richards DA: Behavioural treatments in post traumatic stress disorder. *Bri J Nurs*, 4(16):934–953, 1995.

Marks IM: Phobic disorders four years after treatment. *Bri J Psychiatry* 118:683–688, 1971.

Marks IM: *Fears, phobias and rituals.* New York, 1987, Oxford University Press.

Marks IM: Blood-injury phobia: a review. *Am J Psychiatry* 145(10):1207–1213, 1988.

Marks IM, Bird J, Brown M, *et al.*: *Behavioural psychotherapy: Maudsley pocket book of clinical management.* Bristol, 1986, Wright.

Marks IM, Hodgson R, Rachman S: Treatment of chronic OCD 2 years after *in vivo* exposure. *Bri J Psychiatry* 127:349–364, 1975.

McNamee G, O'Sullivan G, Lelliott P, Marks IM: Telephone-guided treatment for housebound agoraphobics with panic disorder: Exposure vs. relaxation. *Behav Ther*, 20:491–497, 1989.

Miller N: Learnable drives and rewards. In Stevens S, editor: *Handbook of experimental psychology.* New York, 1951, Wiley.

Mowrer OH: *Learning theory and personality dynamics.* New York, 1950, Arnold.

Öst L-G: A maintenance program for behavioural treatment of anxiety disorders. *Behav Res Ther*, 27:123–130, 1989a.

Öst L-G: One session treatment for specific phobias. *Behav Res Ther*, 27:1–7, 1989b.

Pavlov I.P: *Conditioned reflexes and psychiatry.* (W.H. Gantt, translator). New York, 1927, International Publishers.

Rachman S: Agoraphobia — a safety signal perspective. *Behav Res Ther*, 22(1):59–70, 1984.

Stern RS, Cobb JP: Phenomenology of obsessive–compulsive neurosis. *Bri J Psychiatry* 132:233–239, 1978.

Stravynski A, Greenberg D: Behavioural psychotherapy for social phobia and dysfunction. *Int Rev Psychiatry* 1: 207–218, 1989.

Tarrier N: Management and modification of residual positive psychotic symptoms. In: Birchwood M, Tarrier N, editors: *Psychological management of schizophrenia.* London, 1994, John Wiley.

Welner A, Reich T, Robins I, Fishman R, van Doren T: Obsessive–compulsive neurosis: Record, follow-up and family studies: I. Inpatient record study. *Compr Psychiatry,* 17:527–539, 1976.

FURTHER READING

Baer L: *Getting control: Overcoming your obsessions and compulsions.* Boston, 1991, Little, Brown & Company.

Hackman A: Behavioural and cognitive psychotherapies: Past history, current applications and future registration issue. *Behavi Cognit Psychother*, (supplement 1), 1993.

Price V, Archbold J: Development and application of social learning theory. *Bri J Nurs*, 4(21):1263–1268, 1995.

Rachman S, de Silva P: *OCD the facts.* London, 1992, Routledge.

Richards DA, McDonald B: *Behavioural psychotherapy: A handbook for nurses.* Heinemann Nursing, 1990, Oxford.

Approaches to Therapeutic Groups

Learning Outcomes

After studying this chapter you should be able to:

- Explore the historical developments of group psychotherapy.

- Discuss the concepts of psychoanalytical group therapy.

- Identify and describe phases within the development of a group.

- Describe therapeutic elements occurring in a group setting.

- Analyse group theory and the therapeutic milieu.

- Apply the structure and function of nurse led groups.

- Identify ways of researching the effectiveness of group therapy.

*T*he approach to psychodynamic group therapy could be* broadly described as a non-directive or facilitative paradigm of intervention. However, the term 'unstructured', which is often used when referring to psychodynamic groups, is misleading because the approach takes place within a densely organized milieu following tested axioms that are derived from practitioner experience (see Box 30.1). It would be more apt to described the approach as highly structured.

The first group experiments were carried out by Pratt (1907) in Boston, who formed 'classes' to treat and educate patients suffering from tuberculosis, although the term 'group therapy' was first used by Moreno in the 1920s (Brown and Pedder, 1979: Pines, 1986). However, it is Freud's (1921)*Group Psychology and the Analysis of the Ego*, that has formed the basis of the extensive body of literature about group and social processes that has emerged during this century. Following Freud, in the UK the work of Michael Foulkes and Wilfred Bion is notable, while in the USA, Kurt Lewin has been influential in the development of human relations enquiry, coining the term 'group dynamics' (for a discussion of the influence of Lewin, see Yalom, 1975). It is from these sources that group therapy has developed into an international ambient network mediated by journals, practitioners and professional organizations. Arguably, group therapy has remained one of the most enduring paradigms of psychological medicine of the 20th Century. The proliferation of group therapy has informed the development of many group discourses including the creative psychotherapies (Waller, 1991 and 1994), organizational consultancy (De Board, 1978; Granstrom, 1986; Menzies–Lyth, 1988) therapeutic community and psychiatric and milieu therapy (Hinshelwood, 1987; Jackson and Cawley, 1992; Haigh, 1995) to name but a few. The range of therapies that also incorporate a group dynamic approach includes psychodrama, transactional analysis, gestalt therapy and various counselling approaches (Avaline and Dryden, 1988). Peer evaluation, feedback groups and social skills training groups are all settings where in therapeutic intervention is broadly based on the fundamental principle of sharing, where in there is an 'exchange of information, education, encouragement and mutual support' (Brown and Pedder, 1979).

Box 30.1 — *Summary of psychodynamic group therapy parameters*

Time frames
The length of time over which the group meets is consistent: usually between 1 and 1¹/₂ hours per session. Number of sessions: usually one or two per week for out-patient groups and up to daily sessions in residential or day programme settings. The group meeting takes place at the same time and on the same day each week. Breaks in continuity are planned weeks in advance whenever possible. Out-patient groups usually run as closed groups for a set time (often for 1–2 years). Groups in residential and day settings may operate more fluidly as open groups where admission to the group is an integral part of the treatment programme on the unit.

The setting
Wherever possible the same room is used by the group, with chairs set out symmetrically (usually in a circle or oval depending on the shape of the room).

Facilitator's role
The same facilitator(s) run(s) the group each session. In ward or day settings, where there are daily groups, there is more interchange of group facilitators but even here continuity is helpful where possible. Precise techniques are employed and developed with practice and experience. Specialist nurse practitioners may have training beyond their core nurse training (Pedder, 1993). The facilitator style encourages sharing and attempts to foster an atmosphere of open discussion, in settings where patient-to-patient learning is considered pivotal to the therapeutic encounter.

Patient role
Beginning with the premise that patients are capable of mutual learning and reciprocal help, group member-to-member attachment is considered primary in establishing a secure base (Glenn, 1987).

In many psychiatric settings group approaches have also been found to be useful in facilitating staff working together. For instance, group supervision and staff support or sensitivity groups are settings where group theory is applicable. Group supervision has been found to be helpful in the therapeutic milieu, in alleviating some of the stress associated with clinical work (Hardy *et al.*, 1995). In group supervision the complex dynamics of the nurse–patient relationship can be untangled through a collaborative process of pooling and sharing information (Main, 1983; Fabricius, 1995; Winship, 1995). Supervision is integral to helping nurses think about their work and where the impact of the work is difficult to measure; 'The help of another in the review of one's unconscious processes is a ...safeguard' (Main, 1988). Supervisory support, as Peplau (1994) has recently suggested, is clearly indicated if unspoken or unconscious dynamics are to be understood. Supervision should offer a sense of holding and offer an opportunity to process subjective experience, enhancing the clinician's capacity to find creative solutions to clinical problems (Pedder, 1986).

HISTORICAL DEVELOPMENTS IN GROUP APPROACHES

The key texts that map out the historical development of group therapy in the UK are *The Evolution of Group Analysis* and *Bion and Group Psychotherapy* (both edited by Pines, 1983b and 1985, respectively). Foulkes and Bion are the central proponents in the development of group psychotherapy in the UK. Both began their group experiments treating neurotic soldiers at the famous Northfield Hospital near Birmingham during the Second World War. The work of other group theorists also emerged from the wartime experiments at Northfield. Notable is the work of Tom Main who went on to develop the psychoanalytic approach at the Cassel, thereby influencing psychosocial nursing. Maxwell Jones' interest in group approaches also began during the war when he found mutual learning to be beneficial in the treatment of shell-shocked soldiers at the Mill Hill Hospital in North London (Jones, 1942a, b). Jones went on to further develop group approaches at the Belmont Social Rehabilitation Unit and later at the Henderson Hospital in Sutton.

FOULKES
Foulkes, approach to groups differed from Jones, insofar as he emphasized emotionality and unconscious phenomena. Whereas Jones (1942a) discouraged discussions about abstractions, in favour of giving factual information to the patients, Foulkes (1948) accepted exploration and uncertainty in discussions more readily. Foulkes found that events that were apparently unexplainable, were discernible through a collaborative process of discussion employing the psychoanalytic technique of free association. He was freer about the interplay of opinion, either consensual or oppositional, between group members 'Disruptive forces are consumed in mutual analysis, constructive ones utilized for the synthesis of the individual and the integration of the group as a whole' (Foulkes, 1948).

Foulkes went on to develop an approach to group therapy that conceived of group relations in terms of a social model of consciousness that was determined by the capacity of a person to hold two other interns in mind at the same time. This triadic model, the 'Model of Three' (Foulkes, 1948), was the basis for understanding the dynamics of group interrelations. Foulkes' approach was one that interlaced sociological understanding with psychodynamics. He described the basic building blocks of society as 'root groups' (1957a), for instance families, institutions and communities and he contested that the network of other groups later in life featured aspects of interdependence that were a re-enactment of the earliest experiences of infancy. For Foulkes, the group therapy experience extended the interrelations of the classic psychoanalytic dyad, emphasizing the necessary process of psychotherapeutic exploration of transference phenomena.

On the primacy of the social nature of man, Foulkes (1957b) found common ground with the work of WRD Fairbairn (1952) suggesting that small-group analysis represented an avenue for the furtherance of object relations theory, something which Balint (1950) also asserted. (For a discussion of the concept of object relations theory see Grotstein and Rinsley (1994) and for a perspective for nursing see Fabricius (1993). Foulkes saw that small group psychoanalytic study enabled the enactment of the 'Model of Three' and therefore the interplay of internal object relations through transferential interchange

> In the microsphere the child knows and understands objects beyond his body, but he knows them mainly in terms of his own fantasies and wishes. He endows objects with qualities projected from his own mind, the sofa becomes a boat, the doll an angry mother, the mother a witch, as need arises... Relationships in terms of the microsphere do manifest themselves in the group. This is the sphere, par excellence, of transference relationships. The group can come to represent, in the minds of its members, the community as a whole or social conscience, and an individual will feel ashamed, embarrassed, or rejected if the group judges him. Not only can the conductor in his person come to represent these things but the whole group can do so.

> *(Foulkes, 1957a)*

The concept of 'microsphere' is coined from Erikson (1951). Foulkes conceived of a fluid collective group phenomenon, describing it as a matrix, 'the network of all individual mental processes, the psychological medium in which they meet, communicate and interact...' (1957). Foulkes saw the matrix as constituted by a healthiness where the distress of an individual could be held by the group as a whole.

Foulkes' contribution to the development of group psychotherapy is enormous. In 1952 he founded the Group-Analytic Society and was President until 1970. During this time he achieved the distinction of becoming the Physician Emeritus of the Maudsley Hospitals. From a historical perspective, Foulkes' part in the therapeutic and group experiments at Northfield also placed him in the context of the decisive and influential social psychiatry and therapeutic community movements. The emergence of these approaches meant that group therapy became grounded in general psychiatry as practitioners developed the application of group skills in the context of many large psychiatric hospitals (Hinshelwood and Manning, 1979). Foulkes (1969) later in his career developed the synthesis between group analysis and social psychiatry in his position as chairman, during 1964–1965, of the Psychotherapy and Social Psychiatry Section of the Royal Medico–Psychological Association (forerunner of the Royal College of Psychiatrists) thus ensuring the furtherance of group approaches in psychiatry. For an abridged history and discussion of Foulkes' contribution to group psychotherapy see Main (1983).

BION

While Foulkes' views about groups could be described as optimistic (outward looking and positivistic), conceiving of the group as having a healthy wholeness at its core, Bion's views about groups have been described by Pines (1985) as simply mystical, illuminating 'beams of darkness'. Bion (1961) observed predictable patterns of group behaviour or phenomena that he called basic assumptions. The first of these was the attachment to or dependence on the leader: basic assumption *leader dependence*. Bion saw that the task of the group was to overcome its fantasy of the power of the leader, that the members of the group, through a process of self-exploration, had the capacity to realize their own potential and find mutual solutions to their problems. The second basic assumption was that of *pairing*. Bion noted that often the group would allow two members to dominate the proceedings; thus the pair was left to the work that ordinarily would be carried out by the whole group. Thirdly, Bion noted how often the group would regress to attacking objects outside of the group. This process of vilifying an external body served to create a false feeling that inside the group everything was ideal. This process of projecting out of the group Bion called basic assumption *fight–flight*.

Bion saw the key aim of small-group psychotherapy as helping the patients to observe themselves and others in the group process and therefore to learn about their regressive behaviour. The role of the facilitator was to hold in mind the leader dependence fantasies of the group (the unconscious process of constructing an unspoken narrative) and so help the group to see when it is acting in a basic assumption position. Bion noted that the group leader may be fantasized as a magical authority, as the person with the answers or power to solve the group's problems. For a summary of Bion's basic assumption theory see Menzies–Lyth (1988).

Reflecting on the difference between Bion and Foulkes, Sutherland (1985) noted that Bion restricted his study of others' work:

> I never heard Bion discuss Foulkes, and I do not think he knew much about his work because he had left groups by the time Foulkes was publishing his accounts of it. He was not given to disparaging the work of others if it differed from his own; for him, experience would eventually find its survival value. Foulkes was convinced the total group interactions had to be used in therapy, and I believe that Bion, had he done more group therapeutic work, would have accepted that position though he would have insisted on what might be loosely put as more rigour and more depth, more attention to the primitive relationships.

In attempting to integrate the ideas of Bion and Foulkes, Brown (1985) draws attention to the textual polarities of their theories: 'Bion's seems two-dimensional — individuals are either alienated or falsely cooperative, the group is either working on some superficial or imposed task or is avoiding genuine encounter....Foulkes's picture is multidimensional, complex.....lacking the bite of paradox and pessimism'. Brown (1985) believes that the ideas of Bion and Foulkes would only be integrated through the establishment of a metasociology, where clinical experience is integrated with a wider view of man in relation to society and culture.

CONCEPTUAL OVERVIEW OF GROUP DYNAMICS

From the beginning of life, relationships with others are primary and individuality emerges from an intricate process of moving from a state of dependence on others, to a maturing state of interdependence (Rustin, 1991). Stern (1985) has described the various stages of infancy on the path towards maturity, noting at each stage that the infant is not existing in an isolated world but that development from the very beginning is inextricably interpersonally organized (i.e. in relation to parents in the first place and then to an extending network of others). In considering these developmental stages, Ahlin (1995) has mapped Stern's (1985) developmental theory of patterns of self-relatedness in infancy (core self, emergent self etc.) to stages in group-relating capabilities (dyad, subgroup, family triad, family as-a-whole) (see Box 30.2).

In other words, growing up involves moving in and through a network of relationships. One way of beginning to locate developmental basic faults (Balint, 1968) is through an examination of the patient's group-relating capabilities with recourse to a theory of group-relating capabilities. The predication here is that there is a developmental resonance for the patient in a therapy group, where past relationships are recapitulated in the here and now. The group therefore acts as an interface between an inner world experience and an experience of otherness (including physical and psychical proximity to others). This experience enables patients to develop an understanding of themselves in relation to others, this being a fount of insight but also an inter-subjective process that has been appropriately described as outsight (Pines, 1984).

We might see the group as a type of dramatic mini-laboratory or microcosm that resonates with a universal experience of gregariousness (no person is an island, so to speak). The group viewed in this way becomes a rich environment for psychosocial investigation, a tool for researching how a patient interacts with others. Difficulties that the patient may have in the group situation may be a manifestation of previous relationship problems. However, further to this diagnostic role, the group experience may offer at the same time a reparative experience for the patient, where old unhelpful forms of

interacting with others can be replaced by new and more benign patterns of interaction. Yalom (1975) calls this process of recapitulating and reparation of previous developmental conflicts the corrective experience of the family group. The here and now experience in the group is therefore of primary importance, not secondary as is usually thought. The focus on past relationships is considered as a template for the immediacy of current relations. With this developmental model in mind, a theoretical overview of some of the key events in group dynamic therapy will be considered.

PHASES IN GROUP PROCESSES

OPENING PHASE

Group therapy usually takes place in a circle. The opening phase of the group may feature an anxious silence, which Pedder (1977) compares to the silent apprehension felt when waiting for a theatrical play to begin. During the early stage of the groups life, its space may feel quite contrived as a social milieu. Many patients complain that sitting in silence in a circle is a false social experience. They may believe that the therapist has a special set of notions about how the group should develop. Indeed, many patients who have had no previous experience of non-directive therapy may be quite fearful of the apparent boundlessness of the group. The therapeutic task for the facilitator is to bear the uncertainty of the group members' anxiety and, without attempting to 'rescue' the group, to consider how to foster an atmosphere of containment and holding.

COHESION, ATTACHMENT AND CONTAINMENT

The concept of group cohesion is most commonly associated with Yalom's ideas (Yalom, 1975). It refers to the context of new members of a group coming together, getting to know each other and thus forming the basis of a working relationship. The quality of cohesiveness is apparent in the atmosphere of belonging, membership and acceptance in the group and there is evidence to suggest that a cohesive group is favourable to a positive therapeutic outcome (Budman *et al.*, 1989). Yalom (1975) posits cohesiveness as a stabilizing milieu quality that allows the expression of hostility in the group. Although cohesion may be associated with the early 'forming' stage of a group's life, as in Tuckman's (1965) model, it is more the case that cohesion is something that waxes and wanes at stages in the group's life. Initially, the group needs to become cohesive to establish a secure base but then it needs to become cohesive as the patients establish themselves as separate from the therapist, identifying themselves with each other. Finally, the patient becomes once again identified with the group leader in a more adult way, which may result in the loss of cohesion in the group before moving towards the end of therapy. This fragmentation may feature a phase of disappointment and disillusionment (a kind of

---

Box 30.2 *Epistemological compatibility between individual developmental stages and group relating capacities* (derived from Ahlin, 1995)	
Group	Relational
Cultural	Societal
Large	School and friends
Median	Extended family
Small	Child–family
Triadic	Infant–parents
Dyadic	Infant–mother

collective non-cohesion) although this phase is nonetheless an important part of the final process of detachment (Pedder, 1988).

The term 'cohesion' is used to describe a process of sticking something together or a process of unification. Cohesion in individual therapy might be considered as the process of a patient becoming attached to their therapist. While this is an inner experience for the patient, the real relationship with the therapist acts as a conduit for the experience. Winnicott (1965) describes the patient's relationship with their therapist as a prerequisite to the creation of a temporary environment or transitional space, where the patient can experience emotional growth. Bowlby (1973) draws a parallel between the necessary development of a secure base in therapy and the development of a secure base in the infant–mother couple. In other words, the establishment of a facilitating environment in therapy can be understood in the same way that secure mothering can help a child grow emotionally. However, the need for attachment is not necessarily confined to childhood–adults continue to have a need to feel attached although in more mature ways, e.g. membership of clubs and organizations etc.

What is distinctive in the process of attachment in therapy is the apparent difficulty that many patients have in becoming attached to their therapist. The process of attachment then, might be said to repeat difficulties pertaining to attachment difficulties experienced in relation to parental figures. Most attachment theories, even though they have emerged from separate schools of thought, have tended to overlap on this point, that is to say attachment as recapitulating an experience from the past usually associated with a parental attachment. Pedder (1976) examined the attachment theories of Balint and Bowlby and found common ground in their formulations of the link between attachment difficulties in childhood and adult depression. Pedder concluded that therapy was an opportunity for repeating these developmental faults but also an opportunity for a new beginning.

In applying attachment theory to groups, Pedder (1994; personal communication) has made a useful distinction between attachment and cohesion in the group, based on Foulkes' (1964) model of transference relations in the group. Pedder posits that attachment in the group refers to a regressed position of reliance on (an)other(s) where a child to parent attachment is enacted, whereas cohesion in the group refers to maturing relations with others in the context of adult to adult relations (Figure 30.1). Pedder's formulation here seems to bear some parity to Bion's (1961) distinction between a work group (a mature well functioning group) that is engaged well in its task and a basic assumption *leader dependent group* that which is functioning at a more regressed level.

The process of attachment to the group therapist, then, is laden with meaning, but it is seen as prerequisite to the later process of separation from the therapist and individuation. The group leader, therefore, needs to be skilled to recognize the group's propensity to dependence and then be skilled enough to help the group realize its potential for inter-

dependence. For Bion (1961) the transferential relationship between the group and the analyst was the major focus of therapeutic exploration, interpretation being directed mainly towards the whole group and rarely towards individuals.

Certainly, the aim of the group is to create a cohesive experience, where adult relations are fostered. However, the process of fostering these mature relations is often a difficult one and necessitates patients initially becoming attached, recapitulating a regressive position in relation to the group and the therapist, before moving to a more mature position. The very nature of the difficulties that bring the patients to therapy means that attachment is a necessary part of the group process. Attachment theory, within the framework of a psychodynamic approach, implies that dependency may occur in the course of relationships. Criticisms of a such as approach tend to imply that a psychodynamic approach creates false dependence whereby the patient becomes over-reliant on the therapist. The fear of dependence in psychiatric settings is arguably manifest in aspects of organizational systems that have evolved to prevent patients becoming too dependent, for instance short rotational systems for students and trainees (Pedder, 1991). The term 'dependence' has come to represent something that is seen as bad, whereas the concept of attachment is viewed all together more benignly. There may be a case for working with a nomenclature that is acceptable to all, for instance using the word 'attachment' rather than 'dependence'; however, the reality of dependency and its psychopathological nuances should prompt us to consider the concept directly. When considering loss and separation at the end of therapy, Pedder's (1988) paper is a helpful summary of some of the main theories about ending a therapeutic relationship. Pedder contests that ending is not necessarily 'termination' and may be considered more positively as a 'graduation'. Bowlby's (1973) work examining the breaking of affectional bonds is a seminal piece of work on ending, where he argues that the experience of loss and separation is not always pathological. Ending is an unavoidably painful and distressing phase in the therapeutic process.

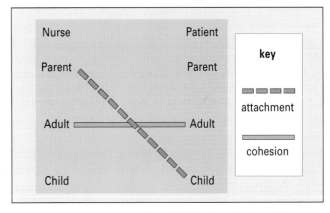

Figure 30.1 Pedder's adaptation of Foulkes' levels of transference relations in a group

APPLYING GROUP THEORY TO THE TOTAL WARD MILIEU

There is a case that can be made for thinking about the total ward milieu from a group dynamic perspective. Peplau (1989) has suggested that, in a psychiatric ward milieu where individual therapy happens every day for, say, 1 hour, we still need to think about the other 'twenty-three hours of the day' (Peplau, 1989) lest they should go missing. The construction of a total ward or psychiatric milieu (e.g. day hospital, hostel etc.) might be conceptualized in terms of a group dynamic perspective where constructs such as transference and counter-transference theory are helpful in understanding relations between clinicians and patients (Jackson and Cawley, 1992; Winship *et al.*, 1995).

The psychiatric milieu often has at its core a struggle with a basic assumption *leader dependent* culture (Bion, 1961). Patients are in a state of dependence initially, psychotic illness, severe depression and suicidality necessitating an appropriate responsiveness from the nursing staff. However, many aspects of the treatment setting seem unnecessarily to disempower patients (for instance patients not being allowed to cook their own food, be in charge of their linen). The task is one of distinguishing between the dependency that arises out of a patient's real dependence (Winnicott, 1965) and those aspects of dependence that arise from a stagnant ward culture that is defensively organized and where patients are prevented from taking responsibility for themselves, for instance in self-medicating or being involved in organizational discussions. In many cases it is necessary to explore those aspects of ward organization (see Case study) that do not challenge the parent–child attachment and do not foster the potential for cohesive adult relations (see Figure 30.1).

Exploration of transference relations needs to be a continuing process if the group and organizational dynamics of staff–patient relations are to be understood and challenged. In this example, the traditional approach was replaced by a peer system of co-operation that was equally as effective, if not more effective than the staff doing this job. The approach and principles of the therapeutic community are probably the most advanced in conceiving a total treatment milieu that offers a living–learning experience that attends to the group dynamic relations between the patients and the staff (Hinshelwood and Manning, 1979). In most psychiatric ward settings, most patients are prevented from making their own meals, not encouraged to self-medicate, or not allowed to take responsibility for cleaning their own environment. Group collaborative activities, beyond formal therapy groups, are helpful here in a whole range of areas, from maintaining the ward environment cleanly and safely (Bjorndal, 1992) to cooking (Flyn, 1993) and leisure activities. The collective approach of the therapeutic community is developing its theoretical base from a robust model of group analysis (Haigh, 1995). In the coming years, the therapeutic community movement will be re-aligning itself with the British Association of Social Psychiatrists (BASP) (1995) and these developments, along with the efficacy and cost-effectiveness of working with a group approach, are likely to make therapeutic communities a most viable treatment paradigm (Knowles, 1995).

WHAT HAPPENS IN GROUPS

The following section outlines some clinical examples of experiences and situations commonly encountered in group therapy situations. The list is presented alphabetically. The examples are discussed drawing upon group theory. The term 'therapist' is used throughout although this should be considered as interchangeable with clinical nurse practitioner and group facilitator, leader or conductor.

ABSENTEEISM

In the following example, the group members experience the absence of their peers as denigrating and trivializing the whole group's existence.

Setting: The group begins with a few patients coming into the room. Several chairs are left empty so that the patients are spaced about the room. Conversation begins tentatively, picking up the threads of the previous week's group. This soon ends and silence falls over the group.

Therapist: 'I wonder if the large number of people missing this week has affected our ability to talk to each other'.

Case study: **Group theory in ward organization**

A charge nurse with experience in working with groups was asked to help out a locked acute psychiatric ward one morning because the ward was short-staffed through sickness. The staff that were on duty on the ward were quite unsettled because the ward had been particularly busy and violent during the week. It was 8.30 a.m. and medication time. The charge nurse and a staff nurse met to do the medication. The staff nurse said rather anxiously that medication always took a long time and tended to be one of the most volatile times of the day, with patients refusing to take their medication. The staff nurse said that it was usual for two staff to dispense the medication and another member of staff to prompt the patients. However, this was going to be difficult on this particular morning because there were no staff available to do the prompting.

The charge nurse suggested that, instead of a member of staff prompting patients, it would be possible for one of the less ill patients to do it. The staff nurse was unsure but said Patient B was quite settled. The charge nurse was introduced to Patient B. The charge nurse asked if Patient B would help by calling the other patients. Patient B was rather pleased to oblige and appeared to have very little difficulty prompting the patients to come. Indeed, very soon other patients were joining in the prompting. This peer system of organization was most effective and the staff nurse reported that the medication round was completed in record time.

Patient A: 'Why should the group be spoiled like this just because they can't be bothered to come?'

Patient B: 'This is all a waste of time nurse, why don't we finish early this week?'

The group may experience itself as fragmented, as if the empty chairs somehow represent a tear in the skin or outer boundary of the group. This experience is characterized by anger and anxiety and the patients attempt to project the unwanted feelings of loss, hurt and fragmentation onto the therapist or the group-as-whole, by assigning blame, saying the group is worthlessness. The therapist may indeed experience a sense of responsibility for the poor attendance. Part of the therapist's role at this stage is to recognize the process of projection and, by making a process comment, help the group to see for itself that it is confronted with a difficult situation that evokes difficult and painful feelings. The therapist may respond to this situation by making a process comment such as, 'It is clear that it is difficult experience for people being in the group at the moment'. The aim of this process comment is to help the group to stay with the experience, and therefore develop a capacity to survive the experience of fragmentation, discovering that such feelings are not necessarily calamitous. It is important to foster a sense that the validity of the group and the contributions that members make are not necessarily destroyed by those who are absent.

Resistance in therapy may be seen as one way of countering unpleasant or dangerous self-truths (Yalom, 1970). Patients may be resistive to communicating verbally and non-verbally within the group. In an extreme form, resistance can be seen in absenteeism or lateness. It remains an important element of the therapist's role to make conscious that which unconsciously may lie at the root of the resistance, thereby enabling patients to modify their relation to the group.

ANXIETY
In the following scenario there are a number of dynamics operating upon the group.

Setting: A weekly, small, closed group on an in-patient acute psychiatric ward. A female patient brings a pillow from her bed with her and sits huddled with it throughout the session. A male patient stands in the centre of the group and speaks loudly and emotionally about his childhood and upbringing. He says he feels under pressure to perform and conform to his family's demands. The female patient stoops lower and lower behind her pillow and begins to shake visibly with fear and anxiety as the male patient speaks.

It is possible that the experience described by the male patient resonated with something in the female patient's history. As he talked about his experience, she became visibly shaken.

However, it is possible also that she was experiencing some of the anxiety that the male patient was not expressing. Indeed, he talked loudly of his experience in a way that perhaps masked some of his underlying anxiety and fear. In this way, the anxiety may have been unconsciously communicated and felt by the female patient instead, as the male patient projected his anxiety. The process of unconscious communication often exerts a great deal of disturbance, by virtue of the fact that it is unseen, uncertainly acknowledged and often only felt. The task of the group facilitator is to monitor how members of the group are reacting as others are speaking, based on the premise that feelings are commonly shared where difficult feelings may be assigned to others. The facilitator, by inviting others to share how they are feel, is able to help orientate the projected feelings towards their true object. That people have similar feelings, such as anxiety and fear, is perhaps the most salient, curative factor in a group therapy setting. When it is acknowledged that these difficult feelings exist and that anxiety or fear can be survived without destruction or catastrophe always resulting, the experience for group members is triumphantly valuable.

Anxiety is on the rise in Western culture (Abse, 1974). The vicissitudes of personal change, like social and cultural change, are often uncomfortable, leaving people feeling disorientated and anxious. This type of experience is a particular phenomenon of Western culture, which breeds high levels of anxiety (Abse, 1974). Group therapy is a particularly potent form of social and cultural investigation, where personal experience can be put in context by patients sharing their view of their world with others and where the group might come to be an interface between personal and social experience.

CLOSING

Setting: A weekly small group for in-patients. Five minutes before the end of the session, one of the female patients discloses that she was assaulted by her father in the past. She says she fears leaving the ward and therefore being exposed to that abuse again. The patients console her and a discussion ensues. The group therapist realizes the group has run over time by five minutes and brings the session to end by saying; 'It seems very hard to close the group, but it is time to finish for today'.

Some very important and sensitive material came up at the end of the session, making it difficult for the group to end. It is possible that the patients wished the intimate and safe experience of the group to continue. It is not unusual for such material to emerge right at the end of a session. The therapist needs to consider how to draw the group to a close in a way that is sensitive to the needs of the patients while maintaining the sense of time structure.

Consistency in starting and ending on time is symbolic of creating the safe containing space in which therapy may take place. This setting of boundaries to experience is the foundation of a therapeutic milieu where a sense of holding in time and space may provide a safe and consistent arena in which the patient may feel able to explore intimate details about his or her life. While it is important for the therapist to maintain this time boundary, the task of bringing material to a group and monitoring the tempo (having an intuition of when is a good time to bring in material and when is not) is part of the learning experience for the patients in the group too.

There is an interchange in the group experience where the process of re-establishing *ego-boundaries* (a secure sense of self grounded in lifeworld reality) may be a derivation of the experience of the group in having a secure group ego boundary. It is important for the therapist to maintain the boundary of the group in the earlier forming stages of the group and *one* way of providing a safe structure is to ensure the group starts and closes on time. Others aspects of the establishment of firm group boundaries consist in the establishment of agreed ground rules around behaviour, confidentiality etc. Patients will test the therapist by pushing for the group to be extended or sometimes shortened. When these ordinary boundaries of the group become twisted, as in the example given below, it can result in barriers being constructed or a sense of fragmentation and diffusion that then hinder the group's work (Hinshelwood, 1987).

CONTAINMENT

Setting:	A weekly group in a mental health day centre. Membership consists of men with serious mental illness. A new member, Sean, joins the group and sits silently throughout, while other members spend time discussing their medication. One of the side-effects a number of the men were concerned about was weight gain. The next week Sean does not attend and his absence is addressed. He returns the following week and the group express their relief that he felt able to return.
Sean:	'This group is useless, I don't see what sitting around here does for anyone'.
Patient A:	'I'm glad you were able to come back to the group as I thought you weren't coming back at all'.
Patient B:	'The group has helped me'.
Sean:	'I don't need this group, I need individual therapy'.
Therapist:	'Perhaps you need to consider what can be learnt from the group and what you are able to bring yourself, so that others can share and learn from your experiences'.

Rivalry may be a source of conflict in the group, as members compete for attention and affection. This appeared to be the case in this example. The group were ambivalent about accepting Sean into their midst. By their silence, that is by neither encouraging Sean to participate nor inquiring after his silence, the group enacted an unconscious wish for Sean not to exist. He represented a risk to the group's equilibrium. There were, perhaps, concerns that Sean might be a new needy patient who would take up the group's or the therapist's time. When Sean did not turn up for the second group, the members were remorseful about how they had excluded him from the first group. When Sean spoke of how difficult he anticipated it would be sharing the therapist with the whole group, and that he would prefer to have the therapist all to himself, he appears to have identified something that was a universal feeling in the group. The conflict in the group about Sean's arrival was denied or repressed and it is invariably the case that it manifests itself in an oblique and destructive way. The members talked about their medication and their fears about greed (apparent in their discussions about becoming fat). The destructive wish to exclude Sean from the group was apparent and felt by Sean, as he was excluded from the group.

ENACTMENT

Setting:	The morning community group welcomed a new member; Steve. He sat in a corner of the room with his headphones on. As the group talked the sound of muffled music became louder and Steve's foot began to move up and down with the music, in an agitated way. His eyes were in a fixed stare on the group leader.
Therapist:	'Steve, are you able to hear me?'
Steve:	'Huh?'
Therapist:	'I'd appreciate you turning off your music, it is distracting'.
Steve:	'Make me'.
Patient A:	'Don't be such an ass man, you're missing out here, not us'.
Steve:	'Shuv it'.
Therapist:	'It seems you're out for a fight, but I think you are frightened of what is happening and this new experience'.
Steve:	'Frightened?'
Patient:	'You look very frightening, 'cos you're frightening me'.

Group situations often stimulate hostility. This may be linked to the fact that the experience of the group is unfamiliar and the sense of alienation and persecution is heightened by the experience of sitting in a circle simply facing others. For patients with mental health problems, the intimate experience of sitting in close proximity to others can be very anxiety provoking. (It can be argued that it is no less so for staff although the response may be tempered by more mature levels of social restraint and self-control.) It is common that the enacting of destructive patterns of behaviour may be symbolic of the threat experienced by the group therapy situation itself. In the example, Steve defends himself against the experience, nullifying his contact by blocking out his capacity to hear what is happening. For Steve this response may be a re-enactment of a past pattern of behaviour. It is helpful for the therapist to note from whom these patterns emerge in the group and to explore if they are familiar. For instance, the therapist may enquire 'In what situations have these patterns occurred before?' or 'What previous significant persons can be remembered in light of what is happening now?'.

Recourse to the theory of transference is useful here where old patterns of familial interaction can be noted if they are recapitulated in the group (Yalom, 1975). The term 'acting out' is often considered in a negative light. However, Freud (1940) described this type of enactment as clarifying an aspect of a patient's life history 'as the patient acts before us, as it were, instead of reporting it to us'. In this example, Steve quickly re-enacted a scenario where the therapist and the group became representative of an authority that needed to be shunned and attacked. In turn, he was attacked by another patient who responded similarly. It is apparent that the therapist's attempt to engage Steve in the group was perceived in a hostile way. (Equally, it could be said that the therapist was irritated by Steve's rebuttal of group norms and acted in an authoritarian manner.) The other group member was irritated by Steve's unwillingness to engage in the group. It is apparent that the therapist in this example may have unwittingly taken on the role of authority although this may have served to isolate Steve further rather than to embrace him in the group.

HOPE

Setting:	A patient is preparing to leave a group and expresses her fear of coping outside it. A new member of the group expresses a wish that they were in the position of leaving rather than just arriving.
Patient A:	'I wish it were me going'.
Patient B:	'I was like you, I couldn't wait for my time to be up and the nightmare to end but I want you to stick with it; it's tough but there is hope. I am frightened of the journey I have ahead of me, without all of you, but if you hang on in there, you'll get over it, but not without other people's help'.

In the early stages of group development, members are chiefly concerned with survival and establishing the boundaries of the group. Factors such as the instillation of hope are especially important at this time (Yalom, 1975). Not only is it required to keep the patient in therapy but also having some faith in the possibility that an experience may be therapeutic is likely to enable the patient to be more open to change. It is perhaps one of the enduring values of group therapy that patients are able to see each other stumble as well as progress through various stages of therapy.

LEADERSHIP DEPENDENCE

Setting:	An afternoon ward business meeting at a day hospital. The consultant attends this one-weekly group meeting and all the patients attend (on average 20 patients, six staff, the consultant, the Registrar and four nursing staff).
Patient A:	'I've been thinking doctor, I should get myself a pet, what do you think?'
Consultant:	'That sounds a good idea, what do other people think?'
Patient B:	'I had a dog once but it got run over; we lived on a busy road'.
Patient A:	'Pets are supposed to be calming, aren't they doc?' [The patient sounds increasingly anxious]
Registrar:	'Are you needing something to help you stay calm?'
Patient A:	'Well, my tablets certainly aren't working, I told you that weeks ago'.

Fear in a group can manifest itself in a number of ways. It may be a reaction to a situation that has occurred in the group or it may be in anticipation of an event that has a memory trace of a previous unresolved fear. Bion (1961) describes fearfulness as predominant in a leader dependent group. The group often structures itself as a dependent group in order to avoid emotional states; members expect the leader to act as the authority figure and sit back and wait for the leader to solve all the problems.

Bion's basic assumption theory incorporates a system of diagnosis whereby the activities that obstruct and divert the group from its therapeutic task can be identified. Basic assumption leader dependence was noted in the above group when Patient A specifically allocated the doctor a role of advice giver. In this group, Patient A, who was dissatisfied, perhaps was elevated to a position of anti-leadership. By deprecating the care received the patient was perhaps perceived by the other patients as representing a view more widely held by the group. The reaction of the Registrar was an essentially defensive one, wishing to medicate away any sense of discontent that might disrupt the group.

PAIRING

Setting:	A twice weekly evening group held in the out-patients department. Two members in the group have an extended interchange and there appears to be little chance for others to feel included. The latter part of the interchange is conducted thus:
Sonjia:	'I had real problems getting here tonight, I just couldn't get going, and at work they kept giving me these little jobs to do, as if they knew I wanted to leave on time but were deliberately stopping me coming'.
Stacey:	'I have that too'.
Sonjia:	'Do you, does your workplace plague you about coming here?'
Stacey:	'Oh no, I haven't told them.'
Sonjia:	'What do you mean then, you have "the same as me"?'
Stacey:	'Well I was supporting you in not wanting to come here, I'll do anything to avoid the thought of what's going to be said or done here every week'.
Sonjia:	'Are you saying I don't want to be here?'
Therapist:	'It seems difficult for others to take part in this conversation'.

Pairing is described by Bion (1961) as a means of avoiding the emotional demands of a group setting and of forming close links with the group as a whole, by finding a single other person who feels similarly. As in the leader dependent group, the creation of a pair in a group means that a wider network of intimacy can be avoided. Emotional contact and the development of relationships is then halted as the focus of the group remains wholly on the pair. The pair may become inward looking, thereby excluding the rest of the group. The pair may then become experienced as an enemy within the group. In the above example, the group appeared to be content to allow the two members to carry on their lengthy interchange. This basic assumption position needs to be questioned and the group needs to see whether it has the capacity to allow certain people to speak to the exclusion of others. Bion's theory is helpful; however, it is important that reasonable interchange and dialogue in a group is not mistaken for pathological and defensive functioning. Indeed, it might be argued that, to some extent, all defences may have a function in allowing some more reticent and anxious members to join in a group. In the above example, both Stacey and Sonjia were new to the group. Their experience of a basic assumption pairing may have contributed to them feeling more secure in the group, adumbrating an anxiety that may have been otherwise unbearable. In other words, we may see basic assumption functioning not only as regressive but also as a necessary process in forming and securing emotional bonds in the group.

The task for the group therapist when faced with basic assumption functioning, whether leader dependence, pairing or flight/flight, is to enable the group to see itself operating. This does not mean that the group therapist necessarily hastily challenges or confronts the behaviour of the group. Rather the therapist needs to create something of an atmosphere where a culture of inquiry in the group may reign, where members begin to feel secure enough to wonder about themselves and each other. Rather than describing this as encouraging a process of insight, Pines (1983) has described that seeing ourselves in the context of others is the real value of the therapeutic exchange, a process of gaining 'outsight', which is possible in a group setting especially, where the emphasis is on the sharing of personal space with others.

PROJECTION

Setting:	A twice weekly closed small-group psychotherapy session on an acute unit.
Steve:	I can't keep going like this, I bring everyone else down with me; all the people I come into contact with and develop a relationship with either leave me or are left damaged somehow. As if I've contaminated them with my sadness'.

Guilt may spring from fantasies about contaminating or poisoning others which is also associated with a low self-esteem. These fantasies may be manifest in the relationships in a group (Hinshelwood, 1987). Retreat into a mournful inner world was apparent in Steve's experience in the group, where his past relationships were experienced in the here and now. His demoralization was apparent and could be seen infiltrating his interrelations with other community members. The experience of interpersonal intimacy evoked strong feelings for Steve. These offer the opportunity for exploring false and illusory pre-occupations about the self, when group interchange may be the basis of forming a new sense of self. The process of splitting between a good and bad self inside, may be manifest in external relations where others may become involved in splitting process. These self-images (true and false) may need to be explored before a more integrated sense of self can emerge.

It is common to externalize unacceptable feelings and then attribute them to others; a very human but tragic state (Brown and Pedder, 1991). In a group setting this can manifest itself in the representation or belief that some kind of transfer of feeling from one person to another has occurred. What is transferred is important, as it can be a relocated piece of personal experience, the end result being the realization that someone else has experienced it. In this example, the experience is one of the whole group feeling the anxiety of some feared and potential pain. Projection can involve one or two people but it is also apparent when the whole group is assumed to take on a quality which is an externalization of an inner mental state.

FIGHT–FLIGHT

Setting:	An in-patient, weekly, small closed group.
Amanda:	[After several minutes, silence] 'What we need is a holiday; can't we organize a day trip out somewhere, nurse?'.
Sue:	'Oh yeah! brilliant idea, get away from the smog and fumes for a while will do us all good'.
Peter:	'I went to Wales once with my parents after my A levels and it was terrible, we all rowed all the time and it rained most of the time. I ended up reading in my room, which I could have done at home anyway'.
Amanda:	'Don't be such a killjoy, it would be good'.
Therapist:	'I wonder whether people are avoiding looking at what is making it so unbearable to be here at the moment?'
Betty:	'Here we go, a little bit of light discussion and we are accused of avoiding the issue'.
Joseph:	'A holiday always used to work for me, get my mind off things, nothing wrong with it I don't think'.

One of the patterns of group behaviour that Bion (1961) noted was that of a group focusing its concentration entirely upon events external to the group space. This pattern of behaviour Bion named basic assumption *fight–flight*. Bion conceived this externalizing of experience as a defence against the immediacy of contact in the group. It would appear that the group in the above example found that they were able to relieve the long and difficult silence at the start of the session by talking about a group holiday. The group fantasized itself into another psychical space, one that was far happier than the space they experienced in therapy. However, while this flight of fancy would seem to be an exemplar of Bion's basic assumption *fight–flight*, treating the material as only a defensive regression from the therapeutic task of the group would be a mistake. To some extent the flight in this case enabled some of the patients to reconnect with previous experiences that, while beyond the inner life of the group, would be valuable to examine. While the therapist in this group would appear to be following Bion's theory correctly, Betty's criticism might indeed be fair. The timing or tempo of a therapist's interpretation is important. In this example it may have been helpful to allow the group to associate freely with their fantasies for a while. The process of drawing the group's attention inwardly to itself needs to be undertaken carefully so as not to compromise its capacity for outwardness.

RIVALRY

Setting:	A large community group attended by all patients, held every morning on an in-patient unit.
John:	'Well it's nice to see everyone here again this morning. How are you Deidre?'
Deidre:	'Leave me alone'.
John:	'Oh, touchy are we? I was only being friendly'.
Bert:	'She doesn't like to be given such attention, John mate, leave her alone'.
Sylvie:	'How can you say that; what do you know she wants or doesn't want?'
Deidre:	'Oh, for God's sake, all of you just shut up!' [Leaves the group and slams the door]

Groups can provide an opportunity to revisit many feelings and sibling rivalry is one such dynamic that may re-emerge in relationships among group members, where members may attempt to claim attention from the group leader. Hatred in siblings is an important factor in the pathogenesis of neurosis, as becomes evident when looking at the effect of birth order. The hate components of the Oedipus complex are a normal consequence of the intense love felt for the parent of the opposite sex and the hate towards a sibling rival for parental attention. The claims of one sibling on the affection of a parent come into conflict with the claims of other siblings. Much of the curiosity children show about gestation, conception and parturition arises from events connected with the arrival of a new member, who threatens to deplete the stores of attention and affection on offer, in this case from the therapist (Abse, 1974).

Scapegoating of a peer member often arises when there are feelings of rivalry underpinning events in a group. Commonly, scapegoating acts as a cover to other hidden conflicts in the group (Loomis, 1979). Unless the facilitator intervenes, scapegoating can isolate and drive the individual member from the group.

SUBSTANCE ABUSE

Setting:	A patient returns from leave in time to attend the group but smells of alcohol and is slurring her speech and giggling inappropriately.
Therapist:	'I think you should leave until you feel more yourself again, Judy'.
Judy:	'No, no, I'm well and truly myself at the moment, thank you'.
Patient A:	'Judy love, go and sleep it off'.

The suitability of different groups of patients for group therapy continues to be debated. Patients who are abusing substances or alcohol, who are excessively intoxicated or under the influence of a substance at the time of a group session should be encouraged not to attend or possibly be excluded. Invariably, policies are formed to say that patients should not attend a group until they are sober. The group should return with the message that members are wanted for who they are, not who they wish to be under the influence of drugs and alcohol. The decision to exclude someone form the group sometimes may need to be taken without prior consultation with the group. Foulkes (1948) indicates the group leader owes the group an opening explanation if someone is banned from the group.

SUICIDE

Setting:	An emergency meeting was called after the news had reached the ward that a patient had been killed at the nearby underground station. The therapist breaks the news about the death.
Betty:	'Has he killed himself?'
Therapist:	'We have to await the coroner's verdict but as far as we know he fell in front of a train'.
John:	'Peter wouldn't kill himself. Only last week he said he was planning to go over to his pool club one night'.
	[silence]
Jason:	Will we have a service for him at the chapel or something like that?'
Therapist:	'That's a lovely idea. I will look into it and arrange something if that's what people want'.
Karen:	'What do we do now then?' [Begins to cry]
Ian:	'I wonder whether we should just think about what this means to all of us, I mean we've lost Peter and that sounds as if that's what he wanted. We have to consider our own lives and where we all hope to be in the future'.
Lionel:	'A bit morbid this'.
Stacey:	'I don't feel comfortable with it either. Do we have to stay in the group, now you've told us? We can discuss it privately and stuff can't we? Let it sink in?'
Therapist:	'It is difficult to know what to say, although I do think that it might be helpful for us to put into words how we are feeling. But it is simply difficult to be here; it might be as much as we can manage just to stay here for a while together'.

Within a group setting, a suicide is a devastating experience. The initial reaction is one of a great shock and the information about a suicide needs to be presented as sensitively as possible. The temptation is to protect the patients from the information. However, as in the above example, there may be much value in sharing the information as it reaches the group, for instance, by calling an emergency meeting as soon as possible. (The same could be said for any shocking or traumatic information.) The notion of being able to protect someone from the sheer horror and shock of suicide is untennable. Secreting such information may well exert greater disturbance as it is leaked unconsciously by the staff. Working with this kind of difficult material is perhaps done most effectively in a group setting. The experience of sharing in sorrow, sadness and loss is often a group experience (e.g. funerals, wakes, memorial services). It is also the case that when faced with trauma people often instinctively huddle together for self-protection and to seek reassurance in others, a type of blitz mentality that group therapy can engender and usefully exploit at difficult times.

Suicide is a highly significant event and its aftermath has the potential to be destructive as a contagion effect. The group will be thrown into disarray by the incident and become disorientated, anxious and isolated. However, if managed openly, the experience can bring people together and offer an opportunity for a depth of learning not previously experienced. Attachments and group affiliation may be enriched as a group survives through such an experience.

REGRESSION

Setting:	A therapy group run by the ward Registrar and clinical charge nurse, once a week. The Registrar had not been able to attend regularly and the charge nurse was about to take two weeks' annual leave.
Therapist:	'I need to let people know I will not be here for two weeks next month, as I'm taking some holiday'.
Susy:	'What will happen to the group while you are away?'
Therapist:	'I have spoken to Dr Roberts and she will be here'.
Clive:	'How can you be sure?'
Susy:	'Yeah, how do we know she'll come at all? We could be sat here all alone'.
Therapist:	'Is that the fear, that I am leaving you all alone?'
Susy:	[Huddled up in her chair, hugging her legs and dropping her head on her knees] 'Well, it wouldn't surprise me. You don't care once you leave the ward at night. I've seen you laughing and smiling as if you're glad to see the back of us in here'.

Regression is a state in which a person may experience feelings that are related to an earlier stage in their development. Quite often, the most regressed feelings are associated with experiences from childhood, where immaturity may be prevalent on the part of the group as a whole or certain individual members. This impedes therapy and achievement of group tasks. It may reveal itself in intense irrational anxiety, a collective murderous rage or severe depression and helplessness. The work of therapy groups is often thwarted by regression phenomena characterized by anxiety, depression and rage. Bion (1961) exemplifies disruptive group behaviour in his basic assumption theory. Considerable effort is needed from the facilitator to provide an environment that is supportive and will result in a reduction of regressive behaviour. Fundamentally, the group experience provides a creative arena for the exchanging of ideas, free verbal expression, symbolism, expressionism and realism by using the related dramas that take place in the sessions. These dramas help patients to explore their characters, conflicts and personal ethical dilemmas. This complex array of experiences needs some form of monitoring from the therapist, whose task it is to safeguard the group from unproductive regression (Abse, 1974). It is not, however, the task of the therapist to lend clarity or understanding to events that are usually very difficult to process at the time. Instead the therapist needs to help the group experience the fullness and variety of its experiences. It is important to note that not all regressive experiences are necessarily pathological. Indeed many normative feelings that are experienced in childhood are just as important to healthy adult functioning.

RESEARCH INTO GROUP PROCESSES

Many people who study groups are themselves practitioners, aiming to help specific groups of people operate more successfully. Most of the discourse in group therapy research relies on information gathered from self-rating and subjective observation. This has been criticized for not seeking to clarify or discover what actually happens in groups or how efficacy can be monitored where research has been poorly designed without experimental controls. However, some of the following studies are exemplars of the possibilities of group research.

Reddy and Lippert (1980) identified the characteristics of members of small groups and found that, in general, people joined a group to achieve some form of remedial change in what they perceived to be as painless and speedy as manner as possible. However, personal change research has shown that group therapy involves a lengthy and often emotionally painful and distressing process.

Yalom (1975) identified 11 curative factors in groups and found that cognitive learning was considered the most important element of group experience. This was further defined as gaining information from the group and insight from the group experience.

When looking at the role of the group leader, Lieberman *et al.* (1973) found that when the leader was seen as caring and able to explain to the group what was occurring, confront emotional situations and maintain the group structure, outcomes were considered more favourable.

A working group has been described as being influential in changing patients' thoughts, feelings and actions (Marcovitz, 1983). People who experience groups learn to relate authentically to each other and to the problems that manifest themselves in the groups' life. The work can be frustrating, enraging, terrifying, humiliating, humbling, painful and sad; it can be full of disappointment, love and hope (Agazarian, 1992). As repeatedly noted by group theorists such as Yalom (1975) the power and centrality of group therapy continually challenges our assumptions about abnormality and intervention. Somehow, the understanding and treatment of inter and intrapersonal events are effective (Slife, 1991).

While research continues into groups and group processes, there is a risk of more rigid and scientific methods being used that will exclude the subtle and more fluid aspects of group therapy. Further research is needed into the outcomes of group therapy and in particular the influential role of the nurse within groups. Many of the elements discussed and presented in this chapter elude accurate forms of measurement but this should not deter nurses from being involved in group therapy, which is a most fulfilling and positive learning experience.

SUMMARY

There are other theories and methods for understanding therapeutic groups but, as the chapter reveals, most have stemmed from a psychodynamic orientation. Groups are extensively utilised and studying them in-depth can reveal as much about oneself as is learnt or observed about other members. All nurses interested in groups should be encouraged to read and learn more and to undertake further study of groups. This will enable nurses to continue learning and increasing nursing's knowledge of the therapeutic effect of groups.

The vignettes given in the second half of the chapter have not captured all the richness of group activity nor all its complexity. The authors have spent many hours themselves in groups and group supervision, both as group members, facilitators and supervisors, yet this chapter has limited the encapsulation of all this experience. What we hope the chapter does do, however, is encourage nurses to remain members, leaders and observers of groups but mostly to consider the therapeutic effect of groups on both themselves and others.

KEY CONCEPTS

- Group therapy remains one of the most frequently used methods of psychological intervention.
- Group supervision is integral to enabling nurses to consider the impact of their work in groups and enhance creative problem-solving.
- Group theory draws on social and behavioural psychology.
- The aim of a group is to provide a corrective experience and better understanding of how one relates to others.
- Groups may present common themes but exhibit unique experiences.
- The here-and-now experience in a group is of primary importance.
- Group work can be highly emotional and needs to be safely facilitated.
- Groups involve long-term commitment and often emotionally painful and distressing work.

REFERENCES

Abse DW: *Clinical notes on group-analytic psychotherapy*. Bristol, 1974, John Wright & Sons Ltd.

Agazarian YM: Contemporary theories of group psychotherapy. A systems approach to the group as a whole. *Int J Group Psychother* 42(2):177–203, 1992.

Ahlin G: The interpersonal world of the infant and the foundation matrix for the groups and networks of the person. *Group Anal* 28:5–20, 1995.

Avaline M and Dryden, W, editors: *Group therapy in Britain*. Milton Keynes, 1988, Open University Press.

Balint M: Changing therapeutical aims and techniques in psychoanalysis. *Int J Psycho Anal* 31:117–122, 1950.

Balint M: *The basic fault*. London, 1968, Tavistock.

Bion WR: *Experiences in groups*. London, 1961, Tavistock.

Bjorndal K: The establishment of a work group on an in-patient drug dependency unit. *Ther Communities* 13(3):179–185, 1992.

Bowlby J: *The making and breaking of affectional bonds*. London, 1973, Tavistock.

British Association of Social Psychiatrists: Official Statement 1995. *ATC Newsletter*, July 1996.

Brown DG, Pedder JR: *Introduction to psychotherapy*, 2 ed. London, 1991, Tavistock.

Brown DG: Bion and Foulkes: Basic assumptions and beyond. In: Pines M, editor: *Bion and group psychotherapy*. London, 1985, Routledge.

Budman SH, Soldz S, Demby A, Feldstein M: Cohesion, alliance and outcome in group psychotherapy. *Psychiatry* 52(3)339–350, 1989.

De Board R: *The psychoanalysis of organizations. A psychoanalytic aspproach to organizations and groups*. London, 1978, Tavistock.

Erikson E: *Childhood and society*. London, 1965, Penguin.

Fabricius J: Psychodynamic perspectives. In: Wright H, Giddey M, editors: *Mental health nursing*. London, 1993, Chapman & Hall.

Fabricius J: Psychoanalytic understanding and nursing: A supervisory workshop with nurse tutors. *Psychoanal Psychother* 9(1)17–29, 1995.

Fairbairn WRD: *Psychoanalytic studies of the personality*. London, 1952, Tavistock.

Flyn C: The patients pantry: The nature of the nursing task. *Ther Communities* 14(4)227–236, 1993.

Foulkes SH: On group therapy. In: Foulkes SH: *Selected papers of SH Foulkes*. London, 1990, Karnac.

Foulkes, SH: *Introduction to group analytic psychotherapy*. London, 1948, Heinemann.

Foulkes SH: Wider theoretical formulations and applications. In: Foulkes SH, Anthony EJ: *Group psychotherapy. The psychoanalytic approach*. London, 1957a (reprinted 1984), Karnacs.

Foulkes SH: Psychoanalytic concepts and object relations theory: comments on a paper by Fairbairn. In: Foulkes SH: *Selected papers of SH Foulkes*. London, 1957b, Karnac.

Foulkes, SH: Two opposed views of social psychiatry: The issue. In: Foulkes SH: *Selected papers of SH Foulkes*. London, 1969, Karnac.

Freud S: *Group psychology and the analysis of the ego*, SE vol 18. London, 1921, Hogarth.

Granstrom K: Dynamics in meetings. *On leadership and followership in ordinary meetings in different organizations*. London, 1986, Artesian Books.

Grotstein JS, Rinsley DB, editors: *Fairbairn and the origins of object relations*. London, 1994, Free Association Books.

Haigh R: *The matrix in the milieu. The ghost in the machine*. Paper presented at the *4th European Congress of Psychology*. Athens, July 11–14, 1995.

Hardy S, Winship G, Crowe M, Caan W: The development of a community atmosphere. 1995. [In preparation.]

Hinshelwood RD: *What happens in groups*. London, 1987, Free Association Books.

Hinshelwood RD, Manning N, editors: *Therapeutic communities: reflections and progress*. London, 1979, Tavistock.

Jackson M, Cawley RH: Psychodynamics and psychotherapy on an acute psychiatric ward: The story of an experimental unit. *Br J Psychiatry* 160:41–50, 1992.

Jones M: Group psychotherapy. *BMJ* 2:276–278, 1942a.

Jones M: Group treatment. *Am J Psychiatry* 101:292–299, 1942b.

Knowles J: Therapeutic communities in today's world. *Ther communities* 16(2)97–102, 1995.

Lieberman MA, Yalom ID, Miles MB: *Encounter groups: First facts*. New York, 1973, Basic Books.

Loomis ME: *Group process for nurses*. Missouri, 1979, Mosby.

Main T: The concept of the therapeutic community: Variations and vicissitudes. In: Pines M, editor: *The evolution of group analysis*. London, 1983, Routledge and Keegan Paul.

Marcovitz RJ, Smoth JE: An approach to time limited dynamic inpatient group psychotherapy. *Small Group Behav* 14(3)369–376, 1983.

Menzies–Lyth I: *The dynamics of the social. selected essays*. London, 1988, Free Association Books.

Pedder J: Attachment and a new beginning. *Int Rev Psychoanaly* 3:491–497, 1976.

Pedder JR: The role of space and location in psychotherapy. *Int Rev Psychoanal* 4(2):215–223, 1977.

Pedder JR: Reflections on the theory and practice of supervision. *Psychoanal Psychother* 2(1)1–12, 1986.

Pedder JR: Termination reconsidered. *Int J Psychoanal* 69:495-505, 1988.

Pedder JR: Fear of dependence in therapeutic relationships. *Br J Med Psychol* 64:117–126, 1991.

Pedder JR: Entrance requirements for psychotherapy training: Rationale and objectives. *Br J Psychother* 9(3)310–316, 1993.

Peplau H: *Selected works. Interpersonal theory in nursing.* New York, 1989, Springer.

Peplau H: Psychiatric mental health nursing: Challenge and change. *J Psychiatr Men Health Nurs* 1:3–7, 1994.

Pines M, editor: *The evolution of group analysis.* London, 1983, Routledge and Keegan Paul.

Pines M: Reflections on mirroring. *Int Rev Psychoanal* 11:27–42, 1984.

Pines M, editor: *Bion and group psychotherapy.* London, 1985, Routledge.

Pines M: Psychoanalysis, psychodrama & group psychotherapy. Step children of Vienna. *Group Anal.* 19:101–112, 1986.

Pratt JH: The class method of treating consumption in the homes of the poor. *J Am Med Assoc* 49:755–759, 1907.

Reddy WB, Lippert KM: Studies of the process and dynamics within experiential groups. In: Smith PB, editor: *Small groups and personal change.* London, 1980, Metheun.

Rustin M: *The good society and the inner world.* London, 1991, Verso.

Slife BD, Lauyon J: Accounting for the power of the here and now: a theoretical revolution. *Int J Group Psychother* 41(2):145–167, 1991.

Stern D: The interpersonal world of the infant. New York, 1985, Basic Books.

Sutherland JD: Bion revisited: Group dynamics and group psychotherapy. In: Pines M, editor: *Bion and group psychotherapy.* London, 1985, Routledge.

Tuckman BW: Developmental sequences in small group psychotherapy. *Psychol Bull* 63:384–399, 1965.

Waller D: Group analysis and the arts therapies. *Group Analy* 23:211–213, 1990.

Waller D: *Group interactive art therapy.* London, 1993, Routledge.

Winnicott D: *The maturational process and the facilitating environment.* London, 1965, Hogarth.

Winship G: The unconscious impact of caring for acutely disturbed patients – a perspective for supervision. *J Psychiatr Men Health Nurs* 2(4)227–232, 1995.

Winship G, Harnimann B, Burling S, Courtney J: Understanding countertransference and object relations in the process of nursing. *Psychoanaly Psychother* 9(2)195–207, 1995.

Yalom ID: *The theory and practice of group psychotherapy.* New York, 1975, Basic Books.

FURTHER READING

Cannard D, Roberts G: *Group analytic workbook.* London, 1994, Routledge.
  An excellent book giving case examples that are then discussed looking at the theory.

Kreiger L: *Large groups.* London, 1975, Constable.
  Deals with large groups comprehensively.

Main T: *The ailment and other psychoanalytic essays.* Free Association Books, 1988, London.

Shermer VL, Pines M: *Ring of fire.* London, 1994, Routledge.
  Another excellent text.

Stock Whitaker DS: *Using groups to help people.* London, 1985, Routledge.
  A much-referred-to book by nurses, filled with interesting concepts.

Wright H: *Group work. Perspectives and practice.* London, 1989, Scutari.
  An excellent and comprehensive study of groups for psychiatric nurses. A must.

Working with Informal Carers and Families of Schizophrenia Sufferers

---

Learning Outcomes

After studying this chapter you should be able to:

- Describe the concept and characteristics of expressed emotion.

- Define a psychosocial and psychoeducational approach that draws on a cognitive–behavioural model.

- Provide a comprehensive rationale as to why this empirically based approach is effective with mental health service users who suffer from schizophrenia.

- Describe how psychological interventions can be used to reduce stress and burden in family environments.

- Relate these interventions to use in routine clinical practice.

---

*S*ince the mid-1980s, considerable research has been conducted to find psychological interventions to help clients and their families to cope with the symptoms, stressors and effects of schizophrenia. Family intervention studies based on the concept of expressed emotion (EE) have considerable clinical significance (see, for example, Leff *et al.*, 1982 and 1989; Falloon *et al.*, 1982 and 1985; Hogarty *et al.*, 1986 and 1991; Tarrier *et al.*, 1988). These are reviewed in this chapter because they provide considerable evidence that a combination of psychosocial, cognitive–behavioural interventions, education and family support in the community helps to reduce incidents of relapse in schizophrenia.

This chapter describes the cognitive–behavioural approach devised to reduce the burden and address the needs of clients and their families. It presents an overview of the concept and characteristics of EE, and reviews the main schizophrenia family work intervention studies. To increase awareness of those families that are in need of help and support, it identifies ways of assessing clients and their families' needs prior to working with them, and goes on to describe the cognitive–behavioural skills and interventions Mental Health Nurses (MHNs) require to work more effectively with this group of clients and their families.

EXPRESSED EMOTION

In the 1960s, researchers started to investigate why some clients with schizophrenia relapsed after discharge despite regular medication while others did not (Brown *et al.*, 1972). The purpose of these investigations was to understand what happened to discharged patients and to explore the effects of the family environment on the course of schizophrenia. Early findings suggested that family influences might affect the course of the illness. Some clients returning to live with spouses or parents seemed to do worse than those returning to other environments. These studies found that clients living with critical, hostile or over-involved relatives were more likely to relapse. In comparison, those who took regular medication and were surrounded by accepting, supportive but realistic relatives tended not to.

The term 'expressed emotion' (EE) was coined and families were designated High EE or Low EE (Table 31.1) using a semi-structured interview known as the Camberwell Family Interview (CFI). The CFI (Box 31.1) is a research instrument that records a range of feelings and emotions contributes little to understanding the aetiology of schizophrenia. However, it has been found to be a robust predictor of relapse when someone with schizophrenia lives with relatives (Kuipers *et al.*, 1992). Its aim is to obtain objective information about events and circumstances in the home and ascertain relatives' feelings and attitudes towards the client in the months before admission (Vaughn and Leff, 1976). The interview takes at least 1½ hours to conduct and a further 1½ hours to rate (Leff and Vaughn, 1985). The measurement and interview technique is therefore intensive and, to become proficient in its use, researchers have to attend a 2-week, full time course.

EXAMPLES OF EXPRESSED EMOTIONS

As Kuipers (1992) points out, particular attributes and comments are not specific to schizophrenia, nor do they occur solely in relatives or in a specific culture or group. EE characteristics have been found in a variety of psychiatric and medical disorders, such as depression, bipolar affective disorder (Miklowitz *et al.*, 1988), anorexia (Szmukler *et al.*, 1987) and obesity (Fischmann–Havstad and Marston, 1984). These studies provide further evidence of the robustness of this concept but, as illustrated earlier, to become proficient in rating, EE researchers have to be intensively trained. Therefore, it must be emphasized that EE is a research concept that helps in understanding of familial attributes but the term should never be used loosely. All too often professionals in the clinical area have been heard to say, 'Oh, she's an over-involved mother' or, 'He's a critical father'. These statements are a criticism in themselves and must always be avoided. Likewise, it is not acceptable to tell people to stop doing something or behaving in a critical manner, as this does not take into consideration the caring emotion behind the perceived criticism. Indeed, being critical is sometimes the only way a family can tell their relative that they really care.

Some of these statements are completely understandable when one considers how difficult it is to cope with schizophrenia and its consequences. Observe your colleagues' and your own interactions with clients and note whether they exhibit similar characteristics to the examples given. To enhance your insight, role-play being a client and relative in a critical or over-involved scenario with a colleague, discuss what it felt like and feed back to each other.

Critical and Hostile Comments

He should be at college like other kids his age, but he *never* does anything, he just sits around all day, doing nothing — absolutely nothing!

Box 31.1 The Camberwell family interview schedule

Critical comments
Unfavourable comments about a person's behaviour or personality.

Positive remarks
Expresses praise, approval, or appreciation of the person's behaviour or personality.

Hostility
Present when a person is attacked for what s/he is rather than for what s/he does.

Emotional over-involvement
Exaggerated emotional response; self-sacrificing and devoted behaviour or extremely overprotective behaviour.

Warmth
Refers only to the warmth expressed in the interview about the person. Tone of voice, sympathy, concern and interest in the person is very important.

If person being interviewed makes 6 or more critical comments, or there is hostility, or 3 or more on over-involvement, they are designated High EE

TABLE 31.1 Response characteristics of low and high expressed emotion

	Low EE	High EE
Cognitive		
	Genuine illness	Legitimacy of the illness in doubt
	Lower expectations	Expectations unchanged
Emotional		
	Other-focused Empathetic } Calm} Objective}	Self-focused Intense anger or distress
Behavioural		
	Adaptive Problem-solving approach Non-intrusive Non-confrontational	Less flexible Intrusive Confrontational

(adapted from Leff and Vaughn, 1985)

She's so lazy, she's unkempt and dirty. Just look at her, she never, ever washes — no wonder she's lost all her friends!

He's so stupid — just look at him now, he's not taking the blindest bit of notice of what you're saying; he's always doing that — off in his own world!

She says the silliest of things — and goes on and on about them, over and over again. It makes me so angry — she never shuts up and it never makes any sense. I tried listening at first, but now I just tell her to get lost or shut up!

He's a no-hoper, we've tried everything; he won't even go to the day centre regularly and that's hardly taxing. I referred him to a rehab place once, but that didn't work, he refused to go — I haven't got the time to take him or sit and hold his hand — you wouldn't believe he's 28, he's like a child.

Over-Involvement

I worry all the time; I just don't know what's going to happen to him. It makes me ache with sadness, when I think of what he's lost — he was such a beautiful, beautiful child.

I have to stay with her all the time; she'd never eat or do anything if I wasn't there.

It's very, very difficult; John's a good boy, but he'd never get dressed if I didn't help him. I lay his clothes out, get a wash bowl and help him shave and once a week we wash his hair — that way he still looks good.

We never go out together, we used to, but he'd get into a terrible mess — once he left the gas on and nearly blew the kitchen up, so one of us is always there now, in case anything should happen!

I'm very frightened of him, he has such violent outbursts; but I'm his mother, so I have to go twice a day to take food and check he's OK.

Warm and Positive Remarks

Sandra's had some very difficult times coping with all this, I am very proud of her.

He always helps out, you never have to ask; he's always been very good at knowing when to help others — he's very caring.

Sometimes Sarah doesn't want to go out, so I give her time and then say 'OK, what would you like to do instead?'

We have good times together, we learn a lot from each other; there are times when I have to be there to hold her hand, but other times she's there for me — so it's a good partnership.

Sometimes you have to let this schizophrenia thing take its course. John and I have decided not to push too hard and to take each day as it comes, but we're always there for Susan if she needs us.

THE ELEMENTS OF FAMILY INTERVENTIONS IN SCHIZOPHRENIA: RESEARCH FINDINGS

It was assumed that schizophrenia has a defined genetic component and is exacerbated by stressful life events and emotional environments (Zubin and Spring, 1977). The Family Intervention studies (summarized below) were designed to promote a low EE environment in the home and address the problems faced by families after the discharge of relatives. The study conditions vary but generally they have either included regular medication or involved other interventions. These interventions are psychosocial in nature because, unlike traditional family therapy, they involve engaging families in the treatment process, teaching communication skills, problem-solving and managing relatives' concerns in a non-blaming atmosphere (Barrowclough and Tarrier, 1992). All packages had a continuing educational component and thus also may be described as psychoeducational (Anderson *et al.*, 1980). Both these approaches have been drawn from a cognitive–behavioural model, which is a relatively new approach. It has been described as a structured form of psychotherapy that incorporates problem solving strategies to alleviate clients' symptoms by helping them to learn more effective ways of coping with the difficulties and distresses they are experiencing (Blackburn and Davidson, 1990). That is, clients and their families can learn to deal with the symptoms of schizophrenia more effectively if they master methods to objectively identify and eliminate the thinking errors that cause them to feel upset. Clients and their relatives will feel more positive about the illness and its outcome.

The studies reviewed were undertaken in a variety of settings and cultures around the world (for example, Vaughn *et al.*, 1984; Leff *et al.*, 1987) and all used the EE selection criteria. This has resulted in their being criticized for negatively labelling families as hostile or over-involved, reinforcing the need for neuroleptic medication and neglecting to examine the impact of these interventions on clients living in low EE environments (Johnstone, 1993). To overcome such misconceptions, and to make family selection simpler, Kuipers *et al.* (1992) now advocate using 'rule of thumb' criteria (Box 31.2).

However, at the time the studies were undertaken there was an assumption that high EE environments were the highest risk situations for clients. Therefore, a number of research teams started to investigate which interventions were most successful at reducing clients' relapse rates.

In their first study Leff *et al.* (1982) compared a number of social intervention methods. These consisted of two, brief

Box 31.2 *The rule of thumb for family intervention*

- Relatives living with clients who relapse more than twice a year despite taking regular medication.
- Relatives who frequently contact staff for reassurance or help.
- Families in which there are repeated arguments leading to violence.
- Any family that calls the police.
- Any relative who is looking after a schizophrenic client on their own.

education sessions about schizophrenia, a relatives' support group and family sessions conducted in the home, with routine out-patient care. The goal was to reduce the amount of contact clients had with relatives and the level of EE. At 9-month follow-up Leff *et al.* (1982) found that the home family sessions had been the most successful in bringing about a change in the levels of EE and the amount of contact, as no client had relapsed. This was a positive outcome but they remained keen to ascertain which aspects of the social intervention were the most successful. In 1989, Leff *et al.* conducted a further study, to compare a relatives' group with home-based family sessions. All the families received two formal education sessions about the effects of schizophrenia and its causes and treatments. The family sessions were carried out in the home, using a structured model of intervention. The model involved two researchers visiting the families every 2 weeks and incorporated a problem-solving and psycho-educative approach. The relatives' group used the same intervention but it ran from a local community centre in London. At 9 months only 8% of the clients from the family sessions had relapsed, compared to 36% in the relatives' group. These two treatments can be compared favourably in efficacy where the relatives actually attended the group. However, the family sessions did appear to be more successful. Perhaps this was because families were less worried about exposing their problems to others in their own homes and the researchers had taken the time to visit them and give them a sense of being valued.

In comparison, Falloon (1988) in California, USA used a behavioural model of intervention that emphasized the importance of teaching clients coping skills to help them deal with stressful environments and family situations. Over a 9-month period, home-based behavioural family management (BFM) was compared with individual supportive therapy for the client. Families were selected because they were either rated as high EE or considered to be 'acutely stressed'. The families all received two education sessions about schizophrenia, the BFM then focusing on educating families in general communication skills and problem-solving. The behavioural-problem solving strategy involved working through six steps, which ranged from initially identifying a specific problem or goal, listing a variety of solutions and selecting the optimal solution, to implementing it and reviewing its outcome

(Falloon, 1988). Using this approach Falloon reported only 1 of the 18 BFM cases relapsed at 9-month follow-up. In comparison, 8 of the 18 in the individual therapy group relapsed. This suggests that relapse rates remained minimal in the BFM, while continuing to rise in the individual intervention group (Falloon, 1985).

In Pittsburgh, USA, Hogarty *et al.* (1986) used four different groups in their study: psychoeducational family treatment plus medication; individual social skills training plus medication; family treatment and individual skills training plus medication and medication alone. All the clients involved lived in high EE environments. The psychoeducational family sessions aimed to reduce family stress, increase their tolerance and re-integrate the client into society. They involved working in collaboration with families by giving them social skills training once each week for 6 months, followed by bi-weekly or monthly sessions for the remainder of the year. The individual social skills training centred upon teaching clients how to interact with their families and went on to emphasize the importance of pursuing independent activities. After 1 year, no one had relapsed following the combined family and individual social skills treatments. From these findings it was deduced that the prophylactic effects of family and individual treatment were equivalent. Subsequently, Hogarty *et al.* (1991) reported that relapse rates had increased in all the groups. Nevertheless, the results are still significant and there appears to be a definite advantage in continuing with family intervention, either alone or by combining it with social skills training.

The cognitive–behavioural trial of Tarrier *et al.* (1988) differed from the three previous studies because they compared two 9-month cognitive–behavioural family treatments for acutely ill clients from high EE homes. In one group, coping skills were taught, using discussion and instruction; in the other, coping skills were taught using role-play, behavioural rehearsal and guided practice. These interventions were again designed to reduce EE and enhance clients' and their families' ability to cope. Two other comparison groups were also included. These included a sample of clients from low EE homes and a sample of high EE families, all receiving either out-patient care or two education sessions. At 9 months the two Family Interviews were comparable, as the relapse rates were minimal in the groups that had received instruction and had been involved in role-play. In contrast, relapse rates were significantly higher in the high EE groups that received education and routine treatment.

In complete contrast to these studies, Kottgen *et al.* (1984) selected young clients who lived in high EE environments and had recently experienced their first or second onset of schizophrenia. Over a 12-month period they compared the use of psychodynamic therapy with no treatment at all. This study resulted in no significant outcome, as the relapses rates were high in both groups. It was concluded that focusing on the family dynamics and analysing their interactions appeared to exacerbate stress in the clients involved and therefore the psychodynamic therapy was counterproductive for anyone suffering from schizophrenia. This study is particularly important, as it helps to reinforce the reason for not using psychoanalytical theories and treatments with this type of client group and their families. Indeed, Hirsch and Leff (1975) attempted to establish the existence of 'schizophrenogenic mothers' but despite the theory's popularity could find no justification for it. Furthermore, researchers such as Lidz *et al.* (1965) and Laing (1970) and their concepts of dysfunctional parent–child relationships and interactions, stigmatized families and led the researchers to believe that their behaviour induced or caused schizophrenia in their relatives (Harding and Zahniser 1994).

SUMMARY OF REVIEWED STUDIES

If the overall findings from the studies are examined (Table 31.2) it is possible to deduce that over a 1-year period, the control groups all had significant relapse rates, in comparison to the experimental groups where they can be seen to be minimal. If continued over a 2-year period, the interventions were more effective than routine generic care in reducing relapse rates. In addition, although educating families about schizophrenia was not particularly effective in changing families' behaviours or delaying relapse (Smith and Birchwood, 1987) it did appear to help engage them in intervention programmes, which reinforces the need for such use in routine clinical work.

Furthermore, it can be concluded that the interventions used all have common themes (Lam, 1991; see Box 31.3) and over-

all they help to reduce relapse further than the protection afforded by medication and to provide families and carers with the skills necessary to cope more effectively with the clients' illness (Bellack and Mueser, 1993). These goals are achieved through educating the family about the illness, teaching techniques to cope with symptomatic behaviour and reinforcing family strengths.

In general, a comprehensive family intervention programme should include the following components:
- A didactic element that provides information about schizophrenia and the mental health care system.
- A skills element that offers training in communication, conflict resolution, problem-solving, assertiveness and behavioural and stress management.
- An emotional element that provides opportunities for airing views, sharing and mobilizing resources.
- A process element that focuses on coping with schizophrenia and its effects on the family.
- A social element that increases the use of informal and formal support networks.

Although it should be recognized that no single intervention programme will suit every situation, it is possible to modify the described approach to suit individual families. It is important that the interventions meet their needs and that there is an opportunity for families and clients to ask questions, express feelings and socialize with others including mental health professionals.

These intervention methods emphasize the importance of empowering families and clients. Indeed, as Brooker (1990) has reported, family input from MHNs improves relatives' mental health and their satisfaction with services. However, the interventions are not perceived to be an alternative to community mental health services. They should exist within the sphere of comprehensive community care (Barrowclough and Tarrier, 1992) as individuals suffering from serious mental illness need continuous support .and a high intensity of care to function successfully in the community. Nevertheless, their use will increase awareness of factors relevant to coping with

Box 31.3 *Common themes of family intervention methods*

- Positive approach and empathetic working relationship.
- Cognitive re-structuring.
- Here-and-now focus.
- Problem-solving approach.
- Provision of education.
- Communication and coping skills.

TABLE 31.2 Research findings compared

Relapse rates	6–12 months		2 Years	
Study	Control	Experimental	Control	Experimental
Leff *et al.*(1982)	50%	8%	75%	33%
Fallon *et al.* (1982, 1985)	44%	6%	83%	12%
Hogarty *et al.* (1986, 1991)	41%	0%	67%	25%
Tarrier *et al.* (1988)	53%	12%	59%	33%
Leff *et al.* (1989)	36%	8%		33%

schizophrenia, facilitate positive alliances between families and health care professionals and ultimately enhance the delivery of services (Table 31.3).

IDENTIFYING CLIENTS, FAMILIES AND CARERS IN NEED OF SUPPORT

In the author's opinion, every client with schizophrenia, their families and informal carers are in need of some sort of help and support. They are searching for recognition, a sense of value and practical help from professionals. However, there is currently increasing emphasis being placed upon the cost-effectiveness of services (Onyett, 1992). Therefore, realistically, there have to be criteria for family intervention. As described earlier Kuipers *et al.* (1992) now advocate selecting families who need intervention through the use of the 'rule of thumb' (see Box 31.2). However, Barrowclough and Tarrier (1992) go further and have devised a Relative Assessment Interview (RAI) which is an adapted clinical version of the Camberwell Family Interview. It aims to obtain information about the relatives' behaviours, beliefs and subjective feelings towards the client, and about their illness and its consequences. The RAI should be perceived as an information-gathering process, which elicits clients' and relatives' positive and successful coping strategies and resources, as well as information on their difficulties. The RAI covers seven main areas, which are summarized in Box 31.4.

The information gained from the interview helps to identify areas of need and can also help MHNs gain a full picture of what the family has experienced and what to expect when they commence family work. It is an important process, because if it is completed at baseline and post-intervention, it allows the efficacy of family work to be assessed. Furthermore, in line with the Care Programme Approach (Department of Health, 1995) it formalizes the assessment and interventions strategies and provides a structured method of reporting about family work to the rest of the multidisciplinary team (Barrowclough and Tarrier, 1992).

However, the interview process can be time consuming and its content has to be intensively analysed. This may prevent it being used routinely by MHNs in clinical practice. Therefore, Brooker and Baguley (1990) have devised a simpler formula to plan and implement care for people with schizophrenia and their families. The Schizophrenia Nursing Assessment Protocol (SNAP) adopts a holistic view of families. This allows nurses to obtain a wide picture of their clients' abilities and to make informed decisions about the interventions they use to strengthen them. Within the context of the stress vulnerability model of schizophrenia (Zubin and Spring, 1977), the formula covers four main assessment areas:

1. Personal history and significant life events.
2. relationships within the household.
3. psychiatric history
4. Understanding and knowledge of schizophrenia and its medication.

Nurses should comprehensively address and explore all these areas, so that strategies and goals can be devised to help families and clients find more productive methods of coping with the major stressors in their lives. SNAP, therefore, helps to improve care planning for families, as its effective use can improve understanding of the illness and family relationships and increase clients' social functioning (Brooker and Baguley, 1990).

Box 31.4

Structure of the relatives' assessment interview

- Background of the patient and his or her family.
- Other background information and contact time.
- Chronological history of the illness.
- Current problems and symptoms.
- Irritability or quarrels in the household.
- Relative's relationship with patient.
- Effect of the illness on relatives.

adapted from Barrowclough and Tarrier, 1992

TABLE 31.3 Summary of interventions and expected outcomes

	Interventions	Outcomes
Relatives and carers + Clients + Mental Health Nurses	Education Coordination of treatment Assessment strategies Problem solving Assertive crisis support Medication	Enhanced social functioning Enhanced quality of life Family and client empowerment Greater independence Reduced relapse rates

To ensure that a comprehensive assessment is completed, it is also recommended that nurses measure their clients' mental states using a reliable standardized psychiatric symptom scale, such as the eponymous KGV devised by Krawiecka, Goldberg and Vaughan (1977). In addition, it is important to assess clients' social functioning, before and after the intervention (Birchwood *et al*., 1990), as social functioning is important in aiding the diagnosis of schizophrenia (Morrison and Bellack, 1987). However, it is acknowledged that standards of social functioning vary considerably between cultures and between social classes within a culture. To avoid imposing a generalized standard upon clients, these factors must be considered when conducting this assessment. It is recognized that further research is needed to understand how social functioning can be measured realistically (Gamble and Midence, 1995).

CULTURAL AWARENESS IN FAMILY WORK

When one thinks of 'cultural awareness' one tends to think in terms of 'ethnic minorities'. Family workers (FWs) should be aware that every family has its own unique culture, class and history. Sensitivity to this fact is essential. It will only emerge through interactions that allow families to express *their* view of themselves. There will be cases when the class and cultural differences between the family and FWs are extremely obvious. In such situations, FWs should openly address the issues and invite the family to place the information gleaned into its own unique context. In the author's experience working with different cultures has been a rewarding and enlightening learning experience. However, to enhance this process, FWs should seek advice and information on such issues such as cultural etiquette from those of a similar background (Kuipers *et al*., 1992).

BEGINNING THE PROCESS

To provide education about schizophrenia appears to help engage relatives and clients in the treatment process. In addition, it is recognized to be a positive way of improving optimism and reducing relatives' criticisms of clients, as many of the myths and misunderstandings about schizophrenia are caused by lack of knowledge (Leff and Vaughn, 1985). Examine the examples of critical and hostile statements given earlier. From these it is noticeable that the majority concern people's lack of motivation and inability to concentrate. These are recognized by mental health professionals as negative (rather than positive) symptoms of schizophrenia but most relatives are usually unaware that they have anything to do with the diagnosis (Box 31.5).

Therefore, education sessions can provide the first step in reducing criticisms and EE, because the formalized approach increases relatives' and clients' understanding of schizophrenia and provides them with the opportunity to recognize these difficult or bizarre behaviours as part of the condition (Berkowitz *et al*., 1984). Indeed, Ewles and Simnet (1992) argue that knowledge is power and without it people are unable to change their behaviour or make informed health choices. Empowerment of the client is now stipulated in present Government policy via the Patient's Charter (Department of Health, 1991). Health education is seen to be an integral part of that process, because it can enhance people's motivation and compliance and enables them to have more control over their health and the factors that affect it (Close, 1988). Therefore, provision of education is important, as clients and relatives have a right to know about the illness, and the process enhances insight and allows individuals to make independent, informed health choices (Catford and Nutbeam, 1984).

Achieving empowerment seems simple, initially. However, it should be seen as a continuing process involving the nurse, client and their family. Gibson (1991) states that for empowerment to operate, nurses need to respect individuals as people who have a capacity for growth, and cultivate an equal, respectful relationship, so that the client and their family feel trusted and accepted and part of the health care team.

ASSESSING FAMILIES' AND CLIENTS' KNOWLEDGE AND UNDERSTANDING

Barrowclough and Tarrier (1992) advocate that to gain relatives' cooperation and maximize the benefits of the education process, it is important to understand how lay people make sense of mental ill health; symptoms are often seen as changes in behaviour rather than physical signs of pathology. These subjective opinions, therefore, have to be acknowledged before giving information, because relatives may assimilate knowledge differently from mental health professionals and interpret it based on their own experiences and subjective opinions on the occurrence of the illness. That is, relatives can be told that hallucinations and delusions are symptoms of schizophrenia but they may find casual reasons for their appearance (Tarrier and Barrowclough, 1986). For example:

> He's always been shy, he never really made friends as a child, so he made up imaginary ones and talked to them. He

Box 31.5 *Symptoms of schizophrenia*

Positive symptoms
Auditory or visual hallucinations or both.
Delusions.
Thought disorder.

Negative symptoms
Loss of motivation, volition, will power, concentration and drive, leading to isolation and withdrawal.

has less and less to do with anyone now — including us; he's shut himself in his bedroom and doesn't really come out. It's understandable that he is like this, because he was bullied at school, so we don't pressurize him. My wife leaves food at his door, as neither of us like to disturb him.

Therefore, the education process should be preceded by assessing relatives' understanding of the illness. The Knowledge about Schizophrenia Interview (KASI, see Box 31.6) is conducted informally, rather then as a test and it aims to examine relatives' knowledge, beliefs and attitudes about six areas of schizophrenia (Barrowclough *et al.*, 1987).

The following Case study (page 503) has not included KASI scoring criteria. If a detailed knowledge of this is required, readers should refer to Barrowclough and Tarrier (1992). Nevertheless, from this assessment it is possible to conclude that Rachel is very supportive of Sam and has a relatively good understanding of schizophrenia. However, although she realized that she had not caused the illness, she was concerned that her divorce had made Sam's problems worse but was not able to attribute this to the fact that schizophrenia can be exacerbated by stressful life events. Therefore, it could be deduced that she felt responsible for inducing Sam's symptoms. Rachel was also unclear about the effects of Sam's medication and whether it would make any difference to the course of the illness if he stopped taking it. This was surprising, as professionals had seen the link between Sam's decision to stop taking medication and his subsequent relapses but his mother had never made the connection. The information obtained from this KASI highlighted two main areas to focus on during the education sessions, i.e. to educate Rachel about the purpose and effects of medication and to increase her understanding and awareness of what could exacerbate Sam's symptoms.

COMMENCING EDUCATION SESSIONS

When starting education sessions it is important to acknowledge and respect the family's subjective opinions on the occurrence of the illness, because this may influence the way they assimilate new information. Hence, it is important to work with these views, as well as providing new information about the illness and how to manage it.

There are no particular rules about how the sessions should be conducted. Indeed, they may be facilitated on an individual basis or as part of a group education programme. In a busy, under-resourced clinical setting, the latter may be a more viable and cheaper option, as more relatives and carers can be involved at any one time. Atkinson and Coia (1995) outline a 10-week educational programme; the sessions cover areas ranging from 'what schizophrenia means to you', 'identifying relatives' problems' and 'creating a low stress environment' to 'using services and dealing with crisis'. These sessions provide essential information, support and mutual aid. However, although the evidence suggests that clients and families want such information–and practical help–it must be recognized that they are often dissatisfied with the way it is presented, and when it is provided they often have difficulty remembering

Box 31.6 *Knowledge about Schizophrenia Interview (KASI)*

- Diagnosis
- Symptomatology
- Aetiology
- Medication
- Prognosis
- Management

adapted from Barrowclough et al., 1987

or understanding what they receive (Ley, 1988). To overcome these problems, Ewles and Simnett (1992) point out that it is important to know how to conduct such sessions. They advocate that facilitators should avoid using medical jargon. To reinforce what is said, education packages, handouts and leaflets written in plain, simple language are also useful.

To engender a collaborative, mutual learning experience, nurses should always plan education sessions carefully and facilitate them in an open, friendly manner. In addition, they should pay particular attention to what may hinder or help the learning process. Some family members may feel awkward about saying things in front of each other, as there may be some questions, such as 'Will she ever get better?' or 'will he ever be able to stop behaving like this?', that they feel frightened of asking with their relatives present. Likewise, some clients may find it too stressful to participate, as they have difficulty concentrating or sitting for long periods. Indeed, the whole engagement process could be affected, if they are distrustful and do not want to disclose their psychotic experiences to their family or they are initially unable to express themselves coherently in front of their relatives. In such cases, it is advisable to conduct the sessions separately, procure the client's consent to participate, then work towards bringing everyone together at a later date. This is highly recommended, because no one knows more about the illness than clients themselves and they rarely get the opportunity to share this knowledge or talk about the experience with their families. Nurses also learn from families about the realities of living with schizophrenia, making it a rewarding two-way exchange of information and knowledge. One particular comment (made by a family member) highlights this point:

> It was a good idea, us all meeting in the comfort of our own home to discuss my sister's illness. We were all able to say how it felt and for the first time I realized that I knew very little about what she was suffering from or how much — the word schizophrenia meant nothing to me before, but its much clearer now. I used to think she was just being lazy until she told me in the meeting what it was really like.

A MODEL FOR EDUCATING CLIENTS AND FAMILIES

- Assess the clients' and families' beliefs and knowledge about the illness and its treatment (perhaps using KASI).
- Plan an education strategy to meet the client's and family's needs for information or skills. Get the client to talk about what it is like to have schizophrenia — they are the expert.
- Acknowledge and reinforce areas of strength.
- Have good, simple, jargon-free literature available, e.g. National Schizophrenia Fellowship's *Notes for relatives and friends* by Leff and colleagues (1996), MIND's publications by Birchwood and colleagues(1985) and SANE publications.
- Go through the education packages together in a structured manner but do not overload; break frequently for questions to clarify what has been covered.
- Draw parallels between medication regimes in schizophrenia and diabetes — as this can be useful in helping the client and family understand their use in health maintenance and lifestyle change (Torrey, 1983).
- Do not assume that everyone will assimilate the information at the same rate — it takes time to change, therefore the education process should be ongoing.
- Get feedback to ensure everyone has understood.
- If you have left an education leaflet with the family to read between sessions — take more copies to your next one. They get lost!

Overall, the education process gives you the opportunity to engage families, prepare the ground for change, assess problem areas and explain how the subsequent family management sessions and are going to run, that is, give information on their time span, duration, structure and those who would be willing to attend.

INTERVENTIONS USED

In addition to providing education about schizophrenia there are a number of other interventions used in family work (see Box 31.3) which can be clinically applied. These are now described.

PROBLEM-SOLVING

As stated previously, most of the criticisms that families express about clients often reflect unrealistic expectations and goals (Cozolino *et al.*, 1988). One of the main aims of the family intervention is to modify these expectations and thereby reduce the family's distress and dissatisfaction. Overly ambitious or intensive interventions are known to increase the risk of exacerbating positive symptoms, but if the goals are too low the client's progress is slow and negative symptoms may be seen. Therefore, it is important to get the balance right and devise interventions that are tailor-made for clients and their families, so that they are more able to cope with the effects and consequences of schizophrenia. A structured method of problem-solving aids this progression (Box 31.7) and is a collaborative, therapeutic

process, which involves respecting and listening to all the view-points expressed and having a clear idea of how to negotiate, set an agenda, prioritize, agree on goals and plan homework tasks with families (Kuipers *et al.*, 1992).

Effective problem-solving relies heavily upon family members objectively communicating their thoughts and feelings to each other. Indeed, it is recognized that expression of negative emotions decreases in direct communication, e.g. it is much more difficult to say directly to someone, 'Joe, you behave so badly', than to say 'He behaves badly'. To aid this process, Kuipers *et al.* (1992) advocate establishing a number of 'ground rules', as they recognize that it is impossible to address families' issues or sort out problems, if everyone disregards what is said or talks over each other. These rules apply to everyone present including those who are facilitating the session, and are summarized as:

1. Talk *to* the person, not *about* them, and encourage the use of names, rather then using he or she.
2. Speaking time should be shared out equally, so that each person's view can be heard, listened to and respected.
3. Only one person may speak at a time and interruptions are to be avoided.

Once these rules have been established, it is possible to address the family issues, identify the family's needs and begin problem-solving.

Box 31.7

Problem-solving with families

- Provides a framework that helps them to define their problems more clearly, as most of the problems faced by families are ill defined.

- By generating ideas on possible alternative solutions to problems, it encourages family members to participate, understand and communicate.

- Helps to develop alternative positive behaviours, exert situational control and apply alternative consequences.

- Helps individual family members manage their own behaviour.

- By initially tackling simple, non emotive problems, clients' information processing abilities are not overwhelmed, which helps to increase their confidence.

- Helps family members focus objectively upon the problem identified, which helps to reduce conflict when tackling more difficult family issues.

- Helps families and clients to practise overcoming the problem outside of the family sessions.

(adapted from Bellack et al., 1989)

The first step is to ascertain from each family member and the client, what they think the main issues are. This gives them the opportunity to say how things have been in the past, and allows them to talk about their current experiences. This process is enhanced if open questions such as, 'Can you tell us about the things that have recently been a problem for you?' are used. This may take time, because families may have a multitude of problems and concerns that they may never have been asked to disclose before. Therefore, the family should be encouraged to elaborate on them, so that a clear picture is gained from the out-set. Invariably, the problems and concerns they wish to be sorted out will be overwhelming. At this stage, (FWs) may be put under a considerable strain, especially if it is their first encounter with the emotional turmoil that characterizes some family interactions. However, they should avoid being critical, retain their objectivity, lower individual expectations and recall that not all the problems will be solved immediately (Leff and Gamble, 1995). Once this has been established, it is possible to identify the family's strengths and resources, give them positive feedback, identify possible alternatives to the issues raised and negotiate a coherent plan for change.

The problems and burdens that families experience can be awesome and extremely difficult to manage. As suggested by Box 31.7, they can also be ill defined, which is why some families find it very difficult to generate their own solutions to them. Therefore, FWs can play a central role in helping to redefine them. They can also help to break them down, so that they become more realistic and achievable (Box 31.8).

Box 31.8 *The problem-solving approach*

Coherent plan for change

Set appropriate, flexible homework tasks that are:
- practical
- measurable
- achievable
- realistic.

Case study: **Problem-solving**

The Jones family have engaged in family work for 6 weeks. The family consists of mother and father, Paul (the client) and his sister Jan. All live in the same house.

The following is the record made after the fourth session. The family workers (FWs) are beginning to explore the family's concept of current problems.

Paul stated that he would 'like to return to work one day' when each family member was asked to take turns in identifying main areas of need. Other members brought up the following statements about Paul: 'Lying in bed till late' 'Not taking an interest in his future' and 'We can't keep paying for his cigarettes and everything' statements. When discussing these statements one of the FW's commented: 'A person needs many skills to work and hold down a job. Firstly, can I ask you Paul, do you get up in the morning at regular times?'

Father and Jan laughed, with Jan commenting, 'Ask him if he can get up at all!'

FWs referred the family to the discussion on negative symptoms given in the education sessions: 'The fact is that many schizophrenia sufferers need support with problems like getting up, remembering to look after their hygiene etc.' to which Paul replied 'It's useless then'.

FW: 'Well, shall we work on that difficulty for a few weeks to see if we can make some change?' The family asked how this could be done.

F W then explored exactly what the family's morning routine was by everyone taking turns to say what each person did. Father and Jan explained that they worked and were out of the house roughly an hour after getting up. Mother stated 'I make everyone breakfast during the working week. I make theirs at 9.30 and wait until Paul gets up, normally at 12.30 or whenever, and then make his. He wouldn't eat otherwise. Then I do the dishes and go shopping. It's inconvenient as I like to go and see my friend if I have time, but if Paul gets up too late I don't get there'.

The mother's statement was focused on as a benefit to another family member if Paul was up earlier. One of the family workers stated that, 'Paul would be helping you if he got up earlier' to which his mother agreed.

When asked if there would be benefits for others, Jan said, ' Well, at least I would get to see him! Sometimes I go to college straight after work and may not see him for two days'.

A discussion followed as to a task definition for Paul and family to be clear on what was being asked.

AGREED TASK
- Paul to get up by 10 a.m. at least four times in 10 days.
- Paul and father to buy alarm clock on Saturday. (Paul requests a radio alarm; his father agrees to contribute £3 towards it. Task to commence the following Monday.)
- If Paul gets up by 10 a.m: Jan to reinforce Paul, by saying 'It's nice to see you' and Paul to have cooked breakfast with family.
- If Paul is not able to get up by 10 a.m: Family to leave Paul; Paul's mum to leave corn flakes for him, if he is not up by 12 noon.

Paul worried he would forget. A written memory aid with the above information was left on the fridge door. Workers ended the session with each member of the family agreeing to do their defined task. The family were reminded that the beginning of the next session would begin with an analysis of how the task went. 'At this stage it is important to remember we are just seeing what happens if we all agree to do something. Think of it as an experiment. Don't worry if things don't go to plan. Next time we meet, we can discuss how it went'.

The problem solving case study shows :

- How Paul's comment 'I'd like to return to work' was valued, yet realistically reframed and accepted as important.
- That the 'ground rules' were established, as individuals can be seen to be taking turns and contributing.
- That education and problem-solving strategies can be effectively combined, for example in the explanation of negative symptoms in this specific problem.
- That changes in Paul's behaviour have positive consequences for other family members: Mum gets the opportunity to see her friend regularly and Jan gets to see more of her brother.
- Jan's comment about seeing Paul in the morning was later reintroduced when the family and FWs negotiated for her to become the positive reinforcer of the homework task. (In this family, mother is usually left with the sole responsibility for the household routine).
- That all family members worked in partnership and now have a clear definition of their own roles in supporting Paul with this task.
- Clear strategies were also identified should Paul find the task too difficult. In many ways for the family to give the responsibility to Paul and not pressurize him to succeed is just as valid (and difficult) as him achieving the outlined task. Hence the workers comment at the conclusion of the session.

Evaluation of outlined problem-solving strategy

With the first problem area and homework task identified, the family and workers have a focus to build upon. Feedback will provide a clear picture of the client's and family's presenting problems and needs. It will also highlight present strengths and weaknesses with regard to problem-solving. The data obtained in feedback give crucial information as to the future direction of the FWs interventions. Let us look at the FWs considerations of possible alternative results.

Non-completion of task: Paul did not get up by 10 a.m. on any occasion

From this it is possible to deduce that this task was too hard for Paul and family. It therefore should be re-analysed by asking each family member to say what actually happened. This gives the FWs the opportunity to see if anything positive had occurred and learn more about what the family feel they can and cannot cope with at the moment. In addition, important clarifying issues can be addressed such as Paul's medication levels, his overall sleep pattern, whether the family were able to leave Paul and if any change was noticed in the family's usual routine.

FWs should take responsibility for the task being too hard and praise the family for giving it their best effort. The re-analysis should lead to a more realistic goal. For example, Paul going to bed earlier, negotiating a reduction in medication, identifying further incentives for him to get up or the need for minimal prompting.

Intermediate completion: Paul got up at 10 a.m. twice

This gives the family and FWs the opportunity to give direct positive feedback. It is important that the workers praise the family for their efforts as well as Paul. The family members should also be praised if they were able to leave Paul on the occasions he did not get up, as this was part of the plan. By asking each individual, it is possible to identify how the family felt when Paul did get up and to ascertain what positive reinforcements were given and noted by Paul. This also gives the FWs the opportunity to reinforce the concept of experimentation and gives them a clear baseline to work from. They can then question everyone as to their willingness to continue with the task. The workers could then see whether there were other factors that contributed to the successes and look at incorporating them in the revised homework task.

Total completion: Paul has achieved the task

Everyone is praised! Humour can be used ('Well that was too easy!', ' I thought you said this was a problem!') but, more seriously, an evaluation of the experience is necessary. The outlined intervention is recognized to be an ongoing learning process, therefore each person is asked to evaluate the experience. The family members need to be reminded that they should continue to exercise the skills they have learnt, so that they become integral to their everyday routine. Benefits and gains are then highlighted, and future goals are explored and identified.

In your own clinical work, identify a client who is having difficulty getting up and negotiate a similar experiment. You need to identify a clear goal, reinforcers and realistic time span. On completion think about how you would reframe your client's efforts in the three feedback scenarios outlined above.

APPLYING A COGNITIVE–BEHAVIOURAL APPROACH

Clients who hear voices or experience strange delusions often have problems making sense of the world and their role within it. Indeed, the situation can be equally as baffling to their families, as they sometimes have great difficulty coping with, and understanding, their relatives' behaviour. This can lead to isolation and misunderstandings. However, with support and training families can not only learn how to interact with their sick relatives but also how to manage and monitor their mental condition. This helps increase everyone's rapport and sense of value. Once a collaborative working partnership has been established, it is possible to achieve this by combining the previous outlined interventions with a cognitive–behavioural approach. Fowler *et al.* (1995) describe a six-stage approach (Box 31.9).

The following Case study shows the family workers working through the first three stages of the outlined cognitive–behavioural approach (see also Box 31.9). They have started to discover how Toby and his family cope with his distressing psychotic experiences and have offered them

Box
31.9

Stages of a cognitive–behavioural approach

1. Developing a collaborative therapeutic relationship. Assessing current problems and obtaining client's and family's perspective.

2. Providing advice and training about cognitive strategies that clients and families can use to cope with distressing psychotic experiences, severe emotional reactions or impulsive actions.

3. Offering a new perspective about the nature of client's experiences and general life predicament.

4. Focusing on specific delusional beliefs and voices. Working with the client's belief system to moderate distress and promote more adaptive response mechanisms. Enlisting family support and understanding.

5. Targeting dysfunctional assumptions about self and others, reducing feelings of worthlessness and raising self-esteem.

6. Consolidation of new perspective, highlighting specific implications for self-regulation of psychotic experiences and developing individualized plans to manage episodes of relapse in the medium- and long-term future.

(adapted from Fowler et al., 1995)

a new perspective about the nature of Toby's experiences and general life predicament (Fowler *et al.*1995). By working through these stages, it is noticeable that the family have already started to piece together how Toby's behaviour changed prior to him relapsing.

These behaviours can be bewildering and frightening. As Toby's sister's reaction shows, they can also become a causal reality, that is, 'When he gets like this he ends up in hospital'. The FWs should be showing, by their ability to frame these events and suggest alternatives, that the consequence of returning to hospital is not a foregone conclusion. Nevertheless, families will only accept this when they experience a similar episode without an admission.

If this meeting is again considered as a data-gathering exercise, then there are a number of cognitive–behavioural assessment strategies that FWs can incorporate. Falloon and Graham–Hole (1994) advocate that families should be encouraged to continue this analysis until such time that they can identify specific early warning signs of relapse and plan accordingly. This procedure is important as it helps the family (and indeed professionals) to intervene at an earlier stage in the relapse process.

Further exploration can also highlight other behaviours that run in parallel to the ones already identified, as common early warning signs usually include functional aspects such as sleep disturbance and an inability to complete simple tasks such as maintaining hygiene, attending day activities or simple budgeting. Furthermore, families often describe intuitive signs, such as a member saying 'I know he is ill when he starts to look vacant, walks or sit funny.' Nevertheless, the exact meaning of these intuitions would need to be clarified, as often behaviours that are not indicators of relapse can be intermingled with true relapse signs; for example, when a mother says, 'He shouts at me when I go into his room without knocking, when he is ill,' It may well be an expression of a natural wish to maintain privacy rather than a sign of relapse.

Toby's family in the Case study were able to examine the sequence of events that led to relapse. However, some families may need more support with this framing. A useful tool to aid this discussion and understanding is to encourage the client to complete a diary, in which they can highlight and record specific stressful events and their responses to them. Alternatively, the FWs could incorporate the Early Warning Signs Interview described by Birchwood *et al.* (1995).

The family's recordings of these early warning signs should always be respected by those who are involved in the client's care. Families often describe frustration when their observations of early stages of relapse are dismissed by professionals as not crucial enough to warrant attention. To overcome such problems, FWs could enhance communication (Table 31.4) and encourage earlier interventions by circulating (Early Warning Signs card) (Figure 31.1) to the members of the multi-disciplinary team.

This would help to acknowledge families as the main care givers and reinforce their expertise. The benefits gained when professionals respond appropriately to these requests cannot be overemphasized, as family empowerment is being shown by action rather than rhetoric. Accurate knowledge of early warning signs also gives the family a clear framework within which to find a voice for their concerns.

Lastly, it is important to build upon these observations, and go on to follow stages 4, 5 and 6 as listed in Box 31.9. In doing so, it will be possible to teach clients how to monitor and gain some control over their symptoms. Indeed, the use of the diary, as quoted above, is a good example of how individual coping strategies can be developed and enhanced. Once this has been accomplished psychological interventions such as thought stopping, focusing versus distraction or belief modification can be incorporated. This will enable clients to gain valuable insight into how to live and cope with their voices more effectively (Romme and Esher, 1993).

DEALING WITH EMOTIONAL INCIDENTS

One of the most difficult aspects of family work is to deal with the emotions generated and experienced in actual family meetings. Many nurses' reluctance to discuss issues with families stems from an awareness that these emotions will be present. The strategies already outlined should give some indications as to how FWs can deal with the traumatic life events caused by severe mental health problems and not become overwhelmed by the emotions generated. The setting of ground rules is important in maintaining boundaries that allow communication to proceed.

Go back and remind yourself of the ground rules. Set up a short role-play between three people who do not obey these rules. Run this for a short period of time. Return to the role-play obeying the ground rules. Ask each person how their feelings changed. If this is not possible, imagine a situation in your own life where someone did not observe these rules. How did it make you feel?

By completing this simple exercise you become aware of how powerful the implementation of these ground rules can be in family meetings. It should be remembered that families can get into patterns of communication that they feel uncomfortable with, but do not know how to change. The setting of ground rules and a firm request that they be respected is also a simple way to begin defusing emotions.

Another aspect contributing to the defusing of emotions is reframing comments positively. Families often can see no positive aspects to their own interactions with clients and therefore expect to be criticized. By lending an empathetic ear to their experiences and highlighting any strengths within the system, FWs can get underneath negative emotion and point out that there is a positive reason for the intensity of the feeling (Kuipers *et al.* 1992). Indeed, it should be acknowledged that the expression of anger is often a cover for fear and sadness. The reality of loss, stigma, grief and isolation felt by families and clients should never be underestimated. For example, a wife who shouted, 'Sometimes I just think a divorce would be the answer to all my problems' was able to reframe this later to, 'The illness makes me feel like I've lost my husband'. The husband was able to respond positively to the second statement, unlike the first where he burst into tears.

Case study: **A cognitive–behavioural approach**

Toby developed schizophrenia during his late teens while he was studying A levels. The illness was characterized by paranoid delusions with persecutory feelings and auditory hallucinations of a derogatory nature. He is an intelligent young man, usually cheerful but during a meeting with his family it was reported that he had recently become verbally aggressive. With support from the family workers Toby was able to tell his parents about these experiences and how he regretted behaving aggressively but did not know any other way of dealing with the derogatory voices when they shouted at him. Toby's mother told him that she wished he could stop shouting, as it was really disturbing to hear him and it was frightening everyone in the house and disturbing them at night.

The FWs recognized that this was a potentially volatile and stressful situation and intervened to ask each family member how they coped with these distressing experiences. Toby's father reported that he left him to it and if it was too disturbing at night he would go downstairs and sleep in the living room. Carol, Toby's sister, said that she was frightened but went on to say that she thought he was getting ill again.

FW: 'Tell us why you think that?'

Carol: 'Well, last time Toby started shouting like this he ended up back in hospital'.

To try to find out whether Toby and his family recognized any other symptoms of relapse, the FWs used this piece of information and asked all the family to return to the time before Toby was readmitted. 'Did you, or anybody else Toby, notice any other changes in your behaviour at that time?'

Toby: 'No, not really, I just remember feeling terrible and I couldn't talk to anyone. The voices were getting on my nerves, they started to say more and more horrible things about me'.

Carol: 'I remember, you shut yourself in your bedroom for hours and stopped coming down to eat with us — just like you're doing now'.

Mum: 'Yes, but before that, I remember, you were invited to that wedding in Scotland; you got into a panic and you talked incessantly about it; you were really paranoid about what people would think of you'.

Dad: 'Yes, that's right Toby, we all thought it would be too much for you, what with the travelling and everything — so you didn't go in the end did you?'.

FW: 'To help us understand more about the symptoms that led up to your readmission to hospital, let's try to summarize the sequence of events. Firstly, you were invited to a wedding, which worried you, as you thought you wouldn't get on with the people there. Is this when the voices started to say horrible things to you, Toby?'

Toby: 'Mm, yes I suppose it was'.

FW: 'So, when the voices got more derogatory you decided to stay in your room, then you started shouting at them?'

Mum: 'Yes, that's nearly right, but he doesn't just stay in his room and shout now; Toby you do it everywhere, at any time of the day or night'.

Carol: 'He's staying in his room, and shouting again. Oh no, Toby, that means you're going to end up in hospital again!'

Toby: 'But I don't know any other way of handling this!'

FW: 'Well, it does seem as through you have already found a number of ways in which to cope. Firstly, it seems that you are affected by stressful events, like the wedding, which you were right not to attend, as it would have been too difficult for you at the time. Secondly you have learnt that it is useful to retreat to your room when the voices get too much for you. Perhaps we could now find some additional ways to help you learn about what triggers these symptoms, so that you can manage them more effectively, then perhaps you won't have to go back into hospital in the future'.

TABLE 31.4 Early Warning Signs interview

Stage 1
Establish date of onset or admission to hospital and behaviour at the height of the episode.
What kind of things was the relative doing or saying? When was it decided to get help?

Stage 2
Establish the date and time of change. When was a change first noticed in him or her?

Stage 3
Establish the sequence of changes up to relapse. What happened? When? How? Find examples.

Stage 4
Find out anything not previously elicited, e.g. Was the relative unduly anxious, aggressive, excitable, drinking, taking unprescribed drugs; did the relative seem suspicious or say or do strange things?

Stage 5
Summarize this information and collaborate on what all have learnt about the client's condition. Utilize this and formally record it with the family, for the future use of both therapist and family.

(adapted from Birchwood et al., 1995)

Name ....
I have a risk of developing episodes of schizophrenia **My early warning signs are:**
1
2
3
If I experience any of these signs I/we will respond by:
1
2
3
My doctor is: .... **phone:** .... **My relative/carer is:** .... **phone:** ....
If I/we have any concerns about my disorder I will
Contact .... **immediately**

Figure 31.1 Example of an early warning signs card

Barrowclough and Tarrier (1992) acknowledge that one of the most difficult problems families have to face is a relative becoming either verbally or physically aggressive. FWs need to consider how to manage these situations, by being able to, families have direct access to interventions modelled by the workers, which they can then emulate. One comment a mother made highlights this, 'I watched his nurse talking to him. He was very angry but she was gentle and patient and got through to him in a way I never could. He really listened to her'. Using a here-and-now focus, FWs can also explain their actions, so that their skills are translated and not perceived as being something 'only professionals can do'.

Emotional tension is a common feature in family meetings. Violence is not. However, in extreme circumstances, it is essential for the FW to use professional judgement. The following is a tool to help frame thinking and interventions:

- Take control but not responsibility. Say to the family, 'We need to work together to keep this safe; I would like everybody to sit down and remember the ground rules'.
- Verbalize concerns calmly and openly. Say, 'I am worried that someone may get hurt', etc.
- Disengage from proceedings and use time out if necessary.
- Plan a course of action with responsive family members.
- Ensure the situation is as safe as possible before leaving.

To sum up, the main priority is the saftey of the FW and the family. Even in extreme circumstances the above should give you the space and time to plan. However, if this is not effective then you should not tackle something that is outside your sphere of competence. The multidisciplinary team members should be informed and the police should be involved if necessary.

CLINICAL SUPERVISION

As indicated, family work can sometimes be very frustrating and stressful, as some families' experiences and interactions can be overpowering. When working with these particular mental health users, it is essential that nurses avoid being critical of them, because staff criticism and hostility has been shown to increase the risk of relapse (Moore *et al.*, 1992). Therefore it is important that nurses study use of a low EE approach with their clients and families (see Table 31.1). To help foster these attributes it is essential that nurses receive ongoing clinical supervision. It is envisaged that if nurses can air their frustrations, in the supportive, sympathetic environment of supervision, then it is less likely that these feelings will emerge in family sessions (Leff and Gamble, 1995).

Family work supervision in its traditional format has, in the past, been put into operation using group experiential role-play (Gamble, 1993). Its aim is to help individuals gain valuable insight into the needs of their clients and families, deal with their feelings towards their encounters with them, review the progress of individual sessions and engage in therapeutic interventions. This method of supervision enables nurses to

Case study: Use of KASI

Sam is a 35-year-old single man, who was diagnosed with schizophrenia 8 years ago. He lives with his mother and younger sister in a council flat. Sam reached all the normal milestones during his childhood and at school and had no significant problems during his adolescence. He left school, aged 16 and worked in a local supermarket for 7 years until it closed in 1983.

Sam's first schizophrenia episode was in 1987. He had become increasingly withdrawn over the previous 6 months and had developed concerns about his physical health. He believed that he had a distasteful body image, which he thought people laughed and talked about when he was in the street. Over a 6-month period Sam stopped going out and continually did physical exercise to improve his physical image. Sam was admitted to the local psychiatric hospital for a period of 4 weeks and was treated on neuroleptic medication. Subsequently, Sam had two serious breakdowns, both of which have occurred after he decided to stop medication.

Rachel, Sam's mother, is 68 and divorced. She has two sons and a daughter. Joe, 41, is married and lives in Wales. Sam, 35, and Sophie, 26, both live at home. Rachel is physically well and there is no family history of psychiatric illness. Prior to commencing family work, Rachel readily agreed to complete the KASI. Although Sophie was interested in participating in the family sessions, she did not have time to complete the KASI and Sam said that he already knew enough about the illness and did not want to participate in another assessment.

Diagnosis
When asked about what the doctors and nurses had told her was wrong with Sam, Rachel knew that it was schizophrenia and was able to say that it was a serious mental disorder that affected all aspects of Sam's life.

Symptomatology
Rachel attributed the symptoms of schizophrenia to an illness and she described how Sam thought people talked about his body. She thought this was what a doctor had once described as a delusion because she could not see what Sam thought was wrong with his body. She believed that Sam was unable to control these feelings and reported the commonest and most significant symptoms of schizophrenia.

Aetiology
When asked about what she thought the cause of Sam's illness was, Rachel said that it had something to do with the way the brain worked but she went on to say that around the time of her divorce things had been very difficult for Sam and she thought this may have caused him to become ill.

Medication
Rachel had a very good knowledge of Sam's medication and was able to name the injection he received, where he obtained it from and how long it lasted for but she was not aware of its side-effects or what to do if they occurred.

Course and prognosis
Rachel did not know whether Sam would have problems again and when asked about whether stressful life problems could make schizophrenia worse, she did not know. Rachel was also vague about whether the medication made any difference to Sam's illness or when he might start to get to worse if he stopped taking it. Therefore, she said she did not know.

Management
Rachel thought there was a lot she could do to help Sam and thought that it was good that he attended the day centre. She also said that sometimes it was helpful to leave Sam to his own devices and not to shout at him.

assess their skills, reflect upon them and identify possible alternatives (Kolb, 1984). Once they have conceptualized an alternative course of action, the interventions can be incorporated into their clinical practice. This helps nurses foster clinical autonomy and retain their clinical competence (Kohner, 1995). Therefore, prior to working with this particular group of users, it is highly recommended that nurses seek out or arrange to recieve this type of supervision.

SUMMARY

Schizophrenia is a serious mental disorder that affects 1 in 100 people in Britain today. Its onset can occur during a formative stage of a person's life, that is, around late adolescence or early adulthood. The positive symptoms of schizophrenia can be extremely distressing, as a person's world can be taken over by strange delusional ideas and vivid hallucinatory experiences. These symptoms can affect the way that person communicates and feels and often results in a loss of motivation and the ability to concentrate. Schizophrenia, therefore can affect every aspect of a person's life and can destroy their own and their family's aspirations for the future. In recent years this devastation has become even more burdensome for clients and their families with the significant shift in treatment philosophy and psychiatric care away from the 19th Century tradition of containment in institutions to a belief in the concept of 'community care' (Ryan, *et al.*, 1991). This change in health care delivery has resulted in more clients with schizophrenia living in the community, which has inadvertently placed the main burden and responsibility of care upon unsupported parents, spouses and informal carers (Hatfield and Lefley, 1987). Families can be an extremely valuable and positive resource for clients and they deserve recognition, support, education and practical help. To promote this approach it is essential that MHNs have a strong appreciation of community management and family relationships and a positive attitude towards schizophrenia. Therefore, to be responsive to the needs of the society in which they live and work, MHNs need to improve their knowledge and competence and become assertive, supportive educationalists, who are able to assess families' needs, work in collaboration with them and use problem-solving techniques skilfully.

KEY CONCEPTS

- The concept of expressed emotion, family work, research and its relevance to clinical practice.
- Empowering relatives and clients through mental health education.
- Assessing families' needs and strengths.
- Collaborating with families to reduce stress and burden using problem solving and cognitive–behavioral approach.
- Working proactively in community settings.
- Supervision and training.

REFERENCES

Anderson CM, Hogarty G, Reiss D.J: Family treatment of adult schizophrenic patients: a psychoeducational approach. *Schizophr Bull* 6:490–505, 1980.

Atkinson JM, Coia, DA: *Families coping with schizophrenia: A practitioner's guide to family groups.* Chichester; 1995, Wiley and Sons Ltd.

Barrowclough C, Tarrier N: *Families of schizophrenic patients: cognitive behavioural intervention.* Chapman & Hall, 1992, London

Barrowclough C, Tarrier N, Watts S, Vaughn C, Bamrah JS, Freeman HL: Assessing the functional value of relatives reported knowledge about schizophrenia: A preliminary report. *Br J Psychiatry* 151; 1–8, 1987.

Bellack AS, Morrison RL, Mueser, KT: Social problem solving in schizophrenia. *Schizophr Bull* 15:101–16, 1989.

Bellack A, Mueser, K: Psychosocial treatment for schizophrenia. *Schizophr Bull* 19(2):17–36, 1993.

Berkowitz R, Eberlein-Fries R, Kuipers L, Leff, J: Educating relatives about schizophrenia. *Schizophr Bull* 10:418–429, 1984.

Birchwood M, Macmillian F, Smith J: *Early Intervention.* In: Birchwood M, Tarrier N: Pyschological management of schizophrenia. London, 1995, Willey.

Birchwood M, Smith J, Cochrane R: The social functioning scale: The development and validation of a new scale of social adjustment for use in family interventions programmes with schizophrenic patients. *Br J Psychiatry* 157:853–859, 1990.

Blackburn I, Davidson K: *Cognitive Therapy for depression and anxiety.* Oxford 1990, Blackwell Scientific.

Brooker C,: The health education needs of families caring for a schizophrenic relative and the potential role for community psychiatric nurses. J Adv Nurs 15:1092–1098, 1990.

Brooker C, Baguley I: Snap decisions. *Nurs Times.* 86(41):56–58, 1990.

Brown GW, Birley JLT, Wing J.K: Influence of family life on the course of schizophrenic disorders: A replication. *Br J Psychiatry* 121:241–63, 1972.

Catford J, Nutbeam D: Towards a definition of health education and health promotion. *Health Educ J* 43(2 & 3):38, 1984.

Close A: Patient education: A review of the Literature. *J Adv Nurs* 13:203–213, 1988.

Cozolino LJ, Goldstein MJ, Nuechterlein KH *et al :* The impact of education about schizophrenia on relatives varying in levels of expressed emotion. *Schizophr Bull* 14;675–685, 1988.

Department of Health: *Patient's Charter.* London, 1991, HMSO.

Department of Health: *Social services departments and the care programme approach: An inspection:* London, 1995, DOH.

Ewles L, Simnett I: *Promoting health — A practical guide,* 2 ed London, 1992, Scutari Press

Falloon IRH, Boyd JL, McGill CW *et al:* Family management in the prevention of exacerbation of schizophrenia. *New England J Med* 306:1437–1440, 1982.

Falloon IRH: *Handbook of behavioural family therapy.* New York, 1988, Guilford Press.

Falloon IRH, Boyd JL, McGill CW: Family management in the prevention of morbidity of schizophrenia: Clinical outcome of a two year longitudinal study. *Arch Gen Psychiatry* 42:887–986, 1985.

Falloon IRH, Graham–Hole V: *Comprehensive management of mental disorders.* Buckingham Mental Health Service, 1994.

Fischmann–Havstad L, Marston AR: Weight loss maintenance an aspect of family emotion and process. *Br J Clin Psychol* 23:265–271, 1984.

Fowler D, Garey P, Kuipers E: *Cognitive behaviour therapy for psychosis: Theory and practice.* Chichester, 1995, Wiley.

Gamble C: Working with schizophrenic clients and their families. *Br J Nurs* 2(17):856–859, 1993.

Gamble C, Midence K: The assessment of social functioning: conceptual and methodological difficulties. *Psychiatr Care* 2(2):52–54, 1995.

Gibson CH: A concept analysis of empowerment. *J Adv Nurs* 16:354–361, 1991.

Harding CM, Zahniser JH: Empirical correction of seven myths about schizophrenia with implications for treatment. *Acta Psychiatr Scand* 90(suppl 384):140–146, 1994.

Hatfield AB, Lefley HP: *Families of the mentally ill: Coping and adaptation.*

Cassell, 1987, Guilford Press.

Hirsch SR, Leff J: *Abnormalities in parents of schizophrenics.* London, 1975, Oxford University Press.

Hogarty GE, Anderson C, Reiss DJ: Family education, social skills training, and maintenance chemotherapy in the care treatment of schizophrenia: I. One year effects of a controlled study on relapse and expressed emotion. *Arch Gen Psychiatry* 43:633–642, 1986.

Hogarty GE, Anderson C, Reiss DJ: Family psychoeducation, social skills training, and maintenance chemotherapy in the aftercare of schizophrenia. *Arch Gen Psychiatry* 7:340–347, 1991.

Johnstone L: Family management in schizophrenia: its assumptions and contradictions. *J Men Health* 2:255–269, 1993.

Kohner N: *Clinical supervision in practice. Nursing Development Units.* London, 1995, Kings Fund Centre.

Kolb D: *Experiential learning: Experience as the source of learning and development.* Prentice Hall, 1984, New Jersey.

Kottgen C, Sonnichsen I, Mollenhauserm K, Jurth R: Group therapy with families of schizophrenia patients: Results of the Hamburg Camberwell Family Interview Study, 111. *Int J Fam Psychiatry* 5:85–94, 1984.

Kuipers L: Expressed emotion in 1991. Social psychiatry and psychiatric epidemiology 27:1–3, 1992.

Kuipers L, Leff J, Lam D: *Family work for schizophrenia: A practical guide.* Gaskell, 1992, Royal College of Psychiatrists London.

Krawiecka M, Goldberg DP, Vaughan M: A standardised psychiatric assessment scale for rating chronic psychotic patients. *Acta Psychiatri Scand* 55:299–308, 1977.

Laing RD: *The politics of experience.* Harmondsworth, 1970, Penguin Books.

Lam D: Psychosocial family intervention in schizophrenia: A review of empirical studies. *Psychol Med* 21:423–441, 1991.

Leff J, Berkowitz R, Shavit N *et al*:A trial of family therapy versus a relatives group for schizophrenia. *Br J Psychiatry.* 154:58–66, 1989.

Leff J, Gamble C: Training of community psychiatric nurses in family work for schizophrenia. *Int J Men Health* 24(3):76–88, 1995.

Leff J, Kuipers L, Berkowitz R, Eberlein–Fries R, Sturgeon, D: A controlled trial of social intervention in the families of schizophrenia patients. *Br J Psychiatry* 141:121–134, 1982.

Leff J, Vaughn C: *Expressed emotion in families.* Guilford Press, 1985, New York.

Leff J, Wig NN, Ghosh A,: Expressed emotion and schizophrenia in North India III: Influence of relatives expressed emotion on the course of schizophrenia in Chandigarh. *Br J Psychiatry* 151:166–173, 1987.

Leff J, Berkowitz R, Eberlein-Fries R, Kuipers L: *Schizophrenia: notes for relatives and friends.* Alderley Park, 1996, National Schizophrenia Fellowship.

Ley P: *Communicating with patients — improving communication, satisfaction and compliance.* London, 1988, Croom Helm.

Lidz T, Fleck S, Cornelison AR: *Schizophrenia and the family.* New York, 1965 International Universities Press.

Miklowitz DJ, Goldstein MJ, Nuechterlein KH, Synder KS, Mintz J: Family factors and the course of bipolar affective disorder. *Arch Gen Psychiatry* 45:225–231, 1988.

Morrison RL, Bellack AS: Social functioning of schizophrenic patients: clinical and research issues. *Schizophr Bull* 13:(4)715–725, 1987.

Moore E, Ball RA, Kuipers L: Expressed emotion in staff working with the long term mentally ill. *Br J Psychiatry* 161:802–808, 1992.

Onyett S: *Case management in mental health.* Chapman & Hall, 1992, London.

Ryan P, Clifford P, Ford R: *Case management and the UK policy context. Case management and community care:* Sainsbury Centre for Mental Health, 1991, London.

Romme M, Esher S: *Accepting voices.* London, 1991, Mind Publications.

Smith J, Birchwood M: Education for families with schizophrenic relatives. *Br J Psychiatry* 156:654–652, 1987.

Szmukler GI, Berkowitz R, Eisler I, Leff J, Dare C: Expressed emotion in individual and family settings: a comparative study. *Br J Psychiatry* 151:174–178, 1993.

Tarrier N, Barrowclough C: Providing information to relatives about schizophrenia: some comments. *Br J Psychiatry* 149:458–463, 1986.

Tarrier N, Barrowclough C, Porceddu K: The community management of schizo-phrenia: a controlled trail of behavioural intervention with families to reduce relapse. *Br J Psychiatry* 153:532–542, 1988.

Torrey E: Management of chronic schizophrenic outpatients. *Psychiat Clin North Am* 9:143–151, 1983.

Vaughn C, Leff J: The influence of family and social factors on the course of psy-chiatric illness: A comparison of schizophrenic and depressed neurotic patients. *Br J Psychiatry* 129:125–137, 1976.

Vaughn CE, Snyder KS, Jones S, Freeman WB, Falloon IRH: Family factors in schizophrenic relapse: a California replication of the British research on expressed emotion. *Arch Gen Psychiatry* 41:1169–77, 1984.

Zubin J, Spring B: Vulnerability — a new view of schizophrenia. *J Abnorm Psychol* 86(4):103–126, 1977.

FURTHER READING

Barrowclough C, Tarrier N: *Families of schizophrenic patients: cognitive behavioural intervention*. London, 1992, Chapman & Hall.

This is a concise logical textbook that describes that describes the history of Expressed Emotion and family intervention work research. Its most relevant chapters are those which describe how to work proactively and effectively with families, and they are reinforced with clinical examples. The appendices include the Relative Assessment Interview, Social Functioning Scale, and Knowledge about Schizophrenia Interview that have been referred to within this chapter.

Deveson A: *Tell me I'm here*. London, 1992, Penguin.

This gives the reader a clear insight into the realities of living and coping with a diagnosis of schizophrenia, as it is a powerful account of how the author managed when her son was diagnosed. This courageous description is presented as a humble story, yet its content is very thought-provoking as it mirrors the way many families present their experiences. It is highly suitable for all nurses who are seeking to enhance their understanding and knowledge of those who experience schizophrenia and the impact this has upon their families.

Hatfield AB, Lefley HP, editors: *Families of the mentally ill: coping and adaption*. New York, 1987, Guilford Press.

Although written by professionals this thoughtful book explores the reality of family situations and looks at how professional carers should function to aid mental health. Of particular interest is section II which moves from general ideas to the impact on families of a severe mental illness. Some chapters could be used as valuable educational aids for carers.

· *Chapter* · 32

Looking Forward

<table>
<tr><td>

Learning Outcomes

After studying this chapter you should be able to:

- Describe a framework for analysis encompassing the context, process and outcome of change.

- Apply constituent elements of this framework to analyse the future of mental health nursing.

- Identify key policy initiatives that set the context for change in mental health nursing and mental health services.

- Understand how mental health nurses can shape the future through understanding and embracing change.

- Identify likely areas of change in relation to practice, research and education in mental health nursing.

</td><td>

CHAPTER OUTLINE

- *The context of change – the why of change*

- *The process of change – the how of change*

- *The content of change – the what of change*

</td></tr>
</table>

*T*his chapter addresses the future of mental health nursing. Emphasis is placed on the importance of understanding the process of change, as it is this that is the most consistent, enduring and predictable factor shaping the future of mental health nursing.

The future will involve major and rapid change. Change is concerned with variation, alteration and substitution; the capacity for change is involved, together with its achievement and maintenance. Change and possible future developments cannot be viewed with a narrow focus but must be seen within a broad holistic and dynamic context.

Pettigrew *et al.*(1992) provide a useful framework for the analysis of change:
- The context of change—the why of change.
- The process of change—the how of change.
- The content of change—the what of change.

These three areas are used in this final chapter as a framework to analyse the concept of change associated with the future of mental health nursing. It is the relationships between these areas and the skills and ideas involved in the regulation of these relationships over time that pose the greatest challenge in understanding change. 'The only way to bring about lasting change and to foster an ability to deal with new situations is by influencing the conditions that determine the interpretation of situations and the regulation of ideas' Norman (1977).

THE CONTEXT OF CHANGE—THE WHY OF CHANGE

What do the notions of revolutionary change and evolutionary change contribute to our understanding of the future of mental health nursing? The rapid-reform characteristic of health care is frequently described in terms of revolutionary change. There are anomalies in this view. For instance, scenes of violence and violent images are often associated with revolution. There can be little doubt that violence has an important bearing on future developments in mental health services. It is a powerful factor in bringing about change. However, it is not the violence of the mass but the violence of the individual that is most likely to bring about change in mental health care, service and policy. Meanwhile, phrases associated with evolutionary change are appearing with increasing regularity in Government discussion and policy documents. For example, 'The environment is changing and it will take time for a new equilibrium to emerge' (Department of Health (DoH), 1995). Terms such as 'ecological balance', 'orderly evolution' and 'evolutionary approach' (DoH, 1995) are not uncommon. But change, in evolutionary terms, is a completely random process. What is likely is that some changes will involve a sudden switch while others will involve a process of more subtle evolution. A better understanding of concepts of major change inform our perspective on the context of change.

EVOLUTIONARY CHANGE

Social change may be understood with reference to evolutionary processes. This perspective owes much to biological theories of evolution, in particular Charles Darwin's *On the Origin of Species* published in 1859. As stated above, evolutionary theory portrays change as a completely random process. There are two central concepts in evolutional theory, differentiation and adaptation. These are associated with natural selection, or survival of the fittest. Evolutionary change involves the development of ever-increasing complexity and differentiation. Biological evolution describes how different species adapt to their environment through mutation or genetic change; particular mutations confer a competitive advantage on certain individuals within a species—this is the advantage of increasing adaptation and greater complexity. The greater the complexity, the greater the capacity to adapt to the environment. Characteristics and attributes crucial for survival of the species are inherited by successive generations through the genes of the living organism.

REVOLUTIONARY CHANGE

The concept of the 'Copernican revolution' has been used to describe changes in mental health services in Britain and North America (Radford, 1992). It adds an interesting perspective to the analysis of current trends and future developments in psychiatric and mental health nursing.

The original meaning of the term 'revolution' is associated with 'rotation' or 'turn', to move in a circle. It was used by the astronomer Copernicus in his *De Revolutionibus* (1543) to describe the regular revolving motion of stars in a theory that the sun, rather than the earth, is the centre of the universe (Bullock and Stallybrass, 1977). The dynamic sense of movement, direction, pattern and purpose is characteristic of the term when used to describe a complete change of method or conditions.

The concept of revolution also captures the notion of turning back in order to progress. The revolutionary ideals of liberty, equality and fraternity are attributes of both the American

Revolution of 1776 and the French Revolution of 1789. Individuals were seen as being born free and equal but increasingly oppressed by powerful authorities. The American and French Revolutions may be seen as campaigns to turn back to a previous order and restore a past form of society. However, many of the changes were permanent and became associated with progress, the establishment of a new, future-oriented social order, and a break with the past. 'The element of novelty is inherent in all revolutions' (Ardent, 1965).

Giddens (1994) defines revolution as 'the seizure of state power through violent means by the leaders of a mass movement, where that power is subsequently used to initiate major processes of social reform'. He identifies a set of three characteristic features of revolutions:
1. Mass social movement—goals are realized through mass action.
2. Major processes of reform or change—new and effective leadership and organization.
3. Violence—either threatened or used by the mass against the pre-existing authority.

Marxist analysts argue that the most significant social change occurs through revolutionary transformations. Social tensions, clashes and struggles, images of violence, conflict and radical change are associated with revolutions.
Conditions for revolutionary change are twofold:
1. A particular revolutionary situation.
2. An appropriate revolutionary agency.

One or other of these conditions may lead the change and take on a greater significance than the other. The revolutionary situation involves the emergence or development of appropriate circumstances which include crisis, conflict and collapse of the established order. This condition emphasizes the inevitable, inexorable and determinist characteristics of change.

The revolutionary agency may be, for example, a militant party or group that leads the revolution rather than waiting for the appropriate circumstances to emerge. This condition emphasizes the important role of new or different ideas and perspectives, innovation, creativity, organization and leadership in an active campaign for change.

SITUATIONAL ANALYSIS

The context of change takes into account wide societal movements and change on a grand scale. It provides the background and setting for an analysis of change. Nevertheless, it may be difficult to see how this affects our immediate circumstances. Both evolutionary and revolutionary concepts of change have a distancing characteristic. They may infer that change, be it sudden or gradual, occurs elsewhere in a different time or place. Change is represented as separate or external to those groups or individuals upon which it has an impact. The concepts of evolutionary and revolutionary change, though useful in understanding the context of change, may tend to emphasize and promote this view of change as external or separate, as inevitable or random.

There is little in these concepts of change that demonstrate how individuals may themselves effect and embrace change. An analysis of the context of change needs to take account of how change may be influenced and shaped. It is essential that mental health nurses understand their role in shaping the future.

The context of change may be addressed in terms of the inner contexts as well as the external or outer contexts for change (Pettigrew *et al.*, 1992). This may be referred to as a situational analysis, focusing on internal and external factors (Skilbeck, 1984). Both inner and outer contexts inform and shape innovation and change.

There is a strong association between the context and the content of change. Skilbeck (1975) describes a model of curriculum planning where both the context and content of the curriculum are key features of the situational analysis. Situational analysis is a prerequisite to development of educational programmes and provides a useful framework to understand factors involved in and influencing change.

A situational analysis involves a critical appraisal of the wider environment as an alternative starting point to setting objectives and goals or specifying outcomes. This appraisal includes consideration of both external and internal factors that affect the functioning of and shape the environment, the relationships, experience and communication patterns between key parties or stakeholders. A situational analysis is a means of analysing change. It may be employed as an initial stage in the implementation of planned change.

The *external analysis* sets the innovation or change in a wider, more general context. It includes the national, economic, political and social context of change, the perceptions and interpretations, actions and events associated with strategy and policy at national and regional levels (Boxes 32.1–32.3). The *internal analysis* is specific to the immediate situation and often cannot be used to generalize about other settings even though those other settings may be influenced by the same or similar external factors. It includes organizational or local strategy, structure, management, chains of command, patterns of communication and culture, and local responses to national policy, meetings and discussion between participants, modes of practice within and across particular settings and services (Box 32.4). The internal and external factors are not mutually exclusive. The interface or boundary between the internal and external factors, the inner and outer contexts is the site of major change. The next section addresses the context for change in mental health nursing.

THE CONTEXT OF CHANGE IN MENTAL HEALTH NURSING

Florence Nightingale (1870) captures the sense of dynamic purpose and direction often associated with revolutionary change in her *Notes on Nursing*. 'No system can endure that does not march....to stand still is to go backwards'.

The means of providing care, the setting of care and the technological, organizational and demographic changes will all shape the future of mental health nursing. The challenges for nursing and midwifery in the 21st Century are identified

in The Heathrow Debate (DoH,1995) in terms of eight strategic issues (Box 32.1).

1. What will be the context in which nurses will work?

The balance of care will continue to shift from hospital to community settings and acute specialist services. A greater range of agencies and venues are likely to provide care. Traditional professional roles will alter in line with these changes, some roles becoming more specialized and focused while others provide a wider range of services to patients and clients in community settings. Continuity and coordination of care provision for individuals and their carers or families across different service boundaries will provide further areas of development in the role of the nurse. With the focus of care moving from illness-oriented hospital services to bases in the community, there is likely to be a greater emphasis on teamwork, delegation of responsibility and accountability and more flexibility across different roles.

2. What will be the contribution of nursing to meeting the needs of individuals?

The contribution of nurses in promoting independence, educating and advising and coordinating care is well established. The close relationship between nurses, patients and clients, their carers and families will continue to be the focus of nursing. There may be more vulnerable people with fewer willing and able carers. Effective needs assessment, communication of information, and care delivery are key tasks.

3. How will substitution impact on the role of nursing?

The term 'substitution' is associated with cost-effectiveness. It refers to the replacement of:
• The more expensive by an equally effective but cheaper equivalent.
• The less effective by the more effective.

Box 32.1 *Eight strategic issues for nursing*

1 What will be the context in which nurses will work?
2 What will be the contribution of nursing to meeting the needs of individuals?
3 How will substitution impact on the role of nursing?
4 How will the public react to the changed role of nursing?
5 How will teamwork be developed with other carers in health and social care?
6 How will professional accountability, authority and responsibility be changed?
7 How will regulation impact on quality?
8 What will be the implications for initial education and training, retraining and continuous training?

(Department of Health, 1995)

Box 32.2 *A vision for the future — twelve targets*

Target No. 1

To assign each patient/client to a named nurse, midwife or health visitor throughout their period of care and monitoring the initiative.

Target No. 2

To complete a consumer satisfaction survey on the quality of the partnership with users and their involvement in care, and convey the findings to the person concerned.

Target No. 3

Provider units should identify outcome indicators responsive to nursing, midwifery or health visiting practice, developing relevant clinical protocols and having in place a framework of clinical audit.

Target No. 4

Purchasers and providers should demonstrate that value for money recommendations are included in contracts for services.

Target No. 5

Clinical and professional leaders should discuss with each professional how they might develop their practice.

Target No. 6

Each nurse, midwife and health visitor should be able to clearly identify the caseload of patients/clients for whom he/she is the named professional and has responsibility for care.

Target No. 7

Employing authorities are to demonstrate what action has been taken to support those with the potential to develop leadership and management skills.

Target No. 8

Professional leaders should be able to demonstrate the existence of local networks to disseminate good practice based on research.

Target No. 9

Providers should be able to demonstrate where clinical practice has changed as a result of research findings.

Target No. 10

To discuss at local and national level the appropriateness of clinical supervision as a means of improving quality of care.

Target No. 11

To demonstrate the input nursing, midwifery and health visiting has to commissioning and purchasing.

Target No. 12

Each provider unit should identify pre and post registration programmes planned to help nurses, midwives and health visitors acquire the necessary skills associated with major policy initiatives, i.e. *The Health of the Nation, Caring for People* and *The Patient's Charter.*

Box 32.3 *Fundamental principles of nursing, midwifery and health visiting education*

Nursing, midwifery and health visiting education should be:

Patient focused

— developing practitioners who constantly strive to improve the care of patients and clients, their families and the wider community;

Practice led

— rooted in the art and science of nursing, midwifery and health visiting as practical activities;

Student centred

— recognizing the individuality of students and harnessing the wealth of experience that they bring to the learning situation, and making programmes accessible, attractive and challenging in terms of both personal and professional development;

Equitable

— providing equality of opportunity;

Appropriate

— preparing practitioners who are 'fit for purpose', with the knowledge, skills, attitudes and commitment to personal professional development necessary to function confidently, competently and with sensitivity;

Effective

— achieving the highest standards while making the most efficient use of resources;

Responsive

— employment focused and capable of adapting to changing health needs with minimum disruption and maximum speed, making full use of research findings to inform curriculum design, delivery and evaluation;

Collaborative

— securing the cooperation of the major stakeholders to work in partnership, to recognize and achieve a common purpose and to create opportunities for shared learning with other professions; and

Accountable

— open to scrutiny, explicable and defensible.

(from Department of Health, 1993b)

Other forms of substitution include substitution of location and task. Examples that involve substitution of one location for another include the substitution of hospital care for community care, day care for home care. Such changes should reflect and be supported by similar changes in resources, as part of a substitution package. The substitution of tasks involves a relocation of tasks between nurses and others. This may ensure that an appropriate level of expertise is applied in care delivery. For example, the most skilled nurses care for the patients and clients with the most challenging or difficult problems. Nurses will need to show that the skills they use are either more effective than or as effective as those used by others and that their employment is less expensive or represents better value than possible alternatives.

4. How will the public react to the changed role of nursing?

The public recognition of the nurse's duty of care for patients and clients has remained a consistent factor throughout a range of changes and reforms. Realistic expectations of the level of service effectiveness, efficiency and acceptability will be enhanced through user involvement and increased availability of comprehensive information about services. Nurses need to take responsibility for educating the public as to the nature of nursing, its strengths and its influence in relation to improvements in care. They must develop a higher profile in addressing public issues and handling public opinion.

5. How will teamwork be developed with other carers in health and social care?

Teamwork is used as an umbrella term for practices that involve working together. Team-working will be needed in and across a range of health and social care, including hospital and acute setting and community services.

A nurse's involvement in teamwork may vary from membership of a formal team to collaboration, consultation and liaison with others in a less formal but structured arrangement. A nurse may also work as an independent practitioner or gatekeeper to other services.

The constitution and definition of the team within which the nurse works will be variable. The patient or client, their carer or family may be seen as part of the team, depending on the basis for team membership. Team roles may conflict with professional roles. Nurses will need to be increasingly familiar with issues such as team leadership and responsibility, purpose and direction.

6. How will professional accountability, authority and responsibility be changed?

Nurses are likely to experience increased responsibility for what they do. They will have more idea of what is efficient and effective, for example, in terms of assessment and intervention. Nursing will become more accountable to those involved in using and funding services, for example, patients and clients, carers and relatives, consumers, purchasers and taxpayers. Systems of audit and accounting will be more open to public scrutiny. Authority may be supported by legislation but will depend on nurses providing an effective service.

Responsibilities may be shared or divided within a team. Issues of shared responsibility for care will need to be addressed. Particular concerns for mental health nurses will include non-compliance with treatment, self-harming behaviours and attempted suicide.

7. How will regulation impact on quality?

Quality is influenced by regulation through professional bodies, individual practitioners, the health market and the law. Regulation offers protection to both the public and professionals. It involves the definition of standards and systems of accreditation. Registration of the professional qualification depends on meeting defined standards. Professional practice following registration is guided by established regulatory arrangements.

Maintenance of professional standards for practice are the responsibility of the individual practitioner. Periodic registration is the mechanism by which these standards are maintained. New systems of regulation and accountability are influenced by competition and market forces. These systems include hospital and service accreditation, Charter Marks, external and internal organizational audits, research and development. The Mental Health Act, employment law, the

Box 32.4 *The internal analysis or inner context*

The inner context for change in mental health nursing includes local initiatives to national policies. Internal factors include:

Local charters for mental health.
Demographic changes.
Education — broader understanding of mental health problems.
Effective evaluation of policy and changes in policy, e.g. Care Programme Approach and supervised discharge, risk assessment, Key Workers, record keeping.
Focus on serious mental illness.
Leadership in nursing.
Media and public concern.
Nurse-led services.
Nursing contribution to national debate.
Prescription of minimum standards for mental health care.
Public mental health education programmes — stigma, improvement in understanding, preventing misinformation.
Recruitment into nursing and in particular to mental health nursing.
Resourcing of comprehensive care packages.
Rising levels of violence.
Roles and models of practice, e.g. liaison, consultation.
Treatment developments.
User involvement in planning, delivery and evaluation of health care.

contract of employment and legislation in relation to professional negligence are examples where legal regulation impacts on the quality of care. Government policy and regulatory mechanisms such as the Care Programme Approach are expected to have a major impact on improvements to service delivery and access to services.

8 What will the implications be for initial education and training, retraining and continuous training?

The Project 2000 approach to pre-registration education is grounded in primary care and health promotion and set at a very general level. The development of skilled interventions and a more focused level of knowledge and expertise must be associated with continuing education programmes. Opportunity for clinical specialization and more focused knowledge must be matched by opportunities in educational awards at diploma, degree, postgraduate diploma and Master's degree level.

Education and training must prepare existing staff to work in new or different settings and equip them with the skills and abilities to commit themselves to various models of practice. Education is a strategic investment. It is an investment in the future. Resources, including teachers, teaching facilities and appropriate training programmes must have adequate funding in order that strategic objectives are met. Service-led education includes practice development sites and use of the new technology for educational purposes. There must be a continuing dialogue at all levels, a range of partnerships between commissioners and providers of education, clinical nurses, nurses teachers and researchers, service users and carers.

GOVERNMENT POLICY

In 1993, the DoH published *A Vision For The Future — The Nursing, Midwifery and Health Visiting Contribution to Health and Health Care* (DoH, 1993). This document sets out the Government's view of the future for nurses, midwives and health visitors. It is a view that is shaped by key policy initiatives including *Working for Patients* (DoH, 1989a) *Caring for People* (DoH, 1989b), *The Health of the Nation* (DoH, 1992) and *The Patient's Charter* (DoH, 1991) along with others such as *Research for Health* (DoH, 1991), *A Strategy for Nursing* (DoH, 1989c), *The Report of the Taskforce on the Strategy for Research in Nursing, Midwifery and Health Visiting* (DoH, 1993a) and *Working in Partnership — A Collaborative Approach to Care* (DoH, 1994a). These policy documents and reports set the outer or external context for change in mental health nursing.

STAKEHOLDERS IN CHANGE

Several of the reports and policy documents identify 'stakeholders' and highlight challenges to particular stakeholders. These include each individual, group or party with an interest or investment in change. Stakeholders include:
• Education commissioners.
• Education providers.

• The Government.
• Health care purchasers.
• Other professionals.
• The National Health Service Executive.
• Nurses, midwives, health visitors.
• Health care providers.
• The public.
• The statutory bodies.

A Vision for the Future (DoH, 1993c) sets out common goals and strategic aims focusing on:
• Patients' and clients' needs.
• Encouraging participation of the service users and their carers in partnership with other professionals and agencies.
• Contributing to improvements in the general health of the population.
• Ensuring a high quality, cost-effective service.

The report identifies the following five broad objectives:

Quality, outcomes and audit — To provide high quality, cost-effective care based on the assessment of individual needs, with nurses', midwives' and health visitors' interventions evaluated and outcomes charted, with the results submitted to professional audit.

Accountability for practice — To develop a clear understanding of the responsibilities and obligations associated with individual professional accountability, clinical and professional leadership, clinical research and supervision and to provide clinical and professional leadership as part of a corporate management agenda.

Clinical and professional leadership, clinical research and supervision — To develop clinical professional leadership in a corporate management agenda.

Purchasing and commissioning — To ensure that clinical and professional expertise feeds into the purchasing and commissioning cycle.

Education and personal development — To recognize and promote the educational and personal needs of nurses, midwives and health visitors as an integral part of the delivery of high quality health care.

The report sets out 12 targets, in addition to these broad objectives (Box 32.2). These objectives and targets are intended as a framework to encourage purchasers, providers and educationalists to shape plans for the future of health care. They provide the context for change and future developments in mental health nursing.

Beardshaw (1990) identifies demographic shifts as the major influence on nursing in the future. There is a very real risk of labour and skills shortages, serious industrial disputes and high wastage, in terms of both money and manpower, if appropriate solutions are not developed within the health service. The main policy challenge involves reshaping nursing to equip nurses to deliver the most effective nursing care. She highlights three key factors for effective nursing care:

1. Improved education and training.
2. Nursing involvement in decision making.
3. Increased opportunities for career development and promotion.

A Vision for the Future also identifies effective education and training as 'the bedrock of professional practice'. This document makes explicit certain fundamental principles that underpin nursing, midwifery and health visiting education (Box 32.3).

THE PROCESS OF CHANGE — THE HOW OF CHANGE

'Perhaps the most critical connection is the way actors in the change process mobilize the contexts around them and in so doing provide legitimacy for change' (Pettigrew *et al.*, 1992). An understanding of how to manage change is essential if mental health nurses are to be involved actively in shaping the future. This section draws on models of change, the characteristics of innovation and successful change and strategies for change that underpin practice and education in mental health nursing.

MODELS OF CHANGE

Several authors describe models of change (Table 32.1). Often these are based on a conceptualization of change as rational, purposeful and linear. For example, Lewin (1951) identifies a three-phase process model incorporating 'unfreezing', 'moving' and 'refreezing'(Box 32.5). Such models help us to understand the role of, for example, purposeful action, power and status as motivating factors and forces for planned, regulated change.

However, change is invariably complex with multiple or simultaneous actions and events. The predicted or anticipated outcome of change may be overshadowed by unforeseen consequences and unanticipated effects. A more eclectic approach to change is required. It needs to encompass not only the rational linear models of change but also competing explanations, the role of chance, surprise and exceptional individuals in relation to innovation.

Box 32.5 *Lewin´s model of changes*

Unfreezing
A 'thawing out' phase where the need for change is recognized by the group or organization. Unfreezing refers to the loss of adherence to established but outdated or otherwise inappropriate attitudes, ideas, beliefs and behaviours. There is a concerted attempt to identify problems and their underlying causes. Motivation, support, encouragement towards the goal of achieving change are necessary components of this initial phase. Trust must be established between all parties involved in identifying and implementing change.

Moving
The second phase involves the group or organization using information to come to a new understanding of their situation and is referred to as cognitive redefinition. Information is gathered and plans for implementation of change are identified. Interventions are employed in attempts to resolve or remove the problem. This involves a heightened awareness of attitudes, beliefs and behaviours.

Refreezing
Newly acquired behaviours are integrated into the group or organizational culture. Reinforcement of new patterns of behaviour, beliefs and attitudes are achieved through feedback and encouragement.

TABLE 32.1 Linear models of change

Havelock (1973)	Lewin (1951)	Lippitt (1973)	Rogers (1983)
1 Relationship building	1 Unfreezing	1 Diagnosis	1 Knowledge
2 Diagnosis	2 Moving	2 Assess motivation	2 Persuasion
3 Available resources	3 Refreezing	3 Assess change agent motivation and resources	3 Decision
4 Choosing the solution		4 Selection of change	4 Implementation
5 Gaining acceptance		5 Identification of change agent	5 Confirmation
6 Stabilization		6 Maintenance of change	
		7 Termination of helping relationship	

CHARACTERISTICS OF INNOVATION AND SUCCESSFUL CHANGE

An alternative approach to these rational, linear models of change involves the identification of characteristics associated with successful innovation and implementation of change. The introduction of an innovation to any setting requires a range of issues to be addressed and understood by participants. These include the nature of the innovation, organizational requirements for the innovation and the need for a planned approach (Docking, 1987) (Box 32.6). Moreover, there are certain characteristics of the environment that will help facilitate change (Rogers and Shoemaker, 1971; Appleby *et al.*, 1995) (Box 32.7).

CHANGE STRATEGIES

Motivation plays a key role in the three types of change strategy identified by Bennis *et al* (1985). These are:

Power Coercive

This approach emphasizes the role of power, influence and authority to ensure compliance with change. Hierarchical authority, legislation and political and administrative policy are examples of different sorts of power that may be brought to bear in effecting change.

Normative Re-educative

Attitudes are changed through personal growth and development and problem-solving. Motivation for change influences commitment to cultural and societal norms. Old systems of values and beliefs are replaced with new and different perspectives.

Rational Empirical

This approach highlights the impact of knowledge and information. Change is motivated by rational self-interest. It is seen as desirable and beneficial.

ACTION RESEARCH

Characteristics of innovation and change and change strategies are useful in describing and informing the change process. They are often derived from action research, which is a collaborative method of studying and implementing change. It can be of direct use to participants, responsive to their needs and foster a sense of empowerment through involvement in the process of change. Action research contributes to the development of theoretical knowledge, planning and decision making through the introduction of innovation and change. Several authors have identified characteristics of action research (Cohen and Manion,1987; Winter, 1989) (Box 32.8).

Box 32.7 *Characteristics of change*

Relative advantage
A change in practice must confer a relative advantage over the present state or status quo. The more advantages or the greater the significance of an advantage, the greater the support for change.

Compatibility
The change is more likely to be implemented successfully if it is compatible with prevailing values, beliefs, attitudes and practices. The size or dimension of the change, i.e. whether it is perceived as a major or a minor change, will influence the implementation. Changes perceived as minor alterations within the prevailing ideology are easier to implement.

Complexity
A change may appear fairly straightforward but be difficult to implement. The complexity of the change refers to the ease with which a change can be implemented.

Observability
A change in practice is more likely to be implemented if the change and the effects of the change can be observed. Identification and acknowledgement, through observation and measurement of the consequences and benefits of the change, lead to more extensive implementation of the change.

Trialability
This is linked to observability but takes it a step further. Rather than observing the change and the effects of change, participants are involved in trying out or testing the innovation, to get a measure of its effectiveness. Implement and see the change.

Understanding
An understanding of the change involves interpretation of information. This is associated with the way the information is communicated and received.

Relevance
To be implemented effectively the change must be relevant to all parties involved.

Appropriateness
The context and timing of the innovation will influence its success.

(Rogers and Shoemaker, 1971; Appleby et al., 1995)

Box 32.6 *Conditions for innovation*

These include:
- An organizational culture that encourages questioning, initiative, problem-solving, openness towards people and problems, the sharing of ideas and a reflective, evaluative approach to practice.
- An opportunity for staff to develop trust, understanding and respect.
- An opportunity to develop individual autonomy, responsibility and accountability.
- Decentralized management.
- Effective channels of communication.
- Constructive conflict management.
- Collaborative working relationships within and between groups.
- A shared ideology and set of core values.
- Acknowledgement of success and achievement.
- An opportunity to give and receive support over difficulties and problems.
- Supportive leadership.

(from Docking, 1987)

The essence of action research is its dynamic, ever-changing nature. It traces the development and forward movement of ideas. Elliott (1982) defines action research in terms of the process involved. 'Action research might be defined as: the study of a social situation with a view to improving the quality of action within it... [The] total process — review, diagnosis, planning, implementation, monitoring effects — provides the necessary link between self-evaluation and professional development' (Elliott, 1982). A greater awareness and understanding of practice develops through this process. Action research may be used to understand, manage and implement change in several different ways. It may be a means of:

- Problem-solving in specific situations, or of improving circumstances.
- Professional or personal development — providing new skills and methods, improving analytical ability and self-awareness.
- Introducing innovation in systems that may be resistant to change.
- Improving communication between service users, practitioners, teachers and researchers — a bridge between theory and practice.

THE CHANGE AGENT

The expression 'collaborative inquiry' is often used in conjunction with action research and is based on the assumption that research and action are inextricably linked through practice (Torbert, 1981). In action research both researcher and participants alike act as agents for change. Research findings and the research process are linked through clinical practice by practitioners who have a vested interest in practice development. They are part of the practice setting. The relationship between the researcher and participants in the action research process is collaborative. This type of relationship is unique to action research, differing from the researcher's role in other types of research.

It has been suggested that action research is 'the antithesis of true experimental research', where randomized controlled trials are set up as the 'gold standard', because the researcher and participants collaborate in the generation of the action research process (Cohen and Manion, 1987). The researcher of the natural and social sciences is usually involved in manipulating, controlling or observing subjects in a one-sided relationship where the power lies with the researcher. The researcher must maintain an objective separateness, viewing the social world as separate from the world of research.

Kurt Lewin, the person most often identified as the founder of action research, states:

> The research needed for social practice can best be characterized as research for social management or social engineering. It is a type of action-research, a comparative search on the conditions and efforts of various forms of social action, and research leading to social action.... This by no means implies that the research needed is in any respect less scientific or 'lower' than what would be required for pure science in the field of social events. I am inclined to hold the opposite to be true.
>
> *(Lewin, 1947)*

Torbert (1981) suggests that in action research the researcher recognizes the nature of enquiry in action and that the researcher is both a practitioner conducting research and a researcher seeking what is going on. The notion of reflective practice is central to the methods of action research. The value of reflection in this context lies in the activity of reviewing a situation, interpretation or attitude. The intention is not merely to confirm what is already known nor to rationalize individual experience. Winter (1989) suggests 'the crucial thing is that it must open up previously neglected possibilities' (Winter, 1989).

The concept of *reflexivity* is often used in action research to describe how the researcher is inextricably linked to the situation they are studying. The change agent is not restricted to a set or single role and may work across traditional boundaries. The vehicle for change may be a collaborative relationship or venture shared between different parties, for example a partnership between practitioner and service user, purchaser and provider, teacher and researcher. Those involved in action research need an awareness of their role in relation to the roles of others in the situation. Individuals may have a multifaceted role as change agent, facilitator, leader, manager, learner, practitioner, researcher, service user and teacher.

Different approaches to action research have been identified (Holter and Schwartz–Barcott, 1993; Titchen and Binnie, 1993). They share many characteristics but vary in their application. Some may be more effective in implementing a desired change than others. For example Titchen and Binnie (1993) suggest that action research that encourages ownership of a change by participants (where implementation of change is the responsibility of the participants) is likely to have a lasting effect, in that participants continue to maintain the change

Box 32.8

Key features of action research

- It may be used to address several issues and problems simultaneously.
- It promotes understanding of change in the social world.
- It provides a vehicle for cooperation, collaboration and partnerships for change.
- It is a practical approach to problem solving.
- It is an extremely adaptable and flexible approach to understanding and working with change in a variety of different contexts.
- It is context specific and situational, focusing on particular problems in particular settings.
- It is self-evaluative. A process of continual evaluation is built into the continuing process.

(Cohen and Manion, 1987; Lewin, 1947)

process after the researcher–leader has withdrawn from the situation.

The objectives of action research are situational and specific, samples used are unrepresentative and little or no attempt is made to control variables. Findings are restricted to the situation in which they are carried out; they are specific to that setting and are not generalizable to other settings. The aim is to generate precise knowledge and evidence for a particular situation and purpose, the principal justification of the method being improvement of practice (Cohen and Manion 1987). This distinguishes action research from other forms of research, which are more concerned with establishing the relationships between variables and theory testing and usually call for large cases, controlled variables and specific sampling techniques.

Action research often takes place within an organizational setting. The formal rules and policies, communication structures and organizational hierarchy as well as the cultural ambience and myriad of social networks provide both backdrop and supporting context. Different parties are likely to have different interests and collaboration between parties is based on finding an overlap in interests. Rapoport (1970) suggests that while an area of overlap may shift and change over the course of the work, an awareness of how, when and why this happens is an important part of the process.

Action research often focuses on improving the functioning and efficiency of professionals, incorporating job or needs analysis into the management of organizational change by addressing characteristics of human relations such as individual functioning, morale, efficiency, motivation and relationships. Box 32.9 gives examples of action research in mental health nursing and mental health services.

The Action Research Process

The research process in action research is usually described as a cyclical or spiral process, where each stage or phase in the cycle builds on the previous stage. Lewin (1947) identifies four steps in this cycle: planning, acting, observing and reflecting (Figure 32.1). Others have developed and elaborated on this basic cycle. Kemmis *et al.* (1982) suggest that the process starts with a general idea for an improvement or change and a plan of action involving a series of steps. The first or initial phase of this process incorporates fact finding, analysis and preliminary surveys and is referred to as the 'reconnaissance' phase (Elliott, 1982; Kemmis *et al.*, 1982). This analysis includes discussion and negotiation and identification of areas for improvement, opportunities, threats and constraints. It may include several key factors identified in a situational analysis.

The first phase in action research involves making a description of the situation prior to the introduction of change (Winter, 1989). Indeed, an understanding of the present situation is crucial where the required changes do not stand out or where the nature of the change required is not clear. Such an analysis may also provide a baseline from which change may be evaluated and maintained.

An overall plan is developed from this initial step and followed by phases of action, reconnaissance and revision.

Box 32.9 *Action research in mental health*

Towell and Harries (1979) used action research to examine the process of change in a psychiatric hospital and found it enabled staff to 'take back the authority for clarifying their own roles and working to establish the conditions required for effective task performance by themselves and others'.

The 3-year management of change project described by Lemer and Smits (1989) focuses on nursing assistants working in a mental health service in transition from a large psychiatric hospital to community based services.

Nolan and Grant (1993) identify basic values and attitudes influencing the quality of care in two continuing care hospitals for the elderly. They required nursing staff to identify the assumptions underlying the care they provided using an action research approach. The process identified the need for change in specific areas leading to an improvement in the quality of care.

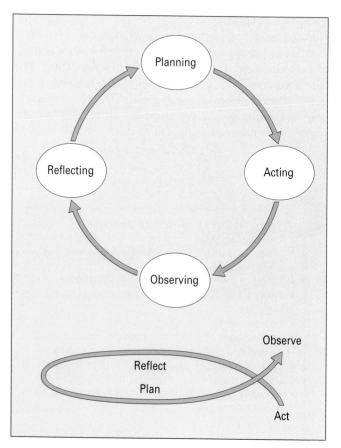

Figure 32.1 The foundation cycle in action research

The means of monitoring the effects of each phase are built into the process as a form of continual evaluation. As data is collected the initial idea is developed. Once the initial cycle is complete it is followed by a continuous repetition of this sequence of events, each cycle involving an analysis, implementation and monitoring of practice (Figure 32.2).

Triangulation

Triangulation involves the use of a variety of different methods of data collection and may be defined as 'the combination of multiple methods in a study of the same object or event to depict the phenomenon being investigated' (Denzin, 1970). The approach involves converging on an interpretation of the situation through validation from a range of perspectives and interpretations. Action research draws mainly on observational data and associated means of data collection, for example transcripts of interviews, questionnaires, field notes and records, diaries, video and tape recordings, photographs, and documents relating to the situation such as agendas and minutes from meetings.

The diagrammatic representation of action research (Figure 32.2) incorporates a feedback loop to emphasize how the process involves reflecting on experience to evaluate practice and changes in practice. The outcome of this process is something tangible, for example, a practical effect, an end product, a model or framework. It arises from the participants' increased knowledge, understanding and awareness of what happens in practice. Action research emphasizes solving specific problems and generates general knowledge and new information through the problem solving-process.

McNiff (1988) exercises caution in representing action research as a model. Using a model may suggest a static state, a linear progression or prescription of actions and instructions. McNiff (1988) applies this criticism to the work of several workers in this field. For example, Kemmis (1982) suggests a model that restricts the process to a single linear tack. This leaves little or no room for creative and flexible manoeuvres in practice associated with the identified idea or problem. Such models tend to organize concepts in phases or stages but offer little by way of explanation. McNiff (1988) argues that in any enquiry there are different functional levels including observation, description and explanation. Systems of action research often lack the power to explain. Approaches to action research that attempt to apply practice to such models, rather than developing or creating a framework from practice, risk being prescriptive and fail to map out the relationship between theory and practice. McNiff (1988) contends that these models are not truly educational because they fail to explain the educational or developmental phenomena with which they are concerned.

A questioning approach

McNiff (1988) provides a list of statements that is a reformation of the action research cycle and associated questions for the teacher–researcher–practitioner to guide developments and to monitor change in practice (Box 32.10) These statements and questions may help to guide the activities and develop the self-awareness of the practitioner. They are based on a set of assumptions about the reflective nature of professional practice.

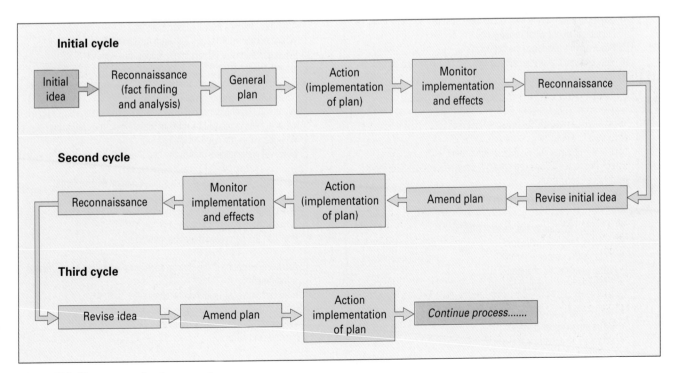

Figure 32.2 The process of action research

Kemmis *et al.*(1982) also identify questions to guide collection of data about the immediate situation (Box 32.11). Winter (1989) and Elliott (1982) describe the intentions of this type of activity as:

1. Identifying and making clear a 'general idea' or problematic situation.
2. Identifying and describing the facts and features of the situation.
3. Explaining the facts and features through the generation of hypotheses.

Docking (1987) takes this further and lists different hypotheses about introducing an innovation. She identifies nine hypotheses, each with associated questions that may be used to guide a rational and planned process of change (Box 32.12). They may form the basis of an action plan where the desired change is identified clearly and key priorities and goals are set out in a timetable (Figure 32.3).

Box 32.10 · *Guiding statements and questions*

Statements
1 I experience a problem.
2 I imagine a solution to my problem.
3 I implement the imagined solution.
4 I evaluate the outcome of my actions.
5 I reformulate my problem.

Questions
1 What is your concern?
2 Why are you concerned?
3 What might you do about it?
4 What kind of 'evidence' could be collected to help make a judgement about what is going on?
5 How can this 'evidence' be collected?
6 How can you check your judgements are quite fair and accurate?

(McNiff, 1988)

Box 32.11 · *Guiding questions*

- What is important in the present situation?
- What is happening already?
- What is the rationale for this?
- What needs to be changed?
- What are considered problems?
- Who is involved?
- Who needs to be involved?
- What are the possibilities?
- What are the obstacles?

(Kemmis et al., 1982)

Box 32.12 · *Hypotheses about introducing an innovation*

Planned, organized and appropriate strategies increase the chances of an innovation being adopted.
What is the state of readiness for the innovation?
What detailed information about the innovation is required?
Where will this information come from?
Who are the stakeholders?
How will the innovation affect them?
Who is likely to accept the innovation?
Why are they likely to accept the innovation?
How can those who accept the innovation support its implementation?
Who is likely to resist the innovation?
Why are they likely to resist the innovation?
What networks and relationships may help or hinder the innovation?
What are the potential problems and possible solutions?
Who will need education and training for what aspect of the innovation?
What other support will be required?
How can effective communication be ensured?
What outcomes can be measured?
How will the innovation be evaluated?

A range of different change strategies will increase the likelihood of the innovation being adopted.
When are power–coercive strategies appropriate?
When are rational–empirical strategies appropriate?
When are normative–re-educative strategies appropriate?
What is an effective combination of strategies?
Which interventions will be used?

Stakeholders will maintain the status quo if it meets their present needs.
Does the innovation match current values and beliefs?
What will convince the different stakeholders that change is needed?
Is the timing right?
Are other changes in progress or planned?
What conditions or factors will help the change?
What conditions or factors might hinder the change?

Resistance to change decreases when stakeholders see relative advantages in accepting the innovation.
What will stakeholders gain from accepting the change?
What are the perceived benefits of maintaining the status quo?
Who identifies the need for change?
How will stakeholders realize the benefits of the innovation?

Resistance will increase if innovation is perceived as a threat.
How is the innovation perceived as a threat?
What degree of choice do stakeholders have?
What is their level of involvement?
How can the perceived threat be minimized?

Active participation in the change decreases resistance and increases commitment.
How can active participation be ensured?
What is the extent of this involvement?
Will some stakeholders be more involved in some aspects of change than others?

(cont.)

THE CONTENT OF CHANGE— THE WHAT OF CHANGE

The content of change refers to what changes take place. It includes the specific focus or area of change. For example, details about changes in educational preparation, changes in patterns of service delivery, changes in client groups. The content of change is inextricably linked to the context and process of change. Education is a key factor shaping the relationships between these three areas.

MENTAL HEALTH NURSING EDUCATION

Education spans the context, process and content of change. It is the single most important factor in shaping the future of mental health nursing. However, mental health nursing education has never properly met the demands of practice and the developing needs of practitioners. Post-registration education has received relatively little attention in spite of the heated debate over the effect of Project 2000 on mental health nursing in Britain (McIntegart, 1990) and surveys of post-registration education and practice in other areas of nursing (Nugent, 1990; Durgahee, 1990; UKCC, 1990). While there are examples of innovation (Barker, 1990) several reports are not so encouraging. White (1991) cites an unpublished report of the Department of Social Security that states that the paucity

Box 32.12

Hypotheses about introducing an innovation (continued)

Effective communication increases the likelihood of the innovation being adopted.
What are the existing channels of communication?
Are they suited to the innovation?
How will stakeholders be fully informed and updated?
What additional means of communication are necessary?

Resistance to change decreases as familiarity with the innovation increases.
Is a practice run of the innovation possible?
Can the innovation be piloted for a limited period?
Can the innovation be initiated in one area and spread or phased-in to other areas?
What resources are needed for such a pilot or trial run?
What are the potential costs of not conducting a pilot or trial run?

The innovation is more likely to be accepted if esteemed, trusted, respected or influential colleagues have accepted it.
Who has formal and informal authority?
Whom do stakeholders trust and respect?
By what means can the support of these parties be directed towards the innovation?

(Docking, 1987)

Figure 32.3 An action plan for introducing innovation

Action Plan	
What are you going to do?	
By when?	
Key people	**Resources:**
What may help this innovation?	**What may hinder this innovation?**

of appropriate post-registration training and education is a severe limitation on new developments and innovation in nursing services. Brooking (1985) describes a 'vicious circle' where inadequate educational provision leads to poorly educated nurses. A lack of research and academic publications means that practice is based on routine and ritual instead of research or evidence-based knowledge. This in turn gives rise to a poor quality of care. Low standards of nursing care lead to loss of prestige and low morale among psychiatric nurses, attracting less well-educated people into the profession. The lack of effective leaders and change agents results in inadequate educational provision, hence the vicious circle. Brooking views education as the most important means of breaking this cycle and notes its role in leading and shaping clinical practice.

Since Brooking described this scenario a number of influential reports and policy documents have completely changed the face of nurse education and practice. Practice leads education in a revised cycle of change. The United Kingdom Central Council for Nursing, Midwifery and Health Visiting (UKCC) *Post Registration Education and Practice Project* (UKCC, 1990) and *Project 2000 – a New Preparation for Practice* (UKCC, 1986) and the English National Board's Higher Award and guidelines for programmes leading to the qualification of Specialist Practitioner (ENB, 1995) have led to radical change from within the profession. External influences include the review of education and service provision (DoH, 1992) and the Government's White Papers *Working for Patients, Education and Training* (DoH, 1989a), *Community Care in the Next Decade and Beyond* (DoH, 1989b) and *The Health of the Nation* (DoH, 1992).

Mental health nursing has influenced other branches of nursing through this period of rapid change. The 1982 syllabus for Registered Mental Nurse training (ENB, 1982) included communication skills and the nature of interpersonal relationships in preparation programmes for psychiatric nurses. Wilson–Barnett (1988) suggests that this focus on communication with patients and therapeutic interactions has resulted in 'a quiet revolution in nursing education'. The common foundation programme of Project 2000 incorporates these elements as essential components for *all* branches of nursing. Such a development illustrates how a specialist or narrow focus in one area of nursing or field of practice can affect change over a wider, more general field of practice. The Thorn Initiative (Gamble, 1995) is an example of a current development in post-registration education for mental health nurses that may have a similar effect on pre-registration mental health nursing education in the future. This programme develops skills in assessment and intervention with people who have serious and enduring mental illness. It may be one of several factors that lead to a shift in the focus of the Project 2000 mental health nursing branch programme and changes in the content relating to mental health in the common core foundation programme. The development and use of skills that are easily defined, open to measurement and transferable across different settings will provide an appropriate focus for the content of mental health nursing programmes and the activities undertaken by mental health nurses.

In 1980 Auld (1980) addressed future challenges for psychiatric nursing education. Many of these seem to have been realized (Box 32.13). Calling for educational programmes that emphasize a holistic approach to the concept of health, encompassing the social and economic context, she advocates a common core preparation (including a module of psychiatric nursing for all nurses) prior to specialization and identifies the major challenges facing mental health nurses in the future.

The UKCC (1995) acknowledge that pre-registration education does not prepare practitioners to meet specialist needs. Further preparation and training is required to equip some practitioners with a higher level of competence necessary to deliver specialist health care. The UKCC's *Standards for Specialist Education and Practice* (UKCC, 1994) are designed to facilitate improved patient and client care and to shape programmes of education leading to the qualification of Specialist Practitioner.

Specialist preparation will enable practitioners to exercise a higher level of judgement, discretion and decision making in clinical care, to monitor and improve standards of care through supervision, clinical audit and leadership and to develop practice through research and teaching.

The specialist education programme covers four broad areas: clinical practice, care and programme management, clinical practice development and clinical practice leadership. All programmes of specialist education must comply with defined standards, including approval by a National Board for Nursing, Midwifery and Health Visiting and association with a higher education accreditation system at a minimum of degree level.

The Council only defines particular areas of specialist practice in relation to community nursing. Community Mental Health Nursing is one of eight areas of specialist community

---

Box 32.13 **+*Future challenges***

- Obtaining the right mental health nursing personnel, in the right numbers, at the right time.
- To provide sensitive care and an acceptable quality of life to the increasing numbers of elderly mentally ill.
- To involve the local community in providing a more homely environment for long-stay patients.
- Appropriate preparation for clinical roles and definition of the necessary skills and knowledge.
- To promote psychiatric nursing as an exciting and worthwhile career for young men and women to pursue.
- To convince other professionals and service planners of the unique skills of the psychiatric nurse in managing complex situations, handling difficult patients and the development of programmes for patients in their daily living, working and recreational activities.

Auld (1980)

nursing practice. The programme consists of a common core of learning outcomes associated with each of the four broad areas, followed by specific learning outcomes for each of the eight specialist areas. Box 32.14 shows the learning outcomes for Specialist Community Nursing Education and Practice — Community Mental Health Nursing (UKCC, 1994). The English National Board for Nursing, Midwifery and Health Visiting (1995) set out the indicative content relating to specific specialist modules for each of the eight areas of specialist community nursing education and practice specified by the Council. Box 32.15 shows the indicative content for the Community Mental Health Nursing programme.

Dissemination of research findings and the incorporation of existing knowledge and information into practice will be more closely linked to the development of educational programmes and will influence the pace and direction of change. Evaluative research, for example on the most effective problem-focused interventions, will increasingly inform the content of education programmes.

The International Congress of Nurses (ICN) (1991) identifies key areas for future development of mental health nursing (Box 32.16). The ICN suggest that at a basic level, education for psychiatric nurses would focus on prevention of mental illness and the promotion of mental health in a wide variety of settings. The theoretical and clinical components of these programmes will address public policy, the biological and psychological basis of behaviour, sociology, social psychology and social psychology. A holistic approach to care would underlie all nursing practice.

McEnany (1991) argues that the future course of psychiatric nursing will involve a paradigm shift toward psychobiology. This will promote a new or redefined form of holism that alters significantly the biopsychosocial perspective. It represents a move away from old perceptions and the influence of a false dualism between mind and brain.

McEnany (1991) argues that the increase in psychopharmacological research and discovery of new drugs has advanced our understanding of relationships between brain chemistry, neurological metabolism, psychological factors and behaviour. He identifies five areas of advancement in this field:

Box 32.15 *Specialist community nursing education and practice: Community mental health nursing*

Indicative content:

- A deeper understanding of the impact of mental illness on the functioning of the individual and the family. The use and analysis of the effectiveness of a range of approaches to help the individual and the family.

- Management and nursing care of people with long-term mental illness and mentally disordered offenders.

- Meeting the mental health needs of vulnerable groups, such as the homeless, unemployed and elderly, including people from ethnic minority groups and black communities.

- Crisis identification, prevention and management. Assessment and management of the suicidal patient/client and prevention of suicide.

- The role of the mental health nurse in the prevention and recognition of substance misuse and early intervention in the care of people who misuse substances.

- Management of challenging and violent behaviour.

- Implementation and evaluation of the Care Programme Approach and supervision of discharge planning. Multidisciplinary and multi-agency working. Knowledge of risk assessment methods including the criteria underpinning clinical judgements. Concepts of liaison nursing.

- Analysis of the ethical, legal, cultural, political and environmental issues relevant to mental health nursing.

- Contribution of the mental health nurse to members of the primary health care team. Analysis of the nurse's role as therapist, educator and consultant.

(English National Board for Nursing, Midwifery and Health Visiting (ENB) 1995)

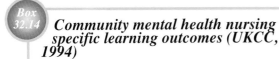

Box 32.14 *Community mental health nursing specific learning outcomes (UKCC, 1994)*

The nurse should achieve the following specific outcomes applied to the area of community mental health nursing practice:

Clinical nursing practice
Assess, plan, provide and evaluate specialist clinical mental health nursing care to meet the immediate, long-term and rehabilitative care needs of patients/clients with a mental health problem/illness living in the community.

Assess and manage clinical emergencies and critical events, including the management of challenging and violent behaviour, to ensure effective care and safety.

Care and programme management
Initiate health promotion and education to facilitate emotional, cognitive and behavioural well-being and play a key role in care management and identify and select from a range of health and social agencies, those which will assist and improve the mental health care of individuals and groups.

1. The development of brain imaging techniques, including magnetic resonance imaging (MRI) scans.
2. The role of neurotransmitters, neurochemical pathways and receptor sites and their role in behaviour and mental illness.
3. The psychobiology of emotion.
4. The improved understanding of brain plasticity.
5. Molecular genetics of psychobiological diseases.

Working in Partnership: a collaborative approach to care (DoH, 1994a) sets out recommendations for the future of all areas of mental health nursing based on the views of the professionals and people who use the services, i.e. the patients and their carers. The recommendations are grouped into six key areas (Box 32.17).

Butterworth (1994) identifies a range of different titles including 'psychiatric nursing', 'mental health nursing', 'psychiatric and mental health nursing' and 'psychosocial nursing'. The variety of titles used by nurses in this field reflects a need to establish a core identity. This has been affected by prevailing influences in nursing generally and the model of psychiatric care practised in a given setting. Current preparation of nurses emphasizes health promotion and prevention of illness, mental health over mental illness. McBride (1990) suggests that this aligns practitioners with the health orientation of nursing rather than the medical model perspective and psychiatric illness.

The Review recommends that the title Mental Health Nurse be assumed by all nurses in this speciality. This serves not only the trend to break down barriers between nursing in hospital and community settings but to promote the community as the usual or expected site of care. Dropping the term 'community' from the title serves to remove any special status. Now that most nursing care is provided in the community such a demarcation is redundant. The mental health nurse is not restricted or linked to a particular location and can work across a range of service settings.

Box 32.17 *Working in partnership*

The relationship with people who use services
Several recommendations address the relationship between nurses and people who use mental health services. They highlight the importance of understanding and awareness of different racial and cultural needs, the need for and use of information and the involvement of patients and their carers in service, education and research.

The practice of mental health nurses
Here recommendations call for the use of the title Mental Health Nurse regardless of the practice setting and emphasize the integral role of clinical supervision in practice.

The delivery of services
Mental health nurses should be involved in policy development and service planning, ensuring that the public and other professionals have direct access to their skills, playing a central role in the care programme approach and supervised discharge.

Challenging issues
These include gender issues, sexual discrimination, sexuality, sexual abuse, women's mental health needs, homelessness, HIV and AIDS, care of the increasing numbers of elderly mentally ill and people with dementia, the mental health care of children and adolescents, the effects of substance misuse behaviours, services for mentally disordered offenders and risk assessment associated with the Care Programme Approach.

Research
Recommendations address local and national research initiatives in mental health. The need for more graduate mental health nurses, potential researchers in mental health, is emphasized, along with the need to develop a 'critical mass' of research activity and a research culture in mental health nursing. Research by mental health nurses and more multidisciplinary research into mental health is called for.

Education
A review of the core skills of the mental health nurse in Project 2000 training should be carried out in conjunction with a review of the common core foundation programme. Service users and their carers should participate in teaching and curriculum development. A national strategy for mental health nurse training is recommended along with more appropriate post-registration education and training being available to all mental health nurses.

Box 32.16 *Recommendations for future developments in psychiatric nursing*

Psychiatric nursing practice
- The development of a psychiatric/mental health framework as the basis for national policy decisions.
- To evaluate, through clinical research, the effectiveness of different psychiatric nursing interventions on patient outcomes.
- To review human resources in psychiatric/mental health nursing at a national level.

Psychiatric nursing education
- To develop and provide all psychiatric/mental health nurses with appropriate programmes that meet their educational needs.
- To build curriculum models that promote cultural awareness and value difference.
- To develop guidelines for both clinical practice for nursing students and for curriculum development.

Psychiatric nursing education and psychiatric nursing practice
- Provide career structures with appropriate educational preparation that recognize and reward psychiatric/mental health nurses at all levels and grades.
- Support the development of psychiatric nurse managers and educators, leaders and role models, particularly in clinical areas.
- Promote involvement of psychiatric/mental health nurses at all levels in policy decision making.

(ICN, 1991)

White (1991) reports on a Delphi study on the future of psychiatric nursing. This addresses questions relating to the future of mental health nursing in three key areas:

1 Community mental health care.
2 Psychiatric nursing practice.
3 Psychiatric nursing education.

The study identifies a 'taxonomy of predictions' where predictive statements from expert panellists are classified according to their likelihood of realization. Each category is divided into further categories indicating the statement's desirability. The study compares the probability and

Box 32.18 Predictive statements on the future of psychiatric nursing

1. *Highly improbable and...*
a) *...highly undesirable:*
'There will be a return to psychiatric nursing courses that lead to two different levels of qualification (Registered and Enrolled).'
b) *...of uncertain desirability:*
'An independent direct-entry initial psychiatric nursing course will be established, as an accredited alternative to Project 2000 preparations.'
2 *Improbable...and undesirable:*
'New psychiatric hospitals will be built'
'Psychiatric nursing will pull out of nursing altogether, to create a separate 'mental health worker' occupation.'
a) *and of uncertain desirability:*
'A single, European-wide psychiatric nursing qualification will be introduced.'
b) *...but highly desirable:*
'The standard of care for chronically mentally ill people will be high.'
3 *Of uncertain probability but ...*
a) *...highly undesirable:*
'The work of community psychiatric nurses will be increasingly controlled by psychiatrists.'
'Psychiatric nursing will increasingly become a 'branch' of general nursing.'
'The training of Health Care Assistants will become the predominant work for Psychiatric Nurse Tutors.'
b) *... desirable:*
'Chronically mentally ill people will attract the largest proportion of available psychiatric resources of any client care group.'
c) *... highly desirable:*
'The community psychiatric nurse will be seen as the key provider of mental health care.'
'Community mental health services will be made available for 24 hours every day.'
'A new post-basic course in Community Psychiatric Nursing will award a qualification which will be the mandatory pre-requisite for practice as a community psychiatric nurse.'
'A coherent post-basic psychiatric nurse education strategy will be developed at a national level.'
4 *Probable and ...*
a) *...highly undesirable:*
'Community psychiatric nurses will increasingly be managed by Social Service Departments.'
'Compulsory psychiatric treatment in community settings will be introduced.'
'In new psychiatric nursing courses, academic achievement will become more important than the acquisition of clinical skill.'
b) *... undesirable:*
'Health care will increasingly be coordinated by personnel from outside the health care professions.'
c) *... of uncertain desirability:*
'A new style Generic Mental Health Worker will emerge, not aligned to a specific discipline.'
'The current English National Board - approved "Community Psychiatric Nursing Certificate" (ENB course 811/812) will be discontinued.'

Box 32.18 Predictive statements on the future of psychiatric nursing (continued)

d) *... desirable:*
'The majority of mental health services will be provided from non-psychiatric hospital settings.'
'The use of alternative therapies (e.g. massage, shiatsu) in mental health care will increase.'
'Appropriately qualified psychiatric nurses will be given licence to prescribe psychotropic drugs from a limited list.'
'A Common Foundation Programme will be introduced for all post-basic community nursing courses.'
e) *... highly desirable:*
'It will become universally accepted that multidisciplinary teamwork is crucial to high quality service provision.'
'There will be a greater determination of community mental health care provision on the part of service consumers.'
'Psychiatric nurses will increasingly provide a "liaison psychiatry" service to nursing colleagues who work in general hospital contexts.'
'A greater emphasis will be placed on linking relevant research evidence to all psychiatric nurse education.'
5 *Highly probable*
a) *....and highly undesirable:*
'The proportion of mentally ill people in prison will increase.'
'Family carers will have an increasing workload caring for dementia patients, without adequate support.'
b) *...but undesirable:*
'Significantly more mental health care will be provided by non-professionally qualified staff.'
c) *...and desirable:*
'There will be an increase in community mental health services provided by the Voluntary Sector.'
'The role of the General Practitioner in the care of mentally ill people will become more important.'
'There will be an increase in the use of non-nurse specialist teachers on psychiatric nursing courses.'
'uncertain probability and highly undesirable'
d) *...and highly desirable:*
'More mental health self-care groups will emerge.'
'More research will be undertaken into psychiatric nursing by psychiatric nurses.'
'Joint training initiatives between psychiatric nursing and other disciplines will increase.'

(White, 1991)

desirability of predictions between psychiatric nurses and non-psychiatric nurses. Box 32.18 gives some examples. (NB. These examples are a small selection of a wide range of statements. Readers are strongly encouraged to read the original report.)

SUMMARY

The advanced and specialized skills and knowledge identified in the preceding chapters build on existing experience and expertise. This enables the mental health nurse to make a confident and constructive contribution to the multidisciplinary team, enhancing multi-agency approaches to care and shaping the mental health services of the future. Our ability to shape the future of mental health care involves not only knowledge and skills in a range of different specialist fields within mental health nursing but an understanding of the context, process and content of change. Mental health nurses have the knowledge and determination to adapt mental health nursing to the future needs of people with mental illness.

Further work is required to improve mental health services. Cooperation and collaboration between health and social care services, mental health and primary care teams is often poor. Primary health care teams often lack the necessary skills and experience to deal with the needs of people with mental health problems. For example less than 20% of practice nurses are qualified mental health nurses and less than 40% of GPs have any experience in psychiatry—even this is experience gained in hospital rather than community settings (RCN, 1995).

Greater emphasis on interagency working, including liaison and mental health consultation, is required along with more interdisciplinary learning. Community general nurses and GPs should be prepared and supported in work with people with common mental health problems. Increasingly, mental health nurses will be integrated within GP practices and primary health care teams. The needs of the severely mentally ill and support of the acutely disturbed patient in the community will be the main focus of mental health nursing practice. Mental health nurses will provide continuity across hospital and acute services and community care in association with the primary health care team. The primary care team, as a whole, need greater human resources in terms of knowledge, skill and expertise to provide high quality mental health services in the community.

The report of the mental health nursing review team (DoH, 1994a) identifies a key role for mental health nurses in the future development of high quality progressive mental health services. Involvement of service users and their carers is the single most important factor in service development and the basis for progress in mental health nursing. A cycle of continual scrutiny and improvement of mental health nursing policy, practice and education is necessary to meet future needs.

KEY CONCEPTS

- Mental health nurses must have a clear understanding of the context, process and content of change.
- A broad perspective of the future of mental health nursing encompasses change in practice, research and education.
- Knowledge of models of change and of characteristics of innovation and successful changes as well as of the principles of action research will help shape the future of mental health nursing.

REFERENCES

Appleby J, Walshe K, Ham C: *Acting on the evidence: A review of clinical effectiveness: sources of information, dissemination and implementation.* Research Paper No. 17, 1995, National Association of Health Authorities and Trusts.

Ardent H: *On revolution.* Harmondsworth, 1965, Penguin Books.

Auld M: Where now for psychiatric nursing? *Nurs Mirror* (supplement)ii–iv, June 26, 1980.

Barker P: Training to meet the new agenda. *Nurs Times* 86(39):71, 1990.

Beardshaw V: *Reshaping nursing for the 1990s: The policy challenge.* London, 1990, King's Fund Institute.

Bennis W, Benne K, Chin R *et al*, editors: *The planning of change,* 4 ed. London, 1985, Holt, Rinehart and Winston.

Brooking J: Advanced psychiatric nursing education in Britain. *J Adv Nurs* 5:455–456, 1985.

Bullock A, Stallybrass D: *The Fontana dictionary of modern thought.* London, 1977, Fontana.

Butterworth T: Working in partnership: a collaborative approach to care: The review of mental health nursing. *J Psych Mental Health Nursing* 1(1):41–44, 1994.

Cohen L, Manion B: *Research methods in education.* 1987, Croom Helm.

Denzin N: Strategies of multiple triangulation. In: Denzin N, editor: *The research act.* New York, 1970, McGraw Hill.

Department of Health: *Working for patients. Education and training.* Working Paper No. 10. London, 1989a, HMSO.

Department of Health: *Caring for people: Community care in the next decade and beyond.* London, 1989b, HMSO.

Department of Health: *A strategy for nursing: Report of the steering committee.* London, 1989c, Department of Health.

Department of Health: *The patient's charter.* London, 1991, HMSO.

Department of Health: *The health of the nation: A strategy for health in England.* London, 1992, HMSO.

Department of Health: *Report of the taskforce on the strategy for research in nursing, midwifery and health visiting.* London, 1993a, Department of Health.

Department of Health: *Research for health: a research and development strategy for the NHS.* London, 1991, HMSO.

Department of Health: *A vision for the future: The nursing, midwifery and health visiting contribution to health and health care.* London, 1993b, Department of Health.

Department of Health: *Working in partnership: A collaborative approach to care: Report of the Mental Health Nursing Review Team.* London, 1994a, Department of Health.

Department of Health: *Nursing, midwifery and health visiting education: A statement of strategic intent.* London, 1994b, Department of Health.

Department of Health: *The challenges for nursing and midwifery in the 21st century — the Heathrow Debate.* London, 1995, Department of Health.

Docking, S: Curriculum innovation. In: Allan P, Jolley M (editors) *The Curriculum in Nursing Education.* London, 1987: 149–163, Croom Helm.

Durgahee T: Directions in post-basic education. *Senior Nurse* 10(7):15–20, 1990.

Elliott J: *Action research: A framework for self evaluation in schools.* Working Paper No. 10: teacher-pupil interaction and the quality of learning. London, 1982, London Schools Council.

English National Board for Nursing, Midwifery and Health Visiting; English and Welsh National Boards for Nursing, Midwifery and Health Visiting. *Syllabus of training: Professional register Part 3 (Registered Mental Nurse).* London, 1982, ENB.

English National Board for Nursing, Midwifery and Health Visiting: *Creating lifelong learners: Guidelines for the implementation of the UKCC's standards for education and practice following registration.* London, 1995, ENB.

Gamble C: The Thorn nurse training initiative. *Nurs Stand* 19(15):31–36, 1995.

Giddens G: *Sociology,* 2 ed. Oxford, 1994, Polity Press.

Havelock R: *The change agent's guide to innovation in education.* New Jersey, 1973, Education Technology Publications.

Holter M, Schwartz–Barcott D: *Action research: What is it? How has it been used and how can it be used in nursing? J Adv Nurs* 18:298–304, 1993.

International Congress of Nurses: *Report on the status of psychiatric nursing education.* London, 1991, ICN/WHO.

International Congress of Nurses: *The current status of psychiatric/mental health nursing and some future challenges.* London, 1991, ICN/WHO.

Kemmis S *et al.: The action research planner,* 2 ed. Victoria, 1982, Deakin University Press.

Lemer B, Smits M: *Facilitating change in mental health.* London, 1989, Chapman & Hall.

Lewin K: Frontiers in group dynamics. *Hum Relat* 1(2):150–151, 1947.

Lewin K: *Field theory in social science.* New York, 1951, Harper & Row.

Lippitt GL: *Visualising change: model guidelines and the change process.* La Jolla, CA, 1973, University Associates.

McBride AB: Psychiatric nursing in the 1990s. *Arch Psychiatr Nurs* 4(1):21–28, 1990.

McEnany GW: Psychobiology and psychiatric nursing: A philosophical matrix. *Arch Psychiatr Nurs* 5(5):255–261, 1991.

McIntegart J: A dying breed. *Nurs Times* 86(39):72, 1990.

McNiff J: *Action research: principles and practice.* London, 1988, Macmillan Education Ltd.

Nightingale F: *Notes on nursing.* London, 1870, Duckworth.

Nolan M, Grant G: Action research and quality of care: a mechanism for agreeing basic values as a precursor to change. *J Adv Nurs* 18:305–311, 1993.

Norman R: *Management for growth.* London, 1977, Wiley.

Nugent AB: The need for continuing professional education for nurses. *J Adv Nurs* 15:471–477, 1990.

Pettigrew A, Ferlie E, and McKee L: *Shaping strategic change.* 1992, Sage Publications.

Radford MD: The Copernican revolution in mental health services: Replacing the revolving door. *J Ment Health* 1:229–239, 1992.

Rapoport RN: Three dilemmas in action research. *Hum Relat* 23(6):499–513, 1970.

Rogers B, Shoemaker: *Communication of innovations: a cross cultural report,* 2 ed. New York, 1971, The Free Press.

Rogers E: *Diffusion of innovation,* 3 ed. New York, 1983, Free Press.

Royal College of Nursing: *Community health care nursing: Challenging the present, improving the future.* London, 1995, RCN.

Skilbeck M: *School Based Curriculum Development.* London, 1984, Harper & Row.

Titchen A, Binnie A: Research partnerships: collaborative action research in nursing. *J Adv Nurs* 18:858–865, 1993.

Torbert W: Why educational research has been so uneducational: the case for a new model of social sciences based on collaborative inquiry. In: Reason P and Rowan J, (editors) *Human inquiry, a sourcebook of new paradigm research.* London, 1981, Wiley.

Towell D, Harries C: *Innovation in patient care: An action research study of change in a psychiatric hospital.* London, 1979, Croom Helm.

United Kingdom Central Council for Nursing, Midwifery and Health Visiting: *Project 2000: A new preparation for practice.* London, 1986, UKCC.

United Kingdom Central Council for Nursing, Midwifery and Health Visiting: *The report of the post-registration education and practice project.* London, 1990, UKCC.

United Kingdom Central Council for Nursing, Midwifery and Health Visiting: The Council's standards for education and practice. London, 1994, UKCC.

White E: *The future of psychiatric nursing by the year 2000: A Delphi study.* Research Monograph, Department of Nursing, University of Manchester, 1991.

Wilson–Barnett J: Lend me your ear. *Nurs Times* 84(33):51–53, 1988.

Winter R: *Learning from experience — principles and practice in action research.* UK, 1989, The Falmer Press.

FURTHER READING

Beck E, Lonsdale S, Newman S, Patterson D: *In the best of health? The status and future of health care in the UK*. London, 1992, Chapman & Hall.

> *This excellent text identifies a broad range of technological, ethical, social and professional issues and their impact on the process of continuous adaption to change in the NHS. It reviews policy initiatives over the last 10 years and sets out policy options for the future examining the effects of, for example, consumerism, financial constraints, competing resources and changes in demography.*

Pettigrew A, Ferlie E, McKee L: *Shaping strategic change*. London, 1992, Sage Publications.

> *This book provides an in-depth analysis of different kinds of change strategy identifying a new model of strategic change that focuses on receptive and non-receptive contexts for change. It addresses issues of strategic management, organizational change and public service management in relation to the NHS. It reviews the relative success of different approaches in various contexts and includes the effects of organizational culture and inter-organizational relations, leadership and sustainable action.*

Baker M, Kirk S: *Research and development for the NHS: Evidence, evaluation and effectiveness*. Oxford, 1996, Radcliffe Medical Press.

> *The book is aimed at clinicians and service managers and will also be of great interest to academics and researchers. It is a clear account of research and development in the NHS and makes research accessible and understandable. It covers strategic initiatives for all disciplines in a research based NHS. The content includes the NHS research and development strategy, the use of research information for evidence based practice and implications of research and development for nursing and the professions allied to medicine.*

Fullan MG: *The new meaning of educational change*. London, 1991, Cassell

> *This book contributes to our understanding of the change process. It is aimed at teachers but contains much of interest to managers and practitioners interested in managing change. Providing new insights, it identifies effective strategies for innovation and improvement. It sets an agenda for future enquiry and provides a guide to action.*

Author Index

Subject Index